Orthopaedic Knowledge Update 5

Home Study Syllabus

American Academy of Orthopaedic Surgeons

Orthopaedic Knowledge Update 5 Home Study Syllabus

Published by the
American Academy of Orthopaedic Surgeons
6300 N. River Road
Rosemont, IL 60018
February 1996

The material presented in this *Orthopaedic Knowledge Update 5: Home Study Syllabus* has been made available by the American Academy of Orthopaedic Surgeons for educational purposes only. This material is not intended to present the only, or necessarily best, methods or procedures for the medical situations discussed, but rather is intended to represent an approach, view, statement, or opinion of the author(s) or producer(s), which may be helpful to others who face similar situations.

Some drugs and medical devices demonstrated in Academy courses or described in Academy print or electronic publications have Food and Drug Administration (FDA) clearance for use for specific purposes or for use only in restricted settings. The FDA has stated that it is the responsibility of the physician to determine the FDA status of each drug or device he or she wishes to use in clinical practice, and to use the products with appropriate patient consent and in compliance with applicable law.

Furthermore, any statements about commercial products are solely the opinion(s) of the author(s) and do not represent an Academy endorsement or evaluation of these products. These statements may not be used in advertising or for any commercial purpose.

The material contained in this volume was submitted as previously unpublished material, except in the instances in which credit has been given to the source from which some of the illustrative material was derived.

First Edition

ISBN 0-89203-114-X
Library of Congress Cataloging-in-Publication Number 96-83090

Acknowledgments

Contents

Task Forces

Editorial Board
James R. Kasser, MD, Chairman
James H. Beaty, MD
Steven R. Garfin, MD
John S. Gould, MD
Michael H. McGuire, MD
Thomas J. Moore, MD
John C. Richmond, MD
Aaron G. Rosenberg, MD
Curtis M. Steyers, Jr., MD
Joseph D. Zuckerman, MD

GENERAL KNOWLEDGE TASK FORCE

Section Editors	John C. Richmond, MD Aaron G. Rosenberg, MD Joseph D. Zuckerman, MD
Soft-Tissue Physiology and Repair	Allen F. Anderson, MD Thomas M. Brushart, MD Christopher D. Harner, MD Michael J. Pagnani, MD Jonathan B. Ticker, MD
Bone Healing and Grafting	Alan D. Aaron, MD
Biomechanics and Gait	Thomas P. Andriacchi, PhD Jeffrey Sum, BSE Douglas Yoder, BS
Biomaterials	Frederick J. Kummer, PhD Jeffrey M. Spivak, MD
Blood Transfusions/HIV/Hepatitis	Ralph L. Bernstein, MD Andrew D. Rosenberg, MD Linda Stehling, MD
Coagulation and Thromboembolism in Orthopaedics	William R. Donaldson, MD William N. Levine, MD
Perioperative Medical Management	Harry D. Fischer, MD
Imaging Beyond Conventional Radiography	Javier Beltran, MD Steven Shankman, MD
Clinical Epidemiology	Mary Louise Skovron, Dr PH
Practice Guidelines	Robert J. Marder, MD
Outcomes Assessment	Sally A. Rudicel, MD

Sports Medicine	Gene R. Barrett, MD R. Jeff Grondel, MD Lew Papendick, MD Ashvin I. Patel, MD Mark F. Sherman, MD Preston M. Wolin, MD
Multiple Trauma: Management of the Injured Patient	Lynn A. Crosby, MD Joseph C. Stothert, Jr, MD, PhD
Occupational Orthopaedics and Disability	Paul M. Brisson, MD Margareta Nordin, Dr Sci

SYSTEMIC DISORDERS TASK FORCE

Section Editors	James H. Beaty, MD Michael H. McGuire, MD
Bone Metabolism and Metabolic Bone Disease	Thomas A. Einhorn, MD
Musculoskeletal Neoplasms	James D. Bruckner, MD Ernest U. Conrad III, MD
Infection	John L. Esterhai, Jr, MD Thomas B. Hughes, Jr, BA
Arthritis	J. Urban Lindgren, MD, PhD
Collagen and Connective Tissue Disorders	Allan M. Strongwater, MD
Genetic Disorders and Skeletal Dysplasias	Frederick R. Dietz, MD
Neuromuscular Disorders in Children	John G. Birch, MD, FRCS(C)
Pediatric Hematologic and Related Conditions	John T. Killian, MD

UPPER EXTREMITY TASK FORCE

Section Editors	James H. Beaty, MD Curtis M. Steyers, Jr, MD Joseph D. Zuckerman, MD
Shoulder and Arm: Pediatric Aspects	John F. Ritterbusch, MD William Warner, MD
Shoulder Trauma: Bone	Frances Cuomo, MD Thomas P. Goss, MD
Shoulder: Instability	Evan L. Flatow, MD Roger G. Pollock, MD
Shoulder: Reconstruction	Joseph P. Iannotti, MD, PhD Jerry S. Sher, MD Gerald R. Williams, Jr, MD
Elbow and Forearm: Pediatric Aspects	John F. Sarwark, MD William Warner, MD
Elbow and Forearm: Trauma	J.L. Marsh, MD
Elbow: Reconstruction	Shawn W. O'Driscoll, MD, PhD, FRCS(C)
Wrist and Hand: Pediatric Aspects	Peter M. Waters, MD

Wrist and Hand: Trauma	Brian D. Adams, MD
Wrist and Hand: Reconstruction	Douglas P. Hanel, MD

LOWER EXTREMITY TASK FORCE

Section Editors	James H. Beaty, MD John C. Richmond, MD Aaron G. Rosenberg, MD Joseph D. Zuckerman, MD
Hip, Pelvis, and Femur: Pediatric Aspects	S. Terry Canale, MD Randall T. Loder, MD George T. Rab, MD Paul Sponseller, MD
Pelvis and Acetabulum: Trauma	Gary S. Gruen, MD M.L. Chip Routt, Jr, MD
Hip: Trauma	Kenneth J. Koval, MD
Hip and Pelvis: Reconstruction	Frank DiMaio, MD David G. Lewallen, MD William A. McGann, MD Richard F. Santore, MD
Femur: Trauma	Berton R. Moed, MD
Knee and Leg: Pediatric Aspects	S. Terry Canale, MD Deborah F. Stanitski, MD
Knee and Leg: Bone Trauma	Clayton R. Perry, MD
Knee and Leg: Soft-Tissue Trauma	Bernard R. Bach, Jr, MD
Knee: Reconstruction	David A. Heck, MD J. David Blaha, MD Russell E. Windsor, MD
Ankle and Foot: Pediatric Aspects	Stephen D. Heinrich, MS, MD Robert Dehne, MD S. Terry Canale, MD
Ankle and Foot: Trauma	Robert S. Adelaar, MD James B. Carr, MD James D. Michelson, MD
Ankle and Foot: Reconstruction	Robert B. Anderson, MD Judith F. Baumhauer, MD Susan K. Bonar, MD Melbourne D. Boynton, MD John S. Gould, MD William M. Granberry, MD L. Andrew Koman, MD Daniel D. Lahr, MD Leland C. McCluskey, MD Michael P. Mott, MD Gary T. Schmidt, MD, FRCS(C) James J. Sferra, MD Mark P. Slovenkai, MD James W. Stone, MD Robert J. Treuting, MD

SPINE TASK FORCE

Section Editor	Steven R. Garfin, MD
Pediatric Spine	Henry G. Chambers, MD Scott J. Mubarak, MD Dennis R. Wenger, MD
Spine: Trauma	Jean-Jacques Abitbol, MD Patrick J. Connolly, MD Hansen A. Yuan, MD
Spondylosis: Degenerative Process of the Aging Spine	Sam W. Wiesel, MD
Cervical Degenerative Disk Disorders	Jeffrey S. Fischgrund, MD Harry N. Herkowitz, MD
Thoracic Disk Herniation	George R. Cybulski, MD Srdjan Mirkovic, MD
Lumbar Degenerative Disease	Edward N. Hanley, Jr, MD
Evidence-Based Recommendations for Patients With Acute Activity Intolerance Due to Low Back Symptoms	Stanley J. Bigos, MD
Spondylolysis and Spondylolisthesis: Congenital and Isthmic	Daniel R. Benson, MD Leslie J. Mintz, MD
Adult Scoliosis	Ensor E. Transfeldt, MD
Spinal Infection	John G. Heller, MD
Tumors of the Spine	John G. Heller, MD
Adult Rheumatoid Arthritis	Stephen J. Lipson, MD
Spinal Instrumentation	Thomas A. Zdeblick, MD

REHABILITATION TASK FORCE

Section Editor	Thomas J. Moore, MD
Spinal Cord Injuries and Miscellaneous Neurologic Diseases	Thomas J. Moore, MD
Stroke	Mary Ann Keenan, MD
Traumatic Brain Injury	Thomas J. Moore, MD
Amputations and Prosthetics	Michael S. Pinzur, MD Michael D. Rooks, MD

Contributors

Alan D. Aaron, MD
Instructor
Georgetown University Hospital
Washington, DC

Jean-Jacques Abitbol, MD
Associate Clinical Professor of Orthopedics
SUNY at Stonybrook
Stonybrook, New York

Brian D. Adams, MD
Associate Professor
Department of Orthopaedic Surgery
University of Iowa
Iowa City, Iowa

Robert S. Adelaar, MD
Professor of Surgery
Vice Chairman, Department of Orthopedics
Medical College of Virginia
Richmond, Virginia

Allen F. Anderson, MD
Director, Lipscomb Foundation for Education and Research
Nashville, Tennessee

Robert B. Anderson, MD
Chief, Foot and Ankle Service
Orthopaedic Department
Carolinas Medical Center
Miller Orthopaedic Clinic
Charlotte, North Carolina

Thomas P. Andriacchi, PhD
Professor, Department of Orthopaedic Surgery
Rush-Presbyterian-St. Luke's Medical Center
Chicago, Illinois

Bernard R. Bach, Jr, MD
Associate Professor, Department of Orthopaedic Surgery
Director, Sports Medicine Section
Rush Medical College
Rush Presbyterian St. Luke's Medical Center
Chicago, Illinois

Gene R. Barrett, MD
Mississippi Sports Medicine and Orthopaedic Center
Jackson, Mississippi

Judith F. Baumhauer, MD
Assistant Professor, Orthopaedic Surgery Department
University of Rochester Medical Center
Rochester, New York

James H. Beaty, MD
Professor of Orthopaedics
Director of Residency Program
University of Tennessee
Campbell Clinic
Memphis, Tennessee

Javier Beltran, MD
Chairman, Department of Radiology
Hospital for Joint Diseases
New York, New York

Daniel R. Benson, MD
Professor of Orthopaedic Surgery
UC Davis Medical Center
Department of Orthopaedics
Sacramento, California

Ralph L. Bernstein, MD
Chairman, Department of Anesthesiology
Hospital for Joint Diseases
Orthopaedic Institute
New York, New York

Stanley J. Bigos, MD
Professor of Orthopaedic Surgery
University of Washington
Seattle, Washington

John G. Birch, MD, FRCS(C)
Associate Professor
University of Texas Southwestern Medical Center
Assistant Chief of Staff
Texas Scottish Rite Hospital for Children
Dallas, Texas

J. David Blaha, MD
Professor and Chairman, Department of Orthopedics
West Virginia University
Morgantown, West Virginia

Susan K. Bonar, MD
Rockhill Orthopaedics
Kansas City, Missouri

Melbourne D. Boynton, MD
Assistant Professor
Department of Orthopaedic Surgery
Medical College of Wisconsin
Milwaukee, Wisconsin

Paul M. Brisson, MD
Chief, Lumbar Surgery
Hospital for Joint Diseases
New York, New York

James D. Bruckner, MD
Assistant Professor
University of Washington Medical Center
Seattle, Washington

Thomas M. Brushart, MD
Associate Professor of Orthopaedic Surgery, Plastic Surgery and Neurology
Johns Hopkins Medical Institutions
Baltimore, Maryland

S. Terry Canale, MD
Professor
University of Tennessee
The Campbell Clinic
Memphis, Tennessee

James B. Carr, MD
Medical College of Virginia
Richmond, Virginia

Henry G. Chambers, MD
Associate Clinical Professor
Pediatric Orthopaedic Surgery
University of California, San Diego
San Diego, California

Patrick J. Connolly, MD
Assistant Professor of Orthopedic Surgery
SUNY Health Science Center
Syracuse, New York

Ernest U. Conrad III, MD
Associate Professor
Director, Sarcoma Service
University of Washington
Seattle, Washington

Lynn A. Crosby, MD
Associate Professor
Creighton University School of Medicine
Omaha, Nebraska

Frances Cuomo, MD
Associate Chief, Shoulder Service
Hospital for Joint Diseases
New York, New York

George R. Cybulski, MD
Associate Professor of Neurosurgery
Division of Neurosurgery
Northwestern University School of Medicine
Chicago, Illinois

Robert Dehne, MD
Assistant Professor
Division of Pediatric Orthopaedics
Department of Orthopaedic Surgery
Louisiana State University Medical Center Children's Hospital
New Orleans, Louisiana

Frederick R. Dietz, MD
Professor of Orthopaedic Surgery
University of Iowa Hospitals and Clinics
Iowa City, Iowa

Frank R. DiMaio, MD
Winthrop University Hospital
Mineola, New York

William R. Donaldson, MD
Associate Clinical Professor
Tufts University School of Medicine
Boston, Massachusetts

Thomas A. Einhorn, MD
Professor of Orthopaedics
Mount Sinai School of Medicine
New York, New York

John L. Esterhai, Jr, MD
Associate Professor of Orthopaedic Surgery
Hospital of the University of Pennsylvania
University of Pennsylvania School of Medicine
Philadelphia, Pennsylvania

Harry D. Fischer, MD
Assistant Clinical Professor of Medicine
Mount Sinai School of Medicine
New York, New York

Jeffrey S. Fischgrund, MD
Attending Spine Surgeon
Department of Orthopaedic Surgery
William Beaumont Hospital
Royal Oak, Michigan

Evan L. Flatow, MD
Herbert Irving Associate Professor of Orthopaedic Surgery
Associate Chief, The Shoulder Service
New York Orthopaedic Hospital
Columbia-Presbyterian Medical Center
New York, New York

Steven R. Garfin, MD
Professor, Department of Orthopaedics
University of California, San Diego
San Diego, California

John S. Gould, MD
Professor and Chairman
Department of Orthopaedic Surgery
Medical College of Wisconsin
Milwaukee, Wisconsin

R. Jeff Grondel, MD
Advanced Orthopedic Care Associates
Las Vegas, Nevada

Thomas P. Goss, MD
Professor of Orthopaedic Surgery
University of Massachusetts Medical Center
Worcester, Massachusetts

William M. Granberry, MD
Assistant Clinical Professor
Baylor College of Medicine
Houston, Texas

Gary S. Gruen, MD
Assistant Professor, Department of Orthopaedic Surgery
Chief, Division of Orthopaedic Traumatology
University of Pittsburgh Medical Center
Pittsburgh, Pennsylvania

Douglas P. Hanel, MD
Associate Professor
Orthopaedic Surgery
University of Washington
Seattle, Washington

Edward N. Hanley, Jr, MD
Chairman, Department of Orthopaedic Surgery
Carolinas Medical Center
Charlotte, North Carolina

Christopher D. Harner, MD
Associate Professor, Orthopaedic Surgery
Chief, Division of Sports Medicine
University of Pittsburgh
Pittsburgh, Pennsylvania

David A. Heck, MD
Department of Orthopaedic Surgery
Indiana University
Indianapolis, Indiana

Stephen D. Heinrich, MS, MD
Associate Professor
Section of Pediatric Orthopaedics
Department of Orthopaedic Surgery
Louisiana State University Medical Center Children's Hospital
New Orleans, Louisiana

John G. Heller, MD
Associate Professor, Orthopaedic Surgery
Emory University School of Medicine
Director of Education
The Emory Spine Center
Atlanta, Georgia

Harry N. Herkowitz, MD
Chairman, Department of Orthopaedic Surgery
Director, Section of Spine Surgery
William Beaumont Hospital
Royal Oak, Michigan

Thomas B. Hughes, Jr, BA
University of Pennsylvania School of Medicine
Philadelphia, Pennsylvania

Joseph P. Iannotti, MD, PhD
University of Pennsylvania School of Medicine
Department of Orthopaedics
Philadelphia, Pennsylvania

James R. Kasser, MD
Associate Professor
Harvard Medical School
Orthopaedic Surgeon-in-Chief
Children's Hospital
Boston, Massachusetts

Mary Ann Keenan, MD
Chairman, Department of Orthopaedic Surgery
Albert Einstein Medical Center
Philadelphia, Pennsylvania

John T. Killian, MD
Chief, Pediatric Orthopaedics
The Children's Hospital of Alabama
Birmingham, Alabama

L. Andrew Koman, MD
Department of Orthopaedic Surgery
Wake Forest University
Winston-Salem, North Carolina

Kenneth J. Koval, MD
Chief, Fracture Service
Hospital for Joint Diseases
New York, New York

Frederick J. Kummer, PhD
Associate Director, Bioengineering
Hospital for Joint Diseases
New York, New York

Daniel D. Lahr, MD
Medical College of Wisconsin
Milwaukee, Wisconsin

William N. Levine, MD
Chief Resident, Orthopaedics
New England Medical Center
Boston, Massachusetts

David G. Lewallen, MD
Associate Professor of Orthopedics
Mayo Medical School
Consultant, Department of Orthopedics
Mayo Clinic/Mayo Foundation
Rochester, Minnesota

J. Urban Lindgren, MD, PhD
Professor of Surgery
Creighton University Medical School
Omaha, Nebraska

Stephen J. Lipson, MD
Orthopaedic Surgeon-in-Chief
Beth Israel Hospital
Boston, Massachusetts

Randall T. Loder, MD
Assistant Professor
University of Michigan
Section of Orthopaedic Surgery
Ann Arbor, Michigan

Robert J. Marder, MD
Medical Director, Quality Management
Rush-Presbyterian-St. Luke's Medical Center
Chicago, Illinois

J.L. Marsh, MD
Professor
University of Iowa Hospitals and Clinics
Department of Orthopaedics
Iowa City, Iowa

Leland C. McCluskey, MD
Staff Physician
Hughston Clinic
Columbus, Georgia

William A. McGann, MD
Chief of Orthopaedic Training
San Francisco Orthopaedic Residency Program
San Francisco, California

Michael H. McGuire, MD
Professor and Chairman
Department of Surgery
Creighton University School of Medicine
Omaha, Nebraska

James D. Michelson, MD
Associate Professor and Vice-Chairman
Department of Orthopaedic Surgery
Johns Hopkins School of Medicine
Baltimore, Maryland

Leslie J. Mintz, MD
UC Davis Medical Center
Department of Orthopaedics
Sacramento, California

Srdjan Mirkovic, MD
Assistant Professor
Department of Orthopaedic Surgery
Northwestern University School of Medicine
Chicago, Illinois

Berton R. Moed, MD
Chief, Division of Orthopaedic Traumatology
Department of Orthopaedic Surgery
Henry Ford Hospital
Detroit, Michigan

Thomas J. Moore, MD
Assistant Professor
Emory School of Medicine
Atlanta, Georgia

Michael P. Mott, MD
Assistant Professor
Medical College of Wisconsin
Department of Orthopaedic Surgery
Milwaukee, Wisconsin

Scott J. Mubarak, MD
Clinical Professor
Pediatric Orthopaedics
University of California, San Diego
San Diego, California

Margareta Nordin, Dr Sci
Director, Occupational and Industrial Orthopaedic Center
Hospital for Joint Diseases Orthopaedic Institute
New York University School of Medicine
New York, New York

Shawn W. O'Driscoll, MD, PhD, FRCS(C)
Associate Professor of Orthopaedic Surgery
Mayo Clinic
Director, Cartilage and Connective Tissue Research Laboratory
Rochester, Minnesota

Michael J. Pagnani, MD
Attending Orthopaedic Surgeon
The Lipscomb Clinic
Clinical Assistant Professor of Orthopaedics and Rehabilitation
Vanderbilt University School of Medicine
Nashville, Tennessee

Lew Papendick, MD
Black Hills Orthopaedics and Sports Medicine
Rapid City, South Dakota

Ashvin I. Patel, MD
Sarasota Orthopaedic Associates
Sarasota, Florida

Clayton R. Perry, MD
Associate Professor of Orthopaedic Surgery
Department of Orthopaedic Surgery
Washington University School of Medicine
Chief of Fracture Service
Barnes Hospital
St. Louis, Missouri

Michael S. Pinzur, MD
Professor, Orthopaedic Surgery
Loyola University Medical Center
Maywood, Illinois

Roger G. Pollock, MD
Assistant Professor of Orthopaedic Surgery
The Shoulder Service
Columbia-Presbyterian Medical Center
New York, New York

George T. Rab, MD
Professor, Orthopaedic Surgery
Chief, Pediatric Orthopaedics
University of California, Davis
Sacramento, California

John C. Richmond, MD
Associate Professor, Orthopaedic Surgery
Tufts University School of Medicine
Boston, Massachusetts

John F. Ritterbusch, MD
Carrie Tingley Hospital
University of New Mexico
Albuquerque, New Mexico

Michael D. Rooks, MD
Associate Professor of Orthopaedics
Emory University School of Medicine
Atlanta, Georgia

Andrew D. Rosenberg, MD
Vice Chairman, Department of Anesthesiology
Hospital for Joint Diseases Orthopaedic Institute
New York, New York

Aaron G. Rosenberg, MD
Associate Professor and Director
Orthopaedic Education
Department of Orthopaedic Surgery
Rush Medical College
Chicago, Illinois

M.L. Chip Routt, Jr, MD
Associate Professor
University of Washington
Harborview Medical Center
Seattle, Washington

Sally A. Rudicel, MD
Associate Professor
Tufts University
New England Medical Center
Boston, Massachusetts

Richard F. Santore, MD
Senior Orthopaedic Surgeon
Sharp Memorial Hospital
San Diego, California

John F. Sarwark, MD
Associate Professor
Department of Orthopaedic Surgery
Northwestern University Medical School
Chicago, Illinois

Gary T. Schmidt, MD, FRCS(C)
Missouri Bone and Joint Center
St. Louis, Missouri

James J. Sferra, MD
Associate Staff
Section of Lower Extremities
The Cleveland Clinic Foundation
Cleveland, Ohio

Steven Shankman, MD
Vice-Chairman
Department of Radiology
Hospital for Joint Diseases Orthopaedic Institute
New York, New York

Jerry S. Sher, MD
University of Pennsylvania School of Medicine
Department of Orthopaedics
Philadelphia, Pennsylvania

Mark F. Sherman, MD
Staten Island University Hospital
Staten Island, New York

Mary Louise Skovron, Dr PH
Assistant Professor and Director
Musculoskeletal Epidemiology Unit
Hospital for Joint Diseases
New York University School of Medicine
New York, New York

Mark P. Slovenkai, MD
Department of Orthopaedic Surgery
Medical Center of Central Massachusetts
Worcester, Massachusetts

Jeffrey M. Spivak, MD
Associate Chief of Spinal Surgery
Hospital for Joint Diseases Orthopaedic Institute
New York, New York

Paul Sponseller, MD
Associate Professor and Head
Division of Pediatric Orthopaedics
Johns Hopkins University
Baltimore, Maryland

Deborah F. Stanitski, MD
Asssociate Chief of Orthopaedic Surgery
Children's Hospital of Michigan
Detroit, Michigan

Linda Stehling, MD
Vice President, Medical and Regulatory Affairs
Blood Systems, Inc.
Scottsdale, Arizona

Curtis M. Steyers, Jr, MD
Professor, Orthopaedic Surgery
Department of Orthopaedic Surgery
University of Iowa
Iowa City, Iowa

James W. Stone, MD
Assistant Clinical Professor of Orthopaedic Surgery
Medical College of Wisconsin
Milwaukee, Wisconsin

Joseph C. Stothert, Jr, MD, PhD
Professor of Surgery
Creighton University
University of Nebraska Medical Center
Omaha, Nebraska

Allan M. Strongwater, MD
Director, Orthopaedic Surgery
Maimonides Medical Center
Brooklyn, New York

Jeffrey Sum, BSE
Research Engineer
Rush-Presbyterian-St. Luke's Medical Center
Chicago, Illinois

Jonathan B. Ticker, MD
Island Orthopaedics and Sports Medicine
Massapequa, New York

Ensor E. Transfeldt, MD
Associate Professor and Director
Twin City Scoliosis Spine Center
Spine Surgeons of Minnesota
Minneapolis, Minnesota

Robert J. Treuting, MD
Medical College of Wisconsin
Milwaukee, Wisconsin

William Warner, MD
Campbell Clinic
University of Tennessee
Memphis, Tennessee

Peter M. Waters, MD
Assistant Professor, Department of Orthopaedic Surgery
Harvard Medical School
Clinical Director, Hand Surgery Clinics
Children's Hospital Medical Center
Boston, Massachusetts

Dennis R. Wenger, MD
Clinical Professor of Orthopedics
Pediatric Orthopedic Surgery
University of California, San Diego
San Diego, California

Sam W. Wiesel, MD
Professor and Chairman
Department of Orthopaedic Surgery
Georgetown University Medical Center
Washington, DC

Gerald R. Williams, Jr, MD
Associate Professor, Orthopaedic Surgery
University of Pennsylvania School of Medicine
Philadelphia, Pennsylvania

Russell E. Windsor, MD
Associate Professor, Orthopaedic Surgery
Hospital for Special Surgery
Cornell University Medical College
New York, New York

Preston M. Wolin, MD
Director
Center for Athletic Medicine
Chicago, Illinois

Douglas Yoder, BS
Research Engineer
Rush-Presbyterian-St. Luke's Medical Center
Chicago, Illinois

Hansen A. Yuan, MD
Professor of Orthopaedic and Neurological Surgery
Director, Division of Spinal Surgery
Syracuse, New York

Thomas A. Zdeblick, MD
Associate Professor, Division of Orthopedic Surgery
University of Wisconsin
Madison, Wisconsin

Joseph D. Zuckerman, MD
Chairman, Department of Orthopaedic Surgery
Hospital for Joint Diseases
New York, New York

Preface

This is the fifth *Orthopaedic Knowledge Update.* As always, this text represents a balance between core information and new material, presented in an unbiased fashion in hopes of providing the basic information with which all orthopaedic surgeons should be familiar. Since the publication of *OKU 4,* the Academy has begun to publish subspecialty *OKUs,* which cover all areas in greater detail than is possible in this text. Each subspecialty *OKU* should serve as an additional resource for those interested in more information in a specific area. In compiling this text, the editorial board has taken great effort to try to avoid presenting data or opinions that conflict with the content of the subspecialty *OKUs.*

In *OKU 5,* you will notice that there are two sections that were not in previous volumes: "systemic disease" and "rehabilitation." Diverse conditions, such as bone dysplasias, neuromuscular disease, and arthritis, are discussed with the hope of providing a general refresher in each of these important areas. The orthopaedic issues surrounding rehabilitation are of major significance to the population as a whole and, therefore, a section on rehabilitation considering such issues as stroke, amputations, and head and spinal cord injury was warranted. Topics not included in this volume of *OKU* include pain management and orthopaedic anesthesia, and I have reduced markedly the content on Epidemiology. *OKU 4* should continue to be used as a resource for information in these areas.

The anatomic organization has been continued with sections in upper extremity, lower extremity, and spine. Pediatric and adult conditions are included together. This organization is meant to reinforce the continuum in management between the pediatric and adult patient. There traditionally has been a positive response to annotated bibliographies. Although these short summaries of papers published in the last 4 years take up considerable space, I think you will find that they provide a "rapid fire" literature update worthy of your attention.

I would like to thank members of the Academy staff, including Marilyn Fox, Joan Abern, and Bruce Davis for their help in compiling this text. Generous contributions of over 100 authors form the bulk of the text. The Editorial Board worked diligently in the organization and editing of these materials. My thanks go out to all those who participated in this effort. While the pressures of orthopaedic practice escalate, the authors and Editorial Board willingly gave unselfishly of their time and intellect. I am grateful to them for this considerable effort.

Just as the pace of orthopaedic practice continues to escalate for the authors, it does for the readers as well. You as a reader of this text are to be commended for your efforts in participating in an update and self-study program. Please continue your efforts at ongoing orthopaedic education with my best wishes. May you learn as much reading this book as I did editing it. Best wishes to you, your families, and your patients.

James R. Kasser, MD

I

General Knowledge

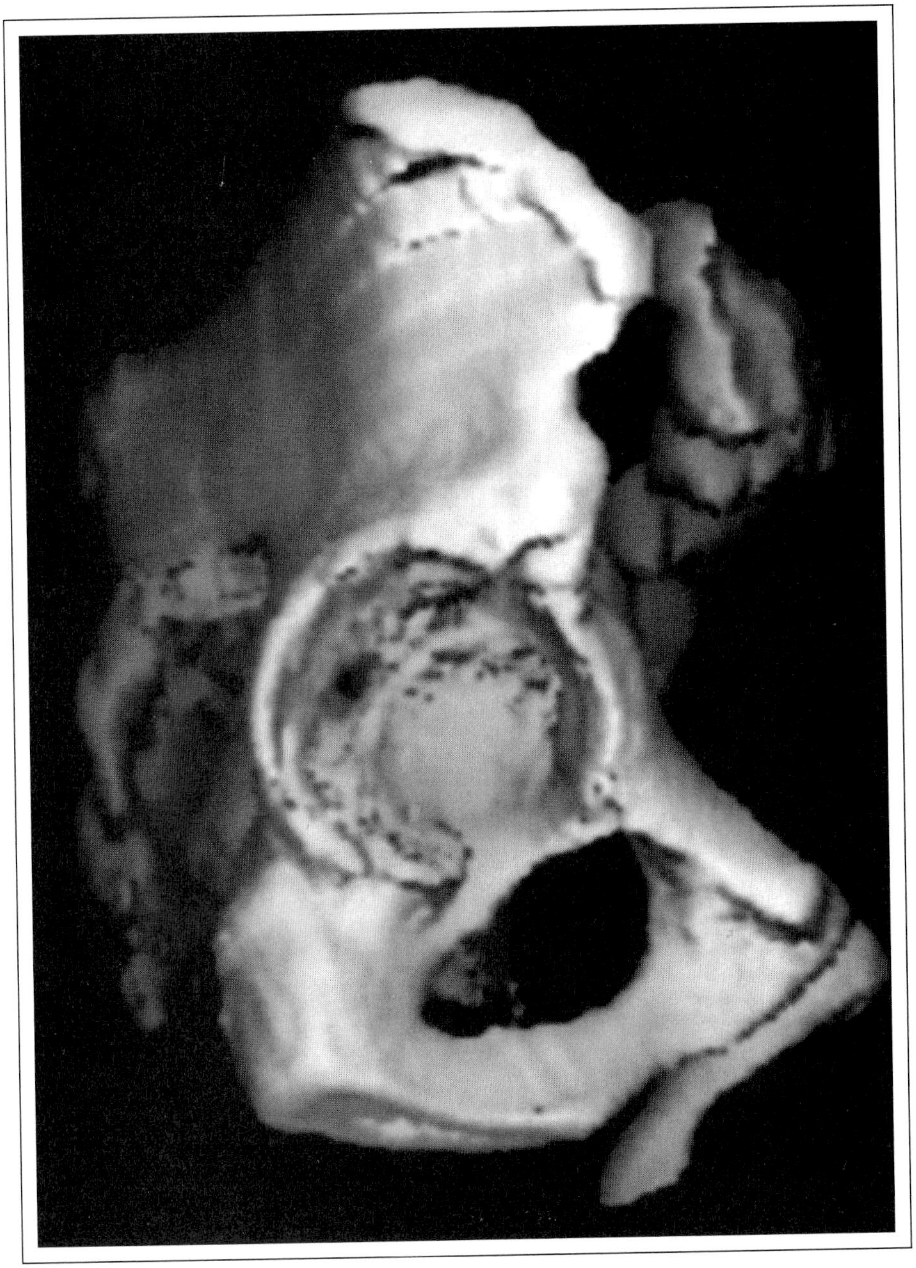

1

Soft-Tissue Physiology and Repair

Cartilage

Articular Cartilage

Structure Normal articular cartilage is composed of a large extracellular matrix (ECM) with a sparse population of cells (chondrocytes). The principal components of the matrix are proteoglycans, collagen, and water. The matrix is generated and maintained by chondrocytes. Metabolic activity within articular cartilage is controlled by chondrocytes in response to environmental stimuli (eg, growth factors, mechanical loads). Mature articular cartilage has no nerve supply and contains no blood vessels.

Over 50% of the dry weight of articular cartilage consists of collagen. The major collagen in articular cartilage is known as type II. With its characteristic triple helical structure (Fig. 1), collagen provides tensile properties to the tissue and acts as a framework to immobilize proteoglycans within the ECM.

Proteoglycans are complex macromolecules that consist of a protein core linked to long-chain, unbranched, polysaccharide (glycosaminoglycan) chains (Fig. 2). Chondroitin sulfates are the most prevalent glycosaminoglycans in cartilage. All glycosaminoglycans in cartilage contain carboxyl (COO^-) and/or sulfate (SO_3^-) groups that become ionized in solution. To maintain electroneutrality within the tissue, free-floating positively charged ions must also be present. These free-floating ions create an osmotic pressure effect within cartilage. In addition, the proximity of the ionized fixed-charged groups within cartilage results in strong repulsive forces. Together, the osmotic and repulsive forces contribute to the swelling pressure of the cartilage.

Normal articular cartilage has water contents ranging from 65% to 80% of its total wet weight. Most of the water is contained in the ECM. The affinity of water is primarily derived from the hydrophilic nature of proteoglycans. There is frictional resistance to flow of this water through molecular-size pores in the ECM. Pressurization of the water in association with this frictional resistance allows cartilage to support very high joint loads. Flow of the water permits transport of nutrients through the cartilage and into the joint. Thus, water flow also contributes to joint lubrication.

Articular cartilage may be divided into four zones (Fig. 3). The superficial zone is the uppermost zone and forms the gliding surface of the joint. Collagen fibrils are arranged parallel to the joint surface in this zone. The superficial zone is rich in collagen and relatively lacking in proteoglycans. Tensile stiffness is greater here than in the middle and deep zones because of the high concentration and orientation of collagen fibrils. The middle (transition) zone contains collagen fibers with a larger diameter and less apparent organization than in the superficial zone. The concentration of proteoglycans increases in this zone. The deep zone has the highest concentration of proteoglycans and the lowest water content of the four zones. In this region, collagen fibers are oriented perpendicular to the joint surface. The zone of calcified cartilage is the deepest layer. It separates the hyaline cartilage from underlying subchondral bone. In this zone, the matrix is heavily encrusted with apatite salts. The tidemark, a wavy blue line seen with hemotoxylin and eosin staining, separates the deep and calcified zones.

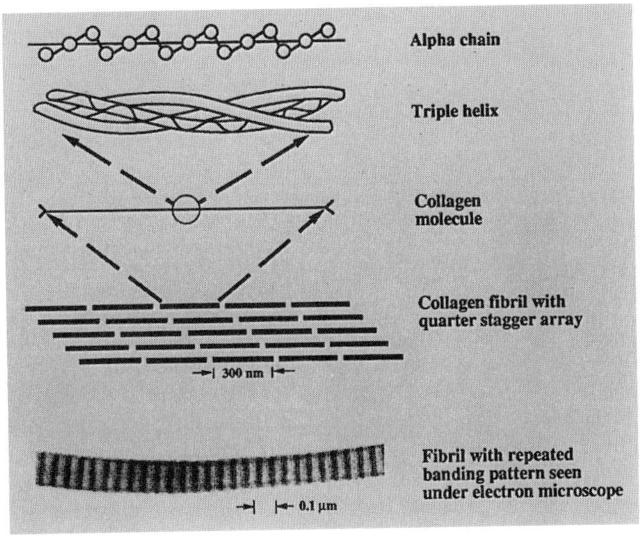

Fig. 1 Basic structure of collagen fibrils. (Reproduced with permission from Mow VC, Zhu W, Ratcliffe A: Structure and function of articular cartilage and meniscus, in Mow VC, Hayes WC (eds): *Basic Orthopaedic Biomechanics.* New York, NY, Raven Press, 1991, pp 143–198.)

The organization of collagen in the middle and deep zones of cartilage contributes significantly to the shear properties of the tissue. The resistance of cartilage to shear stress increases with compression. Shear stress attains a maximal value at the tidemark.

Physiology and Biomechanics Because articular cartilage is avascular, energy production within it is generated primarily through an anaerobic pathway. The energy pro-

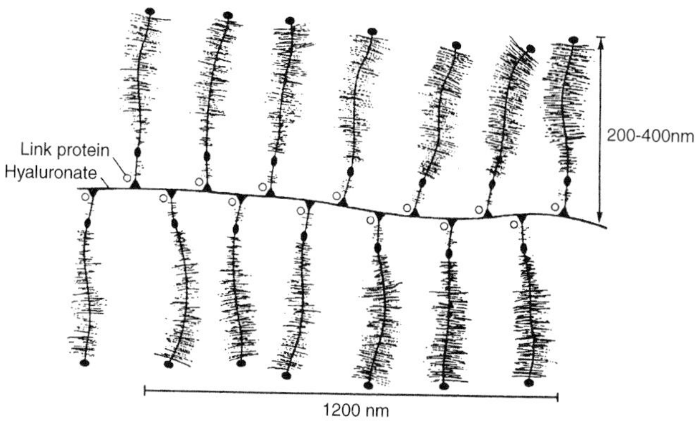

Fig. 2 Basic structure of proteoglycan with extended polysaccharide chains linked to a protein core. (Reproduced with permission from Buckwalter JA, Kuettner KE, Thonar EJ: Age-related changes in articular cartilage proteoglycans: Electron microscopic studies. *J Orthop Res* 1985;3:251–257.)

duced allows chondrocytes to maintain a normal ECM through the synthesis and degradation of matrix components. Metabolic activity is determined by a cellular response to soluble mediators (eg, growth factors, interleukins), matrix composition, mechanical loads, hydrostatic pressure changes, and electric fields. Because adult articular cartilage is avascular, most investigators believe that nutrients diffuse through the matrix from the surrounding synovial fluid. Articular cartilage is also aneural, but chondrocytes are believed to be sensitive to pressure or deformation. Data from recent studies have indicated that mechanical stimuli can alter cartilage metabolism and lead to rapid remodeling.

Articular cartilage is subject to high loads applied repetitively for the lifetime of an individual. The cartilage matrix must be able to resist these loads. The biomechanical properties of articular cartilage are best understood when the tissue is viewed as a biphasic material that has a solid phase and a fluid phase. The cartilage matrix is a porous and permeable material. Water resides in the microscopic pores, and the flow of this water through the permeable matrix may be induced by a pressure gradient or by matrix contraction. High hydrodynamic pressures are required to maintain a significant flow. These high fluid pressures provide a significant component of total load support and, therefore, minimize the stress on the normal cartilage matrix. The permeability of cartilage decreases nonlinearly with compression. Because permeability is strain-dependent, excessive fluid exudation does not occur instantly with joint compression, and load support is maintained. Fluid pressurization appears to be the dominant physiologic load support mechanism.

Joint loading and motion are required to maintain normal adult articular cartilage. Immobilization of a joint will cause a rapid loss of proteoglycans from the cartilage matrix. Proteoglycan content is affected to a greater extent

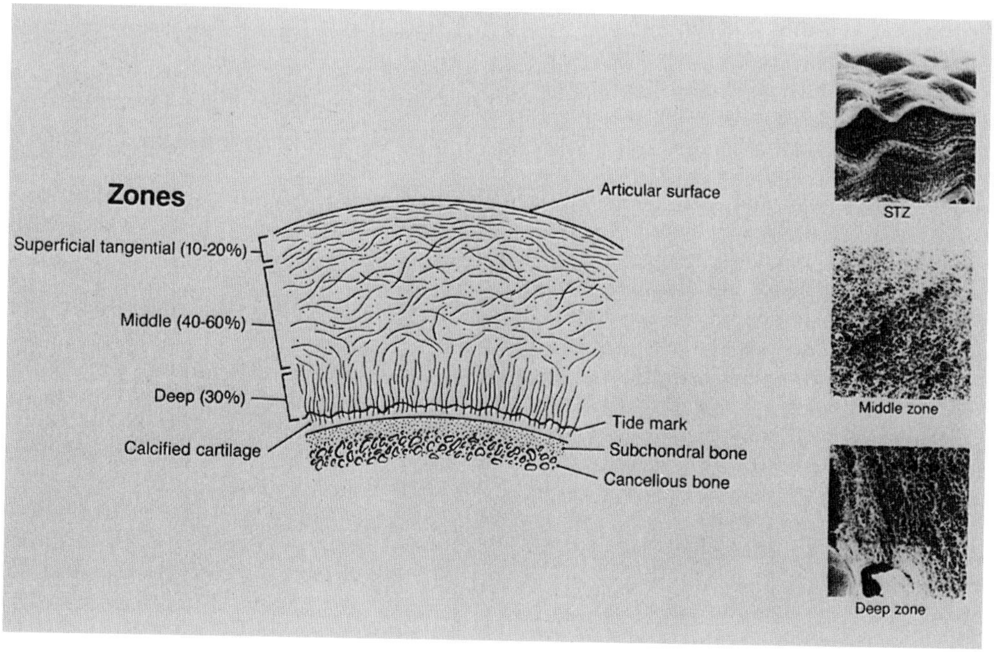

Fig. 3 Collagen fiber architecture in the four zones of articular cartilage. (Reproduced with permission from Mow VC, Proctor CS, Kelly MA: Biomechanics of articular cartilage, in Nordin M, Frankel VH (eds): *Basic Biomechanics of the Musculoskeletal System,* ed 2. Philadelphia, PA, Lea & Febiger, 1989, pp 31–57.)

than collagen composition. Because proteoglycan is lost, fluid flux and deformation in response to compression will increase. Tensile properties, which depend primarily on collagen, are maintained. These biochemical and biomechanical changes are, at least in part, reversible with the restoration of motion. The extent of recovery decreases with increasing periods of immobilization.

Increased joint loading, either through excessive use or increased magnitudes of loading will also affect articular cartilage. Disruption of the intra-articular structures, such as menisci or ligaments, will alter forces acting on the articular surface. In experimental animal models, responses to transection of the anterior cruciate ligament (ACL) or meniscectomy have included fibrillation of the cartilage surface, increased hydration, and changes in proteoglycan content. Significant and progressive decreases in the tensile and shear modulus have been observed in response to transection of the ACL.

Articular Cartilage Repair Although articular cartilage is a metabolically active tissue, it has a limited capacity for repair. Most connective tissues repair damaged areas with new cells and an ECM that closely resemble the original tissue. In these cases, normal or near normal function can be restored. Repair of significant defects of articular cartilage is rarely this successful.

Superficial laceration injuries to articular cartilage that do not cross the tidemark generally do not heal. These superficial lesions do not cause hemorrhage or initiate a bleeding response, and chondrocytes do not migrate to the injured region. When cartilage injury penetrates the subchondral bone, cells pass through subchondral vessels and can initiate a healing response. These full-thickness lesions result in hemorrhage, fibrin clot formation, and inflammation at the site of injury. This fibrinous arcade is believed to act as a "scaffold" that directs mesenchymal cells (derived from marrow) to produce a fibrocartilaginous matrix at the surface edge. In addition, such lesions result in the release of growth factors (eg, platelet-derived growth factor and transforming growth factor-β) that may stimulate migration of undifferentiated mesenchymal cells into the fibrin clot.

Unfortunately, the repaired tissue often lacks the unique composition of normal cartilage. In most cases, the subchondral portion of the defect is repaired with a tissue that consists primarily of bone, but also contains some regions of fibrous tissue and hyaline cartilage. In contrast, the chondral portion of the defect is rarely repaired completely. In many instances, the composition and structure of chondral repair tissue are intermediate between those of hyaline cartilage and fibrocartilage. Chondral repair tissue contains a higher proportion of hyaline cartilage than the bony portion of the defect, but it also contains substantial amounts of fibrous tissue. In a recent study of osteochondral healing in a primate knee joint, repair tissues were noted to have a solid matrix with lower elastic modulus and higher permeability than normal tissues. The orientation of collagen fibrils in repair cartilage does not follow the pattern seen in normal cartilage. In repair cartilage, fibrils are randomly arranged. Swelling is increased in repair cartilage in part because of the loss of the collagen meshwork. These changes tend to remove the fluid-pressure load-carrying capacity of cartilage. The inferior material properties of repair cartilage may make it more susceptible to structural damage when the joint is loaded. In addition, gaps may form between the new cartilage and the adjacent cartilage, suggesting a lack of firm physical interdigitation between the old and repaired cartilage. Micromotion could result as mechanical stresses are applied to the new cartilage, By 1 year after injury, loss of the hyaline-appearing matrix usually occurs in larger defects, and progressive deterioration may ensue.

Articular Cartilage Lesions Current treatments of isolated chondral injuries in adults include debridement of chondral flaps and removal of loose chondral fragments from the joint. Abrasion chondroplasty with drilling of the subchondral bone has been advocated for full-thickness articular cartilage defects despite evidence that the fibrocartilaginous tissue that results from this treatment has inferior biomechanical properties. There is no evidence to suggest that the common practice of arthroscopic shaving of partial-thickness lesions has any beneficial response on tissue healing.

Experimental data suggest that replacement of chondral defects with subchondral bone grafts or tissue adhesives or with chondral or osteochondral allografts may be beneficial. As of yet, there are insufficient long-term studies of the outcome of such procedures. Large osteochondral fractures can often be treated by early open reduction and internal fixation of the fracture. Allograft osteochondral transplantation has been used successfully in the late treatment of selected osteochondral defects. In one series of 91 patients with posttraumatic osteochondral defects of the knee, the implantation of fresh osteochondral allografts was reported to be successful in 75% at 5 years, 64% at 10 years, and 63% at 14 years. Joint alignment should be corrected with osteotomy in conjunction with the placement of the allograft.

Several encouraging experimental techniques to stimulate cartilage repair are currently being investigated. Packing a full-thickness cartilage defect (in a canine knee model) with exogenous fibrin clot led to a more organized and advanced healing response compared to control defects during the first 8 weeks of the process. At 12 and 24 weeks, this difference in healing response was less pronounced. The clot-filled defects tended to heal more uniformly and with less surface depression, particularly if they were located in an unloaded site on the knee.

The experimental use of perichondrial and periosteal allografts stimulated short-term success with regard to cartilage repair. Such tissues have the capacity to form hyaline cartilage. The results indicate that chondral defects can be filled with a tissue that resembles hyaline cartilage, both histologically and biomechanically. Clinical results with these techniques have been variable, with some evidence that younger individuals fare better. Periosteal explants also have the capacity to form cartilage in vitro where they can be treated with growth factors or other chondroinductive agents prior to implantation.

Mesenchymal stem cells and chondrocytes can be maintained in culture and induced to form a matrix that closely resembles that of normal cartilage. Swedish investigators recently reported on a group of 23 patients who were treated with autologous chondrocyte transplantation for deep cartilage defects of the knee. Chondrocytes were obtained arthroscopically from an uninvolved area of the injured knee and cultured for 14 to 21 days. An arthrotomy was then performed, and the chondrocytes were injected into the area of the defect and covered with a periosteal flap taken from the proximal tibia. The authors reported good to excellent clinical results in 14 of 16 patients with femoral condylar lesions and in two of seven patients with patellar transplants at 16- to 66-month follow-up. Hyaline cartilage was noted in biopsy specimens of 11 of 15 femoral transplants and one of seven patellar transplants.

Other investigators have examined the effects of growth factors and hyaluronic acid derivatives on articular cartilage. These substances may protect cartilage against biochemical injury and stimulate its repair. Although these techniques are promising, longer follow-up and further investigation is warranted before any of them can be generally recommended.

Meniscal Cartilage

Structure The meniscus is a fibrocartilaginous structure composed of an interlacing network of collagen fibers, proteoglycans and glycoproteins, and interspersed cells. The cells of the meniscus have been termed fibrochondrocytes and are responsible for the synthesis and maintenance of ECM. The ECM is composed primarily of type I collagen. These collagen fibers are generally oriented in a circumferential direction, although a few small fibers are oriented radially (Fig. 4). The concentration of proteoglycans and glycoproteins is only about 10% of that in hyaline cartilage. The matrix is a biphasic structure composed of a solid phase (eg, collagen, proteoglycan), which acts as a fiber reinforced porous-permeable composite, and a fluid phase, which may be forced through the solid matrix by a hydraulic pressure gradient. Although these properties are shared with articular cartilage, the meniscus is more elastic and less permeable than articular cartilage.

The peripheral borders of the menisci obtain their blood supply from a circumferentially arranged perimeniscal plexus. Radial branches from this plexus penetrate 10% to 30% of the width of the meniscus. Innervation of the meniscus is restricted to the peripheral two thirds of the structure. The menisci contain both free nerve endings and corpuscular mechanoreceptors. Thus, the menisci may act as a source of proprioceptive information for muscular tone and coordination. A deficiency in this proprioceptive input may contribute to articular degeneration after loss of meniscal tissue.

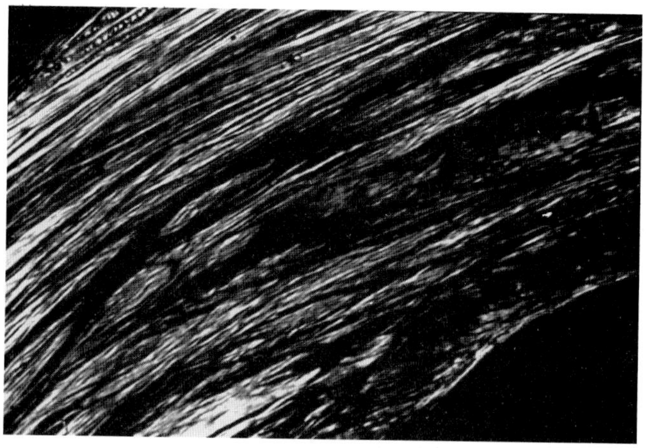

Fig. 4 Photomicrograph of a meniscus under polarized light demonstrating circumferentially oriented collogen fibers. (Reproduced with permission from Woo SL-Y, An K-N, Arnoczky SP, et al: Anatomy, biology, and biomechanics of tendon, ligament, and meniscus, in Simon SR (ed): *Orthopaedic Basic Science.* Rosemont, IL, American Academy of Orthopaedic Surgeons, 1994, pp 45–87.)

Kinematic analysis of the knee has demonstrated that the menisci move anteriorly with extension and posteriorly with flexion. The lateral meniscus is more mobile than the medial meniscus, and the anterior horn of the lateral meniscus has the greatest mobility.

Biomechanics The menisci contribute to knee load distribution, shock absorption, and joint lubrication. Normal menisci transmit 50% to 90% of knee joint force, and the medial meniscus acts as a secondary stabilizer against anteroposterior translation of the tibia on the femur. Loss of meniscal tissue increases the load on the underlying articular cartilage, predisposing to joint degeneration. At heel strike, the meniscus attenuates stress waves, which pass through the knee, by as much as 20%. Compression of the meniscus is thought to cause extrusion of free water into the joint space, increasing the available joint lubricant.

With weightbearing, centrifugal radial forces are resisted by the firm attachments of the anterior and posterior horns of the menisci to the tibia. This situation produces large circumferentially oriented hoop tensile stresses, which are countered by the circumferential arrangement of most collagen fibers in the meniscus. Proteoglycans contribute to the compressive properties of the menisci through their ionic repulsive forces, which increase matrix stiffness, and by contributing to the osmotic pressure within the meniscus.

Compressive forces in the knee generate tensile stresses in the meniscus. There are significant regional variations in the tensile strength and stiffness of differing anatomic portions of the menisci. These variations appear to be a result of differences in collagen ultrastructure rather than of biochemical variations. The presence of radial fibers in a particular portion of the meniscus may increase tensile stiffness and strength under radially applied tension.

Loss of Meniscal Tissue Data from several long-term follow-up studies have confirmed that meniscectomy, either total or partial, commonly results in the development of degenerative change. These findings underscore the importance of preserving meniscal tissue whenever a reparable lesion is encountered. Partial meniscectomy is not necessarily a benign procedure; meniscal function may be compromised despite judicious resection. Stable tears should not be resected. Patients with malalignment or large body mass appear to be at especially increased risk for the development of arthrosis.

Meniscal Repair The vascular portions of the meniscus are capable of a repair response. In contrast, the avascular region does not have reparative abilities. In the vascular zone, a fibrin clot forms after injury. The fibrin scaffold becomes populated with vessels and undifferentiated mesenchymal cells. Remodeling of this fibrovascular scar into normal-appearing fibrocartilage takes several months. Use of an exogenous fibrin clot has been reported to enhance the healing process.

Meniscal Replacement The development of arthrosis after meniscal resection has led to a search for a method of meniscal regeneration or replacement. Two preliminary animal studies illustrate this ongoing quest. One group implanted a Dacron meniscal prosthesis with a polyurethane coating into rabbit knees. Synovial tissue ingrowth was noted in 93% of the prostheses. The prosthesis decreased joint stiffness to values that approached normal, but it was ineffective in dissipating energy under load and it was associated with a high incidence of osteophyte formation and severe synovial reaction.

Another group of investigators implanted absorbable, copolymeric, collagen-based meniscal scaffolds in dog stifle joints. Substantial meniscal regeneration was noted in 63% of the knees. By 9 to 12 months after implantation, the "successfully regenerated" menisci resembled the normal canine meniscus on histologic and biochemical examination. The authors felt that the scaffolds supported meniscal fibrochondrocyte ingrowth and may provide an avenue to permit complete meniscal regeneration. However, it has not been shown that these scaffolds can reproduce normal meniscal mechanics and kinematics.

Meniscal Allografts As the development of a synthetic meniscus or meniscal scaffold evolves, a great deal of interest is being directed toward meniscal transplantation using allograft tissue. The indications for meniscal transplantation are not well-defined. Generally, postmeniscectomy patients who are considered for the procedure should be younger than 45 years of age and should have normal knee alignment, minimal to moderate cartilage wear, and debilitating pain localized to the involved compartment. Early clinical results of such procedures have been promising, but no long-term (> 2 year) outcomes are available. The experimental nature of the procedure and the risks of disease transmission should be carefully explained to patients who are candidates for the procedure. Freeze-dried menisci undergo significant shrinkage after implantation and should not be used.

Recent basic science research has contributed to identification of some inherent difficulties of meniscal transplantation. In one study, deep-frozen dog menisci were reimplanted and were found to be repopulated with cells that seemed to originate from the adjacent synovium. The phenotype of these cells was unclear, but they appeared to resemble meniscal fibrochondrocytes. The cells migrated over the superficial surface of the menisci and began to invade the deeper portions of the menisci. However, the central core of the meniscus remained acellular at 6 months after reimplantation. In addition, there were histologic alterations in the normal collagen architecture of the menisci. The authors felt that this finding was consistent with a remodeling phenomenon that accompanied cellular repopulation and cautioned that similar processes may render allograft menisci more susceptible to injury.

In another study, autografts, fresh allografts, and cryopreserved allografts were analyzed after meniscal transplantation in a goat model. There were few gross or microscopic differences between transplanted and control menisci. The viability of the autograft menisci approached 100% while that of the allografts was found to be 71% to 83%. Analysis of the water and proteoglycan content of the allograft menisci (both fresh and cryopreserved) revealed substantial changes in the biochemical makeup of the menisci. The authors expressed their concern over the long-term function of meniscal allografts. In a follow-up study using the same goat model, the investigators found that viable cells in meniscal allografts do not survive transplantation. Instead, the meniscus is repopulated entirely by host cells. The authors concluded that grafts containing living cells (cryopreserved) may not offer any advantages over those in which the cells are not present (fresh frozen). Cryopreservation also increases cost and, theoretically, the risks of disease transmission. In summary, meniscal allograft transplantation is an experimental and technically demanding procedure with, as yet, unproven clinical efficacy.

Ligament

Structure and Function

Optimal joint function depends on the complex interaction around the joint of ligaments, which act as static restraints, and muscle-tendon units, which act as dynamic restraints, as well as other factors, including articular geometry. When they are under tension, ligaments act as static restraints by maintaining the relationship of the two opposing articular surfaces. In some joints, ligaments function throughout the range of motion (eg, ACL), while in other joints, ligaments function to stabilize the joint at an end range of motion (eg, inferior glenohumeral ligament). Furthermore, different portions within one ligament can have separate functions. For both the ACL and the posterior cruciate ligament (PCL), the anterior component is tight in flexion and the posterior portion is tight in extension. Similarly, different regions of the inferior glenohumeral ligament have been shown to have differences in function, as well as differences in biomechanical characteristics.

Ligaments are dense connective tissue that link bone to bone. These band- or cord-like structures are defined by their anatomic location (eg, anterior talofibular ligament) and appearance (eg, cruciate ligaments, anterior and posterior). The gross structure varies with the location (eg, intra-articular, capsular, and extra-articular) and function. Ligaments appear to have an ultra-, micro-, and macrostructural organization similar to that of tendons. In addition, the structure of the collagen fibril found in ligaments, beginning with a polypeptide chain and a triple-stranded helical formation, is consistent with that found in all tissues in which collagen is present (Fig. 1). This arrangement, along with covalent cross-links between collagen molecules, adds to the strength of collagen. Collagen fibers and bundles are aligned along the axis of tension of the ligament. Under microscopic examination, the collagen fibers are relatively parallel; however, they demonstrate a more interwoven arrangement than that found in tendon. Characteristic sinusoidal patterns, or crimp, are routinely observed within the bundles and may vary between and within ligaments. Fibroblasts, which are relatively low in number, are responsible for producing and maintaining the extracellular components.

The morphologic characteristics vary between portions of a ligament substance and at the insertion sites. Two distinct areas within one ligament may demonstrate different patterns of collagen alignment or crimping, as well as variations in fiber diameters. Two types of insertion sites have been described based on their microscopic appearance. The direct insertion, which is the most common, can be found in the femoral attachment of the medial collateral ligament (MCL) and the ACL (Fig. 5). It is also found in tendons, such as at the insertion of the supraspinatus tendon into the greater tuberosity of the proximal humerus. The collagen, primarily the deep fibers, inserts at right angles to the bone through four zones of transition within a distance of less than 1 mm. Zone I consists of collagen with ECM and fibroblasts. Zone II is represented by the appearance of fibrocartilage with associated cellular changes. Zones II and III are separated by the mineralization front, or tidemark, and zone III is characterized by the presence of mineralized fibrocartilage. Zone IV is distinguished by the abrupt transition to bone. The indirect insertion has a much broader insertion to bone, primarily via the more superficial fibers into the periosteum, as in the tibial attachment of the MCL.

The major biochemical component of ligaments is water, about 60% to 80%. Collagen constitutes approximately

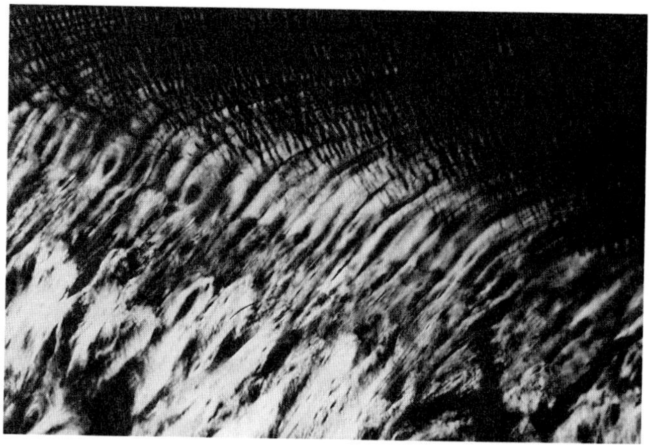

Fig. 5 Photomicrograph of a direct insertion site of the tibial attachment of the canine anterior cruciate ligament, under polarized low-magnification. (Courtesy of Dr. John Matyas, University of Calgary, Alberta, Canada.)

70% to 80% of the dry weight, with type I collagen accounting for approximately 90% of the collagen content and type III and others accounting for the remainder. The formation of cross-links is an important component of the strength characteristics of the collagen fibers. The ground substance includes proteoglycans, which have the capacity to contain water molecules and to affect the viscoelastic properties of soft tissues. The protein elastin, which is present in small amounts, assists with the tissue's ability to lengthen under an applied load by storing energy and return to its original length when the load is removed. Other noncollagenous proteins are found in very low concentrations. The structural and material properties have been reported for a variety of ligaments. The structural properties reflect the mechanical behavior of the tissue as a whole; are influenced by the ligament's geometry, insertion sites, and material characteristics; and are expressed by the load-elongation curve (Fig. 6). The material properties depend on the ligament substance, molecular bonds, and composition, without influence from the geometry or the insertion sites, and are expressed by the stress-strain curve (Fig. 6). Stress is defined as force per unit area, and strain describes the change in length relative to the original length. When a ligament is placed under tension, it deforms in a nonlinear fashion. In the initial stages, or toe region, the coiled nature of the collagen and the crimping are recruited to be more aligned along the axis of tension. In the next stage, or linear region, with continued tension, the collagen fibers become taut and then stretch. The slope of the linear region for the load-elongation curve describes the stiffness of the tissue, and the slope of the stress-strain curve denotes the tensile modulus. Overload occurs at the yield point, where tissue failure is observed. These sinusoidal curves demonstrate the nonlinear nature of soft

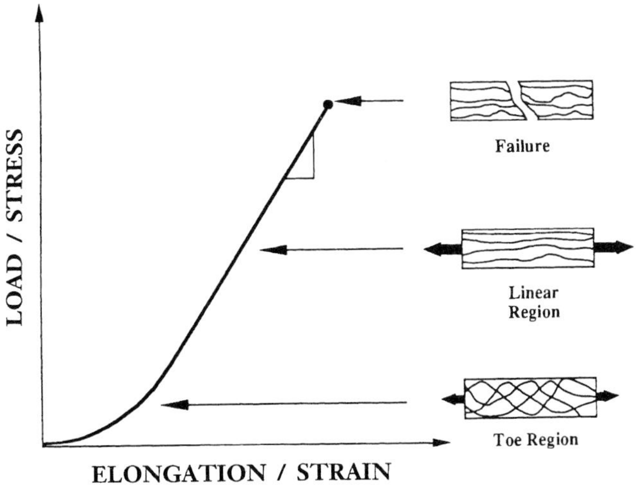

Fig. 6 Typical non-linear curve for structural (load-elongation) and material (stress-strain) properties of a ligament or other collagenous tissue. The behavior of the collagen fibers is shown. (Adapted with permission from Mow VC, Zhu W, Ratcliffe A: Structure and function of articular cartilage and meniscus, in Mow VC, Hayes WC (eds): *Basic Orthopaedic Biomechanics.* New York, NY, Raven Press, 1991, pp 143–198.)

connective tissues. In addition, ligament and tendon biomechanical characteristics demonstrate time-dependent viscoelastic behavior.

The properties of the insertion sites differ from those of the ligament midsubstance, with greater strain found in these areas when tested under uniaxial tension. The failure patterns of bone-ligament-bone complexes change under a variety of circumstances. Age has been shown to be the predominant factor in the rabbit MCL. The skeletally-immature specimens failed at the tibial insertion site, whereas in the mature specimens, failure occurred in the midsubstance. Ligament substance appears to mature earlier than the insertion sites. Strain rate, or rate of elongation, has been shown to affect the failure pattern of both the ACL and the inferior glenohumeral ligament. At higher strain rates, the strength and tensile modulus increased, and failures occurred more in the ligament substance than at the insertion sites. The axis of loading has been shown to affect failure patterns. When the ACL was loaded along the axis of the tibia and not the ligament, the femur-ACL-tibia complex demonstrated decreasing load at failure with increasing flexion angle, and failure was more likely to occur in the ligament substance.

As ligaments age, the structural properties change in response to loading conditions. The load at failure of older specimens is 33% to 50% of that found in younger bone-ligament-bone specimens. In addition, stiffness and elongation at failure are markedly reduced. Diminished material properties have also been shown to occur, with decreases in tensile modulus, stress at failure, and strain at failure. Biochemical changes that occur include a decrease in water and collagen content. In addition, there is a change from a higher concentration of the immature, more labile, cross-links to a higher concentration of the mature, more stable, forms. Fibroblasts are less metabolically active with aging and assume a more elongated shape. It would appear that whereas maturation influences the insertion sites of ligaments as demonstrated in the failure patterns, aging and senescence have a detrimental affect on the ligament substance.

Response to Exercise and Loading

Under conditions in which loading is enhanced for a long period of time, the properties of ligaments demonstrate a modest, yet positive, response. Overall mass increases, and stiffness and load at failure increase. In addition to these changes in structural properties, the material properties are affected with an increase in stress and strain at failure. Similar changes have been shown in the experimental setting when the rabbit MCL was placed under increased tension for a sustained period.

Response to Immobilization and Disuse

These conditions have a much more dramatic effect on ligaments and compromise their structural and material properties. The load at failure decreases by 25% after 4 weeks of immobilization for the cruciate ligaments in rats, and by 66% after 9 weeks of immobilization for the rabbit MCL. A corresponding decrease in the stiffness is also seen after these short time periods, and similar changes in the material properties occur. Thus, changes in both the ligament substance and insertion sites are evident. Subperiosteal bone resorption from increased osteoclastic activity at the insertion sites has been observed; this resorption affects failure patterns. With even longer periods of immobilization, degradation of collagen increases as collagen synthesis decreases, resulting in less total collagen. A decrease in water and proteoglycan content contribute to an overall decrease in ligament mass.

The recovery period following immobilization is more rapid in the ligament substance than at the insertion sites. It may take up to 1 year for the insertion sites to return to a level approaching that of controls. However, following 9 weeks of immobilization and 9 weeks of remobilization, the material properties were similar to those of controls, confirming the more rapid recovery of the ligament substance when motion and loading are permitted.

Response to Injury and Mechanisms of Repair

The MCL in the knee has been studied most extensively following injury. After a rupture in the ligament substance, healing occurs in three histologic phases. During the inflammatory phase, an initial hematoma forms, with cellular invasion to fill the gap. As the reparative phase begins, this is transformed into granulation tissue, and fibroblasts begin to proliferate. Immature type III collagen fibers are found and begin to form a parallel alignment, and the injured tissue is replaced. The biomechanical properties are enhanced as synthesis of type I collagen increases; this phase progresses during the period up to approximately 6 weeks after injury. The remodeling phase, which can last from several months to over a year, involves further maturation and eventual conversion to normal-appearing tissue. Collagen fibrils have a greater diameter and are more densely packed, with an increase in total collagen content. The collagen alignment remains at a less organized level compared with controls. An overall increase in cross-sectional area persists and contributes to the return of the structural properties, which approach normal values. However, the material properties after remodeling do not return completely to preinjury levels.

Various factors influence ligament healing. Degree of injury, location of the ligament, and modes of treatment can influence the repair process. A more severe injury will result in greater damage to the tissue and a larger gap, prolonging and possibly impairing healing. In the case of the MCL, associated injury to the ACL has an unfavorable effect compared with an isolated MCL injury. Reconstruction of the ACL may counteract this effect. Intra-articular ligaments, such as the cruciates, do not heal because they are in an environment that cannot promote the initial phase of healing, unlike the extra-articular and probably intracapsular ligaments. Controlled passive motion leads to a more rapid repair and enhances the collagen alignment and the biomechanical properties of the healing MCL. Immobilization following injury has the opposite effect.

Grafts for Reconstruction

Ligament reconstruction, particularly of the ACL and PCL, is performed to restore joint stability using a graft substitute. Both autograft and allograft tissue have been used successfully under specific conditions. Reported alternatives for autografts include patellar tendon, semitendinosis and/or gracilis tendons, fascia lata, iliotibial band, and achilles tendon. The central third of the patellar tendon is the most commonly used graft, and it is the only autograft that demonstrates a higher load at failure than the ACL when tested experimentally. After implantation in experimental animals, no graft has ever shown biomechanical properties near those of the ACL. Graft incorporation involves an initial phase of ischemic necrosis, followed by revascularization. Remodeling and maturation include a transition of cellularity, distribution of collagen types, fiber size and alignment, and biochemical characteristics that are more ligament-like. Initially, failure after replacement surgery is at the fixation sites. As these attachments heal, failure is more likely to occur within the graft substance, specifically intra-articularly.

Allograft tissue, primarily bone-patellar tendon-bone and achilles tendon, has been used for reconstruction, particularly in the settings of multiple ligament injuries and revision ligament surgery of the knee. Tissue preservation has been an issue, because freeze-drying and high-dose irradiation adversely affect the structural properties. Ethylene oxide sterilization is not well accepted by the host, and use of fresh tissue without freezing results in a substantial inflammatory response. Fresh-frozen tissue and low-dose irradiation are the most accepted methods, and rejection and infection have not been substantial problems. Final allograft incorporation in ACL surgery is similar to that seen with autografts, but occurs at a slower rate. In the animal model, inferior properties are found in allografts at 6 months compared with autografts. Good results have been reported for clinical studies in which allograft tissue was used. Data from the few studies that compare allografts to autografts suggest similar results for the two methods, both subjectively and objectively. A true prospective randomized series has not been conducted. There have been recent reports regarding late failure of allografts (> 1 year), but this has not been shown statistically in a clinical series.

Tendon

Structure and Function

Tendons are dense, primarily collagenous tissues that link muscle to bone. As a highly specialized tissue with parallel-oriented bundles of collagen, the tendon's primary function is to transmit the load generated by muscle to bone. Synovial sheaths surround some tendons (eg, flexor tendons of the hand) to facilitate excursion and gliding. These tendons are not as well vascularized as those without synovial lining, and they require diffusion and specialized vascular channels (vincula) for nutrients in addition to those provided in the regions of the muscle and bone attachments. Tendons comprise individual fibers of collagen that are relatively uniform in alignment and span from the muscle to the bone (Fig. 7). Groups of collagen fibers form microfibrils, which in turn form fibrils. Spindle-shaped fibroblasts are aligned along these subunits and are relatively few in number. The fibrils coalesce to form bundles, which are surrounded by the endotenon. The peritendinous layer of the epitenon and then the paratenon surround a set of bundles to complete the structural anatomy of the tendon.

At the microstructural level, the triple-stranded helical formation within the collagen is present. Histology reveals crimping and low cellular density in addition to the highly uniform, parallel alignment of the fibers. Collagen content of the dry weight is slightly greater than that found in ligaments and is predominantly type I, approximately 95%. Type III collagen, which is a more immature form and often found in greater concentrations in healing tissue, constitutes approximately 5% of the total collagen content. Although there is a very small concentration of proteoglycans in tendons, they serve to support the structure and function of collagenous tissues. Proteoglycans, which influence the viscoelastic properties of tendon by their ability to bind water molecules, have been found in higher concentrations in areas of a tendon experiencing greater compressive forces.

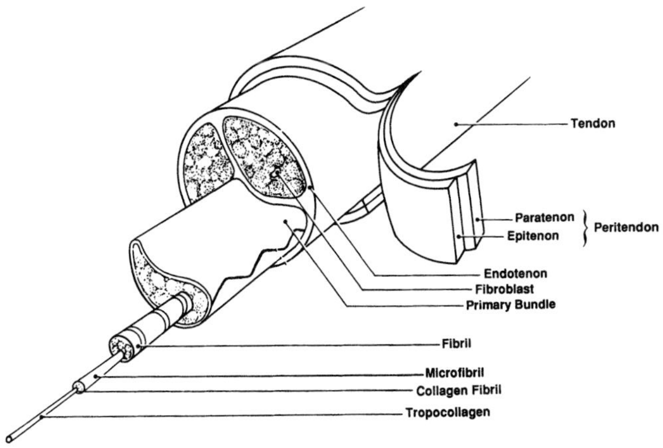

Fig. 7 Structural organization of tendon. (Reproduced with permission from Best TM, Garrett WE Jr: Muscle and tendon, in DeLee JC, Drez D (eds): *Orthopaedic Sports Medicine: Principles and Practice.* Philadelphia, PA, WB Saunders, 1994, pp 1–45.)

The organization and composition of tendons make them ideally suited to resist high tensile forces. Compared to ligaments, tendons deform less under an applied load and, thus, are able to transmit the load from muscle to bone, resulting in motion during concentric contractions or resisting motion during eccentric contractions. Tendons display viscoelastic behavior similar to that of other connective soft tissues, but to a lesser degree, especially in response to changes in strain rate. This difference is likely secondary to a higher concentration of collagen compared with matrix components.

Structural and degenerative changes as a result of aging have been reported. The achilles tendon demonstrates a decrease in its overall diameter. The mean collagen fibril diameter decreases with increasing age, as do total cell count and the amount of crimp. A decrease in the endoplasmic reticulum within the fibroblast suggests diminished cellular metabolic activity. The biochemical composition changes with an increase in collagen content and amount of cross-links and a decrease in glycosaminoglycans. Biomechanically, an increase in stress and stiffness during maturation and then a decrease with senescence have been noted. The rotator cuff, in which mechanical impingement as well as an area of hypovascularity in the supraspinatus tendon have been implicated, and the posterior tibial tendon, which sustains compressive forces from the medial malleolus, have demonstrated degenerative changes that may lead to earlier tendon failure. The effects of decreased activity, or relative disuse, play a role in the changes seen within the tendons of aging individuals.

Response to Exercise and Loading

Controlled increases in training appear to have differential effects on tendons. The biomechanical properties of swine flexor tendons did not change after exercise. However, swine extensor tendons subjected to an exercise regimen responded by developing increased stiffness to the level seen in flexor tendons. This observation suggests that extensor tendons have the capacity to respond to training, whereas flexor tendons function on a regular basis at their peak. Investigators have reported an increase in the number and density of smaller diameter fibrils in response to exercise. Although further investigations are warranted, it may be that the muscle and the tendon-bone insertion site have a greater capability to adapt to an environment of sustained increases in loading than does the tendon itself.

Response to Immobilization and Disuse

Restriction of motion to protect injured tissue or aid in the repair process can affect tendons. Without stress as a stimulus, both the midsubstance of tendons and the insertion sites demonstrate diminished biomechanical properties. After immobilization, stiffness decreases within the tendon. Presumably, other biomechanical as well as biochemical and histologic changes occur, but these have yet to be demonstrated specifically for tendon. It also has not been demonstrated whether such changes are reversible.

Response to Injury and Mechanisms of Repair

Injury or damage to tendons can result from one of three mechanisms: (1) transection within the substance (direct injury); (2) avulsion from bone at the insertion (indirect injury); or (3) intrasubstance damage from intrinsic or extrinsic factors and subsequent failure. Transections or partial lacerations are associated with trauma and are most common in the flexor tendons of the hand. Bone avulsions can occur following overwhelming tensile loads, as seen in the flexor digitorum profundus insertion into the base of the distal phalanx of the ring finger. Degenerative changes within tendon can arise from repetitive tensile loading during the life of an individual; however, impingement of tendon by a rigid surface, such as with the rotator cuff beneath the acromion, is an important factor leading to tendon failure. At the point where the tendon is overloaded, individual fibers can fail, transferring the load to adjacent collagen fibers. Continued loading will lead to further failure until the applied load ceases or the tendon ruptures. If the injury is incomplete and the healing process is interrupted, episodes of microtrauma will result in a weakened tendon structure. Repetitive microtrauma to the tissue are seen in overuse injuries. The bone-tendon junction may also be involved in the injury process.

Tendon healing after an acute injury follows phases similar to those of other soft tissues: inflammatory, proliferative or reparative, and remodeling. The inflammatory response provides an extrinsic source for cellular invasion to promote granulation tissue and vascular ingrowth during the first few days following tendon injury. By the end of the first week, fibroblasts that have migrated to the wound site begin the reparative process, with collagen synthesis noted. The orientation of the cellular and collagen components is random. As the remodeling phase begins, these components become more organized and aligned parallel to the axis of the tendon. This final phase can continue for up to 6 to 12 months, with collagen turnover and tissue maturation proceeding as the repair process is completed. For injury to avascular tendons within a synovial sheath (ie, flexor tendons of the hand), an intrinsic mechanism for tendon healing has been proposed. This mechanism appears to be modulated by the stress of passive motion, thereby bringing the impact of the extrinsic inflammatory response in question. Cells from within the tendon proliferate at the wound site along with increased vascularity, leading to collagen synthesis and further tissue maturation with time. Evidence for both intrinsic and extrinsic mechanisms of healing has been supported. Other factors may determine which is the primary mechanism for healing, such as the local environment, vascularity, or stress.

In the initial phase of healing after tendon repair, the tensile strength is significantly less than for controls. At 3 weeks, the tensile strength increases progressively. Controlled passive motion has been shown to decrease adhesions, lead to a stronger repair, and accelerate gains in tensile strength. Collagen reorganization and alignment, as well as maturation, appear to benefit from controlled application of stress. Active motion, however, results in gap formation at the suture repair site without a positive effect on the biomechanical characteristics or adhesions.

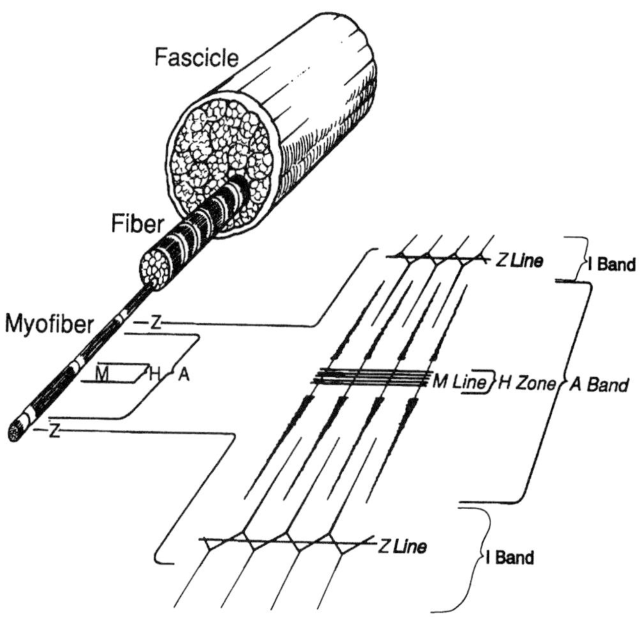

Fig. 8 Organization of skeletal muscle from the micro- to macrostructural level. (Reproduced with permission from Garrett WE, Best TM: Anatomy, physiology, and mechanics of skeletal muscle, in Simon SR (ed): *Orthopaedic Basic Science.* Rosemont, IL, American Academy of Orthopaedic Surgeons, 1994, pp 91–125.)

Muscle

Structure and Function

Skeletal muscle is composed of individual myofibrils in a muscle fiber, which is enclosed by the endomysium (Fig. 8). A group of fibers, termed a fascicle, are surrounded by a connective tissue layer, the perimysium. A number of fascicles, depending upon the size of the muscle, are grouped to form the muscle, which is enclosed by the epimysium. Muscle originates in bone and adjacent connective tissue surfaces, and it inserts into bone via tendon. The myotendinous junction is a highly specialized region for load transmission, which has an increased surface area secondary to membrane infolding (Fig. 9). At the microscopic level, the sarcomere, the contractile unit of the muscle, extends from one Z line to the next Z line (Fig. 8). The thin myofibril protein actin is anchored to the Z line and is the principal protein in the I band. However, the major protein components of the sarcomere are the thick filaments of myosin, which anchor into the M line. In the resting state, the two contractile proteins (actin and myosin) lie adjacent to each other in the A band. Two additional proteins, tropomyosin and troponin, are present on the surface of actin. In the presence of increased calcium, these two proteins promote the binding of actin and myosin, which results in activation of adenosine triphosphatase (ATPase), liberating energy and leading to skeletal muscle contraction. Actin and myosin slide past each

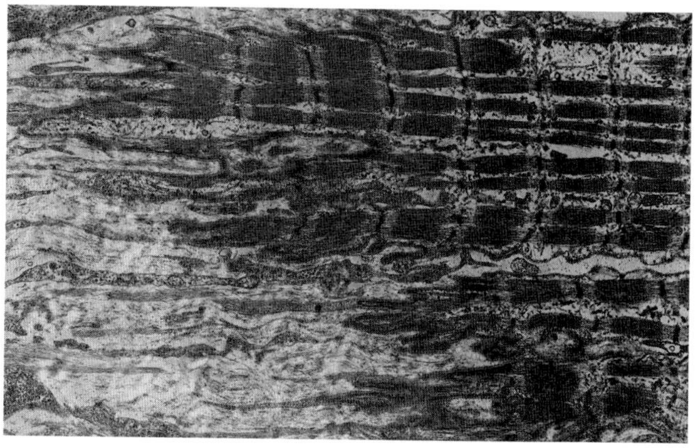

Fig. 9 Electron micrograph of the myotendinous junction demonstrating the transition from muscle to tendon. Examples of the sarcomere, and its components, are shown. (Courtesy of Dr. Morey Moreland, University of Pittsburgh, Pittsburgh, Pennsylvania.)

other while remaining bound together, resulting in a decrease in the I band, while the A band remains unchanged. The muscle fiber shortens, and this shortening is referred to as a concentric contraction. In an eccentric contraction, actin and myosin bind as the muscle generates a force greater in magnitude than that for a concentric contraction, and the muscle fiber lengthens. An important effect of an eccentric contraction is deceleration of the portion of the limb on which the muscle is acting, while acceleration results from a concentric contraction.

The characteristics of the muscle contraction depend on the muscle fiber types. Most muscles in the body are comprised of equal amounts of two types of fibers, type I and type II (Table 1). Type I, or slow-twitch oxidative fibers, predominate in postural muscles and are well suited for endurance by an aerobic metabolism, an ability to sustain tension, and relative fatigue resistance. In general, type II, or fast-twitch fibers, are more common in muscles that rapidly generate power, but have a greater dependence on anaerobic metabolism and are less capable of sustaining activity for prolonged periods due to buildup of lactic acid. The characteristics and composition of the type IIA muscle fiber subgroup are intermediate between those of types I and IIB. Type IIC, or undifferentiated super fast-twitch fibers, are present in very low concentrations, but can increase as a result of training. The alpha motor neurons appear to dictate the fiber type of the motor unit. Type I fibers have smaller motor units with a lower threshold for activation than type II fibers, but force generation occurs more slowly in type I fibers due to the slower conduction velocity. Recruitment during a contraction is based on the size of the motor unit and begins with the smaller motor units of type I fibers, as is seen in a low intensity activity such as jogging. When additional force is required, the larger motor units of the type II fibers are added, such as with sprinting. At the myotendinous junction, the contracting muscle cells attach directly into the tendons to transmit their force. It is at this transition zone that the majority of micro- and macrofailures occur in an otherwise normal muscle that is overloaded.

Like other tissues in the body, skeletal muscle undergoes changes with aging. Muscle mass decreases slowly between 25 and 50 years of age. From this point, the rate of muscle atrophy increases, but the loss of muscle size and strength can be diminished with strength training. With aging, the total number of muscle fibers decreases and muscle stiffness increases. These effects may be related to the increase in collagen content seen with aging. Furthermore, muscle fiber diameter decreases with aging, primarily in type II fibers. These effects may also be the result, in part, of decreased activity and mobility with increasing age.

Table 1. Characteristics of human skeletal muscle fiber types

	Type I	Type IIA	Type IIB
Other Names	Red, slow twitch (ST)	White, fast twitch (FT)	
	Slow oxidative (SO)	Fast oxidative glycolytic (FOG)	Fast glycolytic (FG)
Speed of contraction	Slow	Fast	Fast
Strength of contraction	Low	High	High
Fatigability	Fatigue-resistant	Fatigable	Most fatigable
Aerobic capacity	High	Medium	Low
Anaerobic capacity	Low	Medium	High
Motor unit size	Small	Larger	Largest
Capillary density	High	High	Low

(Reproduced with permission from Garrett WE, Best TM: Anatomy, physiology, and mechanics of skeletal muscle, in Simon SR (ed): *Orthopaedic Basic Science.* Rosemont, IL, American Academy of Orthopaedic Surgeons, 1994, pp 91–125.)

Response to Exercise and Loading

Training and exercise can stimulate alterations in skeletal muscle if the activity is sustained and/or of sufficient load. Under an appropriate program of exercise and loading, muscle can increase its functional capacity to respond. For example, "low tension, high repetition" training of a relatively long duration results in greater endurance, which is to the advantage of the long-distance runner. An increase in capillary density and mitochondria concentration is associated with greater capability for oxidative metabolism, which primarily affects slow-twitch fibers. Furthermore, resistance to fatigue is increased by these adaptations. Exercise also benefits the cardiovascular and respiratory systems, with changes that maximize oxygen intake, facilitate transfer of oxygen to muscle tissue for energy production, and remove waste products, including lactate.

"High tension, low repetition" training emphasizes development of greater muscle strength and power. When loads are progressively increased, muscle size increases, mostly from muscle hypertrophy of primarily type II fibers. This mode of training benefits the sprinter, who requires short and powerful bursts of speed to achieve higher performance. Unlike endurance training, which can be performed more frequently, strength training requires a period of rest, or recovery, for the muscle tissue and should not be performed daily. Under this regimen, anaerobic metabolism is maximized and tissue injury avoided. Stretching has been shown to be useful to facilitate these changes as well as to diminish injury by leading to a decrease in total load at any given length.

Response to Immobilization and Disuse

When stimulation to the muscle fibers is withdrawn, the adaptations in skeletal muscle can be reversed. If muscles are further unloaded, either by disuse or immobilization, the effect on skeletal muscle is magnified. Loss of endurance and strength is observed in the muscle groups affected. As muscle atrophies, these changes are observed at both the macro- and microstructural levels, with decreasing fiber size and number, as well as changes in the sarcomere length–tension relationship. Changes at the cellular and biochemical level occur and may affect the aerobic and anaerobic pathways of energy production. Immobilization of muscles in a lengthened position has a less deleterious effect than immobilization in a shortened position. This difference is a result of the relatively greater tension placed on the lengthened muscle fibers and their physiologic response to the load.

Response to Injury and Mechanisms of Repair

Muscle injury can result from an indirect overload, which overwhelms the muscle's ability to respond normally, or a direct injury, such as a contusion or laceration. The indirect mechanism of injury includes muscle strains and delayed-onset muscle soreness. Injury from muscle strains, in which muscles are unable to accommodate the stretch during either eccentric or concentric contractions, is commonly reported from sports activity. Muscles are at greater risk for strain injury during function in an eccentric manner when the forces involved are greater and during action across two joints, as with the hamstrings. Fatigue has also been associated with increased rates of injury, because fatigued muscle has a diminished ability to perform and to act as an energy, or shock, absorber.

The spectrum of muscle strain injury can range from microscopic damage or partial tears to complete tears and disruption, with a palpable defect within the muscle. The degree of injury from a tensile overload will dictate the potential of the host response and the time course for repair. The status of muscle contraction at the time of overload is usually eccentric, and failure most often occurs at or near the myotendinous junction unless there is previous injury to the muscle. Swelling from hemorrhage occurs initially in the inflammatory phase. The cellular response is more rapid and repair is more complete if the vascular channels are not disrupted. Cell death, with necrosis and degeneration, ensues, and then regeneration proceeds. The muscle fiber type formed depends on the motor nerve type. Delayed-onset muscle soreness (within 24 to 72 hours) is another form of indirect injury to the muscle. However, this occurs within the muscle fibers as a result of intense training or exercise to which the individual, and therefore the muscle, is unaccustomed. The cellular and microstructural changes that occur and the weakness that results are reversible.

Muscle contusions result from a direct blow, usually to the muscle belly. The degree of hematoma formation, subsequent inflammation, and delay in healing is directly related to the compressive force absorbed. The amount of force will also affect the amount of scar formation and muscle regeneration. A more rapid recovery is observed under conditions that limit hematoma formation and promote increased vascularity, as seen in limbs that are initially rested in flexion and undergo early motion and, possibly, in a younger age group. Heterotopic bone, or myositis ossificans, is not an infrequent finding following a more severe injury, but this should not be surgically addressed until healing is complete and the bone fully matured. Repair and recovery following muscle laceration depend on regeneration across the site and reinnervation. Muscle distal to the site of injury that regenerates, but is incompletely reinnervated, has diminished function.

Nerve

Physiology

Epineurium is the connective tissue layer that defines the gross structure of peripheral nerve (Fig. 10). External epineurium forms the outer covering of the nerve, and internal epineurium surrounds and cushions fascicles, permitting them to move on one another in response to external forces. These primarily collagenous tissues absorb longitudinal stress before it is transmitted to the perineurium and, through the proliferation of epineurial fibroblasts, generate scar in response to nerve injury. Perineurium is a peripheral extension of the blood–brain barrier that surrounds individual fascicles and maintains the intraneural environment. Concentric layers of flattened cells linked by tight junctions form this vital physiologic barrier, which limits the spread of infection and maintains a slightly positive intrafascicular pressure. Perineurium is also mechanically important, providing the nerve's strongest resistance to longitudinal stretch. Endoneurium is the loose collagenous packing that surrounds individual axons within the perineurial fascicle (Figs. 10 and 11). It forms the endoneurial or Schwann cell tube, the longitudinally oriented cylinder of basement membrane that surrounds the myelinated axon in normal nerve and serves as the conduit for regenerating axons after nerve injury.

The axon (Fig. 11) is the peripheral process of a central neuron. Motor neurons are clustered in pools within the anterior horn of the spinal cord. Sensory neurons lie adjacent to the spinal cord in dorsal root ganglia, and autonomic neurons are nearby in paravertebral ganglia. The

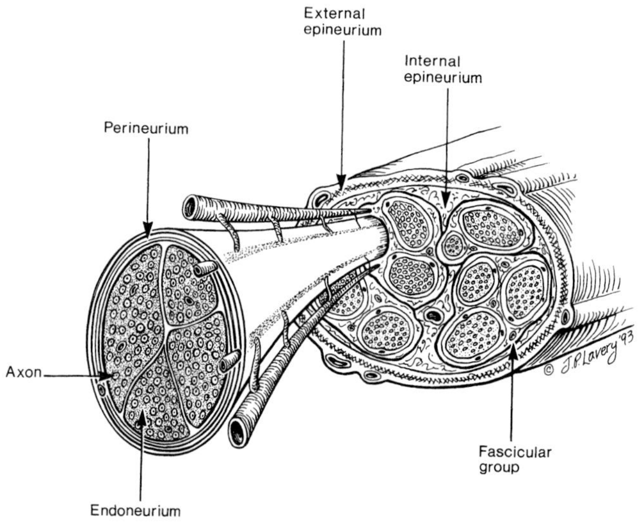

Fig. 10 The macroscopic and gross microscopic organization of peripheral nerve. (Reproduced with permission from Brushart TM: Peripheral nerve biology, in Manske PR (ed): *Hand Surgery Update*. Englewood, CO, American Society for Surgery of the Hand, 1994, pp 20-1 to 20-14.)

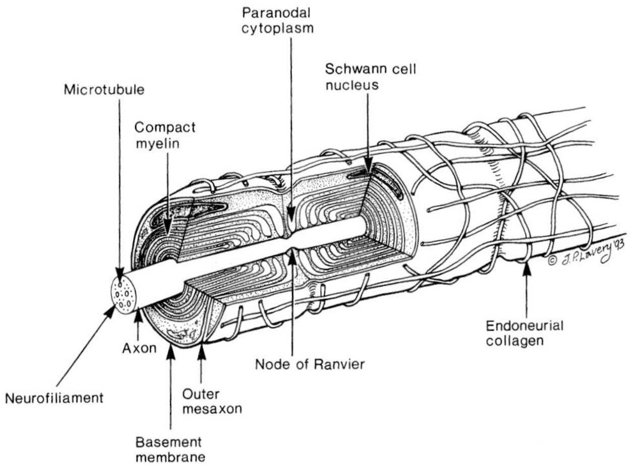

Fig. 11 The Schwann cell tube and its contents. (Reproduced with permission from Brushart TM: Peripheral nerve biology, in Manske PR (ed): *Hand Surgery Update.* Englewood, CO, American Society for Surgery of the Hand, 1994, pp 20-1 to 20-14.)

neuron, containing the Golgi apparatus, ribosomes, and endoplasmic reticulum, is specialized to produce structural components and neurotransmitters. The axon, in contrast, contains a structural framework of neurofilament proteins and a network of microtubules that provide the pathway for axoplasmic transport. Fast anterograde (central to peripheral) transport carries subcellular organelles down the microtubules at up to 400 mm/day. Slow anterograde transport carries cytoskeletal and soluble proteins at 0.2 to 5 mm/day. Fast retrograde (peripheral to central) transport returns scavenged cellular components to the neuron, as well as conveying information about the axon's peripheral connections.

All peripheral axons are associated with neuroglia, the Schwann cells (Fig. 11). Several small (1 μm diameter or less) axons may be wrapped by the cytoplasmic extensions of a single Schwann cell and remain unmyelinated. In contrast, each larger axon is myelinated by a series of dedicated Schwann cells, arrayed longitudinally like beads on a string (Fig. 12). During development, the Schwann cell surrounds the axon, spiraling its tongue-like mesaxon concentrically around the axon to form myelin. This insulation, which facilitates neural conduction, is 70% cholesterol and phospholipid and 30% protein. The junction between adjacent Schwann cells is called the Node of Ranvier; the basement membrane that surrounds them is the endoneurial or Schwann cell tube, which was alluded to previously as a component of the endoneurium.

The fascicle, bounded by perineurium, is the smallest surgically identifiable unit of peripheral nerve (Fig. 10). Fascicles do not maintain their separate identity from one end of the nerve to the other, but are interconnected by intraneural plexi. As a result of this axonal mixing, the contents of individual proximal fascicles do not correspond precisely to those of their distal counterparts. However, in spite of this fascicular intermingling, axons themselves tend to remain localized to a given portion of the nerve's cross section throughout their course. Adjacent fascicles are often bound together by internal epineurium to form fascicular groups (Fig. 10). Intrafascicular connections are much more frequent within a fascicular group

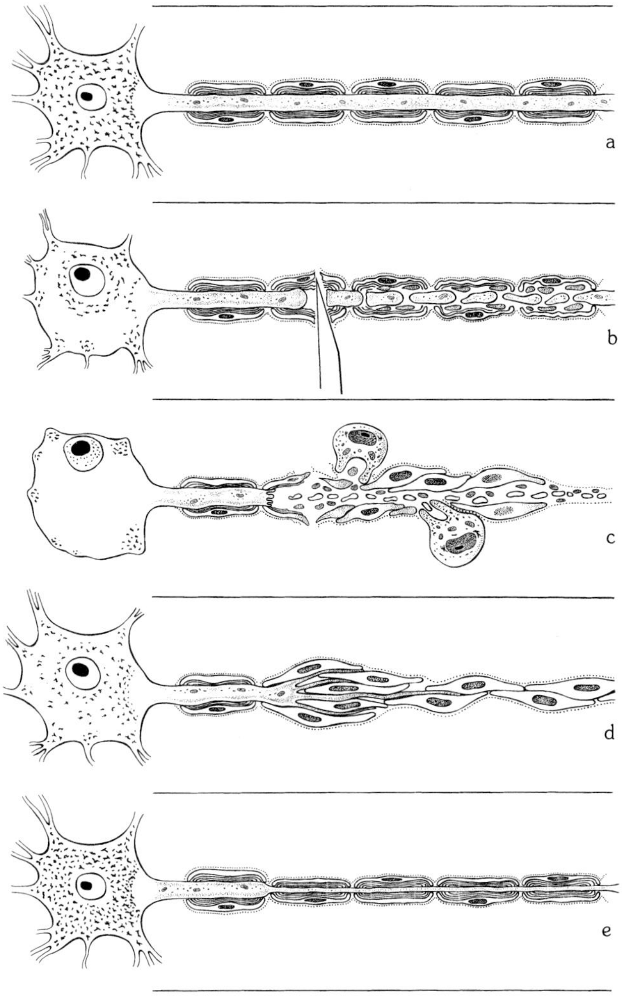

Fig. 12 Degeneration and regeneration of a myelinated axon. (**a**) Normal appearance, with myelinating Schwann cells strung along the length of the axon. (**b**) Axon transection is followed by granular degeneration of the axoplasm and neuronal swelling with nuclear eccentricity. (**c**) Macrophages enter the degenerating segment, digesting myelin and stimulating proliferation of Schwann cells. (**d**) Schwann cells have proliferated to form the Band of Büngner. The injured axon has generated several collateral sprouts that course distally as the regenerating unit, traveling along the Band of Büngner within the Schwann cell tube. (**e**) A single collateral sprout remains at the completion of regeneration. It is smaller in diameter, less well myelinated, and conducts less rapidly than the axon it replaces. (Reproduced with permision from Lundborg G: *Nerve Injury and Repair.* New York, NY, Churchill Livingstone, 1988, p 151.)

than between it and its neighbors. Fascicular groups thus maintain their functional identities over much greater distances than do individual fascicles.

The blood supply of peripheral nerve is remarkable for its flexibility. Segmental vessels supply longitudinally oriented vascular plexi within both epineurium and perineurium. These plexi interconnect with a network of endoneurial arterioles, venules, and capillaries whose direction of flow can be rapidly adjusted in response to injury. This flexibility in the routing of blood renders the nerve relatively resistant to surgical mobilization.

Degeneration and Regeneration

After peripheral nerve transection, the portion of the axon proximal to the injury remains in contact with the centrally located neuron. Because the bidirectional axoplasmic transport of materials continues, this part of the axon remains viable (Fig. 12*b*). The parent neuron responds to injury by increasing production of materials needed for axon elongation: growth-associated proteins; actin, a protein needed for growth cone function; and tubulin, the subunit of microtubules. Conversely, production of neurofilament, a structural protein, is decreased. These molecular changes result in the cell body reaction manifest at the light microscopic level by increase in size of the nucleolus, eccentricity of the nucleus, and clumping of chromatin (Fig. 12*b* and *c*).

Distal to the site of transection, the axon no longer communicates with the parent neuron, and viability is lost. Axoplasm and myelin are cleared from the Schwann cell tubes through the process of Wallerian degeneration (Fig. 12*b* and *c*). Influx of calcium triggers granular degeneration of the axoplasm, then circulating macrophages are recruited to aid the proliferating Schwann cells in digestion of myelin (Fig. 12*c*). At the completion of this process, the Schwann cell tube is empty except for a longitudinally arranged chain of Schwann cells, the Band of Büngner, which serves as an ideal substrate for axon regeneration (Fig. 12*d*). Each transected axon forms multiple collateral sprouts, the regenerating unit, which cross the site of nerve repair and enter the Schwann cell tubes of the distal nerve stump (Fig. 12*d*). These collateral sprouts regenerate distally at the rate of 1 to 2 mm/day in primates. More than one collateral sprout may become myelinated, raising the number of myelinated axons in the distal stump above normal levels for several months. Most often, only one collateral sprout from each axon survives (Fig. 12*e*). Motor axon collaterals are more likely to survive in Schwann cell tubes that previously contained motor axons and lead to muscle, and to be pruned from tubes that lead to skin. The process of collateral pruning may thus be used by the organism to save collaterals that will restore function at the expense of those that will not. At the completion of regeneration, the surviving axon will be smaller than normal caliber and will be less thickly myelinated (Fig. 12*e*), so conduction velocity will be reduced.

Techniques of Nerve Repair

The goal of peripheral nerve repair is to restore the maximum number of functional connections between central neurons and peripheral end organs. This process has two components: delivery of axons from the site of transection to the periphery and reinnervation of end organs that are functionally related to the parent neuron. For instance, a motor axon that previously innervated fast muscle can make a functional reconnection with slow muscle or a related end-organ, but it will be wasted if it reinnervates a sensory receptor in the skin. Delivery of axons to the periphery is influenced more by physiologic factors than by the fine points of surgical technique. The most profound of these factors is patient age. Normal function may be restored in children, with a linear relationship between age and two-point discrimination up to age 20 years and deterioration thereafter. The severity of injury is also im-

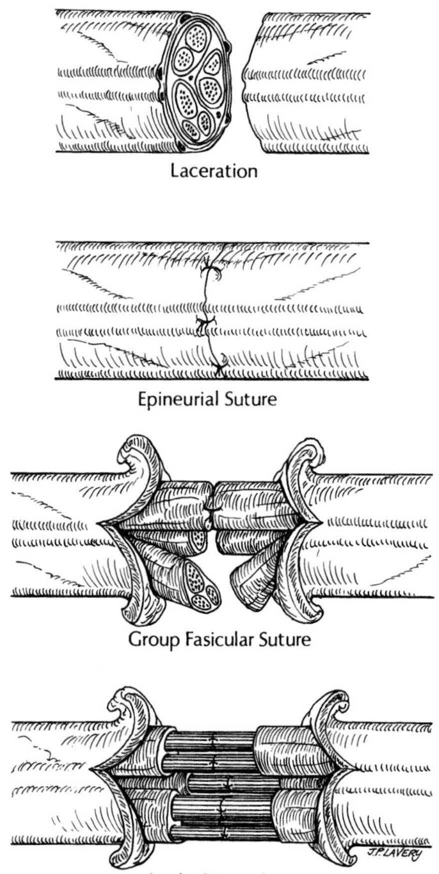

Fig. 13 Techniques of nerve suture. (Reproduced with permission from Brushart TM: Peripheral nerve regeneration: Strategies to augment specificity, in Stauffer R (ed): *Advances in Orthopaedics.* St. Louis, MO, Mosby Year Book, 1994, pp 205–225.)

portant because it determines the nutrition of the nerve and its bed, as well as the amount of nerve tissue that must be resected before repair or grafting can be undertaken. The more proximal the injury, the less likely axons are to continue elongating until they reach the periphery. Delay between injury and repair of more than a few weeks is also associated with diminished recovery.

In contrast to generic delivery of axons to the periphery, the specificity of axon regeneration may be influenced by the choice of suture technique. Two basic techniques of end-to-end nerve repair are available (Fig. 13). Epineurial suture is minimally invasive, but provides only limited control over the alignment of individual fascicles within the nerve. Proximal and distal stumps are trimmed perpendicular to the long axis of the nerve, cleared of epineurial fat, and joined by microsutures placed in the external epineurium. Epineurial vessels and fascicular group patterns are used to align the stumps. Although some tension may be tolerated, inability to hold the stumps together with two 8-0 sutures is usually an indication for nerve grafting. Techniques that take advantage of intraneural anatomy—group and individual fascicular suture—provide improved fascicular alignment at the expense of increased intraneural dissection and scarring and require positive identification of the fascicles to be matched. Higher magnification is required, and less tension is tolerated by 10-0 sutures in the internal epineurium of the fascicular group or the perineurium of the individual fascicle. After clean, sharp lacerations with no substance loss, it is often possible to visually identify and match fascicular groups in the proximal and distal stumps. Two other techniques of fascicular matching are available when visual matching is not possible. In acute injuries, fascicular stimulation in the awake patient will identify the distal termination of both proximal sensory and distal motor fascicles. Additional information may be obtained on the peripheral destination of distal sensory fascicles by surgically tracing them through the nerve. Alternatively, at any time after injury, a section of the proximal stump may be reacted to demonstrate the enzyme acetylcholinesterase within motor axons. This technique provides less information because the specific identity of proximal sensory fascicles is not revealed, and both sensory and motor fascicles in the distal stump can only be identified by dissection.

The choice of surgical technique is based on knowledge of the intraneural anatomy at the site of injury. Whenever possible, that is, if they can be positively identified and matched, portions of the proximal and distal stumps that serve discrete functions should be selectively reunited. For instance, for several centimeters proximal to the wrist, the motor fibers of the ulnar nerve are sandwiched between the dorsal cutaneous fibers (ulnar side) and the palmar cutaneous fibers (radial side). These motor fibers will be wasted if they are directed to either cutaneous branch, so meticulous identification and matching of fascicular groups is important. More proximally, in long unbranched segments of nerve, functional subunits are more difficult to identify, and epineurial suture is more appropriate.

Nerve Grafting

Gaps that cannot be closed by bringing the nerve ends together under mild tension, usually 2 to 3 cm, are most often treated by nerve grafting with interfascicular technique. Fascicular groups are microsurgically dissected from one another in both proximal and distal stumps. Matching groups are then individually joined with segments of nerve graft. The sural nerve is often used when longer segments of nerve are needed, and the medial or lateral antebrachial cutaneous nerve is used when shorter segments are required. Immediate microsurgical restoration of blood flow to the graft has been advocated and may be beneficial in special circumstances, such as a severely scarred graft bed.

Annotated Bibliography

General Reference

Simon SR (ed): *Orthopaedic Basic Science.* Rosemont, IL, American Academy of Orthopaedic Surgeons, 1994.

This text offers the most comprehensive review of the basic science of soft tissues, as well as the entire neuromusculoskeletal system.

Articular Cartilage

Buckwalter JA, Mow VC, Ratcliffe A: Restoration of injured or degenerated articular cartilage. *J Am Acad Orthop Surg* 1994;2:192–201.

This is a review of recent developments in the treatment of articular cartilage damage.

Mankin HJ, Mow VC, Buckwalter JA, et al: Form and function of articular cartilage, in Simon SR (ed): *Orthopaedic Basic Science.* Rosemont, IL, American Academy of Orthopaedic Surgeons, 1994, pp 1–44.

Current knowledge of the structure and biomechanics of articular cartilage is summarized by experts in the field.

Shapiro F, Koide S, Glimcher MJ: Cell origin and differentiation in the repair of full-thickness defects of articular cartilage. *J Bone Joint Surg* 1993;75A: 532–553.

A histologic study of articular cartilage repair in a rabbit model is presented.

Brittberg M, Lindahl A, Nilsson A, et al: Treatment of deep cartilage defects in the knee with autologous chondrocyte transplantation. *N Eng J Med* 1994;331: 889–895.

This is an early clinical report of a clinical trial on treating articular surface defects with autologous cultured chondrocytes and periosteal flaps.

Meniscal Cartilage

Jackson DW, McDevitt CA, Simon TM, et al: Meniscal transplantation using fresh and cryopreserved allografts: An experimental study in goats. *Am J Sports Med* 1992; 20:644–656.

Analysis of the allograft menisci revealed substantial changes in the biochemical makeup of the menisci.

Jackson DW, Whelan J, Simon TM: Cell survival after transplantation of fresh meniscal allografts: DNA probe analysis in a goat model. *Am J Sports Med* 1993;21:540–550.

Menisci were repopulated entirely by host cells.

Stone KR, Rodkey WG, Webber R, et al: Meniscal regeneration with copolymeric collagen scaffolds: In vitro and in vivo studies evaluated clinically, histologically, and biochemically. *Am J Sports Med* 1992;20:104–111.

The authors felt that the scaffolds supported meniscal fibrochondrocyte ingrowth.

Ligament

Engle CP, Noguchi M, Ohland KJ, et al: Healing of the rabbit medial collateral ligament following an O'Donoghue triad injury: Effects of anterior cruciate ligament reconstruction. *J Orthop Res* 1994;12:357–364.

The addition of an anterior cruciate ligament reconstruction led to increased joint stability and improved healing in the medial collateral ligament as determined by histologic and biomechanical properties. The earlier onset of osteoarthrosis seen with this injury in the untreated setting may be averted.

Fu FH, Harner CD, Johnson DL, et al: Biomechanics of knee ligaments: Basic concepts and clinical applications. *J Bone Joint Surg* 1993;75A:1716–1727.

The principles of basic science research of knee ligaments and how these concepts have been applied to clinical practice are reviewed.

Jackson DW, Grood ES, Goldstein JD, et al: A comparison of patellar tendon autograft and allograft used for anterior cruciate ligament reconstruction in the goat model. *Am J Sports Med* 1993;21:176–185.

At 6 months after anterior cruciate ligament reconstruction in the goat model, the bone-patellar tendon-bone autograft demonstrated increased strength and stiffness, more rapid maturation including collagen fibril adaptation, and less instability compared with the bone-patellar tendon-bone allograft.

Ticker JB, Flatow EL, Pawluk RJ, et al: Abstract: The inferior glenohumeral ligament: A correlative biomechanical, biochemical, and histological investigation. *Trans Orthop Res Soc* 1993;18:313.

The structure–function relationship of the inferior glenohumeral ligament was investigated in human cadaver shoulders. The superior band, particularly its insertion sites, exhibited viscoelastic behavior, which correlates with the histologic observations of increased collagen interweaving and the biochemical findings of increased proteoglycan content in this region.

Tendon

Carlson GD, Botte MJ, Josephs MS, et al: Morphologic and biomechanical comparison of tendons used as free grafts. *J Hand Surg* 1993;18A:76–82.

The human palmaris longus, plantaris, extensor digitorum longus of the fourth toe, and flexor digitorum profundus of the index were studied to determine graft length, cross-sectional area, volume, stiffness, and tensile modulus. Potential advantages and disadvantages of the graft substitutes studied are discussed.

Clark JM, Harryman DT II: Tendons, ligaments, and capsule of the rotator cuff: Gross and microscopic anatomy. *J Bone Joint Surg* 1992;74A:713–725.

The structure of the tendons of the four rotator cuff muscles are described in detail. Fibers from tendinous portions all four muscles interdigitate as they coalesce to form the cuff over the humeral head prior to inserting into the tuberosities. Five distinct layers within the tendons were defined.

Rodeo SA, Arnoczky SP, Torzilli PA, et al: Tendon-healing in a bone tunnel: A biomechanical and histological study in the dog. *J Bone Joint Surg* 1993;75A: 1795–1803.

Failure patterns of tendon healing in a bone tunnel in adult mongrel dogs occurred by pull-out from the tunnel up to 8 weeks after placement. After 12 weeks, when histology revealed collagen fibers clearly connecting tendon to the surrounding bone, pull-out from the tunnel no longer occurred. These findings should be considered during postoperative rehabilitation for anterior cruciate ligament reconstruction using soft tissues.

Muscle

Taylor DC, Dalton JD Jr, Seaber AV, et al: Experimental muscle strain injury: Early functional and structural deficits and the increased risk for reinjury. *Am J Sports Med* 1993;21:190–194.

A severe muscle strain injury was created using a rabbit model, and the injured muscle was tested to failure. Compared to control specimens, the injured muscles failed at a mean peak load of 63% and a mean elongation to rupture of 79%. These data suggest that when treating severe muscle strain injuries in the early postinjury period, the weaker properties and increased susceptibility to reinjury must be considered.

Nerve

Brushart TM: Peripheral nerve biology, in Manske PR (ed): *Hand Surgery Update.* Englewood, CO, American Society for Surgery of the Hand, 1994.

This is a current summary of peripheral nerve anatomy, pathology, and physiology.

Wilgis EFS, Brushart TM: Nerve repair and grafting, in Green DP (ed): *Operative Hand Surgery,* ed 3. New York, NY, Churchill Livingstone, 1993, vol 2, pp 1315–1340.

This is a concise summary of current techniques of nerve repair and grafting with discussion of surgical indications.

Classic Bibliography

Anderson AF, Lipscomb AB, Coulam C: Antegrade curettement, bone grafting and pinning of osteochondritis dissecans in the skeletally mature knee. *Am J Sports Med* 1990;18:254–261.

Arnoczky SP, Warren RF: Microvasculature of the human meniscus. *Am J Sports Med* 1982;10:90–95.

Beaver RJ, Mahomed M, Backstein D, et al: Fresh osteochondral allografts for post-traumatic defects in the knee: A survivorship analysis. *J Bone Joint Surg* 1992;74B:105–110.

Cannon WD Jr, Vittori JM: The incidence of healing in arthroscopic meniscal repairs in ACL-reconstructed knees versus stable knees. *Am J Sports Med* 1992;20:176–181.

Fauno P, Nielsen AB: Arthroscopic partial meniscectomy: A long-term follow-up. *Arthroscopy* 1992;8:345–349.

Fithian DC, Kelly MA, Mow VC: Material properties and structure-function relationships in the menisci. *Clin Orthop* 1990;252:19–31.

Garrett JC: Fresh osteochondral allografts for treatment of articular defects in osteochondritis dissecans of the lateral femoral condyle in adults. *Clin Orthop* 1994;303:33–37.

Gelberman RH (ed): *Operative Nerve Repair and Reconstruction.* Philadelphia, PA, JB Lippincott, 1991.

Gelberman RH, Chu CR, Williams CS, et al: Angiogenesis in healing autogenous flexor-tendon grafts. *J Bone Joint Surg* 1992;74A:1207–1216.

Gibbons MJ, Butler DL, Grood ES, et al: Effects of gamma irradiation on the initial mechanical and material properties of goat bone-patellar tendon-bone allografts. *J Orthop Res* 1991;9:209–218.

Hede A, Larsen E, Sandberg H: Partial versus total meniscectomy: A prospective, randomised study with long-term follow-up. *J Bone Joint Surg* 1992;74B:118–121.

Irvine GB, Glasgow MM: The natural history of the meniscus in anterior cruciate insufficiency: Arthroscopic analysis. *J Bone Joint Surg* 1992;74B:403–405.

Lundborg G (ed): *Nerve Injury and Repair.* Edinburgh, Scotland, Churchill Livingstone, 1988.

Marandola MS, Prietto CA: Arthroscopic herbert screw fixation of patellar osteochondritis dissecans. *Arthroscopy* 1993;9:214–216.

Mow VC, Ratcliffe A, Rosenwasser MP, et al: Experimental studies on repair of large osteochondral defects at a high weight bearing area of the knee joint: A tissue engineering study. *J Biomech Eng* 1991;113:198–207.

Neyret P, Donell ST, Dejour H: Results of partial meniscectomy related to the state of the anterior cruciate ligament: Review at 20 to 35 years. *J Bone Joint Surg* 1993;75B:36–40.

O'Driscoll SW, Keeley FW, Salter RB: Durability of regenerated articular cartilage produced by free autogenous periosteal grafts in major full-thickness defects in joint surfaces under the influence of continuous passive motion: A follow-up report at one year. *J Bone Joint Surg* 1988;70A:595–606.

Regan WD, Korinek SL, Morrey BF, et al: Biomechanical study of ligaments around the elbow joint. *Clin Orthop* 1991;271:170–179.

Ryan JB, Wheeler JH, Hopkinson WJ, et al: Quadriceps contusions. *Am J Sports Med* 1991;19:299–304.

Schachar N, McAllister D, Stevenson M, et al: Metabolic and biochemical status of articular cartilage following cryopreservation and transplantation: A rabbit model. *J Orthop Res* 1992;10:603–609.

Sommerlath K, Gillquist J: The effect of a meniscal prosthesis on knee biomechanics and cartilage: An experimental study in rabbits. *Am J Sports Med* 1992; 20:73–81.

Sommerlath K, Gillquist J: The long-term course of various meniscal treatments in anterior cruciate ligament deficient knees. *Clin Orthop* 1992;283:207–214.

Tesch GH, Handley CJ, Cornell HJ, et al: Effects of free and bound insulin-like growth factors on proteoglycan metabolism in articular cartilage explants. *J Orthop Res* 1992;10:14–22.

Wroble RR, Henderson RC, Campion ER, et al: Meniscectomy in children and adolescents: A long-term follow-up study. *Clin Orthop* 1992;279:180–189.

2

Bone Healing and Grafting

Fracture Healing

Fracture repair requires at least three events that initiate the six stages of fracture healing. These events include recruitment, modulation, and osteoconduction. Recruitment requires the transportation of systemic osteoprogenitor cells or inducible pro-osteoblasts to the fracture site. In addition, communication with the local cell population (namely, periosteal osteocytes, primitive multipotential cells, and fibroblasts) occurs to stimulate their osteoblastic capabilities. Modulation or activation of these pleuripotential cell populations then follows. In the final event, osteoconduction, collagen and hydroxyapatite surfaces are used to direct bone production into a biomechanically advantageous three-dimensional (3-D) lattice.

Stages of Healing

Fracture healing proceeds through six well recognized phases. Impact occurs when enough energy is absorbed to induce failure of the bone. The amount of energy absorbed until failure occurs is directly proportional to the volume of bone and the rate of loading. The second stage, induction, begins with the formation of fracture hematoma and ends with the appearance of inflammatory cells approximately 48 hours from impact. Bone necrosis of the fracture fragments results, with cell death and release of intracellular by-products. Low oxygen tension and pH and the release of chemical factors, such as bone morphogenic protein, noncollagenous growth factors, and prostaglandins, stimulate the attraction and delivery of inflammatory cells. The third stage, inflammation, begins with the influx of inflammatory cells and ends with the appearance of bone and cartilage production. This inflammatory cell population includes polymorphonucleocytes, neutrophils, macrophages, and mast cells. Osteoclast arrival results in the removal of necrotic bone. Fibroblasts appear, and there is capillary ingrowth into the periphery of the fracture hematoma. Stage four, known as the soft callus stage, is characterized by the development of cartilage and bone and is complete with the cessation of appreciable fracture motion. This stage is marked by the production of subperiosteal new bone adjacent to the fracture ends. The appearance of chondroblasts in the fracture gap precedes the conversion of fibrovascular stoma to chondroid matrix, which clinically stabilizes the fracture. Stage five involves the conversion of the soft, largely chondroid callus to woven bone by endochondral ossification. At the completion of this stage, the fracture is considered healed both clinically and radiographically. Fracture strength is directly proportional to the amount of new bone produced. Bone remodeling, the final stage, is defined by the conversion of woven bone to lamellar bone. The medullary cavity and normal bone diameter are restored during this stage.

Fracture Fixation

The four definable types of fracture healing following surgical repair are largely a result of the method used and the degree of stability achieved following fracture fixation. The first type is termed the primary fracture callus response and is seen in all cases. This response usually occurs 2 weeks following injury, and the hallmark is the production of large amounts of callus beneath the periosteum. This type of healing has little ability to bridge fracture gaps, but is very tolerant of bone fragment instability. The second type of healing response, external bridging callus, forms when cast immobilization or nonrigid bone fixation (such as unlocked intramedullary nails) is used. The osteoprogenitor cell population is recruited from the surrounding soft tissues, with neovascular proliferation occurring. This type of healing is able to bridge fracture gaps and is very tolerant of fracture instability. Late medullary callus formation, the third type, is slow and bridges fracture gaps only if bone stability is maintained. Whereas primary fracture and external callus formation depend on the periosteal vasculature, late medullary callus depends largely on the intramedullary vasculature. This type of healing is seen with rigid fixation, such as cortical plates with imperfect bone end apposition. The fourth type, primary cortical healing, occurs only with absolute mechanical immobilization and direct cortical apposition. This type of healing is seen with rigid cortical fixation with compression plating at the fracture site. Primary cortical healing is extremely slow, cannot bridge fracture gaps, and depends on an intact intramedullary vascular supply. This type of healing represents primary bone remodeling from osteoclastic resorption of cortical bone and subsequent new osteon formation. These osteons develop parallel to the cortical axis and grow across the bone ends to unite the fracture. Fracture healing with external fixation depends on the construct of the fixator and the alignment of the fracture. A locked external fixator applied with compression at the fracture site will result in primary cortical healing. Poor bone to bone contact will lead to late medullary callus formation and possible nonunion. A patient who bears weight with a dynamized external fixator will exhibit external bridging callus formation.

Blood Supply

Three vessel systems are involved in fracture healing. The nutrient and endosteal vessels supply the inner two thirds of the diaphyseal cortex, while the periosteal vessels supply the outer one third. Surgical disruption of these vessel systems, through either intramedullary reaming or periosteal stripping, can adversely impact fracture healing. Disruption of the intramedullary blood supply by reaming has been well documented. In addition, reaming generates large increases in intramedullary pressure, which contribute to inner cortical necrosis. Modifications in fracture fixation, such as unreamed intramedullary nails and low contact cortical plates, have been designed to address these issues.

Growth Factors

Several local growth factors involved in fracture repair have been identified (Table 1). These include transforming growth factor beta (TGF-β), insulin-like growth factor (IGF), platelet derived growth factor (PDGF), fibroblast growth factor (FGF), tumor necrosis factor (TNF), cytokines (eg, interleukin, IL), and seven individual bone morphogenetic proteins (BMP), including osteogenin (BMP-3). These growth factors are secreted by both inflammatory and noninflammatory cells. Macrophages have been identified as a primary source for cytokine and growth factor production in the initial phases of fracture healing. TGF-β1, FGF, and ILs and other cytokines are synthesized by macrophages. Platelet degranulation during hematoma formation is a significant source of extracellular TGF-β1 and PDGF. Other sources include osteoblasts and bone matrix itself. The sequence of growth factor expression or delivery to the fracture callus is often related to the specific histologic stage of fracture repair. TGF-β1 expression is high during chondrogenesis and endochondral ossification, but low during intramembranous bone formation. Extracellular sources of TGF-β1 are immediately available from surrounding platelets during hematoma formation, but intracellular production is absent. Growth factor concentration can specifically direct fracture repair, with artificially increased local concentrations actually impeding fracture healing. Finally, mitogenic growth factors may stimulate bone resorption, with increased bone cell replication being a secondary process.

Table 1. Growth factors involved in fracture repair

Growth Factor	Location	Function
Transforming growth factor-β (TGF-β1, TGF-β2)	Platelets, osteoblasts, chondrocytes, bone matrix	1 Increase osteoblast–chondrocyte proliferation 2 Increase proteoglycan synthesis 3 Decrease collagen synthesis
Insulin-like growth factor (IGF) or somatomedin C	Found in bone and cartilage	Stimulates cartilage growth
Platelet-derived growth factor (PDGF)	Platelets, monocytes, endothelial cells	1 Increase osteoblast–chondrocyte proliferation 2 Increase protein synthesis (collagen and noncollagen)
Fibroblast growth factor (FGF)	Inflammatory cells, osteoblasts, chondrocytes	1 Increase cell replication 2 Indirectly increase collagen production
Tumor necrosis factor (TNF)	Macrophages	1 Increase bone resorption 2 Increase cell replication

Fracture Nonunion

Fracture nonunions occur when the reparative sequence of fracture healing is interrupted, usually in stage IV. The fracture gap usually consists of fibrous tissue with varying amounts of cartilage. Several factors have been shown to play a role in slowing the rate of fracture healing and thus increasing the subsequent risk of developing a nonunion. These factors are systemic (patient age, nutritional status, tobacco use, and activity level) as well as local (soft-tissue trauma, excessive bone loss, inadequate immobilization, infection, and vascular injury). Nonunions, hypertrophic or atrophic, and pseudarthrosis are generally differentiated based on radiographic and histiologic appearance. Hypertrophic nonunions demonstrate increased vascularity and callus formation, with a horseshoe or elephant-foot configuration on radiographs. Atrophic nonunions typically show little callus formation around a fibrous tissue-filled fracture gap. Pseudarthrosis is defined as a nonunion in which a fluid filled cavity with a synovial-like membrane is present at the fracture site.

Pathophysiology

Data from recent studies have indicated that collagenase production by macrophages and fibroblasts residing at the fracture gap contributes to deficient fracture healing. In addition, a relative absence of peripheral nerves has been found in delayed union or nonunion tissue, when compared to their presence in the surrounding bone and periosteum. This absence of nerve tissue may alter proprioceptive signals used to locally monitor bone strain, thereby adversely affecting fracture healing. Nonunions present clinically as either a fibrous nonunion, which can be classified as either hypertrophic or atrophic, or a pseudarthrosis. Histopathologic studies of human nonunion and pseudarthrosis specimens demonstrate that small clefts exist at the site of nonunions. Progressive motion is implicated in converting these minor clefts into the dominant clefts that denote pseudarthrosis. Although they potentially represent a spectrum of deficient fracture healing, nonunions and pseudarthrosis have different surgical treatments.

Treatment

Surgical exposure and resection of the synovial lined cleft plus rigid fixation and bone grafting are necessary to initiate the process of fracture healing. Hypertrophic nonunions require only adequate immobilization to initiate fracture healing. Atrophic nonunions have classically required local bone grafting in conjunction with adequate immobilization. Techniques in which onlay grafts consisting of allogeneic bone in conjunction with BMP are used have proven promising in clinical trials. In addition, percutaneous techniques, in which bone marrow preparations or recombinant BMP (rhBMP) are used, have been shown to effectively heal nonunions in select fractures. Barriers to fibrous tissue ingrowth, which may also serve as scaffold for regenerating periosteum, have also been studied. Use of a biodegradable polyurethane membrane has been reported to prevent nonunions in segmental bone defects in rabbit radii. It is certain that improvements in fracture and nonunion management will parallel the increasing understanding of the fracture reparative process.

Electrical Stimulation

The application of electrical stimulation for fracture healing is still controversial largely due to the lack of well-controlled clinical trials.

Methods of Application There are three types of electrical stimulation: (1) direct current, (2) capacitance coupling (ie, AC), and (3) inductive coupling. Electrical stimulation of acute fractures has been demonstrated to accelerate the early phases of fracture healing by 20% to 25% and therefore is not indicated for routine fracture care. The FDA has approved electrical stimulation for the treatment of nonunion and congenital pseudarthrosis and to potentiate spinal fusions. DC generators require implantation of the cathode (negative pole) directly into the surgical field. DC generators mirror a sustained injury potential, which results in a greater inflammatory response. AC generators use conductive medium (paste) and are placed on opposite sides of the affected extremity. Capacitance coupling affects cyclic adenosine monophosphate (cAMP), collagen synthesis, and calcification during the soft and hard callus stages of fracture healing. Pulsed electromagnetic fields (PEMFs) have gained greater popularity because their greatest effect is during the conversion of soft to hard callus. PEMFs influence cAMP, protein kinases, calcium-dependent intracellular mechanisms, and angiogenesis, which, in turn, function to initiate the calcification of fibrocartilage in the fracture gap. PEMFs are largely ineffective with fully fibrous nonunions until conversion to fibrocartilage occurs. This conversion is generally achieved through immobilization. PEMF units are placed externally and do not require inductive substances to function. The electrodes are placed on either side of the nonunion site and may be incorporated into or on top of a cast or brace. The advantage of PEMFs over other forms of electrical stimulation is that they do not require surgical implantation or direct contact with the skin.

Clinical Use A wide body of experimental data to support the clinical application of electrical stimulation has been generated over the past 20 years. PEMF electrical stimulation was initially thought to require asymmetric pulses to generate therapeutic results. Data from two recent studies demonstrated that asymmetric and symmetric pulses are equally effective in maintaining bone stiffness in an established rabbit fibular osteotomy model. Symmetric pulses can be delivered with one fifth the energy requirements of current units, allowing the use of more self contained electrical generators. The use of capacitive coupling has also been studied with regard to disuse osteoporosis. Capacitive coupling was found to promote new bone formation in a denervated rat tibia model of disuse osteoporosis when compared to controls. This reversal was not due to slowing of bone resorption, but rather to enhanced bone formation.

Even though data from several animal studies promote the efficacy of electrical stimulation, the current literature still reflects a paucity of well-controlled clinical studies. Although initial results of using PEMFs to treat scaphoid nonunions were encouraging (89% success rate), a follow-up review of this patient population generated more disappointing results (69% success rate). The authors felt that use of PEMFs should be a secondary alternative to open treatment with internal fixation and bone grafting. The use of PEMFs to treat congenital pseudarthrosis of the tibia has enjoyed some recent success.

Bone Grafting

Autografts

Currently the most reliable method of supplementing union of damaged bone is via autografts. Bone grafts serve two functions: they promote osteogenesis and they provide structural support. Osteogenesis may be supported initially by transplantation of viable cells, which are maintained by diffusion, and may produce new bone at the site of transplantation. Osteoinduction and osteoconduction contribute heavily to the production of bone formation and to the eventual incorporation of autografts. Osteoinduction is the recruitment of mesenchymal-type cells to form cartilage and bone under the influence of a particular stimulus. Osteoconductive surfaces provide a framework that facilitates the migration of cells used for angiogenesis, chondrogenesis, and osteogenesis.

Pathophysiology of Incorporation The process of autograft incorporation proceeds through sequential phases similar to those seen with fracture healing. Because of its increased surface area, cancellous bone is more rapidly incorporated than cortical bone. Following an initial phase of hemorrhage and inflammation, creeping substitution takes place, with the ingrowth of new vessels and their accompanying primitive mesenchymal cells. These cells subsequently differentiate into osteoblasts and osteoclasts. Cortical and cancellous grafts undergo creeping substitution, but not in the same sequence. This difference results in predictable differences between the strength of these grafts during the period of incorporation.

Cortical Autografts In cortical bone, new vessels use nutrient arteries to initially resorb the haversian systems, with the lamellar bone being resorbed much later. Bone resorption must take place before new bone formation can occur, and it proceeds at a rate 50 times faster than bone formation. Cortical grafts, which are superior in strength to cancellous grafts at the time of implantation, become mechanically inferior for the first 6 months following transplantation. It is estimated that cortical grafts are at 50% strength at 6 months.

Cancellous Autografts Cancellous bone undergoes bone formation before bone resorption. The application of new bone to necrotic trabeculae before osteoclasts resorb the necrotic bone results in initially inferior structural grafts that continue to gain in strength as this process proceeds. Incorporation of cancellous grafts is usually complete at 1 year. Although they are more uniform for cancellous autografts, resorption and formation occur at different rates in different regions of both types of autograft, resulting in an admixture of necrotic grafted donor bone and viable new bone at any one time.

Vascularized Autografts With the advent of microsurgical techniques, vascularized autografts have gained increased popularity. If both the nutrient artery and vein are anastomosed at the time of transplantation, the vascularized autograft does not require creeping substitution to incorporate or heal. Vascularized grafts incorporate and hypertrophy without losing their structural integrity. Three types of vascularized autografts are available: the fibula, the rib, and the iliac crest. Autografts, although superior to other types of bone grafts in the promotion of union, are limited by a finite supply and complications of graft acquisition. This limitation is especially true in cases of bone loss due to periprosthetic osteolysis or of large bone resections due to tumors. One novel approach is to use autoclaved resected specimens to reconstruct difficult regions, such as the hemipelvis. However, autoclaving bone destroys its osteoinductive capacity by denaturing bone proteins, including BMP. This destruction results in a graft that is purely osteoconductive and may be less stimulatory to bone incorporation than a comparably frozen allograft. Attempts to heal fracture nonunions while avoiding the potential complications of acquiring large volumes of autograft have led some researchers to advocate percutaneous aspiration and injection of concentrated bone marrow material into these sites. Bone marrow aspirates do not obviate the need for adequate fracture stabilization, nor do they provide enough material to fill bone defects. Current research is directed toward the mating of osteoinductive aspirated bone material with osteoconductive materials, such as hydroxyapatite ceramics, to produce suitable autograft substitutes.

Allografts

Because of the limitation of autografts, allografts and, more recently, the use of bone graft substitutes have become extremely popular. There are several forms of allograft bone; most currently used allograft material consists of freeze-dried allograft chips (Table 2). Methods of allograft preservation include freezing to −70°C, lyophilization, and demineralization.

Sterilization of Allografts Grafts can either be acquired aseptically and stored (frozen) without additional sterilization by gamma irradiation or ethylene oxide or they can be sterilized. With increased public awareness concerning the risk of disease transmission by transplanted tissues, bone and soft-tissue allograft banking methods have come under closer scrutiny. Bacterial infections secondary to contaminated allografts are rare. In one large series of 324 allografts, only three infections directly traced to the allograft were reported. Hepatitis transmission by nonsterilized allografts has been reported; however, none has been reported for sterilized bone. Although gamma irradiation is known to reduce the risk of bacterial and hepatitis contamination, it is less reliable for human immunodeficiency virus (HIV). The dose required to kill HIV-1 depends on the amount of virus present, with 0.4 Mrad being necessary to reduce the concentration of HIV by 90% (one log reduction). The concentration of HIV-1 in the blood of an acutely infected individual is at least three times the studied dosage, requiring at least 1.2 Mrad to reduce the highest expected virion concentration to a single virion. Chemical processing, primarily with ethanol, has been shown to inactivate the virus. However virions, although inactive, are still measurable by polymerase chain reaction follow-

Table 2. Types of allograft bone

Type	Processing and Storage	Sterilization
Frozen	Frozen and stored at −80° C; suited for large allografts; shelf life of at least 2 years	Aseptic acquisition; gamma irradiation
Freeze-dried	Usually frozen to −30° C and exposed to low atmospheric pressure; indefinite shelf life; suited to small amounts of material	Gamma irradiation; ethylene oxide exposure
Demineralized	Exposure to strong acids; suited for powders and small amounts of material	Gamma irradiation; ethylene oxide exposure
Fresh	Material refrigerated, not frozen	Aseptic acquisition

ing conventional processing. Initial estimates of HIV transmission risk of one in a million will probably remain accurate, even as the infected donor pool increases. This risk maintenance will largely be due to the continued improvement in viral detection and maintenance of strict donor guidelines, which still remain the most effective methods of disease prevention.

Fresh Allografts Fresh allografts, as opposed to the conventional types, have been used to reconstruct intra-articular posttraumatic chondral defects. The primary advantage of this technique is the ability to maintain a high degree of chondrocyte viability by avoiding adverse environmental extremes encountered with deep freezing and chemical cryopreservation. Cartilage support by a thin layer (5 mm) of subchondral bone is necessary to preserve the integrity of the graft. Advocates of this method have reported unipolar (single chondral defect) survival rates of 76% at 5 years and 69% at 10 years. Patients under the age of 60 years appear to do better. Any malalignment of the knee is corrected with an osteotomy prior to transplantation. This type of program is extremely labor intensive. Recipients are required to remain available for surgery whenever a donor is found, because the graft needs to be implanted within 12 to 24 hours of retrieval. The requirements for rapid and careful donor selection and screening during this short incubation period make the provision of fresh osteochondral allografts difficult for most community bone and tissue banks.

Bone Graft Substitutes

Bone graft substitutes generally include inorganic osteoconductive substances as well as organic bone-derived proteins. Inorganic materials serve purely as osteoconductive matrices and include calcium phosphate ceramics and polylactic acid polymers. Bone-derived proteins can either be extracted from human or bovine sources or generated by recombinant DNA technology and are primarily osteoinductive.

Osteoconductive Materials Traditionally, two ceramics have received the most attention: tricalcium phosphate and hydroxyapatite. Structurally analogous to bone, with a pore size ranging from 100 to 300 μm, these ceramics are extremely biocompatible. The rate of resorption by the host bone is directly related to the porosity of the matrix; tricalcium phosphate is considered to be more biodegradable than hydroxyapatite. Both ceramics have been used in limited studies to reconstruct cancellous bone defects. Unfortunately, calcium phosphates are extremely brittle, making them poor substitutes for structural grafts. Collagen-based graft substitutes are also currently under study. Bovine liquid collagen combined with hydroxyapatite–tricalcium phosphate ceramic granules is considered to be primarily osteoconductive. This composite material has demonstrated promising results in multicenter Phase III clinical trials. Because they are purely osteoconductive, calcium phosphate ceramics and collagen substrates make excellent autograft expanders, with the host graft providing the necessary osteoinductive proteins.

Polylactic acid polymers have enjoyed a reliable history as a resorbable suture material that has an average degradation rate of 6 months. The degradation rate can be adjusted by altering the structure of the material and thereby altering the surface area available to the aqueous environment. In addition, the degradation rate depends strongly on the percentage of the racemic form of lactic acid found in the polymer, with l-lactic acid enjoying the longest half-life. Although promising as an osteoinductive factor delivery system, polylactic acid polymers are still largely investigational.

Osteoinductive Materials A large degree of research activity is being directed toward the study and development of osteoinductive bone graft substitutes. BMP clearly potentiates bone healing; seven individual BMPs have been identified, sequenced, and cloned. Recombinant human BMP-2 (rhBMP-2), when implanted in extraskeletal sites, has been found to induce bone formation through endochondral ossification and, therefore, has undergone the most extensive study. Initial studies have been extremely promising; in these, rhBMP-2 used in conjunction with a variety of carriers demonstrates healing of bone defects in a high percentage of animals. However, severe practical difficulties with the initial collagen-based carriers (disease transmission, potential rejection, and supply limitations) have resulted in research directed toward the combining of rhBMPs with noncollagenous matrices. Resorbable poly L-lactic acid lattices and hydroxyapatite ceramics hold the most promise. Unfortunately, neither composite is sufficiently strong to serve as a structural graft. The clinical indications for these types of combined osteoinductive proteins and osteoconductive matrices are similar to those for current applications of cancellous bone graft or freeze-dried allograft. Frozen allografts are still considered the most versatile structural biologic implant available for long-bone reconstruction.

Distraction Osteogenesis

The application of serial distraction to generate new bone formation to accommodate for segmental bone loss or to lengthen shortened extremities has recently gained wide popularity. In this technique, which was developed initially in the former Soviet Union by Gavriil A. Ilizarov, gradual distraction of newly osteotomized bone ends is used to produce bone by intramembranous bone formation.

Pathophysiology Distraction osteogenesis encompasses three phases: a latency period, a distraction phase, and a consolidation phase. Following a controlled osteotomy, commonly termed a corticotomy, a latency period is permitted to enable the bone ends to complete the first three phases of fracture healing. In this osteotomy, the periosteal blood supply is preserved by carefully cutting the cortical bone with a thin osteotome and producing a controlled fracture in the far cortex. The medullary blood supply is minimally disrupted and, in animal studies, has been found to recover fully prior to distraction. The latency period generally lasts between 3 and 10 days, depending on the age and health of the patient or the amount of soft-tissue disruption at the time of osteotomy. Once the inflammatory phase is complete, gradual distraction is initiated using either an external fixator or a combined intramedullary rod and external fixator construct.

Ilizarov determined that a rate of 1 mm a day at a rhythm of one quarter turn every 6 hours produced the most homogeneous regenerate bone. Faster rates result in fibrous tissue production or cyst formation, while slower rates often result in premature consolidation and healing of the distraction gap. Cyst formation in a regenerate region can be treated with a short period of compression to initiate osteogenesis.

Histology During distraction, histologic examination often reveals bone trabeculae oriented parallel to the direction of distraction. Distraction osteogenesis occurs largely via intramembranous bone formation; little cartilage formation occurs during distraction. Occasionally, small islands of cartilage can be identified histologically and contribute to bone formation via enchondral ossification. Histologic examination of the distraction gap reveals a continuum of bone formation (Fig. 1). At the periphery, large osteons are seen; they gradually thin toward the interzone, which consists primarily of fibrous tissue. Collagen formed at the fibrous interzone gradually organizes into new bone trabeculae, which are mineralized at the osteotomized bone ends. This continuum roughly resembles what happens at a growth plate, although enchondral bone formation does not play a large role. Mesenchymal cells, which are delivered to the fibrous zone by newly formed vessels, gradually mature into osteoblasts, which reside on the newly formed bone trabeculae. As distraction continues, organization of the regenerate bone into a cortex and an intramedullary canal takes place primarily at the bone ends.

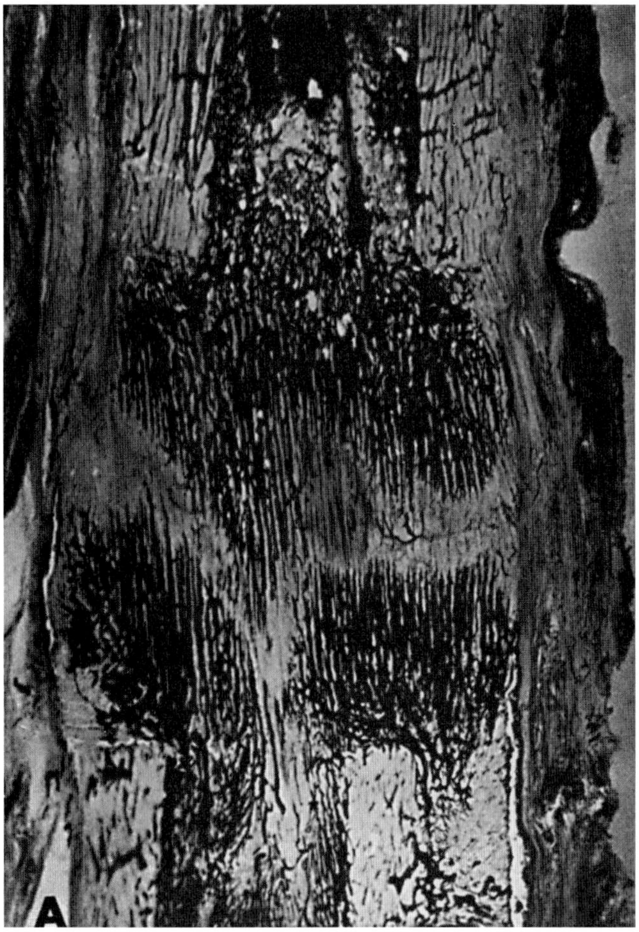

Fig. 1 Whole mount section demonstrating the distraction gap, which represents a continuum of bone formation. The central fibrous region is framed by columns of newly formed osteoid, which becomes increasingly more organized toward the periphery. (Reproduced with permission from Ilizarov GA: The tension stress effect on the genesis and growth of tissue: Part 2. The influence of the rate and frequency of distraction. *Clin Orthop* 1989;238:263–285.)

The final phase, consolidation, initiates once the goals of bone length have been reached and distraction is halted. Gradual organization of the bone takes place at this time, largely in response to the stress of weightbearing. Because patients are encouraged to bear weight during bone transport, bone organization actually begins during the distraction phase. However, it often is difficult for patients to bear weight; this difficulty is due, in part, to the discomfort experienced during lengthening and the occasional development of soft-tissue contractures. Therefore, mineralization and the formal organization of the regenerate bone into a more normal appearing cortex and medullary canal do not take place until distraction is complete. Once the regenerate bone is felt to be biomechanically sound, the distraction apparatus is removed. The bone segment continues to remodel, emulating the final phase of fracture healing. Once complete, distraction osteogenesis influences future bone growth in the immature skeleton.

Lengthening the tibia by up to 20% of the total bone length has been reported to have little impact on future bone growth in rabbits. However, when the bone is lengthened by 30% or more, growth retardation has been demonstrated.

Effect of Fixation Different types of fixators can be used to perform distraction osteogenesis. The type of callus formed often differs depending on the rigidity of the frame and how the regenerate bone is loaded. Circular frames in which small tensioned wires are used deliver uniform loads to bone and are less rigid than half-pin designs. Frames of this nature have been found to generate parallel columns of bone formation, whereas half-pin fixators lead to eccentric angular bone columns. Despite a significant difference in axial rigidity, the circular and half-pin frames induce osteogenesis of equal volume.

Annotated Bibliography

Fracture Healing

Brighton CT, Hunt RM: Early histological and ultrastructural changes in medullary fracture callus. *J Bone Joint Surg* 1991;73A:832–847.

Transformation of capillary and venous endothelial cells adjacent to normal marrow and the appearance of polymorphic mesenchymal cells throughout the medullary callus are described. The early appearance of osteoblasts and new bone formation supports the theory of local endothelial cell transformation to osteoblasts.

Sturmer KM: Measurement of intramedullary pressure in an animal experiment and propositions to reduce the pressure increase. *Injury* 1993:24(suppl 3):S7-S21.

The effect of intramedullary reaming was studied in a sheep model. The disruption of the endosteal and cortical blood supply is directly related to the production of high intramedullary pressure generated during reaming. The use of an irrigation-suction system significantly ($p < 0.05$) reduced the region of necrosis, with the use of an unreamed nail having little effect.

Fracture Nonunion

Milgram JW: Nonunion and pseudarthrosis of fracture healing: A histopathologic study of 95 human specimens. *Clin Orthop* 1991;268:203–213.

Ninety-five human nonunion sites from extra-articular and intra-articular locations were studied. Nonunion sites demonstrated a spectrum of microscopic to dominant clefts on light microscopy. The dominant clefts, which represent pseudarthosis, may not be a separate entity but instead illustrate the most advanced stage of a nonunion.

Electrical Stimulation

Adams BD, Frykman GK, Taleisnik J: Treatment of scaphoid nonunion with casting and pulsed electromagnetic fields: A study continuation. *J Hand Surg* 1992;17A:910–914.

This is a review of 54 patients with scaphoid nonunions that were treated with pulsed electromagnetic fields. A success rate of 69%, documented at 10-year follow-up, was felt to be less successful than that for conventional bone grafting techniques.

Autografts

Connolly JF, Guse R, Tiedeman J, et al: Autologous marrow injection as a substitute for operative grafting of tibial nonunions. *Clin Orthop* 1991;266:259–270.

Twenty tibial nonunions were treated with autologous bone marrow injection and either cast or intramedullary nail fixation. Eighteen of the 20 fractures healed without the need for further bone grafting.

Allografts

Eastlund DT: Bone transplantation and bone banking, in Lonstein JE (ed): *Moe's Textbook of Scoliosis and Other Spinal Deformities*, ed 3. Philadelphia, PA, WB Saunders, 1995, pp 581–595.

This concise review of allograft physiology, bone banking techniques, and processing emphasizes risk of disease transmission.

Bone Graft Substitutes

Cornell CN, Lane JM, Chapman M, et al: Multicenter trial of Collagraft as bone graft substitute. *J Orthop Trauma* 1991;5:1–8.

Collagraft, a composite of suspended fibrillar collagen and porous calcium phosphate ceramic, was mixed with autologous marrow aspirates and compared to autologous bone graft. Collagraft shortened time in surgery and reduced donor site morbidity while demonstrating radiographic union comparable to conventional bone grafting techniques.

Yasko AW, Lane JM, Fellinger EJ, et al: The healing of segmental bone defects induced by recombinant human bone morphogenetic protein (rhBMP–2): A radiographic, histological, and biomechanical study in rats. *J Bone Joint Surg* 1992;74A:659–670.

Forty-five rats were divided equally into three groups consisting of either recombinant human BMP-2 (rhBMP-2) in doses of 1.4 or 11.0 μg, and a control. Implantation of 11.0 μg of rhBMP-2 yielded significant ($p < 0.05$) bone formation; radiographic, histologic, and mechanical evidence of union were greater than for either the lower dose of rhBMP–2 or the control group.

Distraction Osteogenesis

Lee DY, Chung CY, Choi IH: Longitudinal growth of the rabbit tibia after callotasis. *J Bone Joint Surg* 1993;75B:898–903.

Tibial lengthening was found to retard longitudinal growth in rabbit tibias if the tibia was lengthened by 30% or more.

Classic Bibliography

Centrella M, McCarthy TL, Canalis E: Transforming growth factor-beta and remodeling of bone. *J Bone Joint Surg* 1991;73A:1418–1428.

Cornell CN, Lane JM: Newest factors in fracture healing. *Clin Orthop* 1992;277:297–311.

Damien CJ, Parsons JR: Bone graft and bone graft substitutes: A review of current technology and applications. *J Appl Biomat* 1991;2:187–208.

Goldberg VM, Stevenson S: The biology of bone grafts. *Semin Arthrop* 1993;4:58–63.

Ilizarov GA: The tension-stress effect on the genesis and growth of tissues: Part 2. The influence of the rate and frequency of distraction. *Clin Orthop* 1989;239:263–285.

Mahomed MN, Beaver RJ, Gross AE: The long-term success of fresh, small fragment osteochondral allografts used for intraarticular post-traumatic defects in the knee joint. *Orthopedics* 1992;15:1191–1199.

Pienkowski D, Pollack SR, Brighton CT, et al: Comparison of asymmetrical and symmetrical pulse waveforms in electromagnetic stimulation. *J Orthop Res* 1992;10:247–255.

Santavirta S, Konttinen YT, Nordstrom D, et al: Immunologic studies of nonunited fractures. *Acta Orthop Scand* 1992;63:579–586.

Sugioka Y, Hotokebuchi T, Tsutsui H: Transtrochanteric anterior rotational osteotomy for idiopathic and steroid-induced necrosis of the femoral head: Indications and long-term results. *Clin Orthop* 1992;277:111–120.

3

Biomechanics and Gait

Introduction

An analysis of the biomechanics of human movement is fundamental to understanding normal and pathologic function. Although many parameters can be used to describe the biomechanics of human movement, there are several kinematic and kinetic parameters that are particularly relevant to the understanding of the pathomechanics of human movement. This chapter will focus on the description of these kinematic and kinetic parameters and will identify specific applications that have been clinically relevant.

Joint Kinematics

The kinematics of human movement is normally described in terms of relative angles between adjacent limb segments. In practice, human gait is most often described in terms of the sagittal plane motion of adjacent limb segments (flexion–extension). However, some applications call for an analysis of general three-dimensional (3-D) limb motion. The complexity of the kinematic analysis substantially increases when going from a sagittal plane analysis to a complete 3-D analysis. Overall, the relative motion of one limb segment with respect to an adjacent limb segment can be described by six independent parameters. In mechanical terms, this means that there are six independent degrees of freedom (three translational and three rotational) that describe the 3-D motion of a segment.

Flexion–Extension Motion Patterns

Patterns of flexion–extension motion are surprisingly reproducible and consistent among the normal population. Given the complexity of normal human locomotion, a much greater degree of variability among normal subjects would be expected. It is useful to examine these kinematic parameters in terms of the subdivisions of the gait cycle because the timing of deviations from normal patterns often indicate specific pathology.

The stance phase of gait is typically described in terms of five segments: initial contact, loading response, midstance, terminal stance, and preswing. Swing phase has been described in terms of initial swing, midswing and terminal swing. At initial contact, the hip joint is in a flexed position (approximately 30°), the knee joint is near full extension, and the ankle is slightly plantarflexed (Fig. 1). As the limb moves into the loading response phase, the hip joint extends, the knee joint flexes, and the ankle joint dorsiflexes. At midstance phase, the hip joint continues to extend from its initially flexed position, the knee joint reaches a relative maximum, and the ankle remains in a dorsiflexed position. As the limb goes into terminal stance, the hip reaches an extended position, the knee flexes in preparation for swing phase, and the ankle plantarflexes. During initial swing phase, the hip and knee flex while the ankle moves toward dorsiflexion from an initially plan-

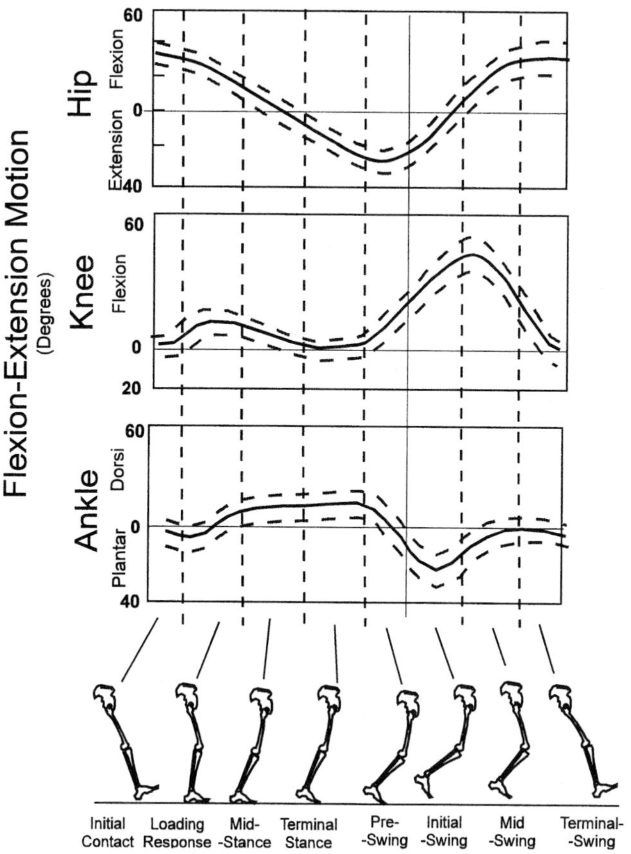

Fig. 1 This figure illustrates the position of the hip, knee, and ankle with the stance phase divided into five segments and the swing phase divided into three segments. The curves represent the normal patterns of motion for the hip, knee, and ankle. The limb below the curves illustrates the position of the pelvis, thigh, and shank as they would be observed during each of these segments of the gait cycle. It is often useful to break up the gait cycle into these segments when evaluating normal and pathologic gait. The normal sequence of events is reproducible as indicated by the relatively narrow standard deviation (dashed-line segments). It is important to note, as illustrated in Figure 2, that these curves can change in magnitude with walking speed.

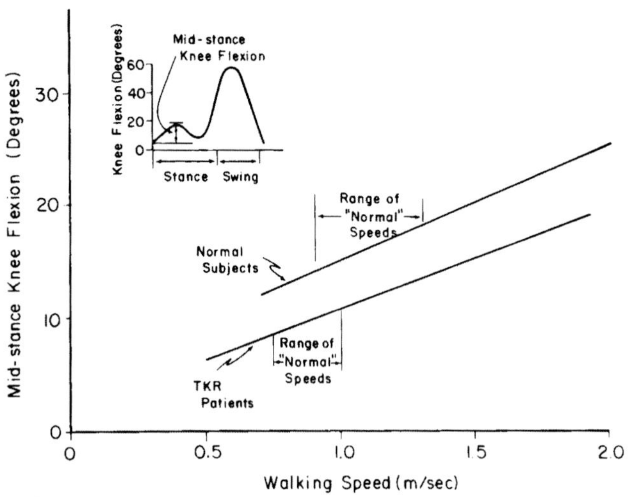

Fig. 2 An illustration of the difference in the change in the relationship between knee flexion during stance and walking speed in control subjects (n = 97 and r = 0.65) and in patients (n = 108 and r = 0.57). (Reproduced with permission from Andriacchi TP: The influence of total knee replacement design on walking and stair climbing. *J Bone Joint Surg* 1982;64A:1328–1335.)

tarflexed position. In terminal swing, the hip reaches maximum flexion, the knee extends for heelstrike, and the ankle plantarflexes.

It is important to note that the narrow band around each of the motion curves (Fig. 1) at the hip, knee, and ankle suggests that the characteristics of these patterns do not vary substantially during normal gait. However, care must be taken in measuring certain peak amplitudes, because it has been shown that these values are related to walking speed (Fig. 2). For example, the maximum stance phase flexion during midstance increases linearly with walking speed and, thus, in attempting to evaluate this parameter between normal controls and patients with walking abnormalities, controlling for walking speed is important. The influence of walking speed is also an important consideration for most aspects of gait analysis.

Gait Analysis

Kinematic variables can be used in clinical applications through gait analysis. Often patients will adapt their patterns of locomotion to stimuli, such as pain, instability, neuromuscular disability, or muscular weakness. Biomechanical analysis of the adaptation can provide more information than conventional clinical measures to reveal the nature of the underlying abnormality. Kinematic measurements can help quantify specific joint involvement associated with a particular type of walking disability. Consider the example of the gait of patients following total knee replacement. It has been shown that these patients have reduced knee flexion during the midstance portion of the gait cycle. Normal midstance knee flexion is approximately 20° at a walking speed of approximately 1 m/s. After total knee replacement, asymptomatic patients tend to walk with less than 10° of midstance knee flexion (Fig. 2). The gait abnormality after total knee reconstruction occurs during the midstance of the gait cycle and involves a subtle adaptation associated with a reduction in the loading response of the knee during the walking cycle. Although this kinematic measure shows where and when the adaptation occurs, it does not provide information on the cause of the abnormality. It should also be noted that the method of analysis shown in Figure 2 accounted for differences in walking speed when comparing normal individuals with patients. The next section will discuss joint kinetics and its value in the identification and interpretation of gait abnormalities.

Joint Kinetics

Kinetics is the study of the relationship between force and motion. The motion of the skeletal system is the result of a balance between external and internal forces. The external forces on the skeletal system include gravity, inertia, and foot-ground reaction forces during walking. Internal forces are created by muscular contraction, passive soft-tissue stretching, and bony contact at joint articulations. At any instant during walking or any activity of daily living, the external forces and moments must be balanced by internal forces and moments.

Interpretation of Joint Moments

External measurements of joint moments can be used to interpret internal forces within the muscles and on the joint surfaces. However, care must be taken in the interpretation of joint moments. For example, consider an external moment (Fig. 3) tending to flex the knee. This external moment would require a net internal moment tending to extend the knee. The term net moment is used because the internal moment is due to the summation of both antagonistic and synergistic muscle forces in the final equilibrium. If antagonistic muscle activity is present (Fig. 3), the net of the balance between the flexor and extensor muscles must still produce a net internal extension moment to balance the external flexion moment. Thus, the moments measured in the gait laboratory (external moments) can be used to infer the net balance between joint flexor and extensor muscles, because these muscles generate most of the internal moment that produces flexion or extension at the joint. Similarly, in the frontal plane, the abduction–adduction moments can be directly related to internal forces from the viewpoint of mechanical equilibrium. When the appropriate care is taken in the interpretation of joint moments, they can be extremely valuable in identifying changes in patterns of muscle activity in joint loading because they are very sensitive to abnormal functional changes.

Normal patterns of net flexor and extensor moments at the hip, knee, and ankle are illustrated in Figure 4. It is

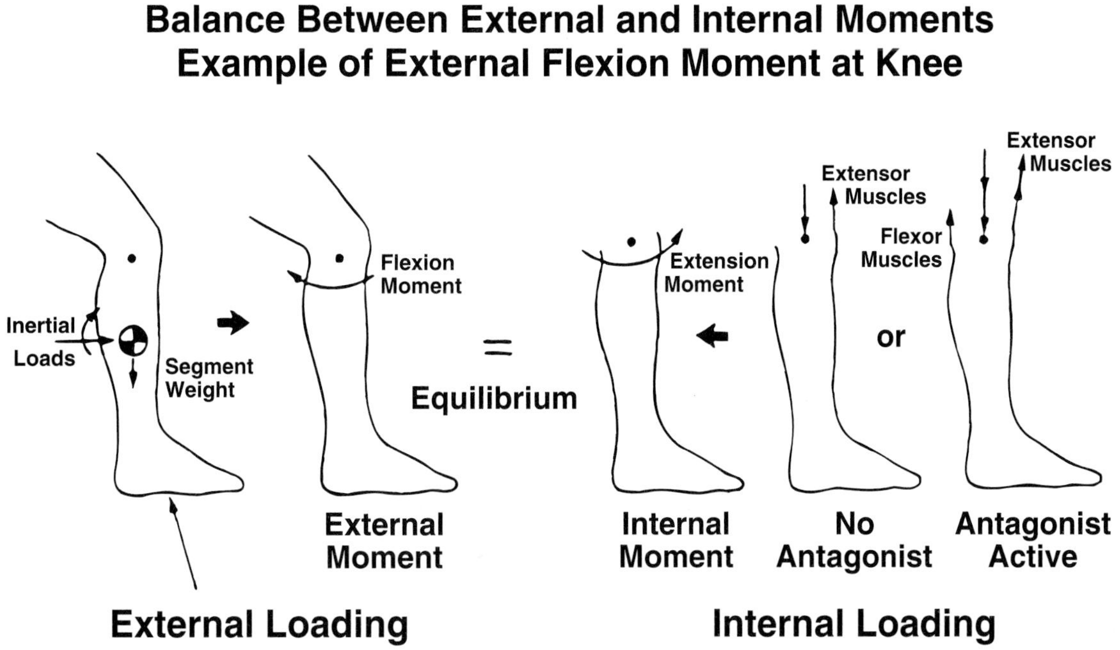

Fig. 3 An example of the balance between external loading producing a moment tending to flex the knee and an equal magnitude (opposite direction) internal moment tending to extend the knee. The internal extension moment is produced by quadriceps contraction (no antagonist) or the net moment produced by the quadriceps and antagonistic hamstrings muscle group. (Reproduced with permission from Andriacchi TP: Dynamics of pathological motion: Applied to the anterior cruciate deficient knee. *J Biomech* 1990;23(suppl):99–105.)

useful to examine the characteristics of the moment curves during the five segments of stance phase. These curves are quite reproducible in a normal population. Typically, at initial contact, the loads acting on the lower extremity require net hip extensor moments, net knee flexor moments, and net ankle dorsiflexion moments for equilibrium. Moving into the loading response phase, there is still a net hip extensor moment, the knee moment reverses to a net extensor moment, and the ankle moment becomes a net plantarflexor moment. In midstance, the net hip extensor moment reduces to zero, the knee moment reverses again to a net flexor moment, and the ankle moment continues as a net plantarflexor moment. During terminal swing, the hip moment reverses to a net flexor moment, the knee moment remains a flexor moment, and the ankle remains a plantarflexor moment. During preswing, only the knee moment changes direction from a flexor to a net extensor muscle moment. It should be noted that the muscle moments depicted in Figure 3 are the net balance between the flexors and extensors. Electromyograph (EMG) activity shows that at heel strike both flexors and extensors are active at both the hip and knee joint. The presence of antagonistic muscle activity at this phase of gait cycle is probably the result of the need to stabilize the limb for initial contact. It should be emphasized that the gait laboratory measurements provide external measures of moments acting at the limb. The internal net moments described here are inferred from these external measurements.

The component of the joint moment tending to flex and extend the joint is very important in the analysis of gait. The flexion–extension component is associated with propulsion during walking, as well as with lowering and raising the body against gravity. Examining the factors that influence the magnitude of the flexion–extension moments is useful, because these parameters can be related to the muscle and joint forces. Walking speed and stature are two factors that influence the magnitude and patterns of the flexion–extension moments.

Factors Influencing Joint Moments

As previously indicated, most gait parameters related to sagittal plane movement change with the speed of walking. It has been shown that the peak magnitudes of the flexion–extension moments at the hip, knee, and ankle are highly sensitive to the speed of walking. This speed dependence is an extremely important consideration when attempting to compare patient populations with normal control groups. Thus, the investigator must be able to separate out the change in moment magnitudes associated with walking speed versus a change in the mechanics of walking. Clearly, a normal subject walking at a slower speed

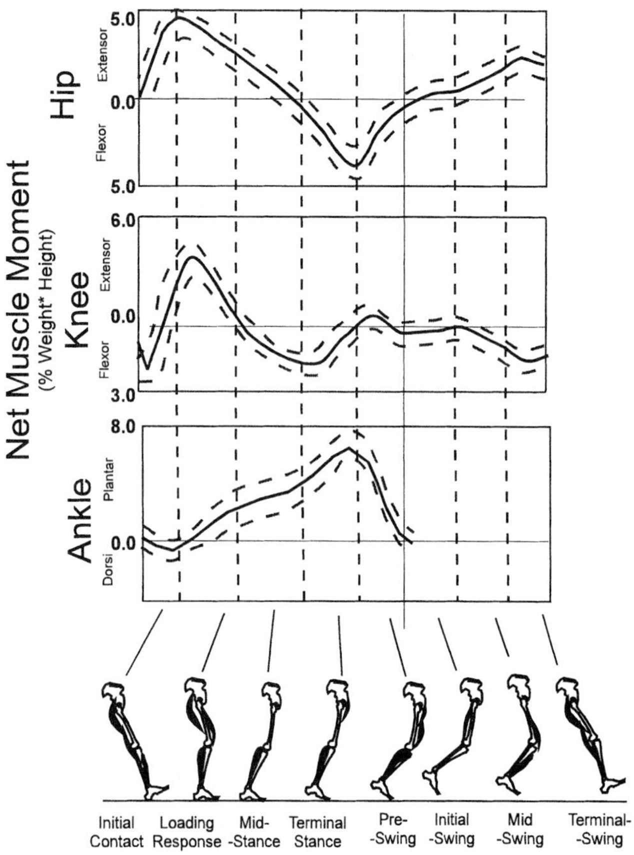

Fig. 4 An illustration of the typical net moments required to balance external loads acting on the limb during walking. The moments are expressed as net muscle moments because they are the minimum internal moments required to balance the externally acting moments in the absence of antagonistic muscle activity. These patterns are typical of a normal gait at an average walking speed. Although these patterns of net muscle moments can be extremely useful in evaluating the presence of pathologic gait, it is important that they do not reflect the presence of antagonistic muscle activity as illustrated in the diagram shown in Figure 3. In addition, the magnitude of the peak values in these diagrams can change substantially with walking speed, and thus, the speed of walking should be taken into consideration when evaluating and comparing these curves.

will have a lower moment magnitude. It is important to always compare moment magnitudes in the sagittal plane (flexion–extension) at nearly the same walking speeds when attempting to identify functional differences. Often, investigators' studies report differences in moment magnitudes at different walking speeds; thus, making it impossible to infer whether the difference was associated solely with the change in walking speed or with a change in function associated with some type of pathology.

The influence of stature can be evaluated by various normalization procedures. Moment magnitudes are often normalized to subjects' body dimensions. The units of a moment are the product of force and distance. Thus, it is possible for two subjects to have different magnitudes of moments based solely on their height and weight being different. To account for the influence of body type on moment magnitudes, moments are often normalized to body mass or the product of height and weight (Fig. 4). The normalization to height and weight is quite practical in the sense that it accounts for variations due to both height and weight. In addition, it normalizes the moment to a nondimensional quantity.

Moment Magnitudes During Activities of Daily Living

A comparison of the maximum flexion moments during walking, ascending stairs, descending stairs, rising from a seated position, and jogging shows a substantial variation in the peak flexion moments at each joint (Fig. 5). It is interesting that the largest flexion moment magnitudes during walking occur at the hip and ankle. The magnitude of the flexion moments at the hip and ankle are more than twice the magnitude of those that occur at the knee for a walking speed of approximately 1 m/s. If it is assumed that muscle lever arms are equal at the hip, knee, and ankle, the difference in moment magnitudes would suggest that during normal walking, the extensor musculature at the hip and the plantarflexor muscles at the ankle would sustain greater forces than the knee extensor muscles. The knee joint, with a relatively small flexion moment during level walking, would sustain substantial increases during

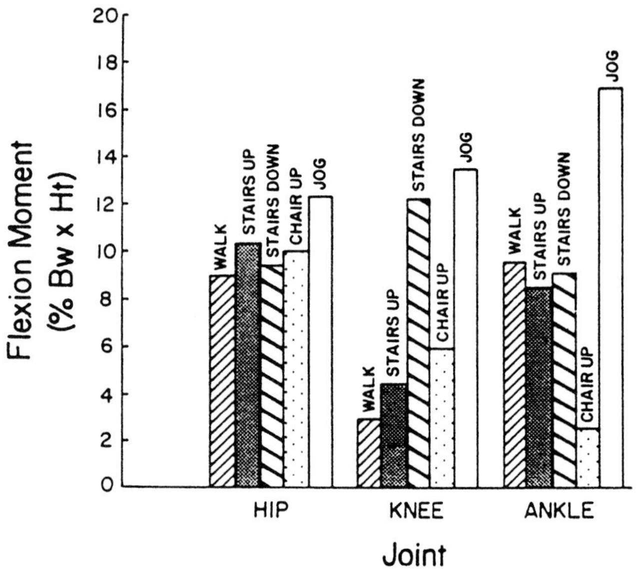

Fig. 5 A comparison of the magnitude of the flexion moments during various activities of daily living. (Reproduced with permission from Andriacchi TP, Mikosa RP: Musculoskeletal dynamics, locomotion and clinical applications, in Mow V, Hayes W (eds): *Basic Orthopaedic Biomechanics.* New York, NY, Raven Press, 1991, pp 51–92.)

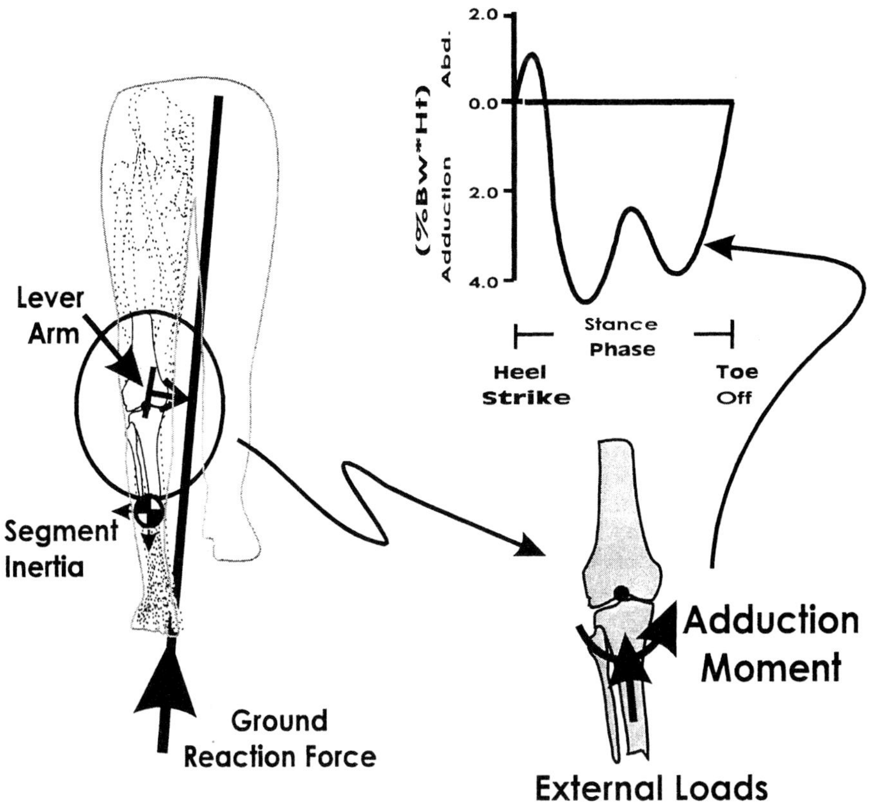

Fig. 6 Knee adduction moment during gait. The ground reaction force acting through a lever arm to the center of the knee joint produces the major portion of the adduction moment during gait. Limb segment inertia properties have minimal effect on this calculation. The adduction moment during gait is an external load tending to thrust the knee into varus.(Reproduced with permission from Andriacchi TP: Dynamics of knee malalignment. *Orthop Clin North Am* 1994;25:395–403.)

several activities, including stair climbing and jogging. The large increases in the flexion moment at the knee joint when jogging is likely associated with the high incidence of patellofemoral problems in middle- and long-distance runners. It is most likely that the relative increase (by approximately a factor of five) in the flexion moment during jogging over the nominal level of walking is more important on a comparative basis than the absolute magnitudes. For example, the ankle dorsiflexion moment during jogging is higher than the flexion moment at the knee. However, the relative dorsiflexion sustained during jogging, as compared with level walking, is increased by a factor of two as compared with the fivefold increase seen in the knee flexion moment.

The moment tending to adduct the limb (adduction moment) during walking is also an important consideration in function and overall joint loading during gait (Fig. 6). This moment magnitude has been particularly relevant for the pattern of loading at the knee joint. The magnitude of this moment is comparable to that tending to flex or extend the knee. The adduction moment is the primary reason for a larger joint reaction force on the medial side of the knee than on the lateral side. Several studies have shown that as much as 70% of the total load that passes through the knee joint is sustained by the medial compartment of the knee. An increase in the adduction moment during walking has been related to an increase in the medial compartment loading on the knee. This information can be generated from basic modeling approaches. Thus, the dynamic adduction moment measured in the gait laboratory can be used as a measure of medial compartment loading. This moment can be applied directly to studies of patients with varus gonarthrosis.

Direct Measurement of Hip Joint Loading During Function

In several recent studies, investigators have made direct measurement of internal joint reaction forces during function. Resultant hip joint force, its orientation, and its moments were measured in two patients during walking and running using an instrumented total hip prosthesis. These data showed peak forces at the hip ranging from 2.8 to approximately 4.8 times body weight when going from a slow to a fast walking speed. Jogging and uncontrolled stumbling increased the forces to between six and nine times the weight of the body. During all types of activities, the direction of the peak force in the frontal plane changed only slightly when the force magnitude was high.

It should be noted that the force measurements generated from the instrumented total hip replacements reflect the sum of all forces, including muscles acting about the hip joint. It is primarily the force generated by the muscles (acting through relatively short lever arms) that produces the resultant forces that are several times the weight of the body. Figure 7 shows the general pattern of the resultant force at the hip and of the three force components acting in an axial direction, anteroposterior direction, and mediolateral direction. As can be seen, the largest reaction force occurs just after heel strike, and as previously noted, this peak increases with walking speed. The second maximum force occurs during the push-off phase of the gait cycle. During swing phase, the minimum forces of both patients were typically between 10% and 40% body weight for all speeds. The angle of the peak force in the frontal plane was typically in the range between 17° and 25°. This force seems invariant and has been described in several studies.

Studies in which instrumented implantable devices such as this are used provide invaluable information that can be used to gain an understanding of the biomechanics of function. This information is useful for comparison to indirect external measurements as described in the early sections of this chapter. The limitations of direct in vivo measurements are, of course, the cost and invasive nature of the test. Thus, providing a statistical basis for the interpretation of the data obtained from instrumented devices is difficult, and information of this nature is best used to complement and interpret measurements obtained from gait laboratories using indirect techniques.

Examples of Clinical Applications for Joint Kinetics

Total Knee Replacement

As previously indicated, the joint moments are excellent indicators of changes from normal function. In addition, because the joint flexion–extension moments can be used to infer changes in muscle activity, these moments provide a basis for the clinical interpretations of abnormal function. A study of patients during stair climbing following total knee arthroplasty illustrates how differences in function based on the flexion–extension moment can be used to evaluate different designs. Patients who were tested had designs that retained or removed the posterior cruciate ligament (PCL) of the knee. The patients were matched for clinical status based on standard clinical assessment. In addition, all patients were tested a minimum of 1 year after surgery. The stair climbing test (Fig. 8) showed a difference in the knee flexion moment between designs that retained the PCL and designs that removed the PCL. The reduction in the moment tending to flex the knee was interpreted based on a reduction in the net quadriceps moment required to balance this external flexion moment. The patients can compensate by thrusting the body forward (Fig. 8) and reducing demand on the quadriceps. The flexion moment pattern during stair climbing was extremely use-

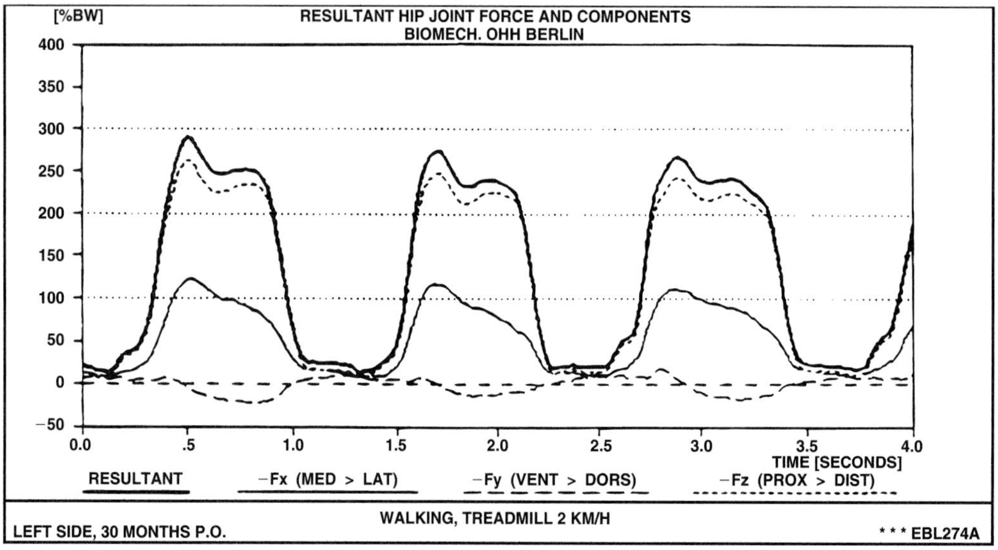

Fig. 7 Hip joint forces for a 30-month postoperative patient during slow walking (2 km/hr). Fx is the medial/lateral force component (thin solid line); Fy, the sagittal force component (long dashed line); and Fz, the vertical force component (short dashed line). (Reproduced with permission from Bergmann G, Graichen F, Rohlmann A: Hip joint loading during walking and runing, measured in two patients. *J Biomech* 1993;8:969–990.)

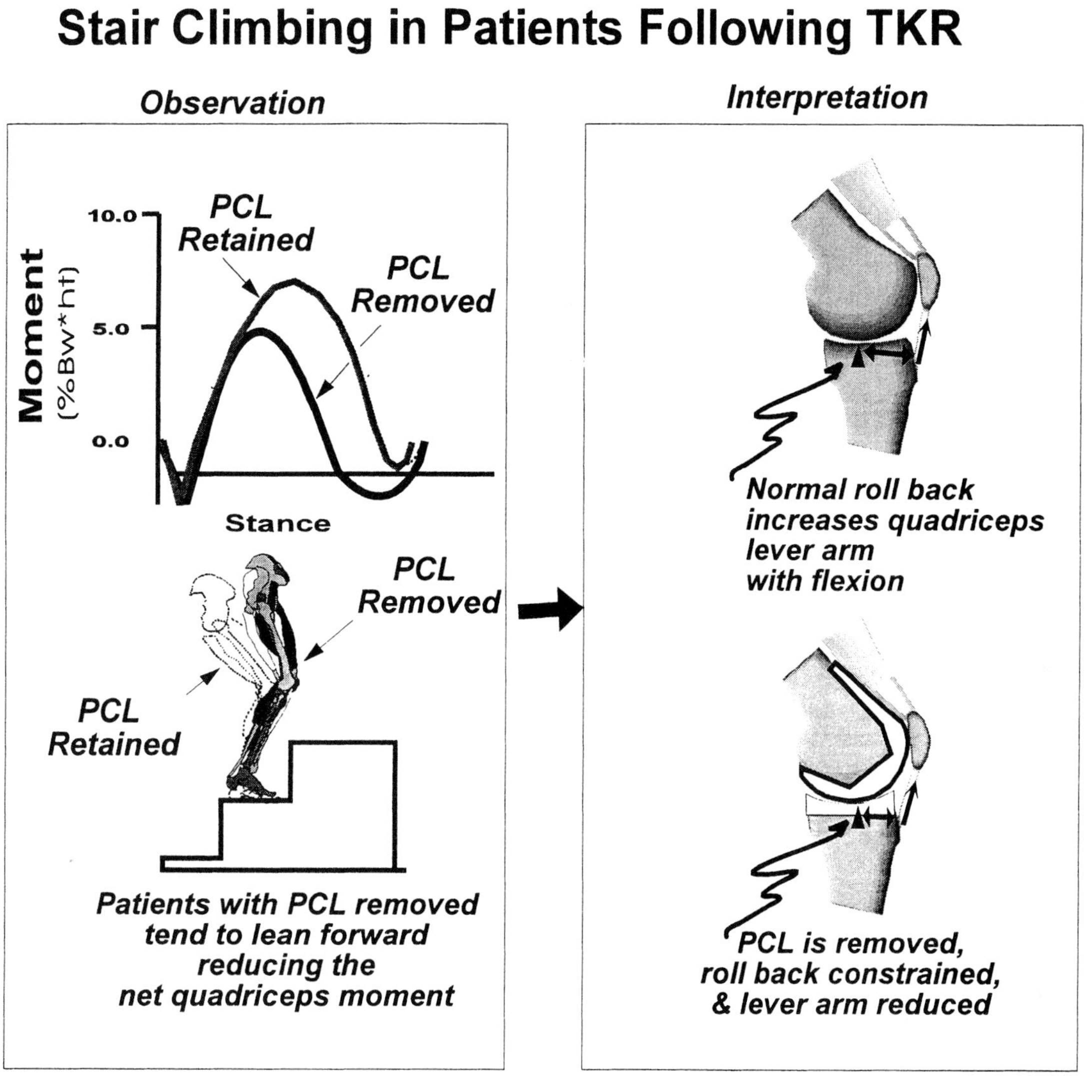

Fig. 8 Patients with designs that remove or substitute for the posterior cruciate ligament (PCL) tend to reduce the knee flexion moment and, thus, the resulting demand on the quadriceps. The mechanism they use for the adaptation is a forward lean of the torso. The biomechanical explanation for the adaptation seen in these patients can be related to the normal posterior movement of the tibiofemoral contact with flexion, which is reduced when the PCL is removed and constraint is added to the articular surface. (Reproduced with permission from Andriacchi TP: Functional analysis of pre- and post-knee surgery: Total knee arthroplasty and ACL reconstruction. *J Biomech Eng* 1993;115:575–581.)

ful in identifying these phenomena because the motion changes were much more subtle than the moment changes.

Anterior Cruciate Deficient Knee

Most studies have shown that the flexion–extension moment at the knee is quite sensitive to subtle changes in motion. For example, in a study of patients with ruptured anterior cruciate ligaments (ACL), it has been shown that a substantial change in the pattern of flexion–extension moment can be seen during level walking. Patients tested in the gait laboratory with ACL-deficient knees have a significantly lower than normal net quadriceps moment during the middle portion of stance phase. Commonly, the net moment reverses from one that demands net quadriceps activity to one that demands net hamstrings activity. This type of gait has been interpreted as a tendency to avoid or reduce the demand on the quadriceps muscle and has been called a "quadriceps avoidance gait." This quadriceps avoidance gait in ACL-deficient patients may seem surprising because the demand on the quadriceps muscles is relatively low during walking. However, despite the rela-

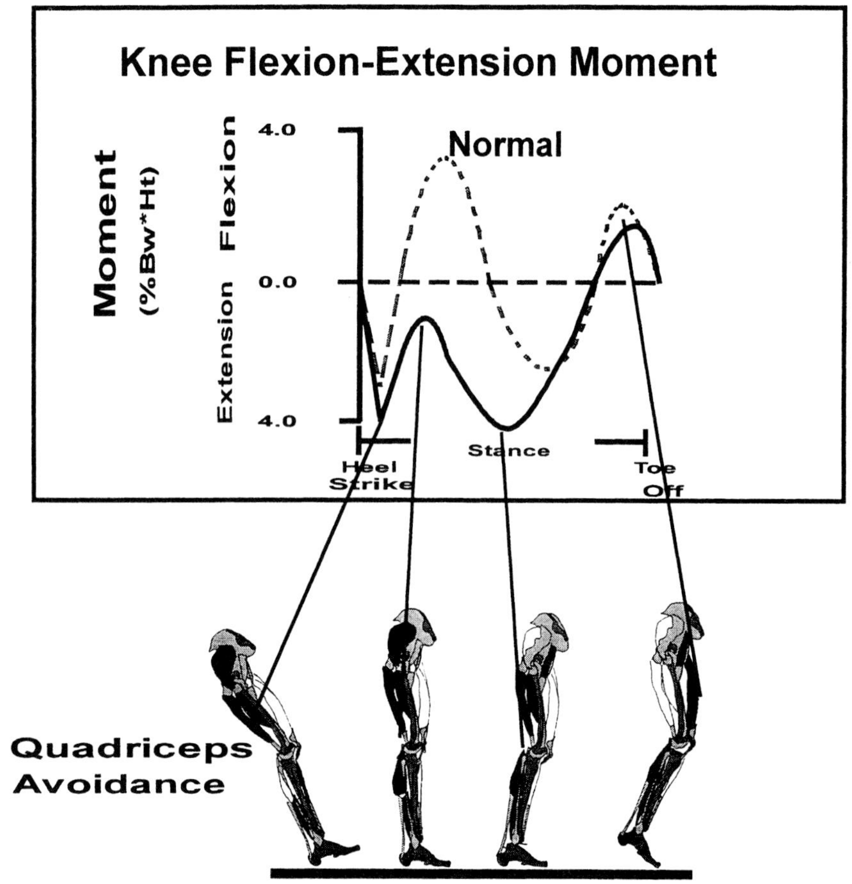

Fig. 9 The normal flexion–extension moment during the stance phase of walking tends to oscillate between flexion and extension as indicated by the dashed line. Patients following total knee replacement with designs that do not include the anterior cruciate ligament (ACL) and patients with ACL-deficient knees tend to have a pattern of knee flexion–extension moment that avoids demand on the quadriceps. (Reproduced with permission from Andriacchi TP: Functional analysis of pre- and post-knee surgery: Total knee arthroplasty and ACL reconstruction. *J Biomech Eng* 1993;115:575–581.)

tively low demands on the knee that occur during level walking, 75% of the patients in a recent report had the quadriceps avoidance gait and 25% had a normal biphasic flexion–extension moment (Fig. 9). It is important to note that the magnitude of the quadriceps moment during walking was changed by more than 100% when compared with the normal value and, thus, was a quite sensitive indicator of functional change. This quadriceps avoidance gait can be associated with the loss of the ACL. Near full extension, the patellar ligament at the knee tends to place an anterior pull on the tibia. The quadriceps avoidance gait seen in patients with ACL deficiencies can be associated with a functional adaptation to avoid this anterior pull on the tibia when the knee is near full extension. The anterior pull on the tibia from the patellar mechanism is reduced as the knee approaches 45° and, thus, the adaptation would be greatest near full extension and most apparent during walking activities.

High Tibial Osteotomy

The clinical outcome of treatment of high tibial osteotomy as treatment for patients with varus gonarthrosis has been related to the magnitude of the adduction moment (Fig. 6). In a large group of patients who were evaluated prior to high tibial osteotomy, one group was considered to have a high adduction moment if it was higher than 4% body weight times height when walking at a speed of approximately 1 m/s. All other patients were classified as having low adduction moments. Approximately one-half of the patients with varus gonarthrosis had moments lower than 4% body weight times height. Thus, it was possible for approximately one-half of the patients to adapt their gait dynamically to reduce the normal loading across the knee. It has been shown that patients with this adaptive gait tend to have better results after osteotomy at long-term follow-up than patients with high adduction moments; when examined between 3 and 8.9 years after surgery, the patients in the low adduction moment group had significantly better clinical outcomes. The passage of time caused a decline in the clinical results in both the high and low adduction moment groups. However, the patients who had low preoperative adduction moments maintained a better clinical result at an average of 6 years than did patients in the high adduction moment group. Further, 79% of the knees in the low adduction moment group had maintained valgus correction, whereas only 20% of the knees in the high adduction moment group remained in valgus alignment despite equivalent alignment correction in both groups immediately after surgery.

The adaptive mechanism used by some patients to reduce the adduction moment has been related to a shorter stride length and an increased external rotation (toe-out) of the foot position during stance phase. The adaptation using the toe-out mechanism greatly affected the reduction of the adduction moment during gait. Gait analysis can be used as an additional means of selecting patients who have a higher probability of good results with high tibial osteotomy. It also potentially is used as a basis for training patients to lower the loads at the knee joint.

Joint Kinetics and Gait Evaluation in Cerebral Palsy

Joint kinetics can be applied in a basic manner by combining the image of the subject with a projection of the ground reaction force. The position of the ground reaction force relative to the joint center can provide a useful estimate of the joint moment. The following is an example in which the visualization of the ground reaction is used to evaluate patients with cerebral palsy (CP).

Hyperextension in the knee during stance phase is a common feature in patients with CP. As previously described (Fig. 3), there is a moment tending to extend the knee during midstance. In patients with a tendency towards hyperextension, this moment can increase the severity of the hyperextension during this phase of the gait cycle. Orthoses that eliminate ankle motion (fixed ankle-foot orthoses or AFOs) can effectively control knee hyperextension during gait. Gait analysis has been used to demonstrate a beneficial effect on performance monitored before and after the use of optimally adjusted fixed AFOs to control knee hyperextension. By examining the moment tending to extend the knee in midstance, it is possible to adjust the brace so that the long-term damage to the knee structures caused by excessive extension moments can be minimized. The effect of the extension moment can be controlled by adjusting the fixed AFOs to control the position of the ground reaction force in relation to the knee. It has been shown that there is significant value in monitoring the moment for subjects treated in this manner. The ground reaction has changed in a way that reduces the tendency to hyperextend the knee.

Annotated Bibliography

Pediatrics/Cerebral Palsy

Butler PB, Thompson N, Major RE: Improvement in walking performance of children with cerebral palsy: Preliminary results. *Dev Med Child Neurol* 1992;34:567–576.

The effect of 4 to 6 months use of AFOs and balance training was determined for six children with CP and spastic diplegia or hemiplegia. Improved foot-ground contact and stance phase posture were noted, although not related to speed or range of motion. The value of monitoring the moment arm is emphasized.

Colborne GR, Wright FV, Naumann S: Feedback of triceps surae EMG in gait of children with cerebral palsy: A controlled study. *Arch Phys Med Rehabil* 1994;75:40–45.

Children with spastic hemiplegia secondary to CP show disrupted patterns of work and power in gait. EMG biofeedback treatment of the triceps surae muscle activity during gait was compared with physical therapy (PT) in a two-period crossover design, with intervening gait analyses to assess treatment. In contrast to the PT, the biofeedback treatment improved gait symmetry and was associated with greater ankle power for push-off, as well as increases in total positive work at the hip and ankle. It is concluded that the feedback protocol might be an effective adjunct to PT in hemiplegic children.

Hazlewood ME, Brown JK, Rowe PJ, et al: The use of therapeutic electrical stimulation in the treatment of hemiplegic cerebral palsy. *Dev Med Child Neurol* 1994;36: 661–673.

The effect of electrical stimulation of the anterior tibial muscles of children with hemiplegic CP was studied. The results showed a significant increase in passive range of motion among the children receiving electrical stimulation. Gait analysis of the knee and ankle motion showed little change.

Hills AP, Parker AW: Gait characteristics in obese children. *Arch Phys Med Rehabil* 1991;72:403–407.

The gait patterns of ten obese and ten normal-weight, prepubertal children were evaluated to provide objective data for a weight status comparison. Obese subjects displayed longer cycle duration, lower cadence, lower relative velocity, and longer stance period than normal weight subjects at all speeds ($p <$ 0.001).

Hoffinger SA, Rab GT, Abou-Ghaida H: Hamstrings in cerebral palsy crouch gait. *J Pediatr Orthop* 1993;13: 722–726.

After observing CP patients with increased anterior pelvic tilt following medial hamstring lengthening, the functional importance of the hamstrings as hip extensors was investigated. EMG analysis showed concentric hamstring contraction in 12 of 16 patients, thus aiding hip extension. Hamstrings may be important hip extensors in some CP patients with crouch gait; however, other deformities contributing to crouch (such as hip flexure contracture) need to be considered before isolated hamstring lengthening is performed in these patients.

Perry J: Determinants of muscle function in the spastic lower extremity. *Clin Orthop* 1993;288:10–26.

The upper motor neuron lesion that causes hemiplegia impairs the patient's selective control and exposes primitive modes of muscle activation. Dynamic EMG revealed the primitive mechanisms leading to these inconsistencies. Using knee flexion to differentiate gastrocnemius and soleus spasticity is not reliable, because the change in neurologic input with flexion may inhibit the extensor muscle's response to stretch so that the soleus is also relaxed.

Sports Medicine

Andriacchi TP, Birac D: Functional testing in the anterior cruciate ligament-deficient knee. *Clin Orthop* 1993;288: 40–47.

Functional testing during stressful activities indicated that some patients with ACL-deficient knees have higher than normal net hamstring moments during the early phase of these activities. Activities included walking, stair climbing, and jogging; patients were tested using gait analysis.

Bobbert MF, Yeadon MR, Nigg BM: Mechanical analysis of the landing phase in heel-toe running. *J Biomech* 1992; 25:223–234.

This study suggests that the three trained heel-toe runners investigated had no opportunity to control the rotations of body segments during the first part of the contact phase, other than by selecting a certain geometry of the body and muscular (co-)activation levels prior to touch-down.

Czerniecki JM, Gitter A: Insights into amputee running: A muscle work analysis. *Am J Phys Med Rehabil* 1992; 71:209–218.

The major compensatory patterns that allow below-knee amputees to run appear to be an increase in stance phase hip muscle work on the prosthetic limb and increased hip and knee muscle work on the intact limb during swing phase.

Devita P, Hunter PB, Skelly WA: Effects of a functional knee brace on the biomechanics of running. *Med Sci Sports Exerc* 1992;24:797–806.

This study assessed the biomechanical effects of a functional knee brace on joint moments and joint powers in the lower limb during the stance phase of running in subjects with a previous ACL injury. The reduction in the extensor moment about the hip and ankle in the previously injured subjects reduced the stresses on the ACL and tibia while at the same time enabling the subjects to run at the required speed.

Lehmann JF, Price R, Boswell-Bessette S, et al: Comprehensive analysis of energy storing prosthetic feet: Flex foot and Seattle foot versus standard SACH foot. *Arch Phys Med Rehabil* 1993;74:1225–1231.

This study compared the mechanical and biomechanical functions, metabolic demand, and shock absorption of two dynamic elastic response (DER) prosthetic foot designs with those of the SACH foot. Because no energy savings resulted for the DER feet, the release of stored energy in the flexible feet may not occur at the proper time to assist in ambulation as a result of the natural frequency of oscillation.

McCulloch MU, Brunt D, Vander Linden D: The effect of foot orthotics and gait velocity on lower limb kinematics and temporal events of stance. *J Orthop Sports Phys Ther* 1993;17:2–10.

In this study, motion analysis was used to investigate the use of foot orthotics to control the mechanics of the foot in ten subjects during walking. The orthotic was found to decrease the degree of pronation during stance.

Messier SP, Davis SE, Curl WW, et al: Etiologic factors associated with patellofemoral pain in runners. *Med Sci Sports Exerc* 1991;23:1008–1015.

Runners afflicted with patellofemoral pain (PFP) and unaffected runners were investigated to determine whether relationships between PFP and anthropometric, biomechanical, muscular strength, and endurance variables exist. The results suggest that Q angle is a strong discriminator. In addition, several muscular endurance and kinetic variables may also be important components in the etiology of PFP.

Noyes FR, Schipplein OD, Andriacchi TP, et al: The anterior cruciate ligament-deficient knee with varus alignment: An analysis of gait adaptations and dynamic joint loadings. *Am J Sports Med* 1992;20:707–716.

Thirty-two patients with an ACL-deficient knee and lower limb varus alignment and 16 healthy controls were analyzed during level walking using a force-platform and optoelectric system. The results show a likelihood of separation of the lateral tibiofemoral joint and condylar lift-off during periods of the stance phase. They also show increased net hamstring muscle activity.

Nyland JA, Shapiro R, Stine RL, et al: Relationship of fatigued run and rapid stop to ground reaction forces, lower extremity kinematics, and muscle activation. *J Orthop Sports Phys Therap* 1994;20:132–137.

The effect of lower extremity fatigue on ground reaction force production, lower extremity kinematics, and muscle activation during the landing phase of a run and rapid stop was investigated. Step-wise multiple regression suggested that the knee may be the primary site of force attenuation following fatigue.

Joint Arthroscopy/Osteoarthritis

Andriacchi TP: Dynamics of knee malalignment. *Orthop Clin North Am* 1994;25:395–403.

The dynamics of malalignment are based on the combination of static limb alignment and the dynamics of loading at the knee during walking and other activities of daily living. The loads that are generated during dynamic activities are substantially greater than the loads during static postures. Therefore, loading at the knee is an important consideration in progression of degenerative processes. Dynamic malalignment that occurs during activities such as walking should be considered in evaluating the progression of disease processes as well as the selection of appropriate treatment modalities.

Bergmann G, Graichen F, Rohlmann A: Hip joint loading during walking and running, measured in two patients. *J Biomech* 1993;26:969–990.

The resultant hip joint force, its orientation, and the moments were measured in two patients during walking and running using telemetering total hip prostheses. The joint loading was observed over the first 30 and 18 months, respectively, following implantation. In the first patient, the median peak forces increased with the walking speed from about 280% of the patient's body weight (BW) at 1 km/h to approximately 480% BW at 5 km/h. Jogging and very fast walking both raised the forces to about 550% BW; stumbling on one occasion caused magnitudes of 720% BW. In the second patient median forces at

3 km/h were about 410% BW, and a force of 870% BW was observed during stumbling.

Brand RA, Pedersen DR, Davy DT, et al: Comparison of hip force calculations and measurements in the same patient. *J Arthroplasty* 1994;9:45–51.

The authors compared mathematical estimates derived from gait laboratory observations made in a patient with an instrumented hip implant. Past models, with appropriate modifications, resulted in force predictions similar to the output of the instrumented implant. The study suggests that previous parametric hip-force predictions resulting from mathematically modeled surgical alterations may be high insofar as absolute peak values are concerned, but that trends are likely correct.

Goh JC, Bose K, Khoo BC: Gait analysis study on patients with varus osteoarthrosis of the knee. *Clin Orthop* 1993;294:223–231.

Thirty-seven knees with varus osteoarthritis were evaluated; 21 were analyzed before and after surgery (average follow-up evaluation: 2 years). Analysis based on moments about the knee showed that 57% of the surgically treated knees with good or excellent clinical results had abnormal load distribution. The abnormal loading was also reflected in the ground reaction force vector diagram. Therefore, the force vector diagram can be used as a quick screening method to detect abnormal joint loading.

Long WT, Dorr LD, Healy B, et al: Functional recovery of noncemented total hip arthroplasty. *Clin Orthop* 1993; 288:73–77.

In 18 total hip arthroplasty patients, EMG and gait analysis patterns were examined preoperatively and up to 2 years postoperatively. This study supports the prohibition of activities that cause high impact loading of total hip arthroplasties and suggests that a prolonged exercise program be used postoperatively.

Messier SP, Loeser RF, Hoover JL, et al: Osteoarthritis of the knee: Effects on gait, strength, and flexibility. *Arch Phys Med Rehabil* 1992;73:29–36.

The results suggest that patients with symptomatic osteoarthritis of the knee have poorer flexibility, increased loading rate, reduced knee range of motion, and are significantly weaker in both legs than unaffected controls.

Schnitzer TJ, Popovich JM, Andersson GB, et al: Effect of piroxicam on gait in patients with osteoarthritis of the knee. *Arthritis Rheum* 1993;36:1207–1213.

Nonsteroidal anti-inflammatory drug treatment in patients with knee osteoarthritis results in a reduction in symptomatic pain and an increase in loading of the knee. Whether the increased loading is due to the analgesic effects of the treatment is unknown, but if so, the development of agents capable of relieving pain while reducing loads at the knee may be desirable.

Amputees

Schneider K, Hart T, Zernicke RF, et al: Dynamics of below-knee child amputee gait: SACH foot versus Flex foot. *J Biomech* 1993;26:1191–1204.

Gait kinematics and dynamics during stance of 12 unilateral, below the knee child amputees were analyzed for the SACH foot and the energy-storing Flex-foot prostheses. This study uses moments and powers to assess energy return. The Flex-foot had a greater potential for reducing the energy cost of walking for the below-knee amputee.

Colborne GR, Naumann S, Longmuir PE, et al: Analysis of mechanical and metabolic factors in the gait of congenital below knee amputees: A comparison of the SACH and Seattle feet. *Am J Phys Med Rehabil* 1992:71: 272–278.

The metabolic test consisted of an 8-min walk around an oval track while expired gases were collected and analyzed. The Seattle foot produced a small increase in stride length, but the overall profile of work was unaffected by the type of foot.

Lemaire ED, Fisher FR: Osteoarthritis and elderly amputee gait. *Arch Phys Rehabil* 1994;75:1094–1099.

A group of transtibial amputees were found to have a significantly higher incidence of osteoarthritis (OA), higher joint impulses, and joint powers that support the hypothesis that these patients have a higher risk of developing OA and experience larger forces at the knee of their nonamputated limb than people without lower extremity amputations.

Basic Concepts

Holzreiter SH, Kohle ME: Assessment of gait patterns using neural networks. *J Biomech* 1993;26:645–651.

A new approach using neural network techniques in gait analysis for the assessment of gait patterns as healthy and pathological is presented.

Livingston LA, Stevenson JM, Olney SJ: Stairclimbing kinematics on stairs of differing dimensions. *Arch Phys Med Rehabil* 1991;72:398–402.

Fifteen women were divided into short, medium, and tall subject groups. Three testing staircases of different riser and tread dimensions were used. Measures of stairclimbing gait cycle duration, swing and stance phase durations, cadence, and velocity appeared to be systematically related to subject height. Individuals appeared to adjust to stair dimensions by varying the flexion–extension patterns of the knee rather than those of the ankle or hip.

Balance: Aging

Hurmuzlu Y, Basdogan C: On the measurement of dynamic stability of human locomotion. *J Biomech Eng* 1994;116:30–36.

The main focus of this investigation was the development of quantitative measures to assess the dynamic stability of human locomotion. The analytical methodology is based on Floquet theory. A stability index based on kinematic data at four instants of the gait cycle was determined as a quantitative measure of dynamic stability.

Winter DA, MacKinnon CD, Ruder GK, et al: An integrated EMG/biomechanical model of upper body balance and posture during human gait. *Prog Brain Res* 1993;97:359–367.

This study developed an inverted pendulum model of upper body balance in both the plane of progression and the frontal plane, and a medial/lateral (M/L) balance model of the total body. Moment and EMG results demonstrated (1) the hip extensor–flexors have an overpowering role in maintaining dynamic balance of the upper body in the plane of progression; (2) the hip abductors are dominant in countering large M/L imbalance of the upper body during single leg support, although assisted by medial acceleration of the hip joint; and (3) the total body M/L balance is achieved by the M/L placement of the foot.

Trauma/Stroke

Olney SJ, Griffin MP, McBride ID: Temporal, kinematic, and kinetic variables related to gait speed in subjects with hemiplegia: A regression approach. *Phys Therap* 1994;74: 872–885.

The gait speed that a patient selects is an indicator of overall gait performance. This study used multiple linear regression to assess the association of temporal, kinematic, and kinetic gait variables with high walking speed in 32 patients with hemiplegia. These results suggest the need for experimental studies to assess effects of treatment aimed at increasing ankle power, hip power, and decreased stance time on the affected side, while obtaining a larger hip flexion moment and larger ankle moment range on the unaffected side.

Miyazaki S, Yamamoto S, Ebina M, et al: A system for the continuous measurement of ankle joint moment in hemiplegic patients wearing ankle-foot orthoses. *Front Med Biol Eng* 1993:5:215–232.

In this paper, a measuring system was developed to assess the effect of dorsi–plantar flexibility of a plastic ankle-foot orthoses (PAFO) on the patient's gait.

Waters RL, Yakura JS, Adkins RH: Gait performance after spinal cord injury. *Clin Orthop* 1993;288:87–96.

Physiologic and mechanical gait parameters were measured in 36 spinal cord injury patients to quantify gait impairment. Compared with able-bodied subjects tested in the same laboratory, the patients walked 52% slower, the rate of oxygen consumption was 23% higher, and the oxygen cost per meter was 240% higher.

Foot and Ankle

McBride ID, Wyss UP, Cooke TD, et al: First metatarsophalangeal joint reaction forces during high-heel gait. *Foot Ankle* 1991;11:282–288.

First metatarsophalangeal joint and metatarsal–sesamoid reaction forces were calculated for 11 normal females during the toe-off phase of gait while walking in bare feet and in high heeled shoes. The results showed these forces to be twice as large in high heels compared to barefoot walking.

Mueller MJ, Minor SD, Sahrmann SA, et al: Differences in the gait characteristics of patients with diabetes and peripheral neuropathy compared with age-matched controls. *Phys Therap* 1994;74:299–308.

This study compares (1) the gait characteristics, (2) the plantarflexor peak torques, and (3) the ankle range of motion of subjects with diabetes mellitus and peripheral neuropathy with those of age-matched controls. The diabetes subjects appeared to pull their legs forward using hip flexor muscles (hip strategy) rather than pushing the legs forward using the plantarflexor muscles (ankle strategy), as seen in the normal group. Implications for treatment are presented to attempt to reduce the number of injuries during walking in patients with diabetes and peripheral neuropathy.

Scott SH, Winter DA: Talocrural and talocalcaneal joint kinematics and kinetics during the stance phase of walking. *J Biomech* 1991;24:743–752.

The talocrural and talocalcaneal joints were each assumed to act as monocentric single degree of freedom hinge joints during the gait of three subjects. The talocrural joint moment was qualitatively similar to the commonly measured sagittal plane moment, but the present results show that the sagittal plane moment overpredicted the true moment by 6% to 22% due to the two-dimensional assumption.

Classic Bibliography

Andriacchi TP, Galante JO, Fermier RW: The influence of total-knee replacement design on walking and stairclimbing. *J Bone Joint Surg* 1982;64A:1328–1335.

Berman AT, Quinn RH, Zarro VJ: Quantitative gait analysis in unilateral and bilateral total hip replacements. *Arch Phys Med Rehabil* 1991;72:190–194.

Dillingham TR, Lehmann JF, Price R: Effect of lower limb on body propulsion. *Arch Phys Med Rehabil* 1992:73:647–651.

Gage JR: An overview of normal walking, in Greene WB (ed): *Instructional Course Lectures XXXVII.* Park Ridge, IL, American Academy of Orthopaedic Surgeons, 1990, pp 291–303.

Inman VT, Ralston HJ, Todd F: *Human Walking.* Baltimore, MD, Williams & Wilkins, 1981.

Jarnlo GB, Thorngren KG: Standing balance in hip fracture patients: 20 middle-aged patients compared with 20 healthy subjects. *Acta Orthop Scand* 1991;62:427–434.

Morrison JB: The mechanics of the knee joint in relation to normal walking. *J Biomech* 1970;3:51–61.

Paul JP, McGrouther DA: Forces transmitted at the hip and knee joint of normal and disabled persons during a range of activities. *Acta Orthop Belg* 1975;41;(suppl 1) 78–88.

Prodromos CC, Andriacchi TP, Galante JO: A relationship between gait and clinical changes following high tibial osteotomy. *J Bone Joint Surg* 1985;67A: 1188–1194.

Radin EL, Yang KH, Riegger C, et al: Relationship between lower limb dynamics and knee joint pain. *J Orthop Res* 1991;9:398–405.

Zangemeister WH, Bulgheroni MV, Pedotti A: Normal gait is differentially influenced by the otoliths. *J Biomed Eng* 1991;13:451–458.

4

Biomaterials

This section will highlight the latest trends in orthopaedic biomaterials and implant processing. New materials will be presented, followed by an update on older materials and implant surface treatments.

New Materials

Metals

Although the currently used metals, 316L stainless steel and titanium and cobalt-chromium alloys, are the materials of choice for most orthopaedic devices, several new alloys have been proposed for hip stems and trauma devices. A Ti-13Zr-13Nb alloy has been shown to have a lower modulus and higher strength than the Ti-6Al-4V alloy currently used, and it addresses the concerns that trace amounts of corrosion products, such as aluminum and vanadium, can interfere with bone growth and healing. High-strength stainless steels, such as 23Cr-13Ni-5Mo stainless steel, have been suggested for use instead of the traditional 316L in weightbearing applications, such as hip stems and femoral fracture fixation devices. These new stainless steel alloys demonstrate approximately 25% greater strength and similar corrosion resistance. However, improved manufacturing techniques, such as cold forging and forming, have been shown to produce equivalent strengths in 316L stainless steel.

Nitinol (~55Ni-45Ti) is currently used for suture fixation devices. Although this is the "metal with a memory" (returns to initial shape after heating to a temperature that depends on specific alloy composition), current applications make use of its high elastic modulus (springiness). Applications suggested for nitinol include mechanisms that can lock a prosthesis in place (by taking advantage of the material's expansion at body temperature) and spinal rods that can be externally heated by radio frequency (RF) power to achieve a gradual correction of curvature for treatment of scoliosis.

Ceramics

The use of partially and completely resorbable calcium phosphate cements has been proposed to address some of the shortcomings of acrylic cements. Some of these new cements harden in a manner analogous to plaster of paris; others incorporate a polyacrylic acid similar to glassionomer dental cements. They use an aqueous base and do not give off appreciable heat during hardening; therefore, they should minimize adverse biologic response. The major problem with these new cements is achieving adequate mechanical tensile strength for weightbearing applications. The most promising current applications are for filling of osseous defects and consolidation of fracture fragments. Clinical studies are in progress for their use in the treatment of Colles' fractures.

Hydroxyapatite ceramic is being used as a bone graft substitute or extender in a variety of clinical settings, including tumors, trauma, spinal fusion, and repair of autologous bone graft sites. It can be used as granules combined with autograft, biodegradable polymers, or ceramics or as a structural block graft (usually porous). In one study of 60 benign bone tumors treated by currettage and implantation of block calcium hydroxyapatite ceramic, the ceramic was found to become well incorporated in almost all cases; late biopsies in several cases showed significant bone ingrowth into the ceramic pore structure.

Polymers

One rapidly expanding area of research and clinical application in orthopaedic biomaterials is the use of biodegradable polymers. Materials such as polylactic acid polymers (PLA), polyglycolic acid polymers (PGA), polycaprolactate, and various polypeptides have been extensively studied in animal experiments. These polymers are based on repeat units of naturally occurring proteins or carbohydrates that revert when the polymer is broken down in the body by enzymatic or hydrolytic processes (Fig. 1). PLA-PGA copolymers have been clinically used for low-demand fracture fixation devices (eg, malleolar screws and Kirschner wires). In one prospective, randomized clinical study, PLA malleolar screws were seen to be clinically equivalent to stainless steel screws in the surgical treatment of displaced medial malleolar ankle fractures; however, approximately 30% demonstrated late tenderness over the implant and some showed cyst formation on radiographic examination. In another clinical trial, PLA-PGA copolymer rods were as clinically effective as stainless steel Kirschner wires (K-wires) when used as intramedullary implants in the surgical treatment of hand fractures.

Concern has recently been expressed over this application of PLA because low-molecular-weight fragments that result from hydrolytic degradation decrease local pH. Some clinical results have shown pain and cyst formation at approximately 1 year. Biodegradable implants containing PGA have been seen to produce surrounding osteolysis in 50% of adults and 14% of children treated. Subcutaneous inflammatory foreign-body reactions with sterile discharging sinuses have been noted in up to 25% of adults.

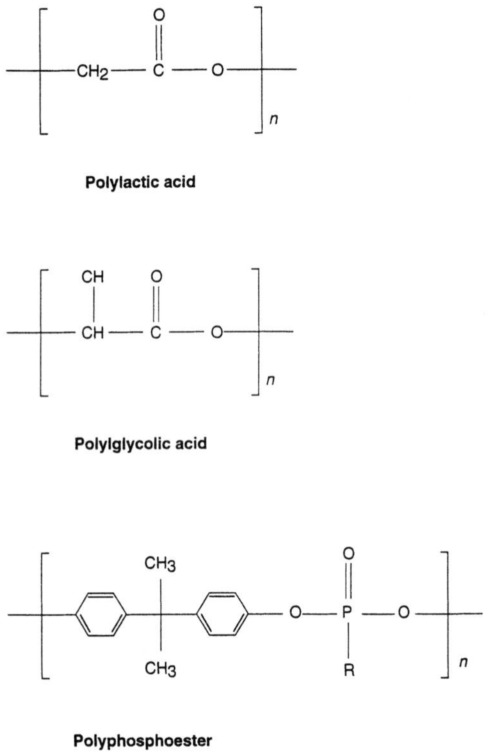

Fig. 1 Types of biodegradable polymers.

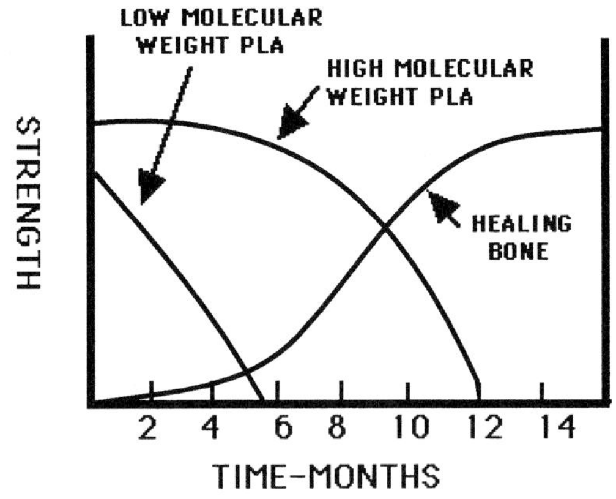

Fig. 2 Schematic representation of polylactic acid degradation showing that the effects of molecular weight on the loss of polymer strength are ideally balanced by an increase in the strength of healing bone.

Most of these biodegradable polymers lack sufficient strength for weightbearing applications; consequently, reinforcement with glass or carbon fibers (composites) and increased device thickness have been proposed as solutions. However, there have been problems with toxicity and migration of the reinforcing components. Processing techniques, such as extrusion, which can orient the polymer chains, can also increase strength and stiffness. Ideally, the biodegradable material should have sufficient strength to stabilize the fracture or osteotomy during healing, degrade quickly enough to prevent stress shielding, and eventually completely disappear without untoward effects (Fig. 2).

Another potential use of these biodegradable polymers is as carriers of antibiotics and growth factors to achieve a controlled localized release. By controlling the types and characteristics of the polymers used and the method of incorporation, it is theoretically possible to construct a carrier that releases several substances at different specified times and/or rates. Such a carrier would be a potential system for release of various growth factors for optimal effect. Polymer carriers have already been experimentally used in bulk form for filling of osseous defects and as coatings on metallic implants. One particular application of interest is the use of PLA or other polymer coatings containing antibiotics and/or silver compounds on cementless prostheses for use in infected patients.

Composites of biopolymers (eg, purified collagen, PLA) and bioceramics (eg, hydroxyapatite), as well as hydroxyapatite alone, have been proposed as bone defect fillers. These materials have been used both in the powdered and bulk form and are free of some of the potential problems associated with allograft materials. Solid ceramic grafts tend to be brittle and take a long time to resorb and be replaced by bone; porous grafts are more readily resorbed but lack appreciable mechanical strength.

Ligaments consisting of a high-strength polymeric core, such as polyester, surrounded by a biodegradable polymer for tissue growth/replacement have been proposed. However, concern has been expressed over the long-term stability of these prostheses. Carbon fibers used for this application eventually fragment, with consequent production of significant particulate debris.

Biologically Derived Biomaterials

Because allografts are costly and carry a risk of disease and immunologic problems, another exciting area of research is the use of biologically derived biomaterials. Recently, artificial cartilage and menisci have been made from a patient's own cells grown in a biopolymer matrix (eg, collagen). Results of numerous animal experiments have suggested the promise of this technique. The report of a recent clinical study indicated a 75% success rate for healing cartilage defects in athletes using reinsertion of externally cultured chondrocytes.

Other potential biomaterials have been derived from biologic sources. Coral has been calcined and used as a porous calcium phosphate substrate for bone repair applications. Glues derived from mussel attachment fibers have been proposed for repair of fractures and meniscal tears. Chitosan (from crustacean shells) has been evaluated for use in sutures and as a substrate for soft-tissue regeneration; purified collagen has been tested for similar applications.

Current Materials: New Data

Metals

Clinical results of using porous metallic surfaces for implant fixation remain mixed. Analyses of retrieved implants indicate that bone ingrowth is never complete and that it occurs primarily in specific locations; 60% to 80% of ingrowth occurs in the acetabular region versus 20% to 40% in the femoral stem and around the pegs in tibial trays. Removal of these devices continues to be a problem. There is also concern that the significantly higher surface area of these devices leads to a greater total release of metallic ions, which leads to problems with metal sensitivity.

Titanium-based metals have become the materials of choice for cervical spinal instrumentation, mainly because they allow improved postoperative magnetic resonance imaging (MRI) of the neural structures with much less artifact than do stainless steel implants. The lower failure strength of titanium wire as compared to 316L stainless steel remains a problem, although braided titanium cables are now available. For the thoracolumbar spine, stainless steel implants remain more common, although full titanium instrumentation is available for most systems and is standard for at least one system.

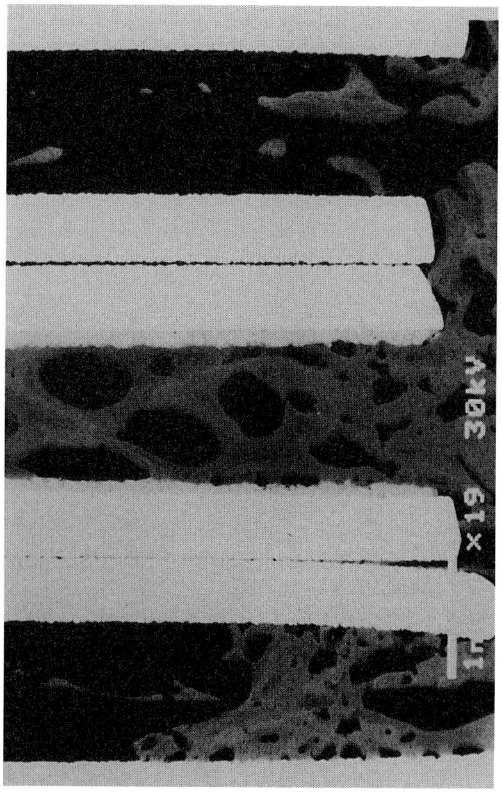

Fig. 3 Bone ingrowth into a multiple-chambered canine medullary implant. The top chamber is Ti-6Al-4V alloy with a smooth surface; bottom chamber is the alloy coated with hydroxyapatite of the same surface roughness.

Ceramics

Clinical data reveal that the use of a ceramic (Al_2O_3) head articulating against polyethylene results in lower wear of the acetabular component than does use of a metal head. Several long-term studies from Sweden have demonstrated approximately 50% less volumetric wear of the polyethylene. Laboratory experiments have demonstrated that zirconia (Th- or Y-dispersed) femoral heads, currently offered by several implant manufacturers, exhibit wear resistance and mechanical properties superior to those of alumina heads because the zirconia has a finer grain size.

Clinical series of alumina–alumina articulating surfaces in total hip arthroplasties have yielded excellent results, with few failures related to wear or to loosening due to wear debris. However, ceramic–ceramic articulations have exhibited severe wear where improper device placement leads to high surface stresses. The ceramic is brittle and prone to local fragmentation of the alumina, which results in third-body wear.

Although hydroxyapatite coatings to enhance initial device stabilization by bone ingrowth continue to be used clinically, some questions as to their long-term stability have arisen as a result of coating delamination and/or osteoclastic resorption (Fig. 3). Data from a canine transcortical plug pushout study have confirmed the superior shear strength of a 50-μm thick coating when compared to a 200-μm coating. However, it has been argued that the implant will remain stable if the coating is resorbed but not if the coating delaminates. Less biologically stable ceramics, such as tricalcium phosphate coatings, have been used to enhance initial bone ingrowth.

Both hydroxyapatite and tricalcium phosphate coatings have been applied to porous metallic implants to enhance bone ingrowth and initial fixation. In one study in rabbits, use of both ceramic coatings resulted in improved implant perimeter bone contact and a higher amount of bone ingrown into the implant pores.

Polymers

There have been increasing concerns that the presence of polyethylene wear debris leads to implant loosening because localized inflammatory processes, which result from the debris, cause bone resorption. Recent studies have shown that there is significant variation in polyethylene quality (molecular weight, inclusions, defects) and that this variation is directly associated with clinical wear behavior. The current use of gamma irradiation for sterilization appears to promote deterioration of the mechanical properties of polyethylene because of continued internal oxidation of the free radicals created during irradiation. As a result, some manufacturers use ethylene oxide for sterilization. A new (extended-chain) polyethylene that has recently been clinically introduced is processed by a treatment of heat and pressure; laboratory tests indicate it has somewhat improved mechanical properties and wear resistance. There is some concern that the increased stiffness can lead to higher subsurface stresses in the polyethylene, and there is no evidence that its clinical wear performance has been enhanced.

In one study of retrieved tibial components in total and unicompartmental knee revisions, 51% of the components were found to have undergone severe wear, which was associated with thin polyethylene, third-body wear, lack of congruency, and the use of heat-pressed material. Delamination was particularly evident in the load-bearing regions of thin polyethylene components. These components also exhibited undersurface cold flow above screw holes in the underlying metal tray. Based on these findings, a minimal tibial tray thickness of 6 mm (8 mm over screw holes) was suggested. For metal-backed modular acetabular components, screw holes have been minimized, and some designs use plugs or pegs instead of screws to minimize the problem of particulate migration or generation. Also, internal metal surfaces have been polished to minimize wear.

Bone Cements

Mechanical mixing techniques, such as vibration, result in improved mechanical properties (compressive strength, shear strength, and modulus of elasticity) when compared to manual mixing techniques. Centrifugation improves static mechanical strength of bone cement when compared to hand mixing but has no significant effect on low-cycle fatigue strength.

Chemical modifications, such as the use of butyl methacrylate, decrease the brittleness of methylmethacrylate and improve resistance to fatigue crack propagation. Additions of water or various low-molecular-weight polyethylenes can reduce the polymerization temperature of methylmethacrylate but deleteriously affect its mechanical properties. Reinforced cement composites formed by the addition of metal, polymer, or ceramic fibers have been shown to increase mechanical properties, particularly fatigue strength. Unfortunately, they increase the viscosity of the cement, thereby creating difficulties in filling and in the penetration of the cement into bone.

Bioceramics such as hydroxyapatite particles and bone chips have been added to cement to improve biocompatibility and promote bone approximation and fixation. However, because these additions are coated by the cement during mixing, their utility appears minimal.

Up to 5 wt% powdered antibiotics can be added to cement without significantly decreasing its mechanical properties and have been shown to deliver effective minimum lethal doses for up to 2 weeks. In one clinical study, tobramycin was shown to sustain adequate local-tissue levels when used in bone cement in total hip arthroplasty, whereas vancomycin exhibited variable elution properties and was otherwise unpredictable as a bone cement additive. Acrylic cement impregnated with methotrexate (MTX) has been studied experimentally in vivo using a rabbit tumor model. The release kinetics resulted in nontoxic systemic MTX levels, and the use of MTX-loaded cement resulted in fewer pulmonary metastases and delayed their onset. In another study of cytotoxic drug release from a series of acrylic cements, it was found that a significantly higher percentage of MTX was released than of either cis-platinum or 5-fluorouracil and that the amount of drug released differed between cements.

Surface Processing

The problem of particulate debris, which was either shed from implant surfaces due to micromotion or resulted from wear, has attracted increased interest. Roughening of metallic implant surfaces by particulate material, such as alumina abrasives during the manufacturing process to facilitate bone attachment has recently been shown to create surface contamination and, thus, to create another concern about debris if these particles are dislodged (Fig. 4).

Another problem of surface roughening is the increased shedding of metallic particles resulting from micromotion of the device against the adjacent bone. To avoid this problem, some manufacturers have returned to highly polished surfaces and have hardened them with a nitriding process. Other manufacturers have hardened the metallic aspects of articulating surfaces by a similar process of nitrogen implantation. Laboratory data for these hardened surfaces show less wear and lower production of metallic and poly-

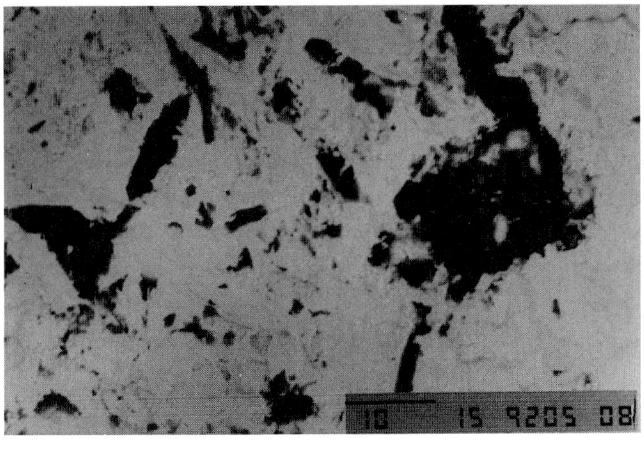

Fig. 4 Roughened titanium alloy implant surface; dark gray regions (25% of total area) are alumina beads impacted into the surface during manufacture of the implant.

meric particulates. The use of experimental coatings of ceramics and carbon on metal to reduce wear is also being investigated. Data showing reduced wear of metal-on-metal articulations have recently been introduced, and initial clinical studies are in progress. Both chemical modification (coatings of prepolymerized methacrylate) and macroscopic surface structuring have been clinically used to improve fixation of bone cement to prosthesis surfaces and enhance load transmission from the implant to the cement.

Modularity

Concern about modular devices has recently increased as a result of findings from examinations of removed implants. Although modularity enables the surgeon to achieve optimal fit intraoperatively and minimizes device inventory, factors such as corrosion (galvanic or crevice) at the interfaces, which results in release of metallic ions, and/or micromotion, which leads to increased debris production, have been clinically demonstrated and have been the subject of numerous laboratory studies. Many manufacturers have responded by narrowing the tolerances of the modular fit to minimize the possibility of creating a crevice between the components, by developing better locking methods, and by improving instrumentation for component assembly prior to implantation. It is critical that the surgeon ensure that the junctions are clean and dry before assembly.

Annotated Bibliography

Metals

Maurer AM, Brown SA, Payer JH, et al: Reduction of fretting corrosion of Ti-6Al-4V by various surface treatments. *J Orthop Res* 1993;11:865–873.

Nitriding and implantation of nitrogen ions into Ti-6Al-4V alloy appreciably increases surface hardness and decreases fretting; corrrosion resistance is not affected.

Rupp R, Ebraheim NA, Savolaine ER, et al: Magnetic resonance imaging evaluation of the spine with metal implants: General safety and superior imaging with titanium. *Spine* 1993;18:379–385.

Titanium spinal implants provide greater MRI with fewer artifacts than stainless steel implants. Both alloys do not show migration or heating due to MRI.

Polymers

Brien WW, Salvati EA, Klein R, et al: Antibiotic impregnated bone cement in total hip arthroplasty: An in vivo comparison of the elution properties of tobramycin and vancomycin. *Clin Orthop* 1993;296:242–248.

Tobramycin elutes from bone cement in patients to provide adequate local tissue levels; vancomycin demonstrated variable elution properties.

Bucholz RW, Henry S, Henley MB: Fixation with bioabsorbable screws for the treatment of fractures of the ankle. *J Bone Joint Surg* 1994;76A:319–324.

Oriented polylactide screws demonstrated no radiographic or functional differences compared to stainless steel when used for medial malleolar fracture fixation in 155 prospectively randomized patients. No adverse effects of the polymer, such as tenderness or drainage, were noted.

Kumta SM, Spinner R, Leung PC: Absorbable intramedullary implants for hand fractures: Animal experiments and clinical trial. *J Bone Joint Surg* 1992; 74B:563–566.

Polyglycolide rods were compared to K-wires for intramedullary fixation of extra-articular hand fractures in 30 patients. No differences were seen radiographically or functionally; no allergic reactions to the polymer were noted.

Lehman WB, Strongwater AB, Tunc D, et al: Internal fixation with biodegradable plate and screws in dogs. *J Pediatr Orthop* 1994;3:190–193.

High molecular weight polylactide plates and screws have sufficient strength weightbearing for implants; they completely degrade in 2 years with minimal tissue response.

Ceramics

Saito M, Saito S, Ohzono K, et al: Efficacy of alumina ceramic heads for cemented total hip arthroplasty. *Clin Orthop* 1992;283:171–177.

Alumina exhibits low clinical wear rates against ultra-high molecular weight polyethylene; movement of alumina against itself can occasionally lead to significant wear.

Hydroxyapatite

Collier JP, Surprenant VA, Mayor MB, et al: Loss of hydroxyapatite coating on retrieved, total hip components. *J Arthroplasty* 1993;8:389–393.

Various forms of hydroxyapatite are used on implants; depending on type and method of coating application, removed implants can exhibit coating dissolution or removal by osteoclastic activity.

Huracek J, Spirig P: The effect of hydroxyapatite coating on the fixation of hip prostheses: A comparison of clinical and radiographic results of hip replacement in a matched-pair study. *Arch Orthop Trauma Surg* 1994;113:72–77.

Bilateral Mecron total hip replacements having one side with and one without hydroxyapatite coating were implanted in 80 patients. The hydroxyapatite-coated prostheses demonstrated less pain and migration, fewer radiolucent lines, and significantly better 4-year clinical results.

Tisdel CL, Goldberg VM, Parr JA, et al: The influence of a hydroxyapatite and tricalcium-phosphate coating on bone growth into titanium fiber-metal implants. *J Bone Joint Surg* 1994;76A:159–171.

A combined hydroxyapatite and tricalcium phosphate coating on porous implants promotes greater and more rapid bone infiltration in porous surfaced implants and provides better initial fixation and long-term results.

Wang BC, Lee TM, Chang E, et al: The shear strength and the failure mode of plasma-sprayed hydroxyapatite coating to bone: The effect of coating thickness. *J Biomed Mater Res* 1993;27:1315–1327.

Fifty- and 200-mm hydroxyapatite coatings on titanium alloy cylinders were implanted in canine femurs. The thinner coating was stronger during the 12 weeks evaluated; defects in the thicker coating reduced its strength.

Wear Debris

Shanbhag AS, Jacobs JJ, Glant TT, et al: Composition and morphology of wear debris in failed uncemented total hip replacement. *J Bone Joint Surg* 1994;76B:60–67.

Wear debris in the interfacial membranes from 11 failed uncemented total hip replacements was analyzed. Most particles were polyethylene of submicron size. Little debris was generated from the titanium stems.

Classic Bibliography

Feng EL, Stulberg SD, Wixson RL: Progressive subluxation and polyethylene wear in total knee replacements with flat articular surfaces. *Clin Orthop* 1994;299:60–71.

Iyoda K, Miura T, Nogami H: Repair of bone defect with cultured chondrocytes bound to hydroxyapatite. *Clin Orthop* 1993;288:287–293.

Jasty M, Rubash HE, Paiement GD, et al: Porous-coated uncemented components in experimental total hip arthroplasty in dogs: Effect of plasma-sprayed calcium phosphate coatings on bone ingrowth. *Clin Orthop* 1992;280:300–309.

Ji H, Marquis PM: Effect of heat treatment on the microstructure of plasma-sprayed hydroxyapatite coating. *Biomaterials* 1993;14:64–68.

Knowles JC, Hastings GW, Ohta H, et al: Development of a degradable composite for orthopaedic use: In vivo biomechanical and histological evaluation of two bioactive degradable composites based on the polyhydroxybutyrate polymer. *Biomaterials* 1992;13:491–496.

Korkusuz F, Uchida A, Shinto Y, et al: Experimental implant-related osteomyelitis treated by antibiotic-calcium hydroxyapatite ceramic composites. *J Bone Joint Surg* 1993;75B:111–114.

Lewis G: Effect of lithotriptor treatment on the fracture toughness of acrylic bone cement. *Biomaterials* 1992;13: 225–229.

Linden U: Mechanical properties of bone cement: Importance of the mixing technique. *Clin Orthop* 1991; 272:274–278.

Maistrelli GL, Mahomed N, Garbuz D, et al: Hydroxyapatite coating on carbon composite hip implants in dogs. *J Bone Joint Surg* 1992;74B:452–456.

Saito M, Maruoka A, Mori T, et al: Experimental studies on a new bioactive bone cement: Hydroxyapatite composite resin. *Biomaterials* 1994;15:156–160.

Soballe K, Hansen ES, Brockstedt-Rasmussen H, et al: Hydroxyapatite coating converts fibrous tissue to bone around loaded implants. *J Bone Joint Surg* 1993;75B: 270–278.

Tateishi H, Iwata Y, Futani H, et al: Clinical experience of ceramic cementless total knee arthroplasty in RA and a histological study of the bone-ceramic interface in revision cases. *Bull Hosp Jt Dis* 1993;53:35–40.

Uchida A, Shinto Y, Araki N, et al: Slow release of anticancer drugs from porous calcium hydroxyapatite ceramic. *J Orthop Res* 1992;10:440–445.

Wasserlauf S, Warshawsky A, Arad-Yelin R, et al: The release of cytotoxic drugs from acrylic bone cement. *Bull Hosp Jt Dis* 1993;53:68–74.

5

Blood Transfusions/HIV/Hepatitis

Blood Transfusions

A New "Transfusion Trigger"?

Orthopaedic surgeons have been at the forefront of minimizing homologous (allogeneic) transfusions. They have done so by accepting lower perioperative hemoglobin (Hb) and hematocrit (Hct) levels, as well as by using predonation and perioperative blood salvage. Although many patients have successfully undergone surgery as well as postoperative recovery and rehabilitation with Hb and Hct levels well below the "10/30 transfusion trigger" of the 1980s, the current intent is to enhance understanding of the physiologic basis for transfusion requirements rather than to define a new transfusion trigger.

The etiology and chronicity of the anemia, the ability to compensate for diminished oxygen-carrying capacity, the actual and anticipated blood loss, the baseline medical condition, and oxygen use by vital organs must be considered when determining the minimal acceptable Hb and Hct for a given patient. Transfusion is indicated to improve oxygen delivery. It is important that this requirement be differentiated from hypovolemia, because volume depletion can result in hypotension and complications unrelated to anemia. In fact, normovolemic anemia is well tolerated by many.

Oxygen delivery and tissue oxygen consumption are important determinants in considering red blood cell (RBC) transfusion requirements because inadequacies in either can lead to vital organ ischemia and complications, such as myocardial infarction or stroke. Oxygen delivery (Do_2) is a reflection of hemoglobin level, inspired oxygen concentration, arterial oxygen concentration (Cao_2), cardiac output (Qt), and pulmonary gas exchange. The equation that expresses this relationship is $Do_2 = Cao_2$ (Qt) where $Cao_2 = \%\ o_2$ saturation $\times$ (1.34 $\times$ Hb) + (0.0031 $\times$ Pao_2).

Whereas a young healthy patient can adequately compensate for lower arterial oxygen carrying capacity by increasing cardiac output, older patients, patients on beta-blockers, or patients with myocardial disease or pulmonary disease cannot adequately compensate and, thus, oxygen delivery decreases.

Adequate RBC oxygen content can be determined by considering how much oxygen is consumed at the tissue level and by determining how much oxygen is extracted from what is delivered. Normally, of the 1,000 ml of oxygen delivered per minute, 250 ml/min is consumed. This consumption results in a normal systemic extraction ratio (ER) of 25%, which leaves a reserve of 75%. Extraction ratios for different organs vary. For example, at normal Hb levels, the ER in the myocardium is so high (55%) that marked decreases in Hct may not be tolerated. Increases in overall systemic ERs to greater than 50% can be deleterious. Recent data demonstrate that when critical coronary artery stenosis exists, decreases in Hb concentrations may result in increases in systemic ER above 50%, thereby indicating marginal myocardial reserve.

Considering the above, when should a patient receive a transfusion? Transfusing patients with Hb levels of 10 g/dl often results in unnecessary transfusions. Unanswered questions include how low a Hb value is safe, is hemoglobin level itself an important indicator of outcome, and are orthopaedic surgeons pushing these lower limits in the desire to avoid a transfusion. Based on individual considerations, the range for considering a transfusion is probably between 6 and 10 g/dl in most individuals. In a study of patients who would not accept blood transfusions and who were undergoing surgery, mortality was 7% when Hb levels were > 10 g/dl and 62% when Hb levels were < 6 g/dl. Data generated by a Medline search involving such patients from 1970 to early 1993 demonstrated that except for three patients who died after cardiac surgery, all patients who died secondary to anemia had hemoglobin levels ≤ 5 g/dl. Data from other studies demonstrate that Hb levels of 6 to 8 g/dl are well tolerated. In 332 patients who underwent primary total hip replacement (THR), there was no correlation between Hb level at discharge, preoperative Hb, or decreases in Hb concentration and the number of days to discharge from the hospital. Discharge Hb levels ranged from 9 to 12 g/dl.

Low Hb and Hct levels are not without risk. In a study involving perioperative electrocardiographic monitoring of 27 high-risk patients undergoing infrainguinal arterial bypass, ten of 13 patients with Hct levels < 28% demonstrated postoperative myocardial ischemia, with six sustaining either a myocardial infarction, unstable angina, cardiac death, or ischemic pulmonary edema. Among the 14 patients with Hct levels > 28%, there were none of the more serious cardiac events, although two developed myocardial ischemia. There was a significant correlation between anemia on day one and both postoperative myocardial ischemia ($p = 0.001$) and morbid cardiac events ($p = 0.0058$). In a study of patients undergoing cardiac revascularization, those patients with postoperative Hb levels of 12.1 g/dl demonstrated better myocardial metabolism than patients with mean levels of 8.0 g/dl. In patients with coronary artery disease, there was a higher incidence of perioperative ischemia in those with left ventricular dysfunction at mean Hb levels of 9.6 g/dl than in patients with coronary artery disease who did not have left ventricular dysfunction.

In summary, when considering whether to transfuse, consider each patient's physiologic state, underlying medical condition, ability to compensate for diminished oxygen-carrying capacity, and oxygen requirements of vital organs, as well as actual and anticipated blood loss.

Adverse Effects of Homologous Transfusions

Fear of human immunodeficiency virus (HIV) transmission is now a major reason for many physicians and patients to avoid homologous transfusions. Although blood is tested for HIV prior to release for transfusion, reports exist, which document transmission of HIV to recipients from blood that tested negative. Transmission can occur because testing is performed for HIV-antibody, and a delay exists from the onset of infectivity and HIV antigenemia to the development of detectable antibody. This delay creates a critical time period, known as the window period, in which blood will test negative but be infectious. In a 1994 report, 39 HIV seropositive recipients were identified who received blood from 182 previously seronegative donors (now seropositive) whose donated blood tested seronegative at the time of donation. Analysis of both donor and recipient HIV seroconversions led to construction of a mathematical model, which demonstrated a window period averaging 45 days. A more recent study demonstrates that with newer assays the window period has narrowed to approximately 22 days. Newer diagnostic tests that can identify the actual virus rather than antibodies to it may decrease this window even further.

Additional concerns about administering transfusions include transmission of other viral (hepatitis, cytomegalovirus), bacterial, and parasitic infections; immuosuppression; increased incidence of postoperative infections; septicemia; allergic reactions; hemolytic transfusion reactions; fluid overload; and, in some cancer patients, an increased risk of recurrence, metastases, and decreased survival.

Homologous transfusions impair immunologic response. This immunosuppressive effect decreases the patient's ability to combat infections or, in the case of tumor patients, to fend off recurrence or metastatic disease. In a study of 155 patients who had nonmetastatic osteosarcoma treated with amputation and adjuvant chemotherapy, perioperative blood transfusion was associated with a significant decrease in disease-free state and decreased overall survival.

An increased incidence of postoperative infection (urinary, respiratory, fever of unknown origin, or surgical infection site) has been noted in THR patients who received homologous blood. Homologous blood transfusion was associated with a 32% rate of proven or suspected infection (16/50) compared with a 3% (1/34) incidence in patients receiving autologous blood ($p = 0.0029$).

In a review of 376 orthopaedic patients, significant predictors of postoperative infection included homologous whole blood transfusion, increasing age, spinal surgery, high admission Hct, and greater time in surgery. In another clinical and immunologic study of patients undergoing spine surgery, homologous blood transfusion was a significant predictor of in-hospital infection ($p = 0.016$), days on antibiotics, and length of stay.

In a recent study of 5,366 trauma patients, homologous blood transfusion was identified as an important independent statistical predictor of infection. A report detailing 484 acute injuries indicates a relationship between transfusion and infectious morbidity independent of other significant factors, such as Injury Severity Score, age, and surgical procedures. In another study, after adjustments for age, sex, and severity of injury, a higher incidence of infection was noted in 236 patients who survived at least 7 days after trauma and received seven or more units of blood.

Perioperative Techniques to Avoid Transfusion

Various methods, either individually or in combination, can be employed to avoid homologous transfusion. These methods include: (1) autologous predonation in which the patient predonates a number of units of blood at intervals starting as long as 4 to 6 weeks ahead of time; (2) acute normovolemic hemodilution (ANH) in which the patient has blood withdrawn just prior to incision and has his or her circulating blood volume replaced with crystalloid or colloid (Blood with a lower Hct is lost during the course of the operation, and at the conclusion of surgery, the blood that was withdrawn prior to incision, which has a high Hct, is reinfused into the patient.); (3) perioperative blood salvage by intraoperative use of a cell salvage device in which wound blood is salvaged, washed, and reinfused into the patient; and (4) salvage and postoperative reinfusion of blood that usually drained out into the wound and was discarded. Additional methods to conserve blood and avoid homologous transfusion include hypotensive anesthesia, surgical technique, proper patient positioning, and pharmacologic means to reduce bleeding.

Predonation Predonation appears to play a pivotal role, alone or when combined with other techniques, in preventing the need for homologous transfusions. Prior to donating, a healthy patient should have a hemoglobin level above 11 g/dl. Under appropriate monitoring, pregnant women, as well as patients undergoing cardiac and vascular surgery, can predonate. Patients with unstable angina or severe aortic stenosis are not considered candidates. The risks of preoperative autologous donations are not significantly different from those of regular blood bank homologous donations. The elderly have a lower incidence of reactions during predonation than younger patients. Patients can suffer vasovagal reactions; there is a 3% incidence of lightheadedness, a 0.3% incidence of transient loss of consciousness, and a 0.03% incidence of self-limited seizures. Patients at increased risk are first time donors, women, patients of low body weight, and a patient who has had a prior reaction. In a study comparing 10,200 patients who predonated with 219,307 concurrent homologous donors, there was no significant difference in severe, moderate, or mild reactions among the groups.

Currently, iron supplementation is frequently administered to patients when they predonate. Erythropoietin (EPO) may have a role in certain circumstances. EPO stimulates red-cell production and is available as recombinant human EPO. When patients who received iron and placebo were compared with those who received iron and EPO during predonation, the iron and EPO group was able to predonate more units of blood. Seven of the 24 patients in the placebo group were unable to predonate four or more units while only one in the EPO-iron group was not able to donate four or more units. Red cell mass was significantly higher in the patients who received EPO. It appears that if many units of predonated blood are required, there may be a role for EPO. Autologous predonation is associated with only a moderate rise in systemic EPO levels, and exogenous EPO or aggressive predonations are probably necessary if marked increases in EPO levels are needed.

Many patients requiring orthopaedic surgery, especially those coming in for scoliosis surgery, weigh less than 50 kg. According to many criteria, these patients cannot predonate full units of blood; however, partial units can be withdrawn. Algorithms exist for determining the amount that can be predonated based on body weight. In one study, over 100 patients were able to predonate two or more partial units and 63% of the patients were able to avoid homologous transfusion.

How much blood should be predonated? Generally, it has been found that patients undergoing total hip surgery should predonate two units. This, combined with other salvage techniques, such as cell salvage and wound drainage reinfusion, significantly decreased the risk of homologous transfusion in over 95% of patients. Spine patients at the Hospital for Joint Diseases commonly donate three or more units, especially for anterior and posterior procedures. In combination with blood salvage techniques, over 90% do not require homologous transfusion. Others have reported that predonation of three to eight units, with adequate initial Hb levels, will allow 95% of patients undergoing hip, knee, and spine surgery to avoid homologous transfusions.

Acute Normovolemic Hemodilution In this technique, blood is rapidly withdrawn from the patient while there is simultaneous replacement of colloid or crystalloid, thereby maintaining normovolemia as the Hct is diminished. This technique enables a patient to lose blood at a lower Hct intraoperatively and, at the conclusion of surgery, receive his or her own blood, which was obtained at preoperative Hct levels. For example, if a patient with an initial Hct of 45 is hemodiluted to a Hct of 25 and loses 1 liter of blood, the patient has lost 250 ml of RBC instead of 450 ml. Recent computer models demonstrate that under such circumstances, the actual difference in blood loss is slightly less than 200 ml. However, in addition to the actual RBC savings, the reinfused whole blood also contains fresh clotting factors and platelets. Decrease in arterial oxygen content is compensated for by increases in cardiac output, coronary blood flow, and oxygen extraction; shifting of the oxyhemoglobin dissociation curve to the right (canine model); and decreased viscosity. Experimental models demonstrate that compensatory mechanisms, such as increases in cardiac output and mean coronary flow, can persist for extended periods of hemodilution.

The need for coronary blood flow to increase substantially during ANH raises concern about its use in patients with coronary artery disease. Significant decreases in Hct in the presence of a stenosed left anterior descending (LAD) coronary artery result in regional myocardial dysfunction. Although earlier studies in canine models with stenosed LADs have demonstrated myocardial dysfunction at Hcts of 35%, more recent studies demonstrate myocardial preservation in some models at Hb levels of 7.5 g/dl. When contractile function deteriorated, it was restored with only slight increases in Hb level. This variability in deterioration of cardiac function from one canine model to another is probably true in humans as well. If coronary stenosis is not critical and ventricular function is good, patients with coronary artery disease may tolerate Hct levels of 25%. However, the surgeon must be aware of heart rate, ventricular function, severity of cardiac disease, and coronary stenosis. Multiple vessel cardiac disease will impair the patient's ability to compensate for ANH.

By use of the following formula the amount of autologous blood volume to be withdrawn can be determined.

$$\frac{EBV(Ho-Ht)}{(Ho+Ht)/2}$$

where EBV is the estimated blood volume of 70 ml/kg, Ho is the starting Hct, and Ht is the target Hct. For example, in a 25-kg female with a starting Hb of 12g (Hct = 36%) and a target Hb of 9g (Hct = 27%), the calculation would be:

$$\frac{1750\ (36-27)}{(36+27)/2} = 500\ \text{ml}$$

Blood donation bags prepared to collect 450 ml of blood are available. After the patient is anesthetized, blood is withdrawn by gravity drainage through an arterial line. While blood is withdrawn, the patient receives crystalloid or colloid replacement in a 3:1 or 2:1 ratio, respectively, to maintain normovolemia.

Intraoperative Cell Salvage In this technique, blood that is usually lost in the wound is collected and reinfused after it has been appropriately washed to remove debris and anticoagulant. Cell salvaging generally is avoided in situations in which there is infection or a malignancy at the site of the surgery, although it is used by some when performing tumor surgery. Cell salvage is not used for patients with sickle-cell disease. A heparinized solution to avoid clotting is added as the blood is collected in a reservoir.

The blood is then pumped into a centrifuging bowl. As the bowl spins, the supernatant waste, surgical debris, free hemoglobin, and anticoagulant rise to the top and drain off. With continued spinning, washing, and addition of blood from the reservoir, the Hct of the blood in the bowl can be increased to 50% to 60%. The blood is further washed to ensure removal of free Hb and waste, then it is stored in a blood bag for reinfusion into the patient.

Although this technique is used extensively with success, complications have been noted. Insufficient washing can result in the patient receiving anticoagulant, fat and bone marrow debris, and free hemoglobin. Free hemoglobin can result in kidney damage. In addition there have been a few reports of air embolism, either as a result of incorrectly connecting tubing or of placing blood pumps on collection bags from which air has not been removed. A 1992 article describes two cases of disseminated intravascular coagulation (DIC) that occurred with use of a cell salvage machine. In addition to the patient's underlying medical condition, precipitating factors for DIC may have been that the suction used to collect the wound blood was too high and that not enough wash was being used to clean the blood. In orthopaedic surgery, it is recommended that more wash be used to remove debris, bone, cement, and fat than in most other surgical procedures.

Postoperative Salvage Device Blood that is ordinarily discarded as it drains out of the wound is now being reinfused. A sterile reinfusion device is connected to the wound drain. A 265-μm filter is used during collection of wound drainage, and a 40-μm filter is used during reinfusion into the patient.

Concern exists about the debris and other material that may enter the postoperative reinfusion device and then the patient. Analysis of the fluid demonstrates a low platelet count, increased fibrin degradation products, low fibrinogen levels, an elevated prothrombin time (PT) and partial thromboplastin time (PTT), and some free Hb. Because the PT and PTT are elevated, some physicians do not add anticoagulant to the collection device. The Hct of reinfused blood is slightly lower than the patient's current intravascular Hct.

Although some potential complications exist, many have used postoperative reinfusion devices both with and without washing without complication. Potential risks when using these devices include a dilutional coagulopathy, reinfusion of anticoagulants, DIC, complement activation, adult respiratory distress syndrome and renal insufficiency due to hemolyzed cells and free Hb. Upper airway edema, which possibly indicates complement activation to the presence of C3a and C5a fragments, has been described in a patient after reinfusion of unwashed cells.

There is a question as to whether or not this salvaged wound drainage should be washed. In one study, there were four complications in 16 patients who received unwashed reinfused blood while there were no complications in 19 patients who received washed blood. Two patients had acute hypotension when the unwashed reinfusion was started, one patient had hyperthermia that remained unexplained, and 5 hours postoperatively, one patient had hypotension, which was due to a myocardial infarction and was unrelated to reinfusion of blood. Despite this report, which involved only a small number of patients, many patients have received unwashed reinfused blood without complication.

Human Immunodeficiency Virus (HIV)

HIV is a human retrovirus that synthesizes DNA from its own RNA genome via a process called reverse transcription. Duplication of HIV occurs within the CD4 lymphocyte, which is an integral part of the immunologic defense mechanism of the body. Continued retrovirus replication leads to CD4 lysis and an impaired immunologic state. CD4 counts are indicative of the activity of the disease, with low counts denoting an advanced disease state. Loss of CD4 cells results in an immunocomprised patient who is susceptible to opportunistic infections and to the development of acquired immunodeficiency syndrome (AIDS). Although a long latency period may exist between infection and signs and symptoms of AIDS, the ultimate prognosis is poor. Thus, it is a major concern of all physicians who are in close contact with blood and body fluids as well as sharp objects contaminated with blood and body fluids that they not become infected with the HIV virus.

Needlestick injuries are considered a major potential source for transmission of HIV from patient to physician. Other possible modes of transmission in the surgical setting include blood contamination of open cuts, sores, and mucous membranes and exposure from splashes, aerosol sprays, power tools, and laser plumes. Whereas the incidence of infection after needlestick exposure is "considered" low (~ 1/200), the cumulative or lifetime risk of a surgeon becoming infected may range from 1% to 4% or higher. Even in a low prevalence area, the cumulative HIV occupational risk during a surgical career was calculated at 1%. The variation in incidence may be multifactorial, including prevalence of HIV in the patient population, surgical technique, type of needlestick (hollow needle worse than solid needle), the number of surgical procedures performed per week, amount and site (subcutaneous vs deep muscle) of innoculum, and the surgeon's use of universal precautions.

Contact with blood is common among orthopaedic surgeons. A 1991 survey of orthopaedic surgeons demonstrated a high incidence of blood-skin contacts (87.4%) and percutaneous exposures (39.2%) within the month prior to the survey, while 3.2% reported an injury with a sharp object known to be contaminated with blood from an HIV-positive patient at some time in their career. HIV testing in the entire study group demonstrated no seroconversions in 3,267 physicians who did not have risk factors for HIV. Two of 108 physicians who had nonoccupational risk factors were seropositive. One critique of the study stated that the results may be flawed because the study only included 48% of orthopaedic surgeons who attended the national meeting, physicians may not have participated if they were concerned about being HIV positive, some physicians with HIV may have been too sick to attend the meeting at which the survey was conducted, and it may be too early to define the cumulative risk to an orthopaedic surgeon.

Recent articles point out the possibility of HIV transmission via respiratory size virus particles in aerosol sprays, laser plumes, and surgical power tools (bone saws, drills). HIV can remain viable in cool aerosols generated by power tools. Although no documented cases of transmission from patient to surgeon have occurred via aerosols, it is of concern that the virus remains viable with these techniques.

While physicians are concerned about acquiring HIV from patients, patients are worried about the possible physician-to-patient mode of transmission. The incidence of transmission from surgeon to patient appears to be exceedingly low, and whatever cases might have occurred are probably secondary to breaks in proper technique. In a 13-year "look-back study" of an infected orthopaedic surgeon's patient population published in 1993, 1,174 former patients (50% of the surgeon's patients) all tested seronegative. In another study involving an HIV seropositive surgeon, 413 patients were recalled for testing and all but one were seronegative. Nucleotide sequencing demonstrated no evidence of HIV transmission from physician to patient in that case.

Proper implementation of universal precautions is crucial to minimize physician exposure. Universal precautions are barrier precautions implemented to isolate the physician from potentially infectious blood and body fluids or sharp objects contaminated with blood and body fluids. These precautions should be used for all patients, even in low-prevalence areas. Data demonstrate that physicians do not use universal precautions at all times; the greatest breaks in techniques occur under stressful situations, such as with multiple trauma patients in the emergency room. Recent surveys of orthopaedic surgeons show frequent noncompliance with universal precautions. The face, including the eyes, should be shielded from splashes. Head covers should be used. Impervious gowns or aprons should be worn when there is a chance of gown contamination with wet fluids. Double gloving is advantageous, and in some cases triple gloving may be indicated. An electronic device used to detect glove perforations or physician contact with wet fluids from the patient through soaked gowns during orthopaedic surgery demonstrated frequent occurrences of both.

The American Academy of Orthopaedic Surgeons has published recommendations that call for the use of universal precautions as well as methods to avoid sharp injuries, which include not passing sharp instruments hand-to-hand and not performing digital examinations when examining sharp fracture fragments or when working with sharp instruments. Exposed pins should be covered. Additional recommendations include not suturing with a needle in the surgeon's hand. Consideration should be given to wearing space-suit equipment when high-impact instruments and power equipment are used. In addition to regular glove use, certain cases may necessitate using stronger impervious gloves. Others recommend chain-link gloves to protect against cutting fingers on bone. It is important that physicians use appropriate precautions to protect themselves and their patients from infection.

Hepatitis

Hepatitis B

Hepatitis B virus (HBV) can be transmitted more easily than HIV. In fact, prior to the introduction of hepatitis B vaccine, some physician populations had incidences of hepatitis B infection exceeding 40%. A single needlestick exposure to hepatitis B virus in a nonimmunized recipient can result in transmission in up to 30% of cases. Compared to HIV, which has a relatively short survival on environmental surfaces, HBV can survive in dried blood for up to 1 week. Transmission from infected patient to physician as well as infected physician to patient has been well documented. This transmission usually occurs when universal precautions are not properly observed.

The introduction of recombinant hepatitis B vaccine has made hepatitis B a preventable disease. Unfortunately, not all physicians have taken advantage of available vaccine, needlessly placing themselves at risk for fulminant hepatitis (1% of cases), death, chronic active hepatitis, or becoming a carrier, which can occur in 10% of cases. A controversial area is the infected physician who is a carrier and whether or not he or she places his patients at risk for infection and should be required to curtail his surgical practice.

Hepatitis C

Currently Hepatitis C virus (HCV) is responsible for the majority of cases of posttransfusion hepatitis. Up to 50% of patients who have HCV infection develop chronic hepatitis. Unlike HBV, no vaccine is available to protect against HCV infection. With the introduction of antibody testing for the presence of hepatitis C in blood, the incidence of posttransfusion hepatitis has decreased to 3 per 10,000 units transfused. Although presence of antibody to hepatitis B indicates that the person is noninfectious, this is not considered to be the case with people having antibody to hepatitis C. Therefore, a patient with hepatitis C antibody may still be infectious.

Annotated Bibliography

Blood Transfusion

Nelson AH, Fleisher LA, Rosenbaum SH: Relationship between postoperative anemia and cardiac morbidity in high-risk vascular patients in the intensive care unit. *Crit Care Med* 1993;21:860–866.

In 27 high risk surgical patients undergoing infrainguinal arterial bypass procedures, there was more cardiac morbidity in patients who had hematocrits < 28% than those with hematocrits ≥ 28%.

Seltzer DG, Brown MD, Tompkins JS, et al: Toward the elimination of homologous blood use in elective lumbar spine surgery. *J Spine Disord* 1993;6:412–421.

This study demonstrates how the combined use of autologous predonation and intraoperative blood salvage can help to markedly decrease the need for homologous transfusion.

Stehling L, Simon TL: The red blood cell transfusion trigger: Physiology and clinical studies. *Arch Pathol Lab Med* 1994;118:429–434.

This article reviews the considerations for determining when a transfusion is appropriate, including the etiology, chronicity, and severity of anemia as well as the patient's ability to compensate for the anemia.

Triulzi DJ, Vanek K, Ryan DH, et al: A clinical and immunologic study of blood transfusion and postoperative bacterial infection in spinal surgery. *Transfusion* 1992;32: 517–524.

This study demonstrates a strong relationship between transfusion of homologous blood and the risk for in-hospital postoperative bacterial infection in spine-surgery patients.

Human Immunodeficiency Virus (HIV)

Johnson GK, Robinson WS: Human immunodeficiency virus-1 (HIV-1) in the vapors of surgical power instruments. *J Med Virol* 1991;33:47–50.

Although transmission has not been documented to occur via this route, this study shows that HIV-1 can remain viable in cool aerosols generated by certain surgical power tools.

Petersen LR, Satten GA, Dodd R, et al: Duration of time from onset of human immunodeficiency virus type 1 infectiousness to development of detectable antibody: The HIV seroconversion study group. *Transfusion* 1994;34: 283–289.

People who recently acquired human immunodeficiency virus (HIV) may be infectious but not have developed detectable antibody to HIV. This creates a window period in which HIV-infected blood can be donated, test negative for HIV-antibody, and infect a recipient. The window period averages 45 days and in most people is less than 6 months.

von Reyn CF, Gilbert TT, Shaw FE Jr, et al: Absence of HIV transmission from an infected orthopedic surgeon: A 13-year look-back study. *JAMA* 1993;269:1807–1811.

This 13.5-year retrospective study demonstrated that there was no transmission to his patients of HIV from an HIV-infected orthopaedic surgeon who utilized infection-control practices. Proper use of infection-control precautions can decrease the risk of transmission of HIV from an infected surgeon to extremely low levels.

Wright JG, McGeer A: Human immunodeficiency virus transmission between surgeons and patients in orthopaedic surgery. *Clin Orthop* 1993;297:272–281.

Occupational exposure to HIV and cumulative risk of seroconversion are discussed. Strategies to prevent transmission are outlined.

Hepatitis

Donahue JG, Munoz A, Ness PM, et al: The declining risk of post-transfusion hepatitis C virus infection. *N Engl J Med* 1992;327:369–373.

With the implementation of donor screening for surrogate markers and antibodies to hepatitis C virus (HCV), there has been a marked decline in posttransfusion hepatitis C. Current risk is about 3 per 10,000 units transfused.

6

Coagulation and Thromboembolism in Orthopaedics

Coagulation

Normal Hemostatic Mechanisms

Hemostasis is caused by the interaction of four physiologic events: vascular constriction, platelet plug formation, fibrin formation, and fibrinolysis. Vasoconstriction is the first response to injury and depends on the local contraction of smooth muscle. This contraction occurs prior to platelet aggregation at the site of the injury. Thereafter, vasoconstriction is closely involved with platelet plug and fibrin formation. Thromboxane A2, a potent vasoconstrictor, is released from platelet membranes during aggregation. Serotonin is also released from platelet membranes and serves as a vasoconstrictor.

Platelets are fragments of megakaryocytes and have a 7- to 9-day life span in circulating blood. If vascular disruption occurs, platelets form a plug that preliminarily stops or reduces the blood loss. Platelets adhere to the exposed intima within 15 seconds of the traumatic event, a step that requires von Willebrand factor. The platelets then expand and recruit other circulating platelets, thereby forming the platelet plug.

Fibrin formation relies on an intricate cascade of circulating proenzymes that are converted in a precise sequence that eventually ends in fibrin (Fig. 1). This cascade follows two pathways: the intrinsic pathway, which involves components normally found in blood, and the extrinsic pathway, which is initiated by tissue lipoprotein. Both pathways

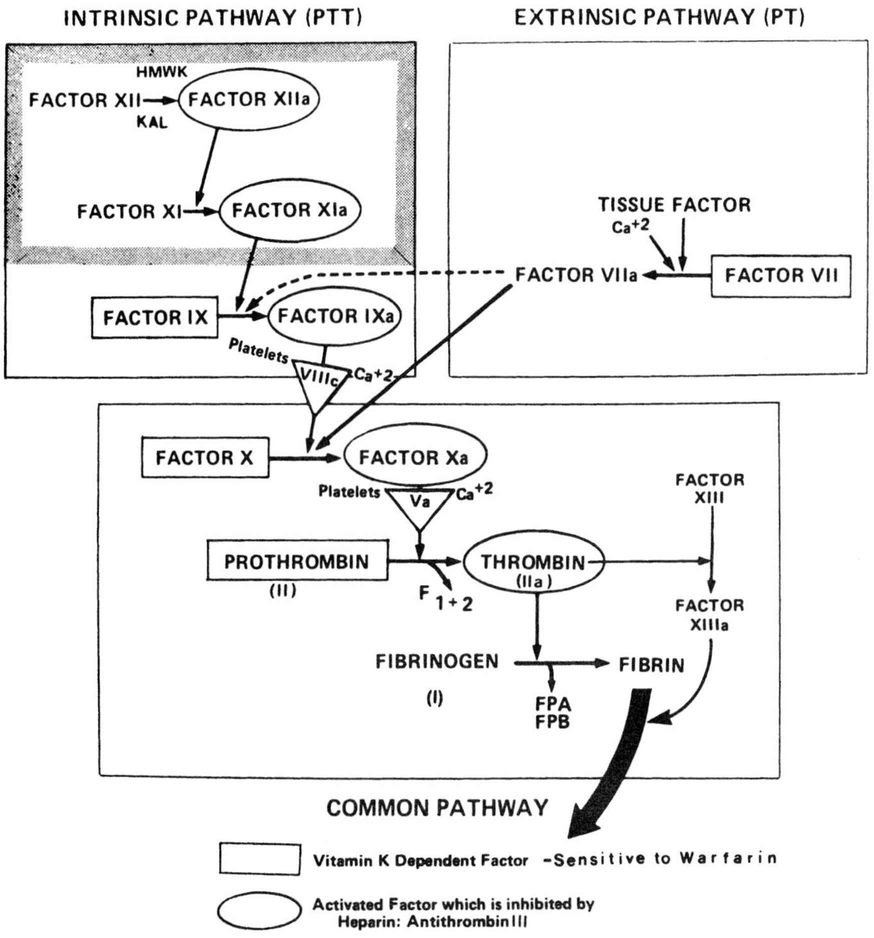

Fig. 1 The coagulation pathways. Important features include the contact activation phase, vitamin K-dependent factors (affected by warfarin), and the activated serine proteases that are inhibited by heparin-antithrombin III. Prothrombin time measures the function of the extrinsic and common pathways; the partial thromboplastin time measures the function of the intrinsic and common pathways. (Reproduced with permission from Stead RB: Regulation of hemostasis, in Goldhaber SZ (ed): *Pulmonary Embolism and Deep Venous Thromboembolism.* Philadelphia, PA, WB Saunders, 1985, p 32.)

lead to activated factor X (Xa), which activates prothrombin to form thrombin. Thrombin, in turn, acts to form fibrin from fibrinogen (factor I) and to activate the fibrin stabilizing factor (XIII). Fibrin cross-links with activated factor XIII (XIIIa) and forms a stable clot, thus supplanting the loose platelet plug.

The final event is fibrinolysis, which acts to maintain blood vessel patency by removing fibrin deposits. Antithrombin III assists in this process by counteracting thrombin and other proteases in the cascade. Fibrinolysis is initiated at the same time as the clotting mechanism. Plasmin lyses fibrin and acts on other coagulant proteins as well.

Coagulopathies

Congenital defects of coagulation factors can lead to severe coagulopathies, which must be addressed preoperatively. The most common defects are of factor VIII, factor IX, and von Willebrand factor.

Classic Hemophilia (Hemophilia A or Factor VIII Deficiency) Hemophilia A is the most common form of hemophilia. It is inherited as an X-linked recessive trait and therefore affects males almost exclusively. Females are carriers and not clinically affected. The severity of clinical manifestations is related to the degree of factor VIII deficiency. Severe hemophilia occurs with $< 1\%$ factor VIII in the plasma. Patients with moderate hemophilia have 1% to 5% factor VIII and rarely experience spontaneous bleeding but are at high risk after trauma or surgical intervention. Mild hemophilia is defined as greater than 5% factor VIII. Severe hemophilia is characterized by spontaneous bleeding episodes, hemarthroses, and eventual joint destruction with repeated bleeds. The knees are involved most frequently, followed by the elbow, ankle, and less commonly the wrist, shoulder, and hip.

The half-life of factor VIII is 8 to 12 hours. Only 7% to 8% of administered factor VIII remains within the circulation after 24 hours. Either low or high purity pasteurized factor VIII or recombinant factor VIII products are the current standard and have largely replaced cryoprecipitate as the appropriate replacement product. The minimum hemostatic level of factor VIII for mild hemorrhage is 30%. Fifty percent is required for treatment of joint and muscle bleeding or major hemorrhage. For major surgery and life-threatening bleeding, 80% to 100% factor VIII should be reached preoperatively and factor VIII should be maintained above 30% for 10 to 14 days. Surgery should be performed in a hospital with a hemophilia center or where personnel are experienced in the care of patients with hemophilia. It must be kept in mind that once a hemophiliac patient has achieved normal factor VIII levels, the risk of deep venous thrombosis is equivalent to that for normal patients.

Complications of replacement therapy include hepatitis, human immunodeficiency virus (HIV) transmission, and the appearance of factor VIII inhibitors. Approximately 10% to 15% of patients with hemophilia A will develop circulating inhibitors if exposed to factor VIII over a long period of time, most commonly patients with severe hemophilia A. There is some evidence for genetic predisposition for development of inhibitors. Although the newer high-purity pasteurized concentrations have greatly reduced the incidence of viral transmission, they have an increased frequency of acquired IgG (immunoglobulin G) antibody inhibitors against factor VIII. The management of patients with factor VIII inhibitors poses serious clinical problems and is more expensive than treatment for patients who do not develop inhibitors.

Christmas Disease (Hemophilia B or Factor IX Deficiency) Hemophilia B is clinically indistinguishable from classic hemophilia. It is also transmitted in a sex-linked recessive fashion. Factor IX deficiency accounts for nearly 20% of all hemophiliacs. Like classic hemophilia, Christmas disease occurs in severe, moderate, and mild forms based on the circulating level of factor IX in the plasma. Patients with 1% or less have severe involvement; 1% to 5%, moderate; and 5% or greater, mild.

Factor IX has a half-life of 18 to 40 hours. A variety of factor IX concentrates are available, and good results have been achieved with few side effects. In patients undergoing surgery, a plasma level of 50% to 70% of normal should be achieved preoperatively. Approximately 10% of patients with Christmas disease develop antibodies against factor IX.

von Willebrand's Disease This disease is the most common hereditary bleeding disorder. It is usually transmitted in an autosomal dominant fashion, but recessive inheritance can occur. The disease is characterized by a reduction of the factor VIII (procoagulant) activity that corrects the clotting abnormality in hemophilia A plasma. Bleeding may be minimal in these patients and is often overlooked. Epistaxis and menorrhagia may be the first clinical signs of the disease. Spontaneous hemarthroses are rare except in the most severe form.

Treatment is directed at correcting the abnormal bleeding time and von Willebrand factor (vWF). Although cryoprecipitate was once the mainstay of treatment, factor VIII concentrates have supplanted this due to several distinct advantages: (1) markedly reduced potential for transmission of viral diseases; (2) decreased volume of infusions; (3) easier home use; and (4) minimal fibrinogen present in newer concentrates. Cryoprecipitate can cause undesirably high levels of fibrinogen if large doses are used. Pasteurized human antihemophilic factor has been successful in shortening the bleeding time, correcting laboratory parameters, and halting bleeding in patients with von Willebrand's disease. Replacement should begin 1 day prior to surgery and be continued for at least 10 days following major surgical procedures. Aspirin must be discontinued 10 days prior to an elective procedure.

Desmopressin (1-desamino-8-D-arginine-vasopressin) causes a sustained increase in factor VIII and vWF concentrations in normal volunteers. It is delivered intravenously, intranasally, or subcutaneously. Desmopressin may be given to a von Willebrand's patient electively to measure responsiveness including factor VIII activity, vWF antigen concentration, and ristocetin cofactor activity. Desmopressin treatment is usually ineffective, although it may correct bleeding time transiently and has been used successfully to treat minor bleeding episodes.

Hypercoagulable States

In 1856, Virchow described three factors leading to thrombosis: stasis, endothelial damage, and hypercoagulability. Patients who develop spontaneous venous thrombosis at an early age, who have a strong family history of deep venous thrombosis (DVT), or who develop recurrent DVT should be considered hypercoagulable and warrant further investigation for predisposing conditions.

DVT may also be the first clue to occult malignancy. This association has been confirmed in autopsy studies. Patients who present with DVT and are 65 years of age and older have a much higher likelihood of malignancy.

Patients with systemic lupus erythematosus (SLE) are at high risk for thromboembolic disease and must be monitored closely. SLE patients with lupus anticoagulant and anticardiolipin have a statistically significant increased risk of developing thrombosis.

Thromboembolic Disease

Prevention

Prevention of thromboembolic disease (TED) remains one of the most controversial issues in orthopaedics. The prevention of proximal DVT and pulmonary embolism (PE) are the goals of prophylactic intervention. If prophylaxis is not used, DVT will develop in 40% to 60% of patients undergoing total hip or knee arthroplasty. Asymptomatic pulmonary embolism will occur in 10% to 15% of patients and fatal pulmonary embolism in 1% to 3% of patients. Patients with hip fractures who are not treated prophylactically face a 3% to 12% mortality rate. Both mechanical and pharmacologic measures have been recommended to prevent TED. Mechanical modalities include compression stockings, continuous passive motion machines, and external pneumatic compression devices. Pharmacologic intervention includes dextran, aspirin, heparin, warfarin sodium, hypotensive epidural anesthesia, and low-molecular-weight heparins.

Mechanical Modalities

Mechanical modalities are attractive options because they do not require laboratory monitoring and have few, if any, side effects. However, they have not proven to be successful in reducing the incidence of TED when used alone. Compression stockings alone do not decrease the risk of TED and should not be used without concurrent pharmacologic prophylaxis.

Continuous Passive Motion Continuous passive motion (CPM) has been reviewed prospectively and found not to lower the risk of TED in patients undergoing total knee arthroplasty. Another study found that there was no difference in the incidence of clots, with or without CPM, for total hip or knee arthroplasty.

External Pneumatic Compression External pneumatic compression devices decrease venous stasis by improving peak venous flow. They also increase local and systemic fibrinolysis. One author advocates the use of thigh-high pneumatic compression beginning intraoperatively for total hip arthroplasty because data from several studies suggest that twisting of the femoral vein during hip dislocation and femoral canal preparation causes isolated femoral thrombosis. The incidence of proximal DVT was 12% and was not statistically altered by the addition of aspirin or low-dose warfarin. A second study also showed significant decrease with intraoperative thigh-high compression. However, 97% of these patients also had hypotensive epidural anesthesia. Although pneumatic compression devices have been shown to be as effective as aspirin in the prevention of TED, several studies have shown that they do not provide as much protection against proximal DVT as does warfarin. Intermittent plantar venous compression has been used in conjunction with pharmacologic prophylaxis and found to significantly decrease the incidence of DVT following total hip arthroplasty. This was a small study, and further conclusions concerning this modality cannot be made at this time.

Pharmacologic Intervention

Dextran Dextran prevents TED by decreasing blood viscosity and platelet aggregation. However, it delivers large amounts of intravenous fluids and has a high association with congestive heart failure, pulmonary edema, hypersensitivity reactions, and bleeding. It is also quite expensive. It should not be considered as a first-line prophylactic drug.

Aspirin Aspirin inhibits the aggregation of platelets and inhibits cyclooxygenase. It has not been as effective for the prevention of proximal DVT and PE as other pharmacologic approaches. One author recommends its use; however, it is used in association with hypotensive epidural anesthesia, which has been shown to lower the risk of TED and may, therefore, be a confounding variable. Another author recommends its use based on the very low rate (0.5%) of symptomatic PE in a review of 920 patients. Most authors, however, do not recommend aspirin as the prophylactic treatment of choice for DVT/PE prophylaxis following total hip or knee arthroplasty.

Heparin Heparin binds to and enhances the activity of the endogenous anticoagulant, antithrombin III. Heparin and antithrombin III then act together to inhibit a number of the activated clotting proteins, including thrombin, factors IXa and Xa. Antithrombin III levels drop dramatically during hip surgery in comparison to abdominal surgery. This drop may explain why standard low-dose heparin has been ineffective in orthopaedic surgery. One study reported significant TED prophylaxis when heparin was given in conjunction with antithrombin III. Low-dose heparin should not be used after hip surgery because of its low efficacy in preventing proximal DVT. In one study, a significant reduction in the incidence of TED was found after intraoperative administration of heparin. However, hypotensive epidural anesthesia and aspirin were used in this group. Heparin-related bleeding should be reversed with protamine sulfate. In general, standard adjusted dose heparinization is not used routinely because of the need for daily monitoring of prothrombin time (PT) and concerns about increased bleeding complications. Heparin-induced thrombocytopenia is a rare complication.

Warfarin Warfarin inhibits the production of the vitamin-K-dependent clotting factors II, VII, IX, and X. Warfarin is rapidly absorbed from the gastrointestinal tract and reaches maximal blood concentrations in healthy volunteers in 90 minutes. It has a half-life of 36 to 42 hours. The dose-response relationship of warfarin differs between healthy subjects, and is even greater among sick patients. Many drugs influence the pharmacokinetics of warfarin by either reducing its absorption from the gut or altering its metabolic clearance. Metronidazole, trimethoprim-sulfamethoxazole, and cimetidine all prolong the PT by pharmacokinetically interacting with warfarin.

The PT is the most commonly performed test for monitoring warfarin therapy in North America. The PT is performed by adding thromboplastin and calcium to citrated plasma. Thromboplastin is an extract of tissues (brain, lung, or placenta) that contains both the tissue factor and the phospholipid required to promote factor X activation by factor VII in the intrinsic pathway. However, thromboplastins have markedly variable responsiveness to the anticoagulant effects of warfarin, depending on the tissue of origin and mode of preparation. Because of this variability, PT results from differing laboratories should not be considered interchangeable. The international normalized ratio (INR) was developed in 1982 to attempt to universalize the monitoring and reporting of anticoagulant therapy. The INR is defined as:

$$\text{INR} = (\text{observed prothrombin ratio})^{\text{ISI}},$$

where ISI is the index of sensitivity for the thromboplastin reagent used for the test. The use of an index of sensitivity is what gives the INR values their inter- and intra-observer consistency. The observed prothrombin ratio (INR) is **not** the same as PT and the INR values **do not** correlate to PTs or to patient-to-control ratios.

Unfortunately, North American physicians have been reluctant to adopt the INR, which is now accepted internationally. In 1985, a joint policy statement of the International Committee for Thrombosis and Hemostasis and the International Committee for Standardization in Hematology recommended that editors and reviewers of scientific papers should not accept PT results unless they are accompanied by the INR. This policy should be adopted by North American physicians.

Low-dose warfarin therapy (PT 1.3 to 1.5 times normal; no INR reported) has gained support based on several studies. One study reported a decrease in proximal thrombi in total hip patients treated with low-dose warfarin when compared to external pneumatic compression. Low-dose warfarin was associated with major bleeding complications in only three of 195 patients. Warfarin continues to be the most widely used prophylactic agent following total hip and knee arthroplasty. Over 50% of all orthopaedic surgeons in the United States use warfarin.

Although low-dose warfarin therapy has gained popularity, 1 mg/day dosing has been shown in one randomized study to be ineffective in preventing postoperative venous thrombosis in patients undergoing hip and knee surgery. Monitoring continues to be problematic in patients taking warfarin postoperatively.

Duration of anticoagulation prophylaxis also remains controversial. The current recommendation is that anticoagulation should be continued for a minimum of 3 weeks postoperatively keeping the INR between 1.8 and 2.5.

Low-Molecular-Weight Heparin Low-molecular-weight hepabrins (LMWH) are derived from standard heparin by depolymerization with the final molecular weight averaging 4 kd (compared to 15 kd for unfractionated heparin). Both standard heparin and LMWH enhance the activity of antithrombin III. Their primary effect, however, is through inhibition of factor Xa.

LMWH have reduced inhibition of platelet function and, therefore, produce less bleeding than unfractionated heparin. LMWH have a longer plasma half-life and a more predictable anticoagulant response to weight-adjusted doses than subcutaneous heparin. LMWH are, therefore, more clinically stable than unfractionated heparin, allowing for consistent dosing in all patients (based on kilogram body weight), once or twice/day administration, and no need for laboratory monitoring.

LMWH have been studied in comparison to placebo, to unfractionated heparin, and to low-dose coumadin, and they were found to be more efficacious than placebo or unfractionated heparin. Bleeding complications were decreased with LMWH when compared to unfractionated heparin. Recently, two prospective studies have compared LMWH to warfarin. There were no statistically different findings in DVT, proximal thrombosis, PE, or major bleeding complications. In patients undergoing total hip arthroplasty, DVT was reduced from 51% to 11% with LMWH (compared to controls). In another study, there also was a significant reduction in proximal DVT when LMWH was compared to unfractionated heparin (13% to 3%).

LMWH have also been compared to placebo in the treatment of patients with hip fractures. Although it reduced the incidence of DVT by 50% compared to the control, there was still a 30% incidence of DVT in these high-risk patients. Limitations of LMWH include cost, limited long-term studies to date, and the parenteral route of administration, which makes it more difficult to treat patients after they leave the hospital.

Diagnosis of Deep Venous Thrombosis

Clinical findings, such as swelling, pain in the calf, palpable cord, and pain on passive dorsiflexion (Homans' sign), are notoriously poor indicators of DVT. The sobering fact remains that PE often is the first clinical sign of TED. Therefore, clinical suspicion should lead to further definitive evaluation. Diagnostic tools available include impedance plethysmography, radioactive fibrinogen, venography, and ultrasonography.

Impedance Plethysmography Impedance plethysmography measures changes in blood volume after deliberate temporary venous obstruction. If there is a thrombus, the outflow rate decreases to the increasing volume challenge of impedance plethysmography. It is an attractive modality because it is noninvasive. However, it has been shown in several studies to have an unacceptably low sensitivity and specificity.

Fibrinogen I 125 Scanning Circulating fibrinogen labeled with iodine 125 is incorporated into a thrombus and creates an overlying area of surface radioactivity measurable by a radioisotope detector. This modality has been shown to be effective in diagnosing calf vein thrombosis but fails to detect proximal vein thrombosis. In addition, the fibrinogen injection is obtained from pooled human serum donors and poses the risk of transmission of hepatitis or HIV.

Venography Venography has been the standard for diagnosis of DVT. However, it is not without controversy. It is invasive and uncomfortable, expensive, and nearly 5% of patients are poor candidates due to insufficient venous access. In a recent review of 32 institutions, the variance in venography readings was impressive. In addition, venography can cause DVT in 1% to 5% of patients.

Duplex Ultrasonography Duplex ultrasonography may become the standard for detection of DVT. Duplex ultrasonography refers to simultaneously viewing the vein in three dimensions and listening to the blood flow. Direct compression in the suspicious area can indicate whether or not a clot is present. Its advantages are that it is noninvasive, painless, portable, and readily repeatable.

Several recent studies have shown that duplex ultrasonography is 100% specific, sensitive, and accurate for proximal DVT only. The accuracy of detecting distal clots remains disappointingly low. Duplex ultrasonography is very technique dependent. At this time, duplex scanning is not a test that can be duplicated in every hospital with specificity.

Diagnosis of Pulmonary Embolism

Routine diagnostic tests, including physical examination, chest radiograph, electrocardiography, and arterial blood gases, for PE are insensitive and nonspecific. The standards for diagnosis of pulmonary embolism are ventilation-perfusion scanning and pulmonary angiography.

Ventilation-Perfusion Scanning Ventilation-perfusion (V/Q) scanning is used to look for a segmental perfusion defect in which no blood is flowing because a clot is obstructing the pulmonary artery. Ventilation, however, remains normal to this unperfused area. V/Q scans are subjectively graded as low-, intermediate-, or high-probability that a PE is present. Although this modality is safe, simple, and relatively fast, it is also highly user-dependent and may be nonspecific.

Pulmonary Angiography Pulmonary angiography remains the standard in the detection of PE. When V/Q scanning yields a low or intermediate probability of PE, pulmonary angiography can be used to confirm the diagnosis. In some centers, angiography is used initially when the suspicion of PE is high.

Treatment of Thromboembolic Disease

Deep Venous Thrombosis

Controversy still exists as to which clots should be treated, choice of anticoagulation, and the duration of treatment. Data from one study demonstrated that the size and location of the clot has a significant correlation with the likelihood of having an intermediate or high probability V/Q scan. The treatment of calf vein DVT remains a controversial issue. Data from one study demonstrated that although there is significantly more calf vein DVT in patients after total knee arthroplasty than in patients following total hip arthroplasty, their rates of symptomatic PE are equivalent. The authors concluded that the presence of calf thrombi does not increase the risk of symptomatic PE. Treatment for symptomatic calf vein DVT and proximal DVT has traditionally been 3 months with warfarin. A recent study has shown that this may be excessively long in nearly 50% of patients with DVT. Nonetheless, heparinization should begin concurrently with warfarin therapy until the INR is in a therapeutic range. Heparin therapy should be continued for 5 days. A randomized study showed that there was no added benefit to treating with heparin for a longer period than this. The current recommendation is to maintain the INR between 2.0 and 3.0.

Pulmonary Embolism

Patients with documented PE should be treated initially with intravenous heparin for 5 days and concurrent oral warfarin until the INR is therapeutic. Duration of anticoagulation for a documented PE is not well established in the literature. However, a minimum of 6 months is recommended. The INR should be kept between 2.0 and 3.0. If the patient cannot tolerate anticoagulation therapy, a vena caval filter is recommended. However, these devices are also associated with severe complications, which include the need for continued anticoagulation, filter migration, and the recurrence of clots at the filter site or beyond.

Annotated Bibliography

Bradley JG, Krugener GH, Jager HJ: The effectiveness of intermittent plantar venous compression in prevention of deep venous thrombosis after total hip arthroplasty. *J Arthroplasty* 1993;8:57–61.

Intermittent plantar venous compression was effective in reducing the incidence of deep venous thrombosis in this small study.

Colwell CW Jr, Spiro TE, Trowbridge AA, et al: Use of Enoxaparin, a low-molecular-weight heparin, and unfractionated heparin for the prevention of deep venous thrombosis after elective hip replacement: A clinical trial comparing efficacy and safety. *J Bone Joint Surg* 1994; 76A:3–14.

Low-molecular-weight heparin was found to be more effective and safer than unfractionated heparin in this review of 604 patients.

Hirsh J, Dalen JE, Deykin D, et al: Oral anticoagulants: Mechanism of action, clinical effectiveness, and optimal therapeutic range. *Chest* 1992;102(suppl 4):312S–326S.

This excellent supplement updates the recommendations from the National Heart, Lung and Blood Institute (NHLBI) from 1989 and strongly advocates the use of INR (international normalized ratio) instead of prothrombin time for warfarin monitoring.

Huo MH, Salvati EA, Sharrock NE, et al: Intraoperative heparin thromboembolic prophylaxis in primary total hip arthroplasty: A prospective, randomized, controlled, clinical trial. *Clin Orthop* 1992;274:35–46.

Intraoperative heparin in conjunction with hypotensive epidural anesthesia and postoperative aspirin was effective in reducing proximal deep venous thrombosis.

Jorgensen PS, Knudsen JB, Broeng L, et al: The thromboprophylactic effect of a low-molecular-weight heparin (Fragmin) in hip fracture surgery: A placebo-controlled study. *Clin Orthop* 1992;278:95–100.

Fragmin (low-molecular-weight heparin) was associated with a 30% incidence of deep venous thrombosis.

Lieberman JR, Huo MM, Hanway J, et al: The prevalence of deep venous thrombosis after total hip arthroplasty with hypotensive epidural anesthesia. *J Bone Joint Surg* 1994;76A:341–348.

Hypotensive epidural anesthesia and aspirin is effective prophylaxis against deep venous thrombosis in patients who have a primary total hip arthroplasty.

Lotke PA, Steinberg ME, Ecker ML: Significance of deep venous thrombosis in the lower extremity after total joint arthroplasty. *Clin Orthop* 1994;299:25–30.

Total knee arthroplasty is associated with a higher risk of large and small calf thrombi than total hip arthroplasty.

Paiement GD, Schutzer SF, Wessinger SJ, et al: Influence of prophylaxis on proximal venous thrombus formation after total hip arthroplasty. *J Arthroplasty* 1992;7:471–475.

Low-dose warfarin provided a statistically significant reduction in deep venous thrombosis compared to aspirin, dextran, or external pneumatic compression and had a tenfold reduction in bleeding complications compared to higher dose warfarin.

Paiement GD, Wessinger SJ, Hughes R, et al: Routine use of adjusted low-dose warfarin to prevent venous thromboembolism after total hip replacement. *J Bone Joint Surg* 1993;75A:893–898.

Low-dose warfarin was given for 12 weeks postoperatively after total hip arthroplasty, was not associated with major bleeding complications, and was more cost-effective than routine screening with either phlebography or duplex ultrasonography.

Wells PS, Lensing AW, Davidson BL, et al: Accuracy of ultrasound for the diagnosis of deep venous thrombosis in asymptomatic patients after orthopaedic surgery: A meta-analysis. *Ann Intern Med* 1995;122:47–53.

A meta-analysis is performed of articles comparing venous ultrasound to venography for diagnosing venous thrombosis after hip or knee replacement surgery. The authors conclude that these noninvasive tests may be only moderately sensitive in detecting venous thrombosis and, thus, may have limitations as a screening test.

Wolf LR, Hozack WJ, Balderston RA, et al: Pulmonary embolism: Incidence in primary cemented and uncemented total hip arthroplasty using low-dose sodium warfarin prophylaxis. *J Arthroplasty* 1992;7:465–470.

Uncemented total hip arthroplasty does not offer any additional protective value against pulmonary embolism when using low-dose warfarin prophylaxis.

Woolson ST: The resolution of deep venous thrombosis that occurs after total joint arthroplasty: A study of thrombi treated with anticoagulation and observed by repeat venous ultrasound scans. *Clin Orthop* 1994;299: 86–91.

The standard duration of anticoagulation therapy for documented postoperative deep venous thrombosis may be excessively long.

Classic Bibliography

Eriksson BI, Kalebo P, Anthymyr BA, et al: Prevention of deep-vein thrombosis and pulmonary embolism after total hip replacement: Comparison of low-molecular-weight heparin and unfractionated heparin. *J Bone Joint Surg* 1991;73A:484–493.

Haas SB, Insall JN, Scuderi GR, et al: Pneumatic sequential-compression boots compared to aspirin prophylaxis of deep-vein thrombosis after total knee arthroplasty. *J Bone Joint Surg* 1990;72A:27–31.

Hull RD, Raskob GE, Rosenbloom D, et al: Heparin for 5 days as compared with 10 days in the initial treatment of proximal venous thrombosis. *N Engl J Med* 1990;322: 1260–1264.

Love PE, Santoro SA: Antiphospholipid antibodies: Anticardiolipin and the lupus anticoagulant in systemic lupus erythematosus (SLE) and in non-SLE disorders: Prevalence and clinical significance. *Ann Intern Med* 1990;112:682–698.

Lynch AF, Bourne RB, Rorabeck CH, et al: Deep-vein thrombosis and continuous passive motion after total knee arthroplasty. *J Bone Joint Surg* 1988;70A:11–14.

Woolson ST, Watt JM: Intermittent pneumatic compression to prevent proximal deep venous thrombosis during and after total hip replacement: A prospective, randomized study of compression alone, compression and aspirin, and compression and low-dose warfarin. *J Bone Joint Surg* 1991;73A:507–512.

7

Perioperative Medical Management

Medical consultation on orthopaedic surgical patients has become an essential part of the perioperative process. Although no surgical procedure can be entirely free of risks, appropriate medical consultation can help to identify potential perioperative problems and reduce perioperative risks considerably.

Preoperative Medical Evaluation

Medical consultants play an important role in elective, as well as emergency orthopaedic procedures. For elective procedures, preoperative medical consultation is ideally an outpatient office-based activity. Patients who are at an increased perioperative risk can be identified early, and attempts can be made to better manage poorly controlled medical problems prior to surgery. Medical consultants can help to coordinate preadmission testing and may order additional noninvasive as well as invasive tests that may help in the evaluation process. Medical consultants should discuss with both the patient and the surgeon the specific potentials for increased perioperative risk. This information can help patients better make an informed decision whether to proceed with an elective procedure.

Patients requiring emergency surgery need rapid inpatient consultations. Patients should be quickly evaluated and poorly controlled problems rapidly stabilized. Attempts should be made to proceed with surgery as quickly as possible because delays may increase chances of perioperative complications and poorer outcomes.

In recent years, the number of elderly patients undergoing orthopaedic procedures has increased steadily. Those with osteoarthritis of the hips and knees are opting for total joint replacement. Those with spinal stenosis are having decompression laminectomies. Falls can result in hip fractures that require emergency repair. Elderly patients may offer special challenges to medical consultants.

Elderly patients may have multiple preexisting medical problems as well as a decreased functional reserve, which may result in significant increased surgical risks and perioperative complications. In addition, emergency surgery in and of itself increases surgical risk. Nonetheless, many elderly patients, particularly those who are closely followed by medical consultants, do quite well with both elective and emergency surgery.

Preadmission Testing

Preadmission testing has often included a complete history and physical examination, electrocardiogram (EKG), chest radiograph, and comprehensive laboratory testing, including complete blood count, coagulation tests, liver function tests, and measurement of electrolytes, creatinine, blood urea nitrogen, and glucose. In recent years, this sort of comprehensive preoperative workup has been criticized as being costly and of limited benefit in identifying patients who will develop perioperative problems. The results of this testing rarely change surgical or medical management. It has been suggested that much more limited preoperative testing is appropriate for many patients. In general, patients who are elderly and have significant preexisting medical problems should have more comprehensive preadmission testing that is geared more toward involved organ systems. Younger, healthier individuals, particularly those who have had relatively recent physical examinations, may have much more limited testing. Both the surgeon and the medical consultant should review the results of the preadmission testing in a timely manner.

The timing of preadmission testing varies by hospital from a few days to 2 weeks prior to surgery. In general, elderly patients, as well as patients with multiple and labile problems are best evaluated and tested closer to the time of surgery. This approach, however, may result in limited time available to perform additional testing, if necessary.

Assessment of Cardiac Disease

Assessment of cardiac risk is of prime importance in any preoperative medical evaluation. Coronary artery disease is extremely common, and patients with it may be at significant increased risk. In addition, cardiac problems contribute significantly to perioperative morbidity and mortality. Patients who have unstable angina, decompensated congestive heart failure, severe aortic stenosis, or recent myocardial infarction are at greatest risk. The Goldman point system (Table 1) is widely used to help predict cardiac complication in patients undergoing noncardiac surgery. Based on the points assigned to various clinical syndromes and findings, patients can be placed in low-, medium-, and high-risk groups. Many of the problems listed in this system can be treated and controlled, thus improving a patient's status. It should be noted that patients with chronic stable angina, controlled hypertension, left ventricular hypertrophy, and nonspecific EKG changes do not appear to be at an increased surgical risk. Preoperative echocardiograms and stress tests are sometimes necessary to fully evaluate a patient's cardiac status.

Although mild to moderate hypertension is not associated with increased surgical risk, hypertensive patients should be evaluated for known associated risk factors and

Table 1. Calculation of multifactorial cardiac risk index

Variable	Points*
S3 gallop or jugular venous distention	11
Myocardial infarction in the past 6 months	10
Rhythm other than sinus or premature atrial contractions on last preoperative electrocardiogram	7
Age more than 70 years	5
Emergency operation	4
Intraperitoneal, intrathoracic, or aortic operation	3
Suspected critical aortic stenosis	3
Poor general medical condition†	3

*Surgical risks, from lowest to highest, may be classified as: I (0 to 5 points); II (6 to 12 points); III (13 to 25 points); IV (> 25 points)

†Electrolyte abnormalities (potassium <3.0 mmol/l or HCO_3 <20 mmol/l), abnormal arterial blood gases (PO_2 <60 mm Hg, or PCO_2> 50 mm Hg), renal insufficiency (blood urea > 17.85 mmol/l [blood urea nitrogen >50 mg/dl], or creatinine >265 μmol/l [>30 mg/dl]), abnormal liver status (elevated transaminase or physical signs of chronic liver disease), or patient bedridden

(Adapted with permission from Goldman L: Cardiac risks and complications of noncardiac surgery. *Ann Intern Med* 1983;98:504–513.)

end organ damage. Most antihypertensives can be continued up to the time of surgery. Patients on diuretics need to be monitored closely for volume status and electrolyte disorders.

Assessment of Pulmonary Disease

Anesthesia and surgery can stress lung function, and patients with underlying pulmonary disease may be of increased risk for postoperative pulmonary complications. Preoperative evaluation of pulmonary function should be performed in patients with a history of heavy smoking, asthma, obesity, and chronic pulmonary disease. Preoperative evaluation should include pulmonary function studies and measurement of arterial blood gases. The results of these studies cannot precisely predict which patients will develop pulmonary complications. However, patients with significant hypercapnia and reduction in FeV_1 to less than 1 liter are at greatest risk.

Determination of preoperative baseline arterial blood gases should be considered in patients with underlying lung diseases. If postoperative pulmonary complications are suspected, comparison of blood gas values is often very helpful. Obtaining baseline blood gases in patients considered at high risk for pulmonary embolus should also be considered. If postoperative pulmonary embolus is suspected, pre- and postoperative blood gas values can be compared.

Attempts should be made to optimize pulmonary function in those patients who have underlying lung disease. Smoking should be stopped in the weeks prior to surgery. Patients should be instructed in deep breathing exercises and coughing. Any respiratory infection should be aggressively treated.

Asthmatic patients should receive bronchodilators and inhaled corticosteroids in the perioperaive period. Strong consideration should be given to the preoperative use of oral as well as intravenous corticosteriods. Asthmatics receiving these medications appear to have low levels of postoperative complications.

Finally, attempts should be made to limit postoperative narcotic analgesics, which can depress respirations. Through the use of these methods, postoperative pulmonary complications can be minimized.

Renal Disease

Patients with chronic renal insufficiency and end-stage renal disease may be at a higher risk for postoperative complications. These patients may be more susceptible to the stresses of volume changes and potassium loads that can occur during surgery. These patients require close attention to volume status and blood pressure monitoring. They are susceptible to changes in serum sodium concentration, as well as hyperkalemia. Hyperkalemia can lead to cardiac arrhythmias. Patients with end-stage renal disease are also at increased risk for infection and bleeding from uremic platelet dysfunction. Patients with chronic renal insufficiency may progress to end-stage renal disease postoperatively. Doses of renally excreted medications need to be adjusted in the setting of renal insufficiency. In addition, potentially nephrotoxic medications should be avoided.

Acute renal failure can occur in the postoperative setting. Volume depletion and hypotension during surgery predispose patients to this complication. Elderly patients and patients with diabetes, congestive heart failure, and preexisting renal disease seem to be most susceptible to postoperative renal failure. Trauma patients are at risk for myoglobinuric renal failure secondary to rhabdomyolysis. In all patients undergoing surgery, attempts should be made to insure normal volume status and both excessive hypo- and hypertension should be avoided.

Liver Disease

Patients with liver disease may be at an increased risk for perioperative complications. The greatest surgical morbidity and mortality occurs in patients with acute viral and alcoholic hepatitis, as well as those with cirrhosis. Patients with evidence of hepatic decompensation as manifested by hypoalbuminemia, coagulopathy, ascites, and encephalopathy are at the greatest risk. Patients with chronic hepatitis who are asymptomatic and have no evidence suggesting hepatic decompensation or cirrhosis generally tolerate surgery well. All patients with liver disease need close perioperative monitoring of fluid status, electrolytes, and blood pressure. Any nonessential and potentially hepatotoxic medications should be avoided.

Routine preoperative liver function studies are generally not recommended in healthy patients whose preoperative history and physical examination do not raise the suspicion of liver disease. However, when abnormal liver function studies are found, it is judicious to thoroughly investigate these abnormalities prior to elective surgery.

Diabetes Mellitus

Patients who have diabetes mellitus require special attention in the perioperative period. These patients are best prepared for elective surgery when their diabetic care is optimized. Patients who have diabetes may have coexisting cardiac, renal and neurologic disease, which can increase surgical risks. Cardiac disease can be silent and not manifest itself until the postoperative period. Surgical stress can result in significant hyperglycemia. Patients with diabetes may be at increased risk for postoperative infection and poor wound healing.

In the perioperative period, blood glucoses are ideally maintained between 150 and 250 mg/100 ml. Patients treated with diet alone or oral hypoglycemic agents are managed in a similar way. Oral agents are discontinued prior to surgery and glucoses are determined four times daily. Small doses of regular insulin are given for glucoses over 200 mg/100 ml. Insulin-dependent patients require much closer monitoring of glucoses in the perioperative period. On the day of surgery, they can be given one half the usual dose of long-acting insulin while 5% dextrose is running intravenously. Glucoses should be monitored carefully and small doses of regular insulin given as needed. Alternatively, patients can be placed on a continuous insulin infusion during surgery. Five percent dextrose is infused through a separate line. The rate of insulin infusion is increased and decreased depending on the blood glucose determination.

Rheumatic Diseases

Patients who have rheumatic diseases frequently undergo orthopaedic surgery. Those with rheumatoid arthritis may have atlantoaxial subluxation; therefore, hyperextension of the neck during endotracheal intubation may be extremely hazardous. It is judicious to obtain preoperative cervical spine films in all patients with rheumatic disease to evaluate for this problem.

Patients with rheumatic disease are often on steroids and require perioperative steroid management. Patients on steroids or who have been on steroids for the past year may have suppression of the hypothalamic-pituitary-adrenal axis (HPA) or an impaired HPA responsiveness to stress. Normal adrenal glands respond to major surgical stress by producing corticosteroids equivalent to 300 to 400 mg of hydrocortisone daily on the day of surgery and for the next 48 hours. The adrenal glands of patients taking exogenous steroids are considerably impaired in their ability to respond to surgical stress. The potential for HPA insufficiency needs to be considered in all patients who have used oral steroids in the year prior to surgery. Those who have received repeated intramuscular injection may also be at risk. Patients using inhaled or topical steroids generally do not have HPA suppression. All patients taking daily prednisone doses of 7.5 mg or greater have HPA suppression. In addition, those taking less than 7.5 mg may have decreased HPA responsiveness to stress. Risk of HPA insufficiency can also be seen in patients who have taken high-dose steroids (20 mg prednisone daily) for a week or more in the year preceding surgery. When doubt exists regarding the use of stress steroids, a cosintropin stimulation test can determine whether adrenal insufficiency is present. A serum cortisol level of greater than 20 mg/dl 1 hour after injection with 25 units of cosintropin (synthetic adrenocorticotropic hormone) excludes adrenal insufficiency.

Perioperative stress doses of steroids should be given as hydrocortisone hemisuccinate, 100 mg by intravenous bolus every 6 to 8 hours. It should be started preoperatively and continued for 72 hours postoperatively.

Surgery may precipitate attacks of gout and pseudogout. Accurate diagnosis can be made by identification of crystals by polaroid microscopy. Treatment needs to be individualized to the patient, depending on the ability to tolerate oral medications, as well as renal function. Treatment options include using nonsteroidal anti-inflammatories, oral or intravenous colchicine, and intra-articular corticosteroids. Postoperative gout can often be prevented through the use of prophylactic colchicine, as well as continuing a patient's own gout medications throughout the perioperative period.

Postoperative Delirium and Confusion

Postoperative delirium and confusional states are often encountered and need to be fully evaluated. Elderly patients and patients with significant medical problems may be more susceptible to this complication. These high-risk patients should be monitored closely for the development of this problem. Knowledge of baseline mental status can help in the assessment of any postoperative confusional states. Patients with postoperative delirium have overall higher rates of major complications. They have higher mortality rates, longer lengths of stay, and are more likely to be discharged to a chronic care facility.

Patients with postoperative behavioral changes need careful neurologic, mental status, and medical evaluation. Although delirium may result from the effect of postoperative stress on a vulnerable patient, it may also be the earliest manifestation of a serious medical problem. Careful neurologic examination can expose serious problems, such as stroke and Wernicke's encephalopathy underlying the delirium. Patients with vivid hallucinations should be evaluated for drug reactions. Alcohol and drug withdrawal syndromes should also be considered.

Delirium may be the first manifestation of fat embolism, pulmonary embolism, infection, or electrolyte abnormalities, particularly hyponatremia. Elderly patients often have very nonspecific presentations for serious medical problems. Confusion in the elderly could signal the development of pneumonia or congestive heart failure. In the intensive care unit, delirium may be a response to pain and deprivation—the so-called "ICU-psychosis."

The treatment of postoperative confusional states should be directed to treatment of any underlying problems. Attempts should be made to have patients in a quiet and reorienting environment with 24-hour attendants if needed. Attempts should be made to limit postoperative narcotics, perhaps through use of nonnarcotic pain medications. In some cases, antipsychotic agents may be needed.

Annotated Bibliography

Assessment of Cardiac Disease

Hollenberg M, Mangano DT, Browner WS, et al: Predictors of postoperative myocardial ischemia in patients undergoing noncardiac surgery: The Study of Perioperative Ischemia Research Group. *JAMA* 1992; 268:205–209.

Clinical and laboratory features of patients who developed evidence of postoperative myocardial ischemia are identified.

Assessment of Pulmonary Disease

Kabalin CS, Yarnold PR, Grammer LC: Low complication rate of corticosteroid-treated asthmatics undergoing surgical procedures. *Arch Intern Med* 1995;155:1379–1384.

The authors find low incidence of pulmonary and nonpulmonary complications in asthmatics treated with corticosteroids perioperatively. They provide recommended dosages of corticosteroids for mild, moderate, and severe asthma.

Assessment of Renal Disease

Kellerman PS: Preoperative care of the renal patient. *Arch Intern Med* 1994;154:1674–1688.

This review article discusses perioperative management of patients with chronic renal insufficiency and end-stage renal disease. Risk factors for postoperative renal failure are also discussed.

Patients with Diabetes Mellitus

Hirsch IB, McGill JB, Cryer PE, et al: Perioperative management of surgical patients with diabetes mellitus. *Anesthesiology* 1991;74:346–359.

This is an up-to-date review discussing management of diabetic patients in the perioperative period.

Postoperative Delirium and Confusion

Marcantonio ER, Goldman L, Mangione CM, et al: A clinical prediction rule for delirium after elective noncardiac surgery. *JAMA* 1994;271:134–139.

This study identifies preoperative factors that can be used to identify patients at increased risk for postoperative delirium.

Williams-Russo P, Sharrock NE, Mattis S, et al: Cognitive effects after epidural vs general anesthesia in older adults: A randomized trial. *JAMA* 1995;274:44–50.

This study looks at elderly patients undergoing elective total knee replacement and finds no difference in cognitive effects of epidural versus general anesthesia.

Classic Bibliography

Burke JF Jr, Francos GC: Surgery in the patient with acute or chronic renal failure. *Med Clin North Am* 1987; 71:489–497.

Friedman LS, Maddrey WC: Surgery in the patient with liver disease. *Med Clin North Am* 1987;71:453–476.

Goldman L: Cardiac risks and complications of noncardiac surgery. *Ann Intern Med* 1983;98:504–513.

Gustafson Y, Berggren D, Brannstrom B, et al: Acute confusional states in elderly patients treated for femoral neck fracture. *J Am Geriatr Soc* 1988;36:523–530.

Jackson CV: Preoperative pulmonary evaluation. *Arch Inter Med* 1988;148:2120–2127.

Macpherson DS, Snow R, Lofgren RP: Preoperative screening: Value of previous tests. *Ann Intern Med* 1990; 113:969–973.

Merli GJ, Weitz HH: Preoperative consultation. *Med Clin North Am* 1987;71:353–590.

Podolsky S: Management of diabetes in the surgical patient. *Med Clin North Am* 1982;66:1361–1372.

White RH: Preoperative evaluation of patients with rheumatoid arthritis. *Semin Arthritis Rheum* 1985; 14:287–299.

8

Imaging Beyond Conventional Radiography

The utility of the numerous imaging modalities available is always a function of the appropriateness of a given examination to a given clinical situation. Such a patient-specific approach becomes more crucial as imaging technology and applications grow, not necessarily replacing older technology but adding to the imaging armamentarium. The more recent advances in orthopaedic imaging are reviewed in this article, and include computed tomography (CT), ultrasound (US) and magnetic resonance imaging (MRI).

Computed Tomography

Advances in CT include two- and three-dimensional (2- and 3-D) reconstruction capability, the use of direct nonaxial imaging planes, CT-guided intervention, and the development of spiral or helical technology. One of the significant disadvantages of CT scanning is the radiation exposure to the patient. In general, radiation exposure with CT is higher than with other radiographic examinations, and it is recommended that it should be minimized as much as possible. Calculations of the skin dose and organ dose for a particular CT study depend on many factors (equipment, technical parameters, slice thickness, size of the patient) and can be calculated with good approximation for each individual circumstance. Published measurements of radiation obtained experimentally show that the mean dose received by the skin is 22 to 36 mGy (1 Gy = 100 rad; 1 rad = 0.01 Gy); the lungs, less than 1 to 18 mGy; the kidneys, 7 to 24 mGy; and the ovaries, less than 1 to 19 mGy, depending on the type of CT performed (abdominal versus pelvic).

The addition of orthogonal planar sections and 3-D reconstruction to routine axial imaging enhances the appreciation of curved or parahorizontal structures, which are underrepresented on transaxial images because of partial volume effects. Such capabilities are readily applied to ankle trauma, pilon fractures, pelvic and acetabulum fractures, tibial plateau fracture, and injury to the shoulder girdle. The edit function allows removal of any structure in the image for direct visualization of a single part, eg, removing the hip so that the acetabulum may be seen directly (Fig. 1). Rotation of the 3-D image allows inspection of the bone from all angles. In addition, 3-D reformation allows for surgical simulation. Osteotomies may be simulated and osteotomized sections discarded, rotated, or translated. Hardware and/or graft material may be added. Similarly, such 3-D models allow for designing prosthetic implants to achieve optimal fit.

Direct nonaxial scanning is now used in certain circumstances, depending on the patient's ability to tolerate different, somewhat awkward positioning in the CT gantry. Direct sagittal and coronal imaging of the wrist, for example, is replacing conventional tomographic imaging. Assessment of scaphoid fracture, arthritis, and fusion are all easily achieved. Direct coronal imaging of the shoulder, following arthrography, provides dramatic evaluation of the rotator cuff.

CT-guided intervention continues to be an effective mode of tumor biopsy and septic aspiration. The latter has been especially helpful in cases of suspected septic spondylitis. CT guidance is also used for treatment of osteoid os-

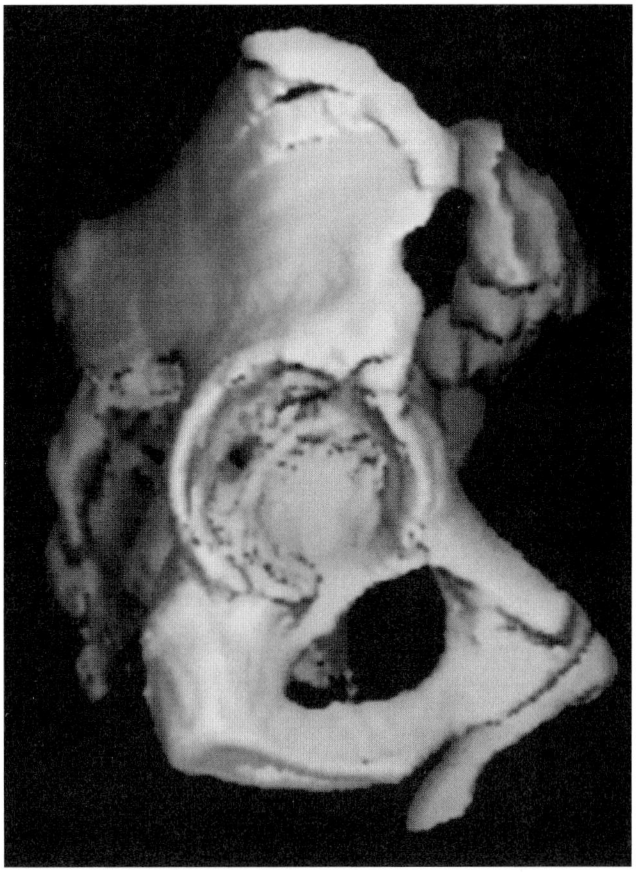

Fig. 1 Computed tomography of the pelvis displayed in three-dimensional surface reconstruction, showing the right acetabulum after removal of the femur. Note the presence of an acetabular fracture.

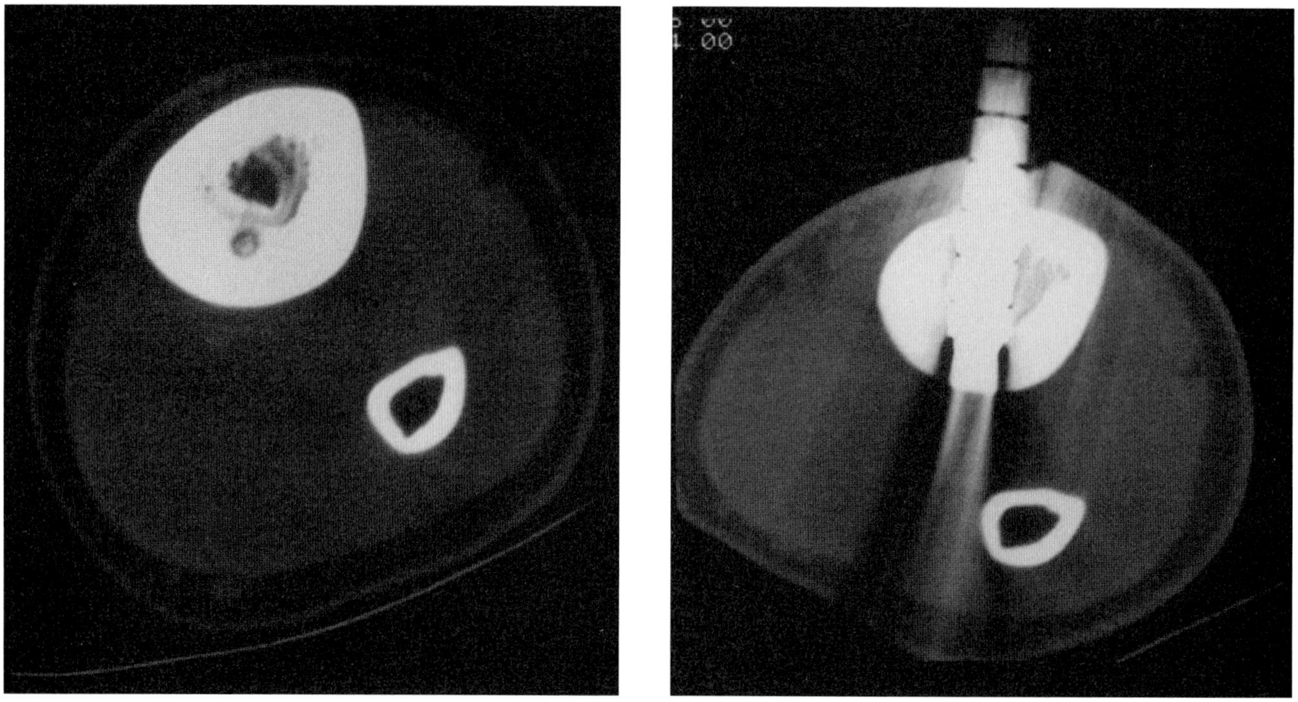

Fig. 2 **Left,** Axial computed tomography (CT) of the left leg shows a small osteoid osteoma at the posterior cortex of the tibia. There is marked reactive sclerosis. **Right,** Excisional biopsy with core drill is performed in the CT suite with CT guidance.

teoma. The difficulty involved in locating the tumor nidus, often hidden in dense reactive sclerosis, repeatedly leads to excessive bone excision, which does not always include the lesion itself. Attempts to localize the nidus have included tetracycline labeling and preoperative technetium administration, both of which yield varying if not poor results. Because an osteoid osteoma is best defined with CT, it is logical to use this modality for treatment. Methods range from needle localization in the CT suite prior to more traditional intraoperative excision to drilling and/or ablating the lesion in the CT suite itself (Fig. 2).

Spiral or helical or volume acquisition CT involves simultaneous radiographic exposure and patient translation during data acquisition and is the latest technological advance in CT scanning. After acquiring the raw data, transaxial as well as multiplanar and 3-D images may be generated. Advantages include decreased scan time, improved lesion detection with elimination of respiratory motion, optimization of enhancement with decreased amount of intravenous contrast, and improved multiplanar and 3-D reconstruction. These advances are most applicable to imaging of the chest, abdomen, and vasculature. However, decreased scan time with improved 2- and 3-D reconstruction certainly benefits orthopaedic patients unable to lie still for longer periods. Currently, there is investigation of the efficacy of spiral CT in the diagnosis of pulmonary embolism, which certainly would aid in the postoperative management of the orthopaedic patient.

Ultrasound

Although real time, gray scale, and color US techniques have been used for diagnostic purposes for more than a decade, new applications in musculoskeletal lesions have become more clinically prolific during the last few years. The advantages of US over other imaging techniques include low cost, general availability, capability to detect very small amounts of fluid collections, and lack of ionizing radiation. Relatively poor spatial resolution, impossibility of imaging through cortical bone, and lack of operator dependability are significant disadvantages.

The most frequent clinical application of US in the field of musculoskeletal imaging is in the evaluation of tendon lesions, such as rotator cuff and Achilles tendon tears. The accuracy of US in the diagnosis of rotator cuff pathology has been the subject of intense debate, probably because it depends on operator expertise. In experienced hands, the sensitivity of US for large, full-thickness rotator cuff tears is probably in the range of 90%, with a specificity in the range of 80%. For partial or small tears and tendinitis, the specificity drops significantly. In general, it is accepted that US is a good screening technique for large rotator cuff tears.

US has also been applied to the diagnosis and follow-up of developmental dysplastic hip (DDH) in patients under the age of 6 months, before ossification of the femoral heads is visible on plain films. Dynamic and static US evaluation provides assessment of the position of the femoral head with and without stress and of the shape of the acetabulum, labrum, and pulvinar (Fig. 3).

New technical developments allow soft-tissue imaging with high resolution in areas such as muscle tears and synovial proliferation, and in the detection of periosteal reaction. The facility of US to discriminate clearly between fluid-containing and solid lesions and its ability to detect blood flow using color Doppler technology has been used clinically to assess the internal characteristics of palpable soft-tissue masses.

Bone Scintigraphy

Bone scintigraphy with technetium Tc 99m diphosphonate compounds has been the mainstay of bone scanning for decades; it has high sensitivity for bone lesions such as metastasis, fractures and infections, but has limited specificity. The addition of gallium citrate Ga 69 scanning and indium 111-labeled leukocyte scanning to the armamentarium of radioisotope imaging has improved significantly the specificity of these techniques, especially when dealing with bone or soft-tissue infection. Combining technetium and indium scanning has been shown to increase the accuracy of evaluating suspected infection in prosthetic joint replacements.

From the technologic point of view, the ability to obtain data in two projections simultaneously (anteroposterior and posteroanterior) with dual head scanners has considerably decreased scanning times. In addition, modern gamma cameras are equipped to perform single photon emission computed tomography (SPECT). With this technique, after injection of the technetium compound, sectional images of the body can be obtained in the sagittal, coronal, and axial planes in a manner similar to MRI. SPECT is used effectively in the evaluation of osteonecrosis and of pseudoarthrosis following spinal fusion, and in the search for small lesions, such as osteoid osteomas.

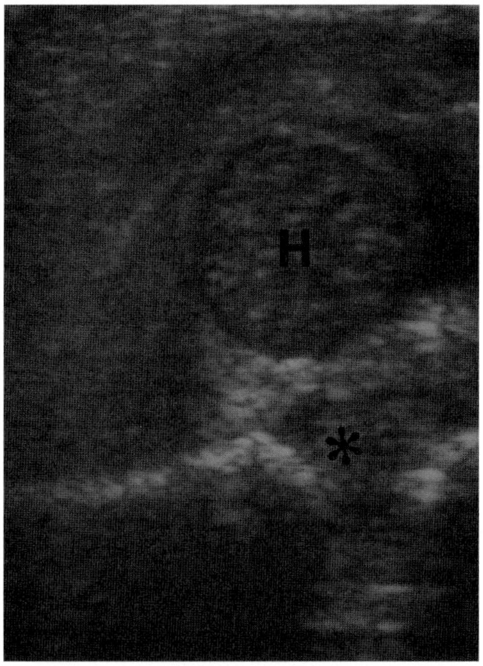

Fig. 3 Ultrasound of the developmental dysplastic hip. Coronal flexion view shows the cartilaginous femoral head dislocated posteriorly, laterally, and slightly superiorly. H = dislocated femoral head. ★ = posterior lip of the acetabulum.

Magnetic Resonance Imaging, Angiography, and Spectroscopy

MRI is the newest and more sophisticated imaging technology. Early after its clinical inception, MRI was used to depict the normal anatomy and pathology of the musculoskeletal system by virtue of its unprecedented soft-tissue contrast resolution and multiplanar imaging capabilities.

MRI is based on the use of magnetic fields, radio frequency (RF) waves, and complex image reconstruction techniques. If an object with abundant protons (eg, the human body) is placed within a high magnetic field, the protons will align themselves with the direction of the magnetic field or against it. Protons have a natural spinning motion at a specific frequency (Larmor frequency). Application of an RF pulse of the same frequency as that of the spinning protons within the magnetic field can deflect the protons from the magnetic field by a specific angle, which depends on the strength of the RF pulse. The protons, now spinning synchronously or coherently at an angle with the magnetic field, can induce a current in a coil or antenna placed nearby. This small signal can then be recorded, amplified, measured, and localized in the space to create a clinically useful image.

Due to existing inhomogeneities of the magnetic field and interactions between adjacent protons, the signal begins to decay as soon as the RF pulse is discontinued. The decaying of the signal is related to two factors: one is the realignment of the protons with the magnetic field, and the other is the loss of coherence or synchrony of the protons as they spin at an angle with the magnetic field. These two phenomena, called relaxation times T1 and T2, respectively, are specific for different types of tissue and their molecular composition; they can be measured independently to create images that depend on different T1 values of the tissues (T1-weighted images) or on different T2 values (T2-weighted images). Images containing T1 and T2 information are called balanced images or proton density (PD)-weighted images.

Contrast between tissues depends on the differences between T1, T2, and PD values on T1-, T2-, or PD-weighted images. These different types of images can be obtained by changing imaging parameters such as the repetition time (TR), echo time (TE), or angle of defection or flip angle (FA). By changing these parameters, it is possible to control the rate of repetition of the RF pulses, the time elapsed between an RF pulse and the production of a signal or echo, and the intensity of the applied RF pulse, which determines the FA. Images obtained using short TR and short TE will produce T1-weighted contrast. Images obtained with long TR and long TE will produce T2-weighted contrast, and images obtained with long TR and short TE will produce PD-weighted contrast. These are the main parameters governing a common pulse sequence design called spin echo (SE). Other clinical useful pulse sequences combine different TRs, TEs, and FAs to provide other types of information, such as blood flow. These are called generically gradient echo pulse sequences. Other sequences use another parameter called inversion time to create images with suppression of the signal intensity (SI) from the fat to enhance contrast between water-rich tissues and fat.

Tissues with high water content (free fluid, edema, infection, effusion, tumors) will show low SI on T1-weighted images and high SI on T2-weighted images. Fat-containing tissues (subcutaneous fat, bone marrow, fat-containing tumors) will demonstrate high SI on T1-weighted and low SI on T2-weighted images and fat suppressed images. Tissues with more than 30% to 40% of calcium content, ligaments, tendons, menisci, and fibrous tissue will demonstrate decreased SI in most pulse sequences. Extravasated blood may show different SIs depending on the location (intra-articular versus intramuscular) and the age of the hemorrhage. Other parameters to take into consideration, when evaluating image contrast and image quality, are the strength of the magnetic field and the use of surface coils. Low field magnets (0.2 Tesla) and medium field magnets (0.5 Tesla) produce less signal than the high field magnets (1.0 to 1.5 Tesla); therefore, image quality is superior at high field strengths. Surface coils are used very frequently in musculoskeletal imaging because they produce significant improvement of the signal-to-noise ratio when imaging small areas such as the joints. Most manufacturers of MRI devices include a variety of surface coils designed for specific joints.

MRI is now being used routinely to evaluate large joints, such as the knee, shoulder, and ankle. In the knee, meniscal tears, anterior cruciate ligament injuries and other soft-tissue lesions can be diagnosed with an accuracy close to 95%. More importantly, occult bone lesions and osteochondral injuries, which are not detectable radiographically or even with arthroscopy, can be diagnosed with confidence. Recent reports of clinical outcomes studies indicate that preoperative MRI evaluation of patients with suspected internal derangement prevented unnecessary surgery in about 50% of the cases.

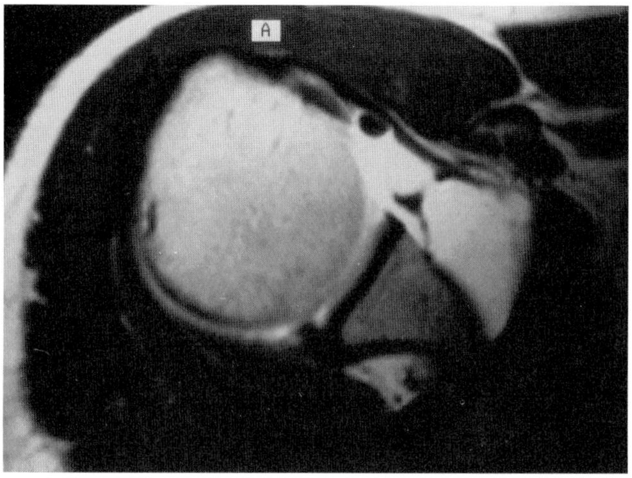

Fig. 4 Magnetic resonance arthrogram of the shoulder in a patient with an anterior superior labral tear. The displaced labrum is attached to the superior glenohumeral ligament.

In imaging of the shoulder, MRI and more recently MR arthrography is considered to be the technique of choice for detection of complete and partial rotator cuff tears, as well as for the evaluation of capsulolabral lesions in patients with glenohumeral joint instability. The addition of intra-articular contrast material (gadolinium-diethylenetriamine pentaacetic acid) has improved the accuracy of MRI in the diagnosis of rotator cuff lesions and capsulolabral lesions (Fig. 4).

In imaging of the ankle, MRI has been also established as an accurate modality to detect osteochondral lesions, tendon tears, and ligamentous injuries. A recent report indicates that the addition of intra-articular contrast improves the sensitivity of MRI in detecting ligamentous tears in patients with chronic ankle pain following injury.

Bone marrow imaging has become one of the most prominent indications for MRI of the musculoskeletal system; its uses include early diagnosis of osteonecrosis of the femoral head, assessment of the presence and extension of osteomyelitis and soft tissue abscesses, detection of non-displaced femoral neck fractures in the elderly, and early diagnosis of bone marrow tumors. Soft-tissue tumor staging is also one of the most important indications for MRI.

Magnetic resonance angiography (MRA) is finding its role as a screening method for problems in the carotid arteries and intracranial circulation, replacing conventional angiography. In the extremities, MRA has been applied with some success to determine patency of the peripheral circulation, based on the principle that MRA is very sensitive to even minimal amounts of flowing blood, which sometimes are not detectable with angiography in distal stenotic arteries (Fig. 5). However, conventional angiography still remains the standard.

One of the latest applications of MRI is in interventional studies. New open magnet designs combined with MR fluoroscopy using ultrafast data acquisition (Echo Planar Imaging, EPI) and nonferromagnetic instrumentation allows performance of MRI-guided procedures, such as biopsies of lesions in the brain and the liver, which are not visualized with other imaging modalities. In the musculoskeletal system, this technique has been used experimentally for MRI guidance to surgically repair meniscal tears.

Finally, magnetic resonance spectroscopy (MRS) of phosphorus and hydrogen using commercial magnets has been extensively investigated for clinical use in the central nervous system, in some metabolic conditions (McArdle syndrome), and in oncology. In the musculoskeletal system, phosphorus spectroscopy has been used to assess tumor response to chemotherapy, mainly in osteosarcoma, demonstrating changes in the phosphomonoesters and phosphodiesters ratio in responding tumors. However, further clinical testing of this technique is necessary before clinical implementation.

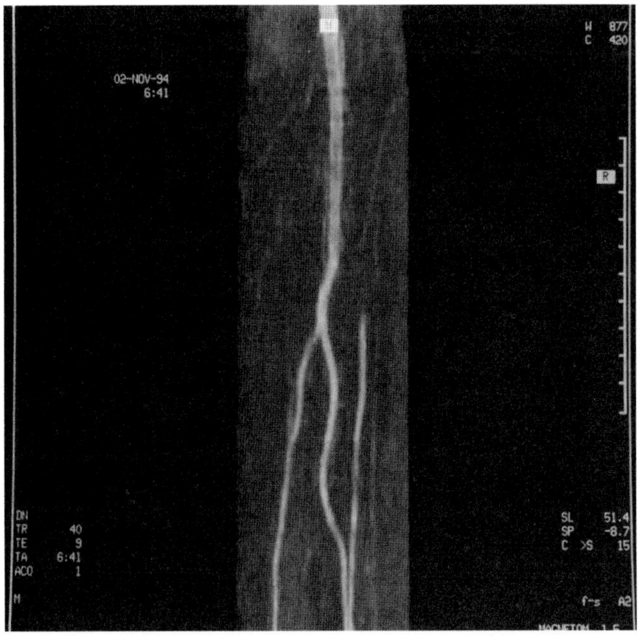

Fig. 5 Magnetic resonance angiogram of the lower extremity. This image was obtained without intravascular injection of contrast material, using the signal produced by the moving protons within the arteries and canceling the signal from the surrounding soft tissues.

Annotated Bibliography

Abiri MM, DeAngelis GA, Kirpekar M, et al: Ultrasonic detection of osteomyelitis: Pathologic correlation in an animal model. *Invest Radiol* 1992;27:111–113.

The authors demonstrated for the first time that very early soft-tissue swelling and periostitis can be shown with US under experimental circumstances. Clinical experience later confirmed their findings.

Blum A, Boyer B, Regent D, et al: Direct coronal view of the shoulder with arthrographic CT. *Radiology* 1993;188: 677–681.

In cases of suspected rotator cuff pathology, where MRI is not available or contraindicated, CT arthrography can replace it. Conventional axial images are limited in showing the rotator cuff pathology. This article describes a new patient position that allows direct oblique coronal CT imaging of the rotator cuff following intra-articular contrast injection.

Chandnani VP, Harper MT, Ficke JR, et al: Chronic ankle instability: Evaluation with MR arthrography, MR imaging, and stress radiography. *Radiology* 1994;192:189–194.

This is the first and only published article comparing the use of three techniques for obtaining images in the same subjects with ligamentous injuries of the ankle and chronic instability. MR arthrography is significantly superior to any other method. The question now is whether the information obtained with MR arthrography will alter treatment or patient outcome.

Heiken, JP, Brink JA, Vannier MW: Spiral (Helical) CT. *Radiology* 1993;189:647–656.

This is one of the more comprehensive reviews of the physics and image reconstruction techniques of spiral CT.

Imamura K, Ashida H, Nakajima H, et al: Reproducibility of magnetic resonance spectroscopy in patients undergoing dialysis and evaluation of the therapeutic response of tumors. *Invest Radiol* 1994;29: 758–765.

The authors address the problem of reproducibility of MRS when data is obtained in different equipment, and using different techniques. MRS is long overdue for its clinical use, beyond the preliminary testing.

Klein MH, Shankman S: Osteoid osteoma: Radiologic and pathologic correlation. *Skeletal Radiol* 1992;21:23–31.

This is an up-to-date review of the radiographic manifestations of osteoid osteoma, with pathological correlation.

Magid D: Computed tomographic imaging of the musculoskeletal system: Current status. *Radiol Clin North Am* 1994;32:255–274.

This review article describes the indications for CT in orthopaedics. Emphasis of the article is placed on postprocessing techniques that allow reconstructions in orthogonal and nonorthogonal planes, as well as 3-D reconstruction techniques.

Rosenthal DI, Alexander A, Rosenberg AE, et al: Ablation of osteoid osteomas with a percutaneously placed electrode: A new procedure. *Radiology* 1992;183: 29–33.

This article describes a new technique for percutaneous ablation of osteoid osteomas using CT guidance. This invasive procedure solves the problem of localization of the nidus in open surgery for this type of tumor.

Spier AS, Meagher T, Ostlere SJ, et al: Can MRI of the knee affect arthroscopic practice? A prospective study of 58 patients. *J Bone Joint Surg* 1993;75B:49–52.

This article addresses the controversy of knee MRI versus diagnostic arthroscopy.

Stewart NR, Gilula LA: CT of the Wrist: A tailored approach. *Radiology* 1992;183:13–20.

This article reviews the different options for CT imaging of the wrist. Up to six different positions of the wrist can be used, allowing excellent visualization of the complex bone anatomy of the wrist, with better detail than conventional tomography.

9

Clinical Epidemiology

Introduction

Clinical epidemiology is the study of the presentation, prognosis, diagnosis, and treatment of disease in groups of patients. It consists of a developed methodology for testing scientific hypotheses in groups of individuals rather than in a laboratory setting. With knowledge of the intrinsic strengths and limitations of the design and execution of studies reported in the literature, the orthopaedic surgeon can evaluate the strength of the evidence derived from these studies and can usually make sense of apparently conflicting results from different studies on the same topic. This chapter is an overview of basic terminology used in epidemiology with emphasis on clinical epidemiology.

There are several types of epidemiologic studies. Descriptive epidemiology is a means of monitoring the health of a population, identifying health problems, and developing information that can be used for the development of causal hypotheses. Analytic epidemiology is the use of epidemiologic study methods to test specific hypotheses, regarding either disease causality or efficacy or effectiveness of prevention, treatment, or rehabilitation, and validity of screening and diagnostic procedures.

Measures of Disease Frequency

Epidemiologic data consist essentially of relative and absolute measures of disease frequency and the characteristics of individuals with and without disease in the population of interest. The most obvious measures of frequency of diseases or disorders in a population are case counts and their variations, which are often referred to as numerator data because they describe the frequency of the disorder without reference to the population at risk or the background against which the cases arise. In population health studies, the case count may be derived from cases of diseases reported to a health agency by office practitioners, from administrative records of hospital admissions or surgical procedures, or from insurance claim records. In clinical practice, the case count is usually derived by a review of charts (retrospectively) or by enrollment of patients seen during a given period (prospectively).

The number of cases of a disorder can be a useful indicator of the demand placed by the disorder on the health care system. Proportionate ratios can provide useful information about the importance of a particular disorder among all disorders of a given type in the population. Without being related to the population at risk, however, these numerator data cannot provide useful information regarding the risk or probability of acquiring the disorder. Without information about the characteristics of the population or, at least, comparison to the characteristics of people without the disorder, descriptions of the characteristics of those with the disorder do not provide sufficient information to test hypotheses about disease causality. For instance, approximately 250,000 hip fractures occur annually in the United States. Without reference to the number of people at risk, it is not possible to estimate the risk of hip fracture in the population or to test hypotheses regarding risk factors for hip fracture. Therefore, rates are used to express disease frequency when the objective is to assess risk of disease or determinants of diseases or their outcomes. Knowledge of how rates can be interpreted is essential to understanding clinical epidemiology.

Rates describe the frequency of a disease or disorder per unit size of the population per unit time of observation. Morbidity and mortality rates are commonly used in epidemiology. The general form of a morbidity or mortality rate is:

$$\frac{\text{Number of cases}}{\text{Number of persons at risk}} \times \begin{array}{l}100\ (1{,}000,\ \text{etc})\\ \text{per unit time}\end{array}$$

Everyone in the numerator is included in the denominator, and everyone in the denominator has a chance to get into the numerator. The rate is usually expressed with reference to a standard number of persons (eg, per 100, per 1,000, etc). A rate of N cases per 100 persons per year is alternatively a rate of N percent per year.

Mortality rates express the number of deaths per unit population per time period and morbidity rates express the number of cases of a disease or disorder per unit population per time period. The most frequently used morbidity rates in epidemiologic research are the incidence rate and the prevalence rate. The incidence rate is based on new cases of a disease or disorder (or new disease events), whereas the prevalence rate is based on existing cases. Therefore, incidence and prevalence rates have different uses and different limitations.

In a sense, the incidence rate is a rate of change, the frequency with which people change from the nondiseased to the diseased state. Thus, the appropriate denominator is the population at risk of acquiring the disease (ie, nondiseased at the start of the time interval). The incidence rate may be quantified, for example, as the number of new events per 1,000 persons per year, when the population is stable and the number of new events is counted each year. Alternatively, it may be quantified as the number of new events per 1,000 person-years, as is done in prospective studies in which a fixed population is followed until acquiring the disease, the end of the study, or loss to follow-up. Another form of incidence rate is the cumulative probability of acquiring a disease; for example, a population of a particular age is followed up through an older age and the total frequency of new cases of the disease expressed. Although the best denominator for incidence rates is the number of people disease-free at the start of the time interval, public-health incidence (and prevalence) rates, which are based on vital statistics or hospital admissions, often use the total population derived from census data.

The prevalence rate is the number of existing cases of disease in a given population in a given time period. Point prevalence is the number of cases per unit population at one moment of counting; for example, all hospitalized cases of hip fracture in New York State on January 1, 1995, expressed per 1,000 population. For point prevalence, because the period of time is effectively instantaneous, the unit of time is often not expressed. Period prevalence is the number of cases existing at one time or another during a definable time interval, such as 1-year, 5-year, or lifetime prevalence. Some epidemiologists do not express prevalence as a rate because in practice it is often derived from surveys, which are difficult to assign to a specific time interval.

The astute reader is always aware that a number of factors other than the actual frequency of a disease in a population may affect the incidence and prevalence rates. These include demographic characteristics of the underlying population, the most obvious of which is age distribution, because age is known to be associated with the onset of almost all diseases. Gender and ethnicity distributions must also be taken into account when interpreting incidence rates. Health-care system influences, which affect the likelihood of coming to medical attention, of being diagnosed with a given disease or disorder, or of having the disorder reported, can distort the apparent incidence rate and should be considered when evaluating these measures of disease frequency, particularly when assessing changes over time or when comparing different populations.

An important consideration when constructing or interpreting measures of disease frequency or estimates of risk is the influence of individual and environmental factors on the risk of disease. The most obvious factors are age, sex, ethnicity, socioeconomic status, education, income, occupation, and place of residence. Indeed, the importance of age, sex, and ethnicity are so prominent that crude morbidity rates (simple number of cases over the population per unit time) are not adequate for comparisons of disease frequency in different populations or for evaluating changes in disease frequency over time. To eliminate the effects of differences in age, sex, or ethnicity on a comparison of morbidity rates in two or more populations, the rates may be adjusted or standardized algebraically. Essentially, the adjusted rates express the risk of acquiring the disease in the populations if they had the same age, sex, and ethnicity distributions. Alternatively, if it is not necessary to have a single summary index of disease risk, the morbidity rates within population strata defined by age, sex, and ethnicity may be compared.

The number of existing cases of a disease or disorder at any time is a function of both the rate of new cases (incidence) and the duration of that disorder. Thus, when a population is stable and the duration of a disorder is also stable, it is possible to estimate prevalence from incidence and vice versa according to the following approximation:

$$\text{Prevalence} \approx \text{Incidence} \times \text{Duration}$$

Thus, a change in prevalence may reflect changes in incidence rate or of duration or of both. It is occasionally the case that improved treatment will paradoxically extend the duration of a disorder, as occurred some decades ago when the prevalence of Down syndrome was observed to be increasing although the incidence was declining as a result of prenatal screening programs. Survival of Down syndrome infants had improved due to improved medical and surgical management of their associated disorders.

Descriptive Epidemiology

The first step often undertaken in epidemiology is the development of the descriptive epidemiology of a disease or disorder. Descriptive epidemiology supports the development of causal hypotheses but does not in itself support conclusions about disease causality or about any hypotheses. In descriptive epidemiology, the frequency of a disorder in the population is characterized in terms of person (age, sex, ethnicity-specific incidence rates, economic, behavioral, occupational, and other factors), place (rural versus urban, type of housing, national variations, type of industry), and time (long-term trend, seasonality, occasionally day of week or time of day). In classic epidemiology, causal hypotheses are developed based on inductive reasoning from the descriptive epidemiology and available information regarding anatomy, pathology, physiology, and so forth. Specific hypotheses are developed and tested by means of analytic studies. As the results of hypothesis-testing (analytic) studies are accrued, they are added to the base for causal inference, depending on their strengths and generalizability, and hypotheses are supported, modified, or negated.

In interpreting the evidence from all scientific sources, rules of causal inference are applied. The orthopaedist may find them useful when evaluating epidemiologic data. Briefly, the hypothesized cause must be demonstrated to have preceded the disease by a length of time sufficient to allow disease development and expression (time sequence of events). The disease should be more common in those with the hypothesized cause than in those without it (increased risk in those exposed to the hypothesized cause), and as the intensity or duration of exposure to the hypothesized cause increases, the frequency of the disease should increase (dose-response relationship). The association between the hypothesized causal factor and the disease should be consistently demonstrated in methodologically sound studies and should be biologically plausible. In addition, the specificity of an association (the extent to which the hypothesized causal factor is associated with only one disease or disorder) lends additional weight to a causal hypothesis, but is not necessary to causal inference; for example, cigarette smoking is accepted as a cause of lung cancer, although the association is not specific. Cigarette smoking is also associated with a number of other cancers, with obstructive pulmonary disease, heart disease, and a variety of musculoskeletal and other disorders.

Analytic Epidemiology

Analytic, or hypothesis-testing epidemiology, relies on two types of study designs: observational and interventional. In observational study designs, exposure to the hypothesized causal factor and development of the disease in the population under study occur in the natural course of events; the investigator does not cause them to occur. The study is designed and executed to maximize the extent to which it can be seen as a natural experiment, ie, the extent to which all extraneous sources of variation are eliminated and only the exposure to the putative cause and the frequency of disease vary between populations being compared. Observational studies are the first undertaken in etiologic epidemiology and it is often the case that, once a substantial weight of observational evidence is accrued, causality is widely accepted, as in the case of smoking and lung cancer. However, it is desirable in etiologic epidemiology and almost universally required in evaluations of treatment in clinical epidemiology that the final test of the hypothesis be in interventional or experimental studies. The hallmark of the experimental study is that the investigator causes individuals or groups of individuals in the population to be exposed to the hypothesized causal factor or to receive the treatment in question. All other factors that might influence the outcome of the study (potential confounding factors) can be eliminated or controlled by the investigator. Because the conditions of the study are much more under the control of the investigator, interventional studies can much more closely approximate true experiments than can observational studies, and when well designed and executed they provide very strong support (or negation) for a hypothesis.

All the analytic study designs present intrinsic problems of internal and external validity that must be solved by the investigator either in the study design or data analysis. The extent to which these problems are solved contributes to the strength of the evidence. Internal validity is the extent to which a study is a true test of the specific hypothesis, that is, the extent to which all possible biases of measurement or information and all possible confounding variables are eliminated as explanations of the observed study result. External validity is the extent to which the study results are generalizable to the population of interest, that is, the extent to which the study subjects are representative of the population at risk.

Because it is not possible to study the entire universe of potentially eligible subjects, epidemiologic studies are conducted on samples of the population of interest. Even an entire city or the workforce of a company constitutes a sample of a larger population. It is essential for internal validity that no selection biases are introduced by the method of sampling. For example, if the study is made up of volunteers, it is potentially susceptible to selection biases, because the health behaviors and health status of people who volunteer for research are well documented to be better than those of refusers. The optimum method of sampling is a probability, or random sample, in which only chance affects whether an individual is selected for study. No characteristics of the individuals, such as their knowledge of the question at issue, their beliefs about the risk factors or about the cause of the disease being studied, or any characteristic such as age, sex, education, and so forth, which could be independently associated with both the disease and the hypothesized causal factor, affect the likelihood of selection for the study.

It is important for the internal validity of the study results that the information collected be accurate and complete. If there is inaccuracy (measurement error) in the information collected, the ability to detect the association of interest will be reduced. If the accuracy of information is worse for one exposure group than for another, the effect on the study results may not be predictable. For this reason, an evaluation of the accuracy (or validity) of measurements is necessary for any study. A number of ways to improve validity of measurements have been described. When reading an article, the clinician may look for descriptions of the reliability or validity of the information, for indications that the information was collected using questionnaires or reporting methods validated in the study population or in similar populations or circumstances, or for study design methods intended to reduce measurement or classification error (misclassification) in the study.

Confounding occurs when the study results, eg, an increase in risk of the disease in the presence of a hypothesized causal factor, can be explained by variation in a factor extraneous to the hypothesis. A potential confounding factor must be associated with both the disease in question and the hypothesized causal factor. That is, the probability of disease and the probability of exposure to the causal factor must be different depending on the presence or absence of the potential confounding variable. Potential confounding factors can be eliminated in the design of the study, for example by restricted or stratified or matched sampling, or in the data analysis phases, for example by stratified or multivariate analysis. In experimental studies, potential confounding should be successfully eliminated by truly random blind assignment of subjects to the different treatments under study.

Confounding is a problem of internal, rather than external, validity. The confounding variable makes the study not a true test of the hypothesis (absence of internal valid-

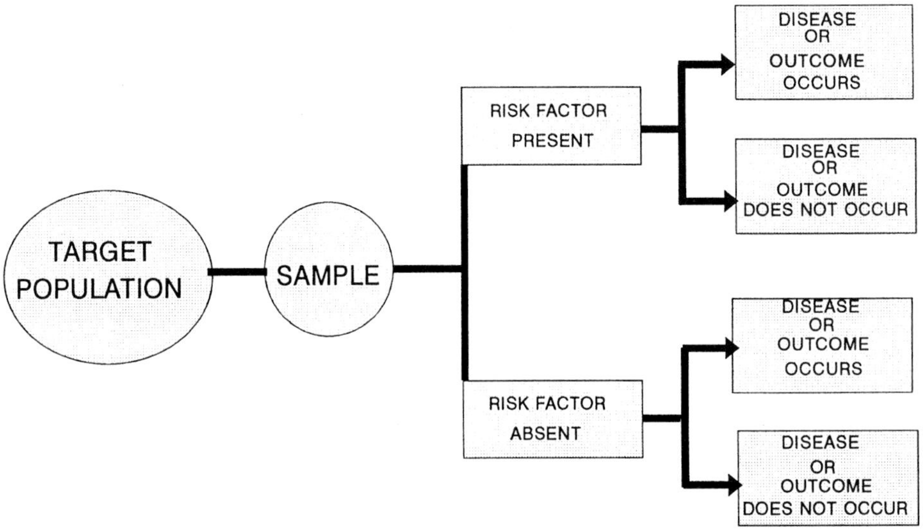

Fig. 1 Cohort study flow chart.

ity). The study's results cannot be taken as evidence of causality or of efficacy of treatment. Lack of generalizability does not invalidate a study's results, but merely means that inference can only be made with respect to populations similar to those under study. Nevertheless, a study's findings are not confounded by the lack of generalizability.

Observational Study Designs

These study designs are applicable in both clinical and etiologic epidemiology; in etiologic epidemiology the investigator tests whether a hypothesized factor is a determinant or cause of disease development in previously healthy people, whereas in clinical epidemiology the investigator tests whether particular characteristics, risk factors, or clinical interventions are determinants of the disease prognosis or outcome in diseased individuals. The classic observational analytic study designs are the cohort study, the case-control study, and the cross-sectional study.

Cohort Study

The cohort study (sometimes called a prospective study) is the design which, when well designed and executed, produces the soundest results in terms of disease etiology of all the observational study designs. In an etiologic cohort study, a nondiseased population is identified and characterized with respect to the hypothesized risk factor, important covariates, and potential confounders. The population is observed for a period of time adequate for disease development, and the new cases of disease (incident cases) are recorded. Because it may take decades for disease to develop, cohort studies are often undertaken by identifying subjects based on existing documentation of their health status and past exposure to the causal factor and ascertaining subsequent exposure and development of disease in the more recent past or in the near future. This type of cohort study is called a historic, or retrospective, cohort study, because at least the exposure and possibly the disease events happened before the study was conducted. When the subjects are enrolled at the time of onset of disease exposure and followed forward in time, the cohort study may be referred to as a follow-up or prospective cohort study (Fig. 1).

Loss to follow-up is a potential problem in cohort studies. If a substantial proportion of subjects are lost to the study for any reason; for example, having moved out of the region, it would be expected that fewer cases of the disease in question would arise in the study than originally planned. The number of study cases may ultimately be too small to yield stable estimates of the incidence rates and, consequently, of the relative risk. When loss to follow-up is selective, it will distort the study results. For example, consider a cohort study examining the causal role of occupational repetitive motion in carpal tunnel syndrome. New workers hired in 1965 to 1970 are enrolled and followed for 25 years, with information on new cases of carpal tunnel syndrome coming from the company medical department records. If 30% of the workers retire, take disability pensions, die, get another job, or leave the company for other reasons, there is a substantial loss to follow-up. Furthermore, if the workers who leave the company are those with the highest exposure to repetitive work movements and if they leave because upper extremity problems consistent with preclinical carpal tunnel syndrome make it more difficult for them to do the job, a bias in loss to follow-up occurs. The observed relative risk is an underestimate of the true relative risk, because the detected incidence of carpal tunnel syndrome among those with repetitive motion jobs is lower than the true incidence, while the detected incidence among the unexposed is not affected. If there have been high proportions lost to follow-up, or higher proportions lost in one exposure category than the other (selective loss to follow-up), biased loss to follow-up with its consequent distortion of the study findings may have occurred.

Another form of selection bias, called selective survival or selective attrition, occurs when people who have both the exposure and the disease have a different probability of dropping out of the population available to be included in the study than do people who are not exposed and get the disease. This type of bias can easily occur in cross-sectional and case-control studies. It can also occur in a particular variant of the cohort study called the prevalent cohort study. For example, a prevalent cohort study examining occupational repetitive motion as a risk factor for carpal tunnel syndrome, which enrolled workers who were first employed between 1965 and 1970 and were still actively employed in 1995, could be affected by selective attrition if carpal tunnel syndrome by and large developed within 15 years of employment, and workers tended to leave the company when they developed it.

Because most diseases or conditions are relatively uncommon or take a long time to develop, cohort studies require enrollment of a large number of subjects who may need years of follow-up. Outcome studies in which the outcome of interest is rare or develops long after the intervention present similar requirements. It can be more efficient in terms of time and number of subjects studied to address the hypothesis by means of a case-control study.

Case-control Study

The essential differentiating feature of the case-control study is that individuals are selected for the study on the basis of the presence of the disease or disorder in question (cases) and compared to individuals selected for the study on the basis of the absence of the disease under study (controls). The presence or absence of the hypothesized causal factor is then ascertained in both case and control subjects (Fig. 2). Although this appears on its face to be a simple undertaking, the case-control study presents a number of methodologic challenges that must be solved in order for the study results to be valid.

One of the principal problems possible in case-control studies occurs when cases and controls do not have comparable exposure opportunity. For example, if in a case-control study of age as a predictor of spinal stenosis, cases with spinal stenosis were identified from Medicare claims and controls were identified from workplace medical facility records, cases and controls would be of different ages because of the way they were selected. It would, therefore, not be possible to assign causality to an association of age and spinal stenosis observed in such a study.

Case-control studies frequently suffer from information biases such as recall bias, in which a case subject is more or less likely to recall an event in the past than is a control subject. There is also the problem of recall failure, which can occur when subjects are asked to recall events or conditions that took place long ago. Establishing that the exposure to the factor of interest took place long enough before the outcome to be a biologically plausible determinant is difficult for certain types of hypotheses. Both of these types of problems are avoided if the case-control study uses exposure or prognostic information that was recorded (for example in medical or prescription records) prior to the development of the disease in question.

Because of the difficulty in avoiding the problems described above, case-control studies often produce weaker causal evidence than do cohort studies. However, well-designed and well-executed case-control studies, which avoid the problems described above, can provide evidence as robust as that of cohort studies at considerably less cost and in considerably less time.

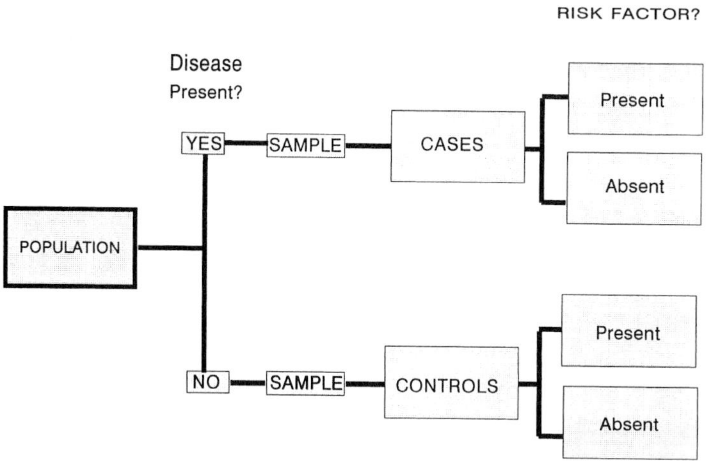

Fig. 2 Case-control study.

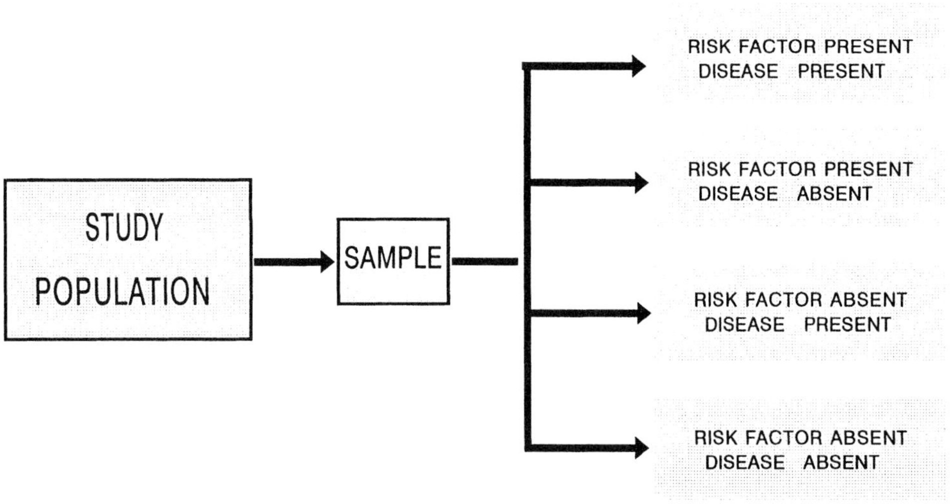

Fig. 3 Cross-sectional study.

Cross-sectional Study

The hallmark of cross-sectional studies is that they simultaneously ascertain exposure to risk factors (or presence of prognostic factors) and presence of the disease (disorder, outcome) in question in a population sampled without regard to the presence of either. This type of sampling is sometimes called naturalistic sampling. In contrast to the cohort study, which follows subjects over time and ascertains incidence, the cross-sectional study ascertains conditions present at the moment of study, that is, the prevalence of the disorders (Fig. 3). The estimates of relative risk derived from cross-sectional studies are, therefore, estimates of prevalence relative risk and are susceptible to distortion by such biases as selective survival or attrition prior to the study, changes in exposure status prior to the study, and others.

Cross-sectional, or survey, studies are often undertaken because, unlike case-control studies, they require few *a priori* decisions with regard to selection of subjects, and, unlike cohort studies, it is not necessary to wait for the study outcome. These advantages are, however, offset by the fact that cross-sectional studies are susceptible to some of the problems of both cohort and case-control studies. When uncommon diseases or exposures are being studied, a large number of people must be included, as in cohort studies. If information on exposures or on determinants of interest is collected at the time of the study rather than from previously existing records, there can be recall biases, recall failure, and problems in establishing the time sequence of events, as in case-control studies. Nevertheless, for relatively common disorders (outcomes) and risk factors (determinants), cross-sectional studies may be a useful first step in exploring a hypothesis. Because of their many limitations, however, cross-sectional studies rarely produce robust results for evaluating the importance of causal or prognostic factors. When the literature on a problem consists predominantly of cross-sectional studies, it is often the case that the analytic epidemiology of that problem is in its infancy.

The intrinsic strengths and limitations of the basic observational study designs are summarized in Table 1. The extent to which a specific study overcomes its intrinsic limitations and embodies the intrinsic strengths of its design, the more robust the evidence from that study.

Interventional (Experimental) Study Designs: Clinical Trials

The distinction between observational and interventional study designs in etiologic and clinical epidemiology is that in observational designs the investigator does not cause the exposure to the causal factor or treatment for the purposes of the study, whereas in the interventional designs, the investigator does cause subjects to be exposed to different factors or treatments. The observational study designs are susceptible to treatment assignment biases in which the treatment the patients receive is influenced by certain patient characteristics (for example, lifestyle or clinical severity) that can confound the results. Treatment trials in which the treating physicians or the investigators control the treatments patients receive are also susceptible to such biases. For this reason, randomized control clinical trials, in which only chance influences which treatment eligible patients receive, are the standard for evaluating therapeutic interventions.

The validity of randomized control trials (RCTs) depends on all the methodologic features described for the observational study designs and more. The study must be confined to those patients who have agreed to participate. Comparisons of treatment outcomes in patients who agree to participate with those in patients who refuse to partici-

Table 1. Strengths and limitations of the observational study designs

	Cohort Study*	Case-control Study*	Cross-sectional Study*
Selective survival	+	−	−
Recall bias	+	−	−
Loss to follow-up	−	+	+
Time sequence of events	+	−	−
Time to complete	−	+	+
Expense	−	+	+/−

*+ = Strength; − = Limitation

pate are not valid. The assignment of patients to treatments must use accepted methods of randomization, which are described in the report, and the resulting comparability of the treatment groups on important covariates should be described, usually in a table summarizing baseline characteristics of the treatment groups. On the occasions when randomization, by chance, does not result in comparable groups, potential confounding must be controlled in the statistical analysis. Figure 4 is a schematic representation of appropriate design in an RCT.

Ordinarily, in randomized trials, the treating physician and the patient should be blind to treatment assignment. Because blinded randomization is not possible in trials of surgical techniques, an independent investigator should assess the study outcome, in order to avoid observer (treating surgeon) biases. This technique is particularly important when the outcome being assessed is subjective. Information should be collected in the same way and with the same frequency in all treatments groups. Eligibility and exclusion criteria should be described and appropriate to the question being addressed. Treatments should be clearly described, and patient compliance, dropouts from the study, and complications should be equivalent in both groups. Finally, the outcomes studied should be appropriate to the treatment or condition in question. Ideally, outcome assessment should go beyond immediate or even short-term assessment of surgical success (eg, by radiologic imaging, measurement of range of motion) and should include measurement of improvement in functional status and quality of life 1 or more years after the surgical intervention. There are a number of general health status assessment measures, such as the SF-36, a standardized multidimensional assessment including functional capacity, pain, locomotion, mental status, and affect. In addition, there are standardized assessment instruments for specific conditions, such as the Oswestry functional disability assessment for back pain.

On occasions when surgeons strongly prefer one surgical technique over another and are more proficient in one technique than the other, it has been suggested to assemble a group of surgeons with proficiency in different techniques and to randomize patients to different surgeons who perform surgery by their preferred technique. When well designed and executed, this randomization can allow comparability of the patients receiving surgery by the different methods being compared, while avoiding confounding by surgeons' skills and avoiding ethical dilemmas for the participating surgeons.

Statistical Issues

Methods of Analysis

The statistical analysis of any study result should be appropriate to the hypothesis and to the structure of the data collected. When the study examines, for instance, the difference in Harris hip scores in patients with two different methods of total hip arthroplasty, comparisons of the mean scores in the treatment groups may be appropriate. If it is necessary to control for pretreatment differences between the groups, the analysis will use multivariate methods, such as analysis of covariance or multiple regression. Occasionally, because of the statistical characteristics

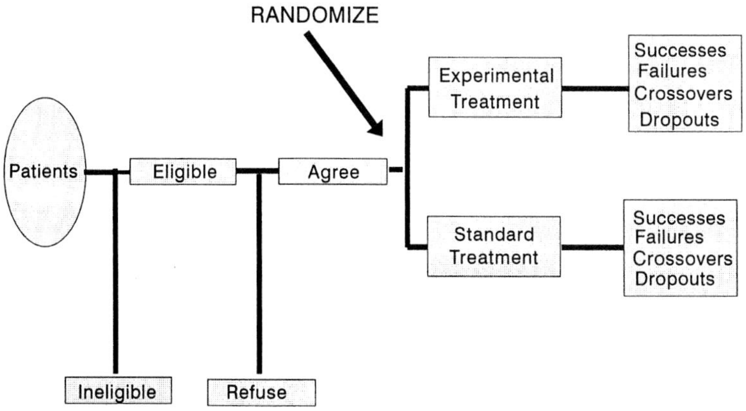

Fig. 4 Randomized controlled trial.

of the outcome being assessed, it may be necessary to transform it (eg, log transformation, square root transformation) and analyze the transformed variable. It is often the case that the outcome variable distribution or the conditions of the study do not conform to the requirements of the usual statistical hypothesis tests such as *t*-tests, analysis of covariance, and regression analysis. In these cases, a nonparametric method of statistical analysis, such as the Wilcoxon method, is appropriate.

When the hypothesis addresses the relative frequency of an event, such as a success rate or a patient mortality rate, the relative incidence of the event in the subjects exposed and those not exposed to the factor of interest is evaluated. A ratio of the incidence rates, called the relative risk, is used to express the association. The larger the relative risk, the stronger the observed association and the stronger the evidence in favor of the research hypothesis. A relative risk of one indicates no effect of the hypothesized causal factor on risk of disease. The relative risk may be adjusted for important covariates or to eliminate potential confounding. There are other statistics that estimate the relative risk. The odds ratio, the ratio of the odds of the disease in the exposed to the odds of disease in the unexposed, provides a good estimate of the relative risk in cohort studies. It also has valuable statistical properties because it can be estimated using logistic regression. The effects of confounding variables can be controlled or the simultaneous effects of several causal variables or covariates can be estimated using multiple logistic regression.

Another way of estimating risk of disease in cohort studies is to estimate the instantaneous probability of acquiring disease at each moment of follow-up over time. The cumulative probability of acquiring the disease is often displayed as a failure–time curve and expressed as the cumulative hazard. The cumulative probability of acquiring disease in the exposed and the unexposed can be similarly displayed; the hazard ratio is an estimate of the relative risk of acquiring the disease. In prognostic or outcome studies, the failure–time curve may be interpreted as a survival curve, so that the hazard ratio is an estimate of the relative risk of death or of recovery associated with the prognostic factor in question. Cox proportional hazards regression, which can be used when there are several predictor variables of interest or when potential confounders must be controlled, is a method of estimating the simultaneous effects of multiple variables.

An advantage of survival analysis is that each study subject contributes information for as long as he or she remains in the study. However, if dropouts during the course of the study are substantial, the estimates of the hazard ratio toward the end of the follow-up period are based on relatively small numbers and are consequently unstable. Furthermore, if dropout is selective, the study results will be distorted.

Estimates and Confidence Limits

Research is conducted on a sample of persons or other units of observation drawn from a target population. The results of any given study, such as the mean difference in Harris hip scores between two groups of patients, the proportions of patients recovering to prefracture ambulatory capacity, or the relative mortality rates of older compared to younger hip fracture patients, are estimates of the true means, proportions, relative risks, and so forth in the population from which the samples were drawn. The precision of a study estimate of the population value, or parameter of a measurement, is described by the standard error of the estimate. The standard error (S.E.) is the square root of the ratio of the variance (s^2), or variability of the measurement in the sample to the number of subjects (N) in the study. For example,

$$\text{S.E.}_{\text{Mean}} = \sqrt{\frac{s^2}{N}}$$

Variance is affected by a number of factors, including interindividual variability, intraindividual variability, such as diurnal variations, and instrument variability. Designing or executing a study to reduce any of these components will reduce the variance of the measurement, thus reducing the standard error and increasing the stability of the estimate of the population parameter. The larger the number of subjects on whom the estimate is based, the smaller the standard error and the more confident it is possible to be in its representation of the population parameter.

Because sample results are estimates of population parameters, it is becoming more and more the standard of reporting to describe the precision of the estimates as a range within which the population parameter probably lies. This is the confidence limit around the estimate, and is by convention expressed as the 95% confidence limit. For example, the 95% confidence limit for a mean is approximated by

$$95\%\ \text{Confidence Interval} = \text{Mean} \pm 1.96\ \text{S.E.}_{\text{Mean}}$$

Statistical Hypothesis Testing

Clinical research is conducted on samples of patients, and the resulting observed relative risks (or differences between treatment groups) are estimates of the true magnitude of an association in the population. Because there is always sampling error, the estimates may be expected to vary from sample to sample. Consequently, study results must be subjected to statistical hypothesis testing, that is, they must be tested to determine the probability that the observed results from a specific study could have occurred by chance alone.

The statistical hypothesis test evaluates the null hypothesis that the observed study results occurred because of sampling error when there was no true association in the population from which the study subjects were sampled. The probability of making this type of error is designated as Alpha. If the observed association is large enough that this kind of error is improbable, the null hypothesis is rejected. The investigators then accept the alternative hypothesis, that the observed estimates of relative risk or differences between treatments reflect the true situation in the population from which the samples were drawn. By convention, the cutoff of Alpha for rejecting the null hypothesis is usually set at 0.05. If the probability (p value) that the observed results are due to sampling error is less than 0.05, that is, less than Alpha, the null hypothesis is rejected, and the results are declared statistically significant. Thus, statistically significant results are simply results that, within an acceptable margin of error, probably did not occur by chance. Further, the larger the observed association relative to the underlying variability of the outcome being measured, the more likely that it will be declared statistically significant.

Statistical Power and Sample Size

Statistical hypothesis tests actually involve two probabilities. Alpha is the probability of making the Type I error by incorrectly rejecting the null hypothesis, or declaring an observed association statistically significant when in fact it is the result of sampling error. Beta is the probability of making the Type II error by incorrectly accepting the null hypothesis, or declaring that the study results are due to sampling error (not statistically significant) when in fact they reflect a true association in the population from which the study subjects were drawn. The complementary probability that a study will be able to correctly reject the null hypothesis when it is false, that is, to detect an association when there is one in the population at large, is referred to as statistical power (1 − Beta). Table 2 illustrates the different conditions and possible results of a statistical hypothesis test.

In the planning phase of clinical research, the investigators should determine how strong an association, ie, how large an estimated relative risk or how big a difference between treatments, would be clinically significant. Because validity of the study requires that it be a true test of the research hypothesis, it is important to design the study so that a clinically significant association will have a good chance of being declared statistically significant, ie, so that the study has sufficient power to detect a clinically significant association. The larger the sample size, the more power the statistical test has to detect associations; in other words, as expected differences or relative risks get smaller, the number of subjects studied has to increase in order to have adequate power to test the hypothesis. Conversely, with very large numbers of study subjects, it is possible to declare trivial associations statistically significant.

Table 2. Conditions in the population, statistical hypothesis tests, and types of errors

	Population	
Test	**Null Hypothesis True (No Association)**	**Null Hypothesis False (Association Exists)**
Accept null hypothesis (No association)	Correct	(Beta) Type II error
Reject null hypothesis (Association exists)	(Alpha) Type I error	Correct

When results that were not statistically significant are reported for studies with small sample sizes, the authors should comment on how strong the association would have had to be to have good power to detect it. The reader should also evaluate whether the observed difference and its upper confidence limit, although not statistically significant, are clinically significant. When statistically significant results are reported for studies with huge numbers of subjects, the reader should decide if the differences are clinically trivial, even though statistically significant.

Conclusion

The validity of clinical research relies on a number of factors. The hypothesis must be formulated specifically enough to be testable. The appropriate study subjects should be eligible, and there should not be differential participation. The information collected should be appropriate to the hypothesis and accurate. The study design and information sources should avoid potential information biases. Potential confounders should be eliminated in the study design or controlled in the statistical analysis. At the time the study is designed, a clinically significant hypothesized result should be defined, the plan of statistical analysis determined, and the necessary number of study subjects defined. Study management should avoid the introduction of differential loss to follow-up, unblinding, and other potential problems. The statistical analysis should be appropriate to the structure of the data and to the hypothesis. Finally, although the discussion should place the study in the context of other work and what is already known about the question, the specific conclusions should not go beyond what was actually tested in the study.

Annotated Bibliography

American Academy of Orthopaedic Surgeons, Department of Research: *Fundamentals of Outcome Research.* Rosemont, IL, American Academy of Orthopaedic Surgeons, 1993.

This collection of papers describes the development, methodologic state of the art, and future directions in outcomes research in orthopaedics. It includes descriptions of instruments for outcomes assessment in different orthopaedic problems.

Deyo RA, Andersson G, Bombardier C, et al: Outcome measures for studying patients with low back pain. *Spine* 1994;18(suppl):S2032–S2036.

This is a description of the validity of health-related quality of life instruments with attention to their applicability for outcome studies in back pain.

Elston RC, Johnson WD: *Essentials of Biostatistics,* ed 2. Philadelphia, PA, FA Davis, 1994.

This is an excellent introductory biostatistics text, written at a level understandable to most readers. It includes a section on critical evaluation of published reports.

Fleiss JL: *The Design and Analysis of Clinical Experiments.* New York, NY, John Wiley & Sons, 1986.

This excellent text concentrates on the statistical issues in clinical trials, including reliability of measurement, variations on the basic two-group design, and statistical methods such as linear regression, analysis of variance, covariance, and repeated measurements, controlling for prognostic variables, sample size determination, and other topics.

Friedman LM, Furberg CD, DeMets DL: *Fundamentals of Clinical Trials,* ed 2. Littletown, MA, PSG Publishing, 1985.

This overview of methods in clinical trials, from defining the question through study planning and management, data analysis and reporting results, is somewhat more detailed than the Hulley text.

Gardner MJ, Altman DG: Confidence intervals rather than p values: Estimation rather than hypothesis testing. *Br Med J* 1986;292:746–750.

The authors present an argument for designing studies to estimate the magnitude of associations (relative risks, mean differences, etc.) with precision (confidence intervals) rather than merely to test whether or not there are associations (*p* values).

Hulley SB, Cummings SR: *Designing Clinical Research: An Epidemiologic Approach.* Baltimore, MD, Williams & Wilkins, 1988.

This is a very readable guide to all phases of research planning and execution. It contains accessible tabular and graphic presentation of important concepts and examples from published studies. It includes all aspects of research design and execution, grant proposal preparation, and appendices with examples of different phases of research design, statistical tables, and randomization procedures.

Morton RF, Hebel JR, McCarter RJ: *A Study Guide to Epidemiology and Biostatistics,* ed 3. Rockville, MD, Aspen Publishers, 1990.

This review guide includes exercises. It is basic.

Rudicel S, Esdaile J: The randomized clinical trial in orthopaedics: Obligation or option? *J Bone Joint Surg* 1985;67A:1294–1297.

This is a discussion of implementation problems in orthopaedic clinical trials, with presentation of randomization to surgeons performing their preferred techniques rather than to different techniques by the same surgeon.

Shekelle PG, Andersson G, Bombardier C, et al: A brief introduction to critical reading of the clinical literature. *Spine* 1994;18(suppl):S2028–S2031.

This is a brief, practical guide to reading the literature with attention to applicability of the results in a physician's own practice.

Troidl H, Spitzer WO, McPeek B, et al: *Principles and Practice of Research: Strategies for Surgical Investigators,* ed 2. New York, NY, Springer-Verlag, 1991.

This is a thorough treatment of research methods, including clinical and animal research, from the surgical perspective. It includes sections on planning, executing, and reporting research, and sections on reliability and validity of measurement.

Classic Bibliography

Altman DC: Analysing data. *Br Med J* 1981;281:1473–1475.

Altman DC: Collecting and screening data. *Br Med J* 1981;281:1399–1401.

Altman DC: How large a sample? *Br Med J* 1981;281: 1336–1338.

Altman DC: Improving the quality of statistics in medical journals. *Br Med J* 1982;282:44–47.

Altman DC: Interpreting results. *Br Med J* 1981;281: 1612–1614.

Altman DC: Misuse of statistics is unethical. *Br Med J* 1981;281:1182–1184.

Altman DC: Presentation of results. *Br Med J* 1981;281: 1542–1544.

Altman DC: Study design. *Br Med J* 1981;281:1201–1203.

Sackett DL: How to read clinical journals: Why to read them and how to start reading them critically. *CMAJ* 1981;124:555–558.

10

Practice Guidelines

Practice guidelines have been given a number of names such as practice parameters, clinical policies, and clinical guidelines. Three important questions must be asked of every guideline: (1) To what extent does the guideline represent a standard of care versus suggestions or options for care? (2) How was the guideline developed? and (3) How has the guideline been evaluated and implemented?

Standards Versus Options

Most guidelines are written so they will not be perceived as standards of care. These guidelines are either vague on specific treatments, or they give multiple options for similar patients. As a result, these guidelines can be difficult to follow and have been found to be ineffective in changing physicians' practices. Guidelines that are more specific (ie, provide only single options for treatment) may potentially be viewed as standards of care. In this case, there is a greater need for scientific evidence to establish that the outcomes achieved through this specific approach are indeed the best outcomes. Because there is a relative paucity of such evidence for most practice guidelines, more specific guidelines are less common than more vague guidelines. Intermediate between these two types would be guidelines that are based on some degree of scientific evidence, which suggests probabilities of effectiveness of specific treatment strategies based on clinical parameters.

Guideline Development

Guidelines may be developed in one of three ways: literature review, expert opinion consensus, and large-scale clinical trials. The most common approach, use of literature review, may take on two forms. In the first case, individual experts or groups of experts may review the literature and determine the best recommendations for the guideline. This approach may be biased because it relies on the individual reviewer to detect the strengths or weakness of the literature. This bias can be reduced to some extent by using rating scales and many reviews. A more sophisticated approach to literature review is through meta-analysis of clinical trials. This method uses statistical techniques that allow data from clinical trials of various sizes and types to be combined to provide recommendations for the guidelines. Although meta-analysis tends to decrease individual reviewer bias, it prevents incorporation of studies that may have practical value but are scientifically flawed in their design. Unfortunately, although literature review provides solid, objective evidence as the basis for guidelines, important aspects of practice are often not dealt with in the scientific literature. This omission may result in an incomplete guideline.

The second approach is to obtain expert opinion consensus. Experts are brought together to discuss their perceptions of the best practice for a given clinical situation. Each expert's perception is based on his or her own experience and knowledge of the literature. The advantage of this approach is that it uses real practice experience apart from clinical trials. The disadvantages are that it depends on which experts are chosen for the group and the dynamics of group opinion expression, both of which can introduce significant bias into guideline recommendations. Although group dynamic issues may be dealt with through use of rating scales and selection bias through broad representation, the tendency for significant bias still exists.

The third approach is to conduct prospective large-scale clinical trials. This is the most desirable and scientifically valid approach to developing guideline recommendations; however, it is also the most expensive and, consequently, the least frequently used. Typically, large scale trials are focused on finding the answers to a few questions that are of particular interest to the investigators. However, such trials may not ask or provide data to answer all of the questions necessary for understanding the complete use of a guideline in the real world where patients have the potential of multiple simultaneous conditions. In summary, each method for guideline development has its flaws, and combinations of approaches often are used to fill the gaps.

The American Medical Association (AMA), through its Practice Parameters Forum, has worked over the past 5 years to develop a framework for guideline development. This process has lead to the development of attributes that can be used either to guide the development of practice guidelines or to judge the developed ones. While these attributes are not absolute, they provide a basis for grading guidelines and a process for improving guidelines in areas that are found to be deficient. The attributes developed by the AMA are as follows. (1) Guidelines should be developed by or with physicians' organizations that have appropriate scientific and clinical expertise. (2) Guideline development should be based on reliable methodologies. This means that the guideline integrates relevant research findings and appropriate clinical expertise, the evidence used for developing the guideline is described, the process by which expert clinical judgment is gathered and review of the literature is performed are adequately described, and the qualifications of the reviewers and experts are provided. (3) A guideline should be comprehensive and specific regarding clinical management strategies, should be based on current information, and should be reviewed within 3 years of its original writing. (4) Guidelines should be widely disseminated with plans to publish in peer review journals and journals with broad circulation.

There is no guarantee that guidelines produced according to these attributes will be valid. However, these attributes do decrease the likelihood that serious errors will be undetected or that serious biases will be introduced. Because there is no perfect method for guideline development and all guidelines will contain some bias, the key feature of these attributes is the adequate description of the development methods so that the guidelines can be interpreted in that light. The actual steps in guideline development have also been described by the AMA in their publications.

Evaluating and Implementing Practice Guidelines

Although many guidelines have been written, the lack of good research on guideline implementation indicates that the effectiveness of those guidelines is unknown. Only recently has more emphasis been placed on the actual methods of evaluation and implementation. The first issue in guideline evaluation is the question of validity.

Guideline Validity

An important question to ask of every guideline is "How valid is this guideline?" In other words, will this guideline produce the best outcomes for the patient population to which it is applied? The first test of validity for most guidelines is what is called face validity, which is an assessment by potential users as to whether the guideline appears appropriate for the clinical conditions it addresses. Although face validity can be quantified by using rating scales, it is essentially a survey of the opinions of potential users that does not truly test the guideline. Although face validity does not provide proof that the guideline is clinically effective, it is an important testing step because the likelihood of successful implementation of a guideline that lacks face validity is relatively low.

Determination of true validity requires measurement of the guideline's ability to achieve its proposed goals. To assess this type of validity, which patients the guidelines should affect and what outcomes the guideline should achieve must be clearly defined. Guidelines are often developed without a clear definition of the expected outcomes. These outcomes may include clinical effectiveness (eg, improved patient function, decreased complications, decreased mortality, return to work), resource effectiveness (eg, decreased tests, decreased length of stay, decreased number of procedures), patient perceptions (eg, patient satisfaction, patient reported functional status), or combinations of these categories. Without a clear understanding of what the guideline is expected to achieve, evaluation of its validity is difficult.

One confounding factor in assessing guideline validity is the practitioners' ability to comprehend the guideline's recommendations well enough to put them adequately into effect. This is an issue of reliability rather than validity. Reliability means the guideline would be applied the same way in the same situations by multiple individuals. Vague guidelines may have reliability problems that make validity assessment difficult. Although the content of a guideline may be highly valid in theory, if it is not presented clearly and easily incorporated into practice, poor reliability will affect the results of validity testing and may make the guideline appear invalid. It is in the area of reliability that the methods of evaluation and implementation interact.

Guideline Implementation

The presumed purpose for developing guidelines is to modify physicians' practice behavior to achieve the best outcomes for their patients. Thus, guideline implementation deals more with issues of sociology and behavioral science than with the "scientific" medical process. The three primary means of guideline implementation are dissemination, monitoring, and feedback.

Dissemination There are three basic mechanisms of dissemination. The first is passive dissemination in which the guideline is simply distributed either generally to all physicians in a group or by physician request. Unfortunately, although this method is the least costly, it also has the least impact on physician practice. Unless the scientific evidence for a guideline is so compelling and so specific that it can be implemented easily, general dissemination does not significantly change physician practice. The second mechanism is active peer education in which guidelines are disseminated through interactions of peers in either education seminars or small groups or by individuals at the local level. This mechanism is found to be much more effective because the guideline takes on the face of a respected colleague rather than being a piece of paper coming from an unknown group. The third mechanism is dissemination through an interactive electronic knowledge basis. This is a new, potentially exciting area in terms of influencing physician practice. In this process, guidelines are incorporated into the process of care through expert systems so that when a particular question or condition arises, the guideline recommendations automatically are presented to the physician for consideration. This process is not the same as having electronic access to a library to do a literature search, which would be merely an electronic version of passive dissemination. This approach requires a sophisticated computer system and an electronic medical record to provide prompting at the time patient-care decisions are being made.

Monitoring The second means of guideline implementation is monitoring. Unfortunately, most guideline processes stop with dissemination, thereby limiting the ability to determine guideline validity. Unless the guideline is monitored to determine its effects on both process and outcome in patient care, its true effectiveness will be unknown. This is the most expensive component of the guideline development and implementation process. Without the data systems and personnel resources to capture and analyze process and outcome information, most guidelines go unmeasured and, therefore, their effectiveness is unknown. At the regional or national level, this lack of data makes guideline revision difficult. At the local level, the lack of good guideline monitoring data deprives the organization of the most effective means for affecting physician behavior—information feedback.

Feedback The third and most critical means of guideline implementation is feedback. Most physicians have been shown to respond very positively when provided with real data about their patients and their treatments. The two main categories of feedback are retrospective and concurrent.

In retrospective feedback, aggregate data are used to inform the physician about his or her degree of guideline compliance over a period of time. Providing performance data to the physician for review and consideration has been found to be reasonably effective if the physician represents a significant outlier relative to his or her peers. However, if the majority of a group of physicians are not compliant with a guideline, individual feedback will have no significant impact unless the physicians get together as a group to discuss the compliance issues.

A second approach to retrospective feedback is to couple the data with peer counseling. This approach, sometimes called "academic detailing," involves engaging the physician in a dialog about why the data indicate his or her practice is different from the norm and what specific ideas might change this. This approach is time consuming, but is quite effective.

A third approach is to use the data in the physician credentialing process. In this situation, the data on the lack of guideline compliance might be used to modify a physician's privileges or to assess the need for greater supervision. There has been a greater emphasis by the Joint Commission and other credentialing bodies to use more specific clinical information in the physician credentialing process. Guideline compliance has the potential for use in this area; however, the real issue for credentialing is patient outcomes. Simply to measure guideline compliance without accurately determining that the guideline produces better outcomes is inappropriate. Thus, credentialing requires measurement of outcomes before guideline compliance can be used as a source of credentialing decision.

A fourth use of retrospective data feedback is the analysis of the guideline performance data by a process improvement team. In this approach, physician behavior regarding guideline compliance is viewed as being influenced by system factors other than willingness to comply with the guideline. Barriers in hospitals and other care delivery systems often prevent physicians from effective guidelines compliance. Looking at guideline data in this mode allows physicians to influence those systems in patient care delivery that are decreasing their ability to comply with guidelines.

The second category of information feedback is in the concurrent analysis of patient care. In this setting, mechanisms are set up to monitor physician guideline compliance concurrent with the patient's actual care. This is usually done either through utilization review authorization screening criteria or through utilization management clinical pathways.

The utilization review approach uses guidelines to determine whether or not care should be granted or authorized. Most physicians find this approach to be the most distasteful and the behavior modification that occurs is done grudgingly. In particular, because many guidelines used in this setting do not have a true scientific basis for prospectively determining the best approach to care, the use of guidelines in utilization review preauthorization is typically grossly unwarranted.

The second area in which utilization review may be helpful is in the development of clinical pathways. In this setting, the guidelines are incorporated into a description or map of the process of care for the typical patient. When followed properly, these guidelines do not restrict the physician's judgment for managing the care of individual patients, but they do set up in advance the plan of care to be provided for the patient if all goes well. Thus, the plan can be followed only when the pathways contain not only what services are to be provided, but also what outcomes are expected as milestones to recognize whether the patient is or is not responding typically to care. If set up properly, clinical pathways are one of the more effective means of implementing practice guidelines into real practice because the entire care team of physicians, nurses, pharmacists, therapists, and so forth are all now aware of the guideline and its potential use and can have a common basis for dialog regarding the appropriate care in a given clinical situation.

Summary

Although the purpose of practice guidelines use is to improve patient care, it is still predominantly a hypothesis requiring proof. To achieve this goal, guidelines must be properly developed, evaluated, and implemented. Unless the last two steps are performed consistently, the potential for misuse of guidelines is as great as the potential for use.

Annotated Bibliography

Audet AM, Greenfield S, Field M: Medical practice guidelines: Current activities and future directions. *Ann Intern Med* 1990;113:709–714.

This article assesses the current state of guideline development, implementation, and evaluation in selected medical societies, health-care organizations, and insurers. The findings indicate that despite the sincere desire on the part of these groups to develop and use guidelines appropriately, significant flaws still exist in guideline development and use.

Dick RS, Steen EB (ed): *The Computer-Based Patient Record: An Essential Technology for Health Care.* Washington, DC, National Academy Press, 1991, pp 8–29.

This book defines the need for a computer-based medical record and its potential applications for studying and improving patient care outcomes.

Eddy DM: Clinical decision making: From theory to practice. Practice policies: What are they? *JAMA* 1990; 263:878–880.

This is the first of a series of articles by David Eddy that appeared in *JAMA* each month for 13 months. In this series, he outlines the critical issues in practice guideline development and the role guidelines play along with other evidence about outcomes in clinical decision making.

Ellrodt AG, Conner L, Riedinger M, et al: Measuring and improving physician compliance with clinical practice guidelines: A controlled interventional trial. *Ann Intern Med* 1995;122:277–282.

This article demonstrates the difficulty in using compliance with practice guidelines as a measure of quality of care. Using a guideline to reduce length of hospital stay in low-risk patients with chest pain, physician causes were the key factor in only a small percentage of patients not treated according to the guideline. Misclassification of patient risk by reviewers and system problems made up the majority of the reasons for failure to comply with the guideline.

Hirshfeld E: Use of practice parameters as standards of care and in health care reform: A view from the American Medical Association. *Jt Comm J Qual Improv* 1993;19: 322–329.

The article reviews the potential problems with the use of guidelines if they are developed improperly to be perceived as standards of care.

Kelly JT: The interface of clinical paths and practice parameters, in Spath PL (ed): *Clinical Paths: Tools for Outcomes Management.* Chicago, IL, American Hospital Publishing, 1994, pp 45–56.

This book provides a theoretical and practical look at the use of clinical pathways. This particular chapter outlines the AMA approach to guideline development. Further information can be obtained via the AMA Office of Quality Assurance.

Lohr KN (ed): *Medicare, A Strategy for Quality Assurance.* Washington, DC, National Academy Press, 1990, vol 1, pp 303–337.

This book outlines how practice guidelines may be used as quality assessment criteria.

Marder RJ: The interface of clinical paths and continuous quality improvement, in Spath PL (ed): *Clinical Paths: Tools for Outcomes Management.* Chicago, IL, American Hospital Publishing, 1994, pp 57–78.

This chapter describes the principles for using clinical pathways to improve overall patient care without restricting physician judgment. This approach is based on a continuous quality improvement model using pathways as a means for describing and improving the systemic causes of problems in the patient care process.

11

Outcomes Assessment

Introduction

The use and delivery of health care differ regionally, often in dramatic ways. Wennberg and Gittelsohn were the first to explore these small area variations and could not explain the differences in usage in terms of medical need or patient benefit. It became clear that physicians often did not arrive at the same answer for the appropriate treatment of a certain medical condition and that responses of physicians were thus variable. It was out of these variations that the outcomes movement developed. There was an obvious need to evaluate health care data collection systems and to determine the effectiveness of many medical interventions. Thus, the impetus of looking at patient-oriented outcomes began.

Certainly medical and especially orthopaedic clinical research has been carried out for a long time. However, that research traditionally has been carried out on a small scale and has focused on the process of the intervention. In orthopaedics, that has meant an inordinate amount of attention was directed at interpreting and evaluating radiographs and determining range of motion of the affected joint, pain, and nonstandardized results of patient function. Orthopaedists rarely asked patients how their life was altered. In fact, objective data were felt to be the only criteria on which to judge success. Subjective data were felt to be too soft for scientific reporting.

The approach of outcomes research is quite different. The focus is on patient-oriented functional outcomes. A truer measure of success is whether the patient functions and feels better rather than whether the patient has a great looking radiograph. Reproducible and scientifically valid methods have been and are being developed to determine subjective patient function information. Outcomes research attempts to determine the effectiveness of a medical intervention, be it surgical or otherwise. There are many components involved in this type of research.

Outcomes research in orthopaedics is of great importance because of the prevalence of musculoskeletal conditions that affect a high percentage of the population and use a significant proportion of health-care resources. Musculoskeletal conditions rank first in frequency of visits to physicians, second in frequency of hospitalizations, and fourth in frequency of surgical procedures performed within hospitals. Injuries in the workplace are a significant source of disability. Musculoskeletal impairments occur at a rate of approximately 124/1,000 population. The impact of musculoskeletal problems on quality of life is very significant. Outcomes research offers the opportunity to find answers for appropriate care, eliminate physician uncertainty, reduce variations, and improve the quality of orthopaedic care.

Small Area Analysis

Wennberg and Gittelsohn described the concept of small area analysis and practice pattern variations in 1973. They used hospital discharge data and population-based analyses to look at utilization of health care. They determined population-based rates of care using the number of people receiving treatment as the numerator and the population that might have been treated as the denominator.

What Wennberg and Gittelsohn discovered was that both medical and surgical problems had very different rates of utilization of medical services from one service area to another. This concept has become known as "small area variation" and has had a tremendous impact on the practice of medicine in the United States. Why should one region, even in the same state, have a rate of tonsillectomies of x and another region a very different rate of y? What is the right rate, and how is it determined?

A few medical diagnoses have similar rates of utilization of hospital services. These include hip fracture, hernia repair, and appendectomy. For these conditions, there seems to be common agreement on the need for hospitalization. However, for most other diagnoses, there is great controversy about medical intervention, and there may be as much as a tenfold difference in utilization from one area to another. This is true for such orthopaedic conditions as total joint arthroplasty, arthroscopy, and spinal procedures. Medical causes for hospitalization vary even more than surgical ones. The financial impact of such variation is obvious. Thus, the need for some attempt to understand these variations and somehow determine what is appropriate is obvious.

There may be multiple reasons for variations in care. One reason may relate to errors in data collection or incorrect analyses of the data. Second, there may be different environmental conditions for patients or differences in disease rates in geographic areas. Other considerations include patient demand for medical care, physician distribution, physician decision making, and the hospital capacity of the community.

Obviously, the human factor of decision making plays a role. Although orthopaedists have fairly standardized training in medical school and residency, physicians develop different practice styles. Consistency is the goal; however, physicians have different thresholds for making a surgical decision and somewhat varying opinions on the best treatment for a particular problem. The variations across four geographic regions nationally show minimal variation for the treatment of hip fractures; total hips vary by a factor of 1.9; total knees by a factor of 2.3, and disk procedures by a factor of 2.4.

There have been two overall responses to this. First, when physicians learn about and analyze variations, they have almost consistently responded by reducing the apparently high rates of utilization. Second, the existence of these variations seems to show the uncertainty of medical treatment and has produced a national initiative for outcomes research. Small area variation does not tell what is the right rate of surgery or of a medical procedure; it only gives the range of variation. These rates may be too high or too low. Outcomes research is an attempt to find the appropriate rate.

Outcomes Research

The Agency for Health Care Policy and Research (AHCPR) was established by the federal government to fund research on the effectiveness of medical interventions and to develop guidelines for medical practice. Patient Outcome Research Teams (PORTs) were established in several medical areas to conduct outcome studies. These are multidisciplinary, multi-institutional groups of physicians, health services researchers, health economists, and statisticians who conduct the research. Three of these outcomes studies center on orthopaedic problems (low back pain, total knee arthroplasty, total hip arthroplasty, and hip fracture patients). The Joint Commission on the Accreditation of Healthcare Organizations is also moving toward quality assessment based on outcomes.

There are several trends that have led to the development of otucomes research in the United States. First is the fear that escalating costs of health care could change the quality of care that patients receive. Second is the need to assess the effectiveness of different interventions and eliminate unnecessary or ineffective procedures or treatment. The third reason relates to the competitiveness of organized health care and the need for payers of health care to get the best "value." The intertwining of these issues has sometimes confused the picture. In its purest form, outcomes research should help answer questions of care in order to give patients the best treatment available and give them the best outcome, regardless of cost. Outcomes research should also help physicians use resources in the most effective manner. Third party payers and the cost of providing the care should take a secondary role.

What is different about outcomes research? Physicians have always been posing questions about their interventions and conducting research to look at the results of those interventions. What is new is the increased focus, improved methodologies, a national effort through the AHCPR, the funding of major projects, and the importance of patient outcomes. The research effort is thus more complex and requires an orderly and statistically sound approach.

Outcomes research is interested in the effectiveness of a medical intervention in the community setting, as opposed to the efficacy of an intervention in the research setting. It not only wants to know what can work but what does work. It encompasses a broader range of patient- and societally-oriented outcomes. Outcomes research is really a more structured approach to answering questions on the appropriateness of care with the patient as the focus.

To determine the appropriateness of care, outcomes research has several components. These include meta-analysis of the available literature, the use of large data bases such as Medicare billing information, the systematic study of patients treated with a particular intervention, decision analysis and information dissemination, and setting guidelines for clinical practice. Not all these components are necessary for every outcomes project, and each may be done individually.

Conduct of Outcomes Research

Meta-analysis of the present literature is a systematic method of aggregrating the literature on a particular topic to find out what is now known on that topic. It was designed for use with randomized clinical trials (RCTs) only, so its use in orthopaedics has been very limited. However, meta-analysis has been modified so that prospective cohort trials have been included in the meta-analysis. This addition, of course, weakens the results but it is the best that can be done given that the orthopaedic literature has few RCTs.

Meta-analysis makes one large cohort out of several smaller cohorts to look at treatment and outcome variables. The studies included in a meta-analysis often have different inclusion criteria and different analyses of outcomes, so criteria for combining results must be clearly spelled out prior to undertaking the meta-analysis. The process is very time consuming and expensive ($30,000 to $50,000 is not unusual), but meta-analysis has been done for some orthopaedic issues (lumbar spine fusions, disk excision, lateral epicondylitis, total knee replacement, closed tibial fractures, hip fractures). Although meta-analysis does not necessarily give definitive answers and is not a substitute for an RCT, it is at least helpful for stating present day knowledge as it is best known to be.

Outcomes research may use large data bases to evaluate area variation in utilization, to determine costs and even length of stay, and to evaluate some easily available patient outcomes, such as death or rehospitalization. The problem with large data bases is that they are usually established for billing purposes and not for clinical research and do not really have the information that is significant for results of an intervention. Outcomes are on a very gross level and give little information on patients' comorbidities or patients' perceptions of outcome. These data bases have large numbers of patients, however, and are often the best that can be done to get these large numbers. Care must be taken in interpretation.

Another component of outcomes research—the evaluation of cohorts of patients—must be done critically and systematically. The physician must understand study design to attempt to answer clinical questions appropriately. Orthopaedic studies have traditionally been small case series that report on observations of a small group of patients. Whereas this type of case is useful in the formative evaluation of a new process or technique, it does not truly give a generalizable result. These studies are usually single observer, unblinded studies without a control group with poorly defined outcome measures. This deficiency in the orthopaedic literature has been discussed by several authors.

Studies may be observational or experimental, and both types are used in outcomes studies. The timing of the studies is important, as well. Cross-sectional studies occur at one point in time, and, while rarely used in orthopaedics, may give a general overview of a condition or specific finding. Otherwise, cohort studies are studies that follow up a group of patients longitudinally over time. Cohort studies are either retrospective or prospective, depending on whether the outcomes of interest have already occurred or will occur after the study begins, according to a specified protocol. Prospective studies, because of their prearranged specifications, are stronger and allow for more control of the design and management of the study. There is much less chance for bias. The RCT, which is a prospective cohort study with concurrent controls and is double blinded, is the strongest study design and should be done whenever possible. Surgery poses some particular problems in conducting an RCT, and there are few examples of RCTs in the orthopaedic literature. However, this design is the best way to answer many surgical questions.

Decision analysis is a concept adapted from the business world to translate the statistical results of clinical research into a series of probabilities of patient outcomes, given various conditions. Outcomes can be weighted and a decision tree created to help a physician and patient consider various options.

The last goal of outcomes research is to disseminate the information learned from the study in hopes of helping to establish practice parameters. With the knowledge of the effectiveness of a procedure and who may benefit, it may be possible to establish some guidelines for intervention to allow those most appropriate for the procedure to receive it. Medicine is not an exact science, however. Patients and disease manifestations are different, and some variation is essential. The concern is that third party payers may use the information inappropriately to deny services. Guidelines are not meant as edicts and must allow room for physician and patient concerns. Patient preferences also must be considered when making therapeutic decisions.

Health Assessment Measures

The assessment of patients' function through the administration of patient questionnaires has been a concern of health research scientists the past several years. There are now several generic health measures that are self-administered questionnaires to quantitatively measure function and quality of life. Several of these questionnaires have been validated; that is, the instrument measures what it is supposed to measure. A good questionnaire should be reproducible; that is, the respondent answers the survey the same today and in 2 weeks, assuming there are no functional changes. In addition, the survey should be responsive; that is, sensitive to clinically important changes. The ideal instrument is expected to be short, simple to use, validated, reliable, responsive, cost effective, and applicable to the presenting problem.

Questionnaires can be either generic health instruments or disease specific. Examples of generic health instruments that have been validated and are reproducible include the SF-36 and the SIP (Sickness Impact Profile). The SF-36 is a series of 36 general health questions that take 15 to 20 minutes to complete, and it looks at health in eight different areas (physical function, physical role function, emotional role function, social function, bodily pain, mental health, vitality, and general health). The SIP consists of 136 questions, takes 30 minutes to complete, and is grouped into 12 categories (sleep and rest, eating, work, home management, recreation and pastimes, ambulation, mobility, body care and movement, social interaction, alertness behavior, emotional behavior, communication).

The AIMS (Arthritis Impact Measurement Scale) is an example of a disease-specific instrument that may be applicable to orthopaedics. This instrument consists of 45 questions grouped into nine sections (mobility, physical activity, dexterity, household activity, social activity, activities of daily living, pain, depression, and anxiety) and takes about 15 minutes to complete.

These types of instruments are critical to outcomes research not only to assess patient function but also to allow comparisons between studies. Health status or quality of life includes the physical, emotional, and social well being of a person. These factors are all important to outcomes research. These instruments are as valid, reliable, and sensitive as traditional measures of outcome. Elaborations on these instruments need to be developed for use in orthopaedic outcomes studies. The AAOS is developing such instruments, which are a combination of a generic health instrument and a regionally specific instrument. The relief of pain clearly needs to be an important component of an orthopaedic questionnaire. Patients' preferences for their satisfaction also need to be incorporated in any assessment. This inclusion implies that the risks and benefits of a procedure need to be understood, and complications after the intervention must be documented.

Conclusion

Much of outcomes research is not new, but the scope is wider and more comprehensive. The focus of this research is more patient-centered and includes information to help improve quality and appropriateness of care. These studies also can focus on the cost effectiveness of care, hopefully without compromising care. However, the possibility of misinterpreting the study findings exists, and physicians must insist on the integrity of the studies and clinical research.

The era of health reform is underway. Orthopaedists must understand and participate in the outcomes movement to help keep it on track. The results of reform will affect both physicians and patients. Orthopaedists must continue to be vigilant in understanding the effects of their interventions and in determining who should receive their treatments. Physicians have the opportunity to improve the delivery of health care. As physicians participate in and do more refined clinical research, they will have a better understanding of how to improve patients' outcomes. By using a standardized, well-thought out approach to a question and using standardized measures and instruments, investigators can compare results in a meaningful and accurate way. Large data bases can be pooled to increase statistical validity.

The ultimate intent of outcomes research is to allow patients more control over their care. With appropriate information about procedures and alternatives, with risks and benefits understood, patients can express preferences about what they want, not what the doctor thinks is best. Outcomes research should also help physicians understand what interventions are effective. Everyone places importance on different aspects of function, and the physician's goal is to provide the most scientific information to patients so that the physician and patient working together can make the most appropriate decisions for the patient.

Annotated Bibliography

Callahan CM, Drake BG, Heck DA, et al: Patient outcomes following tricompartmental total knee replacement: A meta-analysis. *JAMA* 1994;271:1349–1357.

This is a meta-analysis of tricompartmental knee replacement, which shows such surgery is safe and effective, but the limitations of such a meta-analysis are discussed.

Hoffman RM, Wheeler KJ, Deyo RA: Surgery for herniated lumbar discs: A literature synthesis. *J Gen Intern Med* 1993:8:487–496.

This is a meta-analysis of the results of surgery for herniated lumbar disks. The benefits and weaknesses of such a study are discussed as well as the outcomes.

Keller RB, Rudicel SA, Liang MH: Outcomes research in orthopaedics, in Schafer M (ed): *Instructional Course Lectures 43.* Rosemont, IL, American Academy of Orthopaedic Surgeons 1994, pp 599–611.

The origins of the outcomes movement and components of outcomes research are presented.

Lu-Yao GL, Keller RB, Littenberg B, et al: Outcomes after displaced fractures of the femoral neck: A meta-analysis of one hundred and six published reports. *J Bone Joint Surg* 1994;76A:15–25.

A meta-analysis of the treatment of displaced fractures of the femoral neck was performed. The methods of conducting a meta-analysis are discussed as well as results.

Classic Bibliography

Gartland JJ: Orthopaedic clinical research: Deficiencies in experimental design and determinations of outcome. *J Bone Joint Surg* 1988;70A:1357–1364.

Gross M: A critique of the methodologies used in clinical studies of hip-joint arthroplasty published in the English-language orthopaedic literature. *J Bone Joint Surg* 1988;70A:1364–1371.

Labelle H, Guibert R, Joncas J, et al: Lack of scientific evidence for the treatment of lateral epicondylitis of the elbow: An attempted meta-analysis. *J Bone Joint Surg* 1992;74B:646–651.

Rudicel S, Esdaile J: The randomized clinical trial in orthopaedics: Obligation or option? *J Bone Joint Surg* 1985;67A:1284–1293.

Turner JA, Ersek M, Herron L, et al: Surgery for lumbar spinal stenosis: Attempted meta-analysis of the literature. *Spine* 1992;17:1–8.

Turner JA, Ersek M, Herron L, et al: Patient outcomes after lumbar spinal fusions. *JAMA* 1992;268:907–911.

Wennberg J, Gittelsohn A: Small area variations in health care delivery. *Science* 1973;182:1102–1108.

Wennberg JE, Freeman JL, Culp WJ: Are hospital services rationed in New Haven or over-utilised in Boston? *Lancet* 1987;1:1185–1189.

12

Sports Medicine

Introduction

To practice sports medicine, the orthopaedic surgeon must be able to do more than diagnose and treat the musculoskeletal injuries of athletes. The orthopaedic surgeon practicing sports medicine needs an understanding of many other disciplines, including exercise physiology, nutrition, cardiology, and neurology. The orthopaedic surgeon who becomes a team physician must enlist and coordinate the skills of a number of other practitioners. Certain injuries (eg, stress fractures) fall largely to the purview of the physician practicing sports medicine.

This chapter is a space-limited review of the issues of fitness for athletic participation, evaluation of the injured athlete on the field, and return to participation. The scientific basis of rehabilitative techniques is reviewed. Exertional compartment syndromes and stress fractures are also included.

Preparticipation Examination

When conducted in a rigorous and comprehensive fashion with proper emphasis placed on format, scope, frequency, and content, the preparticipation examination can serve as a valuable foundation for the provision of care by either the team physician or the primary care physician.

Examination Setup

Two basic formats of the examination are common: group examination and private examination. The group examination concept has been described as a high volume, expedient, low-cost medical evaluation. When properly done, these assessments are accomplished in a station-by-station fashion that is carefully designed to ensure privacy and are performed by a variety of personnel including primary-care physicians, orthopaedists, athletic trainers, and physician's assistants. The private examination takes place in the primary-care physician's private office. This format has the advantage of the family physician's long-standing relationship with the athlete and thorough knowledge of the athlete's medical history, previous injuries, and level of physical maturity.

Controversy still persists as to the scope of the preparticipation physical examination. Currently, most persons agree that the sports physical is not intended to be a substitute for routine periodic comprehensive health screening or for the relationship between the family physician or pediatrician and the athlete.

Objectives

The preparticipation examination should provide the opportunity for the physician to conduct a rigorous and thorough evaluation of the potential athlete's ability to participate in a sport without undue risk. It should accomplish the following: (1) determine the athlete's general health, (2) assess cardiovascular fitness, (3) evaluate preexisting injuries, 4) assess size and maturation, (5) restrict activity or disqualify from specific activity when contraindicated by physical limitation or disease that would preclude safe participation, (6) recommend appropriate activity when participation has been restricted, and (7) establish a comprehensive data base.

Optimally, an examination should be conducted every 3 to 4 years, and intercedent medical history should be updated on an annual basis. The discovery of a new condition or injury would then trigger appropriate evaluation by the physician. This policy has been adapted by the National Collegiate Athletic Association, is cost effective and efficient, and guarantees that the athlete will be thoroughly evaluated. The content of the examination is summarized by the "Athletic Competition Health Screening Form" developed by The Commission on Public Health and Scientific Affairs of the American Academy of Family Physicians.

The medical history is the cornerstone of the preparticipation evaluation and is best completed by the adolescent athlete and his or her parents. It has been shown that the history can identify 63% to 74% of problems affecting athletes. It has also been shown that a history of injury or illness with incomplete recovery and rehabilitation correlates with increased risk of injury in sports. The examination should focus on identifying potentially disqualifying conditions, with particular attention to cardiovascular and musculoskeletal assessment. Additionally, it should include assessment of physical maturity using standard Tanner staging criteria.

Cardiovascular Assessment The major cause of sudden death in young athletes is cardiac outflow tract obstruction. Therefore, a positive response to the question, "Have you ever felt dizzy, fainted, or nearly or actually passed out while exercising?" should prompt more detailed cardiovascular evaluation. Systolic murmurs are common in athletes, but accentuation of the murmur with Valsalva should alert the physician to the possibility of asymmetric septal hypertrophy and obstructive hypertrophic cardiomyopathy. Unexplained ventricular ectopia should raise the possibility of cocaine abuse. Blood pressure measure-

Table 1. The two-minute orthopedic examination

Instructions	Observation
Stand facing examiner	Acromioclavicular joints, general habitus
Look at ceiling, floor, over both shoulders; touch ears to shoulders	Cervical spine motion
Shrug shoulders (examiner resists)	Trapezius strength
Abduct shoulders 90° (examiner resists at 90°)	Deltoid strength
Full external rotation of arms	Shoulder motion
Flex and extend elbows	Elbow motion
Arms at sides, elbows 90° flexed; pronate and supinate wrists	Elbow and wrist motion
Spread fingers; make fist	Hand or finger motion and deformities
Tighten (contract) quadriceps; relax quadriceps	Symmetry and knee effusion; ankle effusion
"Duck walk" four steps (away from examiner with buttocks on heels)	Hip, knee, and ankle motion
Back to examiner	Shoulder symmetry, scoliosis
Knees straight, touch toes	Scoliosis, hip motion, hamstring tightness
Raise up on toes, raise heels	Calf symmetry, leg strength

(Reproduced with permission from *Sports Medicine: HealthCare For Young Athletes.* Evanston, IL, American Academy of Pediatrics, 1983.)

ment is very important. The upper limits of blood pressure accepted as not requiring further evaluation are 130/75 for children 11 years of age and younger, and 140/85 for children 12 years and above.

Musculoskeletal Assessment This is the most important component of the preparticipation examination, and the examiner should look for preexisting injuries because they are likely to recur. Although a more detailed examination may be required, a screening assessment can generally be done in two minutes or less (Table 1).

Laboratory Studies There are many diagnostic tests which can be implemented in the examination. The complete blood count (CBC) and urinalysis are most commonly recommended, but the consensus is that they should not be done routinely. The routine electrocardiograph and/or echocardiogram are not cost effective. An exercise stress test may be indicated in an adult athlete prior to starting an exercise program. Vo_2max may be helpful in determining performance and training needs of high-level competitive athletes. Drug screening is required at most collegiate and professional levels.

Clearance for Participation

Physicians all too often find it easier to disqualify an athlete from a particular activity than to indicate those athletic endeavors that, in fact, would be permissible and certainly healthier than no activity at all. Although the physician has the responsibility of identifying conditions that contraindicate certain sports activities and of notifying the athlete and the athlete's parents, it is still up to the athlete and/or athlete's parents to make the final decision about participation. Whether an athlete is allowed to play or not is a shared responsibility of the parents, the athlete, the examining physician, and the school. In virtually every disqualifying condition, there are now court cases in which athletes and parents have filed a suit to force schools or leagues to permit participation.

There are three categories of clearance: unrestricted, clear for a specific sports category after complete evaluation and rehabilitation, and not cleared for any sports category. To aid the physician in deciding on clearance, The American Academy of Physicians Committee on Sports

Table 2. Classification of sports

		Noncontact		
Contact/Collision	Limited Contact/Impact	Strenuous	Moderately Strenuous	Nonstrenuous
Boxing	Baseball	Aerobic dancing	Badminton	Archery
Field Hockey	Basketball	Crew	Curling	Golf
Football	Bicycling	Fencing	Table tennis	Riflery
Ice Hockey	Diving	Field		
Lacrosse	Field	Discus		
Martial arts	High jump	Javelin		
Rodeo	Pole vault	Shot put		
Soccer	Gymnastics	Running		
Wrestling	Horseback riding	Swimming		
	Skating	Tennis		
	Ice	Track		
	Roller	Weight lifting		
	Skiing			
	Cross-country			
	Downhill			
	Water			
	Softball			
	Squash, handball			
	Volleyball			

Medicine has designed three categories of sports activities: (1) contact and collision; (2) limited contact and impact; and (3) noncontact activities divided into strenuous, moderately strenuous, and nonstrenuous (Table 2). Disqualifying conditions that constitute absolute or relative contraindications for specific sports activities are delineated based on level of contact (Table 3) and fall into six major categories: (1) neurologic, (2) defects in paired systems, (3) organ enlargement, (4) active infections, (5) vertebropelvic defects, and (6) cardiopulmonary disorders.

Table 3. Disqualifying conditions

	Absolute Contraindications		Relative Contraindications	
Condition	**Contact**	**Noncontact**	**Contact**	**Noncontact**
Seizure within past year	X	X*		X
Concussions with consciousness loss	X			
Solitary functioning eye	X			
Retinal detachment history	X	X		
Pulmonary infection, including tuberculosis	X	X		
Pyelonephritis	X	X		
Bone infection	X	X		
Systemic infection	X	X		
Cardiomegaly	X			X
Aortic or mitral stenosis	X			X
Active myocarditis/ pericarditis	X			X
Major visceromegaly (liver, kidneys, spleen)	X			X
Solitary functional kidney	X			X
Testis overlying pubic ramus	X			
Unhealed fracture	X			X
Spondylolisthesis with back pain	X	X		
Spondylolisthesis without back pain			X	
Painful hip disease	X	X		
Blood coagulation defect	X			X
Uncontrolled asthma			X	X
Skin infection, including herpes	X†		X	X
Active otitis media		X**		
Uncontrolled diabetes mellitus			X	X
Recurrent shoulder subluxation			X	
Uncontrolled hypertension			X	X

*Diving, swimming, high bar, and rings
†Herpes simplex in wrestlers
**Swimming and diving

On-the-Field Evaluation: Return to Participation

Ideally, the team physician should be the leader of an organized sports medicine program composed of an athletic director, team coaches, and an athletic trainer. Close involvement with the team (ie, attending practices and parent meetings and giving lectures) will enhance the athletes' and coaches' confidence in the physician. This relationship will foster a team concept which will ultimately assist the physician with on-the-field evaluations and decisions under fire. Emergency care should be practiced on a regular basis. Prior planning will ensure the availability of all necessary equipment (Outline 1).

The Unconscious Athlete

An unconscious athlete has suffered a serious head and/or neck injury until proven otherwise. Proper precautions must be taken to prevent further injury, and the emergency medical system should be immediately activated. If the athlete is face down, he or she must be brought into the face up position with a logroll. The head and neck must be maintained in a neutral position with gentle longitudinal traction. Do not remove the helmet of an unconscious athlete. If the airway is not open, establish access by removing the face mask with a bolt cutter or screwdriver, performing a chin or jaw lift with the head maintained in traction, or clearing the mouth of foreign material or the tongue. If the athlete is not breathing with an established airway, artificial ventilation should be started using the jaw thrust method. If there is difficulty with ventilation with stridor, hoarseness, bony crepitus, or subcutaneous edema, suspect a laryngeal fracture or edema. A needle cricothyrotomy should be performed if there is laryngeal edema and ventilation can not be established by any other method.

Head and Neck Injuries

The on-field evaluation of head and neck injuries is limited, and thus the physician must have a high index of suspicion. The leading cause of death on the field is head injuries. Concussion syndromes can be graded into three types, with specific guidelines for return to participation based on a sideline evaluation (Table 4). The sideline examination should include a neurologic examination with emphasis on the level of consciousness and memory loss. A grade 1 concussion is most common. There is short-lived confusion and disorientation without amnesia. The athlete may describe it as, "I had my bell rung." Return to play, under the watchful supervision of the medical team, is allowed only if the athlete is asymptomatic during rest and exertion for at least 20 minutes. A second grade 1 concussion in the same contest eliminates the player from competition that day. A grade 2 concussion is characterized by confusion with amnesia. Retrograde amnesia usually develops first and is followed by posttraumatic amnesia in severe cases. A grade 3 concussion is characterized by a loss of consciousness. The presentation of traumatic intracranial hematomas can be variable, and they often cannot be differentiated from grade 2 and 3 concussions

Outline 1. Equipment that should be available

The team physician's bag
Oral airway
Stethoscope
Thermometer
Eyepatches
14-gauge catheters
Scissors (blunt)
Tape (1/2", 1", 2")
Penlight
Ace bandages
Slings
Tongue depressors
Cotton (Q-tip) applicators
Xeroform/Vaseline gauze
Gauze pads (sterile/non-sterile)
Betadyne swabs
Betadyne scrub
Antiseptic ointment (Bacitracin)
Near-vision-card
Suture kit
Adhesive strips (Band-aid, Steri-strip)
Hydrogen peroxide/saline irrigating solution
Albuterol inhaler
Epi-pen (Self-injectable epinephrine)
Plaster of paris/fiberglass
Home care head injury forms
Aluminum splints
Latex gloves (Sterile and non-sterile)
Scalpel

Sideline/Fieldhouse equipment
Spine board
Stretcher
Crutches
Splints (board type)
Sand bags/Philadelphia collar
Bolt cutter/screwdriver
Intravenous/D5 Ringer's lactate, sterile irrigant (saline)
Oxygen tank with mask
Telephone

on the field. Thus, unlike grade 1 concussions, athletes with grade 2 and 3 concussions should not be allowed to return to play and should be suspected of having more serious intracranial injuries. If an athlete is cleared to go home, it is recommended that a home-care guidelines form for head injuries be given and explained to an adult relative.

Athletes who have amnesia should be watched for post-concussion syndrome. This syndrome is characterized by persistent headaches, inability to concentrate, and irritability. Resumption of play is precluded until all symptoms resolve completely because a premature return to contact activity can result in the second impact syndrome. This syndrome results in delayed brain swelling with potential for further neurologic damage or death.

For a conscious athlete down on the field with neurologic symptoms, begin the assessment by determining whether the symptoms are confined to an upper extremity or involve other extremities. Complaints of pain and tenderness in the neck require cervical precautions and immobilization. Included in this group are athletes who have suffered transient quadriplegia. If symptoms and findings are temporary and limited to an upper extremity without neck pain or tenderness, ask the athlete to actively move his head and neck while in his protective gear. If the athlete demonstrates full active painless cervical range of motion, he may be allowed to sit up and is escorted to the sideline for further evaluation. If there is persistent neurologic deficit or if there is guarded or decreased cervical motion, the athlete should be immobilized and transferred to a hospital.

Brachial plexus injuries are relatively uncommon in sports with the exception of transient brachial plexopathy (burner syndrome) in American football. Burner syndrome is characterized by immediate, sharp, burning pain radiating from the supraclavicular area down the arm. Often, the athlete will try to shake the arm to "get the feeling back" or walk off the field holding the involved arm with the contralateral arm. The symptoms frequently resolve in minutes, and transient weakness, most commonly of the deltoid, biceps, and spinatus muscles, may follow the pain. However, the motor deficit may not present at all or it may present several hours or days following the initial injury. Burner syndrome is most commonly an injury to the upper trunk of the brachial plexus involving the C5 and C6 roots. An athlete who has sustained a burner may return to play the same day if he can demonstrate a normal range of painless cervical motion without any residual neurologic deficit. The athlete who has suffered a recurrent burner should not be allowed to play until cervical spine pathology has been excluded.

Table 4. Return to participation for concussions

	Grade 1	Grade 2	Grade 3
Symptoms			
Confusion	+	+	+
Amnesia	−	+	+
Loss of consciousness	−	−	+
Disposition			
Removal from contest	+	+	+
Return to play same day (normal sideline exam)	+	−	−
Home observation program (serial neurologic exams)	+	+	N/A
Transfer to hospital	−	−	+

(Adapted with permission from *Guidelines of The Colorado Medical Society*. Denver, CO, The Colorado Medical Society, 1991.)

Thoracic Injuries

A serious chest injury should be considered when there is any respiratory abnormality. Rib or sternal fractures should be suspected when pain, localized tenderness, and crepitation are present. Athletes who sustain these fractures are excluded from play because damage to the pleura and lung may have occurred with potential for a pneumothorax or a hemothorax. If there is tracheal deviation, chest wall asymmetry, tachypnea, labored respiration, unilateral absence of breath sounds, and distended neck veins with cyanosis, the physician must suspect a tension pneumothorax and begin immediate treatment on the field. Ventilation is reestablished by placing a large-bore needle into the second intercostal space along the midclavicular line. Fractures of ribs seven through nine may be associated with injuries to the liver, spleen, and kidneys. Fortunately, most thoracic injuries are minor and musculoskeletal in nature. An athlete with persistent pain, any respiratory abnormality, or any peripheral evidence of compromised circulation should be referred to a hospital.

Abdominal Injuries

Abdominal and pelvic injuries are most often minor contusions. However, life-threatening injuries can occur and are often subtle in presentation. A blow to the abdomen may result in the athlete's having "the wind knocked out." This is a result of forceful expiration and upward migration of the diaphragm. The discomfort will resolve spontaneously as the abdominal muscles relax. Any athlete that is complaining of continuous and persistent abdominal pain requires serial abdominal examinations and determination of vital signs. Abdominal wall contusions are a common source of pain, and it is often difficult to distinguish them from intra-abdominal injury. Abdominal rigidity, involuntary spasm, guarding, and referred pain are the most common signs of intraperitoneal irritation. Left-sided abdominal pain with associated referred pain to the left shoulder or chest is suggestive of a splenic injury. Similarly, right-sided symptoms may be the result of a liver injury. A kidney injury, the most common abdominal organ injury in sports, should be suspected if the athlete presents with flank tenderness, swelling, and subsequent abnormality such as anuria or hematuria. These athletes should not be given liquids to drink and should be immediately transported to a hospital for further studies.

Extremity Injuries

Initial assessment of an extremity injury on the field is directed towards obtaining the history of the injury from the athlete. With lower extremity injuries, if the athlete gives a history of hearing a pop, falling, and inability to rise unassisted, the magnitude of injury is typically severe. A neurovascular examination is performed. The extremity is examined for evidence of deformity, tenderness, and crepitation. After this initial assessment is completed, the athlete is escorted to the sidelines for a more complete history and physical examination. Athletes with gross deformities are splinted on the field and then transported to the sidelines. Athletes with milder injuries, such as sprains, can often resume play. If the examination reveals a mild sprain, a functional sideline test should be performed. This test includes a short sprint from a stance position, cutting maneuvers, and a hop on the injured leg. If these tests are performed satisfactorily, the athlete may resume play with appropriate taping and splinting. An athlete with a severe sprain will not be able to resume play and should be treated with the RICE (rest, ice, compression, elevation) protocol. The general guidelines for evaluation and treatment of upper extremity injuries are the same as for lower extremity injuries. Dislocations about the hand and shoulder can often be safely reduced with gentle maneuvers. Some hand injuries can be safely splinted and protected so that the athlete may resume play. The position of the player and the sport being played may be a critical determinant on whether an athlete with a hand injury can safely return to play.

Miscellaneous Injuries and Conditions

Testicular Injuries Although uncommon, a ruptured testicle is a surgical emergency. The pain and swelling that often follow testicular injuries can make it difficult to distinguish a contusion from a rupture. If the physician can feel an intact testicle with normal consistency, it is most likely a contusion that can be treated with ice, elevation, rest, analgesics, and scrotal support. However, if the testicle is not palpable and the scrotum does not transilluminate, a testicular rupture should be suspected, and the patient should be immediately referred to a hospital.

Eye Injuries The team physician should stress prevention of these injuries by emphasizing the use of protective eye wear. An eye examination should include a test of the acuity of the vision and an inspection of the pupil, cornea, and conjunctiva with a penlight. The motility of each eye should also be tested, and the eyelid should routinely be inspected for lacerations. Removal of foreign bodies should only be done with sterile irrigating solution or a moistened sterile cotton swab. An eyelid that is swollen shut by edema or hematoma should not be forcibly opened because this could express the eye's contents through an unsuspected laceration. In the presence of a serious eye injury, a firm eye patch should be applied, and the athlete should be referred to an ophthalmologist.

Exertional Heat Illnesses These illnesses have been characterized into three types: heat cramps, heat exhaustion, and heat stroke. Adequate hydration and avoiding excessive exercise in hot, humid weather are key in preventing all these disorders, and the team physician must emphasize this to the coaches and athletes. An athlete with heat cramps generally presents with painful involuntary contractions of large muscles. The core body temperature is normal, and generally, there are no other clinical findings. Treatment consists of stretching and massaging the cramped muscle as well as local application of ice. Fluid replacement should be started, and the athlete may later be able to return to play. Heat exhaustion is a serious heat injury with a wide spectrum of presentation. Commonly, the athlete presents with fatigue, vertigo, profuse sweating, myalgias, nausea, and vomiting. Core temperature is elevated, but is generally less than 104°F (40°C). Sweating mechanisms are generally working, and the mental status is usually normal. The athlete should be treated with fluid replacement and transferred to a hospital for intravenous hydration to prevent progression to heat stroke.

Heat stroke is a medical emergency with a 50% to 70% fatality rate. There is extreme hyperthermia with core temperatures greater than 104°F (40°C) due to failure of thermoregulation. The sweating mechanism may be absent, and the patient may present with dry, flushed skin. Heat stroke may cause a spectrum of signs and symptoms with progressive neurologic and cardiovascular collapse. Treatment consists of external cooling on the field, fluid replacement, and immediate transfer to a hospital for supportive care.

Anaphylaxis Anaphylaxis is the immediate, shock-like, and frequently fatal hypersensitivity reaction that occurs within minutes from exposure to certain allergens, foreign serum, or drugs. It may occur on the field after an insect sting. On-the-field treatment is rapid identification of this disorder and treatment with a self-administrable epinephrine device.

Exercise-Induced Bronchospasm Exercise-induced bronchospasm is a common feature of asthma, which is characterized by airway obstruction following physical exertion. The athlete experiences difficulty breathing, manifested by shortness of breath, coughing, chest tightness, and wheezing. Prophylactic inhalation treatment with a beta receptor agonist such as albuterol is recommended 15 minutes prior to the athletic event and at the time of occurrence.

Table 5. Methods of heat transfer

Type	Description	Example
Conduction	Thermal energy exchange between contacting surfaces	Hydrocolator
Radiation	Heat transfer from a warmer to colder source	Infrared lamp
Convection	Molecular movement causing increased temperature; more rapid than conduction or radiation	Whirlpool
Conversion	Transformation of energy from nonthermal to thermal; allows deep penetration	Diathermy Ultrasound

Rehabilitation

Rehabilitation can be defined as any measure used to restore an injured patient to normal activity as quickly and safely as possible. Physical therapy includes the use of physical agents, therapeutic exercise, and functional exercise. Physical agents include heat, cold, and electricity designed to affect soft-tissue healing; reduce pain, swelling, and spasm; and reduce or increase blood flow. Therapeutic exercises are movements designed to restore or improve range of motion, flexibility, and muscle performance. Functional exercises are movements designed to restore strength and agility.

Physical Agents

Cryotherapy Cold is used to decrease inflammation and pain. The reported mechanisms of action have included vasoconstriction, increased blood viscosity, inhibition of histamine release, increased soft-tissue stiffness, and decreased nerve conduction. Contraindications to the use of cold include ischemia, cold urticaria, Raynaud's phenomenon, cryoglobinuria, and paroxysmal cold hemoglobinemia. Complications from cryotherapy include nerve injury, frostbite, and hunting reaction, which is a secondary vasodilatation following exposure to cold.

Cold may be applied by way of ice packs, ice massage, or commercially available gel preparations. The duration of application is 10 to 30 minutes. More prolonged use can result in the complications listed above, but the cold can be reapplied every 2 to 4 hours. Cold is usually used following acute injuries (along with compression and elevation) to treat strains, sprains and contusions. Cryotherapy can also be used in the initial postoperative period or in combination with therapeutic exercise (cryokinetics).

Although much has been written about the physiologic effects of cold, few controlled studies are available regarding its use. On the basis of experience and physiologic studies, however, cryotherapy does appear to be beneficial within the first 48 to 72 hours following soft-tissue injury.

Thermotherapy Heat has been used to increase temperature in body tissues by various means (Table 5). All heat modalities have similar actions. These include vasodilatation, stimulation of the inflammatory response, increased soft-tissue plasticity, and increased threshold for pain response. Heat is indicated following the cessation of acute inflammation. Used with exercise, thermotherapy can help increase range of motion. It can also be used to decrease subacute–chronic pain and/or muscle spasm.

For heat therapy to be effective, the tissue must be heated to a range of 104° to 113°F (40° to 45°C). This is also the temperature required of each of the superficial heat modalities because none can penetrate greater than 1 cm (some authors say 5 mm). Treatment usually lasts up to 30 minutes.

Contraindications to the use of heat include acute injury (heat will increase secondary hypoxia, edema, and hemorrhage), active bleeding, malignancy, fever, and cardiac insufficiency. Special precautions need to be taken with insensitive or ischemic body parts. Children have an underdeveloped thermoregulatory mechanism, which makes them poor judges of heat.

Diathermy Diathermy uses high frequency electromagnetic currents that vibrate and disturb tissue molecules. The tissue resists the passage of energy, resulting in heat. In patients who have subcutaneous fat that is greater than 1-cm thick, the fat temperature itself will rise to an uncomfortable level before the tissue temperature rises to therapeutic levels.

The special contraindications to diathermy include metal implants (including pacemakers and intrauterine devices), arteriosclerosis, phlebitis, wet dressings, pregnancy, and infection. It should not be used over the gonads or growth plates in children or the pelvic area in menstruating women. Diathermy can heat tissue 3 to 5 cm deep, but does so to an unknown temperature. Specific knowledge about its clinical effects are lacking.

Ultrasound Ultrasound can produce tissue heating to a depth of 10 cm. Pulsed ultrasound uses a lower intensity and has nonthermal effects, which include the possible reduction of inflammation and acceleration of fracture healing. Contraindications to ultrasound use are the same as those for diathermy.

Ultrasound is delivered to the target area by means of a coupling agent, such as glycerine or mineral oil, which is applied to the skin. Treatments last 5 to 10 minutes. Ultrasound may induce cavitation. When gas bubbles are trapped within tissues, ultrasound can cause the bubbles to enlarge and vibrate. This vibration can cause focal high tissue pressure and temperature leading to tissue injury.

Ultrasound has been used in a number of clinical conditions (supraspinatus tendonitis, subacromial bursitis, adhesive capsulitis) with reportedly good results. All of these reports were in an uncontrolled setting. One 20-patient double-blind, randomized study showed no significant difference between use of ultrasound and placebo in treatment of the same disorders. More study is clearly needed.

Phonophoresis uses ultrasound to drive topical medications (usually 10% hydrocortisone) to a deeper tissue location. Data from earlier research on phonophoresis indicated that medication may be delivered to a depth of 10 cm. More recent data have been unable to show penetration beyond the epidermis. Data gathered in two retrospective studies have indicated that clinical improvement occurs in a variety of soft-tissue disorders. Recent work has questioned whether phonophoresis works by systemic absorption rather than by local effects.

Electrotherapy Electrotherapy basically takes two forms: transcutaneous electric nerve stimulation (TENS) and electric stimulation to strengthen muscle (ES). TENS uses electrical stimulation for pain relief. Three theories are used to explain its actions. The first is the gate theory, which postulates that the overexcitement of larger type A sensory nerve fibers can flood the pain pathways to the brain, thus blocking input from the smaller type C fibers. The second theory implicates the electrically stimulated release of endogenous morphine-like substances (endorphins). The third theory states that TENS may modulate midbrain transmission of pain.

TENS can be applied through both high and low frequencies by means of a small, portable radio size unit. Neuroprobe uses electrical stimulation to discover and treat trigger points. Interferential uses a crossing pattern of electrical fields to decrease pain.

Studies do exist that appear to show the effectiveness of TENS for laminectomy and knee patients in the postsurgical setting. Early mobility, decreased hospital stay, and decreased narcotic usage have been reported to occur in TENS-treated patients as compared to controls. There are, however, contradictory studies. Data from one contradictory study indicate that TENS is no more effective than placebo in treating low back pain.

TENS use may be indicated for conditions in which pain limits the patient's ability to comply with therapeutic exercise (eg, adhesive capsulitis). Whether it has advantages over analgesics in acute conditions is not known. TENS should not be used in patients who are pregnant or who have demand (rather than fixed rate) pacemakers, epilepsy, or mental retardation.

In ES, electricity is used to stimulate motor nerve(s), thereby causing muscle contraction. The strength of contraction can be increased by producing multiple, closely spaced stimuli or by increasing the intensity of stimulation and, thus, recruiting more motor units. ES can be applied through both direct (galvanic) or alternating currents. Various wave forms (square, sinusoidal) as well as continuous or intermittent pulses can be used. Frequency and amplitude can also be adjusted.

The use of ES in rehabilitation is controversial; the central issue is whether electrical stimulation can produce results superior to that of voluntary contraction. To have any effect in maintaining or increasing muscle strength, these contractions must be strong enough to produce fatigue (ie, maximal or submaximal contraction). Most of the work done to date involves the quadriceps muscle. ES may have a role in the postinjury/postsurgery model in which voluntary contraction is not possible due to denervation, immobilization, or pain. Unfortunately, the data acquired to date are not conclusive.

ES is applied via electrodes placed to stimulate the motor nerve. The magnitude of the contraction is limited by the patient's pain tolerance. Whether contractions stronger than that produced by maximum voluntary effort are possible is unknown. Also, there is no consistent relationship between current amplitude tolerated and contraction torque. The length and frequency of stimulation and the optimal electrode configuration are controversial. Contraindications to ES use are the same as those for TENS.

Therapeutic Exercise

Therapeutic exercise is designed to promote flexibility and muscular performance. It is also used to counter the response of tissues to injury or immobilization. These responses include contracture, decreased ligament strength, muscle atrophy and strength loss, and decreased bone density.

Flexibility Flexibility can be defined as the full range of motion possible at or in a joint or series of joints. Flexibility training encompasses a variety of techniques. Different sports have different flexibility demands. Controversy exists as to whether flexibility does, in fact, decrease the chance of injury. Nevertheless it has been incorporated into the exercise regimes for various sports.

Flexibility training encompasses static stretching, ballistic stretching, and proprioceptive neuromuscular facilitation. The static method places the muscle tendon unit under a slow gentle stretch for 20 to 60 seconds. This method reduces the intensity of the stretch reflex and the muscle tone of the involved group. Ballistic stretching involves quick, repetitive, and more forceful movements to overcome the muscles to be stretched. Ballistic techniques can, in fact, initiate the stretch reflex, thus countering the stretch.

Proprioceptive neuromuscular facilitation (PNF) aims to stimulate Golgi tendon organs to decrease muscle tone. A slow stretch takes the muscle tendon unit (MTU) to its end range and is held for several seconds. A maximal isometric contraction against a partner's resistance is then performed for 5 to 10 seconds. The MTU is then relaxed and slowly stretched by the partner. It is felt that isometric contraction with the MTU at its greatest length will maximally stimulate the Golgi apparatus. Reciprocal inhibition of the muscle under tension will result and allow further stretch upon relaxation.

Controversy exists as to which method of flexibility training is most effective. Static and ballistic techniques have yielded equal results, but injury risk increases with ballistic stretching. PNF has been found to be superior in some studies but not in others. The partner requirement is another disadvantage. Because pain may increase due to increased muscle activity, PNF must be done in a supervised setting.

Enhancement of Muscle Performance Clearly muscles are involved in any athletic endeavor. There are various parameters of muscular performance (Table 6). Although one or more of these variables may be enhanced by training, the generic term covering all types of such exercise is strength training (Table 7).

Isometric exercise is inexpensive and unlikely to cause injury. If immobilization is required, isometrics can decrease muscle atrophy. This form of exercise can be very useful in the early postinjury/postsurgery period. However, isometrics have serious drawbacks. Strength gains are specific to the joint angle used for the exercise. Because athletic performance requires motion, applicability to functional performance is limited. Multiangle isometrics can be used when exercise through range is limited by pain.

Isotonic exercise can be done with manual resistance, free weights, or machines. Free weights carry a potential for injury if used improperly. Machines have limited availability and adaptability to smaller individuals. Isotonic training can produce strength gains throughout at least part of a range of motion. However, the specific applicability to sports in which explosive strength is required is at issue because most isotonic training occurs at relatively slow speeds.

Table 6. Parameters of muscle performance

Strength	Maximum force generated by a muscle
Work	Force × distance
Torque	Rotational measurement of work: Force × lever arm
Power	Work/unit time
Endurance	Ability to generate force over time without fatigue

Table 7. Types of strength training

Isometric	Muscle contraction against resistance without changing length
Isotonic	Muscle contraction against constant resistance through an arc
Isokinetic	Dynamic muscle exercise at a constant velocity
Eccentric	Contraction occurs while muscle lengthens

Isokinetic machines allow exercise and/or testing up to 300°/s. Studies have established normative date for isokinetic output in athletes, mostly in the upper extremity. These data can be used to measure a patient's progress through rehabilitation. An experienced tester must monitor the patient's position and effort during testing. Isokinetics do have disadvantages. One is the expense of the machine and the requirement for therapist/athletic trainer monitoring. Second is the limited availability and sturdiness of these machines. Most importantly, there are few if any data that correlate isokinetic exercise/performance to athletic performance. Shoulder internal rotation velocity in throwing, for example, is approximately 7,000°/s.

Concentric muscle contraction occurs as the muscle shortens, while lengthening of a contracting muscle is an eccentric contraction. Eccentric exercise can be done isotonically or isokinetically. Sport-related tasks requiring rapid deceleration, such as changing direction, jumping, and throwing, all involve eccentric activity. The basic science of eccentric exercise may not be well understood at present, but strength gains from concentric and eccentric exercises probably occur independently. If needed, eccentric exercises should be added to the overall strength program and can be incorporated in functional exercise. The development of muscle soreness is common. Close monitoring is needed to be sure eccentric exercises are done correctly.

Closed chain exercises are those in which the foot is on the ground and the athlete squats and then straightens. An alternative technique is the leg press. The technique strengthens multiple muscle groups, including the flexors and extensors of the hip, knee, and ankle. It includes eccentric and concentric contractions. The shear forces across the joints are minimized due to cocontraction of opposing muscle groups (eg, anterior shear on the knee by the quadriceps is minimized by coactivation of the hamstrings).

Functional Exercise

Functional exercise aims to restore strength and agility through various techniques that do not require standard strength training equipment. Examples include the improvement of proprioception using tilt boards, core strength by use of the Swiss ball, agility by carioca or single leg diagonal jumps, leap by box jumping, and throwing by high speed elastic tubing exercise. Such exercises have recently gained popularity in places where the need for individual, sport-specific activity is oftentimes counterbalanced by the necessity for cost containment. The role of the athletic trainer/physical therapist in patient instruction and monitoring must not be underestimated, however.

Stress Fractures

Bone is a living tissue with constant turnover of the cellular population. According to Wolff's Law, it also responds to the stress applied to it. When bone fails, a fracture is produced. This failure may be the product of one specific event (macrotrauma) or repetitive small events (microtrauma). A stress fracture can best be defined as a failure of bone due to repetitive small insults.

Stress fractures can masquerade as injuries that produce what are initially relatively minor symptoms, but they can eventually be disabling. Diagnosis should be suspected from the patient's history. There is usually localized pain that worsens with progressive activity. Often it occurs after an increase in training (increased mileage), alteration in technique (new method of serving tennis), change in surface (from natural to synthetic turf), or different footwear. Clinical findings include tenderness over a specific small bone or portion of bone. Limited motion may occur if the fracture occurs about a joint. Nevertheless, certain patients may not have these findings.

Radiographic signs of a stress fracture may include a frank fracture line, yet changes often are limited to periosteal elevation or, in the case of largely cancellous bone, an abnormal trabecular pattern. In the pediatric group, stress fractures may appear as widening of the growth plate or separation of an apophysis. Two thirds of stress fractures have negative plain radiographs acutely, and one third will remain so. Because a large number of stress fractures are radiographically negative, bone scintigraphy has become the imaging technique of choice for diagnosis. It is highly sensitive, but the findings of other hot spots on whole-body images must be interpreted in light of clinical findings. Moreover, the bone scan may remain positive for 12 months or more. Plain tomography, computed tomography scan, or magnetic resonance imaging may be used for diagnosis or to define fracture anatomy or follow healing.

Two important patient groups must be mentioned. The first is pediatric athletes. Children often present late in the course of a stress fracture. The history may be vague, and the patient may have seen multiple physicians before coming to the sports medicine practitioner. Differential diagnosis should include infection and neoplasm—both benign and malignant. Because bone scan may be positive in these conditions, as well, clinical correlation is important. Serial radiographs to monitor bone healing may be required.

The second special patient group consists of female athletes. Several studies have documented an increased incidence of stress fractures in women. While complex, there does appear to be an interplay between dysmenorrhea, exercise, and decreased bone density, especially when combined with eating disorders. These factors should heighten the clinician's suspicions when evaluating female athletes for a stress fracture. A complete menstrual and dietary history should be taken. Hormonal and/or counseling/psychiatric treatment may be indicated.

A number of studies have been done defining fracture frequency. Among the largest studies was that of Matheson, who found the following distribution of stress fractures: 49.1% tibia, 25.3% tarsals, 8.8% metatarsals, 7.2% femur, and 6.6% fibula. It should be noted that this population consisted largely of runners. Other studies including different types of athletes have yielded different numbers.

Treatment must be individualized, but in each case rest should be relative. Alternative exercise such as bicycling or swimming should allow the athlete to maintain cardiovascular fitness. Those stress fractures that present special problems in either treatment or diagnosis are discussed in detail here. Other stress fractures, their typical course, radiographic features, and treatment are listed in Table 8.

Pelvis

Stress fractures of the pelvis occur about the ischium but have been seen in the sacrum, ilium, and the iliac spines. The last usually occurs in the pediatric/adolescent age group. Ischial fractures usually, but not always, present with groin pain and tenderness. Differential diagnosis should include osteitis pubis, adductor muscle injury, hernia, and genitourinary pathology, especially in the female. Treatment is relative rest, but crutches may be required early on.

Femur

Femoral stress fractures occur most commonly about the neck and the shaft. Neck fractures present with groin pain, limited motion, and antalgia. There are two typical fracture patterns. One is the transverse or tension type, which begins as a cortical defect on the superior aspect of the neck. The compression type first appears as a haze of internal callus at the inferior cortex. Failure to diagnose these fractures can lead to fracture displacement, osteonecrosis, nonunion, or malunion, which occurs most commonly in the tension type. Although some fractures of the compression type can be treated with nonweightbearing, any displacement (or any transverse or tension type fracture) requires prompt internal fixation. Multiple screws are usually used.

Other femoral fractures occur in the subtrochanteric region and the diaphysis. The patient usually presents with thigh pain and a limp. Most of the fractures are undisplaced and heal with protection. However, displacement can occur, especially in distal one third fractures, and reduction with internal fixation is required.

Tibia

The location for a stress fracture of the tibia depends, in part, on the sport. Fractures in jumping sports, such as basketball, appear to occur about the proximal metaphysis, whereas those in running sports appear about the diaphysis. Patients present with pain that increases with activity. Tenderness is confined to one specific region of the bone. Differential diagnosis includes compartment syndrome, tendinitis, and shin splints (felt to be due to periostitis, soleal muscle traction, or both). Most fractures of the tibia require limitation of activities for 6 to 12 weeks. Additional protection, such as crutches, orthosis, or cast may be indicated, depending on the patient's symptoms. Most tibial fractures heal uneventfully. One specific frac-

Table 8. Less common stress fractures

Location	Radiographic Features	Common Sports	Treatment
Ribs	Radiographs often negative	Football Weight lifting	Relative rest
Clavicle	Medial to c-c ligaments	Weight lifting Shooting	Relative rest
Acromion	Linear lucency best seen on axillary view; rule out ununited apophysis	Gymnastics	Rest; may require internal fixation
Proximal humerus	Apophyseal widening	Baseball Little League shoulder	Relative rest
Humeral diaphysis	Spiral oblique fracture	Throwing sports	Cast or orthosis until healing
Distal humerus	Apophyseal widening or separation	Baseball Little League elbow	If displaced over 5 mm, internal fixation
Olecranon	May be through apophysis	Baseball	Long arm cast 4 to 6 weeks; if delayed or nonunion, internal fixation
Ulnar diaphysis	Periosteal elevation	Fastpitch Softball	Protection; possible orthosis
Metacarpals	Radiographs often negative	Racquet sports	Padding; relative rest
Patella	Transverse; vertical	Running/jumping sports	Immobilization; may require: internal fixation for transverse fracture or excision of lateral fragment for vertical fracture
Fibula	Periosteal elevation 3 to 7 cm above malleolus	Basketball	Stirrup-type orthosis; activities to tolerance
Medial malleolus	Vertical fracture line	Basketball	If radiograph negative, protection; if radiograph positive, internal fixation
Cuboid/cuneiform	Radiograph often negative	Running	Weightbearing as tolerated; relative rest; may need orthotics after healing
Os calcis	Callus perpendicular to long axis of os calcis on lateral view	Running	Relative rest for about 3 weeks

ture of concern is the isolated stress fracture of the anterior tibial cortex. Radiographs often show only a solitary lucency in the cortex. These fractures are notorious for either delayed healing or nonunion. If the standard treatment fails to produce union, consideration needs to be given to surgical intervention, including localized bone grafting and/or intramedullary fixation.

Fifth Metatarsal

A special area of concern is the stress fracture at the proximal metaphyseal-diaphyseal junction (the so-called "Jones Fracture"). These fractures are commonly seen in jumping sports. Microvascularity studies have indicated that blood supply to this region is tenuous and, therefore, healing is difficult. Treatment options of acute injuries include cast immobilization with strict nonweightbearing for a minimum of 6 weeks or consideration of internal fixation. Although the former may be effective, treatment needs to be continued until healing occurs. Internal fixation offers the possibility for full weightbearing postoperatively and return to sports in 6 to 8 weeks. Delayed or nonunion may require internal fixation and/or bone grafting. Orthotics may be indicated once healing has occurred.

Tarsal Navicular

Persistent medial foot pain as well as localized tenderness draw attention to the possibility of a navicular stress fracture. Fracture through the body of the navicular is notorious for being negative radiographically, at least acutely. The classic configuration is a vertical fracture in the central third of the bone. Once diagnosed, this fracture requires immobilization with strict nonweightbearing for a minimum of 6 weeks. If the symptoms persist, further imaging studies including computed tomography and/or tomograms should be considered. Occasionally these fractures require internal fixation with or without bone grafting.

Metatarsals 2 Through 4

Although most frequent in military recruits, stress fractures of the central metatarsals are common. They usually involve the second or third metatarsals in runners. Because they are diaphyseal in location, routine radiographs may not reveal the typical periosteal new bone formation for 2 to 3 weeks after the onset of symptoms. Treatment can be symptomatic; occasionally a walking cast or orthosis is needed. If excessive callus forms, an orthotic with relief at the site of pain can facilitate the return to athletics.

Distal Radius

Distal radial stress fractures have been described in the gymnastics population. These usually occur in the skeletally immature athlete at the distal radial physis. Radiographs show widening of the physis. Treatment is rest from the offending activity. Whether this fracture can lead to growth abnormalities is currently unknown.

Exertional Compartment Syndromes

Exertional compartment syndrome of the leg presents as pain following exercise. The pain is due to increased intracompartmental pressures, usually in the anterior compartment and occasionally in a separate compartment surrounding the tibialis posterior. Decreasing its intensity or stopping the activity relieves symptoms. A muscle herniation may be noted and often can be found bilaterally. Objective criteria to diagnose an exertional compartment syndrome from intracompartmental pressure measurements using a slit catheter include a preexercise level $\geq$ 15 mm Hg, a 1-minute postexercise level $\geq$ 30 mm Hg, or a 5-minute postexercise level $\geq$ 20 mm Hg. If nonsurgical measures fail to relieve symptoms, an elective fasciotomy of the involved compartment may be indicated.

Annotated Bibliography

Preparticipation Evaluation

Rich BS: Sudden death screening. *Med Clin North Am* 1994;78:267–288.

This is a review of the major causes of sudden cardiac death, the effectiveness of screening studies, and the methods of identifying athletes at risk for sudden death.

Mitchell JH, Maron BJ, Epstein SE: Sixteenth Bethesda Conference: Cardiovascular abnormalities in the athlete. Recommendations regarding eligibility for competition. *J Am Coll Cardiol* 1985;6:1186–1232.

This is a group of articles that arrive at a consensus of opinion for recommendations regarding the eligibility of athletes for competition. Areas covered include congenital heart disease; acquired valvular heart disease; hypertrophic cardiomyopathy, other myopericardial disease, and mitral valve prolapse; systemic arterial hypertension; ischemic heart disease; and arrhythmias.

Head and Neck Injuries

Torg JS, Gennarelli TA: Head and cervical spine injuries, in DeLee JC, Drez D Jr (eds): *Orthopaedic Sports Medicine: Principles and Practice.* Philadelphia, PA, WB Saunders, 1994, vol 1, pp 417–462.

This is a comprehensive review of common head and cervical spine injuries.

Garth WP Jr: Evaluating and treating brachial plexus injuries. *J Musculoskel Med* 1994;11:55–67.

The clinical presentation, differential diagnosis, on-the-field evaluation, and treatment of various brachial plexus injuries are reviewed.

Miscellaneous Injuries and Conditions

Stanitski CL: Enviromental stress: Heat intolerance problems, in DeLee JC, Drez D Jr (eds): *Orthopaedic Sports Medicine: Principles and Practice.* Philadelphia, PA, WB Saunders, 1994, vol 1, pp 374–384.

This is a comprehensive review of the various heat exertion syndromes.

Rehabilitation

Almekinders LC, Oman J: Isokinetic muscle testing: Is it clinically useful? *J Am Acad Orthop Surg* 1994;2:221–225.

The authors review both isokinetic testing and rehabilitation based on current literature. They conclude that the ability of isokinetic testing to identify conclusive muscle weakness as a causative factor in orthopaedic conditions remains uncertain.

Bassett FH III, Kirkpatrick JS, Engelhardt DL, et al: Cryotherapy induced nerve injury. *Am J Sports Med* 1992;20:516–518.

The authors cite six cases and review the mechanisms for cold-induced nerve injury.

Byl NN, McKenzie A, Halliday B, et al: The effects of phonophoresis with corticosteroids: A controlled pilot study. *J Orth Sports Phys Ther* 1993;18:590–600.

This study measures the diffusion of phonophoresed corticosteroid in terms of interference with collagen deposition and change in cellular activity. The results indicate that the corticosteroid is unlikely to reach muscles or tendons and that phonophoresis may work through systemic effects.

Ho SS, Coel MN, Kagawa R, et al: The effects of ice on blood flow and bone metabolism in knees. *Am J Sports Med* 1994;22:537–540.

As shown by bone scintigraphy, all iced knees showed decreased arterial and soft-tissue blood flow as well as decreased bone uptake, indicating changes in bone flow and metabolism. The study provides a scientific rationale for cryotherapy.

Mont MA, Cohen DB, Campbell KR et al: Isokinetic concentric versus eccentric training of shoulder rotators with functional evaluation of performance enhancement in elite tennis players. *Am J Sports Med* 1994;22:513–517.

Thirty elite players were assigned to three types of training: isokinetic concentric, isokinetic eccentric, and control. Serve velocity increased 11% in both training groups as compared to 1% in controls. Subjects in the training group also tended to maintain velocity greater than controls.

Pollock RG, Flatow EL: The efficacy of physical therapy for the shoulder, in Matsen FA III, Fu FH, Hawkins RJ (eds): *The Shoulder: A Balance of Mobility and Stability.* Rosemont, IL, American Academy of Orthopaedic Surgeons, 1993, pp 401–413.

This is a critical review of a number of rehabilitation techniques including both modalities and exercise.

Wilk KE, Andrews JR, Arrigo CA, et al: The strength characteristics of internal and external rotator muscles in professional baseball pitchers. *Am J Sports Med* 1993;21: 61–66.

The authors present an isokinetic performance profile for the professional thrower, which can be used as criteria that should be met before allowing return to competition.

Stress Fractures

Arendt EA: Osteoporosis in the athletic female: Amenorrhea and amenorrheic osteoporosis, in Pearl AJ (ed): *AOSSM: The Athletic Female.* Champaign, IL, Human Kinetics, 1993, pp 41–59.

This chapter details the biochemistry of the problem and reviews the current literature.

De Smet L, Claessens A, Lefevre J, et al: Gymnast wrist: An epidemiologic survey of ulnar variance and stress changes of the radial physis in elite female gymnasts. *Am J Sports Med* 1994;22:846–850.

The authors studied the radiographs of 201 gymnasts (150 with open growth plates). They found a 10% incidence of stress-related changes of the distal physis of the radius. They concluded that repetitive compression leads to premature closure of the distal radial growth plate and secondary ulnar overgrowth.

Eisele SA, Sammarco GJ: Fatigue fractures of the foot and ankle in the athlete, in Heckman JD (ed): *Instructional Course Lectures 42.* Rosemont, IL, American Academy of Orthopaedic Surgeons, 1993, pp 175–183.

This instructional course lecture discusses the history, pathophysiology, biomechanics, presentation, diagnosis, and treatment of these stress fractures.

Johnson AW, Weiss CB Jr, Wheeler DL: Stress fractures of the femoral shaft in athletes more common than expected: A new clinical test. *Am J Sports Med* 1994;22:248–256.

Seven of 34 or 20.6% of all stress fractures in a group of 914 collegiate athletes are found. This is a much higher incidence than previously reported. A new diagnostic test is described.

Kadel NJ, Teitz CC, Kronmal RA: Stress fractures in ballet dancers. *Am J Sports Med* 1992;20:445–449.

This study consists of 54 female dancers with 27 fractures. Metatarsals 63%, tibia 22% and spine 7%, were the most common sites. The incidence of stress fracture increased with greater time of dance per day (5 hours) and longer duration of amenorrhea.

Khan KM, Fuller PJ, Brukner PD, et al: Outcome of conservative and surgical management of navicular stress fractures in athletes: Eighty-six cases proven with computerized tomography. *Am J Sports Med* 1992;20:657–666.

Eighty-six percent of patients treated with immobilization and nonweightbearing returned to sports as compared to 26% allowed weightbearing. Clinical healing as judged by lack of pain and tenderness preceded healing on computed tomography scan.

Mindrebo N, Shelbourne KD, Van Meter CD, et al: Outpatient percutaneous screw fixation of the acute Jones fracture. *Am J Sports Med* 1993;21:720–723.

The authors report on nine patients undergoing the above procedure and early postoperative weightbearing. Average return to running was 5.5 weeks postoperatively and to sports 8.5 weeks.

Compartment Syndrome

Moed BR, Thorderson PK: Measurement of intracompartmental pressures: A comparison of the slit catheter, side-ported needle, and simple needle. *J Bone Joint Surg* 1993;75A:231–235.

In a comparison of three commonly used techniques for intracompartmental pressure measurements, the slit catheter and single-ported needle methods produced similar accurate values. Use of the simple 18-gauge needle with intravenous tubing and a mercury manometer gave inaccurate and falsely elevated values, approximately 19 mm Hg higher than the other two techniques. The use of stiffer arterial line tubing with the simple needle technique needs to be evaluated.

Classic Bibliography

Preparticipation Evaluation

Vinger PF: Editorial: The one-eyed athlete. *Physician Sportsmed* 1987;15:48–52.

Head and Neck Injuries

Cantu RC: Guidelines for return to contact sports after a cerebral concussion. *Physician Sportsmed* 1986;14:75–83.

Hershman EB, Wilbourn AJ, Bergfeld JA: Acute brachial neuropathy in athletes. *Am J Sports Med* 1989;17:655–659.

Kelly J: Guidelines for the management of concussion in sports: The School Health and Sports Medicine Committee, Colorado Medical Society. *Colorado Med* 1990;87:226–227.

Saunders RL, Harbaugh RE: The second impact in catastrophic contact-sports head trauma. *JAMA* 1984;252:538–539.

Torg JS, Pavlov H, Genuario SE, et al: Neurapraxia of the cervical spinal cord with transient quadriplegia. *J Bone Joint Surg* 1986;68A:1354–1370.

Thoracic/Abdominal Injuries

Diamond DL: Sports-related abdominal trauma. *Clin Sports Med* 1989;8:91–99.

Rehabilitation

Akeson WH, Amiel D, Abel MF, et al: Effects of immobilization on joints. *Clin Orthop* 1987;219:28–37.

Amiel D, Woo SL, Harwood FL, et al: The effect of immobilization on collagen turnover in connective tissue: A biochemical-biomechanical correlation. *Acta Orthop Scand* 1982;53:325–332.

Arvidsson I, Eriksson E: Postoperative TENS relief after knee surgery: Objective evaluation. *Orthopedics* 1986;9: 1346–1351.

Arvidsson I, Arvidsson H, Eriksson E, et al: Prevention of quadriceps wasting after immobilization: An evaluation of the effect of electrical stimulation. *Orthopedics* 1986;9: 1519–1528.

Cohn BT, Draeger RI, Jackson DW: The effects of cold therapy in the postoperative management of pain in patients undergoing anterior cruciate ligament reconstruction. *Am J Sports Med* 1989;17:344–349.

Gieck JH, Saliba E: Therapeutic ultrasound: Influence on inflammation and healing, in Leadbetter WB, Buckwalter JA, Gordon SL (eds): *Sports-induced Inflammation: Clinical and Basic Science Concepts.* Park Ridge, IL, American Academy of Orthopaedic Surgeons, 1990, pp 479–492.

Hartsell HD, Kramer JF: A comparison of the effects of electrode placement, muscle tension, and isometric torque of the knee extensors. *J Ortho Sports Phys Ther* 1992;15:168–174.

Knapik JJ, Bauman CL, Jones BH, et al: Preseason strength and flexibility imbalances associated with athletic injuries in female collegiate athletes. *Am J Sports Med* 1991;19:76–81.

Labelle H, Guibert R, Joncas J, et al: Lack of scientific evidence for the treatment of lateral epicondylitis of the elbow: An attempted meta-analysis. *J Bone Joint Surg* 1992;74B:646–651.

Morrissey MC, Brewster CE, Shields CL Jr, et al: The effects of electrical stimulation on the quadriceps during postoperative knee immobilization. *Am J Sports Med* 1985;13:40–45.

Reid DC, Burnham RS, Saboe LA, et al: Lower extremity flexibility patterns in classical ballet dancers and their correlation to lateral hip and knee injuries. *Am J Sports Med* 1987;15:347–352.

Selkowitz DM: High frequency electrical stimulation in muscle strengthening: A review and discussion. *Am J Sports Med* 1989;17:103–111.

Stress Fractures

Barrow GW, Saha S: Menstrual irregularity and stress fractures in collegiate female distance runners. *Am J Sports Med* 1988;16:209–216.

DeLee JC, Evans JP, Julian J: Stress fracture of the fifth metatarsal. *Am J Sports Med* 1983;11:349–353.

Drinkwater BL, Bruemner B, Chesnut CH III: Menstrual history as a determinant of current bone density in young athletes. *JAMA* 1990:263:545–548.

Fullerton LR Jr, Snowdy HA: Femoral neck stress fractures. *Am J Sports Med* 1988;16:365–377.

Giladi M, Milgrom C, Simkin A, et al: Stress fractures: Identifiable risk factors. *Am J Sports Med* 1991; 19:647–652.

Hershman EB, Mailly T: Stress fractures. *Clin Sports Med* 1990;9:183–214.

Johansson C, Ekenman I, Tornkvist H, et al: Stress fractures of the femoral neck in athletes: The consequence of a delay in diagnosis. *Am J Sports Med* 1990;18:524–528.

Matheson GO, Clement DB, McKenzie DC, et al: Stress fractures in athletes: A study of 320 cases. *Am J Sports Med* 1987;15:46–58.

Mandelbaum BR, Grant TT, Nichols AW: Wrist pain in a gymnast. *Phys Sport Med* 1988;16:80–84.

Rettig AC, Shelbourne KD, McCarroll JR, et al: The natural history and treatment of delayed union stress fractures of the anterior cortex of the tibia. *Am J Sports Med* 1988;16:250–255.

Shelbourne KD, Fisher DA, Rettig AC, et al: Stress fractures of the medial malleolus. *Am J Sports Med* 1988;16:60–63.

Tanabe S, Nakahira J, Bando E, et al: Fatigue fracture of the ulna occurring in pitchers of fast-pitch softball. *Am J Sports Med* 1991;19:317–321.

Torg JS, Pavlov H, Cooley LH, et al: Stress fractures of the tarsal navicular: A retrospective review of twenty-one cases. *J Bone Joint Surg* 1982;64A:700–712.

13

Multiple Trauma: Management of the Injured Patient

Trauma remains a leading cause of death, especially in the younger segments of the population. In the United States alone, over 130,000 deaths occur annually as a result of trauma. Treating these injuries accounts for up to 40% of US health care costs. Because trauma is primarily an urban disease process and is viewed as a social indicator rather than a health-care problem, it is often ignored. Trauma care appears to be one of those areas of medicine that would benefit from national health insurance, because the reimbursement rate for much of trauma care is low. Financial problems have led to the closing of a number of trauma centers and of several trauma systems. Current knowledge concerning the management of the acutely injured patient has largely come from these systems. Organized trauma systems need to be supported and developed across the United States.

Trauma systems have been shown to be effective in saving lives. However, a real effort at cost containment must be made, if the trauma systems are to survive. The most effective methods of controlling costs focus on injury prevention, coordination of care, elimination of needless tests, and aggressive rehabilitation.

Injury Prevention

The effectiveness of seat belts in preventing ejection from a motor vehicle and severe injuries has been known for many years. Despite that, fatalities increased until 1992 when usage was made mandatory in many states. Safety belts decrease the incidence of injuries and deaths by lowering the gravity forces of deceleration and by eliminating the risk of ejection from the initial collision. Air bags prevent further injury and deaths from the second collision of the victims and the interior of the car. They also prevent the secondary contusion and the resulting head and chest injuries. The next motor vehicle safety device, which already has been installed in some automobile models, is the side-impact air bag.

Helmet use has dramatically decreased the death rate in bicycle and motorcycle accidents. States that have made helmet use mandatory have seen a 60% decrease in the number of deaths among motorcycle riders.

General

Responses of patients who have been injured vary only according to the organ system injured and the degree of injury. The degree of injury, therefore, becomes important in separating the physiologically unstable multiple trauma victim from a stable trauma patient with a single system or minor injury. Several scoring systems, including the Revised Trauma Score (RTS) and the Glasgow coma scale (GCS), are used in the initial assessment of the injured patient. These systems, which determine the degree of injury and the resulting physiologic impairment, are used in organized trauma systems to triage patients to comprehensive trauma care facilities. Data suggest that if the Glasgow coma scale is less than 13 or if the trauma score is less than 11, patients should be transported to comprehensive facilities. The immediate care of the unstable, multiply-injured patient has been outlined by the American College of Surgeons Advanced Trauma Life Support course. This course divides the care of the patient into four stages, which provide a template for trauma management. The initial care stage is the primary survey phase, in which immediately life-threatening injuries are identified and treated. The resuscitation phase, which includes placement of various lines and tubes for monitoring and resuscitation, begins simultaneously. The third phase of management of the critically injured patient includes the secondary survey or history and physical evaluation of the patient, which are used to identify any injuries that the patient has as a result of the accident. The final phase is the definitive care consisting of surgical intervention or chronic monitoring.

Fluid resuscitation is guided by the patient's vital signs and by estimates of fluid loss. Treatment techniques now used in the prehospital setting include administration of hypertonic saline and dextran solutions and low-volume fluid resuscitation. These techniques are not currently advocated once the patient has been admitted to the hospital or during preparation for surgical intervention.

It is important to emphasize that not all trauma patients require the services of a specialized trauma center. It is primarily the multiply-injured patient with unstable physiologic parameters that requires such expertise. The vast majority of patients can be treated in a less urgent fashion when competent personnel are available.

Patient Response To Injury

Following injury, all patients respond in a similar fashion. The degree of response is related to the severity of the injury and the number of organ systems involved. Major mechanical or thermal injuries result in tremendous increases in caloric requirements (as much as 150% of normal in the severely burned patient). Provision of adequate nutrition to support this requirement has been a major advance in the field of trauma care. Similarly, major injuries resulting in tissue damage and shock have been shown to markedly stimulate the stress response and alter the endocrine balance of the patient. There is an increased secretion of the hormones related to mobilization of fats and glucose. Insulin secretion appears to be elevated during the stress response. Other factors, including tumor necrosis factor and many of the interleukins, are also released into the general circulation. The role of these cytokines in sepsis and in organ failure has been studied. The release of agents from the gastrointestional tract may contribute to developing sepsis and organ failure in the multiply-injured patient. This translocation involves the release of endogenous bacteria or their products into the circulatory system.

Wound Care

Local factors in the wound affect the patient's systemic response. Therefore, early local wound care remains the hallmark of treating injury. Early stabilization of the fractured extremity and the excision of devascularized tissues remove cytotoxic agents. The main therapeutic intervention for soft-tissue injuries includes local wound care and debridement of the devitalized tissue, coupled with antibiotics directed at surface organisms. These concepts are also true for either penetrating or blunt injuries to the brain, thorax, and abdomen. Antibiotic coverage is usually directed toward surface organisms in these areas as well as toward potentially contaminating organisms from the region (eg, in the gastrointestinal tract, antibiotic coverage may be directed toward bowel flora).

Prophylaxis Against Complications

The immediate care of the multiply-injured patient consists of determining what is injured and repairing those injuries in the correct order of importance and in a timely fashion. The subsequent care involves monitoring the patient and preventing complications. Prophylactic therapies indicated in the care of the acutely injured patient include determining nutritional needs; preventing stress bleeding, venous thrombosis, and pressure sores; and assessing antibiotic coverage.

Early nutrition in the injured patient is a critical part of the care. Ideas concerning surgical nutrition have actually come full circle. Following the development of the techniques of parenteral nutrition, surgeons advised early institution of parenteral alimentation in the care of these patients. This concept has gradually been revised. The current recommendations are to provide early enteral nutrition to patients who have a functional gastrointestinal tract. Several new immune-enhancing formulations have shown great promise by increasing the number of calories provided to the acutely injured patient and decreasing the complications associated with immune suppression, which may occur with parenteral nutrition or no nutrition at all. Support of the early hypermetabolism associated with injury and prevention of the protein calorie malnutrition that occurs within a day or two of injury are the goals. The data suggest that many septic complications can be minimized if patients are begun on early enteral nutrition. Even following abdominal procedures, feeding directly into the small bowel (by nasoduodenal or jejunostomy tubes) is tolerated without significant ileus. Similarly, it appears that early enteral nutrition (using the newer formulations) does not result in significant diarrhea. This diarrhea appears to be more related to the prolonged absence of enteral feeding, and early feeding appears to limit its subsequent development.

The severely injured patient exhibits a stress response that includes the release of hormones that stimulate gastric acid production. The introduction of agents to decrease acid secretion has decreased the number of patients requiring treatment of stress bleeding. Prevention of stress bleeding by the use of histamine blockade or mucosal barrier protection is required in any significantly injured patient and is especially required in those not being fed enterally.

Deep venous thrombosis and pulmonary embolism are major concerns in the patient with multiple trauma. Some form of prophylaxis or treatment is required. The best form of therapy remains full anticoagulation; however, anticoagulation frequently is not indicated because of the multiple sites of injury and the potential for bleeding, especially in the central nervous system. Appropriate forms of prophylaxis, which depend on the types of injury, should include one or a combination of the following: (1) passive motion of lower extremities, (2) segmental compression devices for the extremities, (3) vitamin K antagonist (warfarin, Coumadin), (4) low dose or minidose heparin, (5) early ambulation, or (6) placement of a vena cava filter. These have been shown to be effective in reducing the incidence of pulmonary embolism. The indications for insertion of prophylactic inferior vena cava filters are currently being debated.

The development of pressure sores frequently adds $50,000 or more to the cost of caring for injured patients. Therefore, interventions to reduce the incidence of decubital pressure sores are vital. In the multiply-injured patient (especially patients with interference of movement secondary to paralysis or prolonged procedures), attention is directed to preventing prolonged pressure on dependent areas. Preventive measures include obtaining the appropriate bed, removing the patient from rigid spine boards as rapidly as possible, and mobilizing the patient as early as is feasible. It is unfortunate that this is often a low priority item in the critically ill or injured patient and frequently is addressed only after the problem is noted.

The final prophylactic regimen that should be addressed early in patient care is the choice of antibiotics. The care of the multiply-injured patient frequently includes the neurosurgery, plastic surgery, general surgery, and orthopaedic surgery services. Prophylactic antibiotics are chosen based on the needs of each of the individual services. Fortunately, most studies indicate that for closed injuries to many different organ systems, prophylaxis against surface organisms requires only a first generation cephalosporin. The choice of prophylactic antibiotics becomes more challenging when open injuries exist. Coverage against gram-negative and anaerobic organisms may be suggested by the type of wound and the patient's location when the injury occurred.

Trauma Injury Management

Head

The classic approach to the management of the multiply-injured patient with significant head trauma has been stabilization using appropriate fluid management and rapid computed tomography (CT) scan to define the extent of injury. Treatment is designed to reduce cerebral hypertension and includes hyperventilation ($Paco_2$ of 26 to 28 mm Hg), head elevation, and osmotic diuresis. However, lowering $Paco_2$ to these levels may contribute to cerebral ischemia. Similarly, controlling the arterial blood pressure and reducing cerebral hypertension may injure the patient. Some neurosurgeons are now suggesting that $Paco_2$ be maintained between 32 and 35 mm Hg. Osmotic diuresis, using mannitol or urea, remains helpful in treating patients with acute cerebral edema. The role of agents that reduce cerebral activity (such as phenobarbital) has been studied. Few data exist as to the benefits of reducing cerebral metabolism in the face of acute brain injury.

Spine

Cervical spine radiographs are routinely obtained during the evaluation of the trauma patient. The consequence of missing a fracture of the cervical spine justifies this radiography, despite a very low true positive rate. Thoracolumbar spine fractures are associated with a neurologic deficit in approximately 45% of cases. Because of the consequence of a missed fracture of the thoracic or lumbar spine, surveillance radiographs are now recommended for the trauma patient with multisystem blunt injuries, a fall equal to or greater than 10 ft, ejection from a motor vehicle or motorcycle, a Glasgow coma score less than or equal to 8, a neurologic deficit, or back pain or tenderness on physical examination.

The initial (field) care and stabilization of patients with spine injuries is outlined for prehospital personnel in *Emergency Care and Transportation of the Sick and Injured* (American Academy of Orthopaedic Surgeons, 1995). With 14,000 new spinal cord injuries occurring each year, the initial care is important to prevent further injury and functional loss.

High-dose methylprednisolone is recommended in the care of acute injury to the spinal cord. A multicenter national acute spinal cord injury study reported improvement in motor scores in patients with incomplete spinal cord injuries after treatment with high-dose methylprednisolone within 8 hours of injury. These results were compared to those of a similar group of patients treated with naloxone (opiate receptor antagonist) and with a placebo. There was no significant difference between groups when treatment was begun after the initial 8 hours after injury. One year after the injury, the group treated with high-dose methylprednisolone had a higher probability of improved motor function.

The current recommendation is to give methylprednisolone by intravenous administration to all acute spinal cord injury patients. The recommended dose is 30 mg/kg of body weight over 15 minutes followed by an infusion of 5.4 mg/kg/hr for 23 hours.

Chest

In the multiple trauma patient with thoracic injury, the major concern is lung damage with resulting hypoxia. Pulmonary contusion, hemothorax, pulmonary laceration, and pneumothorax all may result in significant hypoxia. Usually these problems can be treated by airway maneuvers such as intubation, mechanical ventilation, or tube thoracostomy. Historically, this type of patient has not been a good candidate for open reduction and internal fixation of long-bone injuries. However, early open reduction and internal fixation of long-bone fractures may enhance the pulmonary status and should make the nursing care of the patient easier.

Controversy remains regarding the best way to evaluate a patient with suspected injury to the thoracic aorta. Several studies have confirmed aortography as the standard against which other diagnostic modalities (such as dynamic CT) should be compared. A patient with a wide mediastinum must be studied prior to repair of long-bone injuries.

The ventilation management of the critically injured patient in the intensive care unit includes refinements of technique such as pressure support and permissive hypercapnia. These modifications lower energy use by the patient and reduce the potential for barotrauma.

Abdomen

Evaluation of the acutely injured multiple-trauma victim still includes peritoneal lavage for those unstable patients suspected of having intra-abdominal injury; however, reasonably stable patients with suspected abdominal injuries are more often evaluated via a CT scan. Several large series have demonstrated that this is appropriate and appears to be much more specific than diagnostic peritoneal lavage. The use of CT has reduced the number of patients requiring urgent laparotomy secondary to positive lavage. A number of patients revealed by CT to have injured livers and spleens and who are stable are now observed. The one injury that CT appears to miss is small perforations of the gastrointestinal tract. Close observation and serial examinations are, therefore, mandatory when diagnostic peritoneal lavage is not used and CT scan is the primary mode of evaluation of the abdomen.

Pelvis and Lower Extremities

The occurrence of fat embolism during intramedullary fixation of the femur has been studied intraoperatively.

Reaming of the intramedullary canal causes fat and bone marrow extravasation into the lymph system and bloodstream. The intramedullary nailing process in itself does not lead to an increase in lung permeability, although it does cause an increase in pulmonary pressure. Postoperatively, hemorrhagic shock does lead to an increase in lung permeability. At the same time, translocation of bacteria and endotoxin secondary to gut damage caused by hypovolemic shock has been implicated as a source of posttraumatic sepsis. The endotoxin may reach the pulmonary bloodstream unfiltered and cause an increase in permeability in the lung. There are no clinical studies that completely explain the cause of fatal fat embolism syndrome in the trauma patient.

An improved mortality rate is noted when major pelvic and long-bone fractures are stabilized early in the care of the multiply-injured patient. It now is recommended that all fractures of long bones and the pelvis should be stabilized within 48 hours in this patient group.

Vascular

Vascular injuries may be obvious or may be suspected by the mechanism of injury. They are known to occur with fractures and dislocations about the elbow and knee. When evaluating a suspected arterial injury secondary to a penetrating wound, noninvasive duplex scanning may be a good alternative to angiography. Several large series have demonstrated that arteriography is no longer indicated for all penetrating injuries. The majority of penetrating injuries do not require arterial evaluation if an obvious vascular injury exists; however, blunt or closed injuries frequently require further evaluation after reduction of any obvious deformities. Contrast arteriography remains the standard for the evaluation of these injuries. As duplex scanning becomes more readily available and accurate, it may add to the initial evaluation of the injured extremity. This addition is important due to the difference in time required to obtain a color flow Doppler and a contrast arteriogram, not to mention the cost involved.

Future Trends In Trauma

Several areas of trauma management are being studied. The use of shock trousers (Military Anti-Shock Trousers, MAST, or Pneumatic Anti-Shock Garments, PASG) for prehospital patient care has been questioned. One large series documented that they were of little use in penetrating injuries that occurred close to an urban hospital. Recently, a similar study from the same institution questioned treating hypotensive patients with fluid in the prehospital setting. Large volumes of fluid may not be necessary and, in some instances, may cause greater overall bleeding. Both of these studies were performed in limited populations with specific injuries and cannot be applied uniformly to all injured patients. Further studies will have to be performed to determine the circumstances under which MAST as well as prehospital fluid administration are to be used for various types of injured patients.

Future directions of trauma care will be dependent on funding for trauma centers and systems.

Annotated Bibliography

Introduction

Eastman AB, Bishop GS, Walsh JC, et al: The economic status of trauma centers on the eve of health care reform. *J Trauma* 1994;36:835–846.

A comprehensive description of many of the problems facing our leading trauma centers and systems.

Injury Prevention

Gokcen EC, Burgess AR, Siegel JH, et al: Pelvic fracture mechanism of injury in vehicular trauma patients. *J Trauma* 1994;36:789–795.

A retrospective review to investigate the correlation between motor vehicle crash mechanisms and pelvic injury in front-seat occupants. The conclusion was made that there is a need for additional side impact protection in motor vehicles based on the direct correlation between pelvic injury and vehicular mechanism of injury.

Swierzewski MJ, Feliciano DV, Lillis RP, et al: Deaths from motor vehicle crashes: Patterns of injury in restrained and unrestrained victims. *J Trauma* 1994;37:404–407.

A time comparison study of motor vehicle crashes. The incidence of major head, thoracic and abdominal injuries in unrestrained and restrained fatally injured victims was the same. This suggests that severe collisions with crushing, intrusion, or significant deceleration exceed the ability of restraints to prevent many fatal injuries.

Prophylaxis Against Complications

Alexander JJ, Yuhas JP, Piotrowski JJ: Is the increasing use of prophylactic percutaneous IVC filters justified? *Am J Surg* 1994;168:102–106.

Retrospective review of 150 patients who had insertion of an IVC filter for prophylaxis. High morbidity and mortality in this group of patients allows the authors to question the indications for the procedure.

Geerts WH, Code KI, Jay RM, et al: A prospective study of venous thromboembolism after major trauma. *N Engl J Med* 1994;331:1601–1606.

Natural history of patients unprotected from the development of venous thromboembolism is examined in consecutive trauma patients with an ISS > 9. This study documents the need for effective regimens for prophylaxis.

Grant JP: Nutritional support in critically ill patients. *Ann Surg* 1994;220:610–616.

Excellent review article documenting some of the new enteral and parenteral preparations being used in modern surgical nutrition.

Moore FA, Moore EE, Kudsk KA, et al: Clinical benefits of an immune-enhancing diet for early postinjury enteral feeding. *J Trauma* 1994;37:607–615.

Clinical evaluation of 98 patients receiving either an immune-enhancing diet or standard enteral feedings in the postinjury period. Data suggest that the immune-inhancing formula lessens the risks of sepsis.

Weinmann EE, Salzman EW: Deep-vein thrombosis. *N Engl J Med* 1994;331:1630–1641.

An excellent review article describing the various techniques of treating or providing prophylaxis for venous thrombosis.

Trauma Injury Management

Bone LB, McNamara K, Shine B, et al: Mortality in multiple trauma patients with fractures. *J Trauma* 1994:37:262–264.

A multicenter study performed to determine the mortality rate of patients with multiple injuries with major pelvic and long bone fractures who had early total care of their injuries. This study clearly revealed the benefit of early fracture stabilization in reducing mortality rates in the young as well as patients over 50 years old.

Dubick MA, Wade CE: A review of the efficacy and safety of 7.5% NaCl/6% Dextran 70 in experimental animals and in humans. *J Trauma* 1994;36:323–330.

Review article which documents the effacacy and safety of hypertonic/Dextran solutions in the acute resuscitation of experimental animals and human trauma patients.

Frankel HL, Rozycki GS, Ochsner MG, et al: Indications for obtaining surveillance thoracic and lumbar spine radiographs. *J Trauma* 1994;37:673–676.

Thoracic and lumbar spine fractures may be associated with a neurologic deficit 45% of the time. As has been found in reviewing the cervical spine screening data, the yield is extremely low but the consequence of missing a fracture is unjustifable. This article reviews the indications for obtaining lumbosacral spine films in the trauma setting.

Liu M, Lee CH, P'eng, FK: Prospective comparison of diagnostic peritoneal lavage, computed tomographic scanning, and ultrasonography for the diagnosis of blunt abdominal trauma. *J Trauma* 1993;35:267–270.

Prospective series from Taiwan examining the relative merits of two scanning techniques (CT and USG) and peritoneal lavage. Stable patients had all techniques. The sensitivity, specificity and accuracy were similar for all techniques. The authors felt that in selected patients the modality of assessing injury was complementary.

Marshall JC, Christou NV, Meakins JL: The gastrointestinal tract: The undrained abscess of multiple organ failure. *Ann Surg* 1993;218:111–119.

The GI tract is an important reservoir of organisms which may contribute to postinjury or ICU acquired infections, thus contributing to the development of multiple organ failure.

Simon RJ, Mawilmada S, Ivatury RR: Hypercapnia: Is there a need for concern? *J Trauma* 1994;37:74–80.

The authors studied the effects of moderate hypercapnia (Paco_2 = 63.3 + 15.7 mm Hg) on patient parameters and found no adverse effects. These data suggest that allowing higher levels of Paco_2 may not adversely affect patients and, therefore, physicians may be able to lessen pulmonary pressures that contribute to barotrauma.

Slucky AV, Eismont FJ: Treatment of acute injury of the cervical spine, in Jackson DW (ed): *Instructional Course Lectures 44*. Rosemont, IL, American Academy of Orthopaedic Surgeons, 1995, pp 67–80.

This is a review of the current pharmacological treatment to include the use of methylprednisolone in the treatment of acute spinal-cord injuries.

Wozasek GE, Thurnher M, Redl H, et al: Pulmonary reaction during intramedullary fracture management in traumatic shock: An experimental study. *J Trauma* 1994:37:249–254.

Intramedullary nailing of sheep was carried out while monitoring the pathophysiologic events in the lung. The conclusion was made that intramedullary nailing of long bones does not lead to increased lung permeability but the addition of hemorrhagic shock postoperatively does lead to lung disturbance.

Future Trends in Trauma

Bickell WH, Wall MJ Jr, Pepe PE, et al: Immediate versus delayed fluid resuscitation for hypotensive patients with penetrating torso injuries. *N Engl J Med* 1994; 331:1105–1109.

In a highly selected group of trauma patients with gunshot wounds to the trunk who are close to a trauma center, it appears that field resuscitation with fluids is not warranted. Survival was better if fluid resuscitation was delayed until patients were in the operating room.

Cayten CG, Berendt BM, Byrne DW, et al: A study of pneumatic antishock garments in severely hypotensive trauma patients. *J Trauma* 1993;34:728–733.

In a series of 142 severely hypotensive patients (BP < 50 mm Hg) patients with MAST support had a better survival than patients without MAST.

14

Occupational Orthopaedics and Disability

Introduction

Each year, there are some 11 million work-related injuries, 19% of all injuries reported in the United States. The direct cost of workplace injuries is estimated at $111 billion, an amount equal to 3% of the US gross national product. Indirect costs are probably more than $111 billion.

Occupational orthopaedics is gaining special attention because workers' compensation care is in a financial crisis: the current cost of medical care in the United States is close to 13% of the gross national product, and increases in expenditures related to workers' compensation exceeded the national rate of increase in medical care costs. The direct and indirect costs related to workers' disability have risen by 1,200% since 1970, with most of the increase dating back to 1985. Medical costs are now becoming equal to indemnity payments.

Over 60% of all disabling (3 or more lost workdays) work-related injuries are musculoskeletal. The two costliest work-related musculoskeletal disorders (WRMD) are low back pain (LBP) and cumulative trauma disorders (CTD). The major effort of governmental, industrial, and labor organizations to focus on prevention results from the fact that more than 25% of disability cases are accounted for by these two disorders.

The solution to the problem is not simple, but possible partial solutions could result in a significant decrease in morbidity, disability, and monetary costs. First, the excessively bureaucratic workers' compensation system procedures that impose a lengthy delay in the delivery of care need streamlining. This delay is an important contributor to the onset of chronic occupational low back pain (COLBP). Second, medical care for occupational disorders needs to be better organized because poorly organized delivery may promote the worker's belief that he or she suffers from a serious condition that cannot be cured. Third, the treatment of occupational disorders and injuries requires special medical expertise.

The orthopaedist is an essential participant in the delivery of workers' compensation care, especially for more severe cases. This participation is in collaboration with other professionals and bureaucrats who can impact on the patient's medical outcome. Despite their good intentions, inexperienced physicians may increase the cost of the patient's medical care simply by promoting fear through the use of medical terminology that the patient cannot understand. Formal education in the special medicoadministrative rules and terminology that govern work injuries is essential.

One national trend in response to the crisis is the involvement of Health Management Organizations, in which the primary focus is cost. These organizations keep the injured worker from unnecessary care and shorten the duration of disability. This managed care model may work, particularly if the injured worker obtains care from experienced "occupational" orthopaedists and/or trained occupational health physicians.

Occupational Orthopaedics

WRMD and injuries are not simple orthopaedic entities. For instance, outcome studies of spinal surgery reveal that patients receiving workers' compensation have poorer outcomes than uncompensated orthopaedic patients. The biopsychosocial model adapted by Waddell shows the multifactorial causes for nonspecific low back pain with more accuracy than the classic disease model. Only a fraction of the health professionals involved with workers' compensation patients search actively for those uncustomary risk factors. The consequence is inefficient care and increased costs.

Workers' compensation care is painfully bureaucratic, difficult to understand, and with all its decision makers—health and other professionals, legislators, and civil servants—bound to remain so for the near future. Totally opposing interests, many related to matters other than health, burden the medicoadministrative process of the compensation law. Finally, the injured worker who carries with him or her a deep suspicion of the entire process, fearing injustice and needing to show solidarity to labor, may not participate to the extent required for rapid recovery, especially if his or her employer is not progressive in preventing injury and correcting dangerous work practices.

The orthopaedic surgeon treating compensation cases has to deal with these external factors. He or she should understand federal and state regulations, general work rules of employers, legal practices of compensation attorneys, and some societal values of the patients. Such knowledge will influence the outcome favorably for all parties involved in the process.

Occupational orthopaedics is different from general orthopaedics. In addition to the medical history, knowledge of the workplace and understanding of the factors leading to work-related injuries and disorders are part of the initial assessment. The orthopaedist has to strongly enumerate the reasonable expectation of a full return to work with the appropriate treatment and/or workplace modification.

Agencies Involved with WRMD

Several federal and other agencies have special interest in occupational LBP and CTD. The Occupational Safety and Health Agency (OSHA) classifies LBP as an injury and CTD as a disorder. It also drafts ergonomics protection standards to prevent the occurrence of WRMD. The National Institute of Occupational Safety and Health (NIOSH) does research primarily in the prevention of WRMD and injuries. The International Standard Organization (ISO) provides performance-oriented rules and incorporates concepts of continuous improvement in working conditions. ISO standards exist as examples for vibration exposure and ergonomic principles in the design of work systems. The American National Standards Institute (ANSI) of the National Safety Council is currently working on standards for "Control of Work-Related Cumulative Trauma Disorders" of the upper extremity through the draft report ANSI Z-365. The US Agency for Health Care Policy and Research (AHCPR) has issued guidelines on LBP that are discussed in detail in Chapter 51 of this book. Finally, the American Medical Association has written the third edition of their "Guides to the Evaluation of Permanent Impairment." Other agencies, guidelines, and standards exist, but they are not as pertinent to the practicing orthopaedic surgeon interested in WRMD.

Occupational Low Back Pain

Industry is particularly interested in risk factors for occupational low back pain (OLBP) because it is one of the costliest problems for workers, industry, and society. OLBP is: (1) the second most common cause of absenteeism in industry; (2) the number one reported impairment in occupational musculoskeletal injuries; (3) the second most costly occupational medical problem after lung diseases and influenza; (4) a disorder that affects up to 50% of the workers in the United States; (5) the leading cause of disability in persons 19 to 45 years of age; (6) the most common complaint treated by primary care physicians; and (7) an expensive disorder that has a median cost of $6,800 per occurrence.

The occupational risk factors for developing LBP are heavy work, repeated lifting, lifting while twisting, whole body vibration, and static postures. However, recent studies have shown that work satisfaction and poor appraisal ratings by supervisors are equally important (Fig. 1). The occupational risk factors for chronicity are a lack of alternative placement, poor job satisfaction, high psychologic work stress, and earnings of less than a $1,000/month (Fig. 2).

The individual risk factors affecting outcomes of COLBP are previously reported LBP, age, inappropriate health beliefs or misconceptions, and cigarette smoking. Health care factors affecting the outcome include doctor shopping, inadequate and/or passive treatment, and overall poor understanding by health care professionals of what is good care in the treatment of OLBP.

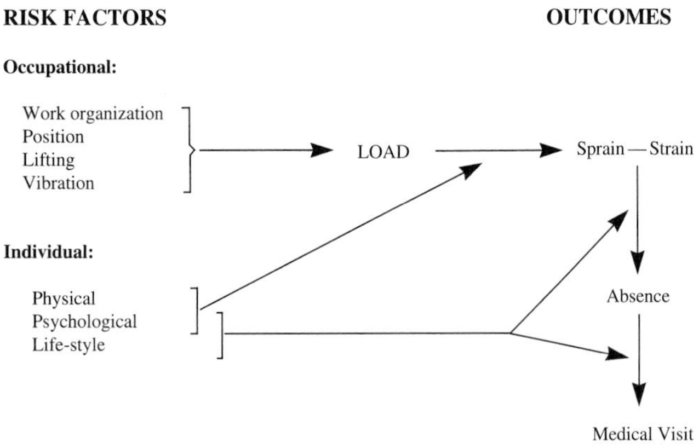

Fig. 1 Possible relationships between risk factors and patients with low back pain (LBP) seeking health care. (Reproduced with permission from Skovron M: Epidemiology of low back pain. *Baillieres Clin Rheumatol* 1992;6:559–574.)

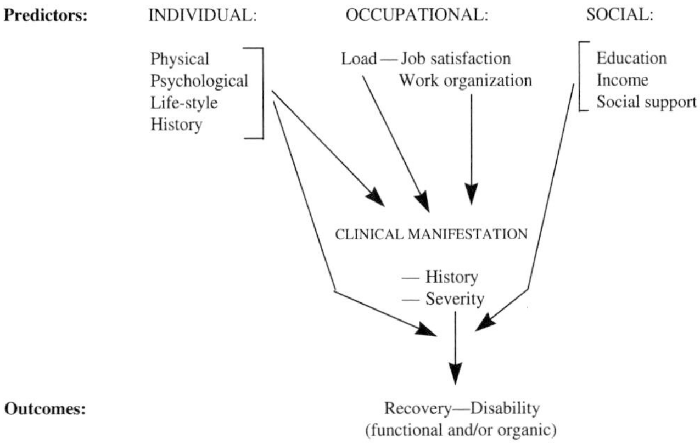

Fig. 2 The possible relationship between predictors and outcome of chronicity of low back pain. (Reproduced with permission from Skovron M: Epidemiology of Low Back Pain. *Bailleres Clin Rheumatol* 1992;6:559–574.)

The success of modern orthopaedic surgery in treating serious spinal pathologies is evident when reviewing the management of disk prolapse, spinal stenosis, and spinal tumors. Disk surgery survived the test of time for more than half a century because 70% to 90% of the carefully selected patients obtain excellent results. These conditions fit in the disease model; the underlying pathology permits physical treatment.

However, the partial failure of current medical management of OLBP is due to inaccurate diagnoses: OLBP is seldom an injury and is not a disease, not a disorder, nor a diagnosis; it is a symptom. Sacroiliac disorders, coccydynia, lumbosacral anomalies, fibrositis, disk degeneration, facet joint pain, and myofascial pain are used repeatedly to describe OLBP. Scientific evidence does not support any of these diagnoses as the basis of OLBP, but physicians treat patients with OLBP by relentlessly searching for structural pathology. Computed tomography and magnetic resonance imaging (MRI) discriminate poorly between normal subjects and patients with acute or subacute backache. The high incidence of lumbar disk degeneration in patients over 35 can be interpreted as falsely positive.

Additional psychologic distress and illness behavior common in patients with OLBP confuse the clinical assessment while applying a pressure to do something. If both patient and clinician are desperate to find a cause for the problem, the risk of overdiagnosis is real. Orthopaedists must recognize these limitations. The regrettable formulation of nominal diagnoses may be no more than convenient clinical labels, and these may compromise the recovery of patients with psychosocial issues. An important discovery is that most OLBP patients present a physiologic impairment rather than structural pathology. A professional approach that focuses on physical findings can aggravate the fear-avoidance behavior and lead to definite iatrogenic disability.

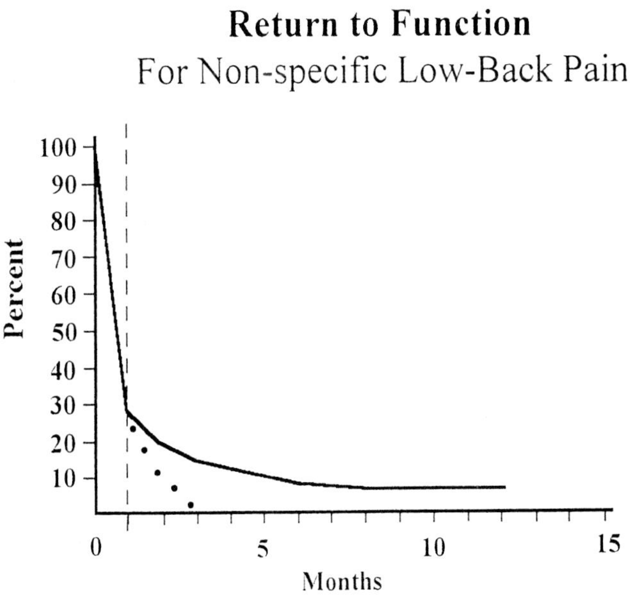

Fig. 3 The natural history of occupational low back pain (solid line). Dashed line represents time line for slow-to-recover patients at risk for chronicity. An agressive multidisciplinary program should be considered. Dotted line represents result of active intervention program at 4 to 6 weeks.

Treatment of Occupational Low Back Pain

OLBP is by far the most frequently reported workplace injury and makes up approximately 80% of all the reported occupational musculoskeletal injuries. The natural history of OLBP is very good: 60% are better within 4 weeks and 80% within 6 weeks (Fig. 3).

The first encounter with the patient complaining of OLBP is crucial. It is during this interview that a physician establishes a relationship with the patient, rules out any serious pathologies, and sets the expected outcome through reassurance and education. The orthopaedist must take sufficient time to obtain a medical history and do a complete physical examination with the patient undressed. The initial focus is on the neurologic examination. The physician must provide an accurate expectation of the outcome based on the natural history of LBP. Proper symptom control (no narcotics or sedative drugs), safe and reasonable modifications of activities (no lifting, some activity), and general recommendations against bed rest and overuse of modalities can possibly limit the number of recurrences. It is wise to resist the temptation to order lumbar MRI with common OLBP unless the patient has one of the red flags, which are fever, unexplained weight loss, major trauma, cauda equina, bowel or bladder dysfunction, and/or a history of cancer.

Eighty percent to 85% of the LBP patients need a second visit in 10 to 12 days. Physical therapy, a brief program of manipulation, or even benign neglect is sufficient during this interval, principally to minimize pain. A good tracking system identifies the patients with a risk of prolonged disability. Those patients complain excessively without serious underlying disease. They should be singled out during the window of opportunity, which is 4 to 6 weeks after the onset of the episode. At this point, a well-organized multidisciplinary treatment team can substantially change the course of the LBP episode. Such intervention, including return-to-work programs, has been shown to be highly effective in preventing the acute-to-chronic conversion of disabling OLBP when multifactorial risks become operational. At this point, early intervention has the best cost/benefit ratio while promoting patients' satisfaction and health. According to the AHCPR Guidelines, early promotion to normal activity within 4 weeks of the onset of LBP is effective and may prevent LBP from becoming a chronic disorder.

Figure 4 presents the algorithm proposed in the AHCPR Guidelines for the treatment of acute low back problems on initial and follow-up visits. At the initial visit, the individual with LBP has been screened and no underlying serious condition has been found. At this time, the important role of the orthopaedist is to provide information and reassurance. If the patient requires help to relieve his or her symptoms, treatment and pain medication should be kept to a minimum. The physician should reinforce the importance of returning to normal activity to the extent possible and as soon as possible. At the follow-up visit within 10 to 12 days, the procedure is repeated, with additional reassurance. If symptoms recur or do not abate, further testing may be indicated to enable the patient to return to work and a normal, active lifestyle.

Figure 5 demonstrates the algorithm after 4 weeks. This is the patient who is slow to recover. The patient is at risk

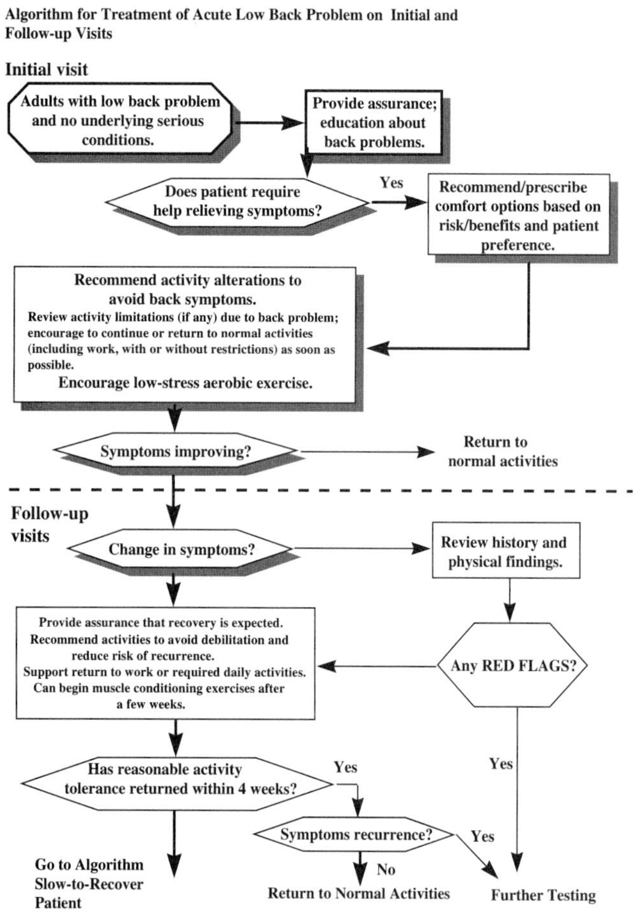

Fig. 4 The medical standards for early care of acute low back pain (LBP). (Adapted with permission from the United States Agency for Health Care Policy and Research: Acute low back problems in adults, in Bigos SJ (ed): *Series: Clinical Practice Guideline No. 14.* Rockville, MD, U.S. Department of Health and Human Services, AHCPR Publication No 95-0642, 1984.)

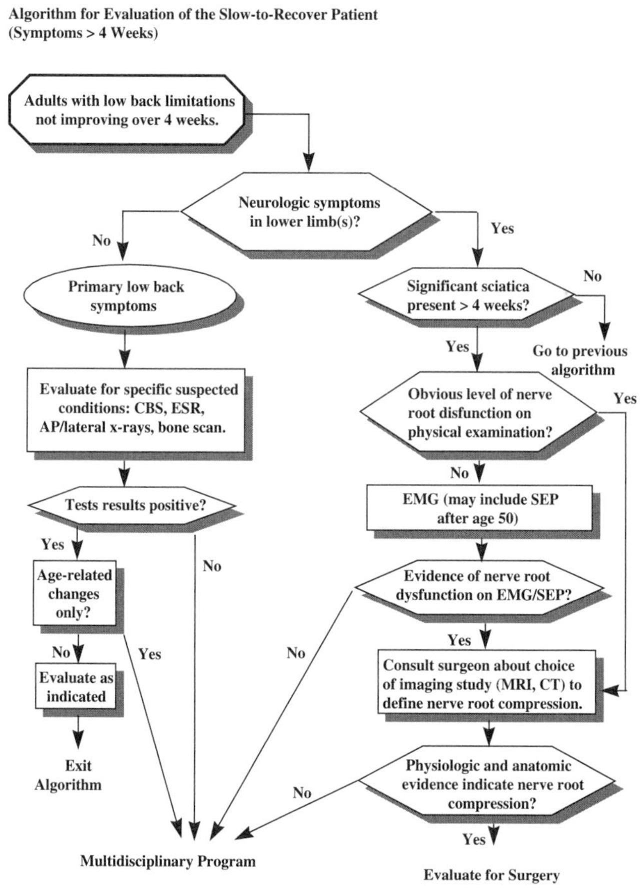

Fig. 5 The medical standards for slow-to-recover patients (symptoms > 4 weeks). (Adapted with permission from the United States Agency for Health Care Policy and Research: Acute low back problems in adults, in Bigos SJ (ed): *Series: Clinical Practice Guideline No. 14.* Rockville, MD, U.S. Department of Health and Human Services, AHCPR Publication No 95-0642, 1984.)

for chronicity. Again, the standardized evaluation is performed for neurologic symptoms in the lower limb(s). At this point, the physician should evaluate the patient for specific suspected conditions if indicated. If the test results are negative, the patient will need a more intensive program to return to full activity. If neurologic symptoms and signs are positive and significant sciatica is present, the patient should be evaluated to determine the level of neurologic compromise. If the special diagnostics are negative, the patient may be referred to a multidisciplinary, intensive treatment program that includes fitness, stress management, and education. A period of 2 to 4 weeks is usually sufficient. The goal to return to full duty has to be carefully explained to the patient. This approach has rendered up to 98% return to full duty if implemented at 6 to 8 weeks postinjury. The longer the sick absence, the less the possibility to return the employee to work. Beyond 4 months of passive treatment and inactivity, the success rate of these comprehensive programs drops to 67% to 82%.

Cumulative Trauma Disorders

CTD are likely to be musculoskeletal. This definition is hardly exclusive; some repeated trauma can be acoustic in nature. According to the Bureau of Labor Statistics there was an 800% increase in all reported cumulative trauma from 1982 to 1992. CTD serves as a descriptor for work-related symptoms in the neck and upper limbs and is an umbrella term for the many specific and nonspecific diagnoses used by health care providers. Hand and wrist symptoms account for the majority of CTD in the upper extremity. The highest rate of hand, wrist, and forearm disorders are found in the food industry (oyster, crab, and clam packing; meat and poultry processing; fish canneries). High rates also are found in the textile industry, fine electrical and mechanical production, and computer users.

A precise epidemiologic model for CTD is lacking. However, there is a consensus that the development of CTD involves multifactorial causes rather than a single stimulus. The outcome of these stimuli may or may not lead to a disorder. Symptom severity seems to be modified by work-organization factors, ie, cognitive demands and possible employee autonomy. The current epidemiologic models are predominantly biomechanical and inherently difficult to generalize because of the wide variation in interpreting the results of exposure measurements. Exposure factors defined as risk factors for CTD are the rates of repetition of body movements of a given segment, the duration of the exposure of static or dynamic muscle work, the time of recovery of muscle work, applied forces (external, internal, or contact), posture, the organization of work, and the environment at work (vibration, cold temperatures). Definitions for rates of repetition, durations of a task, and rest period with time of recovery are lacking. Problems of weak definitions create appreciable methodologic limitations in the measurement of exposure. Despite these problems, high exposure to mechanical factors seems to outweigh individual and work: organization factors. There is, however, a lack of prospective longitudinal studies.

The recent consensus reached by the ANSI Z-365 committee, which included scientists, representatives of industry and labor, and clinicians, offers recommendations for prevention. The committee formulated recommendations for surveillance factors, job analysis and design, medical management, and training. The recent OSHA recommendation is only a partial solution to the definition of exposure. These efforts are directed to a more standardized nomenclature that should help the busy orthopaedic surgeon communicate with industry. These disorders can be categorized as tendon-related disorders, nerve-related disorders, joint-related disorders, muscle-related disorders, circulatory/vascular-type disorders, and bursa-related disorders (Table 1).

Perhaps the most challenging task for the orthopaedic surgeon is to decide whether or not the symptoms are work-related. The second challenge is to decide criteria for safe return to work. The third challenge is to follow up the patient to avoid recurrence of the symptoms. Medical management of CTD of the upper extremity and neck follows current practice and scientific knowledge. Occupational medical management includes a detailed review of the job tasks, which is essential to understand the work-relatedness. Information on prior and current occupations is imperative for the physician to determine whether reported risk factors are in accordance with the patient's symptoms. Important factors are consistent exposure to repetitive tasks, high force exertion, long exertion time, and the use of hand-held vibrating tools. Use of a standardized inquiry into symptoms—onset, quality, intensity, site, radiation, evolution over time, exacerbating and relieving factors, effect of recreation activities, and prior treatments—contributes to an improved differential diagnosis. Finally, an understanding of psychosocial factors influencing and modifying pain behavior is essential.

Table 1. Disorders considered as cumulative trauma disorders

Type	Disorder
Tendon-related disorders	Tendinitis/peritendinitis/tenosynovitis
	Epicondylitis
	De Quervain's
	Dupuytren contracture
	Trigger finger
	Ganglion cyst
Nerve-related disorders	Carpal tunnel syndrome
	Cubital tunnel syndrome
	Guyon canal syndrome
	Pronator teres syndrome
	Radial tunnel syndrome
	Thoracic outlet syndrome
	Cervical syndrome (radiculopathy)
	Digital neuritis
Joint-related disorders	Osteoarthritis of most joints
Muscle-related disorders	Tension neck syndrome
	Muscle sprain and strain
	Myalgia and myositis
Circulatory-related disorders	Hypothenar hammer syndrome
	Raynaud's syndrome
Bursa-related disorders	Bursitis of most joints

(Adapted with permission from Kuorinka I, Forcier L: *Work-related Musculoskeletal Disorders: WMSDs. A Reference Book for Prevention.* London, England, Taylor and Francis, 1995, pp 323–348.)

Three levels of evaluations—musculoskeletal, ergonomic, and psychosocial—have been suggested (Outline 1). In a study of 50 employees, these evaluations could predict return to work. The authors found that when the subjective pain, tenderness, weakness, and sensory loss described by the patient were consistent with the clinical examination and the history of injury, the patient responded to treatment in a predictable way. The ergonomic classification did not independently determine a patient's ability to resume work. The authors concluded that any rating greater than minor psychosocial issues was a major hurdle to a patient's return to work. Although it is one of very few outcome studies and needs further validation, this study underlines the importance of using a biopsychosocial model. CTD in the upper extremity, even with unspecific symptoms, needs a multidisciplinary approach if the patient does not respond to conventional treatment within a certain time frame.

An algorithm for CTD that is currently being tested is designed to provide industry with a standardized clinical/ergonomic approach that includes a tracking system. Employees in a specific company who present with a CTD complaint are screened. Criteria for referral to a physician have been developed, and three levels of treatment are offered depending on the employee's symptoms and work ability. All employees with a complaint receive a workplace evaluation within a couple of days. Work is rarely

Outline 1. Suggested evaluation for upper extremity cumulative trauma disorders

Musculoskeletal disorder

Objective findings: swelling, joint or tendon crepitation, limited joint motion, abnormal radiographic or electromyographic findings.

Reasonable subjective findings: pain, tenderness, sensory loss or weakness appropriate and consistent with the injury and the history.

Unreasonable subjective findings: diffuse, vague unreproducible pain and tenderness not corresponding to anatomic distribution or inconsistent with history of injury.

Ergonomic issues

Minor issues: correctable work station problems or minor ergonomic instruction.

Moderate issues: high repetition, high force or abnormal position that are correctable.

Major issues: high repetition, high force or abnormal positions that are not correctable.

Psychosocial issues

Minor psychosocial issues: usually administrative issues such as providing temporary modified duty or minor conflicts with supervisor.

Moderate psychosocial issues: job frustration, job stress, management insensitivity. Employee anger that is treatable.

Major psychosocial issues: long-standing unresolved frustration, anger, job stress plus degrees of depression that are untreatable.

(Adapted with permission from Bonzani P, Mangieri M, Keelan B, et al: Factors prolonging disability in work-related cumulative trauma disorders. *J Hand Surg,* in press.)

suspended, and short, temporary job restrictions are promoted. The fitness club of the company is involved with special training programs and set goals. This model is not validated and should be seen as an attempt to prevent chronicity in a proactive industrial setting (Fig. 6). The program is supported by management.

Only one multidisciplinary rehabilitation program for chronic work-related upper extremity disorders is reported in the literature. Two groups with nonspecific CTD that were equivalent on measures of duration of work disability, fear of reinjury, pain severity, psychological distress, age, education level, and perceived work environment were studied. The usual care provided was compared to a comprehensive multidisciplinary approach, which included physical generic conditioning, work-related conditioning, pain and stress management, ergonomic consultation, and vocational counseling and placement. The results indicate that 74% of the experimental group returned to work or were involved in some vocational training. The control group achieved only 40% with similar activities. The ergonomic component of treatment was important to facilitate return to work.

Most CTD fall in the category of nerve entrapment or soft-tissue inflammation. The recommended treatment in the early stage is rest of the symptomatic area. However, few outcome studies or randomized controlled trials suggest that any form of treatment is superior in the early stage. The natural history of these different disorders is virtually unknown. This lack of knowledge creates a dilemma for the treating physician and the patient. Patients with symptoms of the upper extremity or neck, whether occupational or not, are treated similarly. A recent published reference book for the prevention of WRMD of the upper extremities and the neck provides evidence for ergonomic intervention in primary prevention. Unfortunately, it does not provide much help for clinical intervention and management. Ergonomic interventions need further evaluation if they are to be used as clinical tools to reduce symptoms and to enhance the rate of return to work. Simple work modifications can alter such components of exposure as loads, repetition, recovery time, reach, etc. The orthopaedist may incorporate an ergonomist in the treatment team to enhance success and treatment outcomes. Perhaps more importantly, the ergonomist can work with local industry to enhance the medical management of injuries if he or she is part of a multidisciplinary team working with an orthopaedist to prevent occurrence and chronicity of CTD.

Ergonomics and Occupational Orthopaedics

Medical management of occupational ailments infers familiarity with the job. In a clinical setting, workers convey information that relates to their work, job tasks, and work environment. The orthopaedic surgeon considers this information while making a final determination for better clinical care. A questionnaire completed by the worker while in the waiting room is often sufficient, although structured computerized data collection is the best method. However, more extensive data collections imply the participation of workers, management, and union representatives. The ergonomic information delivers insightful information on work methods that is valuable to the orthopaedist. Relationships between risk factors and workplace injuries and disorders enhance medical care and may instigate prevention programs.

Successful management of occupational musculoskeletal problems goes beyond the medical dimension. The orthopaedic community has to realize the major efforts by the ergonomists to improve the workplace. Orthopaedic surgeons have to realize that their interventions often come late, after the onset of symptoms. The "ergonomic" responsibilities of the orthopaedic surgeons include proposing to industry the redesign of tasks or tools that could better fit the worker, encouraging the formulation of training programs to reduce hazards of work and to improve work techniques, proposing modifications or transfers to other tasks for workers with particular diagnoses, and, finally, formulating clear and logical disability ratings. The first two items are attractive because the orthopaedist has a major role in the process. But they are time-consuming and force a more thorough understanding of the workplace than most physicians can obtain. Orthopaedists also need a network of trained health professionals to participate in the evaluation and treatment protocol (including nurses, physical therapists, occupational therapists, ergonomists, and/or psychologists). A positive attitude by company managers to improve the safety of the returning worker is essential.

There are many barriers acting against a rapid return to

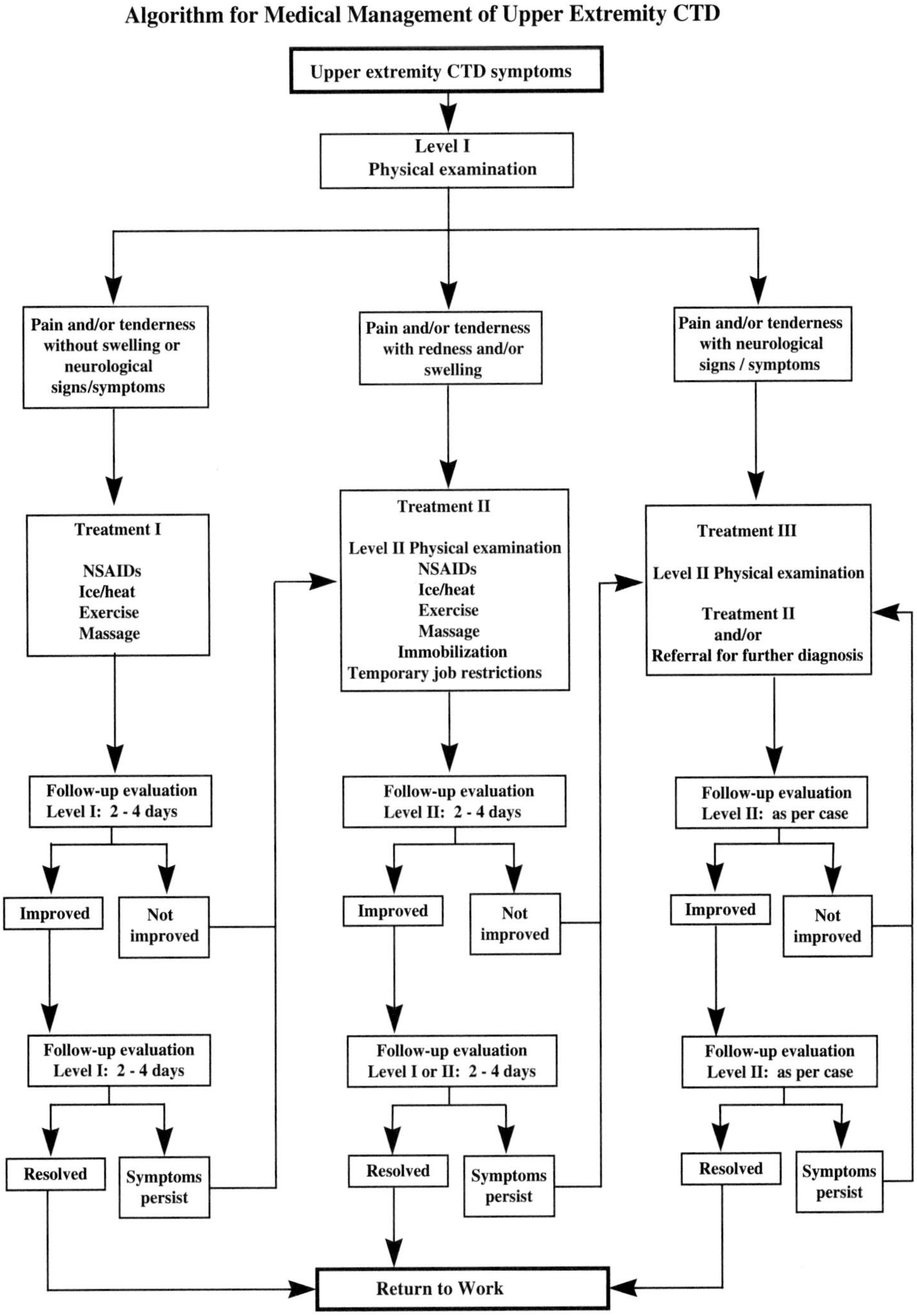

Fig. 6 Algorithm for prevention of chronicity of cumulative trauma disorders (CTD).

work. The complicated compensation system does not ease efforts toward injury prevention and quick delivery of care. The underlying cause of nonspecific work-related musculoskeletal disorders and injuries is related to exposure to loads. But other factors are equally important. It is necessary to determine how much physical load exposure is healthy and necessary, and when the exposure may become a risk to the musculoskeletal system. Epidemiologic data are still lacking and are currently under scrutiny. Simple, low cost, valid, and reliable exposure tools are missing, except for surveys, interviews, and questionnaires. Therefore, it is necessary to take the practical approach when dealing with a patient who is complaining of pain when no organic reason is detectable. Two such approaches include enhancing the patient's physical and/or psychologic ability, and/or evaluating the work demands to better understand the hurdles of returning to a productive lifestyle.

Training in Occupational Orthopaedics

Most medical schools in the United States currently offer no formal training in occupational orthopaedics. It is seldom part of the residency training. This lack poses a problem for the new orthopaedist unless a senior colleague is present who has a special interest in the field. There are educational courses in the workers' compensation system, but the intricate knowledge of work-related symptoms is acquired only with clinical experience and work with a multidisciplinary team in collaboration with industry.

Four strategies for improving this situation are suggested: (1) include occupational orthopaedics in the residency curricula; (2) provide increased funding for outcome studies and randomized controlled trials related to work injuries and disorders; (3) provide continuing education through the American Academy of Orthopaedic Surgeons; and (4) actively involve industry in the discussion and promotion of health programs for the prevention and treatment of work-related musculoskeletal disorders and illness.

Annotated Bibliography

Abenhaim L, Rossignol M, Gobeille D, et al: The prognostic consequences in making the initial medical diagnosis of work-related back injuries. *Spine* 1995;20: 791–795.

A cohort study of 1,848 workers was followed over 24 months. The prognostic value of the physicians' initial diagnosis was analyzed. The results indicate a strong association with initial diagnosis and risk of chronicity. The labeling effect is raised.

Andersson GBJ: Sensitivity, specificity, and predictive value: A general issue in the screening for disease and in the interpretation of diagnostic studies in spinal disorders, in Frymoyer JW, Ducker TB, Hadler NM, et al (eds): *The Adult Spine: Principles and Practices.* New York, NY, Raven Press, 1991, vol 1, pp 277–287.

This is an overview chapter on screening spinal disorders and on the interpretation of spinal diagnoses. Predictive values, sensitivity, specificity of spinal disorders, and diagnostic tools are reviewed.

Frymoyer JW: Predicting disability from low back pain. *Clin Orthop* 1992;279:101–109.

Factors contributing to LBP and disability due to LBP are reviewed. Psychosocial factors and work environmental factors are better predictors than physical findings. A predictive risk model of chronic LBP is offered.

Kuorinka I, Forcier L: *Work-related Musculoskeletal Disorders: WMSDs. A Reference Book for Prevention.* London, England, Taylor and Francis, 1995, pp 323–348.

This is a literature review on the prevention of CTD of the upper extremity and the neck. A critical review of the current knowledge with an excellent bibliography makes this book very informative.

Lindström I, Öhlund C, Eek C, et al: The effect of graded activity on patients with subacute low back pain: A randomized prospective clinical study with an operant-conditioning behavioral approach. *Phys Ther* 1992;72: 279–293.

This reports a prospective randomized controlled trial of graded activity to restore function in blue collar workers who were sick-listed for 8 weeks due to OLBP. Patients were examined by an orthopaedist and a social worker. The patients had to participate in an operant conditional behavioral program carried out by a physical therapist.

National Safety Council: *Control of Work-related Cumulative Trauma Disorders: Part I. Upper Extremities.* Itasca, IL, National Safety Council, ANSI Z-365, April 1995.

This is a literature review and recommendations from the multidisciplinary committee sponsored by the National Safety Council. Surveillance factors, job analysis and design, medical management, and training options are described.

Waddell G: Biopsychosocial analysis of low back pain. *Baillieres Clin Rheumatol* 1992;6:523–558.

Historical aspects are presented of the development of OLBP and the compensation system in this thorough review of the medical versus the biopsychosocial model and its importance in the treatment of LBP. It includes an analysis of medical success and failure in low back disorders.

Wiesel SW, Boden SD, Feffer HL: A quality-based protocol for management of musculoskeletal injuries: A ten year prospective outcome *Clin Orthop* 1994;301: 164–176.

A 10-year prospective study to evaluate standardized algorithms for OLBP and knee injuries accomplished quality care, reduction in time lost, and cost savings.

Wyman EA: *Physician's Primer on Workers' Compensation.* Park Ridge, IL, American Academy of Orthopaedic Surgeons, 1992.

This manual is an introduction to the workers' compensation system; it includes definitions, responsibilities of the physician, and a brief description of the law.

II

Systemic Disorders

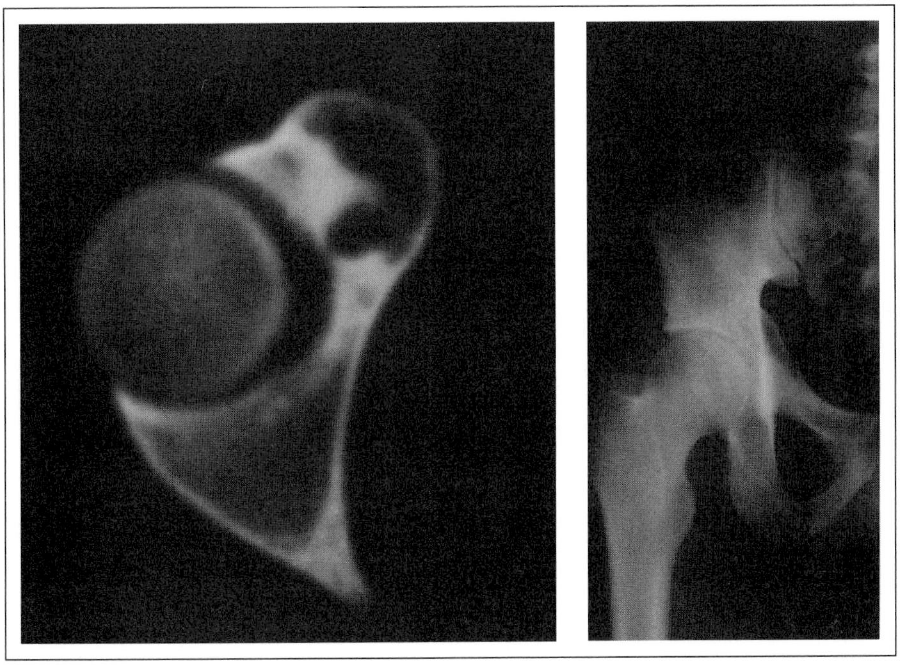

15

Bone Metabolism and Metabolic Bone Disease

Bone metabolism is the study of how bone functions as an integral member of the body's endocrine system. When a failure in hormonal control of bone function occurs, the result is some form of metabolic bone disease or impairment in bone remodeling and repair.

Bone metabolism is regulated by bone cells that are responsive to a variety of environmental signals. Three cell types are found in bone. Osteoblasts are generally regarded as bone-forming cells. Because osteoblasts contain the receptors for most chemical mediators of bone function, these cells also play a critical role in the overall regulation of bone metabolism. Osteoclasts are the active agents in bone resorption and are ultimately responsible for the remodeling of bone. They are the multinucleated cells found at the apex of the cutting cone observed in histologic sections of cortical bone during reparative processes. Osteoclasts also are responsible for the production of resorptive cavities, known as Howship's lacunae, on trabecular bone surfaces. Osteocytes are found in abundance within mineralized bone matrix, but their function is poorly understood. They may be important in receiving mechanical input signals and transmitting these stimuli to other cells in bone. Osteoblasts and osteocytes are derived from the same mesenchymal stem cell precursor (found in bone marrow stroma, periosteum, soft tissues, and possibly peripheral blood vessel endothelium), whereas osteoclasts arise from hematopoietic mononuclear cells.

Mineral Metabolism

Calcium concentration is an important regulator of cellular membrane potentials, blood coagulation, and muscular and cardiovascular functions. It also is a messenger for signal transduction in almost every cell in the body. The normal serum level of calcium is 9 to 10 mg/dl; approximately one half is bound to plasma protein (primarily albumin), a small fraction is associated with phosphate or citrate, and about 45% exists in the form of free calcium ions. The ionized calcium concentration is maintained within very narrow limits, and bone is sacrificed whenever necessary to maintain the ionized calcium level in the physiologic range. At the macroscopic level, calcium homeostasis is maintained by three organ systems—the intestines, the skeleton, and the kidneys.

All calcium intake is from the diet. Calcium absorption varies with the perceived systemic requirements and is under complex hormonal regulation. Approximately 20% of dietary calcium is absorbed; the remainder either is not absorbable or is not absorbed and is excreted in the stool. In the intestines, calcium is actively transported across the duodenum in association with a calcium-binding protein. With low calcium diets, most of the dietary calcium is taken up by this active absorption mechanism. However, in the jejunum, there is passive diffusion of calcium. Under normal conditions, urinary excretion of calcium balances the amount of calcium absorbed. Absorption of calcium from the gut and excretion in the urine averages 150 to 200 mg per day.

It is estimated that, in Western countries, 900 mg of dietary calcium per day is required to maintain calcium balance. Significant variations exist between individuals, however, and dietary calcium requirements are known to be increased both in the very young and in older patients (Table 1). Significantly more calcium is required during growth, and this requirement continues until achievement of the peak level of bone mass, between the second and third decades of life. Later in life, it is necessary to increase dietary calcium intake to counteract the effect of calcium loss caused by increased bone resorption. Unfortunately, the average US diet provides only 450 mg of calcium per day. Recent data show that adolescents consume only 430 mg of calcium per day. This calcium deficiency during growth may adversely affect the peak bone mass attained and, thus, place an individual's skeleton at a higher risk of developing osteoporosis in the future.

Table 1. Optimal calcium requirements recommended by the National Institutes of Health Consensus Panel

Age Group	Optimal Daily Intake of Calcium (mg/day)
Infants	
Birth to 6 months	400
6 months to 1 year	600
Children	
1 to 5 years	800
6 to 10 years	800–1,200
Adolescents/young adults	
11 to 24 years	1,200–1,500
Men	
25 to 65 years	1,000
Over 65 years	1,500
Women	
25 to 50 years	1,000
Over 50 years (postmenopausal)	
On estrogens	1,000
Not on estrogens	1,500
Over 65 years	1,500
Pregnant and nursing	1,200–1,500

(Reproduced with permission from: Optimal calcium intake: NIH Consensus Conference. *JAMA* 1994;272:1942–1948.)

Endocrine Function

The regulation of bone homeostasis depends on the delicate balance between the functions of several endocrine organs including the skin, parathyroid glands, liver, kidneys, gonads, adrenals, and thyroid. In addition, in certain pathologic states, pituitary and hypothalamic function also regulate bone physiology. With respect to bone, the hormonal balance created by the endocrine system serves to maintain normal serum calcium and phosphate levels.

Vitamin D

Vitamin D is a unique steroid hormone that can modulate calcium homeostasis directly or through its effects on the differentiation and development of the various calcium-regulating cell systems. When skin is exposed to ultraviolet light, vitamin D_3 (cholecalciferol) can be formed endogenously from 7-dehydrocholesterol (Table 2). In Caucasians, only 15 minutes of daily bright sunlight exposure to the hands and face is required to produce enough vitamin D_3 to be converted physiologically to the minimum requirement (10 mg) of the active metabolite, 1,25-dihydroxyvitamin D_3 (calcitriol, $1,25(OH)_2D_3$). Dark-skinned people may require longer exposure. The other major source of vitamin D is the diet, which provides ergocalciferol or vitamin D_2. These two isomeric forms have the same endogenous function. Both metabolites are stored in several tissues, with the highest concentrations found in adipose tissue and muscle. All vitamin D metabolites are fat-soluble vitamins. Because certain individuals may lack sufficient exposure to sunlight as well as dietary exposure to vitamin D-containing nutrients, most milk in the United States is supplemented with vitamin D_2. The only significant natural source of vitamin D is cod liver oil.

Vitamin D metabolism begins with a sequence of steps in which precursor molecules are converted to the active physiologic form. Once ultraviolet light acts to convert 7-dehydrocholesterol to D_3 in the skin, this molecule circulates to the liver where it is hydroxylated at its twenty-fifth carbon to produce the major circulating prohormone, 25-hydroxyvitamin D_3 (calcifediol, $25(OH)D_3$). This step is catalyzed by two vitamin D 25-hydroxylases, which are located in hepatic microsomes. Once formed, $25(OH)D_3$ becomes the major circulating vitamin D metabolite and is transported bound to an α-globulin. Conditions that affect hepatic function or drugs that induce P-450 microsomal enzymes (for example, phenytoin) will interrupt this conversion pathway leading to inactive polar metabolites of D_3. As will be discussed later, these conditions can lead to various forms of osteomalacia.

Table 2. Vitamin D and its metabolites

Abbreviation	Vitamin	Drug Name
—	Provitamin D_3	7-dehydrocholesterol
D_2	Vitamin D_2	ergocalciferol
D_3	Vitamin D_3	cholecalciferol
$25(OH)D_3$	25-hydroxyvitamin D_3	calcifediol
$1,25(OH)_2D_3$	1,25-dihydroxyvitamin D_3	calcitriol
$24,25(OH)_2D_3$	24,25-dihydroxyvitamin D_3	—

The next step in the metabolism of vitamin D is the 1-α-hydroxylation of $25(OH)D_3$ to form $1,25(OH)_2D_3$, the physiologically active form of the vitamin. Hydroxylation at this first carbon position is the rate-limiting step in the production of the biologically active form. The hydroxylase enzyme for this reaction is located in the mitochondria of renal tubular cells and is activated by parathyroid hormone (PTH). In the presence of low PTH levels and high $1,25(OH)_2D_3$ levels, alternate hydroxylation of $25(OH)D_3$ occurs at the 24-position, yielding 24,25-dihydroxyvitamin D_3 ($24,25(OH)_2D_3$). Recent evidence suggests that $24,25(OH)_2D_3$ may play a role in cartilage differentiation. The only other tissue that has been shown to participate significantly in this metabolic pathway is the placenta, in which another 1-α hydroxylase has been found. Although parathyroid hormone is the major molecule that controls 1-α hydroxylase function, serum levels of phosphate, ionized calcium, and $1,25(OH)_2D_3$ itself can regulate this activity.

The major target tissues of $1,25(OH)_2D_3$ are kidney, bone, and intestine. In the kidney, it increases proximal tubular reabsorption of phosphate. It also increases 24-hydroxylase activity and reduces 1-α hydroxylase activity, thereby acting as a feedback regulator of its own formation. In the intestine, $1,25(OH)_2D_3$ induces the production of the critical calcium-binding protein that is responsible for active calcium transport. When $1,25(OH)_2D_3$ levels increase, or when $1,25(OH)_2D_3$ is administered exogenously, the first effect observed will be increased intestinal calcium absorption, which leads to increased serum calcium levels.

Bone is the major target tissue for $1,25(OH)_2D_3$; however, here its physiologic role is not as well understood. On the basis of studies with monocytes and macrophages, $1,25(OH)_2D_3$ is thought to promote the differentiation or fusion of osteoclast precursors to osteoclasts. At pharmacologic doses, it can induce accelerated bone resorption by increasing the activity and number of osteoclasts. Because vitamin D receptors have never been shown to exist in the cytoplasm of osteoclasts, but have been demonstrated in osteoblast-like cells, the mechanism by which $1,25(OH)_2D_3$ modulates bone physiology is probably through an action on the osteoblast. Consequently, activities related to mineralization, bone resorption, and cellular differentiation may be osteoblast-regulated.

Circulating levels of the prohormone $25(OH)D_3$ decrease with age. In addition, aging may lead to reduced activity of 1-α hydroxylase as a consequence of impaired renal function and thus result in reduced $1,25(OH)_2D_3$ levels. These alterations in vitamin D metabolism may account for the decreased fractional calcium absorption that has been observed in the elderly.

Parathyroid Hormone

PTH and vitamin D together form an axis, which is the major metabolic regulator of calcium and phosphate fluxes in the body. The three major target organs of PTH are bone, kidney, and intestines. Normally, this peptide hormone is produced in, and secreted exclusively by, the parathyroid gland.

In bone, PTH generally is regarded as a bone resorbing hormone; however, PTH receptors are not found on osteoclasts. Instead, these receptors are found on osteoblasts, osteoblast precursors, and very early osteoclast precursors. The effects of PTH on osteoblasts are to: (1) stimulate the release of neutral proteases that degrade surface osteoid and initiate the bone remodeling cycle; (2) stimulate the release of unknown factors from osteoblasts, which then stimulate osteoclasts to resorb bone; and (3) stimulate osteoblasts to synthesize osteoid and form bone. Osteocytes are assumed to have parathyroid hormone receptors as well, because when osteocytes are stimulated by parathyroid hormone, calcium salts in the immediate surrounding lacunar spaces are mobilized.

The rate of PTH synthesis and its release by the cell are related to the extracellular ionized calcium concentration. Intact PTH is relatively short-lived once it enters the circulation. The liver and kidney rapidly cleave the circulating intact molecule into amino-terminal (N-terminal) and carboxy-terminal (C-terminal) fragments. Both the biologically active N-terminal fragment and the intact PTH have a circulating half-life shorter than that of the C-terminal fragment. When kidney function is impaired, clearance of the inactive C-terminal fragment is prolonged. The N-terminal fragment has a short-half life and thus provides a more accurate measure of PTH activity in the absence of renal function.

Secretion of PTH is a very tightly regulated process. A decrease in the ionized calcium concentration as small as 0.3 mg/dl will stimulate release of the hormone from the parathyroid gland. The adenylate cyclase and cAMP system in cells of the parathyroid gland regulates that secretion. An increase in serum calcium inhibits cAMP formation and decreases the amount of hormone secreted.

In the kidney, PTH activates adenylate cyclases in cells distributed along the length of the renal tubule; in the proximal tubule, PTH decreases phosphorus reabsorption; and distally, it increases the reabsorption of calcium. The activation of tubular adenylate cyclase results in increased cAMP content in the urine. Therefore, nephrogenous cAMP is a good indicator of circulating PTH levels.

Increased levels of PTH have been noted in the elderly, possibly as a consequence of reduced fractional calcium absorption in the intestine. Nephrogenous cAMP levels are increased in these patients as is tubular excretion of phosphorus. These findings support the concept that the parathyroid hormone and $1,25(OH)_2D_3$ axis may have an aggravating (and possibly pathologic) role in the progressive loss of bone mass during the aging process.

Calcitonin

Calcitonin is an important calcium-regulating hormone whose exact physiologic role remains a matter of controversy. It does not directly regulate the functions of PTH or of vitamin D metabolites, but its ability to modulate serum calcium and phosphate levels is significant. Calcitonin is produced and secreted mainly by the C cells (parafollicular cells) of the thyroid gland; however, small amounts of calcitonin are found in the thymus, pituitary, gut, liver, and cerebrospinal fluid.

The major target tissues for calcitonin are bone, kidney, and the gastrointestinal tract. In bone, its major defined action is the inhibition of osteoclastic bone resorption. In vitro, osteoclasts have been shown to lose their ruffled borders and clear zones and undergo considerable contraction within 15 minutes after exposure to calcitonin. Therefore, unlike PTH and $1,25(OH)_2D_3$, osteoclasts do possess specific receptors for this hormone. In the kidney, calcitonin receptors are also known to exist. Calcitonin causes decreased tubular reabsorption of calcium and phosphate. In the gut, pharmacologic doses of calcitonin increase the secretion of sodium, potassium, chloride, and water and decrease the secretion of acid.

Salmon calcitonin, which is available as a drug, differs from human calcitonin at 16 amino acid positions. This alteration is large enough to cause it to be immunogenic. Interestingly, salmon calcitonin is several times more potent than human calcitonin in the treatment of patients.

Calcitonin deficiency states have not been demonstrated to cause a specific metabolic disorder in spite of calcitonin's important physiologic role in calcium homeostasis. Calcitonin does have several proven pharmacologic uses; it is effective in treating patients with Paget disease, in preventing disuse osteoporosis, and in rapidly lowering serum calcium in severe hypercalcemic states. In addition, it has recently been shown to have an important prophylactic role in postmenopausal osteoporosis. Some evidence suggests that calcitonin may have an analgesic effect in controlling the pain in patients with vertebral crush fractures.

Estrogens and Corticosteroids

The association between bone loss, fracture risk, and the postmenopausal state (naturally occurring or surgically induced) is a well-known phenomenon. Many studies have now shown that accelerated bone loss occurs after menopause when ovarian hormone production ceases. Circulating hormone levels fall to 20% of previous levels; the resulting bone loss can be reversed only by administration of estrogen. Obesity can protect against this bone loss, probably because of higher circulating levels of estrogen metabolites from precursor molecules stored in adipose sites. Although estrogens are known to inhibit bone resorption, the mechanisms responsible for this effect are not fully understood. The effects of estrogen on bone may be mediated by interleukins-1 and/or 6. The presence of estrogen receptors in osteoblasts and osteoclasts has been confirmed. Although the levels of such receptors are very low, they appear to be functionally active, thereby providing the first real evidence that bone is a target tissue for estrogen.

Both males and females experience age-related bone loss, particularly from cortical bone. The rate of trabecular bone loss increases in the first few years after menopause and is correlated with decreasing amounts of endogenous estrogens. Estrogen replacement blocks this bone loss in the early postmenopausal years (years 3 to 6), and a decrease in fracture rates in the appendicular skeleton has been documented.

Patients who undergo bilateral oophorectomy before natural menopause also respond to estrogen therapy. This group is especially at risk for developing osteoporosis because a greater period of time is spent with low estrogen levels. To obtain maximal benefit from estrogen replacement therapy, it should be started as soon as possible after surgical or natural menopause and continued indefinitely. A recent study has confirmed that if estrogen replacement therapy is not started within the first 5 years after menopause, it is of limited benefit in preventing future fractures.

Numerous studies have been undertaken to demonstrate the potential risks of estrogen therapy on the induction of cerebrovascular accident, thrombosis, fluid retention, gallbladder disease, and uterine bleeding. More importantly, studies have demonstrated a potentially higher risk of breast cancer and endometrial cancer in women taking estrogens. While the information from each of these studies is extremely valuable, some have suffered from certain flaws in methodology. It is accepted that any factor that increases a patient's exposure to estrogen (eg, early menarche, late menopause, estrogen replacement therapy) may predispose that patient to an increased risk of breast or endometrial cancer. Combination cyclical estrogen-progestin (synthetic progesterone) therapy is believed to decrease the occurrence of endometrial but not breast cancer. In patients who have undergone hysterectomy, unopposed estrogen treatment is indicated.

The most important factors to consider in determining whether a patient should or should not take estrogen is the relative risk-benefit ratio. In general, patients who have a strong family history for breast or endometrial cancer may be at increased risk for developing cancers as a result of estrogen treatment. In addition, estrogen therapy is known to exacerbate benign breast diseases and cholecystitis. On the other hand, estrogen is strongly beneficial not only in the prevention of osteoporosis and hip fractures but in the prevention of heart disease in females.

Less information is available on the role of androgens in maintaining skeletal mass in men. In general, it is assumed that the role of androgens is similar to that of estrogens, and androgen receptors have been identified in osteoblasts. Young men with idiopathic hypogonadotropic hypogonadism have reduced cortical and trabecular bone densities, and delayed puberty is associated with osteopenia in men.

Corticosteroids may lead to bone loss by directly inhibiting calcium absorption, increasing renal calcium excretion, and indirectly stimulating secondary hyperparathyroidism. Their principal effects are to decrease production of the intestinal calcium-binding proteins required for absorption. Very high doses of steroids decrease both bone formation and resorption. Even with doses as low as 10 mg of prednisone per day, significant bone loss occurs.

Thyroid Hormones

Thyroid hormones resemble steroid hormones in that they interact with specific cell receptors and eventually bind to nuclear DNA. The thyroid gland produces two hormones, thyroxine (T4) and 3,5,3′-triiodothyronine (T3). Both hormones are bound to proteins in the plasma.

Patients with hyperthyroidism or who are undergoing exogenous thyroid treatment show an acceleration in their basal metabolic rate. Bone resorption and bone formation in these patients take place at stimulated rates, but resorption seems to occur at a slightly faster rate than formation. Consequently, chronic hyperthyroidism or thyroid supplementation may contribute to osteoporosis. Recent reports have shown that women who use thyroid hormone have lower bone mass in both the axial and appendicular skeletons and have a higher risk for sustaining hip fractures.

Metabolic Bone Diseases

Metabolic bone diseases result from some failure in the normal processes of bone formation, mineralization, and remodeling. They can be broadly divided into the osteopenic conditions, such as osteoporosis, osteomalacia, and hyperparathyroidism, that result in low bone mass or insufficiently mineralized bone and the osteosclerotic conditions, such as Paget disease and osteopetrosis, that result in increased amounts of bone due to abnormal bone remodeling.

Osteoporosis

Osteoporosis is a bone disorder characterized by decreased bone mass and an increased susceptibility to fracture. One major risk factor for osteoporosis is a sensitivity of the skeleton to estrogen withdrawal, whether withdrawal occurs as a result of a natural or surgically induced menopause. Impaired metabolism, long-term calcium deficiency, secondary hyperparathyroidism, and decreased activity levels have also been implicated. Other risk factors include genetic predisposition (individuals who are fair skinned and small, have hypermobile joints, are of Northern European ancestry, or have scoliosis), cigarette smoking, and excessive alcohol intake. Cigarette smokers show significantly increased incidences of bone loss and hip and vertebral fractures. This increase may be due, in part, to the abnormal systemic handling of certain estrogen metabolites. Heavy alcohol users may develop osteoporosis as a result of calcium diuresis or of a direct depressive effect of alcohol on osteoblast function (Outline 1).

Most individuals attain their level of peak bone mass between the ages of 16 and 25 years. This is the greatest amount of bone that the individual will ever have, and the

Outline 1. Osteoporosis risk factors

Genetic and biologic
Caucasian race
Fair skin and hair
Northern European heredity
Scoliosis
Osteogenesis imperfecta
Early menopause
Slender body build

Behavioral and environmental
Cigarette smoking
Alcohol excess
Inactivity
Malnutrition
Caffeine use
Exercise-induced amenorrhea
High fiber diet
High phosphate diet
High protein diet

(Reproduced with permission from Frymoyer JW (ed): *Orthopaedic Knowledge Update 4.* Rosemont, IL, American Academy of Orthopaedic Surgeons, 1993, pp 69–88.)

higher this value is, the less chance there is of developing osteoporosis. The reason for this is simply that the ability of any specific rate of bone loss (from whatever cause) to lead to a critically low level depends on the amount of bone present before bone loss begins. In men, bone is normally lost at a rate of 0.3% of total bone mass per year, whereas in women the rate of bone loss is as high as 0.5% per year. The accelerated rate of bone loss, which occurs at a rate of 2% to 3% of total bone mass per year, begins after menopause and may last from 6 to 10 years. Because they are usually afflicted by this more rapid rate of bone loss, osteoporosis is much more common in women.

For the purposes of description and understanding of the disease, osteoporosis has been categorized into two distinct syndromes. Type I, known as postmenopausal osteoporosis, occurs most commonly in women within 15 to 20 years after menopause. It affects mostly trabecular bone. Type II osteoporosis, known as senile osteoporosis, occurs in men and women over the age of 70 years with a female-to-male ratio of 2:1. It affects cortical and trabecular bone equally. Thus in type I osteoporosis, estrogen deficiency plays a primary role, while in type II osteoporosis, aging and long-term calcium deficiency are more important.

Clinical Presentation and Diagnosis In general, osteoporosis is a silent and progressive disorder that is brought to the attention of the patient or the physician only after a fracture. Occasionally, the condition may be recognized by asymptomatic thoracic wedge or lumbar compression fractures on a routine lateral chest radiograph. Before bone loss is detectable on radiographs, approximately 30% to 50% of the bone mineral must be lost. The differential diagnosis of radiographic osteopenia includes disorders of the cells of the bone marrow, endocrinopathies, primary or secondary osteoporosis, and osteomalacia (Outline 2).

Outline 2. Differential diagnosis of osteopenia

Primary Osteoporosis
- Type I, postmenopausal
- Type II, senile

Osteomalacia

Endocrine disorders
- Cushing's disease
- Diabetes mellitus
- Estrogen deficiency
- Hyperparathyroidism
- Hypogonadism
- Iatrogenic glucocorticoid treatment
- Hyperthyroidism or exogenous thyroid medication

Disuse Disorders
- Prolonged immobilization
- Paralysis

Neoplastic Disorders
- Leukemia
- Multiple myeloma

Nutritional Disorders
- Anorexia nervosa
- High protein diet
- High phosphate diet
- Low calcium diet
- Alcoholism

Hematologic Disorders
- Sickle-cell anemia
- Thalassemia

Collagen Disorders
- Homocystinuria
- Osteogenesis imperfecta

(Reproduced with permission from Frymoyer JW (ed): *Orthopaedic Knowledge Update 4.* Rosemont, IL, American Academy of Orthopaedic Surgeons, 1993, pp 69–88.)

Patient Evaluation The evaluation of the patient with osteopenia is designed to arrive at a diagnosis and to stage the condition for treatment purposes. The medical history is intended to document past and present illnesses, medications, surgery, occupational exposure, nutrition, family history, and social habits, all of which are used to formulate an understanding of the patient's disease risk. Particular attention to specific risk factors (Outline 1), systemic causes of osteoporosis (Outline 2) and known causes of osteomalacia (Outline 3) can be very useful in directing further diagnostic tests.

Serum and urine tests are done routinely to establish the biochemical basis of a patient's condition (Outline 4). A complete blood count and a routine analysis of serum biochemical levels will suggest the presence of hematologic disorders, mineral and electrolyte imbalances, and underlying, unrecognized systemic disease. Renal function can be screened by measuring the blood urea nitrogen and serum creatinine levels, whereas hepatic function is assessed using the aspartate amino transferase, alanine amino transferase, alkaline phosphatase, and γ-glutamyl trans-

Outline 3. Causes of osteomalacia

- Vitamin D deficiency
  - Dietary
    - Malabsorption
    - Intestinal disease
    - Intestinal surgery
  - Insufficient sunlight

- Impaired vitamin D synthesis
  - Liver disease
  - Hepatic microsomal enzyme induction
  - Anticonvulsant
  - Renal failure

- Metabolic acidosis
- Fanconi's syndrome (renal tubular defect)

- Hypophosphatemia
  - Malabsorption
  - X-linked hypophosphatemic rickets
  - Oncogenic
  - Oral phosphate-binding antacid excess

- Mineralization inhibition
  - Bisphosphonate
  - Aluminum
  - Fluoride
  - Iron

- Hypophosphatasia

(Reproduced with permission from Frymoyer JW (ed): *Orthopaedic Knowledge Update 4.* Rosemont, IL, American Academy of Orthopaedic Surgeons, 1993, pp 69–88.)

Outline 4. Laboratory tests

- Routine
  - Serum
    - Complete blood count
    - Electrolytes, creatinine, blood urea nitrogen, calcium, phosphorus, protein, albumin, alkaline phosphatase, liver enzymes
    - Protein electrophoresis
    - Thyroid function tests
    - Testosterone (men only)
  - 24-hour urine
    - Calcium
    - Pyridinium cross-links

- Special
  - Serum
    - 25-hydroxyvitamin D_3
    - 1,25-dihydroxyvitamin D_3
    - Intact parathyroid hormone
    - Osteocalcin (bond Gla protein)
  - Urine
    - Immunoelectrophoresis
    - Bence Jones protein

(Reproduced with permission from Frymoyer JW (ed): *Orthopaedic Knowledge Update 4.* Rosemont, IL, American Academy of Orthopaedic Surgeons, 1993, pp 69–88.)

peptidase values. If the alkaline phosphatase level is elevated, fractionation of this enzyme is helpful because isoenzymes are secreted by several tissues, including bone, liver, kidney, and intestine. In men, measurement of the serum testosterone is part of the routine workup.

The 24-hour urine collection is used to monitor bone resorption. Pyridinoline and deoxypyridinoline are cross-links of bone and cartilage collagen molecules. They are excreted in the urine during bone resorption, and their measurement is a sensitive indicator of bone turnover. In addition, calcium and phosphate excretion remain important ways for determining the rate of bone loss in patients. If calcium excretion is low, there may be insufficient calcium ingestion, defective calcium absorption, or vitamin D deficiency. Phosphorus excretion is indicative of the effects of PTH on the kidney and is usually elevated when PTH activity is high.

Another important marker of bone turnover is the measurement of γ-carboxyglutamic acid in the serum or urine. This molecule, sometimes referred to as osteocalcin or bone Gla protein (BGP), is a low-molecular-weight protein, which is synthesized only by osteoblasts and is secreted directly into the circulation. Although the osteocalcin bound to bone matrix is released from bone during bone resorption, the measurement of the protein in serum or urine is more indicative of bone formation. High levels suggest a metabolic disorder in which bone is being actively formed and degraded (eg, high-turnover osteoporosis, renal osteodystrophy, Paget disease).

Those patients in whom hypercalcemia has been detected should undergo a workup for primary or secondary hyperparathyroidism. This workup requires the measurement of serum PTH and 1,25 dihydroxyvitamin D_3 levels. Although several tests are available for measuring PTH, assay of the intact molecule as opposed to the carboxy or amino terminals is most appropriate. Patients with hypocalcemia, hypophosphatemia, or evidence of renal failure should be checked for vitamin D deficiency by assaying for 25-hydroxyvitamin D.

To complete the biochemical evaluation, a serum protein electrophoresis is performed to rule out multiple myeloma. If there is an elevated γ-globulin region, a serum immunoelectrophoresis is ordered to look for a monoclonal immunoglobulin spike. A urine immunoelectrophoresis may demonstrate the presence of a Bence-Jones protein to confirm a diagnosis of multiple myeloma (Outline 4).

Radiologic Assessment Two forms of radiologic assessment are used in the evaluation of patients with metabolic bone disease: radiographs and densitometric scans. In the workup of patients suspected of having osteoporosis, anteroposterior (AP) and lateral radiographs of the thoracic and lumbar spines are standard. Because the vertebral bodies are the most common skeletal elements at risk, documentation of the fracture status of the vertebrae at the onset of treatment establishes a method for assessing the clinical outcome of any treatment protocol.

Perhaps the greatest contribution to diagnostic efforts in metabolic bone disease has been the development of bone densitometry. At present, the most clinically useful methods are single and dual energy X-ray absorptiometry (SXA

Table 3. Techniques for the measurement of bone mass

Technique	Site	Precision* (%)	Accuracy† (%)	Examination (Time, min)	Dose of Radiation (mrem)
Single-energy X-ray absorptiometry	Distal radius, calcaneus	0.5–2.0	3–5	3–7	1–3
Dual-energy X-ray absorptiometry	Spine, distal radius, hip, total body	0.5–2.0	3–5	3–7	1–3
Quantitative computed tomography	Spine	2–5	5–20	10–15	100–200
Radiographic absorptiometry	Phalanges	1–2	4	2	100

*Precision is the coefficient of variation for repeated measurements over a short period of time in young, healthy persons
†Accuracy is the coefficient of variation for measurements in a specimen the mineral content of which has been determined by other means

and DXA), quantitative computed tomography (QCT), and radiographic absorptiometry (RA). The most important considerations in assessing the utility of each of these methods are the anatomic sites available for study, the radiation dose to the patient, and the precision and accuracy of the test (Table 3).

QCT involves the use of a mineral calibration phantom in conjunction with a computed tomography (CT) scanner. A lateral CT localizes the midplane of two to four lumbar vertebral bodies and quantitative readings are then obtained from a region of trabecular bone in the anterior portion of the vertebra. CT determination of density in the vertebra is then compared to known density readings of solutions in the phantoms. The measurements of the vertebrae are then averaged and used to calculate the density of trabecular bone expressed as mineral equivalents of K_2HPO_4(mg/cm^2). The radiation dose is approximately one tenth of that used in a routine CT study.

The most widely used methods of bone densitometry are SXA and DXA. In these methods, an X-ray tube emits one or two beams, the attenuation of which is detected by an energy discriminating photon counter. The average scan time for the spine is 5 minutes and the radiation dose is so low (1 to 3 mrem) that it is essentially unimportant.

In RA, hand radiographs are taken with an aluminum wedge placed on the films to serve as a density reference. The radiographs are sent to a central facility where they are analyzed using an optical densitometer. The bone mineral density is then averaged for the middle phalanges of the second to fourth fingers and reported as a single value. The advantages of this method are low cost and the fact that it can be performed at a standard radiographic facility without the need for special equipment.

Bone Biopsy An extremely useful test in certain metabolic bone disease workups is the transilial bone biopsy. Although invasive, it is associated with a minimal degree of pain and inconvenience to the patient, can be performed on an ambulatory basis, and has a low complication rate. The biopsy can establish a diagnosis in the patient in whom osteomalacia or an occult malignancy is suspected; the tissue obtained can be used to distinguish between osteomalacia and osteitis fibrosa cystica in certain dialysis patients or to elucidate the cause of severe osteopenia in patients whose blood and urine test results are insufficiently informative.

The biopsy is taken from a point 3 cm posterior and 3 cm inferior to the anterior superior iliac spine. Once obtained, the specimen is embedded in methylmethacrylate and cut, processed, and stained using an undecalcified technique. Unstained sections are examined by fluorescence microscopy to determine the dynamic properties of bone. This is made possible by the presence of the tetracycline labels, which are obtained via the preoperative administration of oral tetracycline in two doses that are separated in time by a specified number of days (eg, 250 mg of oral tetracycline three times a day for 3 days, off for 12 days, repeat for 3 more days, biopsy between 3 and 7 days later). The cellular parameters of bone turnover are assessed by light microscopic examination of hematoxylin- and eosin-stained sections. Differentiation of mineralized from unmineralized osteoid is achieved through the use of a salt stain such as von Kossa, in which calcium and phosphorus salts appear dark, while unmineralized osteoid appears pale (Fig. 1). Through the use of a computer-assisted calculating system, an optical drawing tube, and an integrated ocular eyepiece, a number of quantitative parameters of bone statics and dynamics are measured. This technique, known as histomorphometry, enables the clinician to accurately diagnose the disorder and to determine to what extent resorptive or blastic activities are influencing the disease. In patients with renal disease, special stains are used to identify the presence of aluminum in bone as a cause of osteomalacia. This determination is particularly important because dramatic clinical improvements have been reported after removal of the aluminum from the bone.

Osteoporosis Treatment Regimens The goal of any osteoporosis treatment regimen is to prevent further bone loss. Presently, there are no well-accepted treatment protocols that can be shown to safely increase bone mass to normal levels. If there is no history of breast cancer or thromboembolic or endometrial disease, then estrogen replacement therapy is currently thought to be safe. A gynecological examination is required at the onset of treatment, and an endometrial biopsy is recommended after the first 12 months. If endometrial tissue shows no unusual activity, no further biopsies are required. However, a yearly mammogram is strongly recommended. If the patient is unable to use estrogen, calcitonin therapy at a dose of 50 to 100 U per day, injected subcutaneously, can be prescribed.

Etidronate disodium, a bisphosphonate with a long history of therapeutic use in patients with Paget disease, has been shown to prevent bone loss and provide a small (3% to 5%) increase in bone mass in postmenopausal osteoporotic women. Because the major concern with etidronate therapy has been the development of osteomalacia after chronic use or with high doses, the recommended regimen for using this drug is 400 mg per day in a cyclic fashion. This would mean 400 mg per day for 2 weeks followed by a 10-week period with no medication, and a continuous repetition of this cycle. At a recent Endocrine and Metabolic Drugs Advisory Panel Meeting of the US Food and Drug Administration (FDA), a decision was reached not to recommend approval of etidronate disodium for marketing in the treatment of osteoporosis.

The FDA recently approved two drugs for the treatment of osteoporosis. Alendronate, a bisphosphonate compound, is the first nonhormonal drug approved for the treatment of this disease. It is used in a dose of 10 mg per day, must be taken orally on an empty stomach, and the patient can only drink water (no other food or beverage) at the time of dosing. Because of the low bioavailability of this compound from the intestinal tract (approximately 0.7%), no food can be taken for at least 30 minutes after dosing. Reports show that alendronate prevents bone loss and is associated with gains in bone mass of up to 10%.

Calcitonin, a naturally occurring hormonal compound, has been approved by the FDA for several years in an injectable form. The approved dose of injectable salmon calcitonin is 100 units per day. Recently, the FDA approved a nasal spray formulation of this compound in a dose of 200 units per day. Although it has not yet been approved for marketing by the FDA, an FDA advisory panel has recently recommended approval of a slow-release formulation of sodium fluoride. This drug has been shown to produce substantial increases in bone mass and a reduction in the incidence of new fractures.

If a hypercalciuric component accompanies the active osteoporotic state, one to two daily doses of thiazide can be given to increase total body calcium retention. Studies have shown that an adequate dietary calcium intake in premenopausal women does not, in itself, protect women against the development of osteoporosis. However, in older postmenopausal women (> 6 years postmenopause), dietary supplementation with calcium can protect against bone loss. Moreover, the role of dietary calcium supplementation in the prevention of osteoporosis appears to be most critical during childhood and adolescent years when peak bone mass is being built. An adequate dietary calcium intake (Table 1) is required at all times, however, to prevent the adverse skeletal effects of secondary hyperparathyroidism. For this reason, all patients under treatment for osteoporosis should take 1.5 g of elemental calcium daily plus one or two multivitamins containing 400 units of vitamin D each. Although studies are in progress to determine the best preparation of oral calcium to use in order to enhance intestinal calcium absorption, any calcium is better absorbed when taken with meals. Perhaps the best form of symptomatic relief is achieved through physical therapy and rehabilitation.

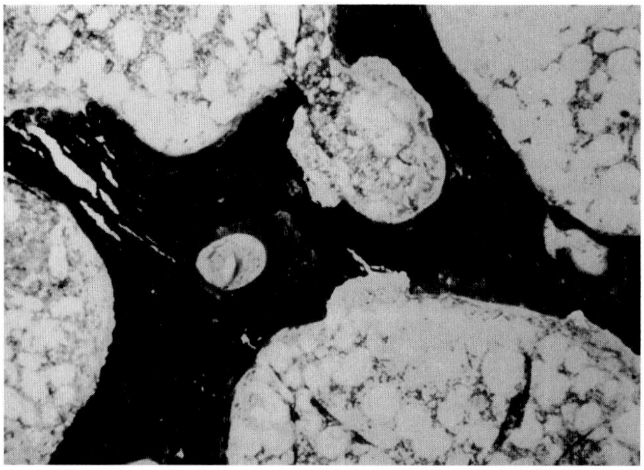

Fig. 1 Low power view of osteomalacic bone from a 25-year-old male with metabolic acidosis. Note that mineralized bone appears dark while unmineralized osteoid fails to take up the stain and appears pale. (von Kossa x 25). (Reproduced with permission from Frymoyer JW (ed): *Orthopaedic Knowledge Update 4.* Rosemont, IL, American Academy of Orthopaedic Surgeons, 1993, pp 69–88.)

Menstrual Function, Exercise and Bone Homeostasis In young women, there is a correlation between abnormal menstrual function and low bone mineral density. It is apparent that several factors contribute to the development of amenorrhea. Runners who begin training on or before the onset of menarche have a higher rate of amenorrhea. Other factors include low body-fat composition, nutritional status, and weekly mileage. Because one third of highly competitive female athletes have some form of an eating disorder, there is a considerable correlation between low calorie intake and amenorrhea. A correlation between anorexia nervosa, amenorrhea, and low bone mineral density has been well established.

Osteomalacia, Renal Bone Disease, and Hyperparathyroidism

Osteomalacia is a metabolic disorder in which there is inadequate mineralization of newly formed osteoid. It can result from vitamin D deficiency, vitamin D resistance, intestinal malabsorption, acquired or hereditary renal disorders, intoxication with heavy metals such as aluminum or iron, and other assorted etiologies (Outline 2). The childhood form of osteomalacia is termed rickets. Rickets of the developing and growing skeleton, which is caused by dietary deficiency of vitamin D, has become rare since the widespread supplementation of dairy products with vitamin D.

The clinical diagnosis of osteomalacia is often difficult because patients usually have nonspecific complaints such as muscle weakness or diffuse aches and pains. Radiographic evidence of osteomalacia can often mimic other disorders including osteoporosis. However, the presence of pseudofractures or Looser's transformation zones is good evidence that some degree of osteomalacia is present. Looser's zones are radiolucent areas of bone that are the result of multiple microstress fractures that heal by the formation of osteomalacic bone, which is not mineralized.

Biochemically, different forms of osteomalacia may present in different ways. However, the orthopaedist can usually be alerted by elevated alkaline phosphatase, low calcium, or low inorganic phosphorus levels. Serum assays for vitamin D metabolites may elucidate the abnormality.

In most patients, transilial bone biopsy is necessary to confirm the diagnosis of osteomalacia. The histologic hallmark of osteomalacia is an increase in the width and extent of osteoid seams (Fig. 1) with evidence of decreased rates of mineral apposition as determined by tetracycline labeling. In normally mineralized bone, tetracycline labels show discrete uptake of tetracycline only at times when mineral is being deposited; however, in osteomalacic bone, the slow rate of mineralization leads to an inability of these labels to appear separated in time and results in a smudged appearance.

Osteomalacia often occurs in patients who are elderly. It has been proposed that the mild malabsorption of the elderly predisposes patients to bone disease. The widespread use of anticonvulsant drugs such as phenytoin has also been shown to cause osteomalacia. The use of these drugs results in the induction of P-450 mixed function oxidases in hepatic cells, and thus the conversion of vitamin D to inactive polar metabolites. This conversion reduces the production of 25-hydroxyvitamin D, which is required for renal conversion to 1,25-dihydroxyvitamin D_3. (Note: A milder form of 25-hydroxyvitamin D synthesis impairment by phenytoin may lead to osteoporosis instead of osteomalacia.)

Osteomalacia is commonly seen in chronic renal dialysis patients. The major cause of the osteomalacia in these patients is the intoxication of the skeleton with aluminum. Aluminum is presented to the body in the form of aluminum-containing phosphate-binding antacids, which are used to control phosphate accumulation in patients with renal failure. Phosphate accumulation lowers the serum calcium level, thereby causing the parathyroid gland to become overactive (secondary hyperparathyroidism). This overactivity can lead to a characteristic destruction of trabecular bone known as osteitis fibrosa cystica. Efforts to develop drugs to control serum phosphate levels may lead to a reduction in the occurrence of this complication. However, if aluminum-containing phosphate-binding antacids are absolutely necessary, aluminum levels can be intermittently controlled with the aluminum chelating agent deferoxamine. It is important to note that, in some cases of severe renal secondary hyperparathyroidism, bone pain can be excruciating, serum parathyroid hormone levels can be difficult to control, and brown tumors can occur (although it is more common to see brown tumors in primary hyperparathyroidism). When this situation is present, a parathyroidectomy (partial or total) may be indicated. If any aluminum is present in bone at this time, the resultant decrease in bone turnover due to parathyroid down-regulation may facilitate aluminum accumulation and exacerbate or cause an osteomalacic state. For this reason, bone biopsy with aluminum staining is indicated in some hemodialysis patients prior to performing parathyroidectomy.

There are several known hereditary causes of renal rickets in growing children. The most common is X-linked dominant hypophosphatemic rickets. If the disorder is detected early in life, the skeleton may develop normally. Treatment with phosphate and 1,25-dihydroxyvitamin D_3 can usually maintain normal growth in these children. Hypophosphatemic rickets is usually due to a renal tubular defect in phosphate reabsorption. In 1948, Albright described a disorder termed "distal renal tubular acidosis." It has a dominant mode of inheritance with variable penetrance. Patients usually show at least one of the three major features: renal stones, hypophosphatemia, and osteomalacia. High doses of vitamin D and sodium bicarbonate are necessary to treat this condition. In addition, a rare form of osteomalacia associated with the presence of a benign tumor has been reported. In most of these cases, the tumor is found in the nasopharyngeal cavity or is never identified. The pathophysiology of this type of osteomalacia involves the secretion by the tumor of a phosphaturic substance. Thus there are a variety of causes of osteomalacia and treatment strategies differ depending on the etiology of the condition (Table 4).

Paget Disease Of Bone

Paget disease of bone is the second most common metabolic bone disease after osteoporosis. The incidence may be as great as 4% of individuals in the Anglo-Saxon population who are greater than 55 years of age. Studies have failed to detect a genetic predisposition or an HLA-antigen association type in Paget disease. However, a viral etiology was proposed in 1974 when virus-like inclusion bodies were found in osteoclasts from affected bone. Since then, researchers have focused on a slow virus as the causative agent.

Histologic analyses of specimens of pagetic bone show resorption by large numbers of osteoclasts. This resorption is followed by activation of osteoblasts and the production of new bone. The new bone produced contains widened lamellae and irregular "cement lines," which produce the characteristic "mosaic pattern" appearance of pagetic bone. The normal fatty or hematopoietic marrow

Table 4. Treatment of osteomalacia*

Disorder	Vitamin D_2 (U)	25-hydroxyvitamin D_3 (ug)	1,25-dihydroxyvitamin D_3 (ug)
Nutritional vitamin D deficiency	50,000 3 to 5 ×/week		
Malabsorption	50,000/day	20 to 200/day	
Anticonvulsant-induced osteomalacia (phenytoin)	50,000/day	20 to 100/day	
**Renal osteomalacia			1 to 2/day
†Metabolic acidosis	50,000/day		1 to 2/day
††X-linked hypophosphatemia			2 to 3/day until healing, then 0.5 to 1.0/day

*All patients receive 1.5 g elemental Ca/day
**Renal patients with bone aluminum intoxication may require deferoxamine
†To correct acidosis, titrate blood pH with sodium bicarbonate
††Add 1 to 2 g/day of phosphorus
(Reproduced with permission from Einhorn TA: Evaluation and treatment methods for metabolic bone diseases. *Contemp Orthop* 1987;14:21–34.)

spaces are replaced by loose, highly vascularized fibrous connective tissue. Ultimately, both the osteoclastic and osteoblastic activities decrease, resulting in a burned-out stage with enlarged and deformed bones that are densely sclerotic.

Biochemically, the high rate of bone turnover in Paget disease results in an immediate increase in the excretion of type I collagen breakdown products. The compensatory osteoblastic state is characterized by an increase in alkaline phosphatase activity, and thus, these two markers, serum alkaline phosphatase and urinary pyridinium cross-links, have been used to follow the course of the disease and its response to treatment.

Paget disease is often discovered as an incidental finding on radiographic examinations. Consequently, clinical experience has shown that most patients who are afflicted by this condition are asymptomatic. Patients who become symptomatic describe bone and joint pain and, later in the disease, may show deformities. One of the most common manifestations consists of low back pain in patients who, on radiographic examination, show pagetic involvement of the spine. The technetium 99m methylene diphosphonate (MDP) bone scan is an excellent method for screening areas of pagetic involvement. When first presented with a patient noted to have Paget disease, a technetium bone scan should be done prior to obtaining any further radiographs. Radiographic examination of areas that show increased isotopic uptake may be needed to determine the extent and nature of involvement of that part of the skeleton.

Most patients with Paget disease do not need pharmacologic treatment. Unless there is pain or significant abnormalities in urinary collagen breakdown products or serum alkaline phosphatase, patients may be followed without the use of drugs. For those patients who do have increased pain and poorly controlled biochemical indices of bone turnover, three classes of drugs are available for use: nonsteroidal anti-inflammatory drugs (NSAIDs), calcitonin, and bisphosphonates. The use of other agents, such as plicamycin, is indicated in more severe states of the disease, such as when there is spinal cord compression or hearing loss. For the management of mild symptoms related to Paget disease, indomethacin and other related NSAIDs have been shown to be useful clinically. Although they do not specifically target metabolic activities, patients usually experience pain relief. Patients who have pain and whose alkaline phosphatase levels are abnormally high may be managed by administration of a bisphosphonate. The only bisphosphonate currently available and approved by the US FDA is etidronate disodium. The mechanism of action of etidronate is to inhibit the ability of osteoclasts to resorb bone. However, with high doses or chronic use, etidronate has been shown to inhibit mineralization. For this reason, most patients treated with etidronate are placed on cyclic programs in which they are on the drug for several months at a time and then taken off the drug for long periods of rest. In the near future, several other bisphosphonates, which are more potent in inhibiting osteoclastic bone resorption and less toxic with respect to inhibiting mineralization, will be available. One of these, pamidronate, is now administered intravenously and is indicated in the treatment of Paget disease that is refractive to other treatments.

Calcitonin is probably the most popular agent for the treatment of Paget disease. This naturally occurring hormone acts via direct inactivation of osteoclasts; however, approximately 60% of patients develop antibodies. As a result, the agent may loose its effectiveness after time. Calcitonin is administered by subcutaneous injection; however, in the near future, a nasal spray may be available. Early studies suggest that nasal spray calcitonin leads to fewer side effects and is better tolerated.

Many patients suffering from Paget disease in the vicinity of joints develop degenerative joint disease, which may result from the biomechanical alteration of subchondral bone. Treatment of degenerative joint disease may involve hip or knee replacement arthroplasty. A 10-year follow-up study of total hip arthroplasty in patients with degenerative coxarthrosis secondary to Paget disease showed the rate of revision was not statistically higher than for patients without Paget disease. Aseptic loosening made revision necessary in approximately 15% of the cases.

The polyostotic form of Paget disease typically involves the pelvis and spine. Pelvic lesions are well tolerated unless the acetabulum is involved. Spinal involvement is not as well tolerated. Low back pain is a frequent complaint and is often associated with symptoms of spinal stenosis. The affected spinal segment may become progressively deformed, leading to a narrowing of static canal measurements and resulting in spinal stenosis. These patients often respond well to pharmacologic therapy; however, decompressive laminotomy may be required in patients who do not respond to medical management.

Sarcomatous degeneration occurs in less than 1% of patients with Paget disease. Osteogenic sarcoma occurs most commonly in association with this condition. Fibrosarcomas, chondrosarcomas, and malignant giant cell tumors have also been reported. A substantial increase in pain secondary to Paget disease is strongly suggestive of the development of a sarcoma. In almost all cases, the prognosis for Paget sarcoma is poor.

A benign tumor associated with Paget disease has been described. Intranuclear inclusion bodies similar to those seen in nonneoplastic pagetic tissue were demonstrated in the nuclei of giant cells associated with this tumor. The epidemiologic aspects of this tumor demonstrate that most cases can be traced to a small town in Italy known as Avellino. This finding further supports an infectious etiology for this condition.

Osteopetrosis

Osteopetrosis (Albers-Schönberg disease or marble bone disease) is a rare metabolic bone disease that is characterized by a diffuse increase in skeletal density and obliteration of marrow spaces. Histologically, the skeleton shows cores of calcified cartilage that are surrounded by areas of new bone; this new bone formation is normal but there is a deficiency of bone and cartilage resorption. The osteoclasts are abnormal and have been noted to lack a functional ruffled border.

In humans, osteopetrosis has traditionally been diagnosed as being either of the congenital (juvenile, malignant, or infantile) or adult (tarda) form. In the juvenile form, the mode of transmission is autosomal recessive, and this condition is characterized by severe anemia, hepatosplenomegaly, thrombocytopenia, cranial and optic nerve palsy, and a compromised immune system. Death usually occurs at a young age from anemia and sepsis. The adult or tarda form of osteopetrosis is inherited as an autosomal dominant trait, but some investigators report that autosomal recessive forms of this disease exist as well. Although osteopetrosis tarda is much less severe than the infantile form, a lifelong history of fractures usually characterizes the clinical picture.

Treatment for infantile or juvenile osteopetrosis is by bone marrow transplantation at a young age with marrow from an appropriately HLA-matched donor. A successful transplant may resolve the hematologic abnormalities including the defect in the immune system and can result in a gradual restoration of patent marrow cavities. HLA-mismatched transplants are unsuccessful in 30% of cases. A few isolated reports have suggested that high-dose 1,25-dihydroxyvitamin D_3 therapy and a low calcium diet can also treat this condition. While the mechanism is unclear, it is possible that 1,25-dihydroxyvitamin D_3 either stimulates the development of a normal ruffled border in osteoclasts, or, more likely, increases the fusion of mononuclear osteoclast progenitor cells to multinucleated bone resorbing osteoclasts.

Annotated Bibliography

Endocrine Function

Cauley JA, Seeley DG, Ensrud E, et al: Estrogen replacement therapy and fractures in older women. *Ann Intern Med* 1995;122:9–16.

The use of estrogen can protect against the risk of hip fracture in older women if it is initiated soon after menopause and continued indefinitely.

Colditz GA, Stampfer MJ, Willett WC, et al: Prospective study of estrogen replacement therapy and risk of breast cancer in postmenopausal women. *JAMA* 1990;264: 2648–2653.

A prospective study of up to 14 years conducted in 121,700 female nurses between the ages of 30 and 55 showed that, in current uses of estrogen, there is a 30% increased risk of breast cancer. However, long-term past use is not related to an increased risk.

Felson DT, Zhang Y, Hannan MT, et al: The effect of postmenopausal estrogen therapy on bone density in elderly women. *N Engl J Med* 1993;329:1141–1146.

This study shows how estrogen affects bone mass as a function of the time after menopause that treatment is begun and the duration over which it is used.

Finkelstein JS, Neer RM, Biller BM, et al: Osteopenia in men with a history of delayed puberty. *N Engl J Med* 1992;326:600–604.

This is a report of the syndrome of osteoporosis in men as a result of delayed sexual development.

Jilka RL, Hangoc G, Girasole G, et al: Increased osteoclast development after estrogen loss: Mediation by interleukin-6. *Science* 1992;257:88–91.

This reports a demonstration of how, in the absence of the ability to produce interleukin-6, estrogen loss will not lead to increased osteoclast activity.

Majeska RJ, Ryaby JT, Einhorn TA: Direct modulation of osteoblastic activity with estrogen. *J Bone Joint Surg* 1994;76A:713–721.

The authors demonstrate the ability of estrogen to directly affect the osteoblast's capacity to mediate bone formation and resorption.

Schneider DL, Barrett-Connor EL, Morton DJ: Thyroid hormone use and bone mineral density in elderly women: Effects of estrogen. *JAMA* 1994;271:1245–1249.

This is a documentation of the relationship between endogenous or exogenous thyroid hormone and the occurrence of osteoporosis.

Silver JJ, Majeska RJ, Einhorn TA: An update on bone cell biology. *Curr Opin Orthop* 1994;5:50–59.

This is an update of bone cell biology.

Silverberg SJ, Shane E, de la Cruz L, et al: Abnormalities in parathyroid hormone secretion and 1,25-dihydroxyvitamin D_3 formation in women with osteoporosis. *N Engl J Med* 1989;320:277–281.

Evidence is provided for an abnormality in parathyroid hormone secretion in addition to a decline in $1,25(OH)_2D_3$ responsiveness in the elderly.

Steinberg KK, Thacker SB, Smith SJ, et al: A meta-analysis of the effect of estrogen replacement therapy on the risk of breast cancer. *JAMA* 1991;265:1985–1990.

This meta-analysis of 16 studies showed a 30% increased risk of breast cancer with or without estrogen use. This risk was higher among women with a family history of breast cancer.

Osteoporosis

Dawson-Hughes B, Dallal GE, Krall EA, et al: A controlled trial of the effect of calcium supplementation on bone density in postmenopausal women. *N Engl J Med* 1990;323:878–883.

This study in healthy older postmenopausal women shows that daily calcium intakes of less than 400 mg lead to bone loss, intakes above 800 mg tend to maintain bone mass, and calcium citrate malate is more effective then calcium carbonate.

Kiel DP, Felson DT, Anderson JJ, et al: Hip fracture and the use of estrogens in postmenopausal women: The Framingham study. *N Engl J Med* 1987;317:1169–1174.

Estrogen supplementation affected the hip fracture rate in the Framingham study.

Johnston CC Jr, Slemenda CW, Melton LJ III: Clinical use of bone densitometry. *N Engl J Med* 1991;324: 1105–1109.

This is a current concepts review of bone densitometry methods.

Liberman UA, Weiss SR, Bröll J, et al: Effect of oral alendronate on bone mineral density and the incidence of fractures in postmenopausal osteoporosis. *N Eng J Med* 1995;333:1437–1443.

This double-blinded, randomized multicenter study established the efficacy of alendronate as a treatment for postmenopausal osteoporosis.

Lindsay R, McDonald EB, Hart DM, et al: Long-term prevention of postmenopausal osteoporosis by oestrogen: Evidence for an increased bone mass after delayed onset of oestrogen treatment. *Lancet* 1976;1:1038–1041.

This is the report of a landmark clinical study that shows that estrogen replacement therapy prevents osteoporosis in postmenopausal women.

Lloyd T, Andon MB, Rollings N, et al: Calcium supplementation and bone mineral density in adolescent girls. *JAMA* 1993;270:841–844.

This is a report of the role of calcium in the acquisition of peak bone mass by teenage girls.

Marcus R, Cann C, Madvig P, et al: Menstrual function and bone mass in elite women distance runners: Endocrine and metabolic features. *Ann Intern Med* 1985; 102:158–163.

This well-designed study shows that the mineral density in the lumbar spines of amenorrheic runners is decreased when compared with that in control runners but increased when compared with that in less physically active amenorrheic runners.

Morton DJ, Barrett-Connor EL, Edelstein SL: Thiazides and bone mineral density in elderly men and women. *Am J Epidemiol* 1994;139:1107–1115.

This is an update of the use of thiazide diuretics in the maintenance of total body calcium.

Pak CYC, Sakhaee K, Adams-Huet B, et al: Treatment of postmenopausal osteoporosis with slow-release sodium fluoride. *Ann Intern Med* 1995;123:401–408.

This randomized, placebo-controlled trial showed that slow-release sodium fluoride and calcium citrate, administered for 4 years, inhibited new vertebral fractures and augmented spinal and femoral neck bone mass.

Prince RL, Smith M, Dick IM, et al: Prevention of postmenopausal osteoporosis: A comparative study of exercise, calcium supplementation, and hormone-replacement therapy. *N Engl J Med* 1991;325:1189–1195.

This study showed that exercise plus calcium supplementation was as effective as estrogen replacement therapy in retarding bone loss.

Prior JC, Vigna YM, Schechter MT, et al: Spinal bone loss and ovulatory disturbances. *N Engl J Med* 1990;323: 1221–1227.

Decreases in spinal bone density in female athletes correlated with asymptomatic disturbances of ovulation and not with physical activity.

Riggs BL, Melton LJ III: Evidence for two distinct syndromes of involutional osteoporosis. *Am J Med* 1983;75:899–901.

This is the first description of the two forms of osteoporosis.

Riggs BL, Melton LJ III: The prevention and treatment of osteoporosis. *N Engl J Med* 1992;327:620–627.

This is an overview of the current management of osteoporosis.

Rigotti NA, Neer RM, Skates SJ, et al: The clinical course of osteoporosis in anorexia nervosa: A longitudinal study of cortical bone mass. *JAMA* 1991;265:1133–1138.

Anorexia nervosa leads to decreased bone mineral density. Bone mass may not be restored to normal when anorexia is reversed.

Riis B, Thomsen K, Christiansen C: Does calcium supplementation prevent postmenopausal bone loss? A double-blind, controlled clinical study. *N Engl J Med* 1987;316:173–177.

Calcium may have had a minor effect on the loss of cortical bone but it has no effect on trabecular bone when used alone in the prevention of postmenopausal osteoporosis.

Sinaki M, Mikkelsen BA: Postmenopausal spinal osteoporosis: Flexion versus extension exercises. *Arch Phys Med Rehabil* 1984;65:593–596.

This important study shows the appropriate use of physical therapy modalities in improving musculoskeletal function in women with existing osteoporosis.

Storm T, Thomsborg G, Steiniche T, et al: Effect of intermittent cyclical etidronate therapy on bone mass and fracture rate in women with postmenopausal osteoporosis. *N Engl J Med* 1990;322:1265–1271.

Uebelhart D, Gineyts E, Chapuy MC, et al: Urinary excretion of pyridinium crosslinks: A new marker of bone resorption in metabolic bone disease. *Bone Miner* 1990;8: 87–96.

This preliminary report describes the use of these two new urinary excretion metabolites, which appear to hold great potential for enhancing the sensitivity of clinical assays of bone resorption.

Watts NB, Harris ST, Genant HK, et al: Intermittent cyclical etidronate treatment of postmenopausal osteoporosis. *N Engl J Med* 1990;323:73–79.

These two reports documented the potential use of this bisphosphonate in the prevention of bone loss in postmenopausal women.

Osteomalacia, Renal Bone Disease, and Hyperparathyroidism

Cai Q, Hodgson SF, Kao PC, et al: Brief report: Inhibition of renal phosphate transport by a tumor product in a patient with oncogenic osteomalacia. *N Engl J Med* 1994;330:1645–1649.

This is an update on the pathophysiology of oncogenic osteomalacia.

Felsenfeld AJ, Harrelson JM, Gutman RA, et al: Osteomalacia after parathyroidectomy in patients with uremia. *Ann Intern Med* 1982;96:34–39.

An important finding is described: the high bone turnover resulting from secondary parathyroidism actually protects the skeleton from osteomalacia in uremic patients, and parathyroidectomy may lead to the development of osteomalacia.

Malluche HH, Smith AJ, Abreo K, et al: The use of deferoxamine in the management of aluminum accumulation in bone in patients with renal failure. *N Engl J Med* 1984;311:140–144.

The importance of diagnosing aluminum-related bone disease is emphasized by the successful treatment that is now possible for this condition.

Mankin HJ: Metabolic bone disease, in Jackson DW (ed): *Instructional Course Lectures 44.* Rosemont, IL, American Academy of Orthopaedic Surgeons, 1994, pp 3–29.

This is an excellent comprehensive overview of metabolic bone disease including the various types of osteomalacia.

Siris ES, Clemens TL, Dempster DW, et al: Tumor-induced osteomalacia: Kinetics of calcium, phosphorus, and vitamin D metabolism and characteristics of bone histomorphometry. *Am J Med* 1987;82:307–312.

This is a careful description of the pathophysiology of this oncogenic presentation of a metabolic bone disease.

Paget Disease

Anonymous: Case Records of the Massachusetts General Hospital: Weekly clinicopathological exercises. Case I-1986: A 67-year-old man with Paget's disease and progressive leg weakness. *N Engl J Med* 1986;314:105–113.

This is a review of the case records of an unusual presentation of giant cell tumor in Paget disease, which suggests a familial form of inheritance traced to the town of Avellino, Italy.

Gabel GT, Rand JA, Sim FH: Total knee arthroplasty for osteoarthrosis in patients who have Paget disease of bone at the knee. *J Bone Joint Surg* 1991;73A:739–744.

The presence of bone with Paget disease did not affect blood loss or rate of loosening. However, multiple technical difficulties resulting in suboptimum varus or valgus alignment were encountered.

Hadjipavlou A, Lander P: Paget disease of the spine. *J Bone Joint Surg* 1991;73A:1376–1381.

Anatomy, physiology, and clinical findings in Paget disease of the spine are discussed.

Mills BG, Singer FR: Nuclear inclusions in Paget's disease of bone. *Science* 1976;194:201–202.

This is a classic study that demonstrates the presence of viral nucleocapsid inclusion bodies in the osteoclasts from patients with Paget disease.

Schajowicz F, Araujo E, Berenstein M: Sarcoma complicating Paget's disease of bone: A clinicopathological study of 62 cases. *J Bone Joint Surg* 1983;65B:299–307.

This is an excellent review of Paget sarcoma.

Osteopetrosis

Kaplan FS, August CS, Fallon MD, et al: Successful treatment of infantile malignant osteopetrosis by bone-marrow transplantation: A case report. *J Bone Joint Surg* 1988;70A:617–623.

This provides five-year follow-up data for a patient who received a bone marrow transplant for osteopetrosis and a review of the subject.

Mills BG, Yabe H, Singer FR: Osteoclasts in human osteopetrosis contain viral-nucleocapsid-like nuclear inclusions. *J Bone Miner Res* 1988;3:101–106.

This report which suggests that, as in Paget disease, viral inclusions are found in the nuclei of osteoclasts from patients with benign osteopetrosis and may be causally related to the disease.

Shapiro F: Osteopetrosis: Current clinical considerations. *Clin Orthop* 1993;294:34–44.

This review of the classification of osteopetrosis includes a description of the physical, biochemical, and radiographic findings.

16

Musculoskeletal Neoplasms

Initial Evaluation

Malignant and benign bone and soft-tissue tumors are uncommon lesions. It is estimated that there are approximately 3,000 new cases of malignant bone tumors in the United States each year. The number of new cases of benign bone tumors is unknown. It is further estimated that approximately 4,000 new cases of malignant soft-tissue tumors are treated in the United States each year.

The evaluation of any patient presenting with a musculoskeletal neoplasm, whether benign or malignant, begins by obtaining a history and performing a physical examination. Pain is the most common symptom elicited in the history of a patient who has a malignant or benign bone tumor. It is important to note the character, location, and duration of the pain. Pain at rest and pain that wakes the patient from sleep at night are thought to be characteristic of aggressive benign or malignant lesions of bone. Activity-related pain is a more frequent complaint and is usually nonspecific.

Important physical findings in patients who have musculoskeletal neoplasms include the presence or absence of associated soft-tissue swelling, warmth, or venous dilation. Notable physical manifestations involving other organ systems should be recorded and may lead to a diagnosis. For example, the presence of a soft-tissue mass in a child with multiple café au lait spots suggests a diagnosis of neurofibromatosis. In addition, the neurologic and vascular status of the involved extremity should be carefully noted at the time of the initial examination. In patients older than 40 years who present with musculoskeletal neoplasms, a careful examination of the breasts in women and prostate in men must be carried out to exclude the possibility of an undiagnosed primary carcinoma.

Routine laboratory examinations are usually obtained at the time of presentation. Although results of these studies are often nonspecific, normal values can narrow the list of possible diagnoses. Furthermore, the studies provide a baseline for comparison with later values during treatment, especially when chemotherapy is indicated. A complete blood count with a differential and sedimentation rate, serum electrolytes, calcium, phosphorus, alkaline phosphatase, blood urea nitrogen, and creatinine are obtained. If prolonged therapy, including hospitalization, is anticipated, a nutritional profile and liver function tests are added. For patients older than 35 years, urinalysis, urine and serum protein electrophoresis, and prostate specific antigen in males are helpful tests that may be used to narrow the differential diagnosis. Finally, in the evaluation of a patient with a musculoskeletal neoplasm a radiograph of the affected portion of the trunk or limb is obtained.

Establishing a Differential Diagnosis

For any bone tumor, a differential diagnosis can be established given the patient's age and the radiographic appearance of the lesion. Most musculoskeletal tumors have a predilection for a narrow age range (Table 1). Important radiographic characteristics include the location of the lesion within the bone, the type of margin between the lesion and the surrounding bone, and the density (or matrix) of the lesion. Almost any primary or metastatic musculoskeletal neoplasm can occur in the metaphysis of a long bone (Fig. 1). Osteosarcoma is an example of a tumor found characteristically in this location. However, the specific location of a lesion within the metaphysis, whether eccentric or central, may provide additional clues to the diagnosis (Fig. 2).

Primary bone tumors of the epiphysis or apophysis are rare. Chondroblastomas are the most common bone tumors that occur in this location. Other conditions that

Table 1. Age predilection of skeletal tumors

1 to 5 years	6 to 18 years	19 to 40 years	40 + years
Osteomyelitis	Unicameral bone cyst	Ewing's sarcoma	Metastases
Metastatic neuroblastoma	Aneurysmal bone cyst	Giant cell tumor	Multiple myeloma
Leukemia	Nonossifying fibroma	Osteosarcoma (rare)	Chondrosarcoma
Eosinophilic granuloma	Ewing's sarcoma		Fibrosarcoma/malignant fibrous histiocytoma
Unicameral bone cyst (rare)	Osteomyelitis		
	Osteosarcoma		
	Enchondroma		
	Chondroblastoma		
	Chondromyxoidfibroma		
	Osteoblastoma		
	Fibrous dysplasia		
	Osteofibrous dysplasia		

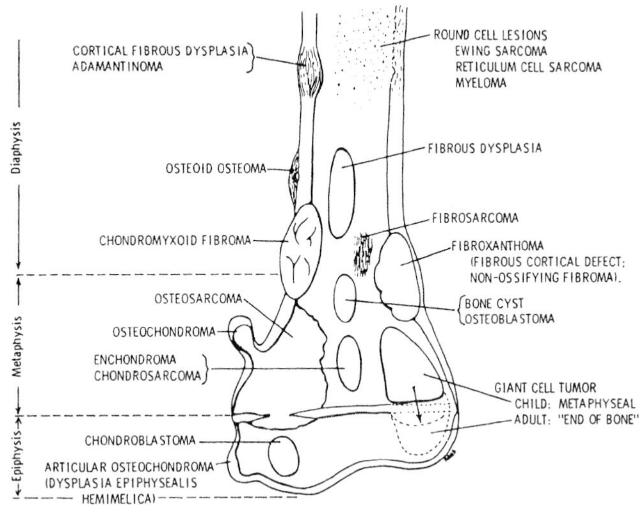

Fig. 1 Composite diagram illustrating the anatomic predilection of the most common primary bone tumors. (Reproduced with permission from Madewell JE, Ragsdale BD, Sweet DE: Radiologic and pathologic analysis of solitary bone lesions: Part I. Internal Margins. *Radiol Clin North Am* 1991;19:715–748.)

may affect the epiphyses and mimic a primary musculoskeletal tumor include degenerative cysts and occasionally osteomyelitis. Diaphyseal primary bone tumors include osteofibrous dysplasia, adamantinoma, Ewing's sarcoma, leukemia or lymphoma, and eosinophilic granuloma.

The best indication of the aggressiveness of any bone tumor is the transitional zone, or margin, that surrounds the lesion within the bone. The size of the lesion within the bone, the presence or absence of cortical breakthrough, the extent of the periosteal reaction, and the presence of a soft-tissue mass are all diagnostic characteristics. Destructive bone lesions are usually described as well-localized, moth-eaten, or permeative. Diagrammatic and radiographic representations of these three types of margins are given in Figure 3. Well-localized destructive lesions are further divided into those with a thick rind of surrounding reactive zone, a well-defined border without sclerosis, and a fading border.

The density, or matrix, of a bone tumor often provides clues to its histogenesis. Certain descriptive terms are applied to tumors that tend to have a consistent radiographic appearance. For example, speckled calcification and rings and arcs are terms given to the calcific densities seen in a typical, maturing, benign enchondroma. Fibrous dysplasia is said to have a ground glass or hazy matrix, which is imparted by the fine spicules of dysplastic bone. A

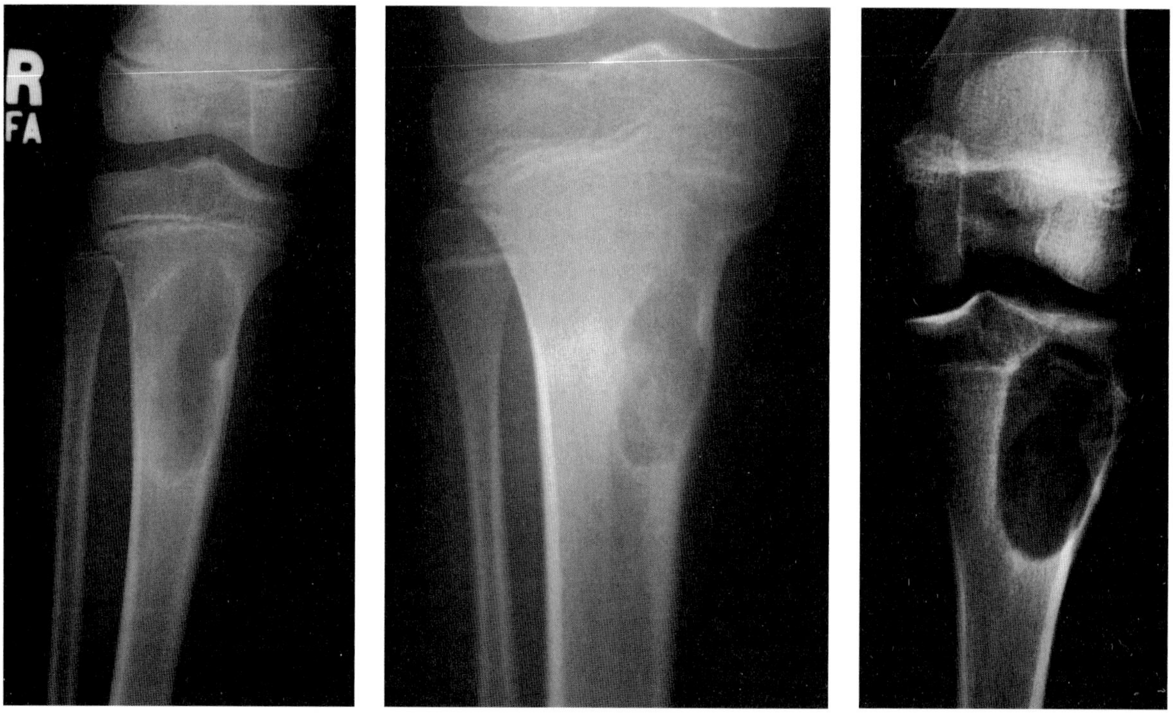

Fig. 2 **Left,** Anteroposterior (AP) radiograph of a proximal tibia unicameral bone cyst demonstrating the tendency of this lesion to occur centrally in the metaphysis. **Center,** AP radiograph of a proximal tibia nonossifying fibroma demonstrating the tendency of this lesion to occur in the metadiaphyseal portion of the bone in a eccentric juxtacortical location. **Right,** AP radiograph of a proximal tibia aneurysmal bone cyst, demonstrating the tendency of this lesion to occur in the subarticular metaphysis in a eccentric location with cortical thinning and expansion.

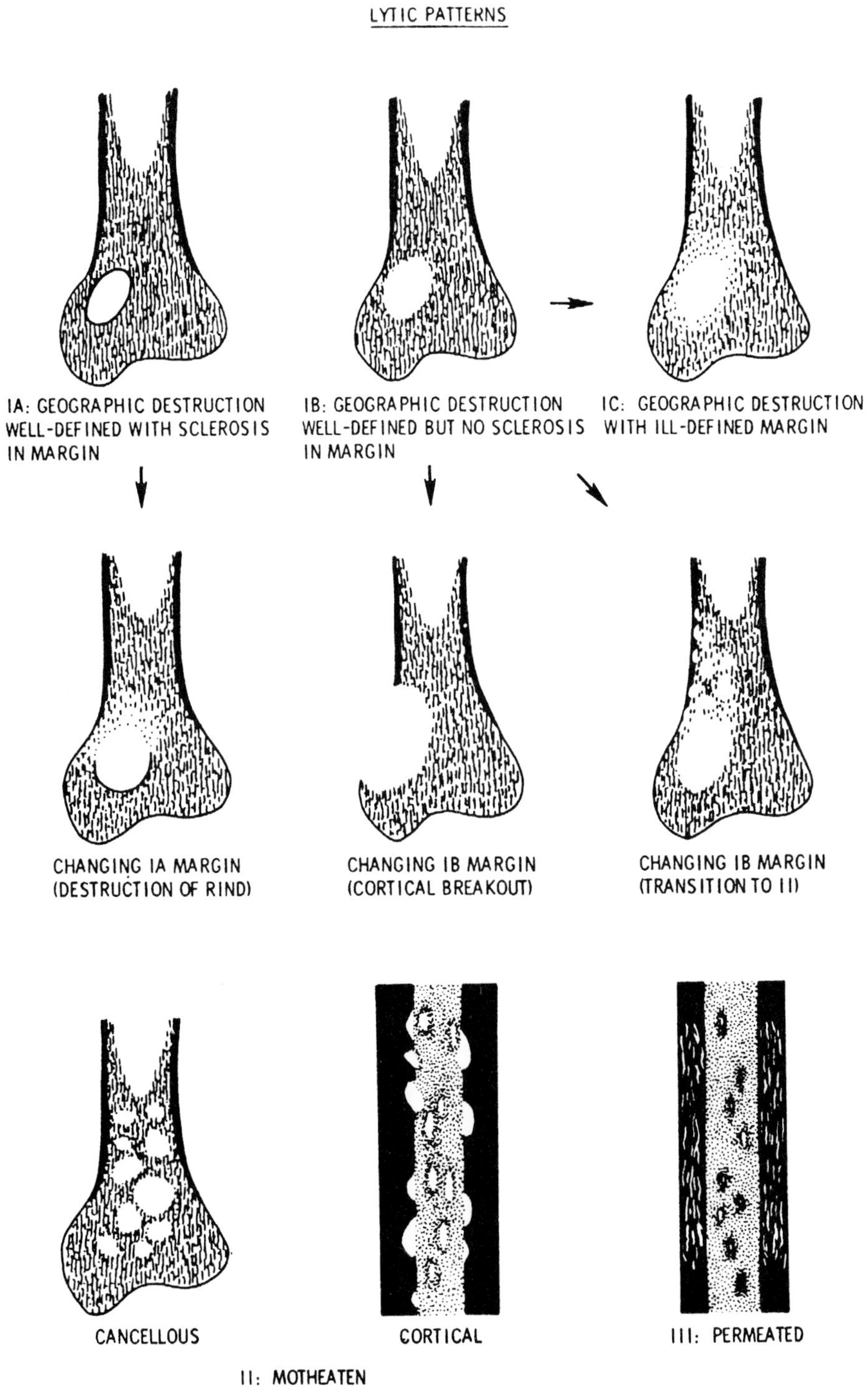

Fig. 3 Schematic diagram of the various patterns of bone destruction caused by primary bone tumors and their typical bony margins. The arrows in the figure indicate the most frequently seen transitional margins. Each transition to a less well defined margin or to a changing pattern of bone destruction indicates a more aggressive and possibly malignant bony lesion. (Reproduced with permission from Madewell JE, Ragsdate BD, Sweet DE: Radiologic and pathologic analysis of solitary bone lesions: Part I. Internal Margins. *Radiol Clin North Am* 1991;19:715–748.)

cloudlike or ivorylike density within bone is most characteristic of osteogenic sarcoma and results from malignant osteoid being produced in a haphazard fashion, mineralizing, and filling the normal cancellous interstices with tumor bone.

The location, margin, and density of a primary bone tumor will allow the clinician to determine whether the lesion is most likely benign or malignant. This finding, in turn, determines the nature and extent of additional staging studies that must be obtained prior to biopsy.

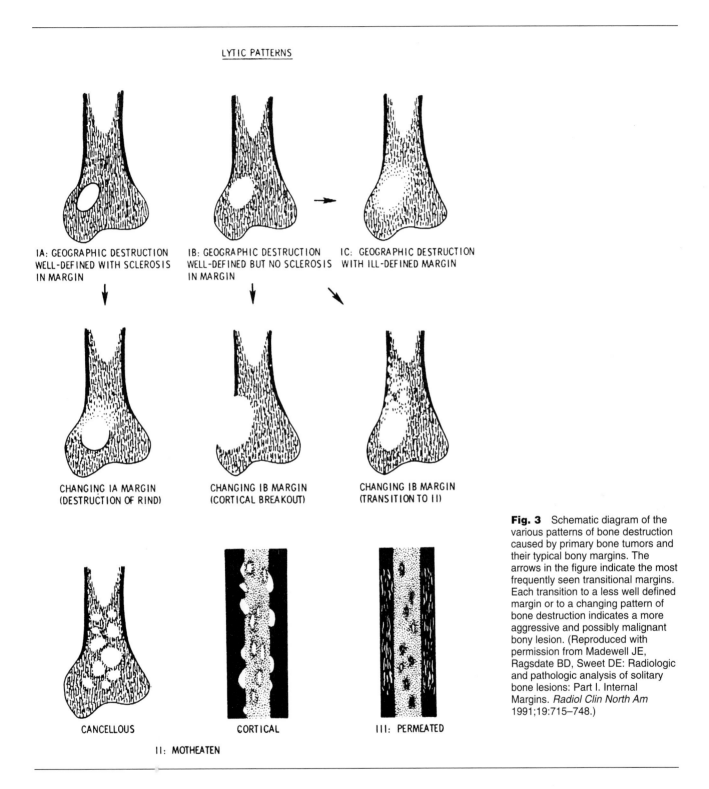

Any malignant lesion of bone in a patient older than 40 years is statistically most likely to be a skeletal metastasis from a primary carcinoma. In the United States, approximately 1 million patients per year are diagnosed with one of the primary carcinomas. Each of these patients is at risk for the development of skeletal metastases. The appropriate diagnostic evaluation of these patients has been established. Primary carcinoma of the lung is best detected by a chest radiograph and chest computed tomography (CT). Primary carcinoma of the breast is best detected by a careful breast examination and mammography; primary carcinoma of the kidneys is best detected with a CT scan of the abdomen; primary carcinoma of the prostate is best detected by a careful digital rectal examination and a serum prostate specific antigen; and multiple myeloma is best diagnosed by serum and urine protein electrophoresis. Therefore, a complete evaluation of a patient older than 40 years who presents with a primary bone lesion includes a careful history and physical examination followed by radiographs of the affected lesion; a laboratory evaluation, which includes serum chemistries, a complete blood count and sedimentation rate, and prostate specific antigen; a urinalysis and microscopic examination of the urine; and serum and urine protein electrophoresis. Advanced diagnostic tests should be limited to a total body technetium bone scan, chest radiograph, CT scans of the chest and abdomen, and mammography. If the primary lesion is not identified by this evaluation, it is not likely to be identified by more invasive and expensive clinical studies.

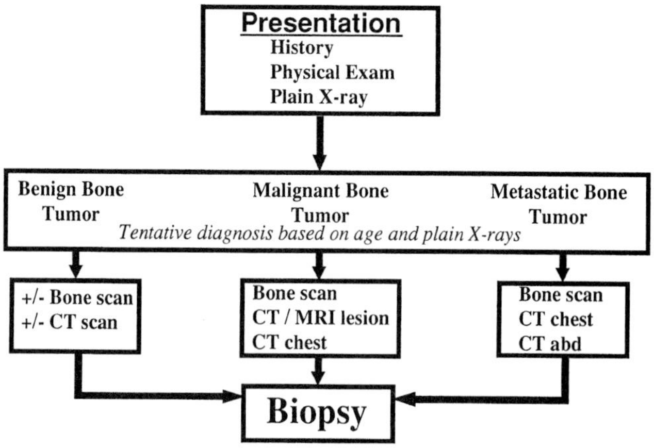

Fig. 4 Algorithm depicting the diagnostic approach to the initial evaluation and advanced diagnostic imaging of patients with osseous musculoskeletal tumors.

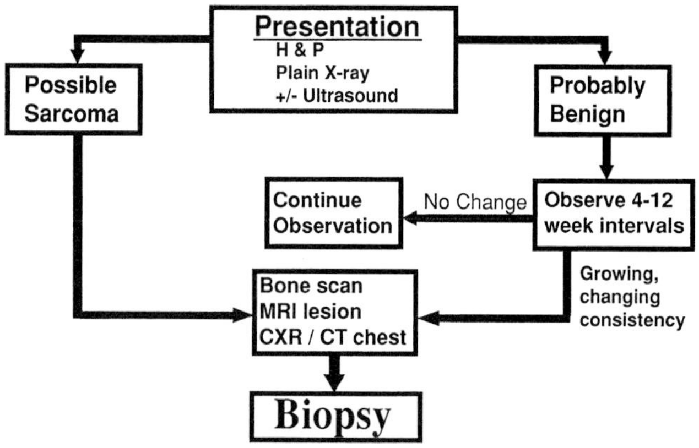

Fig. 5 Algorithm depicting the diagnostic approach to the initial evaluation and advanced diagnostic imaging of patients with soft-tissue tumors.

Staging

The next step in the proper management of a patient with a musculoskeletal neoplasm is accurate staging of the lesion. For both soft-tissue and bone tumors, the extent of this staging depends on whether the tumor is benign or malignant. Guidelines for advanced diagnostic imaging in cases of osseous and soft-tissue musculoskeletal neoplasms are given in Figures 4 and 5. For osseous lesions that are suspected to be benign, a total body technetium bone scan and a CT scan of the lesion are obtained, in addition to the initial radiograph. If the osseous lesion is suspected to be malignant, a magnetic resonance image (MRI) is also obtained of the lesion, and a radiograph and CT scan of the chest are obtained. If a soft-tissue neoplasm is suspected to be benign, appropriate imaging beyond the initial radiograph usually consists of an MRI. For very small (< 5 cm) superficial lesions, MRI is usually not necessary. If the soft-tissue tumor is suspected to be malignant, a radiograph and CT scan of the chest and an MRI of the lesion should be obtained.

The purpose of staging the musculoskeletal neoplasm is to accurately define the extent of the disease prior to proceeding with biopsy and definitive treatment. All staging systems for musculoskeletal neoplasms define tumor stages according to location and size of the primary lesion, the presence or absence of regional or distant metastases, and the histologic grade of the tumor. The relative significance of each of these factors varies from system to system. The Enneking system for staging sarcomas of soft tissue and bone is presented in detail in *Orthopaedic Knowledge Update 3* together with the staging systems developed by the American Joint Commission on Cancer.

The only system for staging of benign musculoskeletal neoplasms is that of Enneking (Table 2). Stage 1 or latent lesions are benign, intracapsular, and without metastases. Their typical clinical course is considered to be unchanging or self-healing. Stage 2 or active lesions are also benign and intracapsular, but their radiographic and clinical characteristics suggest active but contained growth without extracapsular penetration. Typically these lesions have a 5%

Table 2. Staging of benign and malignant musculoskeletal neoplasms

Grade (G)	Site (T)	Metastases (M)
G_0 = Benign	T_0 = Intracapsular	M_0 = None
G_1 = Low-grade malignant	T_1 = Intracompartmental	M_1 = Regional or distant
G_2 = High-grade malignant	T_2 = Extracompartmental	

Benign
1 = G_0, T_0, M_0—Latent
2 = G_0, T_0, M_0—Active
3 = G_0, T_1, M_0—Aggressive

Malignant
I A = G_1, T_1, M_0—Low-grade, intracompartmental, no metastases
B = G_1, T_2, M_0—High-grade, extracompartmental, no metastases
II A = G_2, T_1, M_0—High-grade, intracompartmental, no metastases
B = G_2, T_2, M_0—High-grade, extracompartmental, no metastases
III A = G_{1-2}, T_1, M_1—Either grade, intracompartmental, metastases
B = G_{1-2}, T_2, M_1—Either grade, extracompartmental, metastases

(Adapted with permission from Enneking WF, Spaniar SS, Goodman MA: A system for the surgical staging of musculoskeletal sarcoma. *Clin Orthop* 1980;153:106–120.)

to 10% local recurrence rate after curettage but respond well to wide excision. Stage 3 or aggressive lesions are benign, extracapsular but intercompartmental, and without metastases. The clinical and radiographic growth patterns of these lesions are characterized by extracapsular penetration and destructive growth. These lesions tend to have a 10% to 20% local recurrence rate after interlesional or marginal excision and may even recur after wide local resection.

Biopsy

Once a differential diagnosis has been established, and appropriate staging completed, a biopsy is indicated. The goals of biopsy are to determine whether a lesion is benign or malignant, to determine the specific cell type of the lesion, and to determine the grade of the lesion. This step is perhaps the most crucial, yet remains the most frequent source of error in the management of musculoskeletal tumors. Although this topic has been dealt with in depth in previous *Orthopaedic Knowledge Updates,* the potential for errors in performing a biopsy, which may render a salvageable limb unsalvageable, makes certain principles worth repeating.

Proper biopsy technique for musculoskeletal neoplasms requires that the incision or needle placement be located in such a way as to permit en bloc resection of contaminated and potentially contaminated tissues at the time of definitive surgery. Longitudinal incisions are therefore mandatory; transverse incisions in the extremities must be avoided at all costs. A minimal dissection technique is used; that is, subcutaneous skin flaps are not created. Dissection between muscular intervals also is avoided; the biopsy incision must cross only one compartment of the affected extremity. Dissection near critical neurovascular structures must be avoided. The most peripheral soft-tissue component of an osseous musculoskeletal neoplasm is the most likely to yield an accurate histologic diagnosis and, therefore, is the preferred specimen. Cortical windows should be avoided. Meticulous hemostasis is obtained at the time of wound closure. The wound is closed in layers, with a watertight suture line at each layer. Drains should be avoided. In rare circumstances, highly vascular lesions, such as hemangioendotheliomas, may bleed excessively, and adequate hemostasis may not be possible. In these circumstances, a drain may be used to avoid a dissecting hematoma. If a drain is used for a biopsy of a musculoskeletal neoplasm, it must be brought out in line with and very close to the surgical incision to facilitate complete excision of the drain tract at time of definitive surgery.

Percutaneous needle biopsy is a valuable alternative technique that has specific indications in the evaluation of musculoskeletal neoplasms. It is most useful in the biopsy of extremity soft-tissue masses and certain pelvic and spinal osseous and soft-tissue masses. The technique has the disadvantage of providing less tissue for examination. However, in most large lesions, enough representative specimen can be obtained to facilitate a complete histologic workup. In certain circumstances, needle biopsy can potentially provide a better sampling of a heterogeneous soft-tissue tumor than an incisional biopsy (Fig. 6). There are three basic types of percutaneous needle biopsy: fine-needle aspiration, tru-cut needle, and large-bore needle or trephine biopsy. Fine-needle biopsy is done with a 22- to 23-gauge needle and typically yields material that is suitable only for cytologic examination. It is inadequate for determining histologic grade and more frequently provides inadequate tissue for diagnosis than core needle biopsy. This particular technique is most useful for confirming a suspected diagnosis of metastatic adenocarcinoma. Alternatively, tru-cut and large-bore percutaneous biopsy instruments are available that vary in size from 20 gauge to 3.5 mm (Fig. 7). These instruments are all designed to retrieve a core of tissue for histologic examination. Larger amounts of tissue are obtained with these instruments, facilitating extensive histopathologic evaluations that may

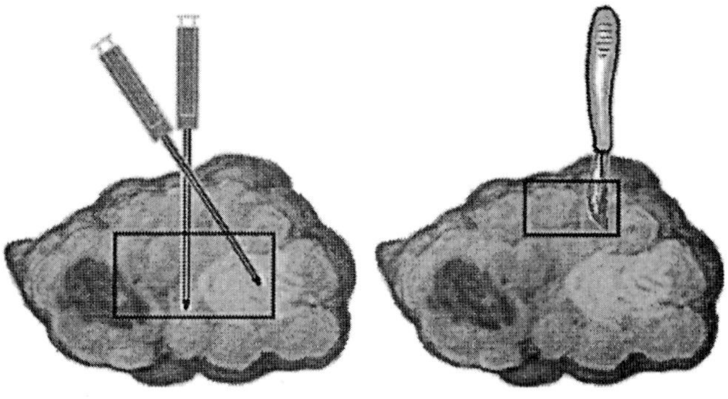

Fig. 6 Diagram illustrating the ability of a core biopsy needle to obtain, in certain circumstances, a more representative sample of a heterogeneous tumor than a limited incisional biopsy. The boxes outline the region of tumor potentially sampled by each biopsy technique.

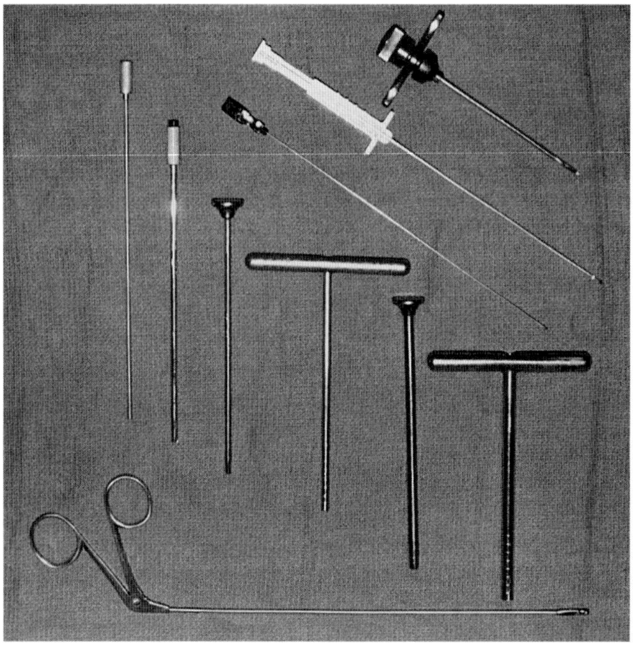

Fig. 7 Representative types of available biopsy equipment for percutaneous biopsy of musculoskeletal neoplasms. Vertically positioned left to right they are: large (3.5-mm) and medium bore (2.0-mm) bone trephines and their trocars; and a 2.0-mm Craig needle biopsy and its trocar. Obliquely oriented from bottom to top are a Jamshidi core biopsy needle, a trucut core biopsy needle, and a 23-gauge needle for aspiration biopsy. The needle employed for fine needle aspiration is the only biopsy instrument in this figure that fails to retrieve a core of tissue suitable for extensive histopathologic evaluation and examination of tumor morphology.

include immunocytochemistry, electron microscopy, and flow cytometry.

The biopsy technique chosen depends on several variables. It is preferable to biopsy all children in the operating room with adequate anesthesia regardless of whether a needle biopsy or incisional biopsy is planned. Incisional biopsies in adults are performed in the operating room, using the technique described above. However, the majority of soft-tissue tumors in adults can be biopsied using a tru-cut needle in the clinic setting. This procedure has the advantage of obviating the need for and expense of a separate surgical procedure, minimizing the amount of tissue that needs to be resected en bloc at the time of definitive surgery, and providing a rapid diagnosis. This biopsy technique does not require image guidance unless the tumor involves the axial skeleton and cannot be readily palpated. The disadvantages of needle biopsy have been previously noted. In certain circumstances, adults who have osseous musculoskeletal neoplasms with a large soft-tissue component may also be biopsied using a tru-cut needle in an outpatient clinic setting. In these cases, the biopsy is often used to confirm an obvious clinical diagnosis and will expedite the institution of appropriate treatment.

Bone Tumors

Benign Bone Tumors

There is a large variety of primary benign bone tumors (Table 3). A review of each of their clinical and pathologic features and treatment is beyond the scope of this chapter. The treatment for most benign bone tumors can be based on the stage of the lesion. Symptomatic latent lesions are best treated with curettage and bone grafting, while most active and aggressive lesions are best treated with curettage, local adjuvant, and bone grafting or en bloc excision. The benign primary bone tumors that are perhaps most commonly encountered by the orthopaedist are the unicameral bone cyst, nonossifying fibroma, enchondroma, and giant cell tumor.

Unicameral Bone Cyst These lesions typically are present in children as solitary fluid-filled cysts in the metaphyses of long bones. The most common locations are the proximal humerus and proximal femur. They frequently abut the growth plate, making aggressive treatment risky for premature epiphyseal closure. In this circumstance, treatment should consist of steroid injection or observation until normal growth increases the distance between the lesion and the epiphysis. These lesions commonly appear after a throwing injury or minor fall with a pathologic fracture and only rarely heal completely as a result of the fracture. Treatment in this circumstance should include immobilization until early fracture healing has occurred followed by methylpronisolone acetate injection, or curettage and bone grafting, which is done more frequently

Table 3. Tumors and tumor-like lesions of bone

Tissue of Origin	Benign Lesion	Malignant Lesion
Bone-forming	Osteoma Osteoid osteoma Osteoblastoma	Osteosarcoma (and variants) Juxtacortical osteosarcoma (and variants)
Cartilage-forming	Enchondroma (chondroma) Periosteal (juxtacortical chondroma) Enchondromatosis (Ollier's disease) Osteochondroma Osteocartilaginous exostosis Chondromyxoid fibroma Chondroblastoma	Chondrosarcoma (central) Conventional Mesachymal Clear cell Dedifferentiated Chondrosarcoma (peripheral) Periosteal (juxtacortical)
Fibrous and fibrohiosticytic	Fibrous cortical defect (metaphysical fibrous defect) Nonossifying fibroma Benign fibrous histiocytoma Fibrous dysplasia Periosteal desmoid Demoplastic fibroma Osteofibrous dysplasia Ossifying fibroma (Sissoris' lesion)	Fibrosarcoma Malignant fibrous histiocytoma
Vascular	Hemangioma Glomus tumor Hemangiopericytoma Cystic angiomatosis	Angiosarcoma Hemangioendrothelioma Hemangiopericytoma Kaposi's sarcoma
Bone marrow (hematopoietic and lymphatic)	Giant cell tumor (osteoclastoma) Eosinophilic granuloma Lymphangioma	Malignant giant cell tumor Histiocytic lymphoma Hodgkin's disease Leukemia Myeloma (plasmacytoma) Lymphangiosarcoma

when these lesions occur in the weightbearing bones of the lower extremities. Incomplete healing is common following either treatment method, and careful follow-up is essential.

Nonossifying Fibroma These lesions typically are seen in the metaphyses of growing children as incidental findings on radiographs taken for other reasons. They usually are eccentric lucent lesions that can occasionally appear multiloculated or bubbly. Smaller lesions will heal over time and do not require treatment. Very large lesions require curettage and bone grafting to prevent pathologic fracture. The decision to surgically treat these lesions must be made on an individual basis, factoring in the patient's activity level, the size of the lesion, and any symptomology.

Enchondroma The solitary enchondroma is a very common bone lesion. It typically presents as a central metaphyseal lesion with a frequently characteristic pattern of calcification, including the so-called rings and arcs, and stippled calcification. Distinguishing a benign latent enchondroma from an active enchondroma or low-grade chondrosarcoma is a commonly encountered and difficult clinical problem. Characteristics of each of these lesions are listed in Table 4.

Biopsy of these cartilaginous lesions is not indicated because the histologic characteristics of a benign enchondroma are indistinguishable from those of an active enchondroma or low-grade chondrosarcoma. The decision to treat these lesions is based on clinical features that suggest the lesion is actively growing or has become frankly malignant (Table 4). For cases of active enchondroma or low-grade chondrosarcoma, intralesional curettage with adjuvant cryotherapy is sufficient treatment. Local recurrence rates may range from 10% to 15% with this treatment. Local recurrences are easily managed with repeat curettage, adjuvant treatment, and additional bone grafting. Alternative treatment for local recurrence is wide resection and limb salvage reconstruction.

Table 4. Clinical features of enchondroma and low grade chondrosarcoma

Enchondroma	Low Grade Chondrosarcoma
Painless	Painful
Bone scan variable	Bone scan variable
Uniform matrix calcification	Lucent regions
No endosteal reosion	Endosteal erosion
Uniform, small, bland cells*	Mild cellular atypia*
Low cellularity*	Moderate to high cellularity*

* Biopsy is usually unreliable in distinguishing these two lesions

Osteochondroma These lesions are actually developmental dysplasias of the peripheral growth plate and are characterized by a sessile or pedunculated outgrowth of trabecular bone with a variably-sized cap of proliferating cartilage. They can occur in any bone formed by enchondral ossification. An osteochondroma is seen clinically as a solitary hard, fixed mass that is not tender; irritation of overlying muscles and tendons with bursa formation is common. On radiographs, the stalk of the lesion is continuous with the underlying normal metaphysis; this often is best seen on axial CT scans. These lesions will grow steadily during childhood and adolescence and cease growing at skeletal maturity. Multiple lesions will develop in individuals with hereditary multiple exostoses, an autosomal dominant genetic disorder. This familial trait often results in short stature, skeletal deformity, and premature osteoarthrosis.

In the adult, symptomatic or enlarging lesions suggest the possibility of malignant transformation to a secondary chondrosarcoma. Evidence of malignant transformation includes a cartilaginous cap thicker than 2 cm, new radiolucencies in previously partially mineralized lesional bone, or a soft-tissue mass. The risk of malignant transformation in solitary lesions is unknown because many solitary lesions are asymptomatic and never diagnosed. In hereditary multiple exostoses, the risk of malignant transformation has recently been shown to be less than 1%.

Symptomatic benign lesions are adequately treated by marginal excision; the local recurrence rate is 5%. Excision of large asymptomatic lesions of the spine and pelvis should be considered because malignant transformation of lesions in these regions tends to go undiagnosed.

Giant Cell Tumor The conventional giant cell tumor (GCT) of bone is a solitary, purely lytic lesion that typically involves the end of long bones, most commonly about the knee, in adults. Osteoclast-like giant cells are a constant histologic finding. These cells, which contain a variable number of nuclei of uniform size and shape, are found in a background of oval to spindle-shaped stromal cells. Mitoses are usually seen, but are generally few in number and are not indicative of malignancy. Osteoid is also commonly seen and may result in a mistaken diagnosis of osteosarcoma. It is important to note that the osteoid seen in GCT of bone is reactive, and it is produced by normal appearing osteoblasts in a reparative response to the destruction produced by these tumors.

Most giant cell tumors are amenable to intralesional curettage. Cryotherapy or other local adjuvant treatment reduces the local recurrence rate after conservative treatment. Giant cell tumors of the sacrum are a very difficult clinical problem. Good results have been obtained with intralesional (if necessary) resection, curettage, and local cryotherapy, sparing sacral nerve roots and the structural integrity of the upper sacral segments.

Malignant Bone Tumors

Osteosarcoma Osteosarcoma is the most common primary sarcoma of bone. It is a heterogeneous disease that is characterized histologically by frankly sarcomatous mesenchymal stromal cells that produce osteoid. Although it may occur in any bone of the appendicular or axial skeleton or even the soft tissues, it has a distinct predilection to occur in the distal femoral and proximal tibial metaphyses of adolescents.

There are numerous clinical and pathologic subtypes of osteosarcoma (Table 5). Treatment, however, is based entirely on the grade of the lesion. High-grade lesions are most commonly treated with neoadjuvant (preoperative) chemotherapy, wide resection with limb salvage reconstruction or amputation, and adjuvant (postoperative) chemotherapy. Low-grade lesions are treated with wide resection and limb salvage reconstruction or amputation. The expected 5-year survival for patients diagnosed with osteosarcoma is now thought to be 50% or more. Aggressive treatment in special centers is producing even higher cure rates for patients with conventional lesions in favorable anatomic locations.

Results of a recent study of the long-term effects of treatment on survivors of primary bone sarcomas suggest that, as adults, these patients have a 7% risk of dying from a second malignancy. These data make continued medical follow-up a necessity. However, despite the impairment resulting from amputation or limb salvage, these patients did not differ significantly from controls in terms of employment status, income, or any other measured psychosocial parameter.

Chondrosarcoma Chondrosarcoma is a malignant tumor, composed of proliferating cartilage, that accounts for approximately 10% of primary sarcomas of bone. It may occur de novo or secondarily from a preexisting enchondroma or osteochondroma. In contrast to osteosarcoma, most chondrosarcomas are very slow growing and histologically low grade. Consequently, they respond poorly to adjuvant treatment modalities such as chemotherapy and radiation therapy. Surgery remains the mainstay of treatment for these tumors. There is a small subgroup of chondrosarcomas that are histologically high grade and carry a very poor prognosis. This subgroup includes dedifferentiated chondrosarcoma and mesenchymal chondrosarcoma.

Table 5. Clinical and pathologic subtypes of osteogenic sarcoma

Type	Grade	Incidence	Location	Histology
Conventional	High	85%	Intramedullary	Osteoblastic Chondroblastic Fibroblastic
Parosteal	Low	3%	Juxtacortical	Fibroblastic
Periosteal	High	Rare	Juxtacortical (Subperiosteal)	Chondroblastic
High grade surface	High	Rare	Juxtacortical	Mixed
Telangiectatic	High	3%	Intramedullary	Hemorrhagic
Low grade intramedullary	Low	Rare	Intramedullary	Fibroblastic
Extraosseous	High	Rare	Soft tissues	Osteoblastic

Ewing's Sarcoma/Primitive Neuroectodermal Tumor The term primitive neuroectodermal tumor (PNET) applies to a group of small round cell tumors that may occur in bone or soft tissue as well as in the central, sympathetic, and peripheral nervous systems. They were first reported by Stout in 1918 and given the name neuroepithelioma. When these lesions occur in the thoracopulmonary region, they are often called Askin's tumor after James Askin, who described 20 such cases in children in 1979.

Ewing's sarcoma was first described by James Ewing in 1921 as an undifferentiated, small, round cell sarcoma of bone. It was later shown to also occur in soft tissue. The true histogenesis of this tumor was unknown for years and was the subject of much debate. It is now generally accepted that these tumors are derived from a mesenchymal stem cell of neural crest origin. Ninety percent of cases occur in the first three decades of life, with the pelvis and lower extremities most commonly affected.

In the past, the relationship of Ewing's sarcoma to PNET has been very controversial. However, recent ultrastructure and immunohistochemical studies have suggested that Ewing's sarcoma and PNET have a similar histogenesis. Therefore, these tumors may share important biologic features that affect their clinical behavior and response to therapy. Optimal treatment of these high-grade undifferentiated lesions includes neoadjuvant chemotherapy and surgical resection, followed by adjuvant chemotherapy and radiation therapy. Disease-free and overall survival rates are similar to those for patients with osteosarcoma and probably exceed 50% at 5 years. Ewing's sarcoma of the pelvis is particularly difficult to treat, and only a few affected individuals survive.

Fibrosarcoma/Malignant Fibrous Histiocytoma Primary fibrosarcoma of bone is a purely fibroblastic malignancy of variable grade that has a skeletal distribution similar to that of osteosarcoma, but tends to occur in an older age group. Histologically, a herringbone pattern of spindle cells is usually recognized, with a variable amount of cytologic atypia and mitotic activity. Malignant fibrous histiocytoma (MFH) of bone is characterized histologically by the presence of round to ovoid histiocytes with foamy or granular cytoplasm in a background of collagen that tends to be arranged in a storiform pattern. The diagnosis of either fibrosarcoma or MFH depends on the absence of osteoid and cartilage in the lesion. The diagnosis of MFH further depends on the absence of significant positive immunohistochemical markers for unusual osseous lesions, such as leiomyosarcoma of bone.

Treatment

Tumor Resection The treatment of any musculoskeletal neoplasm depends on its location and stage. The treatment of benign musculoskeletal neoplasms is outlined in Table 6. In general, latent benign soft-tissue or bone tumors, unless unusually large, may be observed. An example of a latent benign soft-tissue tumor would be a subcutaneous lipoma. An example of a latent benign bone tumor would be nonossifying fibroma. In certain circumstances, surgical intervention may be indicated for these lesions. If the lipoma is unusually large and cosmetically disfiguring, excision may be indicated. If the nonossifying fibroma is associated with a pathologic fracture or is very large and creating the potential for a pathologic fracture, curettage and bone grafting may be indicated.

Table 6. Treatment of benign bone tumors

Tumor Description	Treatment
Latent	Observation
Active/aggressive	Curettage Local adjuvant Reconstruction

Active and aggressive benign soft-tissue and bone tumors require treatment. In the bone, these lesions are best treated with curettage and perhaps a local adjuvant, followed by reconstruction. Reconstruction alternatives following resection of active and aggressive benign bone tumors include allograft, autograft, and polymethylmethacrylate. Prophylactic stabilization of the affected bone may be required, depending on the size and location of the specific tumor. The osteoblastoma shown in Figure 8 is an active benign bone tumor, and the giant cell tumor shown in Figure 9 is an aggressive benign bone tumor.

Treatment for soft-tissue and osseous sarcomas depends on the stage of the lesion. Low-grade sarcomas of bone are treated by wide excision and limb salvage where possible. Wide amputation is indicated if limb salvage is impossible. High-grade sarcomas of bone are treated by a combination of systemic chemotherapy and appropriate local surgery. Radiation therapy is occasionally indicated as a postoperative adjuvant in the management of a high-grade sarcoma of bone, depending on the specific histologic subtype. For example, postoperative radiation therapy may be indicated in same cases of Ewing's sarcoma, depending on surgical resection margins.

One of the more controversial current topics in musculoskeletal tumors is the issue of what constitutes a wide surgical margin. The classic description of surgical margins is shown in Figure 10. An intralesional margin implies that the tumor was removed in a piecemeal fashion or by curettage. It has a potential for leaving gross disease. However, in the case of most benign osseous lesions, intralesional curettage performed through an adequate cortical window will leave only microscopic disease. A marginal margin traverses the pseudocapsule or reactive zone of a musculoskeletal lesion, and it potentially leaves residual microscopic disease that has penetrated the pseudocapsule of the tumor. A wide surgical margin is by definition intracompartmental and passes through normal tissue about the entire three-dimensional surface of the lesion. It generally results in complete removal of the lesion; however, intracompartmental skip metastases may potentially be left behind. A radical surgical margin implies resection of all anatomic compartments that are involved by the tumor.

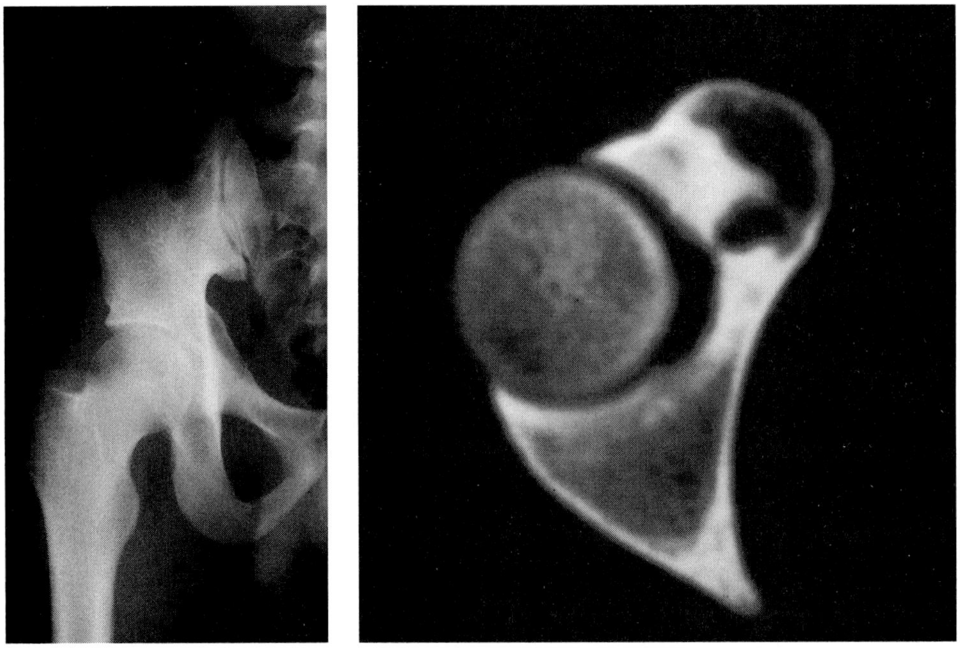

Fig. 8 An anteroposterior radiograph (**left**), and axial computerized tomogram (**right**) of an osteoblastoma of the pelvis presenting as a lytic lesion at the acetabular roof of the superior pubic ramus with minimal expansion of bone and a well-defined sclerotic margin.

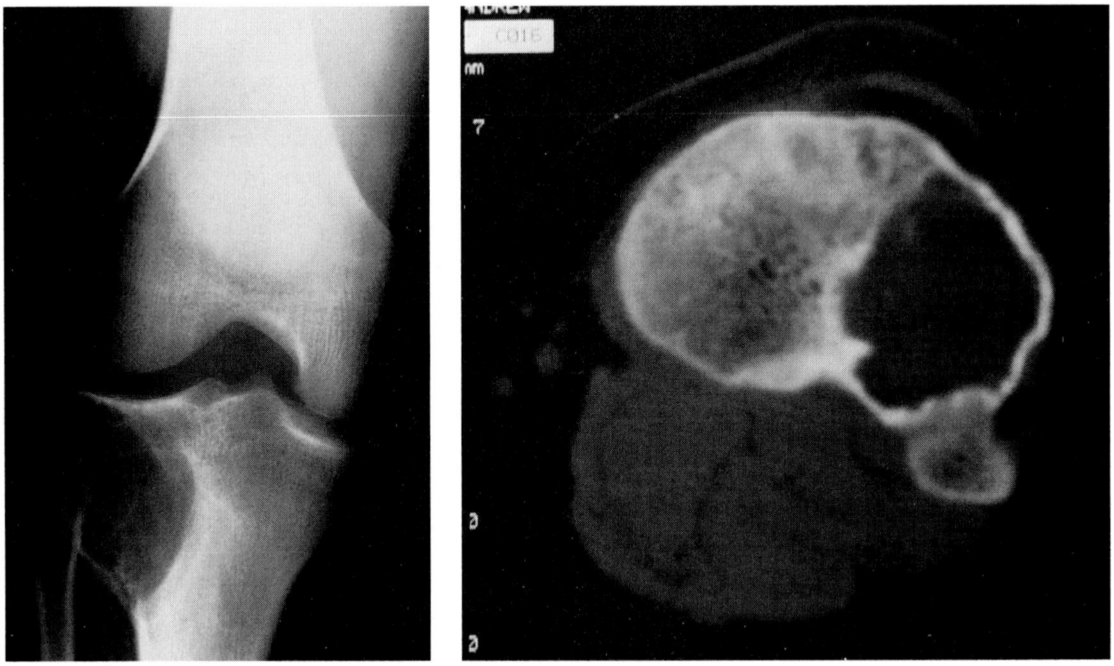

Fig. 9 An anteroposterior radiograph (**left**), and axial computerized tomogram (**right**) of an aggressive benign giant cell tumor of the proximal tibia presenting as a destructive, purely lytic process with cortical thinning and expansion.

This margin results in complete excision of the entire lesion and any possible intracompartmental skip metastases.

In reality, radical surgical margins are rarely used in musculoskeletal tumor surgery. Functional limb salvage is frequently impossible after radical excision. If full compartmental imaging is performed prior to surgical resection, skip metastases can be reliably excluded, making the

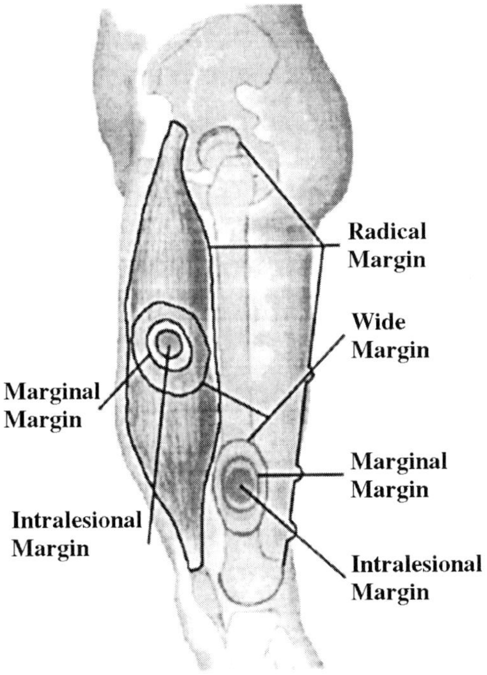

Fig. 10 Surgical margins for bone tumors. (Adapted with permission from Enneking W, Conrad EU: Common bone tumors. *Clin Symposia* 1989;41:29.)

oncologic result of a wide excision equivalent to that of a radical excision.

Chemotherapy Modern adjuvant and neoadjuvant chemotherapeutic protocols for bone and soft-tissue sarcomas use a variety of agents in various combinations. Current research is in part directed at maximizing the efficacy and dose-response curves of these drugs.

Most conventional chemotherapeutic agents belong to one of four general categories: alkylating agents, antitumor antibiotics, plant alkaloids, and antimetabolites (Outline 1). Alkylating agents produce their effect by forming positively charged carbonium ions, which then form covalent bonds at electron-rich sites on nucleic acids and proteins. This alkylation produces cross-linking of DNA and results in single-and double-strand DNA breaks. Most alkylating agents function independently of the cell cycle. Although these various agents share a common mechanism of action, they differ in their pharmacokinetic and biochemical properties. Tumor cross-resistance within this category is unusual, and these agents are not uniformly effective against the same malignancies. The antitumor antibiotics listed in Outline 1 are produced by species of *Streptomyces.* They exert their biologic effects by intercalating between base pairs of DNA, forming a complex that results in both single- and double-strand breaks. The precise mechanism of fragmentation may involve inhibition of topoisomerase II, an enzyme that is capable of cutting double-strand DNA. The plant alkaloids include the vinca alkyloids, which are derived from the ornamental shrub *Vinca rosea.* They bind to tubulin, inhibiting the assembly of microtubules and disrupting the mitotic apparatus. Taxol, a new agent derived from the bark of the Yew tree, also affects tubulin. Rather than inhibiting microtubule assembly, it stabilizes the microtubules in their polymerized form, preventing disassembly and disrupting the cell cycle. Antimetabolites include subcategories of purine antagonists, pyrimidine antagonists, and folate antagonists. These drugs all act as fraudulent substrates for biochemical reactions, interfering with critical cellular functions and/or replication. They act principally during the S phase of the cell cycle and are, therefore, primarily active against replicating cells.

The chemotherapeutic agents most commonly used in bone and soft-tissue sarcomas are indicated in bold print in Outline 1. In the cell, the alkylating agent cis-diaminedichloroplatinum, or cisplatin, loses both of its chloride ions, becoming positively charged and inducing DNA cross-links in the manner described above. Nephrotoxicity, nausea and vomiting, high frequency hearing loss,

Outline 1. Chemotherapeutic agents

Alkylating agents
- Cyclophosphamide (Cytoxan)
- Nitrogen mustard (Mechlorethamine)
- Chlorambucil (Leukeran)
- Busulfan (Myleran)
- Melphlan (Alkeran)
- Nitrosoureas:
  - Carmustine (BCNU)
  - Lomustine (CCNU)
- Cis-diamminedichloroplatinum (Cisplatin)
- Ifosfamide (Ifos)

Antitumor antibiotics
- Anthracyclines
  - Doxorubicin (Adriamycin)
  - Daunorubicin (Daunomycin)
- Bleomycin
- Dactinomycin (Actinomycin D)
- Mitomycin C (Mutamycin)

Folate antagonists
- Methotrexate (MTX)
- Dacarbazine (DTIC)

Plant Alkyloids
- Vinca alkyloids
- Vincristine (Oncovin)
- Vinblastine (Velban)
- Navelbine (Vinorelbine)
- VP-16 (Etoposide)
- Taxol

Antimetabolites
- Purine antagonists
  - Thioguanine (6-TG)
  - Mercaptopurine (6-MP)
- Pyrimidine antagonists
  - Cytarabine (Ara-C)
  - Fluorouracil (5-FU)

anaphylactic hypersensitivity reactions, and hypomagnesemia are potential complications. Renal toxicity can be reduced by adequate hydration. Dose-limiting toxic reactions at high doses are peripheral sensory neuropathy and myelosuppression. The antitumor antibiotic doxorubicin historically is the most active chemotherapeutic agent in the treatment of sarcomas; it has a response rate of over 20% when used as a single agent. The anthracyclines tend to cause significant neutropenia, nausea and vomiting, alopecia, stomatitis, and radiation recall. They also produce three forms of cardiac toxicity. Acute toxicity is manifested by supraventricular arrhythmias and conduction delays. Twenty-four hours after administration, a pericarditis-myocarditis syndrome can occur, which results in congestive heart failure. Finally, a chronic dilated congestive cardiomyopathy can occur, which is dose and schedule dependent. The latter two complications necessitate discontinuation of the drug and may be fatal or require heart transplant. The incidence of congestive heart failure is significantly reduced if doxorubicin is administered by continuous infusion or on a weekly schedule.

Ifosfamide is another alkylating agent that is currently the most active single agent against sarcomas. It causes less myelosuppression than its close relative cyclophosphamide. Ifosfamide is activated by hepatic P450 enzymes, and active metabolites are excreted in the urine. Dose-limiting cystitis is prevented by the concurrent administration of mesna. Methotrexate (MTX) is an antimetabolite; specifically, it is a folate antagonist that inhibits dihydrofolate reductase. The resulting intracellular deficiency of tetrahydrofolate inhibits DNA synthesis. Cellular resistance to MTX occurs through a variety of mechanisms and is countered by the administration of very high doses followed by leucovorin (N 5-formyl-tetrahydrofolate) rescue. Toxicities of MTX include pancytopenia, nausea and vomiting, stomatitis, alopecia, and skin rashes. Nephrotoxicity occurs with very high doses and can be limited by vigorous hydration and alkalinization of the urine. Hepatitis, pulmonary fibrosis, and anaphylaxis can occur.

Chemotherapeutic Adjuvants The art of medical oncology lies in minimizing or preventing the potential complications and known side effects of these very toxic drugs, while maximizing their therapeutic effectiveness. Many medications have been developed that currently are indispensable to the oncologist in achieving this goal. Ondancitron hydrochloride is an antiemetic available both in intravenous and tablet form. It acts as a selective serotonin-receptor antagonist, and it is extremely effective in preventing the nausea and vomiting associated with emetogenic chemotherapeutic agents. Human granulocyte colony stimulating factor, also known as filgrastim, is a 175 amino acid glycoprotein produced by *Escherichia coli* using recombinant DNA technology. It acts by binding to specific hematopoietic cell-surface receptors and stimulating their proliferation, differentiation, and functional activation. It is very effective in reducing the incidence of infection, as manifested by febrile neutropenia, in patients receiving chemotherapeutic agents that tend to cause severe myelosuppression.

Metastatic Disease Treatment of skeletal metastases is individualized to each patient. In the vast majority of cases, treatment will be palliative in nature. Attention to the metabolic and hemodynamic status of the patient is especially important. A number of these patients will be hypercalcemic because of the generalized destruction of their skeleton, and many will be anemic and dehydrated.

Patients who have a pathologic fracture deserve stabilization of that fracture by whatever means seem most appropriate. The use of methylmethacrylate in addition to plates or rods may help stabilize the fracture and the extremity for the life of the patient. Most of the lesions are felt to be radiosensitive, and it is always appropriate to seek consultation from the radiation oncologist in the care of these patients.

Frequently, a patient is evaluated for a skeletal lesion or lesions before development of a fracture. The lesions are discovered because of the patient's complaints of pain, and radiographs are obtained. It is then necessary to decide whether or not prophylactic fixation of the affected portion of the skeleton is required. The decision depends on the likelihood that a fracture would occur and whether the fracture could be prevented by prophylactic stabilization. The size and the location of the lesion are important determinations in the decision-making process. Most observers feel that a skeleton probably has lost as much as 50% of its integrity by the time the lesion is apparent on radiographs. The pain associated with skeletal metastases may often be controlled by the combination of analgesics, chemotherapeutic agents, and local radiation therapy. It seems reasonable for the surgeon to proceed with prophylactic fixation of lesions in a planned and elective fashion where possible, even if the possibility of a pathologic fracture is relatively remote. Again, the appropriate and at times creative use of internal fixation devices and methylmethacrylate will usually suffice for the life of the patient.

Patients with renal cell carcinoma occasionally develop a solitary skeletal metastasis several years after their original diagnosis. In these special cases, it is reasonable to consider treating the solitary metastasis as a primary malignancy. If a successful wide local resection of the tumor can be accomplished, and if a reasonable reconstruction can be performed, the patient may be well served and may be cured.

The orthopaedic treatment of patients with multiple myeloma is similar to that just described. Supportive and compassionate care is required. The management of the patients and the treatment of the disease are best accomplished by a team of caretakers. A cure is most unlikely.

Soft-Tissue Tumors

Patients presenting with a soft-tissue mass may be evaluated with relative accuracy by the assessment of several clinical signs and symptoms that distinguish soft-tissue sarcoma from benign soft-tissue tumors. Those signs include a tumor larger than 5 cm that is deep to the superficial fascia and has a consistency firmer than that of normal muscle. Moreover, most soft-tissue sarcomas in adults are not tender; children may have some tenderness associated with sarcomas. Adults presenting with a soft-tissue mass are more likely to have a tumor than a spontaneous hematoma in the absence of a distinct history of trauma and should be approached appropriately. The appropriate imaging for the vast majority of soft-tissue sarcomas includes an MRI prior to any surgical procedure in order to assess the location, size, and consistency of these lesions.

Diagnostic Subtypes

Benign Soft-Tissue Tumors Benign soft-tissue tumors are more common than sarcomas. In adults, the most common benign soft-tissue tumor is the lipoma, which may be quite large and very difficult to distinguish from a low-grade liposarcoma. Lesions arising out of fibroconnective tissue are also commonly encountered. They exhibit a wide spectrum of biologic activity, from benign reactive processes through aggressive fibromatosis to high-grade malignancies, such as malignant fibrous histiocytoma and fibrosarcoma. Extra-abdominal desmoids or fibromatoses have the highest local recurrence rate of any benign soft-tissue tumor and should be managed with appropriate care. Soft-tissue hemangiomas and ganglions are other benign lesions that typically occur in the lower extremity. Hemangiomas may be diffuse, involving all the soft tissues and bone, and they are occasionally associated with chronic bleeding and infections. In their diffuse form, they often coexist with lymphangiomatosis, resulting in localized gigantism of the extremity, and present significant management problems for young adults. Soft-tissue lesions originating from joint tissue include pigmented villonodular synovitis (PVNS) and synovial chondromatosis. Both of these lesions are associated with chronic local recurrences and are rarely effectively resected with a single surgical procedure. Both PVNS and synovial chondromatosis have been reported to degenerate into higher grade lesions. Although this degeneration is extremely rare with PVNS, long-standing, persistent synovial chondromatosis will give rise to synovial chondrosarcoma in a small number of cases.

Pediatric Benign Soft-Tissue Tumors Hemangiomas, lymphangioma, and fibromatosis are the most common soft-tissue tumors in children. Fibromatosis, or extra-abdominal desmoid, may occur at birth and is usually referred to as congenital fibromatosis. However, it may present with striking cellular pleomorphism and be labeled congenital-infantile fibrosarcoma. Despite their histologic appearance, these lesions only rarely metastasize. Desmoids may be treated with chemotherapy, with variable results; however, the mainstays of treatment are surgical resection and radiation therapy. Children may also develop lipomas, although less commonly than adults, and are treated symptomatically with surgical resection. Other benign soft-tissue lesions peculiar to children include cystic hygroma and pseudorheumatoid nodules (nodular granuloma annulare).

Soft-Tissue Sarcomas Soft-tissue sarcomas are malignant tumors of mesodermal tissues, which may occur in adults or children. They have an incidence of approximately 5,000 or 6,000 lesions per year in the United States. They occur in the extremity in 60% of cases; the trunk, pelvis, or abdomen/retroperitoneum in 30% of cases; and the head and neck in 10% of cases. The overall prognosis for these lesions depends on the age of the patient, the size and grade of the lesion, and to a lesser extent, the specific cell type at diagnosis. Recent results from the intergroup rhabdomyosarcoma study in children show a 5-year survival rate of 65%, while the overall prognosis for high-grade soft-tissue sarcoma in an adult is approximately 50%. Chemotherapy may improve long-term survival in adults and appears to definitely improve survival in children with high-grade soft-tissue sarcomas. Local recurrence is a less significant challenge in both pediatric and adult patients, with local control achievable in approximately 90% to 95% of extremity cases and in 60% to 70% of pelvic cases. Survival for various chemotherapy protocols ranges in adult soft-tissue sarcomas from 40% to 90%, and historic studies are described in Table 7.

Grading and Subtypes

The treatment of soft-tissue sarcomas is based on their stage and histologic subtype. The stage of a particular lesion is determined by histologic grade, size, and the presence or absence of regional (lymph nodes) or distant metastasis. Determination of the precise histologic subtype and grade of a soft-tissue sarcoma often depends on advanced studies, such as electron microscopy, histochemistry, flow cytometry, cytogenetics, and tissue culture. The most common subtypes of adult soft-tissue sarcoma include MFH, liposarcoma, and leiomyosarcoma. Sarcomas of tenosynovial origin include synovial sarcoma, epithelioid sarcoma, and clear cell sarcoma. Other less common histologic subtypes include the peripheral nerve sheath sarcomas and round cell sarcomas, such as primitive neuroectodermal tumors and extraskeletal Ewing's sarcoma (Outline 2).

Management of Soft-Tissue Sarcomas

The appropriate management of soft-tissue sarcomas in adults begins with a detailed history and complete physical examination. The vast majority of patients have a 3- to 6-month history of a nontender, firm, deep mass that is greater than 5 cm in size. With few exceptions, most soft-tissue sarcomas are amenable to needle biopsy under local anesthesia. Percutaneous needle biopsy is facilitated by a staging MRI scan that will demonstrate the location of the lesion, its size and extent, and its relationship to adjacent

Table 7. Randomized adjuvant studies in soft-tissue sarcomas

Regimen*	Median Follow-up (Months)	Number of patients	% Disease-free Survival (Observation)	% Disease-free Survival (Chemotherapy)	% Survival (Observation)	% Survival (Chemotherapy)
CVAD	44	468	61	61	68	74
CVAD	40	59	37	65	43	93
CVAAd	> 120	47	83	76	—	—
ACM	—	85	—	—	—	—
	60	67	28	54	60	54
	36	22	47	77	61	82
	24	15	49	92	100	47
AVCAd	64	61	68	65	70	70
A	60	156	45	60	47	60
A	22	139	44	40	55	52
A	28	119	52	56	70	80
A	47	86	54	71	55	65
A	28	77	44	73	70	91
A	73	46	62	66	72	71
A	105	36	55	68	53	65

C = cyclophosphamide; V = vincristine; A = doxorubicin; D = DTIC; M = methotrexate; and Ad = actinomycin D

Outline 2. Soft-tissue sarcomas with common histologies

- Leiomyosarcoma
- Malignant fibrous histiocytoma
- Liposarcoma
- Fibrosarcoma
- Synovial sarcoma
- Rhabdomyosarcoma
- Carcinosarcoma
- Malignant giant cell tumor
- Malignant schwannoma
- Endometrial stromal sarcoma
- Mixed mesodermal sarcoma
- Angiosarcoma
- Other

neurovascular structures. An adequately performed needle biopsy should retrieve several cores of tissue, and a frozen section should confirm the adequacy of the specimen. If the needle biopsy fails to yield diagnostic tissue, it can be repeated, or the patient can be taken to the operating room for an incisional biopsy, which is best performed by a specialist in the treatment of sarcomas. Following biopsy, the diagnosis, grade, and histologic subtype of the lesion should be determined.

In some sarcoma referral centers, adults with high-grade soft-tissue sarcoma are enrolled in clinical trials of neoadjuvant (preoperative) chemotherapeutic agents. This type of treatment remains controversial, however, and preoperative radiation therapy continues to be the protocol of choice in many institutions. Preoperative chemotherapy is considered useful because it provides systemic treatment early in the patient's course and it may shrink the inflammatory zone of a high-grade sarcoma, thus facilitating a wide resection. Moreover, when the lesion is resected, some chemotherapeutic effect can be measured on the histologic assessment of tumor necrosis.

Soft-tissue sarcomas should be resected with a wide surgical margin. Assessing that margin remains an extremely challenging task for even the most experienced surgeons and pathologists. Careful assessment of the specimen is required to determine the final pathologic margin, and postoperative radiation therapy is indicated for all marginal resections of high-grade or intermediate-grade lesions. Radiation therapy is thought to have efficacy in the treatment of soft-tissue sarcomas when microscopic disease remains likely following resection. The efficacy of radiation in the patient with gross residual disease remains controversial.

Patients should be well-advised regarding the complications of treatment, even with successful treatment for soft-tissue sarcomas. These complications include local recurrence and metastatic disease; wound complications with local wound infections, especially in difficult sites, such as the foot, popliteal fossa, and pelvis; neurovascular injury associated with treatment; pathologic fracture of the adjacent bone following radiation therapy; and the need for amputation regardless of the appropriateness of treatment or control of the disease.

Annotated Bibliography

Evaluation

Barth RJ Jr, Merino MJ, Solomon D, et al: A prospective study of the value of core needle biospy and fine needle aspiration in the diagnosis of soft tissue masses. *Surgery* 1992;112:536–543.

A prospective comparison of fine needle aspirated (FNA) and core needle biopsy in 38 patients with soft-tissue masses demonstrated that the core needle biopsy technique was superior. Diagnoses based on FNA were limited by a high proportion of inadequate samples and the inability to accurately grade many sarcomas.

Nelson TE, Enneking WF: Staging of bone and soft-tissue sarcomas revisited, in Stauffer RN (ed): *Advances in Operative Orthopedics.* St. Louis, MO, Mosby Year-Book, 1994, vol 2, pp 379–391.

This is an update of the Enneking staging system for musculoskeletal sarcomas. The MRI is incorporated into the staging system. Differences between the MSTS staging system and the American Joint Committee on Cancer Staging (AJC) system for soft-tissue sarcomas are emphasized.

Rougraff BT, Kneisl JS, Simon MA: Skeletal metastases of unknown origin: A prospective study of a diagnostic strategy. *J Bone Joint Surg* 1993;75A:1276–1281.

The authors designed a prospective study to test the conclusions of an earlier study. They developed a simple diagnostic strategy for the identification of the site of an occult malignant tumor before biopsy in patients with skeletal metastases of unknown origin.

Saddegh MK, Lindholm J, Lundberg A, et al: Staging of soft-tissue sarcomas: Prognostic analysis of clinical and pathological features. *J Bone Joint Surg* 1992;74B:495–500.

The authors retrospectively analyzed the clinical course of 137 patients with nonmetastatic soft-tissue sarcoma, with respect to several surgical staging systems. Their multivariate analysis identified tumor size and high histologic grade as significant risk factors for metastatic disease and tumor-related death. Sex, age, tumor site, surgical margin, and local recurrence had no correlation with survival.

Benign Bone Tumors

Ahn JI, Park JS: Pathological fractures secondary to unicameral bone cysts. *Int Orthop* 1994;18:20–22.

The authors reviewed a large series of unicameral bone cysts that were complicated by pathologic fracture. In every case of pathologic fracture, the cyst occupied greater than 85% of the metaphysis in both anteroposterior and lateral planes. Cysts recurred in most cases after pathologic fracture and occasionally became larger.

Marcove RC, Sheth DS, Brien EW, et al: Conservative surgery for giant cell tumors of the sacrum: The role of cryosurgery as a supplement to curettage and partial excision. *Cancer* 1994;74:1253–1260.

The authors reviewed the management of seven patients with giant cell tumor of the sacrum treated with curettage and cryosurgery or with limited resection, curettage, and cryosurgery. They limited sacral resection to S3 and below, sparing critical sacral nerve roots and the structural integrity of the sacrum. All patients are free of disease at 12 years follow-up.

Schmale GA, Conrad EU III, Raskind WH: The natural history of hereditary multiple exostoses. *J Bone Joint Surg* 1994;76A:986–992.

The authors established a database of hereditary multiple exostoses for the state of Washington in order to determine the prevalence, range of clinical expression, and rate of malignant degeneration in this disease. They found a prevalence of at least one in 50,000, a wide range of clinical expression, and a secondary chondrosarcoma rate of 0.9%.

Yu CL, D'Astous J, Finnegan M: Simple bone cysts: The effects of methylprednisolone on synovial cells in culture. *Clin Orthop* 1991;262–34–41.

The authors tested methylprednisolone acetate against synovial cells in culture and suggest that it may have a different effect on the cellular component of unicameral bone cysts, based on changes in cell structure, especially with a steroid concentration of 40 mg/ml.

Enchondroma/Chondrosarcoma

Bauer HC, Brosjo O, Kreicbergs A, et al: Low risk of recurrence of enchondroma and low-grade chondrosarcoma in extremities: 80 patients followed for 2-25 years. *Acta Orthop Scand* 1995;66:283–288.

The authors reviewed the outcome of 80 patients treated with intralesional surgery for either an enchondroma or a low-grade chondrosarcoma and found a 10-year local recurrence rate of less than 10%. There were no metastases or amputations.

Ishida T, Kikuchi F, Machinami R: Histological grading and morphometric analysis of cartilaginous tumours. *Virchows Arch* 1991;418:149–155.

The authors performed a morphometric analysis on 25 chondrosarcomas, nine enchondromas, and two chondroblastic osteosarcomas, examining cellularity, nuclear area, binuclear cells, and mitotic activity. They suggested that nuclear area and binuclear cells are useful for differentiation between benign and malignant cartilaginous lesions.

Malignant Bone Tumors

Bacci G, Picci P, Ferrari S, et al: Prognostic significance of serum alkaline phosphatase measurements in patients with osteosarcoma treated with adjuvant or neoadjuvant chemotherapy. *Cancer* 1993;71:1224–1230.

The authors examined serum alkaline phosphatase levels in 656 patients with osteosarcoma. They found some prognostic significance to elevated levels, especially in terms of the relapse rate after treatment in those patients with elevated pretreatment levels.

Davis AM, Bell RS, Goodwin PJ: Prognostic factors in osteosarcoma: A critical review. *J Clin Oncol* 1994;12: 423–431.

This is a critical review of all potential prognostic variables in osteosarcoma. Tumor size and necrosis are significant after univariate analysis. After multivariate analysis, only tumor necrosis remained significant.

Mameghan H, Fisher RJ, O'Gorman Hughes D, et al: Ewing's sarcoma: Long-term follow-up in 49 patients treated from 1967 to 1989. *Int J Radiat Oncol Biol Phys* 1993;25:431–438.

In a retrospective review of 49 patients with Ewing's sarcoma at an average potential follow-up of 12.3 years, almost all patients had radiation therapy as adjuvant or primary treatment. The local control rate was 75%, and disease-free survival was 44% at 5 years. Severe or fatal complications occurred in seven patients, and increased dramatically at 10-, 15-, and 20-year follow-up.

Nicholson HS, Mulvihill JJ, Byrne J: Late effects of therapy in adult survivors of osteosarcoma and Ewing's sarcoma. *Med Pediatr Oncol* 1992;20:6–12.

The authors interviewed 82 osteosarcoma and 29 Ewing's sarcoma patients who had been diagnosed before the age of 20 years and had survived at least 5 years. They found a 7.2% incidence of death from a second malignancy ($p = .002$). Although survivors had some physical limitations, they had no significant deficits in marriage, fertility, or employment status when compared to 151 sibling controls.

Toni A, Neff JR, Sudanese A, et al: The role of surgical therapy in patients with nonmetastatic Ewing's sarcoma of the limbs. *Clin Orthop* 1993;286:225–240.

Approximately half of 131 patients with Ewing's sarcoma of the extremity had radiation therapy alone for local disease control, and the remainder had either amputation (13) or resection (56). Of these patients, 31 (55%) also had adjuvant radiation therapy after surgery. Local recurrences were 5% in patients treated with surgery alone, 1% in patients treated with surgery and radiation therapy, and 24% in patients treated with radiation therapy alone.

Treatment

Black DJ, Livingston RB: Antineoplastic drugs in 1990: A review (Part I). *Drugs* 1990;39:489–501.

Black DJ, Livingston RB: Antineoplastic drugs in 1990: A review (Part II). *Drugs* 1990;39:652–673.

This is an excellent review of the large number of antineoplastic drugs available today. Drugs are categorized according to mechanism of action. Dosage, administration, and toxicities are carefully covered.

Enneking WF, Dunham W, Gebhardt MC, et al: A system for the functional evaluation of reconstructive procedures after surgical treatment of tumors of the musculoskeletal system. *Clin Orthop* 1993;286:241–246.

This article summarizes the revised functional evaluation form for limb salvage surgery developed by the Musculoskeletal Tumor Society and the International Symposium on Limb Salvage. This form is the standard system used by musculoskeletal oncologists and is designed to permit valid comparative studies of a variety of limb reconstructions.

Postma A, Kingma A, DeRuiter JH, et al: Quality of life in bone tumor patients comparing limb salvage and amputation of the lower extremity. *J Surg Oncol* 1992; 51:47–51.

Fourteen patients with limb salvage and 19 patients with amputation following lower extremity bone cancer were studied an average of 10 years after surgery. There were no significant differences in somatic distress, activities of daily living, self esteem, and adjustment to illness.

Soft-Tissue Tumors

Azzarelli A, Quagliuolo V, Casali P, et al: Preoperative doxorubicin plus ifosfamide in primary soft-tissue sarcomas of the extremities. *Cancer Chemother Pharmacol* 1993;31(suppl 2):S210–S212.

Fifty-one patients with high grade soft-tissue sarcomas of the extremities were treated preoperatively with doxorubicin and ifosfamide/mesna. Eighty-seven percent had limb-sparing surgery, and in four cases a response to chemotherapy resulted in avoidance of amputation. Four-year actuarial survival was 91% and 4-year metastasis-free interval was 69%.

Bujko K, Suit HD, Springfield DS, et al: Wound healing after preoperative radiation for sarcoma of soft tissues. *Surg Gynecol Obstet* 1993;176:124–134.

Wound healing morbidity was retrospectively evaluated in 202 patients who had received preoperative radiation therapy for soft-tissue tumors of the extremities, torso, and head and neck. The overall wound complication rate was 37%. Lower extremity tumors, advancing age, and postoperative boost with interstitial implants were statistically significant predisposing factors for wound morbidity.

Coffin CM, Dehner LP: Soft tissue tumors in first year of life: A report of 190 cases. *Pediatr Pathol* 1990;10:509-526.

Benign tumors accounted for 75% of cases; hemangio-endothelioma, lymphangioma, and fibromatosis-myofibromatosis constituted the majority of cases in this category. Embryonal rhabdomyosarcoma and peripheral primitive neuroectodermal tumor were the two principal types (17 of 27) of malignant soft-tissue tumors. The authors discuss the tendency for benign tumors in this age group to appear more histologically aggressive than similar lesions in older patients.

Springfield D: Liposarcoma. *Clin Orthop* 1993;289:50–57.

This is an excellent review of the pathologic features and clinical behavior of liposarcoma.

17
Infection

Introduction

At a time when orthopaedic diagnostic studies and treatment modalities are becoming more sophisticated, old pathogens have reemerged. The microorganisms that produce orthopaedic infections have become more difficult to kill and the cost and effectiveness of treatment regimens have come under increased scrutiny. Therefore, the prevention of microbial infection, the elucidation of the development of resistance to antibiotics, the application of molecular biology techniques to diagnosis and treatment, and the honing of surgical skills are becoming increasingly important. Guidelines to optimize financially responsible care are needed.

Antibiotic Resistance

Methicillin resistant *Staphylococcus aureus* (MRSA), methicillin resistant *S epidermidis* (MRSE), and vancomycin resistant *enterococci* (VREC) have become the microbiologic problem that antibiotic treatment of pseudomonas was in the 1980s. The development of antibiotic resistance and the ability of bacteria to produce a protective glycocalyx present ongoing clinical challenges.

Antibiotic resistance arises by one of two mechanisms: genetic exchange and mutation. Genetic exchange can occur via exchange of either entire bacterial chromosomes or of plasmids. Plasmids are small, independently reproducing strands of DNA. Many plasmids encode a protein, which is responsible for the bacteria's ability to pass the plasmid to other bacteria. The genes that are transferred enable the bacteria to survive in the presence of antibiotics by encoding proteins that (1) degrade antibiotics, (2) modify receptor sites, (3) decrease the bacteria's permeability to the antibiotic, or (4) produce metabolic pumps, which remove the antibiotic from the interior of the cell.

The incidence of antibiotic resistance is increasing; therefore, it is important to select the proper antibiotics. Once the bacterium has been identified, only the most specific chemotherapy should be used. Narrow-spectrum antibiotics decrease the risks that an antibiotic-resistant bacteria will develop or be selected. There are, however, circumstances in which multidrug or wide-spectrum therapy is acceptable.

Enterococci, which are increasingly resistant to antibiotics (even high dose aminoglycosides and vancomycin), are now the third leading cause of nosocomial bacteremia, after *S aureus* and coagulase-negative staphylococci. The most important route of transmission of multiresistant strains is by contact with the hospital environment. The vancomycin resistance of *Enterococcus faecium* is mediated by gene vanA, located on a plasmid. Multiresistant enterococci are becoming more of a threat in that no currently available regimen is reliably bactericidal against such organisms.

Virulence of the Bacteria

Virulence factors are important in the pathogenesis of any infection. These mechanisms circumvent the host's normal resistance. *S aureus* produces leukocidin, a neutrophil toxin. *Pseudomonas aeruginosa* produces an exoprotease that cleaves and inactivates immunoglobulins. A collagen receptor on *S aureus* has been isolated from patients with septic arthritis. This receptor mediates the adhesion of *S aureus* to cartilage that is particularly rich in type II collagen. Other organisms associated with some forms of arthritis, such as yersinieae, *Streptococcus pyogenes,* and other streptococci, have also been found to have a collagen receptor.

In 1987, the first of several outbreaks of rheumatic fever caused by a group A beta-hemolytic streptococci (GABHS) was recorded. In the preceding 40 years, rheumatic fever had all but disappeared. In the last 10 years, however, there has been a resurgence in the incidence of infection with GABHS, especially the M1 and M3 strains. From 1980 to 1988, the M1 strain increased from 18% of all GABHS strains in patients with sepsis to 50%. This strain has always been common, but it has only recently become associated with invasive disease. The recent change in virulence may be due to the production of several virulence factors including streptococcal pyrogenic exotoxins A, B, and C; streptolysin O and S; and streptokinase.

Strains, which are responsible for a streptococcal toxic shock like syndrome and which have not been isolated since the preantibiotic era, have recently appeared and have been shown to produce streptococcal pyrogenic exotoxin A. The streptococcal toxic shock-like syndrome, which was recognized in 1983, has a mortality rate of approximately 30%. The syndrome manifests itself with hypotension, fever, rash, desquamation, and multi-organ failure. The site of infection is usually the skin or soft tissue. The invasive nature of this infection, combined with the extensive tissue necrosis that occurs, prevents this disease from being managed with antibiotic therapy alone. In severe infections, rapid diagnosis and surgical debridement are necessary to decrease mortality. Antibiotics are used in conjunction with debridement. Penicillin is normally effective against streptococci, but it may have limited effect in some virulent GABHS infections. Cephalosporin, vancomycin, or clindamycin may be the agents of choice in some aggressive streptococcal infections.

Direct examination of tissue and biomaterials from infections related to prostheses, internal fixation devices, and percutaneous sutures has shown bacteria enveloped by extracellular material. This exopolysaccharide glycocalyx protects the bacteria from host-defense factors and accounts, in part, for their persistence and resistance to treatment. Many factors affect the adherence of bacteria to prostheses. These factors include the surface charge and surface free energy of the bacteria and biomaterial, the extracellular components of the bacteria, bacterial interaction in mixed infections, and alterations in host immune competence. The extracellular glycocalyx is composed of protein and carbohydrate. Slime-producing strains of *Staphylococcus epidermidis* produce more clinically significant infections than nonslime producers. The interactions between adherent organisms and nonadherent organisms are important because such interactions promote the development of infection. Analysis of joint fluids, of swabs of excised tissue, and of prosthetic surfaces frequently yields only one species of organism from a polymicrobial population. In these instances, suppression of clinical infection can be accomplished, but a long-term cure requires surgical removal of the hardware and glycocalyx.

Antimicrobial Treatment of Osteomyelitis

The mainstay of *medical* treatment of osteomyelitis remains parenteral antibiotics. It is crucial to obtain adequate blood, bone, and tissue samples for culture and sensitivity testing prior to antibiotic administration. If this protocol is followed, antibiotic therapy can be tailored to the specific organism or organisms responsible.

The duration of antibiotic therapy is empiric and, in part, depends on the clinical response of the patient. The standard length of parenteral treatment has been 4 to 6 weeks. There is little evidence, however, that this time period is superior to any other. The ability to continue parenteral antibiotics at home after hospital discharge has led to a significant decrease in the total cost for therapy. Some patients may be transferred to an oral antibiotic after 1 to 2 weeks of parenteral antibiotics without a decrease in efficacy. There is evidence that successful treatment correlates better with blood levels of the drug than with the route of administration. The need for prolonged treatment makes it important for the orthopaedic surgeon to have knowledge about specific antibiotic interactions (Table 1) and toxicities (Table 2).

Antibiotic Polymethylmethacrylate (PMMA) Beads

Gentamicin-impregnated polymethylmethacrylate beads release antibiotics locally, thereby producing high levels of drug in the area of infection (up to 200 times higher than achieved with systemic antibiotics) without increased risk of renal toxicity or ototoxicity. Animal studies have shown that the treatment of chronic osteomyelitis with antibiotic-impregnated beads alone is equivalent to treatment with systemic antibiotics alone. Clinical studies have also confirmed the effectiveness of the beads. The standard protocol for their use includes thorough debridement, perioperative systemic antibiotics, and intraoperative local bead implantation. By postoperative day 5, systemic antibiotics can be discontinued. In particularly severe, extensive infections, physicians frequently choose to keep patients on systemic antibiotics longer, and this seems to be more effective than either local or systemic antibiotic treatment alone. The beads are usually removed from 2 to 7 weeks after implantation.

If the focus of bone infection is local, without significant involvement of the surrounding soft tissue, some physicians believe that systemic antibiotics are unnecessary and that local beads alone are sufficient. If local soft-tissue inflammation or systemic symptoms are present, parenteral antibiotics are indicated. The length of this treatment must be governed by the clinical response. Unresponsive, persistent infection requires further debridement, long-term systemic antibiotics, and consideration of re-implantation of additional beads.

The use of a local antibiotic does not replace the need for thorough surgical debridement. Other factors that affect the success rate of antibiotic-impregnated polymethylmethacrylate beads include bone stability and soft-tissue coverage. If the wound cannot be closed primarily, it is important to use a water-impermeable synthetic wound film to prevent antibiotic loss from the wound site. Suction drains are not used because they decrease the local antibiotic concentration.

Beads can be implanted temporarily or permanently. The use of permanent implantation is reserved for those patients in whom a large cavity, which cannot be obliterated by soft-tissue transfer or bone grafting, remains after debridement. However, in this setting, once the antibiotic has leeched out of the methylmethacrylate, the beads may act as a foreign body for persistent partially treated infection or new hematogenous infection.

Preliminary studies have shown that the treatment of osteomyelitis with debridement, antibiotic beads, and short-duration perioperative systemic antibiotics is cost effective. In one series, total treatment costs were reduced by greater than 30% when compared to debridement and routine systemic antibiotic treatment alone. Total costs were increased only minimally over systemic antibiotic treatment alone when severe cases warranted the use of both antibiotic impregnated beads and systemic antibiotic.

Local Antibiotic Infusion

For several years, implanted pumps have been used to deliver antibiotics for local treatment of chronic osteomyelitis. These are usually continuous infusion, vapor-powered pumps capable of delivering high concentrations of the antibiotic. Amikacin sulfate, the antibiotic most frequently

Table 1. Important antibiotic interactions

Antibiotic	Interacting Agent	Interaction
Aminoglycosides	diuretics	enhanced nephro- and ototoxicity
	neuromuscular blocking agents	enhanced respiratory suppression
Amphotericin B	cyclosporine	enhanced nephrotoxicity
	digoxin	digoxin toxicity/hypokalemia
	diuretics	hypokalemia
	leukocyte transfusions	pulmonary infiltrates
	skeletal muscle relaxants	prolonged muscle relaxation
Beta-lactam antibiotics	alcohol-containing products	disulfiram-like reaction
moxalactam	anticoagulants	hypoprothrombinemia, bleeding
ampicillin	oral contraceptives	possible decreased contraceptive effect
Ciprofloxacin	antacids	decreased drug absorption
	iron and zinc salts	decreased drug absorption
	sucralfate	decreased drug absorption
	theophylline	increased theophylline levels
Clindamycin	neuromuscular blocking agents	enhanced neuromuscular blocking effects
Trimethoprim	methotrexate	megaloblastic pancytopenia
Sulfamethoxazole	oral anticoagulants	increased prothrombin time
	oral hypoglycemic agents	enhanced hypoglycemia
	phenytoin	increased phenytoin levels
Erythromycin	carbamazepine	increased carbamazepine levels
	cyclosporine	increased cyclosporine levels
	digoxin	increased digoxin levels
	oral anticoagulants	increased prothrombin time
	theophylline	increased theophylline levels
Fluconazole	cyclosporine	increased cyclosporine levels
	oral anticoagulants	increased prothrombin time
	oral hypoglycemic agents	enhanced hypoglycemia
	phenytoin	increased phenytoin levels
Metronidazole	alcohol	disulfiram-like reaction
	oral anticoagulants	increased prothrombin time
Rifampin	glucocorticoids	decreased glucocorticoid effect
	ketoconazole	decreased antifungal effect
	oral anticoagulants	decreased anticoagulation
	oral contraceptive agents	increased estrogen metabolism
	oral hypoglycemic agents	decreased hypoglycemic effect
	theophylline	decreased theophylline levels

used with these pumps, has one of the broadest spectrums of the aminoglycosides. It is unaffected by the aminoglycoside degradation enzyme. Levels as high as eight to ten times the minimum inhibitory concentration can be infused locally without the toxic systemic effects frequently observed with aminoglycosides. These pumps have recently been used to treat infected arthroplasties. Local debridement was followed by pump implantation. Several days of postoperative systemic antibiotics are administered along with the local antibiotic delivery. In two studies of 32 patients, 27 had their infection resolved without joint revision. This is a promising result; however, it must be realized that the patients were carefully selected and included only those who had no evidence of prosthetic loosening.

Quinolones

The most significant new antiboitics used in the treatment of skeletal infections are the quinolones. The quinolones are a group of antibiotics related to nalidixic acid. Their usefulness was greatly increased by the development of the fluorinated quinolones, such as ciprofloxacin, ofloxacin, norfloxacin, amifloxacin, and lomefloxacin. These bactericidal drugs interfere with DNA synthesis by specifically inhibiting the A subunit of a bacterial type II topoisomerase, thereby leading to uncontrolled messenger RNA and protein synthesis and cell death. Tissue bioavailability is excellent for these drugs, even with oral administration. The drugs are only minimally bound to plasma proteins, which leads to a higher degree of tissue penetration. In addition, they can penetrate the leukocyte and contribute to intracellular bacterial killing. The fluoroquinolones are active against a wide range of pathogens including gram-negative and gram-positive aerobic and facultative anaerobic bacteria as well as *Mycobacterial, Mycoplasma, Chlamydia,* and *Legionella* species.

One of the concerns with the fluoroquinolones is their toxic effects on cartilage. The administration of fluoroquinolones to developing rats, beagles, and marmosets leads to irreversible erosion of articular cartilage, particularly in major diarthrodial joints. In vitro studies demon-

Table 2. Adverse reactions to antibiotics

Reaction	Frequent	Occasional	Rare
Dermatologic			
rash	ampicillin	cephalosporins	metronidazole
	co-trimoxazole	clindamycin	erythromycin
	penicillins		
	vancomycin		
Gastrointestinal			
abdominal pain/cramping	erythromycin	metronidazole	
diarrhea	clindamycin	all antibiotics	
	ampicillin		
nausea/vomiting	erythromycin (IV and PO)	imipenem (with rapid infusion)	
	co-trimoxazole		
pseudomembranous colitis	clindamycin	beta-lactams	
	ampicillin		
Hematologic			
anemia	amphotericin B	penicillins (hemolytic)	
	(normochromic, normocytic)	co-trimoxazole	
		(megaloblastic)	
hypoprothrombinemia	moxalactam	cefoperazone	
		cefamandole	
		cefotetan	
		cefamandole	
neutropenia		co-trimoxazole	
		vancomycin	
		penicillins	
		cephalosporins	
platelet dysfunction	moxalactam		
	carbenicillin		
	ticarcillin		
Hepatobiliary			
biliary sludging			erythromycin
cholestatic hepatitis			co-trimoxazole
transaminase enzyme elevations		nafcillin	
		ticarcillin	
		aztreonam	
		imipenem	
		co-trimoxazole	
		ceftriaxone	
Neurologic			
neuropathy		metrinidazole	
ototoxicity		aminoglycosides	cancomycin
			erythromycin
		impenem	pencillins
seizures		ciprotloxacin	pencillins
Phlebitis	erythromycin	cephalosporins	
	vancomycin	metronidazole	clindamycin
	amphotericin B		
	nafcillin		
Renal			
acute tubular necrosis		aminoglycosides	beta-lactams
		amphotericin B	
dose-dependent renal insufficiency	aminoglycosides		
	amphotericin B		
hypokalemia	amphotericin B	carbenicillin	aminoglycosides
		ticarcillin	
interstitial nephritis		methicillin	rifampin

strate that these antibiotics reduce synthesis of DNA, collagen, and glycosaminoglycans. However, these articular changes have never been documented in humans.

The clinical data justify cautious use of the fluoroquinolones for the treatment of a specific group of difficult infections. Included in this group is osteomyelitis, particularly the subacute form and cases with atypical sites of infection. However, these drugs are not approved for use in the pediatric population and their use must be limited to control studies in this patient group.

Pediatric Infection

Orthopaedic infections in the pediatric population fall into the same major categories as do adult infections: osteomyelitis and septic arthritis. However, pathogenesis, location, causative organisms, and presenting signs and symptoms of these pediatric diseases make their management unique. Processes such as congenital syphilis are unique to the pediatric population.

Acute Hematogenous Osteomyelitis

Hematogenous osteomyelitis occurs more frequently in children than in adults because of the vascular anatomy of growing bones. Infection begins in the metaphyseal venous sinusoid where there is a change to a low flow state along with increased turbulence and decreased phagocytosis. This anatomy, the more frequent bacteremia, and repeated trauma in the pediatric population are responsible for the higher rate of acute hematogenous osteomyelitis in this age group.

Microbiology *S aureus* remains the most common causative agent, accounting for 80% of all osteomyelitis. Unfortunately, many strains are found to be resistant to penicillin and methicillin. In children younger than 3 years of age, *Haemophilus influenzae* type B (HIB) may be responsible for septic joints and, rarely, osteomyelitis. With the advent of vaccination against *H influenzae,* this organism has disappeared for the most part as a musculoskeletal pathogen. *Pseudomonas aeruginosa* is more commonly found in the peripubertal (9 to 12 years old) age group. These infections are often related to a penetrating foot injury. The patients may have a normal white blood cell (WBC) count and an elevated erythrocyte sedimentation rate (ESR).

Clinical Presentation The clinical scenario remains crucial to the early diagnosis of acute hematogenous osteomyelitis. A history of prior infection, unexplained bone pain, fever, and local inflammation all suggest the diagnosis. Other symptoms include irritability, anorexia, lethargy, and vomiting. It is important to obtain material for culture prior to the administration of antibiotics.

Diagnosis Several laboratory values are helpful in the diagnosis and management of acute hematogenous osteomyelitis. The WBC count is frequently elevated. An elevated ESR is found in most patients, but it takes 3 to 5 days for the ESR to rise to its peak level. Another limitation of the ESR is that it does not fall with the improvement of the clinical condition. Measurement of C-reactive protein (CRP), appears to be a better test for monitoring the course of the infection. The CRP levels are almost always elevated (>19 mg/l) at the time of admission, with the peak level being reached by day 2. The CRP level drops rapidly with treatment, returning to normal within a week. CRP is also useful in the diagnosis of concomitant septic arthritis. In patients with both osteomyelitis and septic arthritis, CRP increases to higher levels and takes longer to return to normal.

Blood cultures and bone aspiration should be done in all cases. Aspiration is the single most valuable test and should be postponed only if a malignant process is suspected. Bone aspirations should not be delayed for a bone scan. Radiographs are frequently of little help in the diagnosis of acute hematogenous osteomyelitis. By the third day, soft-tissue swelling may be evident. More commonly, no changes are seen for up to 2 weeks after symptoms begin. Technetium 99m diphosphonate bone scanning is indicated in most cases of acute hematogenous osteomyelitis. Within 24 hours of infection, this test can detect changes. Unfortunately, when it is performed this early, the test has low sensitivity (missing up to 20% of infections) and low specificity (increased uptake may also indicate either trauma or tumor). Magnetic resonance imaging has been described as having 100% sensitivity with a much greater specificity. MRI may distinguish cellulitis from acute hematogenous osteomyelitis and can locate abscesses, sequestra, and sinus tracts. It may also be particularly useful to differentiate between acute and chronic osteomyelitis.

Treatment After the completion of the required cultures, empiric antibiotic therapy should begin. The choice of first line antibiotics should be based on organism prevalence. In children, it is crucial to cover *S aureus* with an antibiotic such as oxacillin. In neonates, additional coverage of HIB with gentamicin is required. In patients with sickle-cell anemia, both cefotaxime and oxacillin should be used to cover salmonella and *S aureus.* Treatment of infection caused by deep penetrating wounds should include an antibiotic that covers pseudomonas, and tetanus prophylaxis is required. When culture results are available, antibiotic therapy is tailored to the specific organisms found.

Choosing the proper antibiotic dose for the neonatal, infant, and child populations is important. Measurement of serum levels allows estimation of local antibiotic concentration. Close monitoring of peak and trough levels assures that the minimal inhibitory concentration is reached. Initially, all children are started on parenteral antibiotics. While 6 weeks of intravenous antibiotics is frequently recommended, the current trend is to switch to oral antibiotics after 2 to 3 weeks or even earlier. Several criteria can be used to help decide if oral antibiotics will be effective. The most important of these is clinical response as noted by changes in the physical examination, by defervescence, and by evaluation of laboratory values such as CRP and ESR. Other criteria for changing to an oral antibiotic include isolation of a bacterial pathogen that is sensitive to an oral antibiotic, the ability of this antibiotic to reach appropriate serum levels without excessive toxicity, the patient's ability to tolerate the medication, and the assurance of proper patient and parental compliance.

If necrotic bone and exudate have formed an abscess,

antibiotics alone will not be effective. Aspiration of exudate is an indication for surgery. Patients with clinically diagnosed osteomyelitis who remain ill in the presence of appropriate nutrition and hydration or who continue to have local tenderness and fever should undergo surgical debridement.

One useful classification system divides pediatric patients into three groups: early acute osteomyelitis, late acute osteomyelitis, and neonatal and infantile osteomyelitis. The first group includes patients over 1 year of age who have a febrile illness of less than 48 hours duration with localized tenderness, pain, and swelling, but without an abscess. This group is treated successfully with a combination of parenteral and oral antibiotics in approximately 90% of cases. Only about 2% of the early acute osteomyelitis group require surgical intervention. Late acute osteomyelitis defines a group of patients older than 1 year of age who have osteomyelitis with an abscess and radiographic evidence of bone destruction. All patients in this group should be treated with surgical debridement and with antibiotics. Antibiotics may need to be continued for 6 to 12 weeks, although oral antibiotics can be used once a clinical response is achieved.

The final group, neonatal and infantile osteomyelitis, is much more difficult to diagnose. When osteomyelitis is suspected in a patient less than 1 year of age, parenteral antibiotics for 7 to 14 days followed by oral antibiotics resolve greater than 80% of infections. This classification system does not include the group of neonates with bony abscesses. These children are treated similarly to the late acute group.

Once a decision to proceed with surgery has been made, the procedure should include an incision at the point of maximum tenderness, removal of necrotic soft tissue, and exposure and incision of the periosteum. Drill holes in the cortex are made to decrease intramedullary pressure and increase metaphyseal blood flow. However, this decrease in pressure has never been demonstrated, and the usefulness of drill holes is disputed. Alternatively, a window can be removed from the cortex to allow for curettage and irrigation. Care must be taken to avoid damage to the physis.

Septic Arthritis

In the first 6 months of life, *S aureus* is responsible for 80% of septic arthritis. Joint infections in neonates are rare (0.4% of live births). The disease in neonates is frequently hospital acquired and is found in patients with multiple potential sources of infection. When the joint is warm or erythematous, the diagnosis of bacterial arthritis may be easy. However, these signs are not always present. At times, pseudoparalysis secondary to pain may be the only positive physical finding. The prognosis in neonates is poor, and aggressive treatment is required.

In children under 2 years of age, *Haemophilus influenzae* is an important pathogen historically. Onset is usually sudden, with irritability and a decrease in the child's ability to ambulate or bear weight on the affected limb. In more than 50% of these patients, the joint infection is preceded by an upper respiratory infection. Since 1989, vaccination against *H influenzae* has become nearly universal and is protective against this infection.

The length of antimicrobial treatment must be tailored to the patient. *S aureus* and gram-negative bacilli infections require longer treatment than other infections, regardless of clinical response. Some suggest a minimum treatment length of 4 weeks when *S aureus* or gram-negative bacilli are involved, and 14 days if the infection is caused by *H influenzae, Neisseria meningitidis,* or streptococci.

Surgical intervention should first include early drainage for relief of symptoms and organism identification. There has been some suggestion that repeated aspirations lead to a better result than open surgical drainage, although the studies are controversial. Indications for surgery in the pediatric population include infection of the hip joint, loculation of debris within the joint, or continued local or systemic symptoms following 72 hours of treatment. Some physicians advocate surgery in all shoulder infections as well.

The factors that best predict outcome are patient age, causative organism, and rapidity of treatment. Worse prognoses are seen in patients less than 1 year of age, those with infections caused by *S aureus* or enteric gram-negative organisms, and those in whom symptoms were present for 5 or more days before the initiation of treatment.

Osteomyelitis in the Adult

The diagnosis of osteomyelitis is based on the physician's clinical judgment and synthesis of data available from clinical examination, laboratory studies, imaging (Fig. 1), and biopsy.

Indium-labeled leukocyte scintigraphy and MRI have made it possible to diagnose subclinical osteomyelitis and its extent within the medullary canal. Indium-labeled leukocyte scintigraphy is more accurate than plain technetium or sequential technetium-gallium imaging in suspected low-grade infection of a long bone. Sequential technetium-gallium imaging is still preferred if the focus involves the vertebral column, because the hematopoietic nature of the vertebral marrow makes interpretation of indium-labeled leukocyte scintigraphy images difficult.

MRI is superior to indium-labeled leukocyte scintigraphy in defining the extent of infection. An MR image is considered to be consistent with active osteomyelitis when an area of abnormal marrow with low signal intensity on T1-weighted sequences corresponds to an increased signal intensity on the T2-weighted image. Abnormal marrow caused by posttraumatic and postsurgical fibrosis and scarring is defined by a low marrow signal on T1-weighted images with no evident increase in signal on T2-weighted images. Cellulitis is defined by the diffuse areas of interme-

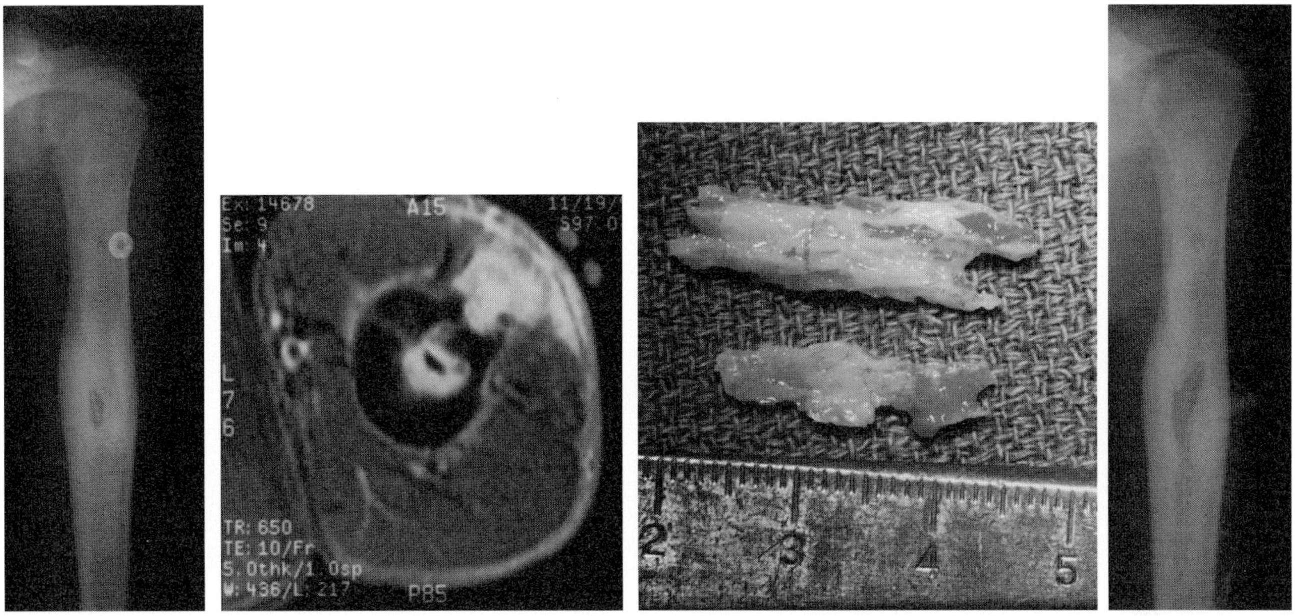

Fig. 1 **Left,** Radiograph of the left humerus of a 17-year-old male immigrant who presented with a history of chronic hematogenous osteomyelitis. Note the sequestrum visualized in the center of the bony cloaca. He denied a history of any prior surgery or antibiotic therapy. **Center left,** T2-weighted magnetic resonance image of the humerus that shows the cortex of the humerus, thickened in response to the chronic inflammation; the intramedullary sequestrum; and intramedullary and subcutaneous exudate accumulation. **Center right,** Intraoperative photograph of fragments of sequestrum. **Right,** Postoperative radiograph showing the extent of the bony debridement and placement of postoperative suction drains. The patient was treated with perioperative, organism-specific intravenous antibiotics followed by oral antibiotics, and remains infection free.

diate signal in the soft tissues on T1-weighted images with similar soft-tissue areas displaying increased signal on T2-weighted images. The extent of intramedullary and extramedullary disease seen on MRI correlates directly with that seen on serial sectioning of amputated specimens. MRI cannot differentiate between edema and bacteria-induced cellulitis; and it differentiates poorly between areas of abnormal marrow resulting from chronic inactive osteomyelitis and areas previously disrupted by trauma or surgery. MRI is unable to define the presence of a cortical osteomyelitis if there is no cortical disruption or medullary involvement.

The evaluation of different treatment regimens is hampered by the absence of a standardized classification and clinical staging system. Considerations include the bone involved, the duration of infection (acute versus chronic), the mechanism of infection (hematogenous versus exogenous), the site of infection (medullary versus cortical, periarticular versus diaphyseal, localized versus diffuse), and the local and systemic quality of the host (Outline 1).

Surgical treatment of osteomyelitis consists of the excision of all necrotic and infected tissue. Management of the resulting cavity may include antibiotic-impregnated methylmethacrylate beads, local or vascularized soft-tissue flaps, autogenous bone grafting (Fig. 2), distraction osteogenesis, or the use of vascularized bone grafts. Aggressive debridement, appropriate antibiotics, and adequate dead space management can eradicate the infection in nearly all patients. Staging of the reconstruction is important. Neither autogenous bone grafting nor vascularized cortical bone grafting is effective if the donor material is placed into an inadequately prepared, inflammatory soft-tissue bed.

A complication of persistent, chronic osteomyelitis is the development of squamous cell carcinoma, which occurs in 0.2% to 1.7% of patients. Treatment in these difficult cases may require amputation.

Outline 1. Classification system modified after Cierny and Mader

Bone involved:
Duration of infection: acute/chronic
Mechanism: hematogenous/exogenous site
Site: periarticular subchondral/metaphyseal/diaphyseal
Extent: medullary/superficial: localized/diffuse

Host characteristics:
- A: Normal host
- B: Systemic compromise (malnutrition, diabetes, renal or liver failure, malignancy, immune deficiency, extremes of age, tobacco abuse, alcohol abuse, intravenous drug abuse)
- B: Local compromise (chronic lymphedema, venous stasis, extensive scarring, diminished local sensation, major vessel compromise)
- C: Severe compromise: treatment worse than the disease

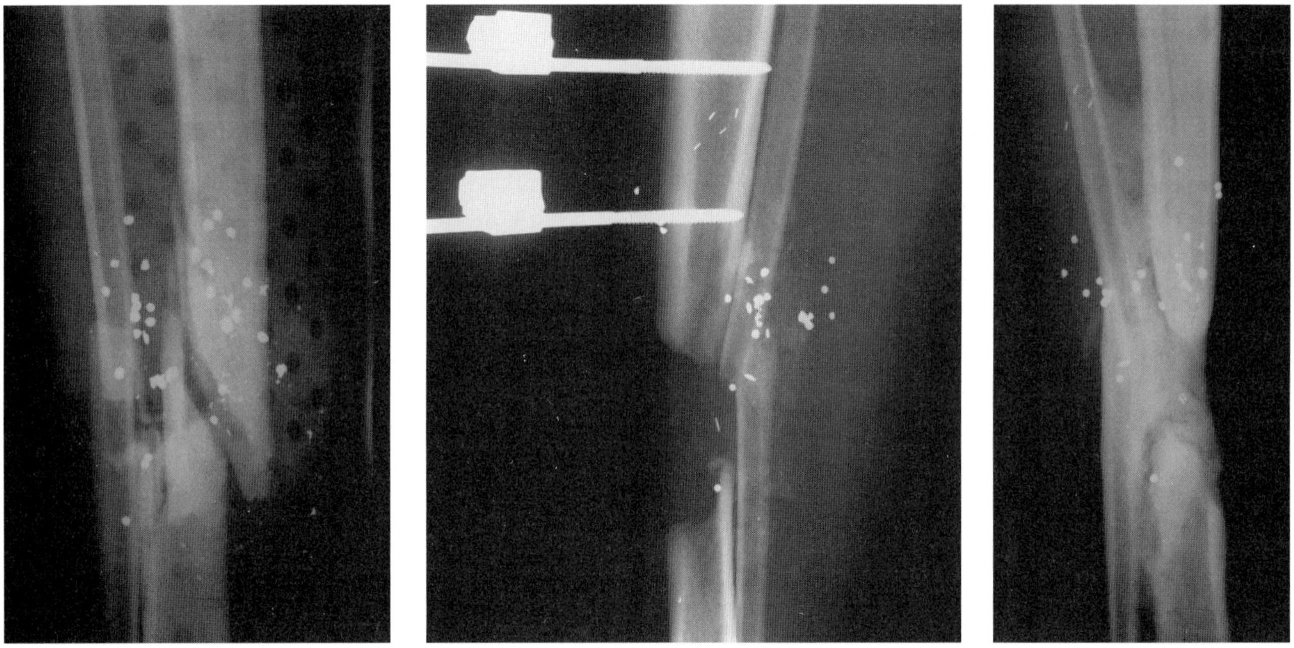

Fig. 2 Left, Emergency room radiograph of right tibia and fibula of 31-year-old male who had just sustained a close-range shotgun injury. **Center,** Lateral radiograph of right tibia after debridement of all necrotic bone and soft tissue, external fixator stabilization, microvascular soft-tissue reconstruction at 5 days, and placement of autogenous cancellous iliac crest bone graft through Harmon posterolateral approach at 7 weeks. **Right,** Anteroposterior radiograph view at 24 months, showing consolidation of fibula-pro-tibia bone graft with reconstitution of infection-free, weightbearing extremity.

Septic Arthritis in the Adult

Nongonococcal Bacterial Arthritis

Bacteria can reach a joint by several routes: bacteremia; direct inoculation; or contiguous spread from adjacent osteomyelitis, cellulitis, or septic bursitis. Once bacteria have gained access, the processes of bacterial phagocytosis, synovial proliferation, granulation tissue formation, and bone and cartilage destruction begin. This destruction is mediated by the direct toxic effects of the bacteria and by the increased intracavitary pressure. Host cell phagocytosis and the release of proteolytic enzymes contribute to the tissue destruction. Lysosomal enzyme release within 24 hours of infection in animal models has been demonstrated. Glycosaminoglycan depletion occurs by day 5. Sterile inflammatory synovial fluids have been shown to contain proteinase capable of destroying articular cartilage.

Most patients with nongonococcal bacterial arthritis present with arthritis in only one joint, monoarticular septic arthritis (MASA). The knee is most affected. Although systemic symptoms of fever and chills are common, the local sign of infection is incapacitating joint pain.

Polyarticular septic arthritis (PASA) is also seen. Approximately one fourth of all septic arthritis patients may have more than one joint involved. In PASA, three to four joints are usually infected, and 40% of patients have extra-articular septic foci, such as pulmonary infections, endocarditis, and subcutaneous abscesses. The greatest risk factor for the development of PASA is the presence of a concurrent rheumatologic disease. Over 50% of patients with PASA have some form of rheumatologic disorder, which is usually in its more severe form at the time that the infection develops. The most common disease is rheumatoid arthritis. Although rheumatoid arthritis affects more women than men, more men than women develop PASA. Those patients with rheumatoid arthritis have a higher incidence of fatality. The overall mortality in patients with PASA ranges from 32% to 42%. One contributing factor to the poor outcome in rheumatoid arthritis patients is the delay in diagnosis that often accompanies these infections because of the difficulty in distinguishing a rheumatoid flare from an acute infection.

An important risk factor for the development of an infection of a joint is the presence of a prosthesis. Approximately 1% to 2% of all hip and knee arthroplasties are complicated by infection. Human immunodeficiency virus (HIV) infection also increases the risk of joint infection, although studies have shown no significant difference in the causative organisms, clinical presentation, treatment, or outcome in this group. However, with the onset of clinical AIDS, the variety of infectious agents increases, while the chance of a successful outcome decreases. Other diseases that predispose to infectious arthritis include rheumatoid arthritis, diabetes mellitus, hemophilia, and sickle-cell anemia. In sickle-cell anemia, salmonella causes more than 50% of the infections. Intravenous drug users are at risk for gram-negative joint infection with involvement of the sternoclavicular, sacroiliac, and manubriosternal joints, or the symphysis pubis.

The diagnosis of bacterial arthritis is based on the physical examination and on the analysis of synovial fluid. Although the WBC count in the synovial fluid can vary, counts above 100,000 cells/ml in the immune competent host strongly suggest the presence of infection.

The coexistence of an acute bout of crystal-induced arthritis and septic arthritis can be missed by the failure to examine synovial fluid for bacteria or crystals if one or the other is found. Crystal-induced arthritis and septic arthritis may occur simultaneously. The decreased joint pH associated with infection decreases the solubility of urate. All patients with an acute arthritis should be screened for both infectious and crystal-induced causes.

Parenteral antibiotics should be initiated as soon as material for culture has been obtained. The goals of treatment include sterilization of the joint; decompression and removal of all inflammatory cells, enzymes, debris, or foreign bodies; elimination of the destructive pannus; and return to full function.

The best methods for drainage, decompression, and cleansing of the joint are debated. Repeated joint aspiration is painful. The physician must weigh the benefit of aspiration versus arthroscopy or arthrotomy. Surgical drainage is indicated for all joints that do not respond to antibiotic therapy and aspiration within 72 hours, for those in which the synovial fluid appears to be loculated, and for infections involving the hip. Arthroscopy of the knee, when technically feasible, seems to be the best treatment to accompany antibiotic therapy.

Gonococcal Bacterial Arthritis

Neisseria gonorrhoeae is the most common cause of septic arthritis among young adults. The disease is four times more common in women than in men. Recent menstruation and the immediate postpartum period increase the risk of gonococcal dissemination. The disease most commonly presents with acute onset of migratory polyarthralgia, low-grade fever, and chills. Tenosynovitis and skin involvement are seen in two thirds of patients. Fewer than 50% of patients develop a true arthritis. The disease is frequently divided into the bacteremic form, characterized by dermatitis, tenosynovitis, fever, and chills, and the less frequent suppurative form in which arthritis is the primary manifestation. In these latter patients, there can be large purulent effusions. In all types of disseminated gonococcal infection, blood cultures are frequently negative and only 50% of joint effusions are culture positive. Frequently, the patient will present without symptoms at the primary site of infection, whereas other patients will complain of vaginal or urethral discharge, urethritis or dysuria.

Synovial fluid aspiration usually yields a WBC count between 30,000 and 100,000, primarily polymorphonuclear neutrophils. Gram stains are frequently negative, although the sensitivity of this test can be increased by concentration of the synovial fluid prior to staining. Gram stains and culture of skin lesions are rarely positive. Blood cultures are positive in only 30% of patients. The best yield for positive cultures is the genitourinary tract. Cultures of the cervix or urethra are positive in 80% to 90% of women and 50% to 75% of men, respectively.

Initial therapy should include hospitalization, especially in patients with purulent effusions. Because most infections are caused by penicillin-resistant strains of *N gonorrhoeae,* a beta-lactamase-resistant cephalosporin, such as ceftriaxone, is usually the first line of therapy. After local signs of infection have subsided, oral antibiotics, such as amoxicillin with clavulanic acid, may be substituted. The total duration of antibiotic therapy should be at least 7 days. Large, purulent synovial effusions may require longer-term antibiotics with repeated aspiration. Open drainage is rarely necessary except with hip involvement. Of crucial importance in the prevention of recurrence is patient education and the treatment of sexual partners.

Lyme Disease

Lyme disease, the most common vector-borne illness in the United States, is carried by the tick *Ixodes dammini* in the eastern and central United States and by *I pacificus* in the Pacific northwest. These ticks carry the causative gram-negative agent, *Borrelia burgdorferi* between humans and their animal reservoirs: deer and rodents. In the United States, the disease is seen in the northeastern, middle Atlantic, north central, and Pacific coastal regions. The disease is divided into the clinical stages of early localized infection (stage 1), early disseminated infection (stage 2), and persistent infection (stage 3). In stage 1, erythema migrans, the characteristic skin lesion, occurs within 3 to 32 days after the tick bite. Stage 2 is the first to have musculoskeletal involvement. Migratory pain without swelling of both articular and periarticular structures is the usual presentation at this stage.

Arthritis is the dominant feature of late Lyme disease. This typically becomes symptomatic 6 months after infection, with intermittent inflammatory mono- or oligoarthritis of large joints, most frequently the knee. Initial attacks present with large effusions but are usually brief in duration. Episodes occurring in the second or third year usually last months. Of untreated patients, 19% progress to chronic Lyme arthritis (one episode of continual joint involvement lasting at least 1 year). Local factors may affect the clinical presentation of the disease. Patients with high concentrations of interleukin-1 receptor antagonist and low levels of interleukin-1 beta had rapid resolution of arthritis attacks in comparison with those with the opposite cytokine profile.

Diagnosis of Lyme disease is complicated by the absence of a readily available, highly sensitive test. Enzyme linked immunosorbent assay (ELISA) is 90% sensitive and specific in late disease. However, in the early stages as few as 26% of patients have an immunoglobulin G (IgG) response. There is also very little standardization between, or even within, laboratories, and false positives and negatives occur. Immunoblotting may be as high as 95% specific, but again there is little standardization. Other possible modalities for diagnostic testing under development include polymerase chain reaction (PCR) and recombinant protein ELISA.

Treatment of Lyme disease is based on the stage of the infection. In early disease, oral treatment with amoxicillin for 10 to 30 days, depending on disease severity and clinical response, is adequate. Lyme arthritis initially should be treated with a course of doxycycline or amoxicillin for 30 days, with parenteral ceftriaxone reserved for nonresponders. In persistent arthritis, other therapies include intra-articular steroid injections or synovectomy.

Reactive Arthritis

Reactive arthritis (ReA), although not a true infection, is believed to have an infectious component. It is defined as an arthritis preceded by an immunologic sensitization. The pathogenesis of the disease is not clearly defined, but it is believed that spondyloarthropathies result from an inherited susceptibility, the HLA-B27 haplotype, combined with an infectious agent that serves as the inciting factor. It was previously thought that the infectious trigger only started the disease process. More recently, detection of DNA from various inciting agents at all stages of the disease indicates some continued role for the trigger. The Yersinia urease B subunit is an antigen that has been identified as one protein responsible for the disease process. It is believed that an interaction between the responsible infectious agents and the HLA-B27 haplotype leads to the progression of the disease via stimulation of CD8+ cytotoxic T cells.

ReA is divided into urogenic, enterogenic, respiratory tract-associated, and idiopathic arthritis. *Clostridia, Salmonella, Shigella, Staphylococcal, Streptococcal, Neisseria* and *Mycobacteria* species all cause ReA. The group of idiopathic causes is decreasing as other causes are discovered. Some of these newly discovered triggers include hepatitis B vaccine, *Chlamydia pneumoniae,* and *Vibrio parahaemolyticus.* It is often difficult to separate ReA from bacterial arthritis, given their similar presentations and causative agents. In patients in whom an organism cannot be identified despite a preceding infection, the diagnosis of ReA should be considered.

The treatment of ReA has long relied on nonsteroidal anti-inflammatory agents (NSAIDs). Intra-articular steroids have also proven useful, as have systemic steroids in severe cases. Recent studies, however, have investigated the use of antibiotics in the treatment of reactive arthritis. Some studies have demonstrated that long-term (3 months) tetracycline therapy shortens the duration of arthritis in patients with *Chlamydia trachomatis*-induced ReA. However, there is some question as to whether the efficacy of tetracycline is due to its anticollagenolytic properties rather than its antimicrobial properties. An investigation of the effectiveness of the quinolones in the treatment of enterogenic ReA showed some improvement in certain categories, but was unable to conclusively demonstrate the antibiotic's efficacy. Sulfasalazine has proven to reduce the occurrence of peripheral joint symptoms in spondyloarthropathy patients, and it may be of some use in ReA.

Human Immune Deficiency Arthropathy

Infection with HIV can lead to a variety of musculoskeletal manifestations. The most common of these is a sterile polyarthritis that is believed to involve a mechanism similar to ReA. HIV itself is believed to be the causative agent in most of these patients, rather than the disease being a result of bacterial infection secondary to decreased immune response. The HIV type of ReA is frequently refractory to treatment. Although NSAIDs are usually administered, they seem to be less effective than in other cases of ReA. Sulfasalazine appears to be beneficial in some patients. Immunosuppressive drugs, such as methotrexate and azathioprine (AZT), should be avoided given the increased incidence of opportunistic infections and Kaposi's sarcoma. Also common in HIV patients is psoriatic arthritis. The disease is almost identical to classic psoriatic arthritis, except that the skin lesions may be found in unusual locations and may be particularly aggressive. Treatment involves the use of NSAIDs, and some patients respond to AZT and etidronate. Other noninfectious bone and joint diseases seen in patients with HIV include non-Hodgkins lymphoma and Kaposi's sarcoma.

These aseptic articular manifestations are much more common than true musculoskeletal infections. Even with HIV's increased incidence of bacterial and fungal infections, the number of infections with bone and joint involvement are few. One study found 0.3% of HIV patients with an infection of the musculoskeletal system; the most common infections were septic arthritis and osteomyelitis. Other infections include bursitis, bacterial myositis, and polymyositis. These infections are caused by both common bacteria such as *S aureus* and by opportunistic infections such as *Cryptococcus neoformans, Nocardia asteroides, Mycobacterium kansasii,* and *Histoplasma capsulatum.*

The diagnosis of musculoskeletal infections in patients with HIV is especially challenging for several reasons. These bone and joint manifestations are rare and, as such, are frequently not considered. This omission is especially true in the patients that are beginning to have multiple systemic problems. Also complicating the diagnosis is the fact that many patients are receiving antibiotics at the time of first presentation with a bone or joint symptom. This fact makes organism isolation and identification an even more difficult problem. The clinical manifestations are also altered by the HIV infection. A low WBC count, for example, cannot be used to rule out an infection in this population. One study contained two patients in whom multiple organisms could be visualized in the synovial fluid, but the fluid itself was clear, with less than 10,000 WBC. Finally, the incidence of a concomitant infection in the HIV-positive patient is high, so systemic symptoms are frequently attributed to the other source.

Although these factors make diagnosis difficult, early diagnosis and aggressive treatment can lead to cure rates approaching 80%. Treatment for these individuals is similar to that for other patients, except that the antibiotic choices will differ, as will the length of antibiotic administration. Prior to identification of the organism and its sensitivities, several antibiotics are given to cover a variety of bacteria that may include the causative agent. It is also important to realize that identification of an organism in the blood does not mean the causative agent of the joint infection has been identified. In several cases, bone and joint infections caused by an opportunistic infection of one type have coincided with bacteremia of a different species. Long-term parenteral antibiotics are required to treat these infections, and data to support a switch to oral antibiotics do not currently exist.

Annotated Bibliography

Microbiology

Delmi M, Vauduax P, Lew DP, et al: Role of fibronectin in *Staphylococcal* adhesion to metallic surfaces used as models of orthopaedic devices. *J Orthop Res* 1994;12:432–438.

Coverslips made of titanium, steel alloy, or titanium-aluminum-niobium (Ti-Al-Nb) alloy were coated with fibronectin and exposed to bacteria. Fibronectin concentration was directly proportional to the amount of bacteria that adhered. The *Staphylococcal* species bound specifically to fibronectin when compared to albumin-coated controls. Of the three metals, the Ti-Al-Nb alloy allowed the greatest adhesion.

Antibiotics

Calhoun JH, Henry SL, Anger DM, et al: The treatment of infected nonunions with gentamicin-polymethylmethacrylate antibiotic beads. *Clin Orthop* 1993;295:23–27.

Fifty-two patients with infected nonunions were treated with debridement and long-term parenteral antibiotics or with gentamicin-polymethylmethacrylate (PMMA) beads. The infection cure rates were 83.3% and 89.3%, with union being achieved in 83.3% and 85.7%, respectively. Although there was no evidence to support gentamicin-PMMA bead superiority to parenteral antibiotics, it was found to be as effective and less expensive.

Henry SL, Osterman PA, Seligson D: The antibiotic bead pouch technique: The management of severe compound fractures. *Clin Orthop* 1993;295:54–62.

The current standard treatment for posttraumatic osteomyelitis consists of irrigation, debridement, skeletal stabilization, soft-tissue coverage, and parenteral antibiotics for up to 6 weeks. An alternative to long-term antibiotics is the use of local antibiotics delivered via a polymethylmethacrylate (PMMA) bead. The bead pouch is formed after external fixation and thorough debridement with removal of all necrotic tissue. Chains of antibiotic beads are placed in the wound and then covered with two layers of a porous wound film. This method reduces infection rates and is particularly effective in the treatment of grade IIIB fractures.

Laurencin CT, Gerhart T, Witschger P, et al: Bioerodible polyanhydrides for antibiotic drug delivery: In vivo osteomyelitis treatment in a rat model system. *J Orthop Res* 1993;11:256–262.

Staphylococcus aureus osteomyelitis was induced in 40 rat tibiae. One group received polymethylmethacrylate (PMMA) with gentamicin, another received the polyanhydride without antibiotics, and one received polyanhydride with gentamicin. Three weeks following cement placement, the fewest colony-forming units remained in this latter group. Polyanhydride with gentamicin was statistically superior to the gentamicin-PMMA cement, and has the additional benefit of being biodegradable, so that no subsequent operation is needed to remove it.

Pediatric Infections

Cushing AH: Diskitis in children. *Clin Infect Dis* 1993;17:1–6.

Fifteen patients with diskitis are presented along with a review of the disease as it is presently understood. The 15 patients fell into two groups, one group of 10 patients younger than 4 years old, and another five who were post-adolescents. In both groups, the course of the infection was similar. The review discusses the suspected pathogenesis of the disease, along with the presentation, laboratory and radiologic findings, and the treatment of the infection.

Dagan R: Management of acute hematogenous osteomyelitis and septic arthritis in the pediatric patient. *Pediatr Infect Dis J* 1993;12:88–92.

This paper reviews the basic guidelines for the treatment of acute hematogenous osteomyelitis and septic arthritis in children. It discusses the importance of *Staphylococcus aureus* and *Haemophilus influenzae* type b in the pathogenesis of acute hematogenous osteomyelitis in the child and infant respectively. Suggested treatment regimens are also presented. Specific information is given on the management of antimicrobial therapy, such as the need for monitoring serum drug levels and the role of outpatient antibiotics. Finally, a discussion of the surgical method of treatment of acute hematogenous osteomyelitis and septic arthritis is included.

Frederiksen B, Chritiansen P, Knudsen FU: Acute osteomyelitis and septic arthritis in the neonate, risk factors and outcome. *Eur J Pediatr* 1993;152:577–580.

Twenty-two neonatal cases of acute osteomyelitis and septic arthritis were studied to discover risk factors and prognoses for these infections. Risk factors included prematurity, respiratory distress syndrome, umbilical artery catheterization, and possibly heel punctures. Diagnosis is difficult given the typical patient's vague symptoms, rare fevers, and normal white blood cell count and erythrocyte sedimentation rate. Common symptoms included pseudoparalysis and soft-tissue swelling. The use of plain radiographs was considered more valuable than scintigraphy in the diagnosis of acute osteomyelitis and septic arthritis in the neonatal population.

Unkila-Kallio L, Kallio MJ, Eskola J, et al: Serum C-reactive protein, erythrocyte sedimentation rate, and white blood cell count in acute hematogenous osteomyelitis of children. *Pediatrics* 1994;93:59–62.

Forty-four children with acute hematogenous osteomyelitis had serial erythrocyte sedimentation rate, white blood cell count, and C-reactive protein levels measured. Erythrocyte sedimentation rate was elevated in 92% of patients to an average of 45 by days 3 to 5, and the levels returned to normal in an average of 18 days. C-reactive protein, however, was elevated in 98% of patients, and it reached its peak levels by day 2. The levels fell from the mean peak of 83 mg/l within an average of 6.9 days. White blood cell count was elevated in only 35% of patients, and therefore was a poor predictor of acute hematogenous osteomyelitis. Additional advantages of C-reactive protein include the laboratory test's simplicity, the need for a finger stick blood sample only, and the elevation of levels within 48 hours from the onset of symptoms.

Imaging

Schauwecker DS: The scintigraphic diagnosis of osteomyelitis. *Am J Roentgenol* 1992;158:9–18.

The three-phase bone scan with technetium 99m-diphosphonate is the suggested procedure for the diagnosis of osteomyelitis. Galium 67-citrate can be useful in some cases, but it is not recommended for the diagnosis of osteomyelitis if indium 111-labeled leukocytes are available. This test is particularly useful when hypermetabolic bone disease is present concurrently. Indium 111-labeled leukocytes have good sensitivity for the diagnosis of infection in diabetic foot disease, while it is a poorer test for the diagnosis of chronic osteomyelitis. A set of guidelines are enumerated for the best use of these imaging studies.

Tehranzadeh J, Wang F, Mesgarzadeh M: Magnetic resonance imaging of osteomyelitis. *Crit Rev Diagn Imaging* 1992;33:495–534.

This is a review of the imaging of osteomyelitis with radiography, scintigraphy, and magnetic resonance imaging. It specifically includes a discussion of the magnetic resonance diagnosis of acute, subacute, chronic, chronic recurrent multifocal, and vertebral osteomyelitis; abscesses; septic arthritis; tuberculosis; and brucellar and coccidoidal spondylitis. In addition, the evaluation of the diabetic foot and the benefit of magnetic resonance enhancement are discussed.

HIV

Malin JK, Patel NJ: Arthropathy and HIV infection: A muddle of mimicry. *Postgrad Med* 1993;93:143–146, 149–150.

The symptoms of human immunodeficiency (HIV) infection can frequently include articular manifestations. They commonly have patterns similar to those of patients with classic rheumatologic disease. HIV can induce a reactive arthritis, with the HIV particle being the suspected causative agent. This presentation of HIV-induced arthropathy is the most common rheumatologic syndrome associated with the disease.

Septic Arthritis

Kalish R: Lyme disease. *Rheum Dis Clin North Am* 1993; 19:399–426.

This thorough review of Lyme disease includes a discussion of Lyme arthritis. Of non-treated patients, 60% develop a mono- or oligoarthritis of the large joints.

Nocton JJ, Dressler F, Rutledge BJ, et al: Detection of *Borrelia burgdorferi* DNA by polymerase chain reaction in synovial fluid from patients with Lyme arthritis. *N Engl J Med* 1994;330:229–234.

Infection with *Borrelia burgdorferi* leads to arthritis in 60% of untreated patients. The ability to detect the infectious agent in the synovial fluid in nonresolving joint effusions would further enhance understanding of the disease as well as assist in decisions concerning antibiotic therapy. The synovial fluid of 88 patients with Lyme arthritis was tested for the presence of *B burgdorferi* by polymerase chain reaction (PCR). The test was 85% sensitive and 100% specific. Most patients with chronic arthritis and adequate antibiotic treatment were PCR negative. This suggests, along with the disease's association with certain markers, that genetic susceptibility may play a role in the pathogenesis of chronic lyme arthritis.

Scopelitis E, Martinez-Osuna P: Gonococcal arthritis. *Rheum Dis Clin North Am* 1993;19:363–377.

Disseminated gonococcal infection is estimated to have a prevalence between 0.5% and 3%. It is caused by *Neisseria gonorrhoeae,* which is a nonmotile, nonsporeforming, gram-negative diplococcus. This review discusses the symptoms, diagnosis, and treatment for this common cause of septic arthritis. Treatment with antibiotics, usually a cephalosporin, is frequently the only treatment necessary.

Osteomyelitis

Evans RP, Nelson CL, Harrison BH: The effect of wound environment on the incidence of acute osteomyelitis. *Clin Orthop* 1993;286:289–297.

Ninety-nine adult New Zealand rabbits with experimentally induced osteomyelitis were studied to determine which local wound factors had the greatest effect on rates of bone infection. The study examined the presence of dead bone, virulent bacteria, hematoma, and internal fixation. The combination of dead bone and virulent bacteria led to a significantly increased incidence of osteomyelitis when compared with wounds with either dead bone or virulent bacteria alone, or when compared with those wounds with hematoma and virulent bacteria. Hematoma with virulent bacteria, however, does increase the incidence of osteomyelitis.

Lerner RK, Esterhai JL Jr, Polomano RC, et al: Quality of life assessment of patients with posttraumatic fracture nonunion, chronic refractory osteomyelitis, and lower-extremity amputation. *Clin Orthop* 1993;295:28–36.

Patients with chronic orthopaedic problems require effective coping skills to deal with treatment outcomes. One hundred nine patients were evaluated using the Arthritis Impact Measurement

Scale (AIMS) and the Psychosocial Adjustment to Illness Scale (PAIS). Patients with osteomyelitis reported poorer psychological adjustment and functional outcome than those patients with fracture nonunion and amputation, while there was no difference in those groups' AIMS scores. There was an increase in both the AIMS and PAIS of all groups as the patients aged.

Levine SE, Esterhai JL Jr, Heppenstall RB, et al: Diagnoses and staging: Osteomyelitis and prosthetic joint infections. *Clin Orthop* 1993;295:77–86.

Osteomyelitis is diagnosed using clinical signs, laboratory data, and radiologic studies. The white blood cell count is rarely elevated. The erythrocyte sedimentation rate is elevated in 71% to 97% of children, as well as in patients with acute posttraumatic osteomyelitis and infected total hip arthroplasties. The earliest radiographic changes in osteomyelitis include soft-tissue swelling and periosteal thickening or elevation. In patients with infected total hip arthroplasties, old radiographs must be compared with the most recent films to assist with diagnosis. Proper classification of both osteomyelitis and infected prosthetic joints aids in selection of an appropriate treatment regimen; however, no unified system exists. Various classification systems are discussed.

Mader JT, Landon GC, Calhoun J: Antimicrobial treatment of osteomyelitis. *Clin Orthop* 1993;295:87–95.

Parenteral antibiotics continue to be critical to the proper treatment of osteomyelitis. There are many issues to consider in order to use antibiotics appropriately. This review discusses the rationale for antibiotic selection, including sensitivity testing, appropriate serum antibiotic levels, and bone antibiotic concentrations. A detailed discussion of the classes of antibiotics is also included.

Patzakis MJ, Wilkins J, Kumar J, et al: Comparison of the results of bacterial cultures from multiple sites in chronic osteomyelitis of long bones: A prospective study. *J Bone Joint Surg* 1994;76A:664–666.

Cultures from osteomyelitic bone are important in the treatment of infection, because they are used to identify the causative organism and subsequently that organism's antimicrobial sensitivities. This study of 36 patients showed that cultures from different sites, including the sinus tract, purulent fluid, soft tissue, bone, and the bone bed, yielded several different organisms. The results showed that while *Staphylococcus aureus* was the most commonly cultured organism (70%), multiple organisms were isolated in as many cases (70%). Cultures produced 10 different organisms from two patients (7%). These organisms included fungi and anaerobes, so it is important to culture specimens on the proper medium to detect these infections.

18

Arthritis

Synovial joints or diarthroses withstand extremely high mechanical stresses. They transmit the stresses caused by gravity and by muscle contractions as well as those caused by the anatomic constraints of the joint. Both stress transfer and motion occur between adjacent surfaces of hyaline cartilage, thereby making joint failure almost synonymous with cartilage failure. Joint failure due to arthritis can be caused by abnormal stresses, by insufficient cartilage, and by inflammatory or infectious disorders. At the cellular level, it involves a change in the cartilage metabolism. Progress in the area of molecular biology has contributed to understanding of the physiology and pathophysiology of cartilage and has also elicited some of the genetic factors involved in the development of arthritis.

Joint Development

Diarthrodial joints develop in the central chondrogenic core as part of the segmentation process. The interzones between two adjacent anlagens form in the shoulder joint by the thirty-sixth day of embryonic development and in the knee by the forty-fourth day. A central loose layer of randomly arranged cartilage cells appears between two more dense zones, and the process of cavitation begins in the loose central portion of the interzone. Small cavities appear and merge into a single larger cavity as a result of the release of lysosomal enzymes from chondrocytes. The formation of the interzone clefts is genetically programmed, but a true joint cavity will not form unless there is motion between the segments. The articular cartilage develops from the dense layers of the interzone. The first synovial lining cells are then formed by surrounding mesenchymal cells. A meshwork of synovial cells (not connected by gap junctions), hyaluronic acid (hyaluronan), and collagen with a vascular stroma create the synovial membrane. Synovial fluid consists of an ultrafiltrate of plasma, the composition of which depends on the size, shape, weight, and electrical charge of the molecules in the general circulation. In addition, the synovial fluid contains hyaluronic acid. The membrane consists of A cells, which are macrophages containing lysosomal enzymes, B cells, which are exocrine cells producing hyaluronic acid, and cells with mixed A and B cell characteristics, which have been called C cells. By the fifth month the joint takes its final shape. There are two zones of cartilage cell replication at the articular end of the bone. One is located within the articular cartilage. The other is deeper and contributes new cells to the proximal expansion of the secondary center of ossification. Once growth ceases, mitotic activity cannot be seen in the cartilage except when there is advanced osteoarthritis (OA).

Joint Physiology

Chondrocyte nutrition is supplied by synovial fluid that, aided by joint motion, diffuses into the cartilage. Articular chondrocytes are unable to repair gross cartilage damage in vivo, but in vitro the cells proliferate and synthesize extracellular matrix.

The anatomic characteristics of the joint create stability while allowing a defined range of motion. Because the muscles act on joints with short lever arms, high forces are necessary to accelerate and decelerate movements, especially under load-carrying conditions. This force would cause extremely high shear forces in the cartilage if the friction were not remarkably low. The coefficient of friction in a normal diarthrodial joint is lower than has been obtained in man-made machines. In addition to the low friction between the cartilage surfaces, there is also a low friction between the hyaline cartilage, the menisci, and the synovial membrane. The lubrication between the joint surfaces includes both boundary and fluid film lubrication. The former is caused by a coating of glycoprotein molecules covering the articular cartilage surface. Fluid film lubrication is caused by joint compression forces resulting in fluid being expressed from the cartilage. Because of the deformation of the cartilage surface, the fluid becomes entrapped and a small volume of fluid is sufficient for lubrication. When the water is expressed, the cartilage also becomes progressively more dense and more resistant to disruption. Hyaluronic acid assists in the lubrication, especially where there is contact with the synovial membrane.

Because synovial fluid is an ultrafiltrate of plasma with the addition of hyaluronic acid, there are no cells, large globulins, or fibrinogen in the fluid. The viscosity is proportional to the concentration of hyaluronic acid and its degree of polymerization. During inflammatory conditions, the synovial membrane becomes more permeable, and cells, fibrinogen, and other molecules penetrate. One such molecule is α-2 macroglobulin, which contributes to the removal of free enzymes from the joint.

Cartilage

The hyaline cartilage that covers the articular ends of the bones forms a low-friction surface. It also reduces peak stresses to the subchondral bone. As a rule, the cartilage is thinner in more constrained joints, such as the ankle, and thicker in more unstable conditions, such as in the patella. It also tends to be thicker on the top of a convex surface and thinner in the center of a concave surface as can be noted in the hip. The cartilage is securely attached to the bone through the zone of calcified cartilage, which on slides stained with hematoxylin and eosin is seen to end with a wavy blue line that is called the tidemark.

The Matrix

The collagen, which is mostly type II, is highly organized so that in the middle layers there are columns of cartilage that are flattened out at the surface to become parallel with the gliding zone. The collagen fibers are finer near the chondrocytes and become coarser more peripherally. At the articular surface, the collagen fibrils are thinner. Collagen constitutes more than 50% of the dry weight of the cartilage. The cartilage-specific collagens are types II, IX, X, and XI. Type XI collagen is hypothesized to be the glue that holds together the type II collagen latticework. The bulk of the fiber is made up of type II collagen with type IX concentrated to the surface of the fiber and type XI to the interior.

The proteoglycans constitute most of the remainder of the cartilage matrix. The largest and most abundant proteoglycan is aggrecan, which consists of a linear protein core to which long chain glycosaminoglycans (GAGs) are linked (see Figure 2 in Soft Tissue Physiology and Repair). The GAGs make up the well-known test-tube brush aggregates. They consist of either chondroitin-4 sulfate, chondroitin-6 sulfate, or keratan sulfate chains. Three globular domains of aggrecan's core protein have been defined (the G1, G2, and G3 domains). Numerous aggrecan molecules interact with a single filament of hyaluronic acid via their amino terminal globular regions to form an aggregate of large size and high anionic charge (the proteoglycan macromolecule). The charge helps the tissue resist compressive loading. Aggregate stability is maintained by the additional interaction of link proteins. The chondroitin sulfate chains of the aggrecan molecule provide the high fixed-charge density required for the tissue material properties. A clear function for the keratan sulfate chains has not yet been established.

Decorin and biglycan are two forms of dermatan sulfate proteoglycans present in the extracellular matrix of articular cartilage (Fig. 1). Decorin is the predominant proteoglycan of fibrous tissue. Biglycan is another common small proteoglycan of connective tissue. They are multifunctional macromolecules that bind to molecules such as fibronectin, collagen, and growth factors and, by doing so, participate in the regulation of their functions. They appear to inhibit processes involved in tissue formation and repair. Decorin binds to the fibrils at the articular surface and may influence their structure and mechanical properties. It has a core protein to which a single dermatan sulfate is attached at residue 4 from the amino acid terminus. Decorin has been shown to reduce collagen fibril diameter when fibrils form. It may account for the presence of smaller fibrils at the cartilage surface. Fibronectin is a glycoprotein that may also have a role in the organization of the collagen network, the links to proteoglycans, and the binding of chondrocytes to the connective tissue matrix via cell surface receptors. Small amounts of other glycoproteins, phospholipids, and lipids are also in the cartilage matrix.

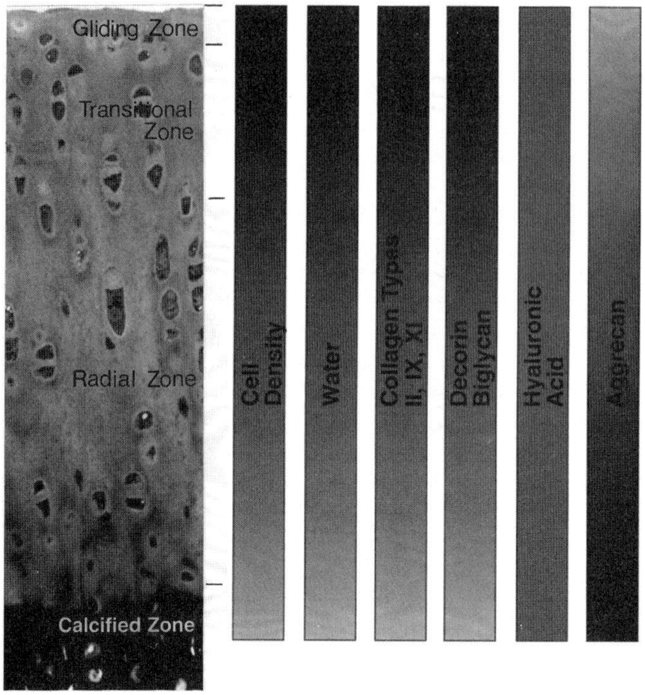

Fig. 1 Section of articular cartilage (von Kossa stain) schematically showing the distribution of some of its components. (Adapted with permission from Williams CJ, Jimenez AJ: Heredity, genes and osteoarthritis. *Dis Rheum Clin North Am* 1993;19:523–543.)

Cells

The matrix of adult articular cartilage is relatively acellular, with chondrocytes occupying about 2% of the total volume. The cellularity is the highest at the surface (Fig. 1). The chondrocytes direct the dynamic and tightly controlled process of cartilage remodeling by synthesizing and secreting extracellular matrix, degradative enzymes, and the activators and inhibitors of these enzymes. These cells have a high level of metabolism and use both anaerobic and aerobic pathways. Many effects of the extracellular matrix molecules on chondrocyte processes are exerted through binding and signal transduction via the integrin receptor family. For example, chondrocytes express fibronectin and vitronectin receptors, which contribute to chondrocyte attachment and cell binding. Via these receptors, the chondrocytes can also interact with extracellular type II collagen.

Degrading Enzymes

Matrix metalloproteinases (MMPs) (ie, collagenase, gelatinase, and stromelysin) are a family of enzymes that contain zinc at their active site and that can degrade most of the matrix macromolecules found in connective tissues. The genes for these enzymes are located on chromosome 11. The MMPs appear to be the principal agents involved in matrix destruction both during skeletal development and in arthritic joints. Cleavage of the interstitial collagens is initiated only by the collagenases (fibroblast collagenase and neutrophil collagenase). These enzymes degrade the native collagen molecule at a single peptide bond in the alpha chain. However, the structural domains responsible for this precise substrate specificity remain to be defined. The MMPs can be secreted by different connective tissue cells and infiltrating leukocytes in response to inflammatory mediators. MMP activity is inhibited specifically by tissue inhibitors of metalloproteinases (TIMPs), whose members TIMP-1 and TIMP-2 show a broad inhibitory activity toward all MMPs. In addition, TIMP-1 is known to be an antiangiogenic factor in cartilage.

Tissue Activators

The matrix hemostasis is controlled by a variety of proteins, growth factors, and cytokines. Growth factors are most commonly associated with the stimulation of matrix formation, whereas cytokines such as interleukin-1 (IL-1), tumor necrosis factor alpha (TNF-α) and tumor necrosis factor beta (TNF-ß) are most commonly associated with the stimulation of matrix degradation. The functions of TNF-α and β overlap those of IL-1 in strongly inducing collagenase and prostaglandin E_2 (PGE_2) production by synovial cells. IL-1 can cause degradation of proteoglycans; this degradation is thought to occur through upregulation of chondrocyte MMP production. It also inhibits proteoglycan synthesis. Apart from a direct effect of IL-1 on chondrocytes, it may play an indirect role by attracting inflammatory cells (eg, polymorphonuclear cells). Chondrocytes that are close to the articular surface and most exposed to synovial fluid are more responsive to IL-1 than chondrocytes located deeper within the joint. The chondrocytes of the superficial zone have also been shown to be especially rich in receptors for IL-1 and to be the most responsive to the cytokines. IL-1 also induces the production of IL-6 in human articular cartilage and inhibits proteoglycan synthesis.

IL-4 is a glycoprotein that was originally described as a B-cell stimulatory factor produced by activated T cells. However, its anti-inflammatory functions can suppress TNF-α, IL-1, and PGE_2 production in human monocytes. Thus, IL-4 appears to be an essential chondroprotective factor in the modulation of cartilage and matrix degradation.

The Role of Nitric Oxide in Cartilage Metabolism

Nitric oxide (NO) occurs in the form of a free radical that is generated by the enzyme nitric oxide synthase (Fig. 2). NO is an important physiologic regulator in cartilage and other tissues. It has an important role in inflammation, but its effects are complex because it has both inflammatory and anti-inflammatory properties. Articular chondrocytes normally produce relatively large amounts of NO and respond to stimulation by IL-1 or TNF-α. However, the role of NO in the breakdown of cartilage matrix has not been established. NO seems to mediate the suppression of proteoglycan synthesis following the administration of IL-1, but it may not be directly involved in the activation of "aggrecanase" (ie, the catabolic process).

Osteoarthritis

Osteoarthritis (OA) is recognized as the most common joint disorder in humans. Age is the strongest and most consistent determinant in epidemiologic studies. There are also distinct patterns of distribution by sex, ethnicity, and geographic location, and there is genetic susceptibility. Mechanical factors associated with wear and tear on the joint have been found to be associated with site-specific OA.

Repetitive, excessive stresses on normal joints or malformations causing compromised joint mechanics may cause OA after a long period of time. However, joint injuries, such as osteochondral or intra-articular fractures, can lead to OA within 1 or 2 years. The length of the delay is, in part, related to the level of activity. Exercise alone has not been found to lead to an increased incidence of OA, although in one study it was concluded that high intensity, high mileage running could be a risk factor for OA of the hip. Athletes in mixed sports and power sports are more often admitted to a hospital for OA than athletes in endurance sports. Below-the-knee amputees experience in-

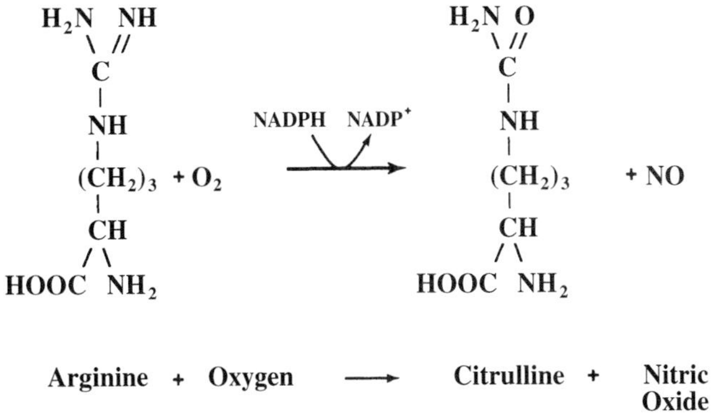

Fig. 2 Diagram showing the synthesis of nitric oxide, which is catalyzed by NO synthases.

creased forces at the knee of the nonamputated limb and are at an increased risk of developing OA. Obesity is a risk factor for OA of the knee, at least in women. The condition is progressive (for example, over one third of middle-aged women with unilateral OA of the knee will progress to bilateral OA of the knee within 2 years). There is, however, a slower progression of the disease after 75 years of age.

Numerous experimental animal models have been designed to mimic OA. Most are joint injury models, but there are also certain animal species with naturally occurring primary OA that morphologically resembles the human disease (eg, Hartley guinea pigs).

Pathophysiology

In OA, changes in the cartilage matrix are caused by several mechanisms, including the induction of metalloproteinase synthesis by IL-1 and by attempted repair. There may be a change in chondrocyte phenotype, a switch in the synthesis of collagen type, increased activity of locally secreted metalloproteinases, and induction of self-proteolytic activities. There is uniform evidence of increased formation of type II collagen fibers and increased degradation and synthesis of aggrecan and collagen. At the time when deep fissuring of cartilage occurs, aggrecan content is clearly reduced.

New bone formation is an important factor in the pathophysiology of OA. Patients with OA have a tendency to have a relatively high bone density, and patients with osteoporosis have less OA than expected. New, subchondral bone formation appears to be an early event in the development of OA. There is an enlargement of the joint from the formation of osteophytes and, in the hip, there is a lateralization of the center of rotation because of new bone formation in the center of the acetabulum. Finally, in advanced OA, there is advancement of the tidemark with new bone formation in the basal layers of the calcified zone.

Cartilage that is supported by abnormally dense bone is subjected to excessive stresses that could contribute to its degeneration. Moreover, degeneration of cartilage decreases its capacity to distribute stress, thereby causing higher peak stresses to the subchondral bone, which make the addition of new subchondral bone a secondary event. The degeneration of cartilage could also lead to the release of growth factors that contribute to new bone formation and to ingrowth of blood vessels into the cartilage. The abnormal cartilage is abraded where the stresses are the highest. Often, the subchondral bone is exposed, and it can have defects filled with fibrous tissue. These defects are often continous with subchondral cysts, which may be formed as a result of joint fluid access. Because of high intra-articular pressures, joint fluid can be forced into the cancellous bone. The cysts weaken the bone and can sometimes even collapse. At the same time, new bone forms in less loaded areas in the form of osteophytes. These may cover part of the intact articular cartilage, thereby forming a new joint surface that, in its turn, is covered with a thin layer of new, more fibrous, cartilage (Fig. 3). The end result is an enlarged, deformed, stiff, and painful joint.

Matrix Degeneration

The degradation of matrix is mediated primarily by proteinases, particularly metalloproteinases such as collagenase, stromelysin, and gelatinase. Collagenase and stromelysin can be activated by the cysteine proteinase, cathepsin-B. In OA, many of the newly synthesized molecules are degraded extracellularly shortly after synthesis. TIMP-1 is increased and TIMP-2 is markedly increased. When collagen is broken down at the articular surface in early OA, decorin and aggrecan have been reported to disappear, but their concentration can at the same time be increased in the deeper regions of the cartilage.

Growth Factors and Tissue Activators

Growth factors such as insulin, insulin-like growth factor-I (IGF-I), basic fibroblast growth factor (bFGF), and transforming growth factor-beta (TGF-ß) can influence osteoarthritic cartilage. Insulin appears to be important in promoting repair of human OA cartilage. In vitro studies have shown that TGF-ß is able to stimulate articular cartilage proteoglycan synthesis and to inhibit proteoglycan degradation, thereby inhibiting the cartilage destructive actions of IL-1. These results have been confirmed in vivo in young, but not old, mice. The addition of TGF-ß to explanted cartilage can trigger an increase in fibronectin synthesis over time. TGF-ß injected into joints of rats caused thickening of the subchondral bone, fibrosis of the synovial membrane, cartilage necrosis with chondrocyte regeneration, cloning of cells, and ingrowth of vessels from the subchondral bone into the cartilage. These changes have similarities with early OA. When bFGF is injected into a rat knee, cells at the edge of the femoral condyle and chondrocytes in the femoral groove proliferate. The IGF family possess both mitogenic and anabolic properties and are active in the degenerative processes. The IGF-I mRNA content of cartilage defects is elevated compared to that of normal cartilage. When added to chondrocytes in tissue cultures, IGF-I stimulates chondrocyte mitogenesis and matrix synthesis.

The cytokines present in the synovial fluid are believed to originate from the synovial cells. IL-1 can increase the degradation of cartilage matrix macromolecules by promoting the synthesis and secretion of MMPs by chondrocytes. The effect is not limited to protein synthesis; the production of PGE_2 is also stimulated. PGE_2 is of particular interest because of the role it may play in exacerbating joint inflammation by stimulating bone resorption and modulating the immune response. IL-1 induces the synthesis and secretion of IL-6 by human chondrocytes. IL-6 appears to act on a variety of connective tissue cells to stimulate the production of TIMPs. In this manner, IL-6 production would counteract the degradative potential of IL-1. TNF-α appears to induce many effects analogous to

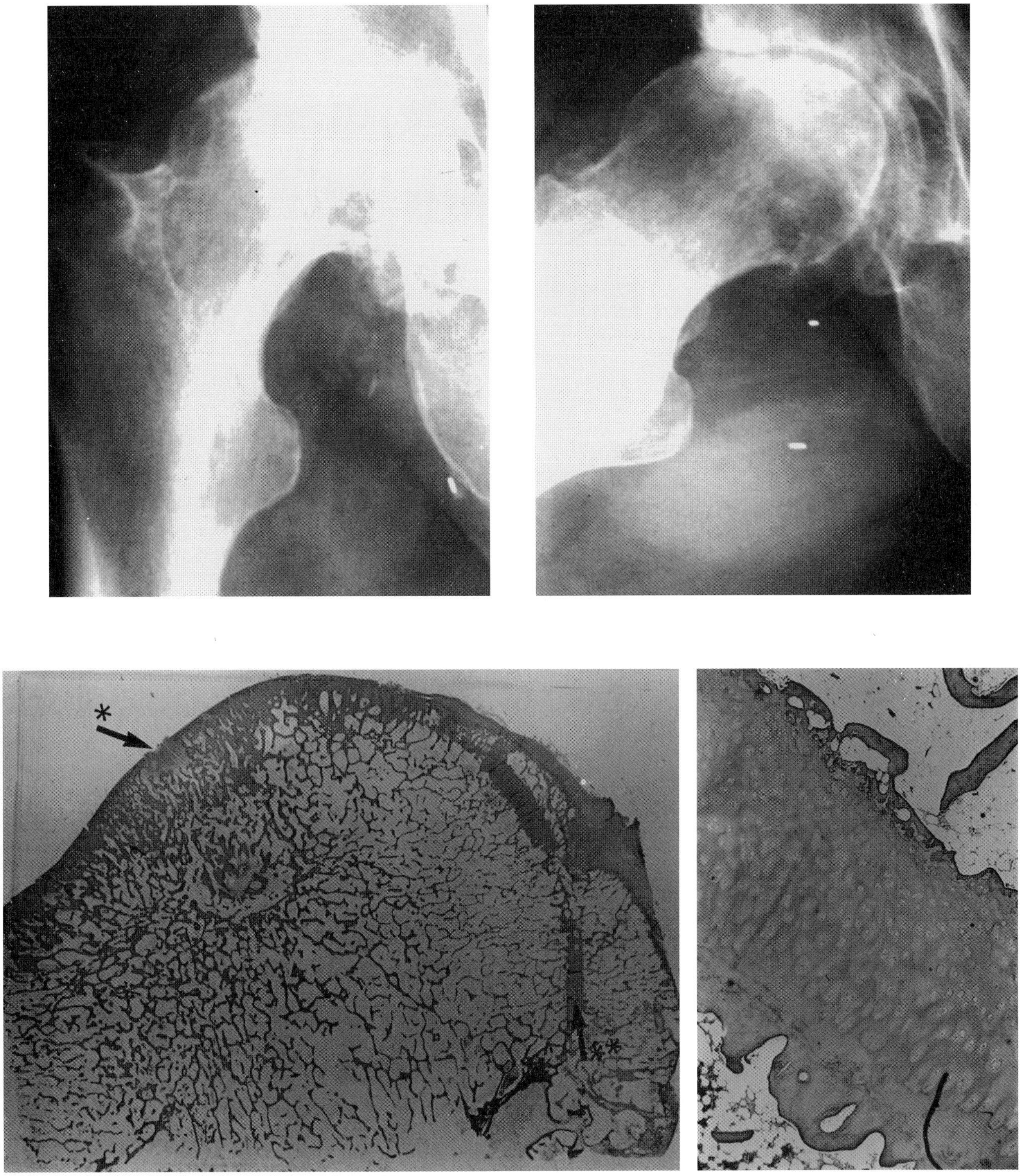

Fig. 3 **Top,** Anteroposterior **(left)** and frog **(right)** view lateral radiographs of the right hip in a patient with advanced osteoarthritis. **Bottom left,** Section of the femoral head showing a fibrous defect in the bone at the joint surface overlying the cyst (arrow with an asterisk). The medial part of the joint surface (arrow with two asterisks) is covered with the new bone of a large osteophyte. **Bottom right,** Micrograph showing the original cartilage of the medial part of the femoral head. The tidemark and bone marrow can be seen at the lower left, and on the upper right, bone can be seen on the original cartilage surface. (Courtesy of MH McGuire, MD)

those generated by IL-1. It is a major cytokine derived from the monocyte macrophage system. TNF-α decreases the production of cartilage collagens and suppresses aggregating proteoglycan synthesis while promoting tissue degradation. In addition, it stimulates the production of plasminogen activator, PGE_2, and IL-6 in chondrocytes. However, TNF-α is less potent than IL-1 and does not act via the IL-1 receptors but through specific receptors.

An increased synthesis of prostaglandins due to IL-1 and TNF-α could be responsible for several of the symptoms observed in patients with OA. However, direct evidence that supports the involvement of either IL-1 or TNF-α in osteoarthritic cartilage degradation is scarce; neither has the role of IL-6 been defined. An increase in the minor types of collagen in OA cartilage is possibly the result of the influence of IL-1, which may stimulate collagen types I and III synthesis while decreasing the synthesis of types II and IX. High levels of IL-1 and IL-1-inhibiting proteins like TGF-ß have been found in OA joints. Chondrocytes from OA joints in patients also have increased levels of inducible NO synthase compared to controls.

Cartilage Repair

As mentioned earlier, decorin content may increase in the middle and deep zones in OA. This increase is thought to reflect new synthesis of collagen fibers as a compensatory response to the collagen damage that is initially most pronounced at or near the articular surface.

In cartilage defects, there is a striking increase in fibronectin. There seems to be an increased synthesis by the chondrocytes and accumulation in the extracellular matrix. Part of the fibronectin is composed of isoforms that are more sensitive to proteolytic cleavage than those in normal cartilage. Whether the increased synthesis of fibronectin is part of the repair process or whether it acts as a deleterious agent of the cartilage is not known. Inappropriate synthesis of nonspecific matrix proteins such as type I collagen is also common. Several embryonic-fetal chondroitin sulfate epitopes also are found in OA cartilage.

The etiology of OA is multifactorial, but there is a common end point (cartilage breakdown). The cartilage appears to be a highly refined tissue that can withstand high pressures during motion by being strong and elastic, and, most of all, by minimizing friction. However, cartilage is formed as a bearing surface devoid of blood circulation and has a relatively low capacity to heal when injured. It is possible that healing cartilage cannot provide the mechanical qualities necessary to maintain its structure during weightbearing and motion. However, immobilization does not provide satisfactory nutrition.

Diagnostic Markers

Immunochemical analysis of macromolecules released from the extracellular matrix of cartilage and bone into synovial fluid and serum offers possibilities to study the tissue turnover in pathologic conditions. Studies of animal models of posttraumatic OA (as well as studies of patients) show that there is an increase in the concentrations of proteoglycan fragments, cartilage oligomeric matrix protein fragments, stromelysin-1, and TIMP-1 in synovial fluid. The molecular fragments that result from matrix turnover are transported via regional lymph nodes to the general circulation. Matrix molecule fragments are eliminated from the blood mainly via a rapid liver uptake and kidney excretion. The half-life in blood varies markedly from molecule to molecule. Many of the markers are present at concentrations below the current limit of detection of the assays.

Animal Models of OA

Experimental monoarticular OA models are essentially joint injury and repair models. For example, joint instability, overloading, or immobilization can cause OA in animals. The type of loading is also important. Exercise on hard concrete surfaces can cause degenerative changes not seen in control animals exercised on softer wood chip paths. Studies of local cartilage injuries have shown that after an injury, the matrix initially consists of a type I collagen fibrocartilage, which under favorable conditions can remodel to hyaline cartilage composed of type II collagen. Where proteoglycans have been degraded by papain injection, repair can occur in the presence of collagen meshwork integrity. Nutritional and endocrine manipulations can also promote the development of degenerative arthritis. For example, mice fed a high-fat diet developed arthritis in the knees and the spine. Finally, spontaneous polyarticular OA develops in several strains of mice, rats, guinea pigs, dogs, and primates.

Genetic Factors

Primary generalized OA (PGOA) occurs in middle-aged women and is manifested by nodular arthritis of the distal interphalangeal joints of the hand, and occasionally by involvement of the knee and other joints. A single mutation that substitutes cysteine for arginine in position 519 in the type II procollagen gene (*COL2A1*) is found in this disorder. Patients with this mutation can also display mild spondyloepiphyseal dysplasia. Because PGOA is a heterogeneous disease, mutations in other genes may also lead to this phenotype. Several other of the chondrodysplasias, including the multiple epiphyseal dysplasias, such as spondyloepiphyseal dysplasia, are commonly associated with OA and have also been linked to mutations in the *COL2A1* gene. They are often inherited in an autosomal dominant manner.

Hereditary pyrophosphate arthropathy is related to the deposition of calcium pyrophosphate dihydrate (CPPD) in cartilage. A large subset of these cases appears to be inherited, mostly in an autosomal dominant manner. The same inheritance pattern seems to occur in hydroxyapatite deposition arthropathy and hereditary arthro-ophthalmopathy (the Stickler syndrome).

Because cartilage contains a large number of collagens and other macromolecules that are important for its mechanical characteristics, in the future it may be possible to link specific genetic aberrations to molecular abnormalities of the cartilage and to the development of OA.

Aging

Old age is the single greatest risk factor for OA. However, OA should not be regarded as simply a result of aging. The aging cartilage with its senescent cells is thinner, its surface is less smooth, and it is usually a dull yellow compared to the shiny white cartilage of the young. Osteophytes often occur in old individuals, but they are smaller than those seen in OA. Examination of aging articular cartilage has revealed evidence for type II collagen unwinding, especially close to the articular surface. With aging there is an increase in chondroitin-6 sulfate relative to chondroitin-4 sulfate and an increase in the size of keratan sulfate chains. There is also a reduction in the molecular weight of the core protein of the aggrecan molecule. There may be multiply sized core protein fragments with attached GAGs in the matrix; however, the tensile strength and stiffness of aging cartilage is only modestly reduced. Aging cartilage also contains senescent cells, but because matrix integrity is maintained, the chondrocytes seem able to control matrix turnover.

In contrast to aging cartilage, the OA cartilage is highly irregular, fibrillated, and hypertrophic in unloaded areas; in the more highly loaded parts of the joints, eburnated bone is seen. Hypertrophic osteophytes usually occur at the joint margins and may lead to deformation of the joint, which is not seen in unaffected joints in old people. In OA, clustering of cells and even cell mitoses can occur.

Treatment

Extensive cartilage defects heal poorly and, if left untreated, can lead to OA. Cartilage grafts applied to articular defects may become clinically relevant in the prevention of OA. Chondrocyte-collagen copolymer grafts have resulted in enhanced cartilage-defect repair in long-term studies using rabbits. Histologic and histochemical examination demonstrate hyaline-like tissue in the deeper zones of chondrocyte-grafted defects compared to poorly attached fibrous tissue in ungrafted defects. However, the surface layers of grafted and ungrafted sites consisted of fibrous tissue.

Advanced OA causes pain, occasional swelling, and effusion. The affected joint has a decreased range of motion, crepitus during movement, tenderness to palpation, bone enlargement, and malalignment. The arthritic process may, therefore, result in deformities, restricted range of motion, and instability. The treatment of established OA is multifaceted and aimed at controlling pain and maintaining function. Commonly used analgesics include acetaminophen and nonsteroidal anti-inflammatory drugs (NSAIDs).

There are no data from controlled clinical trials in humans to indicate that any NSAID favorably influences the progression of joint breakdown in OA. Moreover, NSAIDs may be associated with side effects, such as stomach pain and gastrointestinal bleeding. As is well known, NSAIDs blunt the inflammatory response mostly by inhibiting the formaton of prostaglandins. These are local modulators whose synthesis is stimulated, for example, by vasoactive hormones, cytokines, and local trauma. Prostaglandins also participate in the regulation of renal blood flow, and NSAIDs may, therefore, cause reversible impairment of glomerular filtration, acute renal failure, edema, interstitial nephritis, papillary necrosis, or hyperkalemia. They should, therefore, be used cautiously in the elderly in whom these adverse effects are more common. In spite of the risks, a large number of people over 65 years of age use prescribed NSAIDs. It has been determined that over 90% of primary care physicians would prescribe an NSAID as the initial treatment for an elderly patient with uncomplicated OA of the hip. Although NSAIDs are superior to placebos for symptomatic treatment of OA, they have not been shown to be better than analgesics, such as acetaminophen or dextropropoxiphene. Acetaminophen treatment is less risky and far less costly than treatment with most NSAIDs. However, it should be noted that not only do NSAIDs have peripheral anti-inflammatory effects, but they also have a central analgesic activity. They can be highly potent as analgesics in acute conditions and may be used as an adjuvant to, or even instead of, opioids in the treatment of severe pain immediately postoperatively, especially in younger patients.

Patients with OA of weightbearing joints should be instructed to modify their activity to avoid prolonged standing or carrying. A cane can be remarkably effective, especially in patients with OA of the hip. Often patients with OA of the knee benefit from using shoes with soft soles. Physical therapy can often improve the situation, and it decreases the risk for contractures. Exercises performed in water can be an excellent treatment alternative.

The early correction or even overcorrection of malalignment may delay or prevent the progression of OA. For example, varus alignment of the knee with arthritis of only the medial compartment is likely to progress more rapidly if left untreated than if the knee is put in a moderate valgus position. In addition, joint replacement procedures of the hip and knee offer excellent long-term results and have a low rate of complications. Arthrodesis, therefore, has come to appear less attractive and is now rarely used.

Rheumatoid Arthritis

Rheumatoid arthritis (RA) has an annual incidence of between two and four per 10,000 adult population. It affects women more than twice as often as men and becomes more common with advancing age. The disease affects approximately 1% of the world's population. After 10 years of disease, fewer than 50% of patients can continue to work. About 80% of patients with RA have circulating rheumatoid factor (RF). Among those who are RF-positive there is an increased frequency of patients who are positive for the human leukocyte antigen HLA-DR4 haplotype. This haplotype is, however, less common in blacks with RA. It is believed that RA occurs in genetically predisposed individuals in response to a pathogenic agent or antigen.

Pathophysiology

The major biologic function of HLA molecules relates to the fact that antigens can be recognized only by T cells in conjunction with HLA molecules. Several HLA types are linked to the disease, but the vast majority of patients carry HLA-DR4 or HLA-DR1, or both, although only a small percentage of those who test positive develop RA. The genetic markers can be especially helpful in identifying patients who will have a more severe disease course (ie, it seems that the density of HLA molecules on the cell surface is important for the severity of RA). It has, furthermore, been proposed that the HLA-DR molecule harbors different functional domains that can be involved in distinct functions and distinct autoimmune diseases.

Probably the most central event in the development of RA is the reaction between the antigen presenting cell (APC) macrophages and the T cell, which leads to cytokine production, B-cell proliferation, and antibody production. The APCs may have receptors of the class 2 major histocompatibility complex molecules to which the antigens are bound. These are recognized by the corresponding cell receptors on the helper T cells. The role of the T cells in the progression of joint destruction is substantial. CD4 cells (ie, helper/inducer cells) are the dominant T-cell phenotype in pannus. Depletion of those T cells, such as in thoracic duct drainage or in acquired immunodeficiency syndrome (AIDS), is associated with improvement in symptoms.

Activation of B cells into plasma cells also occurs in RA, with the resultant immunoglobulin production. The predominant immunoglobulins (Ig) produced are IgG and IgM; a substantial portion are RFs.

In chronic RA, there are fibroblast-like cells in the pannus that produce collagenase and stromelysin and contribute to the erosion of bone and to the chronic inflammation. There are also osteoclasts, which are stimulated by PGE_2. The cartilage destruction is mediated especially by the effects of IL-1 on the chondrocytes. There may be a local production of antibodies to type II collagen by synovial B cell populations. Substantial quantities of immune deposits can be found in the articular cartilage. The adherence of antibody to the cartilage matrix occurs by both antigen-antibody complexes and intermolecular disulfide bonds. High titers of antibody to type IX collagen have been found in the serum of patients with RA. Antibodies to the other minor cartilage collagens have also been detected. Cartilage-bound immune complexes could thus augment joint inflammation by activating complement and inflammatory cells. This phenomenon may explain why in a rheumatoid knee the synovitis disappears following removal of the cartilage during a total knee arthroplasty, even though no attempt has been made to perform a synovectomy.

Histamine, serotonin, bradykinin, substance-P, and enkephalin probably contribute to the progression of the disease and to the pain. Prostaglandins, such as PGE_2, participate in the inflammatory reaction, but they suppress T cells, B cells, and natural killer cells and inhibit the proliferation of synovial fibroblast-like cells. IL-1 and TNF-α are found in rheumatoid synovium and synovial fluid. TNF-α appears to regulate the production of IL-1. They both play a central role in activating B cells, thereby increasing the production of RF and other antibodies. TNF-α and IL-1 also contribute to the formation of the pannus by stimulating fibroblast-like synovial cells to proliferate and by promoting angiogenesis. In addition, they activate chondrocytes to release enzymes, which together with PGE_2 degrade cartilage and demineralize bone. IL-1 may also stimulate production of adrenocortical hormone and some of the acute phase proteins. IL-2, IL-3, and IL-6 also contribute to the rheumatoid inflammation.

Granulocyte-macrophage colony-stimulating factor, which is produced by T cells, epithelial cells, and fibroblasts supports the growth, differentiation, and activation of both granulocytes and macrophages. All three types of interferons, alpha, beta, and gamma, are prominent in the disease process. In general, they limit the proliferation of cells.

Platelet-derived growth factor is present in rheumatoid synovial fluids at high concentrations. It is apparently the single most effective stimulator of synovial fibroblast-like cell growth. It acts synergistically with other growth factors such as insulin, IGFs, and epidermal growth factor. TGF-α and epidermal growth factor are probably produced by local macrophages.

Etiology

It has been suggested that RA is a recent disease that has become epidemic, but may now be declining. An environmental factor, such as an infection, seems to be involved in the etiology. It has been suggested that RA, as well as other diseases including sarcoidosis, Crohn's disease, ulcerative colitis, psoriasis, and giant cell arteritis are, in fact, caused by microorganisms, especially mycobacteria. The etiologic role of infection has been established in Lyme disease, and reactive arthritis is known to be related to infections. Mycobacteria can exist in forms that are difficult to detect using conventional histologic techniques, and they are difficult to culture. Infections caused by mycobacteria or spirochetes, for example, seem to have common features with RA, which include arthritis, RA antibodies, and RF. The theory that an infection could trigger RA is supported by the fact that serologic changes have been found in the spouses of patients with RA, and altered antibody and skin test responses to mycobacteria are not infrequently found in RA.

Heat shock proteins (HSP) are a group of polypeptides produced by cells of all species in response to different stressful stimuli, including temperature elevation. Mycobacterial HSP can be used to create arthritis in rodents, and this has lead to their widespread use for experiments in arthritis research. Levels of antibodies against HSP from mycobacteria are increased in RA. It is possible that bacterial HSPs could accumulate in the synovial membrane and interact with specific antibodies or T cells. They could also, by their similarity with molecules of host origin (eg, type II collagen), create cross-reactivity against joint components. However, so far no bacteria have been isolated from rheumatoid joints.

Based on experiments in mice, it has been suggested that RA could be caused by a retroviral agent; however, human studies have also implicated the Epstein-Barr virus (EBV) as an etiologic factor. Similarly to other herpes viruses, EBV can persist in a latent state in an infected individual. It can stimulate intrinsic pathways to form EBV nuclear antigen. EBV infection is often mentioned as a possible etiologic agent for Sjögren's syndrome, especially concerning the lacrimal gland pathology.

Natural History of RA

Most patients will have a progressive disease with substantial morbidity and mortality. Long-term studies of RA in which patients have been monitored for over 10 years have demonstrated the likelihood for significant progression of the disease. More than 90% of those who met the American Rheumatism Association (ARA) criteria for RA have evidence of disease 3 to 5 years later, generally with progression. The RF effectively differentiates patients with a poor long-term outcome, but the titer value does not appear to be of major significance. In one study in patients with seropositive RA, only 24% had no progression in the radiologic destruction of the joints of the hands and feet over an 8-year period. The mean life expectancy is reduced by 7 years for men and 3 years for women. The increased mortality can be predicted effectively by such evidence of more severe disease as the involvement of many joints. Vasculitis (causing skin lesions and neuritis), cardiac involvement, pericarditis, pulmonary disease (pleuritis and pneumonitis), or ocular involvement (scleritis or episcleritis) is more frequent in patients with more severe RA. Comorbid cardiovascular disease is also of significant importance for the increased mortality.

Treatment

Much of the data in the literature suggest that aggressive drug therapy does not improve the long-term prognosis of RA. In fact, the major factor leading to improved outcome in recent studies was surgery and not drugs. There is less doubt that the standard drug treatment for RA relieves symptoms and improves the quality of life in the short-term perspective. First-line drugs for RA include salicylates and NSAIDs; second-line drugs with more or less well-established use in RA include antimalarials, gold salts, d-penicillamine, azathioprine, sulfasalazine, cyclosporin, and methotrexate.

RA is associated with a decreased life span because of the systemic nature of the disease and because of the toxicity of various treatments. Probably as a result of side effects, four-fifths of the patients in one study who had been started on gold, penicillamine, or sulfasalazine were not taking the drug 5 years later.

Newer Treatments

Several studies have shown low dose methotrexate to be a relatively potent and safe drug in the treatment of RA. However, the majority of patients achieve only partial remission. Still, methotrexate has a better record of protracted use than the other so-called second-line drugs.

The therapeutic hopes for the near future seem to be biologic agents that interfere with critical steps in the pathogenesis of RA. Among these are agents that affect cytokine function, such as IL-1 receptor antagonists or soluble cytokine receptors. Substances that affect T cells include anti-CD4 and anti-CD5 agents. The CD5 antibody has been linked to resin toxin, a potent plant toxin that inhibits protein synthesis. It depletes the CD5-positive B cells and it reversibly suppresses T cells, which all express CD5. Anti-CD4 antibody has been tried in RA patients with some symptomatic improvement. DAB486IL-2 is a fusion protein of IL-2 linked to diphtheria toxin. It interacts with the IL-2 receptor and activated T cells, delivering lethal diphtheria toxin to the activated T cells. Early results suggest significant improvement in symptoms in patients with RA. Anti-TNF also appears to have an impressive effect on the disease activity in RA patients. There is also now good evidence that MMPs are the major class of proteinases responsible for the excessive degradation of cartilage that leads to joint dysfunction in RA. They can be inhibited by TIMPs in the extracellular environment, and synthetic inhibitors of collagenase have been shown to exert both anti-inflammatory and cartilage protective effects in rats with inflammatory arthritis.

Menocycline, one of the tetracyclines, has been studied in a few patients with RA. It inhibits collagenase and has an anti-inflammatory effect. Preliminary studies show that it may be beneficial in RA patients.

Seronegative Spondylarthropathies

These diseases include ankylosing spondylitis and juvenile ankylosing spondylitis, psoriatic arthritis, Reiter's syndrome, arthritis of inflammatory bowel disease, and undifferentiated spondylarthropathies. They often include inflammatory arthritis similar to RA, but they also frequently present as inflammation of the entheses (ie, the cartilaginous site of attachment of a tendon or a ligament to bone). The peripheral arthritis is usually pauciarticular. The enthesopathy leads to localized pain, stiffness and often to local bone formation, causing spur formation or even ankylosis. The sacroiliac joint or the spine may be involved as well as other areas, such as the calcaneus where the Achilles tendon or the plantar fascia inserts.

Ankylosing spondylitis causes low back pain and can also involve larger peripheral joints. It is the type of spondylarthropathy that is most associated with an HLA antigen. Ninety percent of patients with this disease are HLA-B27 positive as compared to approximately 8% of the normal population. The disease is more commonly seen in men; however, it may more often be undiagnosed in women because of milder or uncharacteristic symptoms. In either sex, early onset of the disease and peripheral joint inflammation are indicative of a worse prognosis. Up to 25% of patients with ankylosing spondylitis develop iritis, but pulmonary and cardiovascular symptoms can also occur. Ankylosing spondylitis rarely develops after the age of 50 years.

The diagnosis of ankylosing spondylitis can sometimes be difficult, especially in the early stages. Decreased range of motion in the lower spine can usually be seen and thoracic expansion might be decreased. The sacroiliitis is often not apparent on radiographs. It develops on the average 9 years after the onset of the disease. Bone scans may show an increased uptake earlier. In selective cases, HLA-B27 testing may be of diagnostic help.

It has recently been suggested that ankylosing spondylitis is a type of reactive arthritis to *Klebsiella* based on the more frequent findings of the bacterium in the feces of patients with active ankylosing spondylitis compared to controls. However, additional investigations will be needed to confirm this association.

Reiter's Syndrome; Reactive Arthritis

This disease occurs shortly after an infection, but there is no evidence of a true infection of the joint itself. Up to 90% of patients are HLA-B27 positive. The disease occurs frequently after enteric infections caused by *Yersinia, Salmonella, Shigella,* or *Campylobacter* species. It also occurs after venereal infections (eg, infections caused by *Chlamydia*). There is inflammatory arthritis with effusion, particularly in the larger joints in the lower extremities. There are also enthesopathic symptoms and, not uncommonly, the patient may present with a so-called sausage digit. Some degree of back pain is common. Iritis, balanitis, stomatitis, skin rash, and nail lesions can also occur. In Caucasian populations, the incidence of HLA-B27 positivity is high in Reiter's syndrome, although in African Americans and Central Africans there is no apparent association. The course is variable, with recurrences, and occasionally, the arthritis can persist for more than a year.

Enteropathic Arthropathies

Patients with Crohn's disease and ulcerative colitis frequently have arthritis. It is more common in Crohn's disease. The arthritis often parallels the abdominal symptoms. Sacroiliitis is common, and about 50% to 70% of these patients are HLA-B27 positive.

Psoriatic Arthritis

Two-thirds of patients with psoriasis have some degree of joint involvement. Nearly one third have five or more involved joints. Although a symmetric oligoarthritis in the larger joints (eg, the knees, hips, ankles or wrists) is the most common pattern of psoriatic arthritis, the distal interphalangeal joints sometimes are characteristically involved. The arthritis often accompanies pronounced psoriatic nail changes, but it may entirely precede the other manifestations. Spondylitis may occur in some of the patients with psoriasis and they are often HLA-B27 positive. RF or antinuclear antibodies are usually not found in psoriatic arthritis.

Treatment of Spondylarthropathies

NSAIDs, especially indomethacin, are usually effective. Education and physical therapy are equally important. In some patients with ankylosing spondylitis, sulfasalazine may provide significant relief from the peripheral symptoms. In chronic cases of Reiter's syndrome, methotrexate or sulfasalazine can be considered. There is no proof of the value of antibiotics in the treatment of reactive arthritis.

Juvenile RA, Juvenile Chronic Arthritis

There are three types: pauciarticular, polyarticular and systemic (Still's disease). In particular, early onset pauciarticular juvenile RA (JRA) is likely to be associated with characteristic HLA configurations and T-cell receptor genes. There is a recognized association between HLA phenotypes and the presence of antinuclear antibodies. Several studies have shown that the number of T cells of both CD4 and CD8 phenotypes is increased in polyarticular JRA patients. The number of T cells of CD4 phenotypes is increased in systemic JRA. Serum from patients with JRA contains immune complexes, RFs, and other autoantibodies. These autoantibodies include several kinds of antinuclear antibodies in addition to RF. There is a particularly high frequency of the antibody against nucleoprotein in sera from patients with pauciarticular disease who have chronic uveitis.

At least 75% of patients with JRA eventually enter long periods of disease quiescence. Most of these patients have only minimal disability. The treatment should be based on both physical and pharmacologic methods. Aspirin remains the most important anti-inflammatory medication, although NSAIDs should be tried in those who do not respond within 6 to 12 weeks. Systemic corticosteroids should be avoided, but may be necessary in severe polyarticular and systemic disease. Surgical treatment includes joint replacements in long-standing severe joint disease after closure of the epiphyses. Synovectomy is rarely indicated.

Human Immunodeficiency Virus-Related Musculoskeletal Disease

Early in the course of infection, patients infected with the human immunodeficiency virus (HIV) may have transient polyarthralgia, which is felt to represent viral invasion of synovium with an associated host response. It resembles the polyarthralgia frequently seen in other viral diseases, such as hepatitis B or influenza. The polyarthralgia is usually mild and of short duration. It most frequently involves knees, shoulders, and elbows. Some patients will, however, present with established synovitis, usually in one of the joints in the lower limbs. A few may have septic monoarthritis, which sometimes is caused by opportunistic infections.

Reiter's syndrome may occur during the course of established HIV disease. Classically, this syndrome presents as an asymmetric arthropathy most commonly involving large joints together with uroarthritis, cervicitis, and conjunctivitis or other inflammatory eye disease. Psoriasis and associated arthritis are not uncommon in HIV-positive individuals. Rapid onset or worsening of existing disease should alert clinicians to possible HIV infection. HIV infection may also present with proximal muscle weakness and myalgia, together with elevated serum creatine kinase levels, and may be indistinguishable from the primary idiopathic form of polymyositis.

Reiter's syndrome or psoriatic arthritis associated with AIDS may be extremely severe. It is therefore of interest to assess possible risk factors for acquiring HIV infection in this group of patients.

Of note is the universal finding that RA virtually never occurs in the presence of the virus. There have been several reported cases in which patients with RA have gone into remission after infection with HIV. This is further evidence of the central role of the CD4-positive lymphocyte in rheumatoid disease.

Annotated Bibliography

Cartilage Physiology

Buttle DJ, Handley CJ, Ilic MZ, et al: Inhibition of cartilage proteoglycan release by a specific inactivator of cathepsin-B and an inhibitor of matrix metalloproteinases: Evidence for two converging pathways of chondrocyte-mediated proteoglycan degradation. *Arthritis Rheum* 1993;36:1709–1717.

Metalloproteinases are involved in cartilage proteoglycan breakdown, but the lysosomal proteinases cathepsin-B and cathepsin-D also have an important role. In this study, cartilage explants were stimulated to break down proteoglycans, and the effects of inhibitors of metalloproteinases or of cathepsin-B were studied. The results demonstrate two independent pathways of cartilage proteoglycan breakdown that converge at the activation of matrix prometalloproteinase.

Flannery CR, Lark MW, Sandy JD: Identification of a stromelysin cleavage site within the interglobular domain of human aggrecan: Evidence for proteolysis at this site *in vivo* in human articular cartilage. *J Biol Chem* 1992;267: 1008–1014.

This paper shows the cleavage point for stromelysin in the aggrecan molecule and that a proportion of the aggrecan that accumulates in human articular cartilage is generated by cleavage at this point. These data support the view that stromelysin is active in vivo. Furthermore, the study provides indirect evidence that a major cleavage site in aggrecan catabolism is within the so-called interglobular domain.

Kuettner KE: Biochemistry of articular cartilage in health and disease. *Clin Biochem* 1992;25:155–163.

This is an excellent review article. It summarizes current knowledge of cartilage physiology and biochemistry.

Macirowski T, Tepic S, Mann RW: Cartilage stresses in the human hip joint. *J Biomech Eng* 1994;116:10–18.

This is a finite element analysis based on information about stresses that was obtained by using an instrumented hemiprosthesis of the hip. The authors found that when loaded, cartilage consolidates, and interstitial fluid is pressed out into the joint space. Using the normal flow velocities into the gap and the contact network stresses of the cartilage surfaces, it was found that fluid pressure supported 90% of the load while the cartilage network stresses remained well below the drained modulus of the cartilage. The result supports the importance of the weeping mechanism of joint lubrication.

Palmer RM, Hickery MS, Charles IG, et al: Induction of nitric oxide synthase in human chondrocytes. *Biochem Biophys Res Commun* 1993;193:398–405.

This paper provides an excellent review of previous work regarding nitric oxide synthesis. It is the first paper that demonstrates that nitric oxide synthase can be induced in human chondrocytes. As well, the authors have partially characterized this enzyme biochemically, pharmacologically and at the molecular level.

Osteoarthritis: Cartilage

Brittberg M, Lindahl A, Nilsson A, et al: Treatment of deep cartilage defects in the knee with autologous chondrocyte transplantation. *N Engl J Med* 1994;331: 889–895.

In this clinical study of 23 patients who underwent autologous chondrocyte transplantation, chondrocytes from the patient's own knee were cultured, and a cell suspension was injected into the defect, which was covered with a periosteal flap. The patients were allowed active movement without weightbearing beginning at 2 or 3 days after the surgery. Follow-up arthroscopies revealed formation of new cartilage similar to normal cartilage (eg, because of its content of collagen type II). The treatment was more successful when done on the femur than when done on the patella.

Lohmander LS, Hoerrner LA, Dahlberg L, et al: Stromelysin, tissue inhibitor of metalloproteinases and proteoglycan fragments in human knee joint fluid after injury. *J Rheumatol* 1993;20:1362–1368.

The authors point out that injury to the menisci and the ligaments of the knee can lead to osteoarthritis, the incidence of which is 40% to 60% after a total meniscectomy and 60% to 90% after a rupture of the anterior cruciate ligament. Analysis of knee joint fluid samples obtained from patients with a knee injury indicated that the average stromelysin concentrations increased 40-fold in association with the injury and decreased after about 6 months to a plateau level about 10-fold greater than that of a reference group with healthy knees. Tissue inhibitors of metalloproteinase and proteoglycan also increased in similar temporal patterns. These synovial fluid markers were maintained in patients examined up to 17 years after the injury.

Lohmander LS, Saxne T, Heinegard DK: Release of cartilage oligomeric matrix protein (COMP) into joint fluid after knee injury and in osteoarthritis. *Ann Rheum Dis* 1994;53:8–13.

Cartilage oligomeric matrix protein (COMP) is a cartilage specific protein that is found in high concentrations in synovial fluid in connection with knee trauma. It can be detected in knee joint fluid for many years after an injury and is also present in primary osteoarthritis; however, joint fluid COMP concentrations were not increased in cases of advanced osteoarthritis.

Pelletier JP, Faure MP, DiBattista JA, et al: Coordinate synthesis of stromelysin, interleukin-1, and oncogene proteins in experimental osteoarthritis: An immunohistochemical study. *Am J Pathol* 1993; 142:95–105.

The sources and the localization of stromelysin, two interleukins and the oncogene products (*C-fos, C-jun* and *C-myc*) in synovium and cartilage from normal and experimental canine models of osteoarthritis are studied. The study suggests that the metalloproteases, interleukin–1, and oncoproteins in osteoarthritis are actively synthesized in situ. Stromelysin levels are much higher in osteoarthritic cartilage compared to normal.

Osteoarthritis: Epidemiology

Felson DT: The epidemiology of knee osteoarthritis: Results from the Framingham Osteoarthritis Study. *Semin Arthritis Rheum* 1990;20(suppl 1):42–50.

This population-based study focuses on independently living elderly patients in order to document the radiographic and symptomatic prevalence of knee osteoarthritis. The study shows that knee osteoarthritis increases in prevalence throughout the elderly years, more so in women than in men. It also demonstrates several risk factors such as obesity, knee injury, chondrocalcinosis, occupational knee bending under load, and physical labor.

Osteoarthritis: Etiology

Hulth A: Does osteoarthritis depend on growth of the mineralized layer of cartilage? *Clin Orthop* 1993;287: 19–24.

The author has for several years noted a tendency for continued growth at the joint surface in osteoarthritis. He has noted that the subchondral bone has a higher metabolic activity than normal and an increased density compared to normal. The theory is advanced that growth factors released in the joint cause the typical osteoarthritic changes in cartilage, subchondral bone, and joint capsule.

Imeokparia RL, Barrett JP, Arrieta MI, et al: Physical activity as a risk factor for osteoarthritis of the knee. *Ann Epidemiol* 1994;4:221–230.

This is a case control study of the association between osteoarthritis (OA) and physical activity in people 40 years and older. There were 239 individuals with OA of the knee and 239 controls with no radiologic evidence of OA of the knee. There was a statistically significant association between physical activity and knee OA in women only, with an age adjusted odds ratio of 1.66. The patients with OA were more obese than the controls, that is, they had a higher body mass index.

Kujala UM, Kaprio J, Sarna S: Osteoarthritis of weight bearing joints of lower limbs in former elite male athletes. *BMJ* 1994;308:231–234.

The authors compared a cumulative 21-year incidence of hospital admissions for osteoarthritis of the hip, knee, and ankle between former elite athletes and control subjects. They found that athletes from all types of competitive sports are at slightly increased risk of requiring hospital care because of osteoarthritis of the hip, knee, or ankle. They also found that the admissions occurred later in endurance athletes than in the remainder.

Lemaire ED, Fisher FR: Osteoarthritis and elderly amputee gait. *Arch Phys Med Rehabil* 1994;75:1094–1099.

An elderly group of transtibial amputees and a similar control group were compared. There was a greater incidence of osteoarthritis in the contralateral knee in the amputee group than was seen in the normal control group. The amputee group also had consistently larger knee joint reaction forces in the knee of the nonamputated leg.

Osteoarthritis: Animal Models

Carlson CS, Loeser RF, Jayo MJ, et al: Osteoarthritis in cynomolgus macaques: A primate model of naturally occurring disease. *J Orthop Res* 1994;12:331–339.

The authors examined a species of monkeys, which are similar to the rhesus monkeys, for osteoarthritis of the knee joint. The animals had been used in a study of the effects of sex steroids on atherosclerosis. They found the earliest change to be thickening of the subchondral bone plate, followed by fibrillation clefting of the cartilage. The changes were most common and most pronounced in the medial tibial plateau. This species has similarities to other species with the spontaneous development of osteoarthritis (for example, the Duncan-Hartley guinea pigs).

Osteoarthritis: Genetic Aspects

Ala-Kokko L, Baldwin CT, Moskowitz RW, et al: Single base mutation in the type II procollagen gene (COL2A1) as a cause of primary osteoarthritis associated with a mild chondrodysplasia. *Proc Natl Acad Sci USA* 1990;87: 6565–6568.

This study of nine affected members of a family with primary generalized osteoarthritis and signs of mild chondrodysplasia found a single base mutation that converted the codon for arginine at position 519 $\alpha 1(II)$ collagen chain to the codon for cysteine, an amino acid normally not found in type II collagen. The mutation was found in all affected members of the family, but not in unaffected members.

Holderbaum D, Malemud CJ, Moskowitz RW, et al: Human cartilage from late stage familial osteoarthritis transcribes type II collagen mRNA encoding a cysteine in position 519. *Biochem Biophys Res Commun* 1993;192: 1169–1174.

Among the genetic factors which predispose for osteoarthritis is mutation in the gene for type II collagen. It has been shown that this can be the result of a substitution of cysteine for arginine at position 519 in the triple helical region of the gene *COL2A1*. Transcription products of both mutant and normal type II collagen alleles were found in cartilage taken from patients with the Arg-Cys519 mutation at the time of a total knee replacement. The mutant protein was continually synthesized in the cartilage of these patients.

Jimenez SA, Dharmavaram RM: Genetic aspects of familial osteoarthritis. *Ann Rheum Dis* 1994;53:789–797.

This is an excellent article that reviews some of the strategies that have been successfully utilized or may be potentially useful to identify collagen gene mutations in inherited diseases affecting cartilage. Twenty mutations that affect procollagen are listed.

Rheumatoid Arthritis: Etiology

Paliard X, West SG, Lafferty JA, et al: Evidence for the effects of a superantigen in rheumatoid arthritis. *Science* 1991;253:325–329.

The authors state that the pathogenesis of rheumatoid arthritis (RA) is unknown although genetic and environmental factors are implicated. They propose that patients with RA might have encountered a microbial superantigen, which has led to the activation of most of the cells in a certain receptor group, some of which will end up in the joints initiating disease. The reason the cells settle in joints is presumed to be because of cross-reaction with local self-antigens.

van de Loo FA, Joosten LA, van Lent PL, et al: Role of interleukin-1, tumor necrosis factor alpha, and interleukin-6 in cartilage proteoglycan metabolism and destruction: Effect of in situ blocking in murine antigen- and zymosan-induced arthritis. *Arthritis Rheum* 1995; 38:164–172.

The authors describe the effect of blocking endogenous interleukin-1 (IL-1), tumor necrosis factor (TNF), or IL-6 in murine arthritis induced either by antigen or by zymosan, a potent inducer of both IL-1 and TNF in vivo. The results showed that the suppression of prostaglandin synthesis in both types of arthritis in mice is due to the combined local action of IL-1α and IL-1β and neither IL-6 nor TNF is involved. Blocking IL-1-normalized prostaglandin synthesis in antigen induced arthritis.

Rheumatoid Arthritis: Treatment

Brooks PM, Day RO: Nonsteroidal anti-inflammatory drugs: Differences and similarities. *New Engl J Med* 1991;324:1716–1725.

This interesting review article compares currently used nonsteroidal anti-inflammatory drugs.

Horneff G, Burmester GR, Emmrich F, et al: Treatment of rheumatoid arthritis with an anti-CD4 monoclonal antibody. *Arthritis Rheum* 1991;34:129–140.

A monoclonal antibody against the CD4 antigen present on T helper cells was studied in ten patients with severe rheumatoid arthritis. Treatment resulted in a drastic depletion of CD4+ cells, which generally persisted for 3 to 4 weeks and led to improvement in several clinical and laboratory parameters. This new form of immunosuppression may become an alternative to conventional methods.

Kremer JM, Phelps CT: Long-term prospective study of the use of methotrexate in the treatment of rheumatoid arthritis: Update after a mean of 90 months. *Arthritis Rheum* 1992;35:138–145.

This long-term study demonstrates that methotrexate is useful in the treatment of rheumatoid arthritis (RA) and has relatively few side effects in the doses used. The authors consider it to be the most effective and best tolerated drug available for the treatment of patients with RA. The most important side effect is liver toxicity. They also point out that alcohol intake should be completely avoided by patients taking methotrexate.

Seideman P, Muller-Suur R, Ekman E: Renal effects of low dose methotrexate in rheumatoid arthritis. *J Rheumatol* 1993;20:1126–1128.

Renal failure has been reported during treatment with high doses of methotrexate but has not so far been observed with the low doses used for the treatment of rheumatoid arthritis. The authors found that after 4 to 8 weeks, the treatment caused a significant decrease in kidney function, which is important, particularly in situations of combined treatment with other potentially nephrotoxic substances.

Williams RO, Feldmann M, Maini RN: Anti-tumor necrosis factor ameliorates joint disease in murine collagen-induced arthritis. *Proc Natl Acad Sci USA* 1992;89:9784–9788.

Tumor necrosis factor alpha (TNFα) has an important role in the pathogenesis of rheumatoid arthritis. The authors studied the effect of administrating TNF neutralizing antibodies to mice with collagen-induced arthritis. This treatment, given before induction or after development of the disease, significantly reduced paw swelling and histologic severity of the arthritis without reducing the incidence of the arthritis or the level of circulating anti-type II collagen IgG.

Rheumatoid Arthritis: Prognosis

Isomaki H: Long-term outcome of rheumatoid arthritis. *Scand J Rheumatol* 1992;95(suppl):3–8.

This is an 8-year follow-up of 201 patients with rheumatoid arthritis. The course of the disease was influenced by the number of involved joints and whether the patient was seropositive. Thirty-nine percent of the patients showed a linear progression of the disease from their first visit, whereas 38% showed late remission or no progression at all. The remainder, 23%, progressed but in a nonlinear fashion.

Weyand CM, Hicok KC, Conn DL, et al: The influence of HLA-DRB1 genes on disease severity in rheumatoid arthritis. *Ann Int Med* 1992;117:801–806.

The authors examined 102 patients diagnosed with seropositive rheumatoid arthritis. The HLA-DR4 haplotype has been characterized as a susceptibility marker that is present in most patients; however, it is also expressed in normal persons. The study showed that HLA-DRB1 alleles have the potential to be used as markers for disease severity. This finding is important when assessing the results of different treatments, because usually seropositivity has been the only criterion applied.

19

Collagen and Connective Tissue Disorders

Marfan Syndrome

Marfan syndrome is a heterogeneous group of connective tissue disorders that are potentially life threatening and share common physical and genetic findings. The genetic defect has been mapped to a site on the long arm of chromosome 15, the site of a fibrillin gene *FBN1*. The incidence in the United States is estimated to be four to six per 100,000. This incidence is probably an underestimation because the variable penetrance of the disorder results in a group of mildly affected individuals, many of whom are not reported. The syndrome is transmitted as autosomal dominant; however, spontaneous mutation is thought to account for nearly 25% of new cases. Males and females are equally affected by the syndrome.

The diagnosis of Marfan syndrome may be difficult; major and minor diagnostic criteria have been proposed (Outline 1). Several observations have resulted in clinical signs, including Steinberg's thumb sign (positive when the thumb, held in the clasped fist, protrudes beyond the ulna border of the hand), the wrist sign (positive when the thumb overlaps the fifth finger as they encircle the contralateral wrist), and the knee sign (positive when the legs are overlapped and crossed and the toe of the top leg reaches the floor). The three signs are a reflection of ligamentous laxity and arachnodactyly; they are suggestive of, but not diagnostic for, Marfan's syndrome. The diagnosis may be made by establishing two of the following groups of criteria: positive family history and classic orthopaedic, cardiovascular, or ophthalmologic findings.

Individuals afflicted with the syndrome demonstrate dolichostenomelia, an arm span three or more inches greater than their height. A disproportionate upper to lower body length is reflected as a ratio of less than 0.85 in whites or 0.78 in blacks. Variable orthopaedic findings include ligamentous laxity resulting in dislocation or subluxation of the patella, shoulder, and sternoclavicular joints; scoliosis; thoracic lordosis; chest wall deformity (pectus excavatum or pectus carinatum); acetabular protrusion; dural ectasia; and high palate. Ligamentous laxity also is associated with ankle instability and pes planovalgus foot deformity with elongation of the great toe.

Marfan syndrome results in death in as many as 90% of affected individuals due to cardiovascular complications related to collagen deficiency. Pulmonary function may be restricted by thoracic lordoscoliosis. Aortic root dilation and rupture and mitral valve prolapse may be diagnosed by ultrasonography. Bilateral superior lens dislocation occurs in 60% of affected individuals. Most patients are myopic, and premature cataracts are common. Retinal detachment, resulting in a treatable lesion that subsequently may result in blindness, has been reported. Careful cardiovascular and ophthalmologic evaluation is essential.

Marfan syndrome may be confused with other connective tissue disorders, particularly congenital contractural arachnodactyly (CCA) and homocystinuria. It is thought that CCA is the syndrome Marfan actually reported; however, CCA is mapped to a locus on chromosome 5. In addition to arachnodactyly, dolichostenomelia, and scoliosis, CCA demonstrates ear deformities. Homocystinuria, hypermobility syndrome, and Stickler syndrome share some features of Marfan syndrome and must be considered in the differential diagnosis.

Outline 1. **Diagnostic criteria of Marfan syndrome**

Major physical findings
- Aortic dilation
- Ectopic lentis 60%
- Severe kyphoscoliosis
- Chest wall deformity (pectus excavatum > pectus carinatum)

Minor physical findings
- Arachnodactyly
- Knee sign
- Ligamentous laxity
- Mitral valve prolapse
- Myopia
- Tall stature
- Thumb sign
- Wrist sign

Ehlers-Danlos Syndrome

Ehlers-Danlos syndrome (EDS) is a group of no less than 11 genetically distinct disorders (Table 1), plus many additional subgroups that share similar clinical findings related primarily to joint laxity and skin elasticity. There is confusion regarding EDS type 11, because it has been classified as joint instability syndrome. It is seen most commonly in whites of European descent, with a male predominance. The biochemical abnormality in many forms of EDS has not been defined, but the final common pathway is defective elastin and collagen formation, which result in fragile skin that splits open easily with minimal trauma, does not hold sutures well, and forms broad, thin, cigarette paper-like scars. Hyperelasticity of the skin is variable depending on the type of EDS (Table 1). Arterial fragility is common to many forms of EDS, resulting in subcutaneous bleeding. Cholesterol analysis of the subcutaneous lipomatous nodules points to previous hematoma as the source. Occasionally, the tumors may calcify or ossify.

Table 1. Ehlers-Danlos Syndrome (EDS)

Type	Acronym	Transmission*	Biochemistry	Orthopaedic	Miscellaneous
1	Gravis	AD	Unknown	Hyperextensible skin, poor wound healing, scoliosis, pes planus	Bruise easily, varicose veins, miscarriages, prematurity, mitral valve prolapse
2	Mitis	AD	Unknown	Similar to EDS 1	Less severe than EDS 1, no prematurity
3	Benign hypermobile	AD	Unknown	Early onset osteoarthritis, joint dislocations	Skin hyperextensible
4	Ecchymotic	AD and AR	Defective type III collagen	Hands and feet appear prematurely aged, thin skin without hyperextensibility	Uterine, bowel, arterial ruptures; stroke; abnormal facies with large eyes, thin nose, thin lips; short life expectancy
5		XR	Deficient lysyl hydroxylase ??	Joint laxity	Similar to EDS 2
6		AR	Deficient lysyl hydroxylase	Kyphoscoliosis, muscle hypotonia, joint laxity, skin hyperextensibility	Easy bruising, arterial rupture, ocular fragility
7	Arthrochalasis	AD and AR	Abnormal procollagen peptidase affecting collagen formation	Multiple joint dislocations, bilateral hip dislocation at birth, increased skin elasticity without fragility	Easy bruising, short stature
8		AD	Unknown	Joint laxity, increased skin elasticity with fragility	Periodontal disease with early tooth loss, easy bruising
9**	Occipital horn	XR	Deficient lysyl hydroxylase, abnormal copper metabolism	Short humeri, short broad clavicles, increased skin elasticity without fragility	Occipital horns, bladder diverticuli, decreased serum copper and ceruloplasmin
10		AR	Abnormal fibronectin	Mild, similar to EDS 2 or EDS 3 without dislocations	Platelet aggregation dysfunction resulting in poor clotting
11†		AD	Unknown	Joint laxity with dislocation	Skin elasticity normal with easy bruising

* AD = autosomal dominant, AR = autosomal recessive, XR = x-linked recessive
** Type 9 is no longer part of EDS; it has been reclassified as a disease of copper metabolism
† EDS type 11 is now reclassified as a disorder of joint instability

Physical findings frequently associated with and presumptive of EDS are hyperextension of the metacarpophalangeal joints beyond 90°, hyperextension of the thumb to meet the forearm, hyperextension of the knee or elbow beyond 10°, and the ability to flex the trunk forward and place the palms flat on the floor. Other findings less commonly seen are blue sclerae, lipomatous tumors, easy bruising, acrocyanosis, and arterial ruptures. In some forms of EDS, inguinal, diaphragmatic, and umbilical hernias have been reported, as well as rupture of any of the hollow organs such as the bowel and uterus.

Orthopaedic management of most patients with EDS should be conservative, with physical therapy and orthotics, if possible. Surgical wounds tend to heal poorly and may dehisce in severe cases. In a high percent of individuals, joint instability leads to premature arthralgia and osteoarthritis in the third to fourth decade of life. Arthrodesis is preferred to arthroplasty because of joint laxity and instability secondary to poor collagen, depending upon EDS type.

Homocystinuria

Homocystinuria (HCU) is a well-defined disorder of amino acid metabolism, which is caused by deficient cystathionine beta synthase. It is the second most common metabolic disorder resulting in perinatal mental retardation. The disease is transmitted as autosomal recessive, with heterozygote and homozygote forms distinguishable based on enzyme activity. Two forms have been described, sensitive and resistant to pyridoxine (vitamin B6). Urine analyses for homocysteine and methionine are effective screening measures.

Physical findings in HCU include the Marfanoid habitus with arachnodactyly, dolichostenomelia, scoliosis, and pectus excavatum. However, these individuals have tight joints rather than the laxity seen in patients with Marfan syndrome. Additionally, flaring of the distal femur, bowing of the tibia, enlargement of the carpal bones, genu valgum, muscle weakness, gait abnormality, and osteoporosis are common. Fine hair, malar rash, downward dislocation of

Table 2. Osteogenesis Imperfecta

Type	Transmission*	Biochemistry	Orthopaedic	Miscellaneous
I				
A,C	AD	Half normal amount of type I collagen	Bone fragility, osteoporosis, fractures at birth	Blue sclerae, hearing loss, no hearing or dental problems
B	AD		Short stature	More severe than IA or IC with dentinogenesis imperfecta
II	AD and AR	Unstable triple helix	Intrauterine fractures, extreme bone fragility	Usually lethal in perinatal period, delayed ossification of skull, blue sclerae
III	AR	Abnormal type I collagen	Extreme bone fragility with fractures at birth, limb deformity, scoliosis	Hearing loss, short stature, blue sclerae becoming less blue with age, shortened life expectancy, dentinogenesis imperfecta
IV				
A	AD	Shortened pro alpha$_1$ (I) chains	Mild to moderate severity of bone fragility	Normal sclerae, normal hearing, normal dentition, normal life expectancy
B	AD			Similar to IV A with dentinogenesis imperfecta

* AR = autosomal recessive, AD = autosomal dominant

the lens, myopia, cataracts, and glaucoma are present. The major and life threatening problem of HCU is the thrombotic tendency resulting in thrombosis of major arteries and veins. The disorder results in a reduced life expectancy and varying spasticity.

Osteogenesis Imperfecta

Osteogenesis imperfecta (OI) is a group of hereditary disorders of collagen metabolism that affect several tissues including bone. The defective collagen, primarily type I, results in bone fragility, which varies from mild osteoporosis to intrauterine fractures and perinatal death. Males and females are equally affected. The incidence of OI is approximately one in 20,000 births. The older classification of OI of congenita and tarda is being replaced in common usage by the Sillence classification into four groups (Table 2). The long-term prognosis is strongly related to the Sillence grouping.

Patients who have OI share similar physical findings to varying degrees, including bone fragility with numerous fractures and bowing of long bones, scoliosis, wormian cranial bones, a triangular facies, and trifoil shaped pelvis. Orthopaedic treatment is directed toward prevention and treatment of recurrent long bone fractures.

In the young child, lightweight bracing is helpful in the early ambulatory stage. Repeat fractures in the lower extremities with continuous casting is a vicious cycle to be avoided. With two or more fractures of the femur and/or tibia in less than 12 months' time, the use of expandable Bailey-DuBow rods or Rush rods becomes a reasonable option. The rods will assist in fracture management and maintain reasonable lower limb alignment with growth.

Progressive scoliosis may be difficult to control despite internal fixation. Bracing is not recommended due to chest deformity secondary to bone plasticity. Early stabilization with segmental fixation is the procedure of choice.

Annotated Bibliography

Ainsworth SR, Aulicino PL: A survey of patients with Ehlers-Danlos syndrome. *Clin Orthop* 1993;286:250–256.

This review of 151 patients with Ehlers-Danlos syndrome documents physical findings and their incidence as well as specific diagnostic criteria.

Hanscom DA, Winter RB, Lutter L, et al: Osteogenesis imperfecta: Radiographic classification, natural history, and treatment of spinal deformities. *J Bone Joint Surg* 1992;74A:598–616.

This is a review of the orthopaedic manifestations of osteogenesis imperfecta, with emphasis on spinal deformity and its management.

Joseph KN, Kane HA, Milner RS, et al: Orthopedic aspects of the Marfan phenotype. *Clin Orthop* 1992; 277:251–261.

This is a review of the diagnostic criteria of Marfan's syndrome with emphasis on the orthopaedic manifestations of the syndrome and probability of successful diagnosis.

Lieberman ER, Gomperts ED, Shaw KN, et al: Homocystinuria: Clinical and pathologic review, with emphasis on thrombotic features, including pulmonary artery thrombosis. *Perspect Pediatr Pathol* 1993;17:125–147.

This detailed review of the disease contains clinical, including orthopaedic, biochemical, histologic, and genetic analysis.

Tsipouras P, Devereux RB: Marfan syndrome: Genetic basis and clinical manifestations. *Semin Dermatol* 1993; 12:219–228.

This is an excellent review of physical findings and natural history of Marfan's syndrome.

Yeowell HN, Pinnell SR: The Ehlers-Danlos syndromes. *Semin Dermatol* 1993;12:229–240.

This is a review of Ehlers-Danlos syndrome types 1 through 10 with respect to the biochemical, genetic, and physical findings in the complex group disorders.

20

Genetic Disorders and Skeletal Dysplasias

Skeletal Dysplasias

Skeletal dysplasias (osteochondrodysplasias) are inherited disorders of bone and/or cartilage growth and development. Most are chondrodysplasias, a heterogeneous group of disorders characterized by defective cartilage growth and/or development that results in disproportionate short stature and, often, deformity of the extremities and spine. Nonskeletal tissues are involved in some disorders. More than 150 distinct skeletal dysplasias have been described, and most are diagnosed by a combination of physical appearance, radiographic characteristics, and, occasionally, bone or physeal histology. These disorders range in severity from perinatally lethal to so mild that no medical problems occur. Many are apparent at birth, but some do not become evident for several years.

Most skeletal dysplasias are named descriptively based on phenotypic or radiographic features. Some are commonly referred to by eponym. Increased understanding of the cause of these disorders will lead to improved classification in the near future. "Families" of chondrodysplasias with the same known or presumed etiology are being described. For example, disorders with a mutation in the gene for type II collagen include some spondyloepiphyseal dysplasias, hypochondrogenesis, and the Stickler syndrome.

In spite of their heterogeneity, these disorders have in common a group of potential problems in addition to short stature and deformity of the limbs and spine. Patients with many of these disorders have respiratory problems caused by chest wall or upper airway abnormalities, especially during infancy and early childhood. Central nervous system problems include hydrocephaly, spinal stenosis, and spinal cord injury from cervical spine and/or craniovertebral junction instability. Muscle hypotonia, muscle contracture, and intrinsic muscle disease may occur. Hearing loss, dental problems, myopia, and retinal detachment are also more common with some of the skeletal dysplasias.

Achondroplasia

Achondroplasia is the most common form of short-limbed dwarfism. Achondroplastic dwarfs are recognizable at birth by rhizomelic short limbs and a relatively long, narrow trunk; an enlarged head with frontal bossing, depressed nasal bridge, and midface hypoplasia; and short, broad hands with the trident configuration. Most joints are excessively lax (most obvious at the knee), although the elbows have limitations of extension, and forearm rotation is decreased. Most children are somewhat hypotonic and a thoracolumbar kyphosis usually is apparent (Fig. 1). Achondroplasia is an autosomal dominant disorder. Eighty to 90% of affected individuals represent new mutations. The cause of achondroplasia is a point mutation in the gene coding for fibroblast growth factor receptor 3. This mutation causes a single amino acid change (arginine to glycine) in the transmembrane portion of this cell surface receptor. The function of this receptor is not yet known, although it is expressed in all prebone cartilage as well as diffusely in the central nervous system (CNS). A previous report that implicated a mutation of the gene coding for type II collagen as the cause of achondroplasia has been retracted.

Radiographs reveal short pedicles (on the lateral view) and interpedicular narrowing from L1 to L5 (on the AP view) in the lumbar spine. A thoracolumbar kyphosis is present. The pelvis has a champagne glass conformation with short, square iliac wings and horizontal acetabular roofs. All tubular bones are short, with metaphyseal flaring. Genu varum with fibular overgrowth relative to the tibia is present.

Gross motor milestones are delayed, and most achondroplastic dwarfs start walking between 18 and 24 months. Hypotonia, laxity of ligaments, and the problems of balance posed by the enlarged head and the short extremities are believed to cause this delay. However, hydrocephalus and cord compression secondary to foramen magnum stenosis must be considered as possible causes of gross motor delay. Upper cervical cord compression may also manifest itself as failure to thrive, quadriparesis, apnea, and sudden death. The risk of sudden death is more than twice as great in achondroplastic dwarfs under age 4 years than in an unaffected population. Anesthesia and postoperative management may be complicated because of abnormal chest wall configuration, midfacial hypoplasia, and upper airway obstruction, as well as craniovertebral spinal stenosis.

In childhood, the most common orthopaedic problem is genu varum. The femoral bowing is mild, and the major deformity is in the tibia, with the fibula being long relative to the tibia. Although premature osteoarthritis is rare, correction is often indicated for cosmesis and to avoid progressive ligamentous laxity and pain. Proximal tibiofibular osteotomy usually is all that is necessary for adequate correction. Proximal and/or distal fibular epiphysiodesis may result in correction in older childen and preadolescents who have mild to moderate varus deformity.

A less common problem in childhood is the failure of the thoracolumbar kyphosis to resolve after the child begins to walk. The kyphosis gradually corrects in more than

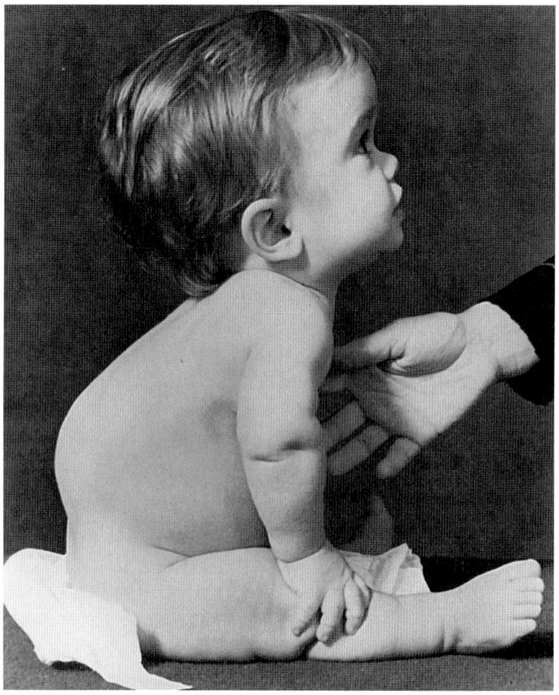

Fig. 1 Thoracolumbar kyphosis in a 6-month-old infant with achondroplasia. Deformity gradually resolves in many children once independent ambulation begins. (Reproduced with permission from Bassett GS: Skeletal dysplasias and other genetic disorders, in Canale ST, Beaty JH (eds): *Operative Pediatric Orthopaedics,* ed 2. St. Louis, MO, Mosby Year-Book, 1995, pp 332–366.)

90% of children. If it is still present at 3 years of age, extension bracing may be tried. If the kyphosis persists and is greater than 40° at age 5 or 6 years, several authors recommend anterior/posterior fusion without instrumentation to attempt to avoid thoracolumbar spinal cord compression. Fusion is most strongly indicated if there is a sharp kyphosis resulting from a single wedge-shaped vertebra. Whether early surgery will, in fact, avoid later problems of stenosis is not known.

Lumbar spinal stenosis occurs most commonly in late adolescence through early adulthood. Forty to 50% of achondroplastic dwarfs develop clinically significant stenosis. Symptoms from lumbar spinal stenosis include exercise intolerance, claudication, paresthesias, and numbness. Symptoms are exacerbated by the erect posture and relieved by sitting, squatting, or bending forward as with other causes of lumbar spinal stenosis. Incontinence, impotence, and paraplegia may result from neglected lumbar stenosis. Degenerative changes in the lumbar spine (intervertebral disk degeneration with narrowing and facet joint arthropathy with joint hypertrophy) further compromise the congenitally narrow canal caused by the short, thick pedicles, narrow interpedicular distance, and thick laminae. Computed tomography (CT) and magnetic resonance imaging (MRI) help to identify the stenotic levels, which often extend from the lower thoracic spine to the sacrum. Posterior decompression of all stenotic levels is necessary for symptom resolution. Fusion is not necessary if the stenotic spine is not kyphotic as well. Instrumentation generally is contraindicated because it further compromises the congenitally stenotic canal.

Symptoms of cervical spine stenosis usually develop in the early to middle adult years. Upper and lower motor neuron signs are present with lower extremity hyperreflexia. Decompression three levels above and below the most stenotic levels without fusion is commonly recommended.

Limb lengthening techniques for treatment of skeletal dysplasias have been performed extensively in the former USSR and Italy. These procedures are useful for achondroplasia and hypochondroplasia, conditions in which the soft tissues initially appear too large for the short bones. Limb contour becomes more normal with lengthening. The callotasis method is preferred for lengthening, but significant and major complications continue to be an issue. Joint contractures require intensive physical therapy and occasional soft-tissue releases. Significant joint limitation occurs infrequently. To maintain proper proportions between the arms and legs, both humeri must be lengthened.

Studies show a high percentage of patient satisfaction with these techniques. However, the ultimate height achieved is still well below that of the average adult, and whether or not functional benefits (the ability to use public facilities and standard equipment such as automobiles) outweigh the considerable expense, morbidity, and risk is questionable. Thus, limb lengthening remains controversial.

Pseudoachondroplasia

Pseudoachondroplasia is one of the more common skeletal dysplasias, and it is characterized by disproportionate short-limbed dwarfism and ligamentous laxity.

Pseudoachondroplasia seems to be a single autosomal dominant disorder with variable expressivity. Histology of the physis shows disorganized columns with a variable reduction in the number of hypertrophic chondrocytes. The cause of this disorder is a mutation in the calmodulin-like calcium-binding region of the gene coding for cartilage oligomeric matrix protein (COMP), which is present at high levels in the territorial matrix of cartilage. The mechanism by which this defective gene causes pseudoachondroplasia is speculative, but may involve disruption of calcium-dependent proteoglycan binding by COMP that results in proteoglycan accumulation in chondrocytes.

Pseudoachondroplasia is not clinically apparent at birth, although platyspondyly is evident on radiographs. Growth retardation becomes apparent between 1 and 3 years of age. The disproportionate limb shortness increases with growth. The hands and feet are short and broad (Fig. 2). The facies are normal but tend to resemble

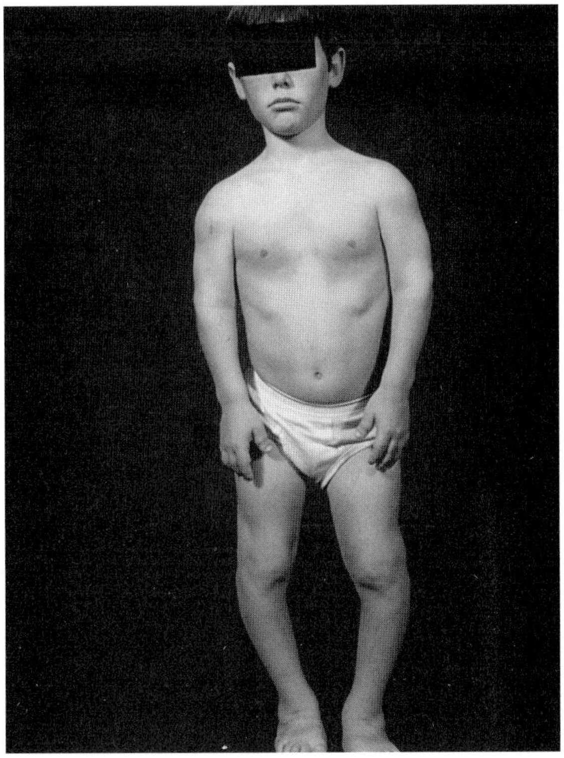

Fig. 2 Rhizomelic shortening of the extremities; broad, short hands and feet with normal head and trunk in a 12-year-old boy with pseudoachondroplasia. (Reproduced with permission from Bassett GS, Scott CI Jr: The osteochondrodysplasias, in Morrissy RT (ed): *Lovell and Winter's Pediatric Orthopaedics,* ed 3. Philadelphia, PA, JB Lippincott, 1990, pp 91–142.)

those of others who have pseudoachondroplasia. Generalized ligamentous laxity is present and is most evident in the hypermobile wrists, fingers, and knees, and markedly flexible flat feet. Although generalized laxity exists, limitation of elbow and hip motion is common. An exaggerated lumbar lordosis is usually present after walking age. Motor milestones are met at the normal ages.

The platyspondyly of infancy develops into ovoid vertebral bodies with an anterior tongue-like projection that is seen on lateral radiographs of the spine in early childhood. This projection gradually diminishes, but end-plate irregularities persist. The metaphyses are flared and irregular. Tubular bones are short. The epiphyses are small and fragmented. Lumbar spine interpedicular distances are not narrowed as seen in achondroplasia. Atlantoaxial instability may be present due to odontoid hypoplasia.

Deformity at the knee is the most common orthopaedic problem requiring treatment. The knees may be in varus, in valgus, or windswept. Recurrent deformity and overcorrection are both common after osteotomy about the knee. Overcorrection usually occurs because of a displacement of the weightbearing line medial or lateral to the knee such that the severe ligamentous laxity allows the limb to fall into an overcorrected alignment. The ligamentous laxity in this disorder requires a restoration of the mechanical axis as precisely as possible. This restoration may obligate distal femoral, proximal tibial, or simultaneous femoral and tibial osteotomies. If the epiphysis is insufficiently ossified to accurately assess the joint surface, arthrography at the time of surgery is useful in obtaining optimal alignment.

The hip presents a difficult problem. Deformity of the femoral head with extrusion, loss of motion, and premature osteoarthrosis is common. Both kyphosis and scoliosis may occur. Instrumentation and fusion may be necessary for severe or progressive deformities. Instrumentation is appropriate because congenital stenosis of the spinal canal is not present. C1 to C2 stability should be assessed before any surgical procedure and as a routine in follow-up, because of the occurrence of odontoid hypoplasia in this disorder.

Spondyloepiphyseal Dysplasia

The spondyloepiphyseal dysplasia (SED) "family" denotes a group of chondrodysplasias that are all caused by a mutation in the gene coding for type II collagen. The most severe disorder in this family is the perinatally lethal achondrogenesis type II. Hypochondrogenesis, SED congenita and tarda, Stickler syndrome, and precocious osteoarthropathy are progressively milder disorders that share a defect in type II collagen. SED congenita is usually inherited as an autosomal dominant disorder, although cases of apparent autosomal recessive inheritance have been reported. The delayed onset SEDs may be inherited as X-linked recessive.

The SEDs are characterized by disproportionate short trunk dwarfing. Most of these clinically heterogeneous disorders are evident at birth and are named congenita. The facies show mild midface flattening, the neck is short, and the chest is barrel-shaped. There is usually a thoracolumbar kyphosis with excessive lordosis in walking age children. Rhizomelic shortening of the limbs is present with fairly normal hands and feet. The vertebral bodies are ovoid in the newborn period and become markedly flattened with irregular endplates during childhood. The iliac bones are short and square. The tubular bones are short with mild metaphyseal irregularity, and the epiphyses show delayed ossification and are usually fragmented in appearance. These changes are most pronounced in the proximal femoral epiphyses. The features of SED become more apparent with growth.

There is marked variability in the severity of SED. The later onset or tarda forms of SED may not be clinically evident until late childhood or adolescence. Patients' complaints include short stature, scoliosis, and hip pain. Mild short-trunked dwarfism is due to platyspondyly. Hip radiographs may be confused with Legg-Calvé-Perthes disease, but the fragmentation changes are symmetrical.

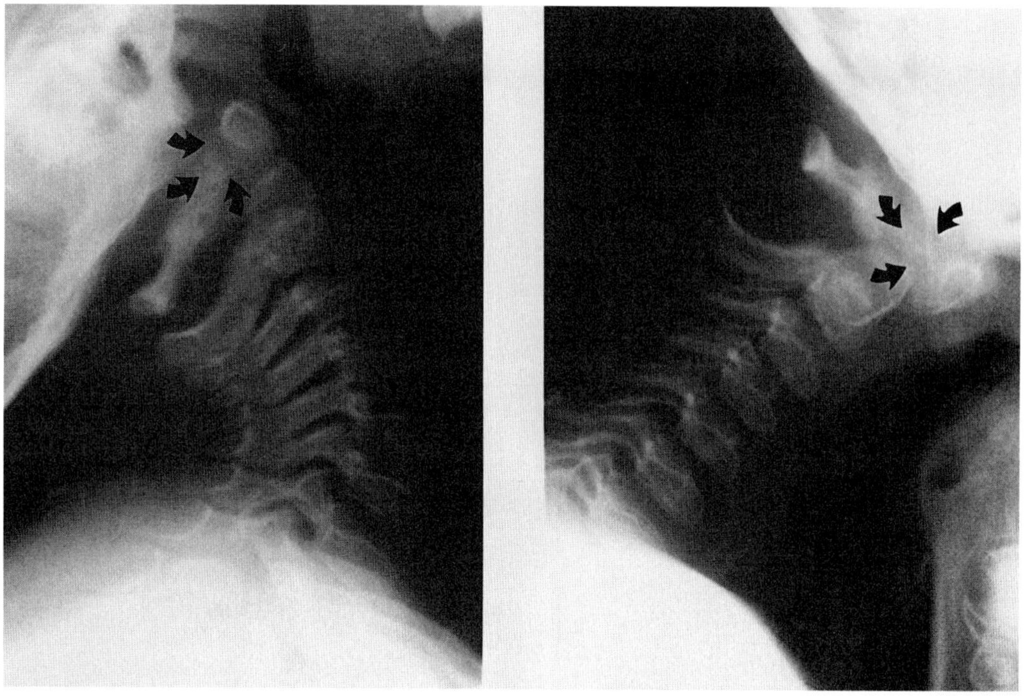

Fig. 3 Extension and flexion views show cervical instability due to odontoid hypoplasia in a patient with spondyloepiphyseal dysplasia. (Reproduced with permission from Weinstein SL, Buckwalter JA (eds): *Turek's Orthopaedics: Principles and Their Application.* Philadelphia, PA, JB Lippincott, 1994.)

Developmental milestones are met at the appropriate time. The children often have a waddling, wide-based gait that may be due to coxa vara and/or hip flexion contracture with resulting lumbar lordosis. Many patients with SED have atlantoaxial instability because of odontoid hypoplasia (Fig. 3), and spinal cord compression may occur as early as infancy. A delay in reaching motor milestones, an abnormal neurologic examination, decreased endurance, or respiratory dysfunction should prompt a search for spinal cord compression. Retinal tears are common and regular ophthalmologic evaluation and treatment are necessary to preserve vision. Premature osteoarthrosis develops in the weightbearing joints.

If spinal cord compromise from atlantoaxial instability is found, a posterior C1 to C2 fusion should be performed. Scoliosis may develop, and standard hardware can be used in surgical treatment of severe curves. Symptomatic genu valgum of more than 20° to 25° may be sufficiently severe that osteotomy is necessary. Severe coxa vara may require valgus intertrochanteric osteotomy with pelvic osteotomy. Whether surgical intervention alters the rate of degenerative arthritis in this disorder is not known.

Diastrophic Dysplasia

This is a rare skeletal dysplasia characterized by severe short-limbed dwarfism and distinctive hands with short digits and the hitchhiker (abducted, proximally displaced) thumb. At birth, babies have a narrow nasal bridge, broadened midnose, flared nostrils, and circumoral fullness. Inflammation of the external ear results in fibrosis and the typical cauliflower ear in 80% to 85% of affected children. Cleft palate and rigid foot deformities (equinovarus and valgus hindfoot with adducted midfoot) are common. Proximal interphalangeal joint fusion (symphalangism) is also common. Motion of the hips, knees, ankles, elbows is limited.

Radiographs show short tubular bones with metaphyseal flaring. The ulna and fibula are disproportionately short. The first metacarpal is ovoid in shape. Interpedicular narrowing from L1 to L5 and clefts of the cervical laminae are found. The epiphyses are delayed in appearance, irregular or fragmented, with a saucer-shaped central defect in the femoral head.

Diastrophic dysplasia is inherited in an autosomal recessive pattern. The etiology is a mutation in a gene on the long arm of chromosome 5, which codes for a novel sulfate transporter. Most people with diastrophic dysplasia have a normal life expectancy, if cardiopulmonary compromise secondary to severe scoliosis or quadriplegia secondary to cervical kyphosis does not occur.

The severity of orthopaedic anomalies is quite variable, even within families. Osteoarthritis is a common sequela of coxa vara and hip joint incongruity, and genu valgum is frequent. Treatment is complicated by the severe flexion

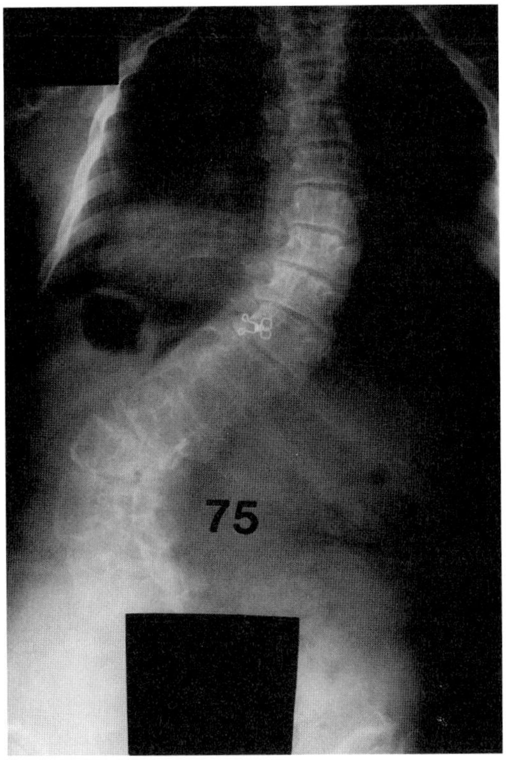

Fig. 4 Seventy-five degree kyphoscoliotic deformity in a young adult with diastrophic dysplasia. (Reproduced with permission from Bassett GS: Skeletal dysplasias and other genetic disorders, in Canale ST, Beaty JH (eds): *Operative Pediatric Orthopaedics,* ed 2. St. Louis, MO, Mosby Year-Book, 1995, pp 332–366.)

contractures that involve most joints and tend to recur after soft-tissue or bony correction. Clubfeet may require extensive soft-tissue release and talectomy to obtain plantigrade feet. Thoracolumbar spine deformity occurs in 83% of patients, with scoliosis, kyphosis, or kyphoscoliosis usually developing before the age of 4 years (Fig. 4). Early orthotic management is considered when the curves are flexible. Surgical treatment is required for curves that continue to progress. When present, cervical kyphosis may resolve or progress to result in quadriplegia. Surgery is indicated for progression or instability.

Multiple Epiphyseal Dysplasia

Multiple epiphyseal dysplasia (MED) denotes a group of disorders with epiphyseal dysplasia of the tubular bones and normal or near normal vertebrae. Dwarfing is mild and symptoms vary from childhood (a waddling gait and difficulties with running or stair climbing) to adulthood (premature osteoarthrosis). Pain, limp, or decreased range of motion in the weightbearing joints may prompt evaluation. One type of MED is caused by a mutation in the gene coding for COMP, which is the same gene that causes the defect in pseudoachondroplasia. Different kinds of mutations in the COMP genes may result in the different phenotypes of these two disorders. Another type of MED is caused by a mutation in the gene coding for the alpha 2 polypeptide chain of collagen type IX.

The ossific centers appear late and are fragmented, irregular, and flattened. The epiphyseal changes are symmetric and more pronounced in the lower extremities. The appearance of the hips may be confused with that in bilateral Legg-Calve-Perthes disease, but the changes are symmetric and epiphyses other than those of the hip are involved. Osteonecrosis may develop in addition to the underlying dysplasia, and it seems to follow the same pattern of evolution as in Legg-Calvé-Perthes disease (Fig. 5). The vertebral bodies are of normal height but may show endplate irregularity.

MED usually is inherited as an autosomal dominant trait with variable penetrance, although recessive inheritance has been reported. The pathologic abnormality is a disturbance in endochondral ossification of the epiphyses.

The natural history of the hips is quite variable. It appears that the severity of the arthritis is reasonably constant within families. Precocious arthritis is more likely when the epiphyseal ossification is fragmented, the femoral head is deformed and poorly covered, and the acetabulum is dysplastic. Whether osteotomies to improve hip biomechanics can alter the natural history of premature osteoarthrosis is uncertain. Genu varum or valgum may be sufficiently severe to warrant osteotomy, but recurrent deformity is common. Shoulder disability also is common, and minor epiphyseal abnormalities can lead to painful osteoarthritis, while severe deformity or "hatchet head" shoulder results in severe joint limitation at an early age.

Multiple Cartilaginous Exostosis

This is one of the most common skeletal dysplasias, with an estimated prevalence of nine per 1,000,000 live births. Inheritance of multiple cartilaginous exostosis is autosomal dominant, and it has been localized to three different chromosomal locations: chromosome 8 (8q24.1), chromosome 11 (pericentric), and chromosome 19 (19p). The specific gene has not been identified in any of these locations.

Most affected individuals are below the mean height for their age. Leg-length discrepancy occasionally is severe enough to require equalization procedures. The most serious potential problem is the development of chondrosarcoma, which has been reported to occur in 0.5% to 40% of patients older than 21 years of age. The true incidence is probably less than 1%. An increase in size of an exostosis or the onset of pain in an affected adult is cause for further investigation.

Cartilaginous exostoses (osteochondromas) are found throughout the endochondral skeleton, predominantly involving the long bones, iliac crests, scapulae, and ribs. They arise from the metaphyses, point away from the epiphyses, and appear to extend down the diaphysis during growth. The exostoses increase in size and number with growth, and cease growth at skeletal maturity. Bones with

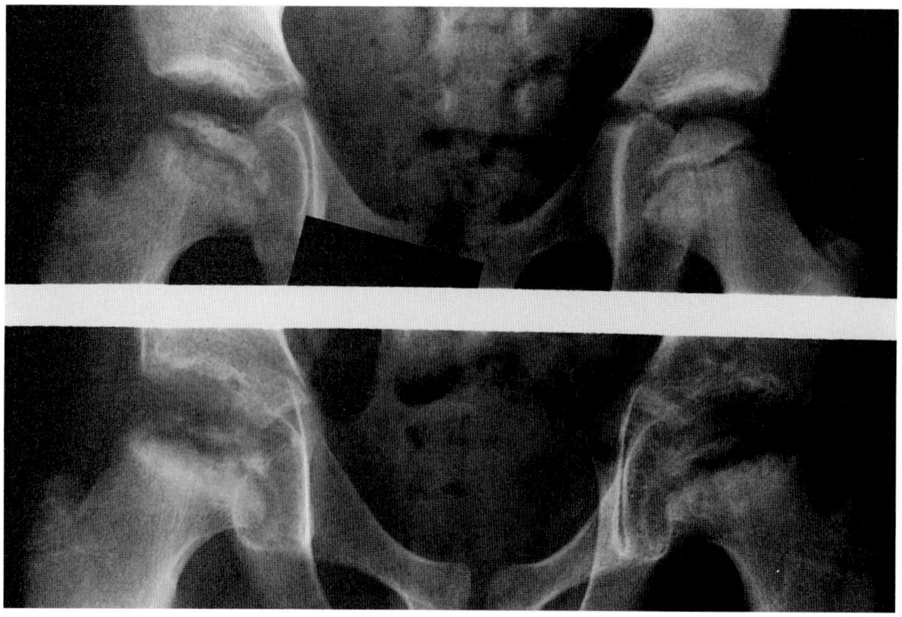

Fig. 5 Bilateral femoral head fragmentation and flattening in a patient with multiple epiphyseal dysplasia. (Reproduced with permission from Balderston RA, Rothman, RH (eds): *The Hip.* Malvern, PA, Lea & Febiger, 1992.)

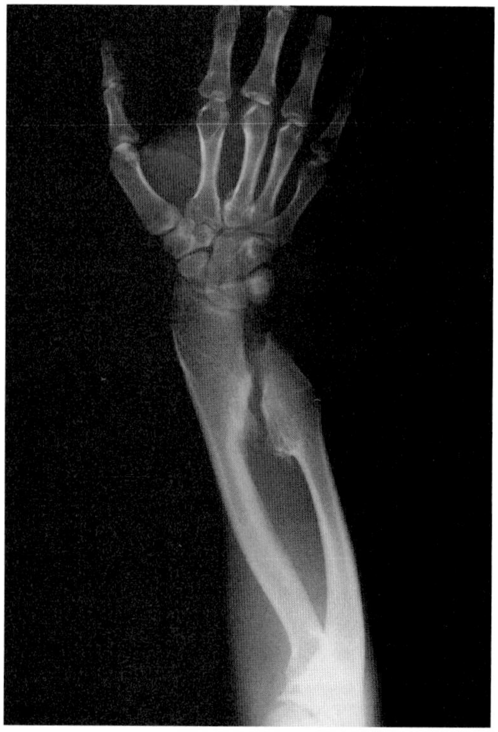

Fig. 6 Multiple cartilaginous exostosis of the distal radius and ulna in a 17-year-old resulting in shortening and bowing of the forearm. (Reproduced with permission from Bassett GS, Scott CI Jr: The osteochondrodysplasias, in Morrissy RT (ed): *Lovell and Winter's Pediatric Orthopaedics,* ed 3. Philadelphia, PA, JB Lippincott, 1990, pp 91–142.)

the smallest cross-sectional area at the epiphyses are more affected. In two bone extremities, differential growth results in angular deformities. In the upper extremities, shortening of the ulna leads to radial bowing, ulnar tilt at the distal radius, ulnar translation at the carpus, and radial head subluxation or dislocation (Fig. 6). Forearm rotation may be limited. In the lower extremity the fibula is more involved, resulting in valgus deformity of the ankle, diastasis of the ankle, and genu valgum.

Surgical excision of the entire osteocartilaginous lesion is indicated when symptoms are caused by pressure on peripheral nerves, vessels, or tendons or when there is interference with normal joint mobility. Excision may also be done if an exostosis is contributing to an angular deformity or if the appearance is cosmetically unacceptable. Osteotomy and/or hemiepiphysiodesis occasionally may be required for valgus angular deformities about the knee and ankle. Surgical options vary for osteochondroma of the ulna with shortening and radial head subluxation.

Metaphyseal Chondrodysplasia

The several metaphyseal chondrodysplasias are characterized by radiographic abnormalities of the metaphyses of the tubular bones. Jansen type, an autosomal dominant disorder of unknown etiology, is a rare, severe disorder characterized at birth by severe limb shortening with a prominent forehead and micrognathia. The tubular bones are short, and the metaphyses are markedly flared with irregular ossification. During childhood, the lower extremities become bowed with enlarged joints. Flexion contractures develop at the hips and knees.

Schmid type metaphyseal chondrodysplasia becomes apparent at 2 to 3 years of age because of mild short stature, genu varum, excessive lumbar lordosis, and a waddling gait (due to coxa vara). The tubular bones are short, with cupping and flaring of the metaphyses and a widened physis. Schmid type is autosomal dominant; a mutation in the gene coding for type X collagen has been found to cause this disorder. Coxa vara, if very severe or progressive, is treated by intertrochanteric valgus osteotomy. The varus bowing of the lower extremities may spontaneously improve in childhood. However, if it is progressive or severe, proximal tibial osteotomy is appropriate.

McKusick type metaphyseal chondrodysplasia (cartilage-hair hypoplasia) also becomes apparent in the second or third year, although the dwarfing is progressive and marked in adults. Children have bowed legs; short, broad hands and feet; and stubby fingers with severe ligamentous laxity. The hair is blond or light compared to relatives and very fine. The knees show metaphyseal cupping and flaring (Fig. 7); the hips do not have coxa vara and are mildly affected. This disorder is autosomal recessive and is especially common in the Amish population. Neutropenia, lymphopenia, immune deficiency, pancreatic exocrine insufficiency, Hirschsprung's disease, and intestinal malabsorption have occurred in people with McKusick type metaphyseal chondrodysplasia.

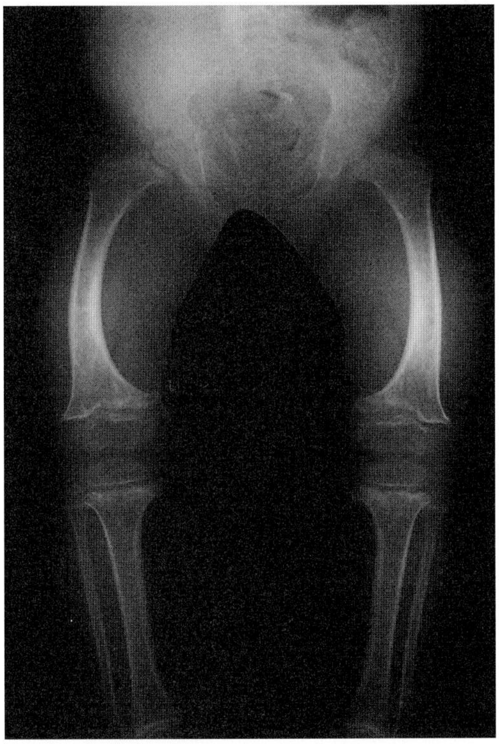

Fig. 7 Metaphyseal cupping and flaring, mild coxa vara, and femoral and tibial bowing in a 4-year-old with McKusick-type metaphyseal chondrodysplasia. (Reproduced with permission from Bassett GS, Scott CI Jr: The osteochondrodysplasias, in Morrissy RT (ed): *Lovell and Winter's Pediatric Orthopaedics,* ed 3. Philadelphia, PA, JB Lippincott, 1990, pp 91–142.)

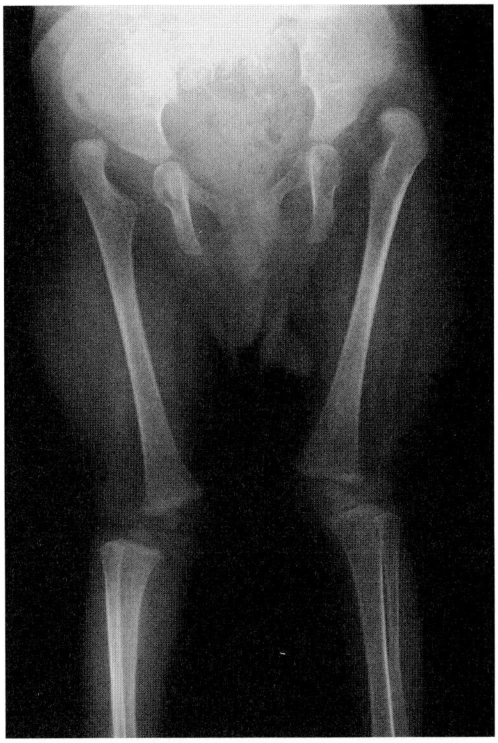

Fig. 8 Bilateral dislocations of the hips and knees in a 9-month-old infant with Larsen syndrome. (Reproduced with permission from Bassett GS, Scott CI Jr: The osteochondrodysplasias, in Morrissy RT (ed): *Lovell and Winter's Pediatric Orthopaedics,* ed 3. Philadelphia, PA, JB Lippincott, 1990, pp 91–142.)

Larsen Syndrome

Larsen syndrome consists of typical facies (a flat face with ocular hypertelorism and a depressed nasal bridge) and multiple congenital joint dislocations. The hips, knees, and radial heads are most commonly dislocated (Fig. 8), although other joints may be affected. Clubfoot deformity is typical, and 25% of affected individuals have cleft palates. A broad thumb may be present. Radiographs are typical for congenital dislocations of the involved joints. Some individuals have an unusual ossification center posterior to the primary ossification center of the calcaneus.

The etiology is unknown, and Larsen syndrome's inheritance may be autosomal dominant or recessive. The differential diagnosis includes arthrogryposis multiplex congenita, skeletal dysplasia, chromosomal anomalies, and Ehlers-Danlos syndrome.

Treatment of dislocations of the knee and hip has mirrored treatment in other teratologic syndromes: serial casting for knee subluxations, surgical treatments of more severe deformities, and, commonly, open reduction of the hip with primary femoral shortening. Foot deformities often are resistant to manipulation and serial casting and require surgical treatment. Spinal anomalies are common and should be detected early. Cervical dysraphism and hypoplasia, thoracic scoliosis, lumbar scoliosis, spondylolysis, and lumbar dysraphism have all been reported. The cervical anomalies may result in a severe kyphosis. Surgical stabilization of progressive kyphosis and scoliosis is warranted.

Enchondromatosis

Enchondromatosis (Ollier disease) is characterized by linear masses of cartilage in the metaphyses and diaphyses of the long bones. The extent of the lesions varies greatly, and distribution is asymmetric and often unilateral. The cartilaginous lesions may expand the involved bone causing deformity and inhibition of growth (Fig. 9). Pathologic fractures may occur. Lesions enlarge during growth, ceasing at puberty.

Most cases of enchondromatosis are sporadic, although familial occurrence has been reported. Orthopaedic treatment often is required to correct limb-length discrepancies and to realign the deformities. Epiphysiodesis can be used when the discrepancies are small. Limb lengthening methods can be used both to lengthen and to realign a significantly shortened and deformed extremity.

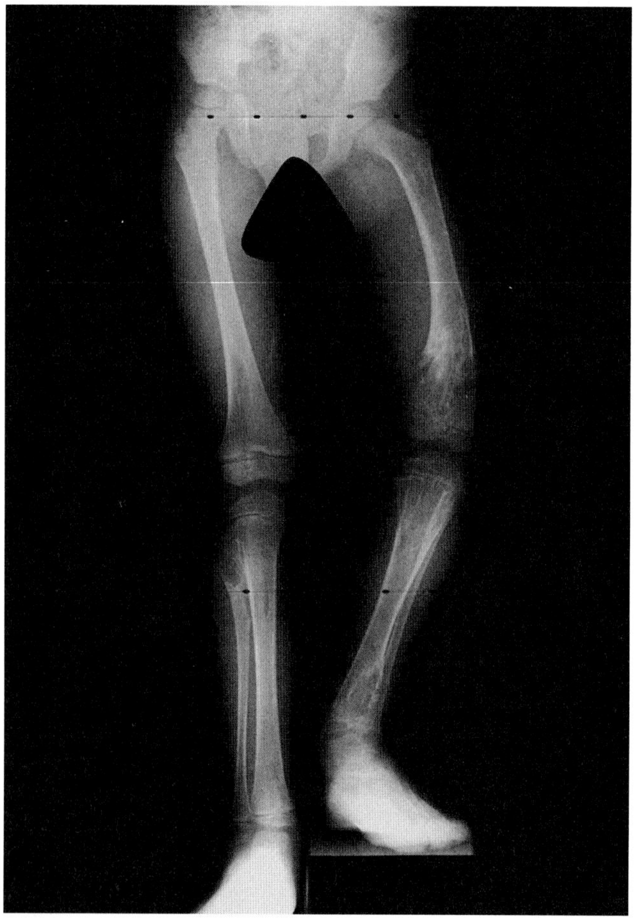

Fig. 9 Limb-length inequality (5 cm) in a 5-year-old boy with multiple enchondromas. (Reproduced with permission from Bassett GS, Scott CI Jr: The osteochondrodysplasias, in Morrissy RT (ed): *Lovell and Winter's Pediatric Orthopaedics,* ed 3. Philadelphia, PA, JB Lippincott, 1990, pp 91–142.)

The incidence of sarcomatous changes, often heralded by localized growth or pain in adults, is unknown. Although malignant degeneration has been reported in up to 25% of lesions, it is believed that selection bias in these series has overstated the incidence. The chondrosarcomas that occur are usually low-grade.

When enchondromatosis is accompanied by hemangiomata it is called Maffucci syndrome. Many malignant tumors have been reported in this syndrome. Although the exact incidence of malignant transformation is unknown, it is probably higher than in enchondromatosis alone.

Mucopolysaccharidoses

Mucopolysaccharidoses are caused by a defect in various enzymes necessary for lysosomal glycosaminoglycan degradation. Accumulation of these substances in different organs results in a variety of phenotypes of differing severity. Most are characterized by short stature, hepatosplenomegaly, corneal clouding, deafness, cardiac disease, and joint contractures. With the exception of X-linked recessive Hunter syndrome, all are inherited as autosomal recessive traits. Diagnosis is difficult and includes urine screening for glycosaminoglycans (dermatan sulfate, heparan sulfate, keratan sulfate and chondroitin sulfate); analysis of blood, bone marrow, skin, and liver samples; and white blood cell (WBC) enzyme analysis. Conjunctival biopsy with ultrastructural evaluation establishes the diagnosis in most cases. These disorders are classified by the specific enzyme involved and the clinical course (Table 1). Different phenotypes may be caused by the same enzyme defect, and different enzyme defects can cause similar clinical disorders. For example, Hurler syndrome and Scheie

Table 1. The mucopolysaccharidoses

Type	Syndrome	Biochemical Defect
I	Hurler, Hurler-Scheie, and Scheie	α-L-Iduronidase
II	Hunter	Sulfoid uronate sulfatase
IIIA	Sanfilippo A	Heparan N-sulfatase
IIIB	Sanfilippo B	N-Acetyl-α-D-glucosaminidase
IIIC	Sanfilippo C	Acetyl CoA: α-glucosaminide-N-acetyltransferase
IIID	Sanfilippo D	N-Acetyl-α-D-glucoaminide-β-sulfatase
IVA	Morquio A	N-Acetylgalactosamine-6-sulfatase
IVB	Morquio B	β-Galactosidase
VI	Moroteaux-Lamy	N-acetylgalactosamine-4-sulfate
VII	Sly	β-Glucuronidase

(Adapted with permission from Frymoyer JW (ed): *Orthopaedic Knowledge Update 4.* Rosemont, IL, American Academy of Orthopaedic Surgeons, 1993, pp 125–140.)

syndrome share the same enzyme defect, but Hurler syndrome is lethal and Scheie syndrome is quite mild. Three are discussed—Hurler syndrome (MPS I-H), Hunter syndrome (MPS II), and Morquio syndrome (MPS IV-A and -B).

Hurler syndrome is characterized by coarse facial features, hepatosplenomegaly, progressive neurologic deterioration, cardiac disease (congestive heart disease or myocardial infarction), and progressive airway obstruction. The hands become broad and stubby, with stiff, flexed interphalangeal joints. Motion of large joints is limited, and equinus of the ankles is common. Genu valgum, coxa valga, and pes planus may develop. Thoracolumbar kyphosis often is present. The tubular bones show thinning of the cortices and an enlarged medullary canal. The disorder is recognizable before 2 years of age and usually is fatal by 10 years of age as a result of cardiac disease or respiratory failure. The only effective treatment is bone marrow transplantation, which must be done early for optimal results, because established brain damage and skeletal malformations are not reversible. Rarely, the thoracolumbar kyphosis may be sufficiently acute and severe to threaten spinal cord compression. Because of the poor quality of the bone, anterior and posterior fusion may be necessary, although success with posterior fusion alone in lesser amounts of kyphosis maybe successful. Anesthesia in these patients has special risks due to airway disease, cardiac disease, and cervical spine pathology. The perioperative mortality is as high as 20%.

Hunter syndrome shares many features with Hurler syndrome: coarse facial features, hepatosplenomegaly, short stature, and stiff joints. However, Hunter syndrome patients lack corneal clouding and the thoracolumbar kyphosis, mental deterioration is slower, and survival is longer. A severe form results in death by 15 years of age, but the milder variant allows survival into early adulthood. Inheritance is X-linked recessive. The joints are stiff and flexed, and movement of all joints is limited and painful. Osteoarthrosis develops in the longer surviving patients. Radiographs show bone changes similar to but less severe than in Hurler syndrome. Occasionally, orthotic treatment for the ankles or tendo Achilles lengthening is helpful. A mild scoliosis is common, but it rarely progresses sufficiently to require treatment.

Morquio syndrome is characterized by short stature, barrel chest with pectus carinatum, and a short neck. Affected people have hyperlaxity of joints, lack organomegaly, have normal facies, and have unimpaired intellect in contrast to most mucopolysaccharidoses. The clinical features, which appear in the second or third year of life, include growth retardation, genu valgum, sternal bulging, flat feet, and thoracic kyphosis. Platyspondyly with kyphoscoliosis is typical. Early development of the hips is normal, but progressive fragmentation and flattening occur. Ligamentous laxity results in C1 to C2 instability in a large number of patients. Symptoms often are nonspecific, such as a decrease in exercise tolerance, diffuse leg aching, or difficulty climbing stairs. A search for atlantoaxial instability may be life-saving because upper spinal-cord compression has been a major cause of death. Fusion is indicated if instability is present. Because growth stops by age 8 years, osteotomy to correct genu valgum should be delayed to this age to avoid recurrence.

Genetic Disorders

Trisomy 21: Down Syndrome

Down syndrome occurs in approximately one of every 700 to 800 live newborns. Growth and development are delayed, and affected children are of short stature. The IQ range is quite wide. Because 50% of children have some hearing loss that can affect intellectual development, audiology examinations are necessary. The onset of ambulation is delayed to between ages 18 months and 3 years, and the characteristic gait is broad based and waddling. Congenital heart defects are present in 30% to 50% of affected individuals. One third are endocardial cushion defects, and one third ventricular septal defects. Gastrointestinal malformations are present in 5%. The mortality rate is increased during the first 10 years, even when deaths resulting from congenital heart defects are excluded. This problem is believed to be caused by an increased susceptibility to infections. Ninety percent of children without significant congenital defects, however, live to adulthood.

Orthopaedic problems are predominantly related to ligamentous laxity. The most significant problem is atlantoaxial instability with an anterior C1 to C2 interval greater than 5 mm, which occurs in approximately 10% to 15%. Recent reviews have demonstrated a very significant complication rate in cervical fusions for instability. Prophylactic fusion is not indicated. Fusions should be reserved for those with neurologic symptoms and findings or severe instability with a marginal space available for the spinal cord.

An idiopathic scoliotic pattern develops in 50% of involved individuals. It should be managed according to the usual criteria with bracing and posterior spinal fusion.

Recurrent subluxations of the patella occur in one third of the individuals, while 10% have recurrent dislocations. Physical therapy is difficult in these children, but surgical results are compromised by recurrence caused by ligamentous laxity. One out of 20 children will be affected with hip instability during the first decade. Acute dislocations, habitual dislocation, subluxation, and progressive instability and dysplasia may continue into childhood. Treatment must be tailored to each anatomic problem, but soft-tissue procedures should be supplemented by correction of bony deformities with femoral and/or pelvic osteotomy to obtain stability.

Slipped capital femoral epiphysis may be seen in these individuals, and screening for hypothyroidism should be performed. Planovalgus deformities of the feet are common but rarely symptomatic. Metatarsus primus varus is often found and may result in a symptomatic hallux valgus deformity.

Neurofibromatosis

Neurofibromatosis is the most common single gene disorder in humans. It is autosomal dominant, with a nearly complete penetrance. Half of reported cases are new mutations.

There are two forms of neurofibromatosis. NF-1 has a gene location on chromosome 17 and an incidence of one in 3,500 live births. The gene responsible codes for the protein neurofibromin, which is a signal transduction protein. The molecular pathology is not yet elucidated. NF-2, with a gene location on chromosome 22, is far less common, with an incidence of one in 50,000 births. The mutant gene codes for schwannomin, which is a protein that links the cytoskeleton to the plasma membrane. The mechanism by which this defect creates the NF-2 phenotype is not yet known. In NF-2 there are fewer peripheral lesions, but more significant intracranial ones, including bilateral acoustic neuromas and other tumors of the meninges and Schwann cells (Outline 1).

Outline 1. **Criteria for NF-1 and NF-2**

Criteria for NF-1 (2 or more of the following):
1. Six or more café-au-lait macules whose greatest diameter is 5 mm in prepubertal patients and 15 mm in postpubertal patients
2. Two or more neurofibromas of any type or one plexiform neurofibroma
3. Freckling in the axillary or inguinal regions
4. Optic glioma
5. Two or more Lisch nodules (iris hamartomas)
6. A distinctive osseous lesion, such as sphenoid dysplasia or thinning of long bone cortex, with or without pseudarthrosis
7. A first-degree relative (parent, sibling, or child) with NF-1 by the above criteria

Criteria for NF-2 (1 of the following):
1. Bilateral eighth nerve masses seen with appropriate imaging techniques (eg. computed tomography or magnetic resonance imaging)
2. NF-2 in a first-degree relative, and either a unilateral eighth nerve mass or two of the following: neurofibroma, meningioma, glioma, schwannoma, or juvenile posterior subcapsular lenticular opacity

(Reproduced with permission from Aoki S, Barkovich AJ, Nishimura K, et al: Neurofibromatosis types 1 and 2: Cranial MR findings. *Radiology* 1989;172:527–534.)

Affected individuals tend to be short with large heads, and they frequently experience precocious puberty. Seizures are another finding, and varying degrees of intellectual deficiency are present in 50%.

The diagnostic clinical appearance of the disease varies widely, and many affected individuals appear normal at birth. The typical neurofibromas begin to appear by age 10 years. They increase in size and number during puberty. Lesions are composed of benign Schwann cells and fibrous connective tissue. They are either sessile or peduncular and may develop along the path of a peripheral nerve or motor root. They rarely cause neurologic deficit.

Plexiform neurofibromas present a much more serious problem. Although histologically benign, they cause the significant problems of limb overgrowth and gigantism, infiltration of the neuraxis, and grotesque facial disfigurement. Because the lesions are highly vascular, surgical removal usually is impractical. Partial gigantism and macrodactyly usually are related to the plexiform neurofibromas. The overgrowth does not symmetrically involve all parts, and the skeleton often is variably involved. Erosion and cystic changes may occur within bones and may mimic other diseases.

Malignancies occur in 5% to 15% of affected individuals. Neurofibromas in adolescence and adulthood may undergo malignant degeneration, or malignant neurofibrosarcomas may appear de novo. Other malignancies, such as rhabdomyosarcoma, are more likely.

A major orthopaedic problem is present in at least 40% of these individuals. Neurofibromatosis must be considered when evaluating a patient with a significant scoliosis or spinal deformity; pseudarthrosis of the tibia, fibula, radius, or ulna; hypertrophy of a part; or an unusual radiographic lesion.

Scoliosis occurs frequently, and it may be the presenting symptom. Curvatures are either idiopathic or dystrophic. The dystrophic type is short (four to six spinal segments) and sharp. The classic radiographic findings are scalloping of the posterior vertebral bodies, enlargement of the neuroforamen, defective eroded pedicles, and thinning or pencilling of the ribs. The enlarged neuroforamen may occur with normal intraspinal contents, but may also be indicative of intraspinal tumor, dumbbell neurofibroma, dural ectasia, and lateral meningocele. The idiopathic variety is treated as such. Dysplastic curvatures usually are progressive with no benefit from treatment. (See Chapter 45.)

Spinal stability often is lost because of the pedicular changes that lead to subluxations or dislocations throughout the spine. Cervical kyphosis commonly is associated with a dystrophic thoracic curve and must be evaluated before using endotracheal anesthesia. Spinal dislocation with minimal or no neurologic defects can occur, because the dural ectasia causes significant erosion, leaving more space for the neural elements. Stabilization alone without reduction, which avoids dissection near the precarious neural elements, may reverse early neurologic findings in selected patients.

Pseudarthrosis usually involves the tibia and appears in infancy with the classic anterolateral bow. The ulna, femur, clavicle, radius, and humerus may also be involved. The relationship of pseudarthrosis to neurofibromatosis is well established, but the mechanism remains unknown. The prognosis for establishing a solid union remains guarded. Recent reports suggest an acceptable union rate with intramedullary rodding and bone grafting; vascularized fibula transfer and Ilizarov technique are reserved for failure of rodding and grafting.

Magnetic resonance imaging studies have demonstrated a high sensitivity and allow the detection of intracranial lesions and the differentiation of type I from type II neurofibromatosis. Such studies of the spine are mandatory before surgery to detect the intraspinal lesions of neurofibroma, dural ectasia, and meningocele can be undertaken.

Annotated Bibliography

General

Bassett GS: Orthopaedic aspects of skeletal dysplasias, in Greene WB (ed): *Instructional Course Lectures XXXIX.* Park Ridge, IL, American Academy of Orthopaedic Surgeons, 1990, pp 381–387.

This is a to-the-point review of the characteristics of achondroplasia, diastrophic dysplasia, pseudoachondroplasia, spondyloepiphyseal dysplasia, multiple epiphyseal dysplasia, and metaphyseal chondrodysplasias.

Bassett GS: Lower-extremity abnormalities in dwarfing conditions, in Greene WB (ed): *Instructional Course Lectures XXXIX.* Park Ridge, IL, American Academy of Orthopaedic Surgeons, 1990, pp 389–397.

This is a practical, concise guide to the treatment of the most common extremity deformities in patients with skeletal dysplasias.

Horton WA, Hecht JT: The chondrodysplasias, in Royce PM, Steinmann B (eds): *Connective Tissue and its Heritable Disorders: Molecular, Genetic, and Medical Aspects.* New York, NY, Wiley-Liss, 1993, pp 641–675.

This chapter from a recent textbook is well organized, thoughtful, and complete for use as a reference or as an easy update on the skeletal dysplasias.

Jacenko O, Olsen BR, Warman ML: Editorial: Of mice and men: Heritable skeletal disorders. *Am J Hum Genet* 1994;54:163–168.

This is a superb and brief review of the state of knowledge of the causation of skeletal dysplasias and the directions of future research. Some familiarity with the vocabulary of molecular genetics is required.

Rimoin DL, Lachman RS: Genetic disorders of the osseous skeleton, in Beighton P (ed): *McKusick's Heritable Disorders of Connective Tissue,* ed 5. St. Louis, MO, Mosby-Year Book, 1993, pp 557–689.

This chapter from a recent textbook gives detailed information on common and rare skeletal dysplasias that was up to date as of publication.

Tolo VT: Spinal deformity in short-stature syndromes, in Greene WB (ed): *Instructional Course Lectures XXXIX.* Park Ridge, IL, American Academy of Orthopaedic Surgeons, 1990, pp 399–405.

This is a practical, reasoned approach to the challenging spinal problems in this patient population.

Achondroplasia

Shiang R, Thompson LM, Zhu Y-Z, et al: Mutations in the transmembrane domain of FGFR3 cause the most common genetic form of dwarfism, achondroplasia. *Cell* 1994;78:335–342.

The cause of achondroplasia is identified as a point mutation in the gene coding for fibroblast growth factor receptor 3, which is expressed in all cartilage anlage and the resting cells of the physis.

Diastrophic Dysplasia

Hastbacka J, de la Chapelle A, Mahtani MM, et al: The diastrophic dysplasia gene encodes a novel sulfate transporter: Positional cloning by fine-structure linkage disequilibrium mapping. *Cell* 1994;78:1073–1087.

The abnormal sulfate transporter probably impairs sulfation of proteoglycans in the cartilage matrix, thereby causing the disease phenotype.

Poussa M, Merikanto J, Ryoppy S, et al: The spine in diastrophic dysplasia. *Spine* 1991;16:881–887.

Spinal problems in 101 patients of varying ages are presented including cervical kyphosis, scoliosis, and spinal stenosis with comments about natural history and treatment.

Ryoppy S, Poussa M, Merikanto J, et al: Foot deformities in diastrophic dysplasia: An analysis of 102 patients. *J Bone Joint Surg* 1992;74B:441–444.

This report of 102 patients with diastrophic dysplasia found 43% of feet had hindfoot valgus and midfoot adductus; 29% equinovarus adductus; 8% equinus; 13% adductus; and 7% normal. Brief observations on natural history and treatment are included.

Multiple Cartilaginous Exostosis

Cook A, Raskind W, Blanton SH, et al: Genetic heterogeneity in families with hereditary multiple exostoses. *Am J Hum Genet* 1993;53:71–79.

Eleven families were studied of which 70% showed linkage to a region of chromosome 8, while the other families did not. This difference demonstrates genetic heterogeneity that may explain clinical heterogeneity among different families.

Schmale GA, Conrad EU III, Raskind WH, et al: The natural history of hereditary multiple exostoses. *J Bone Joint Surg* 1994;76A:986–992.

This longitudinal study of 46 kindreds found 39% with forearm deformity, 10% leg length discrepancy, 8% knee deformity, 2% ankle deformity, 0.9% incidence of chondrosarcoma, and functional ratings of 47% fair or poor, 53% good or excellent.

Metaphyseal Chondrodysplasia

Dharmavaram RM, Elberson MA, Peng M, et al: Identification of a mutation in type X collagen in a family with Schmid metaphyseal chondrodysplasia. *Hum Mol Genet* 1994;3:507–509.

A third family with Schmid metaphyseal chondrodysplasia is reported with a defect in the gene for type X collagen, which is expressed only in the hypertrophic zone of the physis and is probably involved in endochondral ossification.

Larsen Syndrome

Bowen JR, Ortega K, Ray S, et al: Spinal deformities in Larsen's syndrome. *Clin Orthop* 1985;197:159–163.

A review of eight patients reports the common spinal anomalies, including cervical dysraphism and hypolasia, thoracic scoliosis, and lumbar scoliosis, spondylolysis, and dysraphism.

Lutter LD: Larsen syndrome: Clinical features and treatment: A report of two cases. *J Pediatr Orthop* 1990;10:270–274.

Two cases of sporadic Larsen syndrome are reported and their management detailed with emphasis on one patient's several postoperative wound dehiscences.

Mucopolysaccharidoses

Whitley CB: The mucopolysaccharidoses, in Beighton P (ed): *McKusick's Heritable Disorders of Connective Tissue,* ed 5. St. Louis, MO, Mosby-Year Book, 1993, pp 367–499.

This is a recent complete review of the etiology, manifestations, and treatment of these disorders.

Down Syndrome

Shaw ED, Beals RK: The hip joint in Down's syndrome: A study of its structure and associated disease. *Clin Orthop* 1992;278:101–107.

Radiographs of the hips in 114 patients (mostly skeletally mature) with Down syndrome revealed abnormalities in 11 of 228 hips (4.8%) including dislocation, acetabular dysplasia, Legg-Perthes disease, and slipped capital femoral epiphysis.

Neurofibromatosis

Craig JB, Govender S: Neurofibromatosis of the cervical spine: A report of eight cases. *J Bone Joint Surg* 1992;74B: 575–578.

Eight patients, half in the second decade, presented with neurological deficit, mass, or deformity and typically with severe kyphosis who required anterior or combined anterior/posterior fusion for successful treatment.

Funasaki H, Winter RB, Lonstein JB, et al: Pathophysiology of spinal deformities in neurofibromatosis: An analysis of seventy-one patients who had curves associated with dystrophic changes. *J Bone Joint Surg* 1994;76A: 692–700.

Review of spinal deformity in 71 neurofibromatosis patients revealed the following risk factors for progression: early age of onset, a greater curve at presentation, vertebral scalloping, severe apical rotation, apex in the mid or lower thoracic spine, and penciling of ribs.

Gutmann DH, Collins FS: Recent progress toward understanding the molecular biology of von Recklinghausen neurofibromatosis. *Ann Neurol* 1992;31: 555–561.

The gene for type 1 neurofibromatosis codes for a ubiquitously expressed, cytoplasmic protein that may act as a tumor suppresser gene.

Joseph KN, Bowen JR, MacEwen GD: Unusual orthopedic manifestations of neurofibromatosis. *Clin Orthop* 1992;278:17–28.

This is a description of 44 children with three relatively uncommon manifestations of neurofibromatosis—thoracic lordoscoliosis, protrusio acetabuli, and monomelia neurofibromatosis—with recommendations for management.

Classic Bibliography

Aldegheri R, Trivella G, Renzi-Brivio L, et al: Lengthening of the lower limbs in achondroplastic patients: A comparative study of four techniques. *J Bone Joint Surg* 1988;70B:69–73.

Anderson IJ, Goldberg RB, Marion RW, et al: Spondyloepiphyseal dysplasia congenita: Genetic linkage to type II collagen (COL2AI). *Am J Hum Genet* 1990; 46:896–901.

Cattaneo R, Villa A, Catagni MA, et al: Lengthening of the humerus using the Ilizarov technique: Description of the method and report of 43 cases. *Clin Orthop* 1990; 250:117–124.

Crawford AH: Pitfalls of spinal deformities associated with neurofibromatosis in children. *Clin Orthop* 1989; 245:29–42.

Goldberg MJ: *The Dysmorphic Child: An Orthopedic Perspective.* New York, NY, Raven Press, 1987.

Habermann ET, Sterling A, Dennis RI: Larsen's syndrome: A heritable disorder. *J Bone Joint Surg* 1976;58A:558–561.

Hecht JT, Francomano CA, Horton WA, et al: Mortality in achondroplasia. *Am J Hum Genet* 1987;41:454–464.

Horton WA: New insights into the chondrodysplasias. *Surg Rounds Orthop* 1990;4:24–30.

Maffulli N, Fixsen JA: Pseudoarthrosis in the ulna in neurofibromatosis: A report of four cases. *Arch Orthop Trauma Surg* 1991;110:204–207.

McCann PD, Herbert J, Feldman F, et al: Neuropathic arthropathy associated with neurofibromatosis: A case report. *J Bone Joint Surg* 1992;74A:1411–1414.

Narod SA, Parry DM, Parboosingh J, et al: Neurofibromatosis type 2 appears to be a genetically homogeneous disease. *Am J Hum Genet* 1992;51:486–496.

Peltonen JI, Hoikka V, Poussa M, et al: Cementless hip arthroplasty in diastrophic dysplasia. *J Arthroplasty* 1992:7(suppl):369–376.

Price CT: Limb lengthening for achondroplasia: Early experience. *J Pediatr Orthop* 1989;9:512–515.

Robertson FW, Kozlowski K, Middleton RW: Larsen's syndrome. *Clin Pediatr* 1975;14:53–60.

Rogalski RP, Louis DS: Neurofibrosarcomas of the upper extremity. *J Hand Surg* 1991;16A:873–876.

Saleh M, Burton M: Leg lengthening: Patient selection and management in achondroplasia. *Orthop Clin North Am* 1991;22:589–599.

Shapiro F: Light and electron microscopic abnormalities in diastrophic dysplasia growth cartilage. *Calcif Tissue Int* 1992;51:324–331.

Sher C, Ramesar R, Martell R, et al: Mild spondyloepiphyseal dysplasia (Namaqualand type): Genetic linkage to the type II collagen gene (COL2AI). *Am J Hum Genet* 1991;48:518–524.

Segal LS, Drummond DS, Zanotti RM: Complications of posterior arthrodesis of the cervical spine in patients who have Down syndrome. *J Bone Joint Surg* 1991;73A: 1547–1554.

Treble NJ, Jensen FO, Bankier A, et al: Development of the hip in multiple epiphyseal dysplasia: Natural history and susceptibility to premature osteoarthritis. *J Bone Joint Surg* 1990;72B:1061–1064.

Tredwell SJ, Newman DE, Lockitch G: Instability of the upper cervical spine in Down syndrome. *J Pediatr Orthop* 1990;10:602–606.

Vilarrubias JM, Ginebreda I, Jimeno E: Lengthening of the lower limbs and correction of lumbar hyperlordosis in achondroplasia. *Clin Orthop* 1990;250:143–149.

21

Neuromuscular Disorders In Children

Introduction

Neuromuscular diseases represent a substantial proportion of the disorders that confront the orthopaedist who evaluates and treats children. A specific diagnosis should be sought and confirmed as appropriate whenever a clinically significant neuromuscular disorder is suspected. A careful birth and developmental history of the patient, as well as a family history, should be obtained. Physical examination should identify muscle tone and strength, sensory disturbances, and reflexes. The presence of hyperreflexia and pathologic reflexes, such as Babinski and Hoffman, should be determined. Specific signs of neuromuscular disease, such as cavovarus feet in Charcot-Marie-Tooth disease or Friedreich ataxia, Gowers' sign in Duchenne muscular dystrophy, and abnormal grasp and release in the myotonic dystrophies, should be sought. Muscle enzymes, muscle and nerve biopsies, and electrophysiologic investigations in consultation with a neurologist should be obtained as necessary to confirm a specific diagnosis.

Cerebral Palsy

When static encephalopathy is suspected, any possible etiology for the disorder should be elicited from the patient's history. The most common cause of cerebral palsy is premature birth, but prenatal factors, such as drug abuse or maternal infection, or postnatal disorders, such as significant head injury, encephalitis, or meningitis, may all cause central neurologic injury. If no clear cause of gross motor delay or abnormal neurologic findings can be determined from the history, the patient may be evaluated by a neurologist in an effort to identify the etiology.

The goals of orthopaedic intervention in patients with static encephalopathy are to prevent deformity in the nonambulatory patients and to maximize mobility in patients who are capable of ambulation. Nonambulatory patients should be examined periodically for evidence of diminishing hip abduction as a precursor of hip subluxation or dislocation and scoliosis. Diminishing hip abduction, especially in conjunction with radiographic evidence of hip subluxation, should be treated with adductor release and hip flexor lengthening in children 4 years old and younger. In children over 4 years of age, femoral varus osteotomy also may be required. Severe acetabular dysplasia may require shelf, Dega, or Chiari osteotomy to provide adequate coverage of the femoral head (Fig. 1).

Unchecked progressive scoliosis in a wheelchair-dependent child may result in the loss of comfortable independent or even prop sitting. In younger patients, a thoracolumbar orthosis may be tried, but this treatment usually is poorly tolerated. Stable segmental posterior fusion to the pelvis is indicated when loss of sitting balance is evident.

Ambulatory patients with flexible lower extremity deformities can benefit greatly from the use of light-weight lower extremity bracing with upper extremity aid (walker or crutches) as needed for balance. Soft-tissue lengthenings or selected tendon transfers of the hip, knee, and ankle should be considered when contractures are progressive and are interfering with otherwise functionally effective bracing. It is important to evaluate the spine, hip, knee, and ankle in a comprehensive manner. One-level tendon lengthening is uncommon because it may exacerbate the crouched gait; "three-level" lengthening of contractures of the hip adductor and flexors, hamstrings, and Achilles tendon is necessary to correct the crouched gait. Instrumented gait laboratories, where available, may help determine the nature and extent of soft-tissue procedures to be performed.

Alternatives to standard orthopaedic treatment of spasticity include selective dorsal rhizotomy, intrathecal baclofen pumps, and repeated botulinum toxin injections into offending muscles. The exact role of these modalities in conjunction with or in place of traditional orthopaedic procedures is yet to be determined.

Myelomeningocele (Spina Bifida)

Myelomeningocele is a multisystem disorder, which demands a coordinated approach from a large number of health disciplines to maximize each patient's potential. Neurologic dysfunction rarely is limited to that corresponding to the level of spinal column dysraphism. Hydrocephalus, Arnold-Chiari malformations, and tethered cord syndrome all may compromise an otherwise stable neurologic disorder. Patients with myelomeningocele should be screened to confirm maintenance of known neurologic function, and any documented loss of function should be appropriately evaluated by magnetic resonance imaging (MRI) of the brain and spinal cord.

In general, most children with myelomeningocele are able to ambulate with the use of bracing appropriate for the level of paralysis. The initial orthopaedic goal should be to align the limbs for brace fitting; this can be done by releasing soft-tissue contractures or correcting foot deformities when the child is 12 to 18 months of age. All

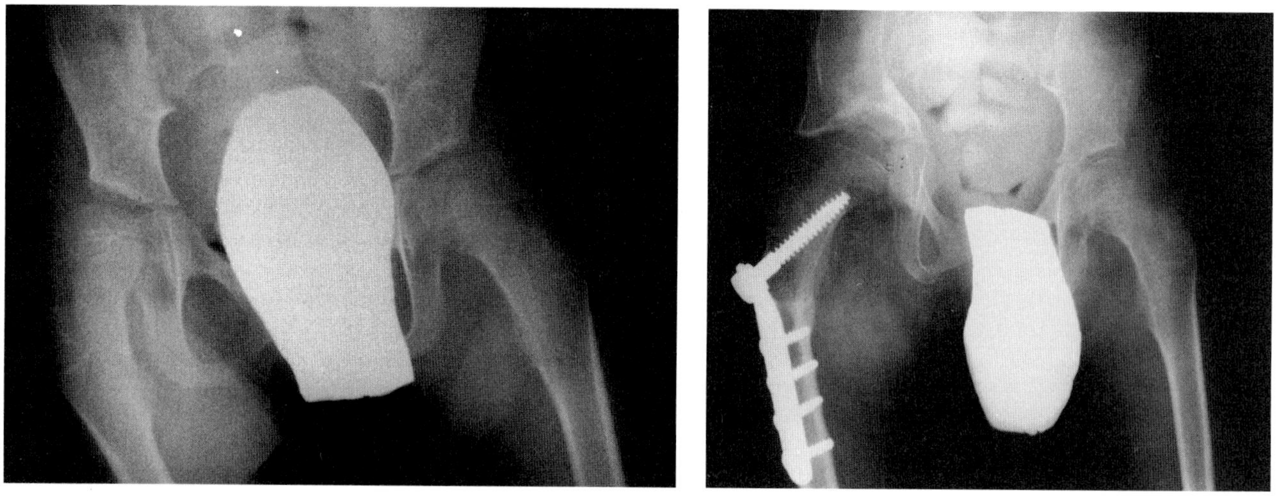

Fig. 1 **Left,** Sublulxation of the right hip in an 8-year-old child with cerebral palsy. **Right,** After femoral varus derotation and Chiari pelvic osteotomies.

patients with myelodysplasia should be assumed to be latex allergic. The need for concentric reduction of the hip, particularly in patients with midlumbar level lesions, remains controversial. Hip dislocations in children with lesions at the thoracic, L1, and L2 levels should not be reduced. Patients with lesions at the L4, L5, and sacral levels who have hip subluxation or unilateral hip dislocations are surgical candidates if they have functional quadriceps and will remain ambulatory. Maintenance of hip reduction may require soft-tissue release or transfer combined with femoral and/or pelvic osteotomy. Whether continued ambulation in adulthood is more related to neurologic level than to reduction of hip dislocations is unclear.

Patients with myelomeningocele have high incidences of both congenital and developmental scoliosis. Children should be screened early, using radiographs to identify any congenital vertebral anomalies, which should be treated the same as any congenital scoliosis. Progressive developmental scoliosis usually becomes problematic in nonambulatory children. When sitting balance is at risk of being impaired, posterior spinal fusion to the pelvis should be performed. Consideration must be given to the dysraphic area, which can be secured by anterior fusion, pedicular fixation, or wire loops to the laminar remnants as necessary. Folate taken by women prior to conception has been shown to decrease the incidence of myelomeningocele.

Poliomyelitis

Poliomyelitis is caused by viral inflammation and necrosis of the anterior horn cells of the central nervous system with subsequent motor paralysis in the affected area. The introduction of vaccines has reduced the frequency of acute poliomyelitis from one of the most common disorders requiring orthopaedic intervention to one that is rarely seen in North America. Occasional limited outbreaks do occur; almost all are due to passive infection of an unimmunized child from another child who was recently immunized with live attenuated oral vaccine. Postpolio syndrome, a late sequelae in poliomyelitis survivors, is covered in Section 6, "Rehabilitation."

The Muscular Dystrophies

Duchenne Muscular Dystrophy

Duchenne muscular dystrophy (DMD) is an inherited progressive disorder of muscle, which is characterized by muscle weakness in childhood with gradual loss of cardiopulmonary function until death in late teenage or early adult years. The disorder is sex-linked recessive and is the second most common lethal genetic disorder in humans, after cystic fibrosis. The incidence is approximately one per 3,300 live male births. The location of the defective gene has been identified as the p21 locus of the X chromosome. The normal gene at this locus produces a protein called dystrophin, the function of which is calcium transport. Patients with DMD have low or absent levels of dystrophin in their skeletal muscle.

An affected patient typically is seen between the ages of 3 and 5 years with a history of clumsiness, frequent falls, and difficulty running and climbing stairs. Pseudohypertrophy of the calves may be present, but this finding is neither pathognomonic nor universal. A child with DMD typically demonstrates a positive Gower's sign, ie, when asked to arise from the floor unaided, the child uses his hands to "crawl up his legs" to compensate for weak quadriceps and gluteus maximus muscles. Serum creatine phosphokinase (CPK) levels should be determined. Very high levels (up to one thousand times normal) are typical in DMD, and in conjunction with a typical clinical picture these levels can be taken as presumptive evidence for the diagnosis of DMD.

Definitive confirmation of the diagnosis can be made by muscle biopsy, which shows necrosis and regeneration of muscle fibers with variable fiber diameter, large hypertrophic fibers, and endomysial fibrosis. The muscle should be examined for dystrophin content and molecular weight. Absent dystrophin indicates typical DMD; decreased amount of dystrophin or dystrophin of abnormal molecular weight may be indicative of DMD or Becker muscular dystrophy (see below).

Patients with DMD invariably develop progressive difficulty walking due to a combination of deteriorating muscle strength and increasing lower extremity contractures. Most patients lose independent ambulation by the age of 8 to 10 years. Almost all patients with DMD have ankle equinus contractures and hip and knee flexion contractures, associated with a contracted iliotibial band. Soft-tissue releases with or without transfer of the posterior tibialis tendon to the dorsum of the foot, followed by lower extremity bracing and physical therapy, can prolong ambulation for an additional 1 to 3 years. Most authors recommend that this procedure be performed before complete loss of independent ambulation and that postoperative immobilization be kept to a minimum both in extent and duration. Occasionally, patients with minor contractures may be braced without soft-tissue release or after heel-cord lengthening alone. Patients with DMD have difficulty with or are unable to use crutches or a walker because of upper extremity weakness or contracture.

Significant scoliosis rarely develops before cessation of walking, but development of progressive lumbar or thoracolumbar scoliosis is inevitable after the child ceases ambulation and is in a wheelchair full time. Bracing to prevent progression of deformity appears ineffective and unwarranted unless surgery is refused by the family, in which case bracing may be used to aid sitting posture. Usually, however, bracing is poorly tolerated by the patient. Posterior spinal fusion with segmental fixation, such as with the Luque technique, should be performed after the scoliosis has reached 30° to halt progression of the scoliosis and maintain comfortable sitting. The impact of spinal fusion on longevity and the rate of loss of pulmonary function is controversial. Cardiac and pulmonary function should be carefully evaluated preoperatively, and postoperative respiratory therapy and ventilatory support should be available. The anesthesiology department and the family must be alerted to the possibility of malignant hyperthermia (See Section 5, "Spine.").

Even with successful surgical management and excellent respiratory therapy, the loss of pulmonary function due to progressive muscular weakness is relentless, and patients typically die from respiratory insufficiency in their late teens or early twenties.

Becker Muscular Dystrophy

Becker muscular dystrophy is an inherited progressive muscular dystrophy that is related to DMD, but it is characterized clinically by a slower, more benign course of muscle deterioration. Patients remain ambulatory until at least age 16 years and often survive into middle adulthood. Evaluation of dystrophin in muscle biopsy material shows a decreased amount of dystrophin or dystrophin of abnormal molecular weight compared to normal; whereas in DMD, dystrophin is absent. It is thought that Becker muscular dystrophy may be caused by a different defect in the same gene that causes DMD.

The orthopaedic approach to patients with Becker muscular dystrophy is the same as in DMD; however, because of the slower rate of progression of clinical weakness, intervention for lower extremity contractures or scoliosis is later and less frequent than in DMD.

Facioscapulohumeral Muscular Dystrophy

Facioscapulohumeral muscular dystrophy is an autosomal dominant disorder that may manifest itself clinically anytime between infancy and young adulthood. Progression of weakness is variable and typically insidious, with long periods of stable strength. Life expectancy is usually normal.

Face and shoulder girdle muscles usually are the first affected. Patients may have a weak, drooping smile, incomplete eyelid closure, and decreased facial wrinkles. Most clinical symptoms are related to shoulder girdle weakness. The clavicles have a horizontal position, and the shoulders are held lower than normal because of trapezius weakness. Scapular winging and decreased abduction of the shoulder due to weakness of the trapezius, levator scapulae, and rhomboids are typical findings. The abductors of the glenohumeral joint (deltoid, supraspinatus, infraspinatus, and subscapularis) remain relatively strong. Lower extremity weakness usually affects the peroneals, causing foot drop or equinus contracture. The pelvis, forearm, and other muscle groups occasionally are affected. Scoliosis is rare.

Orthopaedic treatment consists of stabilization of the scapula to the thorax to assist in deltoid function. Stabilization compensates for scapular muscle weakness and results in greater shoulder abduction because of the relative preservation of abductor strength. The potential gain of abduction usually can be demonstrated by temporarily stabilizing the patient's scapula and asking the patient to abduct the shoulder. Permanent stabilization may be accomplished surgically by soft-tissue arthroereisis (scapulopexy) of the medial border of the scapula to several underlying ribs in the posterior thorax, or by scapulothoracic arthrodesis. Dropfoot can be treated by ankle-foot orthosis or compensatory tendon transfer to the dorsum of the foot.

An autosomal recessive infantile form of facioscapulohumeral dystrophy has been described. This form typically manifests in the first year of life and is characterized by more severe weakness. Weakness of the upper and lower girdle muscles is present, and patients usually lose the ability to walk by the second decade.

Myotonic Dystrophy

This is an autosomal dominant condition characterized by facial myopathy and distal muscle myotonia. The defective gene has been localized to chromosome 19. Clinical forms include slowly progressive myotonia with onset in late adolescence and early adulthood and the more severe form with onset in early childhood.

Clinical findings include delay in relaxation of involved muscle groups, especially the eyes and hands, with the pattern of weakness distally rather than proximally. Foot deformity may require surgical correction. The disease is slowly progressive, often with loss of ambulation within 20 years of onset.

Charcot-Marie-Tooth Disease

Charcot-Marie-Tooth disease is now incorporated in a classification scheme of inherited neuropathies known as hereditary motor and sensory neuropathies (HMSN). There are seven types according to this scheme, but only the first three occur with any regularity in pediatric patients.

HMSN I includes the common, familiar form of Charcot-Marie-Tooth disease (hypertrophic form) characterized by autosomal dominant inheritance, weakness in the hands and feet, absent reflexes, and diminished peripheral sensation. Nerve conduction velocity is markedly reduced and electromyography indicates a neuropathic disorder. Muscle biopsy will also show a neuropathic pattern. The disorder is characterized by demyelination of peripheral nerves and can be confirmed by identifying this demyelination on sural nerve biopsy, when necessary.

HMSN II is a rare neuronal form of Charcot-Marie-Tooth disease characterized by preservation of reflexes, only mildly depressed motor and sensory nerve conduction velocities, and a variable inheritance pattern.

HMSN III (Déjèrine-Sottas disease) resembles HMSN I (Charcot-Marie-Tooth disease, hypertrophic form), but is inherited as an autosomal recessive condition, with onset in infancy, and is typically more severe.

Children with Charcot-Marie-Tooth disease usually have clumsiness or difficulty running. Cavovarus feet are the most common, nearly universal finding in older children and adults (Fig. 2). When cavovarus foot deformities can no longer be controlled with an ankle-foot orthosis, surgical correction is indicated. The Coleman block test is effective for evaluating hindfoot flexibility. For forefoot cavus with a flexible hindfoot, plantar release and first metatarsal osteotomy are appropriate. For a fixed varus hindfoot, Dwyer osteotomy may be added to the procedure. For fixed cavovarus deformity at skeletal maturity, triple arthrodesis may be used to correct all deformities. Transfer of the tibialis posterior tendon anteriorly may assist in ankle dorsiflexion in selected patients.

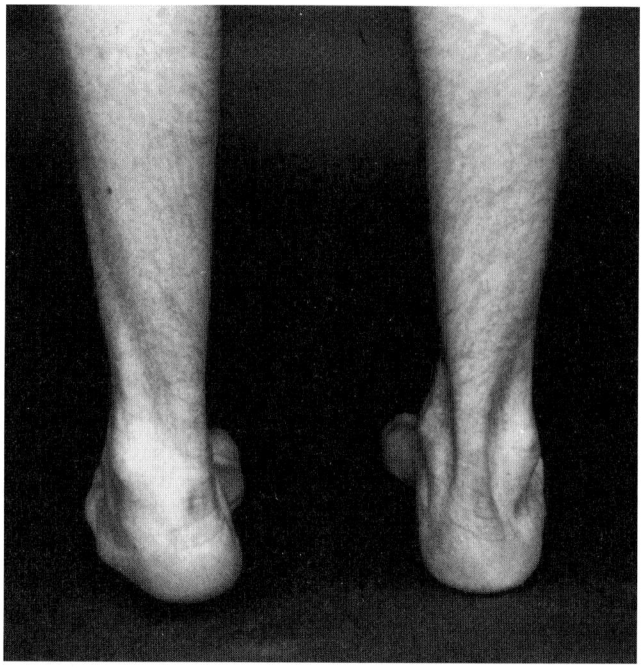

Fig. 2 Foot deformity in a 17-year-old patient with Charcot-Marie-Tooth disease.

Dysplasia of the hip, either discovered incidentally or manifesting itself as increasing pain and limp in adolescence, has been reported in as many as 10% of patients with Charcot-Marie-Tooth disease. Symptoms or progressive deformity may require pelvic or upper femoral osteotomy; however, the results of these procedures may not be satisfactory because of muscular weakness about the hip.

Scoliosis also may occur in up to 10% of patients who have hereditary motor and sensory neuropathy. Patients should be screened for the deformity and treated with observation, bracing, or surgery; treatment is similar to that for idiopathic scoliosis.

Arthrogryposis Multiplex Congenita

The term arthrogryposis implies multiple congenital joint contractures. Unfortunately, the term has been applied to a broad spectrum of genetic and sporadic disorders, some of which are well recognized and others of which are obscure. The orthopaedic manifestations of these disorders are equally broad in nature and severity.

The most common and familiar form of arthrogryposis (myopathic form or amyoplasia) is characterized by severe, generally symmetric involvement of both upper and lower extremities, including adducted, internally rotated shoulders, extended elbows, radially deviated wrists with thumb-in-palm deformity, stiff or dislocated hips, knee hyperextension or flexion deformity, and rigid clubfeet. Decreased fetal movement is associated with the development of arthrogryposis, but the relationship of this finding to the development of deformity is not understood. In this most common form, tendons typically are normally formed and inserted, but there is limited excursion, and the associated muscle usually is fibrotic.

Clubfeet, although typically quite rigid, may improve at least partially with serial manipulation in infancy. Complete surgical correction can be difficult, and recurrence is frequent. Extensive soft-tissue release, which includes excision of tendons and, frequently, removal of cancellous bone from or excision of the talus, is required to obtain a plantigrade foot. Postoperative bracing of the feet for an indefinite time is recommended.

Knee flexion deformity also is difficult to treat. If the deformity impedes walking or effective bracing, hamstring lengthening with joint capsulotomy and femoral shortening to relax the neurovascular structures may be performed. Significant recurrence may require repeated extension osteotomies of the distal femur. Extension deformities of the knee usually do not impede function in childhood, but they become more troublesome in adolescence because of difficulty with sitting.

The management of hip dislocation is more controversial. Open reduction is indicated for unilateral dislocation. Medial open reduction at 3 to 6 months of age has been shown to be at least as effective as closed or anterior open reduction. Bilateral hip dislocations can be similarly treated, but the benefit to the patient with stiff, symmetric deformity is questionable.

Arthrogrypotic patients can adapt to upper extremity contractures quite well, and caution should be exercised in attempting correction. Treatment efforts should be designed to provide independence in feeding and personal hygiene activities. Gentle passive range-of-motion exercise of the shoulders, elbows, wrists, and digits should begin in infancy. If exercise fails, internal rotation at the shoulder may require rotational osteotomy of the humerus. Passive elbow flexion can be improved by triceps lengthening and capsulotomy, but this should be done only if the patient does not require elbow extension for crutch use. Active elbow flexion may be gained by transfer of the pectoralis major or latissimus dorsi muscles. Persistent wrist flexion deformity may require proximal row carpectomy or dorsal closing wedge osteotomy of the carpus or radius.

Arthrogrypotic patients should be monitored regularly for the appearance of scoliosis, which occurs quite commonly. The pattern and severity vary considerably. Bracing is usually difficult in these patients, but spinal fusions are successful and should be carried out when clinically indicated.

Spinal Muscular Atrophy

Spinal muscular atrophy (SMA) is the second most common inherited neuromuscular disorder of children after DMD. The prevalence of SMA is approximately one per 25,000 live births. The disorder is almost always inherited as an autosomal recessive trait, although sex-linked and dominant types have been reported. The defective gene has been localized to chromosome 5q11, although the exact gene product has not yet been identified. It is likely that multiple genetic anomalies occur at this location to account for the variation in clinical severity.

The most commonly used classification system is based on the age at onset of detectable weakness. Acute Werdnig-Hoffmann disease, the most severe form, is characterized by onset of weakness between birth and 6 months of age; patients frequently die before the age of 1 year due to respiratory insufficiency. Children with chronic Werdnig-Hoffmann disease or intermediate type have onset between age 6 months and 2 years; these patients rarely are able to walk, and in the most severe cases, may also die due to respiratory insufficiency. Onset of Kugelberg-Welander disease or the mild type occurs after age 2 years; these patients generally can walk, may be able to run, and can have a normal lifespan. There is overlap in disease severity and in the prognosis of individual patients within this simplified scheme, so that early in the clinical course, rehabilitative programs must be individualized and monitored.

The fundamental pathologic finding in SMA is degeneration of anterior horn (motor) cells. The loss of anterior horn cells is thought to be an acute, nonprogressive event. Consequently, muscular weakness tends to be stable for prolonged periods during growth, rather than relentlessly progressive.

Patients with onset in infancy should begin a program of gentle passive range-of-motion exercises to prevent joint contractures. Patients with milder involvement who show some walking capability may require lightweight lower extremity bracing to facilitate mobility. Contracture release to facilitate bracing is not generally recommended.

The most frequent problem encountered by the orthopaedic surgeon is progressive paralytic-type scoliosis in nonambulatory patients. Custom-molded thoracolumbar orthoses may be used to improve sitting balance or, theoretically, to reduce the rate of progression of scoliosis in young patients, but the efficacy of such braces is not established. When uncontrollable progressive collapsing scoliosis occurs, posterior spinal fusion to the pelvis with segmental instrumentation is recommended to maintain comfortable sitting. Patients may have decreased self-help abilities with activities such as drinking, feeding, and hygiene as a result of altered upper extremity and sitting posture soon after surgery. Although there usually is a gradual improvement in these activities, caretakers should be alerted to these changes before surgery.

Friedreich Ataxia

Friedreich ataxia is an autosomal recessive disorder characterized by loss of cerebellar and spinal function. Onset is between 7 and 15 years, usually manifesting as a triad of ataxia, areflexia, and Babinski plantar response. The abnormal gene has been located on chromosome 9, but the exact gene product has not yet been identified.

Ataxia usually is the first symptom, but dysarthria and symmetric upper and lower extremity weakness follow. Physical examination also reveals areflexia and loss of position and vibration sensation. Weakness is progressive, with patients beginning to use a wheelchair between age 18 and 20 years and complete loss of ambulation ability by age 25 years. Death generally occurs in the fourth or fifth decade due to cardiomyopathy.

Scoliosis and cavovarus feet occur in most patients. Scoliosis with prepubertal onset may progress, and posterior spinal fusion is recommended for deformities of more than 50° or 60°. In some patients with onset after puberty, the deformity may stabilize at less than 40°; surgery is not required in these patients. The effectiveness of bracing has not been established, but bracing is, in general, poorly tolerated.

Cavovarus foot deformity may be adequately symptomatically controlled with the use of ankle-foot orthoses. If surgery is required, triple arthrodesis can provide satisfactory results.

Annotated Bibliography

Cerebral Palsy

Albright AL, Cervi A, Singletary J: Intrathecal baclofen for spasticity in cerebral palsy. *JAMA* 1991:265:1418–1422.

Twenty-three patients with spasticity, including 17 with congenital spastic cerebral palsy, were injected intrathecally with either baclofen or placebo in a randomized, double-blind study. Upper extremity tone and function were not appreciably affected by the injection of baclofen, but lower extremity tone was significantly reduced from 2 hours after injection for more than 8 hours. The authors conclude that intrathecal injection reduces spasticity in children with cerebral palsy.

Boscarino LF, Ounpuu S, Davis RB III, et al: Effects of selective dorsal rhizotomy on gait in children with cerebral palsy. *J Pediatr Orthop* 1993;13:174–179.

The authors performed gait analysis before and 1 year after selective dorsal rhizotomy in two groups of patients: 11 ambulators and 8 nonambulators. Improvement in passive joint range-of-motion and lower extremity spasticity were noted. In the ambulatory patients, step and stride length significantly improved, but gait velocity remained stable. The authors concluded that the relationship between these improvements and functional increase in ambulation is difficult to define, and that further studies will be required.

Calderon-Gonzalez R, Calderon-Sepulveda R, Rincon-Reyes M, et al: Botulinum toxin A in management of cerebral palsy. *Pediatr Neurol* 1994;10:284–288.

Fifteen patients with cerebral palsy and functional deformities of the lower extremities not amenable to bracing and physical therapy were injected with botulinum toxin A. Six patients whose adductors were injected had decreased scissoring in stance, six showed increased knee extension after hamstring injection, and three showed improved dorsiflexion and plantigrade gait after gastrocnemius injection. Five patients showed persistent improvement 9 to 11 months postinjection, while the rest had recurrence of their dynamic deformities. Other than pain at the time of injection, no complications were identified.

Myelomeningocele

Brinker MR, Rosenfeld SR, Feiwell E, et al: Myelomeningocele at the sacral level: Long-term outcomes in adults. *J Bone Joint Surg* 1994;76A:1293–1300.

Thirty-six patients with sacral-level myelomeningocele were reviewed at an average age of 29 years. Eleven of 35 patients who had been community ambulators initially had declined in their ability to walk; the one patient who had been a household ambulator was nonambulatory at follow-up. Fifteen patients had osteomyelitis, and 11 had undergone a total of 14 amputations. The authors concluded that patients with sacral-level myelomeningocele did not always do well after childhood and recommended orthopaedic follow-up of these patients into adulthood.

Broughton NS, Menelaus MB, Cole WG, et al: The natural history of hip deformity in myelomeningocele. *J Bone Joint Surg* 1993;75B:760–763.

The authors studied sequential radiographs of the hips of 802 patients with myelomeningocele from two centers. Patients with an L3 functional level dislocated early, but no further dislocations occurred after age 3 years. Between the ages of 9 and 11 years, patients with thoracic level lesions had significantly greater hip flexion contracture than those with low lumbar and sacral level lesions. The authors concluded that the high incidence of flexion deformity and dislocation in the patients with thoracic level lesions was not explainable on the basis of muscle balance alone, and that sitting posture and spinal deformity may be factors in the development of these deformities.

Phillips DP, Lindseth RE: Ambulation after transfer of adductors, external oblique, and tensor fascia lata in myelomeningocele. *J Pediatr Orthop* 1992;12:712–717.

Thirty-seven of 41 patients undergoing either triple (adductor, external oblique, and tensor fascia lata) or double (adductor and external oblique) transfers were functionally improved in gait at average 4.5 years follow-up. The authors recommend triple transfer in patients with mid- and low-lumbar level myelomeningocele. Poor motivation, obesity, scoliosis, and joint contractures are considered relative contraindications to the procedure. The surgical technique used is described and illustrated.

The Muscular Dystrophies

Bach JR, McKeon J: Orthopedic surgery and rehabilitation for the prolongation of brace-free ambulation of patients with Duchenne muscular dystrophy. *Am J Phys Med Rehabil* 1991;70:323–331.

This is a study of 13 patients undergoing extensive iliotibial band release, rectus femoris and tensor fascia lata release, heel-cord lengthening, and (in four of the 13) posterior tibial tendon transfer to the dorsum of the foot. Patients who were still ambulatory at the time of surgery maintained independent ambulation the longest, had the least frequent number of falls, and expressed the greatest satisfaction with surgery. The authors recommend these soft-tissue procedures prior to loss of effective independent ambulation.

Galasko CS, Delaney C, Morris P: Spinal stabilisation in Duchenne muscular dystrophy. *J Bone Joint Surg* 1992; 74B:210–214.

Fifty-five patients were followed prospectively; 32 agreed to posterior spinal fusion with Luque instrumentation and 23 refused. Forced vital capacity declined an average of 8% per year in the patients treated nonsurgically but remained stable for 3 years with slight decline thereafter in the surgically treated patients. Deformity in the surgically treated patients was 30° postoperatively, declining to 34° in follow-up, whereas the nonsurgery group progressed from an average 37° to an average 93°. Mortality rate was significantly higher in the nonsurgery group in follow-up (17 of 23 versus 12 of 32).

Iannaccone ST: Current status of Duchenne muscular dystrophy. *Pediatr Clin North Am* 1992;39:879–894.

This publication summarizes the history of Duchenne muscular dystrophy (DMD) as well as current knowledge of dystrophin and genetic aspects of DMD. There are good examples of histologic specimens including dystrophin detection. A general approach to both the patient and families regarding genetic counseling, psychological support, respiratory therapy, physical therapy, and orthopaedic management is nicely outlined.

Letournel E, Fardeau M, Lytle JO, et al: Scapulothoracic arthrodesis for patients who have fascioscapulohumeral [sic] muscular dystrophy. *J Bone Joint Surg* 1990;72A: 78–84.

Thoracoscapular arthrodesis using wires and plates was performed in nine patients (seven bilaterally) with facioscapulohumeral dystrophy. At average follow-up of 69 months, patients had gained an average 33° of flexion and 25° of abduction. Results did not deteriorate with time. Complications included pleural effusion, pneumothorax, and one asymptomatic pseudarthrosis of one rib. The authors recommend the procedure for patients with facioscapulohumeral muscular dystrophy, symptomatic limitation of shoulder abduction, and unsightly scapular winging.

Shapiro F, Specht L: The diagnosis and orthopaedic treatment of inherited muscular diseases of childhood. *J Bone Joint Surg* 1993;75A:439–454.

This review article summarizes current knowledge and orthopaedic management of Duchenne muscular dystrophy, Becker's muscular dystrophy, and facioscapulohumeral muscular dystrophy. The authors succinctly overview the rarer myotonias and congenital myopathies. A general diagnostic approach for the orthopaedic surgeon, specific treatment guidelines for the various disorders, and an excellent bibliography make this publication an excellent update source for the muscular dystrophies.

Charcot-Marie-Tooth Disease

Roper BA, Tibrewal SB: Soft tissue surgery in Charcot-Marie-Tooth disease. *J Bone Joint Surg* 1989;71B:17–20.

Eighteen feet in ten patients with Charcot-Marie-Tooth disease were assessed an average of 14 years after soft-tissue reconstruction of cavovarus feet. Surgery consisted of heel cord lengthening, split transfer of the tibialis anterior, Steindler plantar fascial release, and toe tendon transfers. One patient had a Dwyer calcaneal osteotomy. Age at surgery averaged 14 years but ranged from 5 to 36 years. At follow-up, all feet were graded satisfactory, and none had required triple arthrodesis. Two patients had required further soft-tissue procedures for recurrence of the deformity.

Wetmore RS, Drennan JC: Long-term results of triple arthrodesis in Charcot-Marie-Tooth disease. *J Bone Joint Surg* 1989;71A:417–422.

Sixteen patients with 30 triple arthrodeses were followed up for an average of 21 years. Fourteen feet (47%) were rated poor at follow-up, nine were fair, five good, and only two feet were rated excellent. Six patients had undergone ankle arthrodesis secondarily for degenerative changes. The authors conclude that triple arthrodesis should be considered a salvage procedure reserved for only the most severe foot deformities in Charcot-Marie-Tooth disease.

Arthrogryposis Multiplex Congenita

Brown JC, Zeller JL, Swank SM, et al: Surgical and functional results of spine fusion in spinal muscular atrophy. *Spine* 1989;14:763–770.

Patients (34) treated by posterior spinal fusion and Harrington instrumentation, and patients (6) treated by spinal fusion and Luque segmental wire fixation were assessed with regards to the influence of surgery on their ambulatory status, upper extremity equipment use, and functional activities. Postoperative sitting endurance improved in only 10% of patients; patients required mobile arm supports, lapboards, and reachers postoperatively because of the change in their sitting posture, and upper extremity activities had declined at 2 years, but improved at 5-year follow-up.

Sarwark JF, MacEwen GD, Scott CI Jr: Amyoplasia (A common form of arthrogryposis). *J Bone Joint Surg* 1990;72A:465–469.

This article reviews the current thinking on orthopaedic treatment of the manifestations of the most common and familiar form of arthrogryposis (amyoplasia, formerly known as arthrogryposis multiplex congenita).

Solund K, Sonne-Holm S, Kjolbye JE: Talectomy for equinovarus deformity in arthrogryposis: A 13 (2-20) year review of 17 feet. *Acta Orthop Scand* 1991;62:372–374.

Seventeen feet in ten children with arthrogryposis underwent talectomy for severe clubfoot deformity; all but one were treated after at least three previous surgical procedures. At review averaging 13 years, 14 of 17 feet were deemed satisfactory. The authors conclude that talectomy should be performed in children with arthrogryposis and rigid clubfeet at walking age.

Staheli LT, Chew DE, Elliott JS, et al: Management of hip dislocations in children with arthrogryposis. *J Pediatr Orthop* 1987;7:681–685.

The authors reviewed the results of 18 patients with arthrogryposis (exact type not specified) treated for hip dislocations by anterior open reduction, closed reduction, or medial open reduction. Satisfactory maintenance of reduction and subsequent acetabular development occurred in patients treated by medial open reduction; these patients had better range-of-motion compared to patients treated by closed reduction or anterior open reduction. The authors recommend medial open reduction in conjunction with knee and foot procedures between the ages of 3 and 6 months.

Spinal Muscular Atrophy

Merlini L, Granata C, Bonfiglioli S, et al: Scoliosis in spinal muscular atrophy: Natural history and management. *Dev Med Child Neurol* 1989;31:501–508.

This publication is a review of the literature on scoliosis in spinal muscular atrophy as well as a report on the natural history of 109 patients over a 12-year period. All 18 children with the severe form died during the study at an average age of under 6 months. Of the 52 with the intermediate form, whose maximal functional ability was unaided sitting, five died between the ages of 5 and 13 years. Sixteen of the 39 mild cases lost the ability to walk between the ages of 4 and 15 years; the others continued to walk during the period of study (age range 3 to 36 years).

Phillips DP, Roye DP Jr, Farcy JP, et al: Surgical treatment of scoliosis in a spinal muscular atrophy population. *Spine* 1990;15:942–945.

In this retrospective analysis, 31 patients with all three clinical forms of spinal muscular atrophy were treated over a 20-year period with an average follow-up of 11.5 years. Scoliosis was documented at an average age of 8.8 years. Twenty-two patients were treated conservatively and nine surgically. Sitting balance and endurance improved after surgery. Complications of surgery included one each of loss of correction, pseudarthrosis, and prolonged ventilatory support. The authors conclude that the prolonged survival of patients with spinal muscular atrophy justifies aggressive orthopaedic management of scoliosis.

Shapiro F, Specht L: The diagnosis and orthopaedic treatment of childhood spinal muscular atrophy, peripheral neuropathy, Friedreich ataxia, and arthrogryposis. *J Bone Joint Surg* 1993;75A:1699–1714.

This is a review article of spinal muscular atrophy, the hereditary motor and sensory neuropathies, Friedreich ataxia, and arthrogryposis. The role of muscle and nerve biopsy, enzyme analysis, and electrophysiologic investigations in establishing the correct diagnosis is reviewed. Clinical features, natural history, and orthopaedic treatment are summarized. General approaches to the diagnosis and orthopaedic treatment of the most common hereditary motor and sensory neuropathy disorders, Friedreich ataxia, and arthrogryposis are similarly reviewed.

Thompson CE, Larsen LJ: Recurrent hip dislocation in intermediate spinal atrophy. *J Pediatr Orthop* 1990;10: 638–641.

Hip deformity and progressive dislocation are known to occur in patients with spinal muscular atrophy. The authors report four cases treated for unilateral hip dislocation using a variety of methods. In each case, the hip redislocated, and no functional benefit was achieved. The authors concluded that because these patients did not have pain or functional problems due to the dislocations, hip surgery appeared to be unwarranted.

Freidreich Ataxia

Beauchamp M, Labelle H, Duhaime M, et al: Natural history of muscle weakness in Friedreich's ataxia and its relation to loss of ambulation. *Clin Orthop* 1995;311:270–275.

The authors analyzed 170 muscular strength assessments in 33 patients taken over a 13-year period to postulate on the pattern of loss of strength in Friedreich ataxia. Patients in this study began to use a wheelchair at an average age of 18 years, and became totally unable to walk by an average age of 20.5 years. At the time of initial use of the wheelchair, lower extremity strength was still approximately 70% of normal, leading the authors to conclude that loss of ambulation potential was not due primarily to muscular weakness. Rapid loss of lower extremity strength was documented after initiation of use of the wheelchair.

Labelle H, Tohme S, Duhaime M, et al: Natural history of scoliosis in Friedreich's ataxia. *J Bone Joint Surg* 1986; 68A:564–572.

This is a retrospective review of the prevalence and natural history of scoliosis in 56 patients with Friedreich ataxia. Scoliosis of at least 10° was identified in all patients. The authors concluded that curves over 60° should be fused, those under 40° should be observed, and those between 40° and 60° observed or fused depending on age of onset of the disease and identification of the presence of scoliosis.

22

Pediatric Hematologic and Related Conditions

Hemophilia

Musculoskeletal complications and deformities often result from the genetically transmitted deficiency in coagulation factors VIII and IX. Classic hemophilia or hemophilia A (factor VIII deficiency) is transmitted as a sex-linked recessive gene, has an incidence of 1:10,000 live male births in the United States, and constitutes the majority of coagulopathies. Christmas disease or hemophilia B is a similarly inherited factor IX deficiency, which is present in 1:100,000 live births.

Coagulation abnormalities in a child with recurrent bruising or joint bleeds are evaluated by platelet count, Ivy bleeding time, plasma prothrombin time, and plasma partial thromboplastin time (PTT). In both forms of hemophilia, the PTT is abnormal. The severity of the deficiency often is correlated with the incidence of musculoskeletal complications: $< 1\%$ activity, severe; 1% to 5%, moderate; and $> 5\%$, mild.

The medical management of hemophilia is designed to raise the circulating level of the deficient coagulation factor to at least 50% activity for most muscle or joint hemorrhage and to 100% for most surgical procedures. Each unit of factor VIII concentrate provides a 2% increase in the serum activity level per kg of body weight with dosing every 8 to 12 hours. Each unit of factor IX concentrate increases the serum activity level by 1% per kg of body weight with dosing every 18 to 24 hours.

The orthopaedic problems encountered in a child with hemophilia may be grouped as acute or chronic. Acute hemarthroses in children occur typically in the knee, elbow, and ankle in decreasing order of frequency. Acute compartment syndromes, carpal tunnel syndrome, and femoral nerve neuropraxia occur less commonly. Rapid and aggressive medical management is required. Joint aspiration or decompression may be performed following replacement therapy. Splinting for 24 to 48 hours is used for patient comfort, and then rehabilitation starts. Replacement therapy may be continued through the next 5 to 7 days because rebleeds may occur in major joints.

The chronic phase of hemophilia begins with synovial hypertrophy and recurrent small bleeds. Management is aimed at shortening this phase with a prophylactic concentrate transfusion regimen for 4 to 6 months. Persistent synovitis after this point may be handled with open or arthroscopic synovectomy, especially in the knee and elbow (Fig. 1). The relentless arthropathy of hemophilia is seen often by the time a patient is 20 years of age. These patients may need to be managed with physiotherapy and certain nonsteroidal anti-inflammatory drugs (NSAIDs) because factor VIII inhibitors develop in 30% of patients. Total joint arthroplasty may be performed in selected candidates.

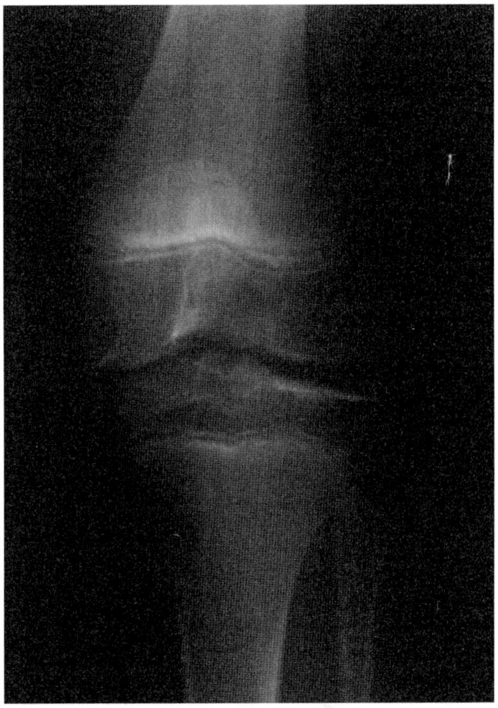

Fig. 1 This patient's hemophilic knee arthropathy was treated with arthroscopic synovectomy, and there was a satisfactory result at 2-year follow-up.

A large percentage of the hemophiliac population are now human immunodeficiency virus (HIV) positive, primarily as a result of having received pooled, untreated factor VIII preparations. Serial examinations of T4 counts are performed, with medical therapies still evolving for the AIDS patient who has hemophilia. (See Chapter 5, "Blood Transfusion/HIV/Hepatitis.")

Sickle-Cell Disease

Approximately 8% to 10% of the United States black population has sickle-cell trait. Each affected individual inherited a hemoglobin S and a hemoglobin A gene, and will, therefore, have few clinical manifestations. A smaller proportion of that population is homozygous; they have inherited both hemoglobin S genes and are referred to as having SS disease or sickle-cell anemia.

Although sickle-cell anemia may have deleterious effects on the central nervous, renal, and hepatic systems, significant morbidity is associated with the osseous system. The osseous changes can be grouped according to whether the pain is from bone infarction or bone infection.

Pain from acute polyarthritis in sickle-cell disease occurs as muscle spasms, joint pain, and effusion. Aspiration of the joint effusion indicates a minimal reactive synovitis. The elbow is predisposed to these episodes, and treatment centers on splinting and physiotherapy. Recovery usually is complete.

Bone infarction occurs as the result of the vascular channels and marrow becoming blocked by the abnormal sickled erythrocytes. In a child as young as 6 to 12 months of age, the hand or foot may display symptoms of sickle-cell dactylitis, which clinically may resemble an infection. The swelling and pain may last for 1 to 2 weeks and the radiographic changes will ultimately demonstrate the infarction in as many as 74% of patients. The femoral head may sustain a partial collapse with osteonecrosis in an adolescent, and treatment options include a regimen of traction and nonweightbearing. Total joint replacement rarely is indicated in young adults with refractory pain from osteonecrosis and degenerative joint disease of the hip. Vaso-occlusive episodes are managed with NSAIDs, oxygen, hydration, and, if anemia is present, transfusion.

Bone infection in this particular disease, which occurs in only one of 50 affected patients, manifests itself with a warm, swollen, painful extremity. Routine evaluation should include blood cultures and needle aspiration of the affected area. Differentiation from a sickle-cell crisis has improved by comparing the results of technetium 99 scans with those of a bone marrow scan. Salmonella along with *Staphylococcus aureus* and *Streptococcus pneumoniae* are typical causative organisms in osteomyelitis. Septic joints are very infrequent in patients with sickle-cell disease. Surgical drainage of infected joints, osteomyelitis, and subperiosteal abscesses is indicated (Fig. 2).

The preoperative use of exchange transfusions in patients with sickle-cell disease is calculated to lower the hemoglobin S to less than 45%. With proper hydration, oxygenation, and maintenance of body temperature, complications associated with intraoperative tourniquet use and postoperative bone crisis may be minimized.

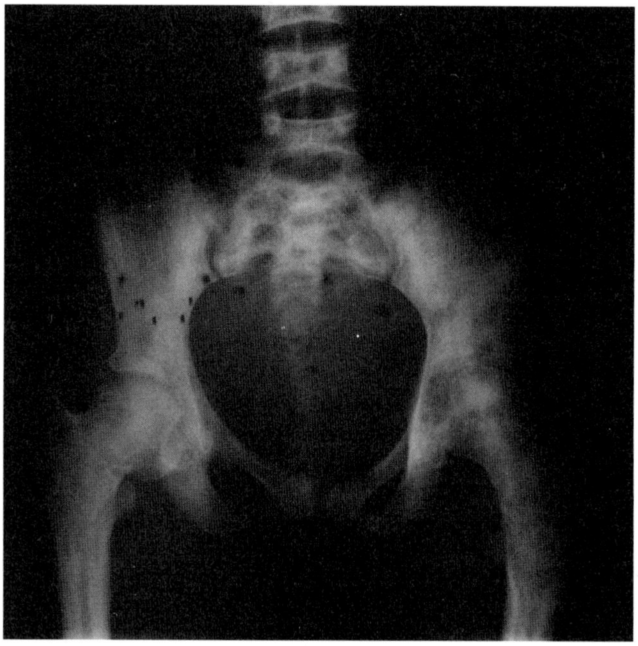

Fig. 2 This 12-year-old, black female with sickle-cell anemia presented with a 2-week history of progressive hip pain and femoral head osteomyelitis due to *Staphylococcus aureus*.

Thalassemia

Thalassemia is an inherited hemoglobinopathy with abnormal hemoglobin A production. Although there are two major sites of altered production, which result in an alpha and beta chain, it is the genetic penetrance that is more important clinically. The homozygous form, thalassemia major or Cooley's anemia, is a severe chronic microcytic hemolytic anemia, which is treated with multiple transfusions. The child develops jaundice and hepatosplenomegaly by 1 year of age. The hyperplastic marrow contributes to the long bone thinning and metaphyseal expansion, and the skull develops a "hair-on-end" appearance. Pathologic fractures and premature physeal closure, especially of the proximal humerus and distal femur, are common childhood problems. With the onset of puberty, the severity of the growth retardation and altered skeletal maturation are more apparent. The altered skeletal formation may predispose these patients to degenerative osteoarthritis in the second and third decades. Paraparesis due to spinal cord compression from extramedullary hematopoiesis usually can be treated with radiation therapy, decompressive laminectomy, or both. The heterozygous form, thalassemia minor, has few symptoms, and children with this disease experience normal longevity.

Leukemias

The leukemias are the largest group of childhood malignancies, making up over 30%. The acute lymphocytic leukemias (ALL) account for over 70% of this group. An etiology has not been established, but there is an increased occurrence of lymphoid leukemias in patients with Down Syndrome, immunocompromise, and ataxic telangiectasia.

Peak incidence is at 4 years of age. An affected child may present with fatigue, fever, or bone and joint pain. In the early phase of the disease, the hallmark laboratory findings of anemia, neutropenia, and thrombocytopenia

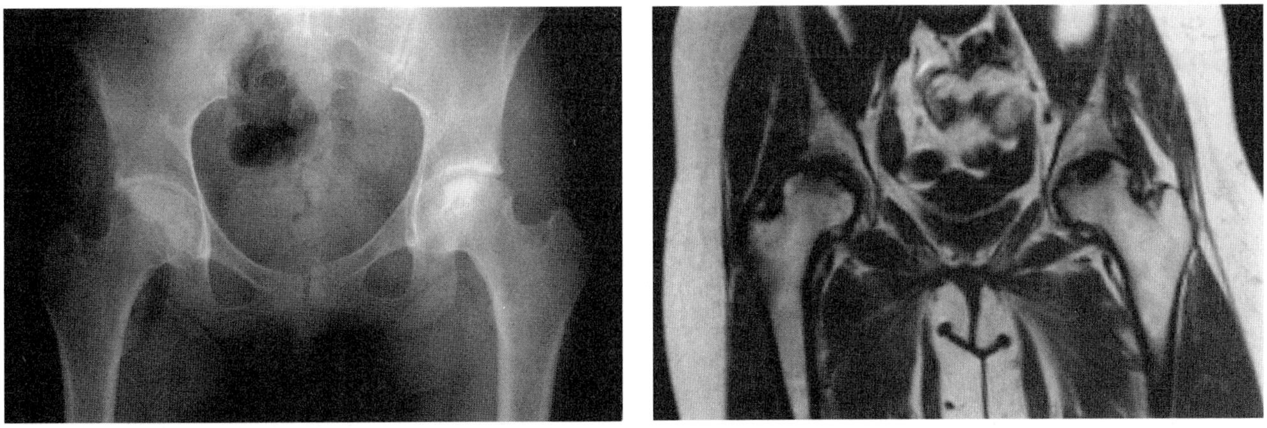

Fig. 3 Bilateral osteonecrosis of the femoral head in a 17-year-old with acute lymphocytic leukemia. **Left,** Radiograph. **Right,** Magnetic resonance imaging scan.

may not all be present. Radiographic findings may mimic osteomyelitis with lytic areas, osteopenia, and periostitis (Fig. 3). The appearance of juxtaepiphyseal lucent lines is caused by the malignancy's destruction of bone trabeculae or alteration of enchondral bone formation; these lines are more typical in older children (Fig. 4).

The diagnosis hinges on the identification of abnormal cells in the peripheral smear or bone marrow. Bone scan may aid in identifying clinically silent areas but may not correlate with areas of obvious destruction on radiographs.

Medical management with prednisone, vincristine, and asparaginase has improved remission rates to 95% of children with standard risk ALL.

Gaucher's Disease

Gaucher's disease is another disease process, which involves the macrophages of the reticulo-endothelial system and their abnormal accumulation of glucocerebroside, caused by an enzymatic deficiency. This autosomal recessive trait has three clinical presentations. Type I represents a chronic, nonneuropathic form with visceral and osseous involvement. Type II is an acute, neuropathic type with central nervous system (CNS) involvement and early death. Type III is a subacute nonneuropathic type with chronic CNS involvement.

The hemopoietic changes that result from replacement of the marrow include anemia, leukopenia, and thrombocytopenia. The osseous lesions resulting from the abnormal accumulation in the marrow include thinning and expansion of the metaphysis, or Erlenmeyer flask appearance; osteonecrosis, particularly of the femoral head; and pathologic fractures, especially of the spine and femoral neck. Magnetic resonance imaging (MRI) is more sensitive than radiographs or computed tomography (CT) in demonstrating the involvement of the marrow.

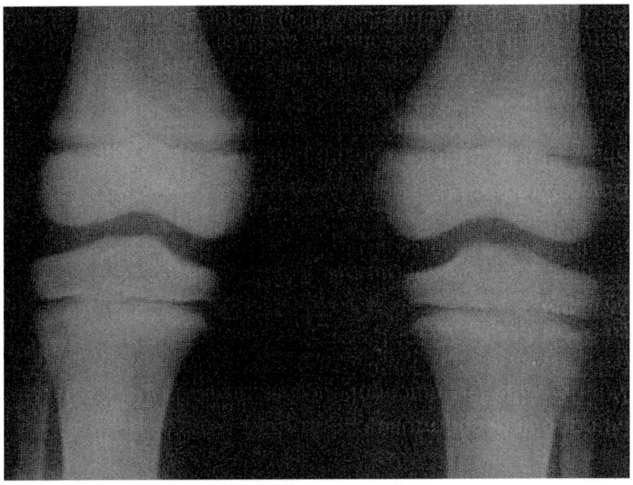

Fig. 4 The juxtaepiphyseal lines are present in this 8-year-old female with acute lymphoblastic leukemia.

Osteonecrosis of the femoral head and humeral head is managed with medications, limitation of activity, and joint replacement. Pathologic fractures, especially of the femoral neck in children and of the spine, are best managed conservatively.

The orthopaedic surgeon is clinically challenged by the similar symptoms in bone crisis and osteomyelitis in patients with Gaucher's disease. With bone crisis, a patient may have severe pain in the extremity, rubor, fever, and an elevated white blood cell count. Radiographs may demonstrate periosteal reaction or lytic lesions, which are difficult to differentiate from osteomyelitis. Technetium 99 bone scan often will not demonstrate increased uptake with crisis but, in difficult cases, gallium 67 scintigraphy may be useful. Acute osteomyelitis confirmed by closed needle biopsy or laboratory tests is best managed conservatively. Open irrigation and debridement of the bone may result in chronic osteomyelitis (Fig. 5).

The medical management of Gaucher's disease with enzyme replacement (alglucerase) is offered to patients with at least moderate disease symptoms. A recent report recommended 2.3 U/kg three times weekly with satisfactory clinical results. The annual cost of treatment was approximately $100,000.

Niemann-Pick Disease

Niemann-Pick disease represents the abnormal accumulation of sphingomyelin in the viscera and ganglioside in the CNS, which is caused by a deficiency of the enzyme sphingomyelinase. The disease has a recessive inheritance pattern in males and females equally. Few children survive the first few years. Patients who survive have progressive marrow cavity expansion and altered remodeling, especially in the femurs and metacarpals. Pathologic fractures and osteonecrosis usually do not occur.

Fanconi's Anemia

Fanconi's anemia is a rare congenital aplastic anemia that is inherited as an autosomal recessive trait. The hematologic problems may not manifest until late during the first year of life. Anemia, granulocytopenia, and thrombocytopenia may be severe, and the prognosis is poor. Anomalies of the upper extremity include the thumb, first metacarpal, or radius. Similar lower extremity deformities described in thrombocytopenia with absent radii (TAR) may be present.

Thrombocytopenia With Absent Radii

TAR is a rare congenital syndrome that usually is transmitted as an autosomal recessive trait. The hematologic findings are hypomegakaryocytic thrombocytopenia, periodic leukemoid reactions, and eosinophilia. Resolution of the thrombocytopenia usually occurs after 1 year of age, but may require medical support. The osseous deformities of complete absence of the radii, with intact thumbs, result in foreshortened forearms and radially deviated hands. Various ulnocarpal stabilization procedures have been described. A persistent genu varum with tibial torsion is present in many patients and is attributed to an intra-articular knee dysplasia. A progressive deformity may be treated with braces, surgery, or both. Because occult hip dysplasia may be present, once children with TAR have reached walking age, screening hip radiographs should be obtained. Cardiac abnormalities (tetralogy of Fallot and atrial septal defect) and cow's milk allergy are included in the clinical features of TAR.

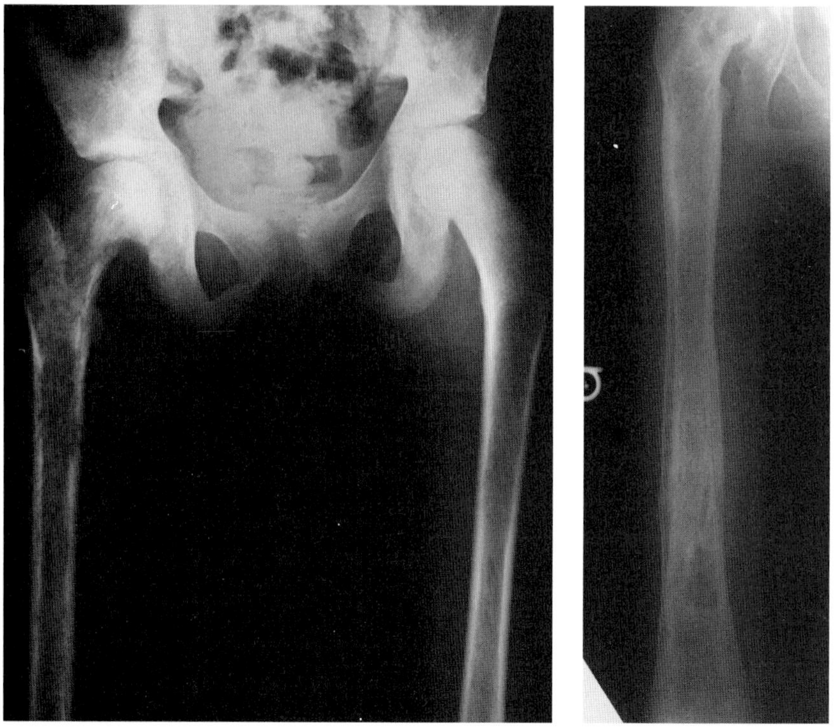

Fig. 5 **Left,** This 10-year-old female has acute Gaucher's disease, bone crisis pain, and biopsy proven *Staphylococcus aureus* osteomyelitis in the left femur. **Right,** The patient's left femur after treatment with parenteral antibiotics and enzyme replacement therapy.

Annotated Bibliography

Hemophilia

Gomperts ED: HIV infection in hemophiliac children: Clinical manifestations and therapy. *Am J Ped Hematol Oncol* 1990;12:497–504.

The article reviews material about children with human immunodeficiency virus (HIV) and hemophilia. Material covered includes epidemiology, clinical manifestations, management, and complications.

Greene WB, McMillan CW: Nonsurgical management of hemophilic arthropathy, in Barr JS Jr (ed): *Instructional Course Lectures XXXVIII.* Park Ridge, IL, American Academy of Orthopaedic Surgeons, 1989, pp 367–381.

This is a good review article on the development, use, and results of factor VIII replacement therapy.

Kitchens CS: Factor IX: A review of its biochemistry and deficiency. *Semin Thromb Hemost* 1991;17:55–72.

This is a review of 25 patients with factor IX deficiency. The biochemistry and physiology of factor IX are presented.

Lusher JM, Warrier I: Hemophilia A. *Hematol Oncol Clin North Am* 1992;6:1021–1033.

This review article details home therapy treatment programs and musculoskeletal problems.

Scharrer I, Neutzling O: Incidence of inhibitors in haemophiliacs: A review of the literature. *Blood Coagul Fibrinolysis* 1993;4:753–758.

Young children with severe hemophilia A are at the highest risk of inhibitor development after relatively few replacement treatments.

Telfer MC: Clinical spectrum of viral infections in hemophilic patients. *Hematol Oncol Clin North Am* 1992;6:1047–1056.

This article discusses the spectrum of infections with HIV, hepatitis B, and hepatitis C in patients with hemophilia.

Triantafyllou SJ, Hanks GA, Handal JA, et al: Open and arthroscopic synovectomy in hemophilic arthropathy of the knee. *Clin Orthop* 1992;283:196–204.

A comparison of techniques demonstrates reduced length of stay and factor replacement with arthroscopic synovectomy but neither technique halts the arthropathy.

Sickle-Cell Disease

Bennett OM, Namnyak SS: Bone and joint manifestations of sickle-cell anaemia. *J Bone Joint Surg* 1990;72B:494–499.

Salmonella was the causative organism in 71% of patients with osteomyelitis and sickle-cell disease.

Huo M, Friedlaender GE, Marsh JS: Orthopaedic manifestations of sickle-cell disease. *Yale J Biol Med* 1990;63:195–207.

A review is presented of the osseous manifestations in sickle-cell disease, including osteomyelitis.

Thalassemia

Giardina PJ, Hilgartner MW: Update on thalassemia. *Pediatr Rev* 1992;13:55–62.

This article outlines the standards for transfusion, splenectomy, prevention of postsplenectomy infection, and effective iron chelation therapy.

Leukemia

Bleyer WA: Acute lymphoblastic leukemia in children: Advances and prospectus. *Cancer* 1990;65(suppl 3): 689–695.

This review outlines the staging and treatment of acute lymphoblastic leukemia.

Heinrich SD, Gallagher D, Warrior R, et al: The prognostic significance of the skeletal manifestations of acute lymphoblastic leukemia of childhood. *J Pediatr Orthop* 1994;14:105–111.

Gaucher's Disease

Beutler E: Gaucher's disease. *N Engl J Med* 1991;325: 1354–1360.

The current recommendations for the medical management of Gaucher's disease are reviewed.

Bilchik TR, Heyman S: Skeletal scintigraphy of pseudo-osteomyelitis in Gaucher's disease: Two case reports and a review of the literature. *Clin Nucl Med* 1992;17:279–282.

Decreased perfusion and impaired uptake on bone scan are suggestive of bone crisis or pseudo-osteomyelitis in Gaucher's disease.

Figueroa ML, Rosenbloom BE, Kay AC, et al: A less costly regimen of alglucerase to treat Gaucher's disease. *N Engl J Med* 1992;327:1632–1636.

The treatment of Gaucher's disease with smaller doses of alglucerase given more frequently yields satisfactory results and greatly reduces the annual cost per patient.

Zevin S, Abrahamov A, Hadas-Halpern I, et al: Adult-type Gaucher disease in children: Genetics, clinical features and enzyme replacement therapy. *Q J Med* 1993; 86:565–573.

The article reviews the hematologic and osseous conditions in Gaucher disease and replacement therapy.

Fanconi's Anemia

Alter BP: Fanconi's anemia: Current concepts. *Am J Pediatr Hematol Oncol* 1992;14:170–176.

Current management techniques including bone marrow transplants are reviewed.

Alter BP: Arm anomalies and bone marrow failure may go hand in hand. *J Hand Surg* 1992;17A:566–571.

This review article outlines the association of Fanconi's anemia, Diamond-Blackfan anemia, thrombocytopenia, and absent radii and congenital anomalies involving the hand, forearm, or both.

III

Upper Extremity

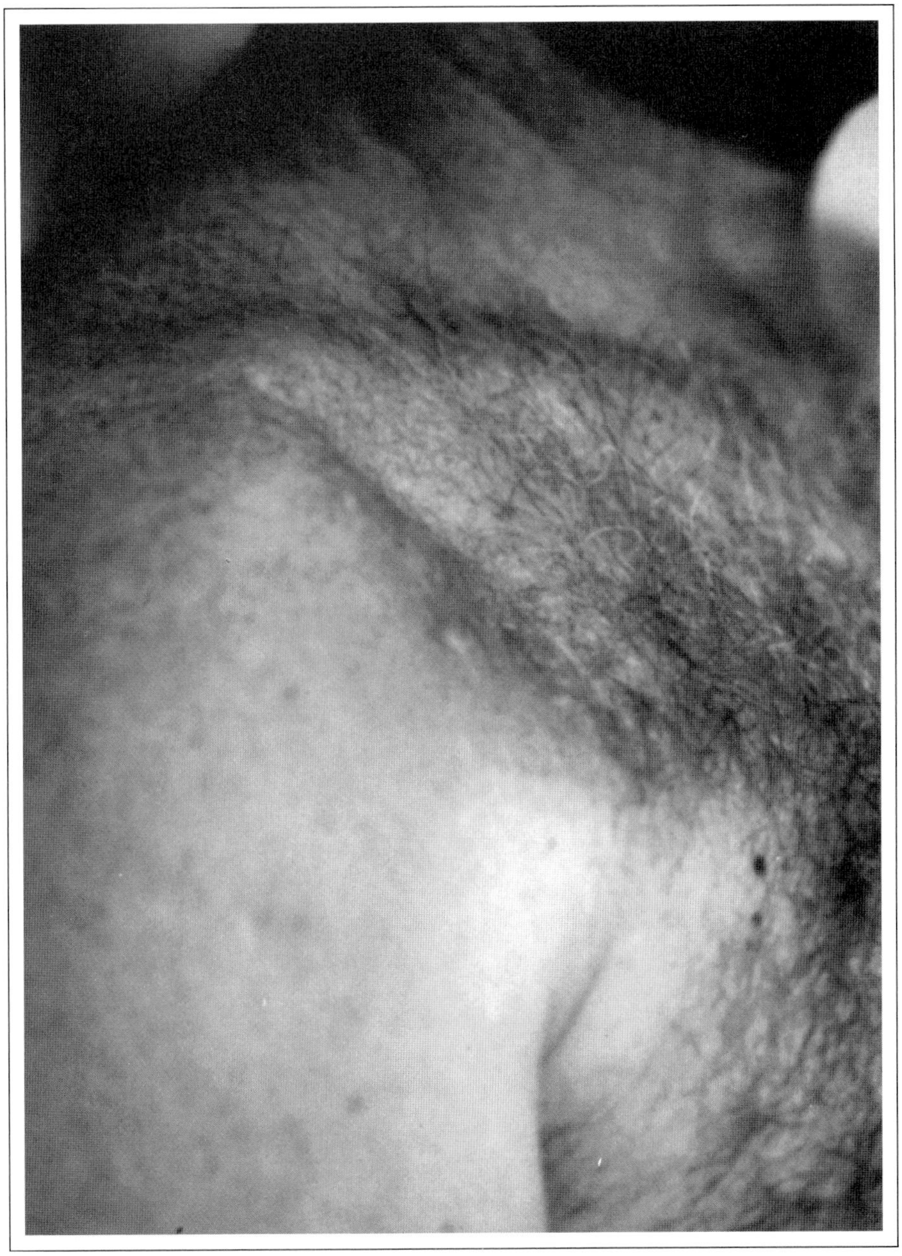

23

Shoulder and Arm: Pediatric Aspects

Congenital Anomalies and Acquired Disorders

Brachial Plexus Injury

Brachial plexus injuries occur in 2.0 to 2.5 of every 1,000 live births in this country. Risk factors for obstetric palsy include high birth weight, prolonged labor, shoulder dystocia, breech presentation, and forceps delivery. The incidence of brachial plexus palsy has remained constant, but fewer severe palsies occur as a result of modern obstetric techniques. These techniques include induction of labor at an earlier gestational age in maternal diabetes when a large infant is expected and cesarean sections for prolonged labor or difficult deliveries. Brachial plexus injuries range in severity from neurapraxia and axonotmesis to complete rupture of roots and avulsion from the spinal cord.

A newborn with a brachial plexus injury may present with a completely flail upper extremity, or the limb may be held in a posture that reflects the imbalance caused by selective paralysis of upper extremity muscle groups. The differential diagnosis includes clavicle fracture with pseudoparalysis, proximal humeral epiphyseal separation, and posterior shoulder dislocation. The most common of these conditions is an isolated clavicle fracture. This condition is easily distinguished from brachial plexus injury because infants with isolated clavicle fractures have an intact Moro reflex and active motion usually returns within 1 week. Clavicle fractures occur in association with a brachial plexus injury in approximately 10% to 15% of patients.

The predominant level of plexus involvement usually becomes apparent within the first 2 to 8 weeks of life. Upper plexus involvement is most common. Infants with C-5, C-6 level lesions typically present with an adducted and internally rotated shoulder, an extended elbow, and normal hand function. If C-7 is also injured, the elbow may be slightly flexed. If the entire plexus is injured, the arm and hand are flail. Isolated involvement of the distal roots is uncommon. A Horner's sign indicates root avulsion from the cord, generally at a C-8 or T-1 level.

The natural history of obstetric brachial plexus palsy remains uncertain. Reports of several studies have noted very high rates of spontaneous, complete recovery, whereas other reports have noted less favorable long-term outcomes. These differences may be explained by differences in the patient populations studied and in the scoring systems used to record results. For studies that emphasize shoulder function, less favorable overall results tend to be reported, whereas for those that emphasize elbow and hand function, more favorable functional outcomes are reported.

There is general agreement that initial treatment should be conservative for at least 2 to 3 months. Most authorities recommend passive range of motion exercises and emphasize shoulder external rotation, shoulder abduction, and forearm supination, although there is little objective evidence that documents the efficacy of these programs.

The indications for and timing of surgical intervention remain controversial. Advocates of early intervention argue that if the deltoid and biceps muscles do not begin to contract by 3 months of age, recovery may be good but not normal and that if biceps function is not normal by 5 months of age, then spontaneous, complete recovery will not occur. Most proponents of early surgery recommend brachial plexus exploration and reconstruction if deltoid and biceps function does not appear by 3 to 5 months of age. Those who advocate a more conservative approach argue that satisfactory, spontaneous recovery occurs in almost all patients and that reconstructive procedures are available for patients with residual deformity and dysfunction. Two recent natural history studies dispute the premise that the presence or absence of biceps function at 3 months of age correlates with eventual spontaneous recovery. In one prospective series, 173 infants were followed up until their neurologic conditions stabilized. Eighty-four percent of the upper plexus injuries that persisted more than 6 weeks ultimately had good or excellent results at final follow-up. Notably, 80% of the children with no elbow flexion at 3 months had good or excellent results. In another study, 92% of 66 patients reviewed recovered spontaneously. The presence or absence of elbow flexion at 3 months incorrectly predicted recovery in 13% of patients.

Lesions found at surgery include avulsion of nerve roots from the spinal cord, ruptures of nerve roots, and neuromas in continuity. Surgical procedures have included neurolysis, end-to-end repair, and nerve grafting. If the C-5, C-6 nerve roots can be reconstructed, biceps reinnervation may occur by the fifth or sixth month postoperatively with good recovery of function.

A total plexus palsy or isolated involvement of the lower plexus that persists beyond 3 months usually results in an unfavorable outcome if treated conservatively. Surgical results are also disappointing, although the results in children far exceed those achieved in adults. Lower plexus injury is more likely to involve nerve root avulsion from the spinal cord, which is not amenable to nerve grafting.

The late sequelae of upper brachial plexus palsy most frequently include an internal rotation contracture of the shoulder caused by an imbalance between normal internal rotators and paralyzed external rotators. Limited abduction and elevation of the shoulder also occurs (Fig. 1) as

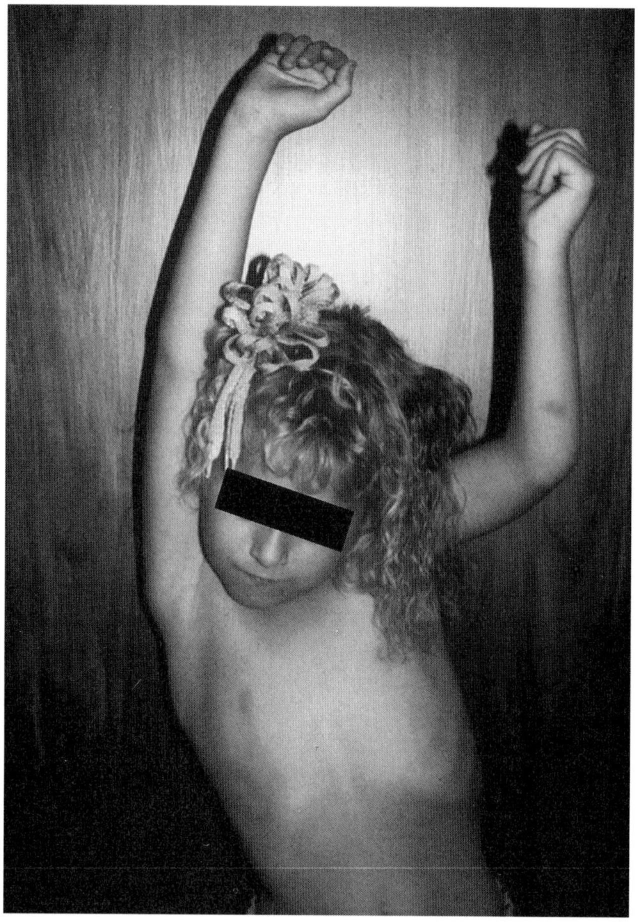

Fig. 1 Limited abduction and shoulder elevation (left) in a child with Erb's palsy.

well as elbow flexion contractures, radial head dislocation, and hypoplasia of the limb. The Sever-L'Episcopo procedure, when performed before the age of 6 years, provides improved external rotation of the shoulder by releasing the internal rotation contracture and transferring the latissimus dorsi and teres major posteriorly to provide active external rotation. Shoulder elevation can be improved if these muscles are transferred to the posterior capsule. Axillary nerve injury has been reported as a complication of the Sever-L'Episcopo procedure. Other authors favor an external rotation osteotomy of the humerus to improve external rotation in older children.

Sprengel's Deformity

Sprengel's deformity is a congenital elevation of the scapula and is the most common congenital disorder of the shoulder. This condition probably is caused by a failure or interruption of the normal caudal migration of the scapula from the lower cervical level to the upper thoracic level. Associated anomalies are found in 70% of patients. The most common anomalies are absent or fused ribs, Klippel-Feil syndrome, congenital scoliosis, and kidney and cardiac anomalies. A connection between the superior border of the scapula and the cervical spine is found in approximately one third of children and, when ossified, is known as the omovertebral bone.

The predominant clinical findings in children with Sprengel's deformity are a web of the neck and limitation of shoulder abduction. In patients with milder grades of this condition, the webbing is invisible when the patient is dressed and shoulder motion is only slightly limited. In more severe grades, the deformity is obvious and total abduction of the shoulder is limited, mainly because of a loss of scapulothoracic motion.

Surgical treatment can improve appearance and function. The Green and the Woodward procedures lower and rotate the scapula and increase abduction as much as 50° to 60°. Most authors agree that the results of surgical treatment are better in children younger than 6 years of age. Patients with milder cosmetic deformities or older children are most appropriately treated with resection of the prominent part of the superior angle of the scapula only. This procedure improves the appearance of the patient but does not change shoulder motion.

Congenital Pseudarthrosis of the Clavicle

Congenital pseudarthrosis of the clavicle almost always involves the right side, although 10% to 15% of cases are bilateral. Pressure exerted by the subclavian artery on the right clavicle during development or a failure of the two ossification centers of the clavicle to coalesce may account for this condition. This condition is distinct from acute neonatal fracture, and spontaneous healing does not occur. Patients with congenital pseudarthrosis of the clavicle present with a lump over the involved clavicle, and the diagnosis usually is made in the first year of life. Radiographs show a pseudarthrosis in the middle of the clavicle with the medial end overriding the lateral end. The ends may be enlarged and bulbous or sclerotic.

Many children are asymptomatic. The principal indications for treatment include persistent pain or an objectionable deformity. Treatment consists of bone grafting and internal fixation with a plate and screws. This has most commonly been done in children older than 4 to 6 years of age. Alternative techniques have been reported in younger patients with favorable results.

Epiphysiolysis of the Proximal Humerus

Adolescents may develop painful widening of the proximal humeral physis with repetitive upper extremity activities. This condition occurs most frequently in adolescent baseball pitchers between the ages of 12 and 15 years and probably represents a stress fracture of the proximal humeral physis. Plain radiographs demonstrate widening and irregularity of the physis. Bone scans are normal. Treatment includes rest and activity modification. Radiographic improvement may lag behind clinical improvement.

Traumatic Injuries

Fractures of the Medial End of the Clavicle and Sternoclavicular Joint

Fracture-separations of the medial end of the clavicle are uncommon and account only for 1% of all clavicular fractures. In children and adolescents, physeal separations usually occur instead of true dislocations of the sternoclavicular joint, because the physis of the medial end of the clavicle does not close until the age of 22 to 25 years, and the strong ligamentous attachments on the medial physis cause it to fracture before the joint dislocates. The mechanism of injury usually is a fall on an outstretched arm or a direct blow to the shoulder or proximal clavicle. Plain radiographs may not show the fracture because of overlapping of the ribs and sternum. An apical lordotic view, with the tube angled 50° to the head and centered on the manubrium, should be obtained. Computed tomography (CT) often is necessary for definitive diagnosis. If the fracture reduces spontaneously, a stress maneuver may be necessary to demonstrate pathology.

Fracture-separations of the medial end of the clavicle displace either anteriorly or posteriorly, and treatment is determined accordingly. Anteriorly displaced fracture-separations are treated with sling immobilization for support and usually heal with little or no functional disability. When the distal fragment is anteriorly displaced, a prominence over the medial end of the clavicle at the junction of the sternum is noticeable and may persist after healing. However, about 80% of the growth of the clavicle occurs from the medial physis, and significant remodeling may occur.

Fracture-separations with posterior displacement of the distal fragment are more serious injuries, because the fragment may impinge on mediastinal structures, causing hoarseness, shortness of breath, dysphasia, vascular compromise, paresthesias, and weakness of the involved upper extremity. Closed reduction should be attempted; if it is unsuccessful, a sterile towel clip can be used to percutaneously grasp the displaced clavicle and bring it forward. Open reduction is indicated only when percutaneous reduction fails. A vascular surgeon should be available at the time of reduction to repair any vessels injured by the posteriorly displaced fragment. After reduction, the patient is immobilized in a figure-of-eight harness. Internal fixation should be avoided because of the danger of implant migration. Posteriorly displaced fracture separations are difficult to reduce by closed methods more than 72 hours after injury, and if there is no evidence of intrathoracic trauma or mediastinal compression they are best treated with simple sling immobilization.

Clavicular Fractures

Displaced and nondisplaced fractures of the midshaft of the clavicle are the most common clavicular fractures in children, and most heal with sling or figure-of-eight immobilization. A noticeable "bump" at the fracture site usually is present after fracture union, but causes little or no functional restriction and will remodel with growth.

Surgical treatment is recommended for open fractures or if severe tenting of the skin indicates impending open fracture. If open reduction and internal fixation (ORIF) are indicated, careful technique is essential to minimize periosteal damage. Acceptable techniques include use of a one third semitubular plate or a small dynamic compression plate for fixation. Intramedullary fixation should be considered very carefully because of the risk for migration that has been reported to cause both minor and major (life-threatening) complications. For nonunions, iliac crest bone grafting should be used at the time of internal fixation.

Fractures of the Lateral End of the Clavicle

Most fractures of the lateral end of the clavicle in children involve stripping of the thick periosteum with herniation of bone through the periosteal sleeve. In adults, acromioclavicular dislocations tear the coracoclavicular ligament, but in children these ligaments usually remain intact and attached to the intact periosteal sleeve, and fracture occurs through the physis of the distal end of the clavicle. Rockwood classified these fractures into six types: type I, a ligamentous strain of the acromioclavicular ligaments without disruption of the periosteal tube; type II, a partial disruption of the dorsal periosteal tube with some instability of the distal clavicle and widening of the acromioclavicular joint, but a normal coracoclavicular distance; type III, a large dorsal split in the periosteal tube with gross instability and displacement of the distal clavicle, and a coracoclavicular distance of 25% to 100% greater than normal; type IV, an injury similar to type III with the distal clavicle buttonholed through the trapezius muscle posteriorly (types III and IV injuries usually are pseudodislocations of the acromioclavicular joints and are Salter-Harris type I injuries); type V, a complete dorsal periosteal split with stripping of the deltoid and trapezius muscle off the clavicle, and a coracoclavicular distance of more than 100% of normal; and type VI, a rare inferior dislocation of the clavicle beneath the coracoid and complete stripping of the tissue off the distal clavicle. Types I through III injuries should be treated nonsurgically with sling immobilization or a clavicular strap for comfort. Because of the excellent potential for remodeling in young children, types IV and V injuries may be treated nonsurgically, but in adolescents ORIF with soft-tissue repair may be required. All type VI fractures require ORIF.

Fractures of the Proximal Humerus

Fractures of the proximal humeral physis are more commonly seen in adolescents than in children because of the increased incidence of trauma from sports and motor vehicle accidents in adolescents. Weakening of the perichondral ring just before skeletal maturity also may be a contributing factor. If this fracture occurs in an infant, the possibility of child abuse should be considered.

Because the periosteum and physis are weaker anterolaterally and stronger posteromedially, these fractures tend to displace anterolaterally. In children younger than 5 years of age, proximal humeral physeal fractures usually are Salter-Harris type I fractures, and in children older than 10 years of age, they usually are Salter-Harris type II fractures. Proximal humeral metaphyseal fractures are more common than physeal fractures in children between the ages of 5 and 10 years, because rapid growth weakens the metaphyseal bone. Salter-Harris types III, IV, and V fractures of the proximal humerus are uncommon.

Dameron and Rockwood developed guidelines for acceptable alignment of proximal humeral fractures in children. In those younger than 5 years of age, 70° of angulation with some apposition is acceptable; in children between the ages of 5 and 12 years, 40° to 45° of angulation with 50% apposition is acceptable; and 40° of angulation with 50% apposition is acceptable in children older than 12 years of age. In adolescents in the last 2 years before skeletal maturity, only minimal (less than 30°) angulation is acceptable. Because of the excellent potential for remodeling, most proximal humeral fractures in children can be managed nonsurgically. Treatment consists of a simple sling and swathe. Open reduction is required for open fractures that require irrigation and debridement, Salter-Harris types III or IV fractures, and fractures in adolescents in whom remodeling cannot be expected.

Humeral Shaft Fractures

Humeral shaft fractures are uncommon in children. In infants and neonates, most are caused by child abuse. Humeral shaft fractures become more common as children approach adolescence because of increased exposure to trauma during sports activities.

Most humeral shaft fractures should be treated nonsurgically. In infants and neonates, a sling and swathe is used. The parents need to be advised that some angulation may be present after union, but remodeling can be expected. In older children, a coaptation splint with the elbow supported in a collar and cuff for 3 to 4 weeks is the usual form of treatment. When callus formation is evident, this treatment can be converted to a sling. If angulation of the fracture site is unacceptable and cannot be controlled, a hanging arm cast can be used. In older adolescents approaching skeletal maturity, a fracture brace can be used to maintain alignment while the fracture is healing.

ORIF generally is indicated for open fractures, although internal fixation is not always necessary. Irrigation and debridement and immobilization in a coaptation splint may be all that is required in a younger child. Internal or external fixation may be required for patients with polytrauma, head injuries, vascular compromise, or ipsilateral forearm fractures.

Humeral shaft fractures may cause radial nerve dysfunction. If the radial nerve is not functional at initial examination, the nerve injury probably occurred at the time of fracture, and a period of observation up to 3 to 4 months is acceptable. If, however, radial nerve function is normal at initial examination but is abnormal after manipulation, exploration is indicated. Spontaneous recovery can be expected in most patients. Nerve severance is reported to occur in 4% to 12% of humeral shaft fractures. Exploration and primary repair of the radial nerve is indicated in an open fracture at the time of debridement. Exploration and delayed repair for a nonfunctioning radial nerve gives results equivalent to primary repair. Overgrowth is reported to occur in about 80% of humeral shaft fractures but usually does not cause a functional problem.

Annotated Bibliography

Obstetric Brachial Plexus Palsy

Gilbert A, Whitaker I: Obstetrical brachial plexus lesions. *J Hand Surg* 1991;16B:489–491.

Fourteen years of experience with 290 surgical cases followed up for 2 or more years are reviewed. The authors outline their indications and report favorable results as well as a 50% complication rate from surgery.

Greenwald AG, Schute PC, Shiveley JL: Brachial plexus birth palsy: A 10-year report on the incidence and prognosis. *J Pediatr Orthop* 1984;4:689–692.

This study reports a retrospective review of 34 of 61 patients with an obstetric brachial plexus palsy. Average follow-up was 4 years 7 months. All but three patients had upper plexus palsies, and complete recovery was recorded in 96% of the 34 patients reviewed. Complete recovery occurred in 92% of the patients by 3 months.

Hentz VR, Meyer RD: Brachial plexus microsurgery in children. *Microsurgery* 1991;12:175–185.

This is an excellent review article in which the authors present a strong argument for early reconstruction of brachial plexus injuries. They present a review of the literature on the natural history of this condition and then describe their strategy for patient evaluation and their indications for surgery. Strategies for managing lesions typically found at surgery are outlined and results from surgery are contrasted with natural history data.

Jahnke AH Jr, Bovill DF, McCarroll HR Jr, et al: Persistent brachial plexus birth palsies. *J Pediatr Orthop* 1991;11:533–537.

Sixty-four children were retrospectively reviewed. Hypoplasia of the limb, internal rotation contractures of the shoulder, and elbow flexion contractures were the most common residual deformities in this group of children who had all been treated with range of motion exercises.

Laurent JP, Lee R, Shenaq S, et al: Neurosurgical correction of upper brachial plexus birth injuries. *J Neurosurg* 1993;79:197–203.

Twenty-four infants with no neurologic improvement in the upper plexus by 4 months underwent surgical reconstruction. The deltoid and biceps were improved to antigravity at 9-month follow-up.

Michelow BJ, Clarke HM, Curtis CG, et al: The natural history of obstetrical brachial plexus palsy. *Plast Reconstr Surg* 1994;93:675–681.

Sixty-six patients with an obstetric brachial plexus palsy were reviewed at a median age of 12 months. Ninety-two percent of patients recovered spontaneously. Although elbow flexion at 3 months correlated with spontaneous recovery at 12 months, use of this parameter alone incorrectly predicted the probability of recovery in 13% of cases.

Strecker WB, McAllister JW, Manske PR, et al: Sever L'Episcopo transfers in obstetrical palsy: A retrospective review of twenty cases. *J Pediatr Orthop* 1990;10:442–444.

Improvement in external rotation as well as subjective functional improvement was seen after the Sever L'Episcopo procedure. Three transient and one permanent axillary nerve palsy occured in this series.

Sprengel's Deformity

Greitemann B, Rondhuis JJ, Karbowski A: Treatment of congenital elevation of the scapula: Ten (2–18) year follow-up of 37 cases of Sprengel's deformity. *Acta Orthop Scand* 1993;64:365–368.

Thirty-seven patients with Sprengel's deformity treated over a 20-year period were reviewed. Thirty-four patients had additional deformities but none had neurologic deficits. Twenty-three underwent a variety of surgical procedures. The Woodward procedure provided the best improvement in function. If the primary indication for surgery is cosmesis, then resection of the superior angle of the scapula provides a suitable improvement in appearance.

Leibovic SJ, Ehrlich MG, Zaleske DJ: Sprengel deformity. *J Bone Joint Surg* 1990;72A;192–197.

Sixteen patients (18 shoulders) were treated surgically at an average age of 3 years and 9 months with a procedure that included release of all muscle attachments to the scapula, resection of the omovertebral band, and displacement of the scapula into a pocket in the latissimus dorsi. Average shoulder abduction improved approximately 60°.

Congenital Pseudarthrosis of the Clavicle

Grogan DP, Love SM, Guidera KJ, et al: Operative treatment of congenital pseudarthrosis of the clavicle. *J Pediatr Orthop* 1991;11:176–180.

Eight young children (ages 1 to 6 years) were treated with a technique that included resection of the fibrous pseudarthrosis and sclerotic bone ends, preservation of the periosteal sleeve, and apposition of bone ends. Internal fixation and additional bone graft were not used. All were solidly healed by 14 weeks after surgery and no recurrences were noted.

Schoenecker PL, Johnson GE, Howard B, et al: Congenital pseudarthrosis. *Orthop Review* 1992;21: 855–860.

Five children with congenital pseudarthrosis of the clavicle were treated with open reduction and internal fixation with contoured plates and screws. Iliac crest or local bone graft was used in all cases. Healing occured in all patients by 3 months and the hardware was removed at an average of 16 months following surgery.

Epiphysiolysis of the Proximal Humerus

Barnett LS: Little league shoulder syndrome: Proximal humeral epiphyseolysis in adolescent baseball pitchers. A case report. *J Bone Joint Surg* 1985;67A:495–496.

The author reports the typical clinical and radiographic findings in patients with this uncommon condition. Anteroposterior radiographs with the arm in external rotation will reveal the characteristic radiographic findings. Comparison views with the opposite side may be helpful and are recommended.

Traumatic Injuries

Baxter MP, Wiley JJ: Fractures of the proximal humeral epiphysis: Their influence on humeral growth. *J Bone Joint Surg* 1986;68B:570–573.

The authors demonstrate the potential for remodeling of proximal humeral fractures in pediatric patients.

Beaty JH: Fractures of the proximal humerus and shaft in children, in Eilert RE (ed): *Instructional Course Lectures Volume XLI.* Park Ridge, IL, American Academy of Orthopaedic Surgeons, 1992, pp 369–372.

This is a review article of the treatment of proximal humeral and humeral shaft fractures in pediatric patients.

Cope R, Riddervold HO, Shore JL, Sistrom CL: Dislocations of the sternoclavicular joint: Anatomic basis, etiologies, and radiologic diagnosis. *J Orthop Trauma* 1991;5:379–384.

The authors describe the plain radiographic views and CT scan stress maneuver to make the diagnosis of sternoclavicular fracture separations.

de Jager LT, Hoffman EB: Fracture-separation of the distal humeral epiphysis. *J Bone Joint Surg* 1991;73B: 143–146.

This is a report of the high incidence of cubitus varus after closed treatment of this injury. Closed reduction and percutaneous pinning are recommended.

de Jong KP, Sukul DM: Anterior sternoclavicular dislocation: a long-term follow-up study. *J Orthop Trauma* 1990;4:420–423.

The authors of this long-term follow-up study of patients with anterior sternoclavicular joint dislocations report good results with nonsurgical treatment.

Lewonowski K, Bassett GS: Complete posterior sternoclavicular epiphyseal separation: A case report and review of the literature. *Clin Orthop* 1992;281:84–88.

This review article describes the anatomy, diagnosis, treatment, and complications of posterior sternoclavicular fracture separation.

24

Shoulder Trauma: Bone

Proximal Humerus Fractures

With increasing life expectancies and concomitant rates of osteoporosis, proximal humerus fractures, which represent 5% to 7% of all fractures and 76% of humeral fractures in patients over 40 years of age, continue to pose challenging management problems. A recent study suggested that the increasing number of osteoporosis-related fractures are related to impaired vision, balance, and decreased muscle trophism, which are due to the overall poor health of the elderly and predispose them to falls. Despite this, these authors were unable to find a difference in the healing rates of minimally to moderately displaced fractures in osteoporotic and normal subjects. Although the mechanism of injury in the elderly still most commonly involves a fall on the outstretched hand, high-velocity injuries are often responsible for the severely displaced fractures in young patients with good bone quality.

An accurate diagnosis is mandatory to classify and successfully treat these injuries. Although recent studies have addressed the issue of inter- and intraobserver reliability when the Neer classification system is used, it remains the standard. It is a comprehensive classification system based on the degree of displacement of the four osseous segments about the proximal humerus: humeral head, shaft, and greater and lesser tuberosities. Fragments are considered displaced if they are separated by at least 1.0 cm or angulated greater than 45°. The displacement is dictated by the deforming muscle forces of the rotator cuff insertions on the tuberosities and the pectoralis major on the humeral shaft. The degree of separation of fracture fragments has prognostic implications because disruption of the local blood supply to the articular segment has been shown to correlate with degree of displacement and subsequent osteonecrosis. Rates of osteonecrosis as high as 94% have been reported for three- and four-part fractures. The anterolateral branch of the anterior circumflex artery provides the main head arterial blood supply via the intertubercular groove and is most often implicated in the development of osteonecrosis. One case of posttraumatic osteonecrosis has been reported in a 28-year-old male 3 years after an anterior dislocation with a nondisplaced greater tuberosity fracture in which the posterior humeral circumflex artery is implicated as the cause.

Radiographs in three planes consisting of scapular anteroposterior (AP), scapular lateral, and axillary views represent the trauma series and are the required minimum to accurately classify these injuries (Fig. 1). It has been reported that additional studies such as computed tomography (CT) scans aid in the determination of the size of artic-

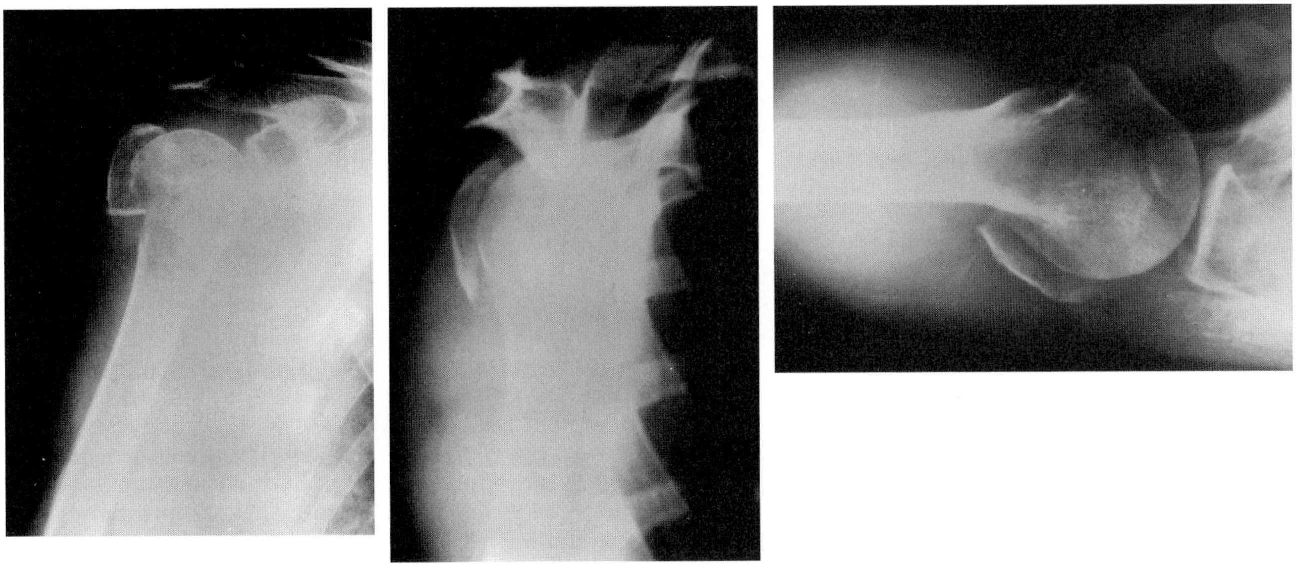

Fig. 1 Trauma series, consisting of (**left** to **right**) scapular AP, lateral and axillary views of displaced two-part greater tuberosity fracture.

ular surface defects, but add little to change the original diagnosis based on the three orthogonal plain films. Further detail to identify all four segments is best sought in the form of oblique plain radiographs. The crucial need for the axillary view has been emphasized in several studies. It is needed not only to describe the glenohumeral articular surface relationships for dislocations and head defects, but also for the ability to identify posterior greater tuberosity and medial lesser tuberosity displacement, both of which may be missed on standard AP films. The axillary view has been found to add significantly more information toward making a definitive diagnosis than the scapular lateral view. Accurate radiographs are required before any type of fracture or dislocation reduction, because further displacement of neck fractures may be caused iatrogenically. One study reported seven such cases, in three of which the surgical neck fracture was unidentified prior to attempted reduction. Five cases led to complete displacement of the head segment. Therefore, the authors advised ruling out neck fractures, especially when tuberosity fractures were also identified. It should be noted that only biplanar (scapular AP and lateral) views were used in this series and that perhaps the addition of the axillary view would have increased the diagnostic accuracy prior to reduction maneuvers.

Upon clinical presentation, immediate neurovascular examination should be carried out in an organized manner. Early detection is required for adequate treatment. Previous studies report neurologic injury rates between 21% and 36%. In a recent prospective study, 45% of 101 patients had electrophysiologic evidence of nerve injury in primary glenohumeral dislocations or humeral neck fractures. Nerves most commonly involved were the axillary, suprascapular, radial, and musculocutaneous. The elderly population was at higher risk, especially when significant hematomas were identified. Most patients recovered partially or completely in less than 4 months, but eight had persistent motor loss. The authors recommended early diagnosis and physiotherapy. Vascular injuries, most commonly involving the axillary artery, remain devastating surgical emergencies that require a high level of suspicion when ischemia is noted, despite the presence of distal pulses, which have been reportedly palpable in 27% of patients with major arterial injuries about the shoulder. It is believed that rigid fixation of the fracture is necessary to protect the site of vascular repair, but this point recently has been debated.

Goals of fracture management include restoring anatomy, obtaining soft-tissue and osseous healing, and maximizing the function of the entire upper extremity. Indications for nonsurgical versus surgical management are dictated by a host of factors, including the degree of displacement of fragments; the fracture type; the patient's physiologic age, general medical condition, ability to comply with intensive rehabilitation, bone quality, concomitant medical problems, associated injuries, and arm dominance; and the surgeon's level of expertise.

The literature contends that 80% to 85% of proximal humerus fractures are minimally or nondisplaced and can functionally do quite well with nonsurgical treatment regimens, which begin with sling and swathe immobilization, until the fracture moves as a unit. Early passive motion remains the treatment of choice at 1 to 14 days postinjury, depending on fracture stability, and treatment progresses to active motion and strengthening only after radiographic union has been achieved. Overly aggressive early passive motion and active motion prior to fracture healing have been correlated with increased rates of nonunion.

Fractures described as displaced require management in the form of closed reduction (with or without percutaneous pinning), open reduction and internal fixation (ORIF), or prosthetic replacement. Although some two-part fractures and fracture-dislocations do well with closed reduction, many displaced two- and three-part fractures will require ORIF. Fracture patterns amenable to ORIF include two-part greater tuberosity fractures, lesser tuberosity fractures involving the articular surface and limiting internal rotation, surgical neck fractures in which reduction cannot be obtained or maintained, and some anatomic neck fractures in which there is adequate head size and quality to allow fixation. Surgical neck fracture-dislocations as well as two-part tuberosity fracture-dislocations with persistent tuberosity displacement after glenohumeral joint reduction warrant surgical intervention. ORIF remains the treatment of choice for most three-part fractures and fracture-dislocations unless the tuberosity and head fragments are too osteoporotic, with frail tendinous insertions, to obtain secure enough fixation to allow early passive motion. In these cases, prosthetic replacement is the better choice. Prosthetic replacement is also indicated in four-part fractures and fracture-dislocations, head-splitting fractures, and in impression defects greater than 40% of the articular surface.

Although plate fixation has been popular in the past, there is a growing trend toward minimal osteosynthesis because of the problems associated with plates and screws. Problems include loss of fixation in soft, osteoporotic bone, osteonecrosis from soft-tissue stripping, and plate impingement on the surrounding tissues and acromion. Various other techniques, such as skeletal traction, external fixation, percutaneous pins, staples, intramedullary nails, wire or suture loops, and tension-band intramedullary nail and wire constructs, have been described. The use of suture or wire fixation is reported to have several advantages in osteoporotic bone: (1) it requires less extensive exposure and soft-tissue stripping and, therefore, may better preserve humeral head vascularity; (2) it allows for incorporation of the rotator cuff tendon insertion, which is often stronger than fixation in osteoporotic bone; and (3) when combined in a figure-of-eight tension-band fashion with intramedullary rods or nails, this configuration can produce extremely solid fixation that allows for early passive motion, which is critical for successful results.

Treatment of two-part surgical neck fractures depends on the inherent stability of the fracture. Fractures in which a stable closed reduction can be achieved may be treated as such with or without the addition of percutaneous pin fixation. If a stable reduction cannot be maintained, the addition of percutaneous pins or ORIF is warranted. Authors reporting a series of 48 fractures treated with closed reduction and percutaneous pin fixation stressed the importance of pin placement using at least three pins, but advised open reduction with limited internal fixation for three-part fractures involving the greater tuberosity. Complications of this technique included pin tract infection with fixation loosening, malunion, and humeral shaft fracture at the site of pin insertion after hardware removal. ORIF is indicated for two-part surgical neck fractures in which soft-tissue interposition of the deltoid or biceps tendon precludes achieving an acceptable closed reduction.

AO plate fixation was compared to Rush pin insertion through the greater tuberosity combined with a tension-band wire to the shaft. Plate fixation was found to achieve good functional results in seven of eight patients under 50 years of age who sustained injuries from high-velocity trauma. However, in the more common low-energy injury, osteoporotic fractures population, results were unsatisfactory in 12 of 14 patients, with failure usually due to loss of fixation. The Rush pin technique produced more reliable results in this age group; satisfactory functional scores were obtained in 16 of 23 patients. The authors suggest that the Rush pin technique is preferable to plate fixation in the more common osteoporotic, insufficiency fracture in the elderly. In another series, ORIF of two- and three-part surgical neck fractures was undertaken using heavy, nonabsorbable suture or wire that incorporated the rotator cuff tendons, tuberosities, and shaft. In cases with significant surgical neck comminution, curved 3.5-mm Ender nails inserted in an antegrade fashion were used in a tension-band construct that was found to give three-point fixation and add longitudinal and rotational stability (Fig. 2). Eighteen (82%) of the 22 patients had good or excellent results. Results were good to excellent for 71% of two-part and 100% of three-part surgical neck fractures, with average active forward elevation of 142°, external rotation to 47°, and internal rotation to the eleventh thoracic vertebra. The authors modified the Ender nail by placing an additional hole above the eyelet for passage of the tension-band suture. This allowed for deeper insertion of the nail well below the surface of the cuff tendons. After this modification, no patient required rod removal due to prominence superiorly. All fractures achieved union, there were no infections, and there was only one partial loss of fixation.

Humeral head replacement remains the preferred method of management in two-part anatomic neck fractures because of the high incidence of osteonecrosis due to disruption of the vascularity to the articular segment. In young, active patients in whom the articular segment is of adequate size and quality, ORIF or percutaneous pin fixation may be attempted despite the potential for a high rate of revision surgery.

Two-part tuberosity fractures may occur as isolated injuries or in conjunction with glenohumeral dislocations.

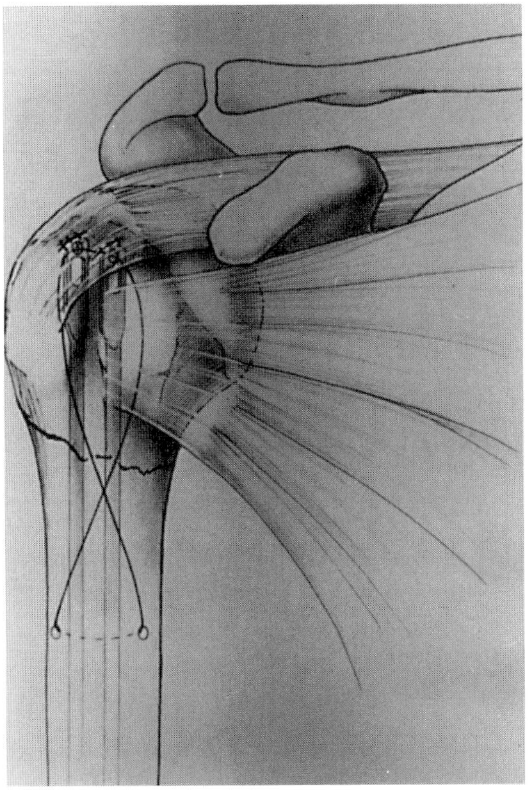

Fig. 2 Figure-of-eight tension band fixation supplemented with Ender nails incorporates strong rotator cuff in repair. (Reproduced with permission from Cuomo F, Flatow EL, Maday MM, et al: Open reduction and internal fixation of two- and three-part displaced surgical neck fractures of the proximal humerus. *J Shoulder Elbow Surg* 1992;1:287–295.)

Anterior and posterior dislocations are associated with greater and lesser tuberosity fractures, respectively. Fracture-dislocations of this type tend to respond well to closed reduction and subsequent immobilization. Redislocation is rare after fracture healing. Up to 80% of posterior dislocations are still missed on initial presentation and require complete radiographs with axillary view to improve diagnostic accuracy. After reduction of the joint, the tuberosity will often return to its cancellous bed in near anatomic position (Fig. 3). If there is significant residual displacement, the anatomy should be restored surgically with open reduction and repair of the rotator cuff tear. Isolated greater tuberosity fractures are pulled superiorly and/or posteriorly by the rotator cuff insertion.

A recent report on ORIF of two-part greater tuberosity fractures indicated that scapular AP and lateral views failed to demonstrate precisely the amount of posterior retraction and overlap of the fragment with the articular surface. The need for surgical intervention was underestimated in four of 16 patients. The authors stressed the importance of the axillary view to accurately assess poste-

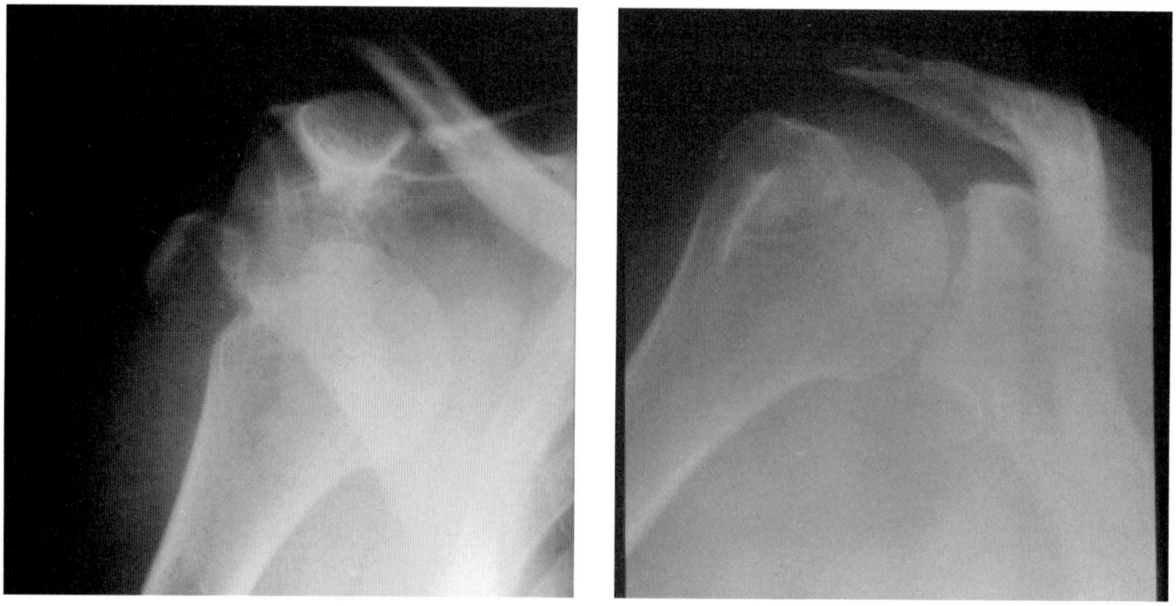

Fig. 3 **Left,** Two part anterior greater tuberosity fracture-dislocation. **Right,** After reduction of the joint, the tuberosity returned to near anatomic position.

rior displacement. In this same series, a deltoid splitting approach combined with heavy, nonabsorbable suture fixation of the tuberosity and rotator cuff repair gave good to excellent results in 100% of 12 patients with average active forward elevation of 170°. Isolated lesser tuberosity fractures are extremely rare, with only 16 cases reported. A review of these cases identified a violent external rotation force while the arm was in abduction as the mechanism of injury in almost all patients. Surgical intervention in the form of ORIF is warranted if a significant portion of articular surface is involved and/or the level of pain and limitation of internal rotation are unacceptable to the patient. Excision of the avulsed lesser tuberosity fragment with repair of the subscapularis and anterior capsule has also been described.

Three-part fractures and fracture-dislocations are often best managed by ORIF. Techniques similar to those discussed for two-part surgical neck fractures are applicable. Figure-of-eight tension-band wiring with and without intramedullary nails has yielded excellent results in several reported series. Standard T-plate fixation has lost favor due to reported high failure rates related to extensive soft-tissue stripping, inadequate screw fixation, and hardware impingement that required further surgery for removal. Treatment of three- and four-part fractures with a modified cloverleaf plate in 26 young patients (19 to 62 years) yielded excellent results in 22, good results in two, and fair results in two. The authors stated that this small malleable plate, which allows placement of four small cancellous screws into the head and tuberosities, could be placed high on the head without impingement. They suggested the results obtained were associated with limited exposure, careful soft-tissue dissection, and stable fixation with less damage to the head fragment than with 6.5 mm cancellous screws used with the T-plates, should it be necessary at surgery to change screw placement. Good bone stock in this youthful population was also a factor. Humeral head replacement may be warranted in cases in which rigid fixation cannot be obtained to a degree satisfactory to allow early passive range of motion.

Immediate humeral head replacement remains the accepted treatment for four-part fractures and fracture-dislocations, although ORIF in young patients with good bone quality and absence of dislocation may be considered. A series of 35 patients with four-part fractures and fracture-dislocations with a mean age of 59 years were treated with Kirschner wires (K-wires) and tension-band fixation. Results were satisfactory for 65%, with 35% unsatisfactory and poor results. Nine patients developed osteonecrosis (25%), and all cases of fracture-dislocations yielded unsatisfactory or poor results and had a 100% rate of osteonecrosis. These data corroborate results of previous studies, which distinguish between four-part valgus impacted fractures and the classic displaced four-part fracture-dislocation. Lower osteonecrosis rates (20% to 25%) and satisfactory results with open reduction and limited internal fixation were seen in the impacted injury. The majority of four-part fractures and fracture-dislocations are best managed by humeral head replacement (Fig. 4). Technical considerations that correlate with successful outcome include the restoration of humeral length and retroversion (35° to 45°), secure tuberosity fixation, repair

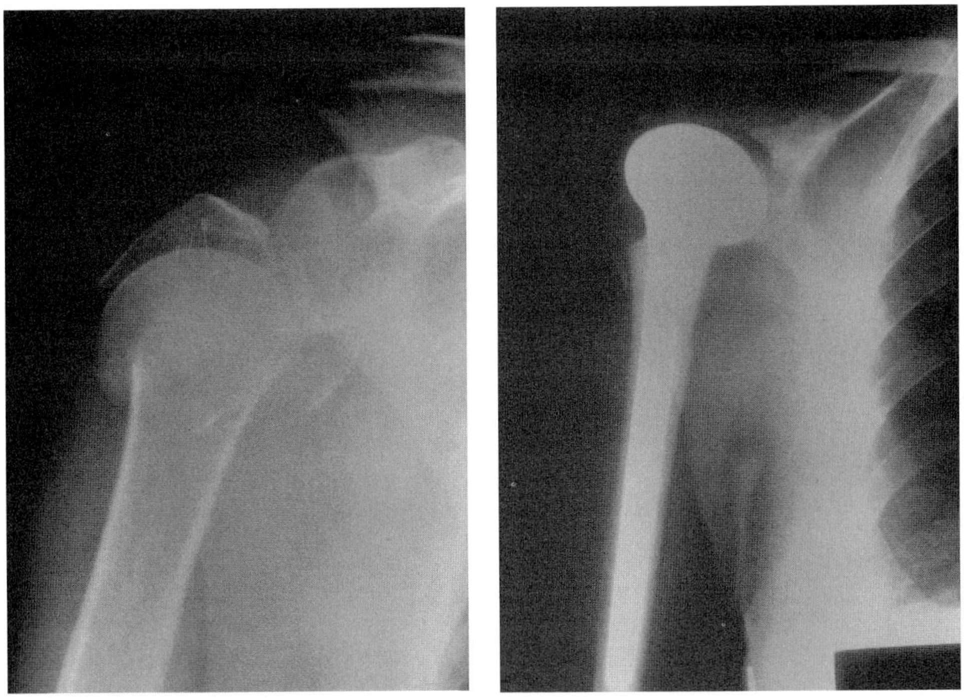

Fig. 4 **Left,** Four-part fracture. **Right,** Following treatment by proximal humerus replacement.

of the rotator cuff, and achievement of anatomic humeral offset. Numerous series have demonstrated consistently reliable results with respect to pain relief. Functional outcome has varied and has been found to be related to age (< 70 yielding superior results), humeral offset > 28 mm, rotator cuff integrity, and individual functional requirements. Humeral head replacement was also deemed to be more successful in three-part rather than four-part fractures.

Articular surface fractures include head-splitting injuries and impression defects and occur secondary to impaction against the glenoid rim. Humeral head replacement is indicated in most head-splitting fractures. Impression fractures most often occur with posterior dislocation; their management is governed by the size of the humeral head defect and the duration of dislocation (Fig. 5). Stable closed reduction can usually be obtained in defects that involve less than 20% of the articular surface and have been present for less than 6 weeks. After reduction, patients are immobilized with the arm at the side in 10° to 15° of external rotation for 4 to 6 weeks. If the dislocation is present for more than 6 weeks, open reduction is indicated. Defects involving between 20% and 40% of the articular surface, which have been present for less than 6 months, can be treated with open reduction and transfer of the lesser tuberosity into the defect through an anterior deltopectoral approach. When the defect is greater than 40% of the articular surface or the dislocation has been present for longer than 6 months, humeral head replacement is indicated with decreased relative retroversion to ensure stability. In a series of chronic anterior dislocations, nine of which were treated with unconstrained replacement arthroplasty, results were satisfactory to excellent in eight of nine. The authors stressed the need for increased humeral retroversion, glenoid bone grafting when anterior bone loss was found to be 50% of the surface, soft-tissue releases, and modified rehabilitation more consistent with an instability repair than with shoulder replacement surgery.

Rehabilitation remains an integral part of postoperative and postinjury management, with optimum results requiring strict attention to protocols. The most useful protocol consists of three phases. Early passive motion is the initial phase and is imperative after ORIF or humeral head replacement. There should be no active motion for 6 weeks or until the fracture or tuberosities have healed. Active and early resistive exercises are then instituted in the second phase. The third phase involves advanced stretching and strengthening exercises with progressive resistance.

Complications of proximal humerus fractures most commonly include osteonecrosis, nonunion, malunion, stiffness, infection, neurovascular injury, and loss of fixation. Nonunion at the level of the surgical neck has been related to soft-tissue interposition, inadequate immobilization, poor patient compliance, excessive soft-tissue stripping, and overly aggressive physical therapy. Treatment includes ORIF with bone grafting or humeral head replacement. In one preliminary report on the operative

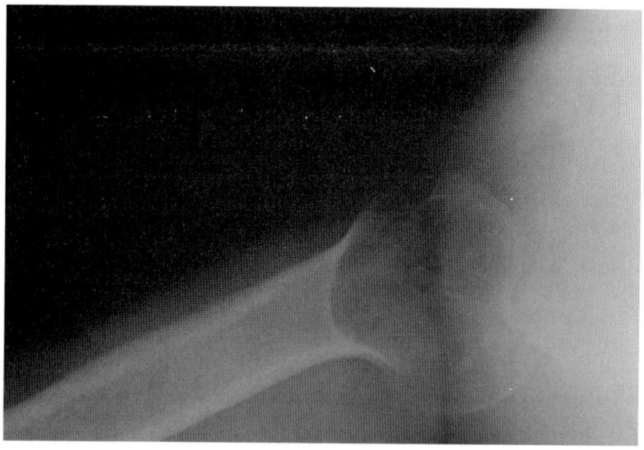

Fig. 5 Axillary view of locked posterior dislocation.

treatment of nonunions of the surgical neck, no significant differences were found between the replacement and ORIF groups with regard to result, although reoperation rates in the ORIF group were higher by fourfold. The high incidence of complications noted with this challenging surgery has led authors to recommend reserving surgical intervention for those patients with significant symptoms.

Fractures of the Scapula

Scapular fractures are uncommon, making up only 1% of all fractures. Disruptions of the scapular body and spine make up approximately 50% of the total, fractures of the glenoid neck approximately 25%, fractures of the glenoid cavity approximately 10%, and fractures of the acromial and coracoid processes approximately 7% each. Scapular fractures are usually caused by high-energy direct trauma. As a result, there is an 80% to 95% incidence of associated injuries, which may be major, multiple, and even life threatening. Consequently, scapular fractures are often diagnosed late and/or definitive treatment is delayed. This delay may compromise the individual's final result. Indirect forces may cause a variety of avulsion fractures at musculotendinous and ligamentous attachment sites. Finally, fatigue or stress fractures are occasionally seen.

Diagnosis is radiographic and the scapular trauma series includes true scapular AP and lateral views as well as a true glenohumeral axillary projection. Due to the complex bony anatomy in the area, however, computed tomography (CT) is generally necessary to accurately detect and define the extent of injury. The scapular body and spine; the acromial, coracoid, and glenoid processes; and the adjacent scapulothoracic, glenohumeral, and acromioclavicular articulations need to be evaluated.

The vast majority (> 90%) of scapular fractures are minimally and acceptably displaced, due primarily to the thick, strong support provided by the surrounding soft tissues. Treatment is symptomatic and nonsurgical. Short-term immobilization in a sling and swathe bandage is provided for comfort. Early progressive range of motion exercises and use of the shoulder out of the sling within clearly defined limits are begun as pain subsides. Most scapular fractures heal completely by 6 weeks, and all external support is discontinued at this time. Progressive functional use of the upper extremity is then encouraged. Physiotherapy continues until range of motion and strength are maximized. The prognosis for these fractures is excellent. Fractures of the scapular body and spine may be severely comminuted and displaced; however, despite sporadic reports describing surgical management, to date there seems to be little enthusiasm for surgery. Fractures of the acromial and coracoid processes, unless severely displaced, are also managed nonsurgically.

There has been increased interest in fractures of the glenoid process (fractures of the glenoid rim, the glenoid fossa, and the glenoid neck). Because these fractures are so rare, large personal series and, especially, strictly controlled studies in which nonsurgical and surgical management of these injuries have been compared are unavailable and always may be. However, relevant case reports and the personal experiences of a number of investigators are available. This information has been summarized in recent papers in an effort to accurately describe these injuries (fracture patterns and mechanisms of injury) and provide therapeutic guidelines (surgical indications and principles as well as postoperative management). Depending on the clinical situation, the glenoid process may be surgically approached anteriorly, posteriorly, and superiorly. Four regions of substantial bone stock are available for internal fixation: the glenoid neck, the scapular spine, the lateral scapular border, and the coracoid process. Fixation can be achieved with a variety of devices; however, the most useful are K-wires, appropriately contoured 3.5-mm reconstruction plates, and 3.5-mm interfragmentary cannulated compression screws. The choice of implant depends on the surgeon's experience and preference as well as the available bone stock.

Surgery is considered for fractures of the glenoid rim if the fragment is displaced greater than or equal to 10 mm and at least one quarter of the glenoid cavity anteriorly or one third of the glenoid cavity posteriorly is involved. The goal is to reestablish osseous stability, thereby preventing chronic glenohumeral instability. Fractures of the anterior rim are approached anteriorly, whereas those of the posterior rim are approached posteriorly. The fracture fragment is reduced anatomically and internally fixed to the glenoid process.

Surgical management is considered for fractures of the glenoid fossa if there is (1) an articular step-off of 5 mm or more; (2) severe separation between the glenoid fragments; and/or (3) significant displacement of the glenoid fragment, such that the humeral head follows and fails to lie

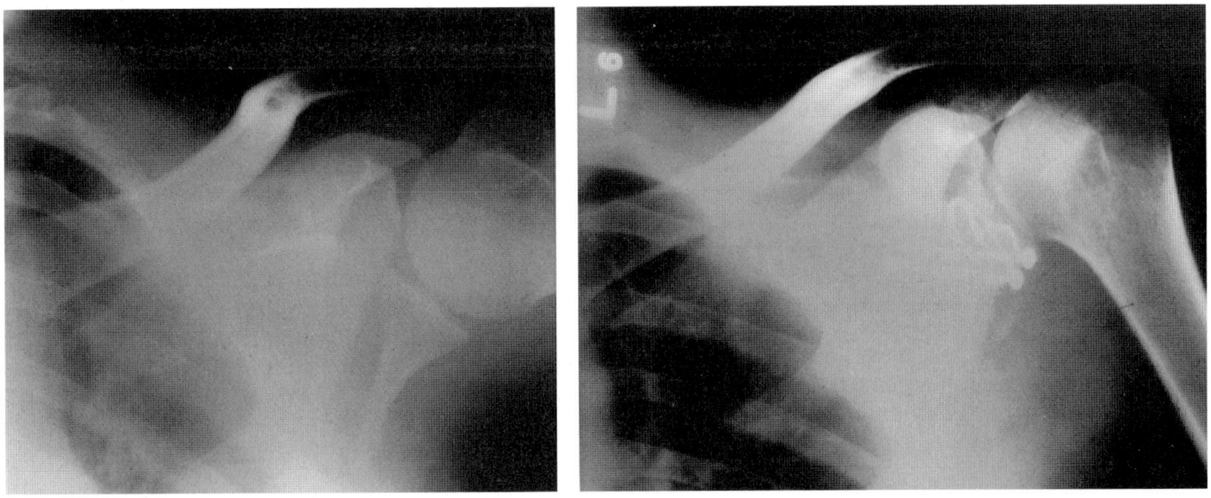

Fig. 6 Radiographs of an individual who sustained a type II fracture of the glenoid cavity. **Left,** A pre-operative AP radiograph showing significant displacement of an inferior glenoid fragment with a severe articular step off. **Right,** Postoperative AP radiograph showing anatomic reduction and stabilization of the inferior glenoid fragment with restoration of articular congruity.

in the center of the glenoid cavity. The goals of operative intervention are to prevent posttraumatic glenohumeral osteoarthritis, to prevent chronic glenohumeral instability, and to prevent a nonunion from occurring at the fracture site. All fractures of the glenoid fossa are approached posteriorly. If a significantly displaced superior glenoid fragment is present, a superior approach is added. The fracture is reduced and internally fixed as anatomically and securely as possible (Fig. 6). Comminuted fractures of the glenoid fossa are managed nonsurgically. The authors of a recent study on ten displaced intra-articular fractures of the glenoid fossa treated with ORIF between 1980 and 1989 found ORIF to be a useful and safe technique for the treatment of selected displaced fractures of the glenoid fossa that can restore excellent function of the shoulder. In another report of 14 displaced intra-articular glenoid fractures treated with ORIF (average follow-up 30.5 months), all shoulders were rated good according to Rowe's scoring system and complications were minimal. The authors concluded that surgical treatment for these fractures gives good and predictable results.

Surgical management for fractures of the glenoid neck has been suggested if there is medial translational displacement of the glenoid fragment of 1 cm or more or angulatory displacement of 40° or more. The goals of surgery are to prevent glenohumeral dysfunction (due primarily to altered mechanisms of the rotator cuff) and glenohumeral instability. All glenoid neck fractures are approached posteriorly, with addition of a superior extension if necessary. The glenoid fragment is reduced and internally fixed as anatomically and securely as possible (Fig. 7). In one recent study, 37 glenoid neck fractures were treated nonsurgically (10 to 20 year follow-up). The functional result was either fair or poor in 32%, leading the authors to conclude that in some fractures early ORIF might have improved the result. In another study, 16 displaced glenoid neck fractures managed nonsurgically (36-month average follow-up) were reviewed retrospectively. Twenty percent were found to have decreased range of motion, 50% had pain (75% night pain), 40% had weakness with exertion, and 25% noted popping. In particular, the authors found these individuals frequently had shoulder abductor weakness and subacromial pain due at least in part to rotator cuff dysfunction. They recommended ORIF for significantly displaced glenoid neck fractures. If comminution precludes internal fixation, overhead olecranon pin traction is a consideration, or displacement of the glenoid fragment must be accepted.

Postoperative management of a surgically treated scapular fracture depends on the degree of stability achieved. Rigidly fixed fractures are protected in a sling and swathe bandage, but early progressive range of motion exercises are begun and functional use of the shoulder out of the sling is permitted (within clearly defined limits) as symptoms allow. If stabilization is less than rigid, full-time postoperative immobilization in a sling and swathe bandage, an abduction splint, or even overhead olecranon pin traction for 7 to 14 days may be necessary, depending on the clinical situation before initiating the rehabilitation program. By 2 weeks, most fractures need only a sling and swathe bandage for protection, progressive range of motion exercises can be prescribed, and gradually increasing functional use of the arm within clearly defined limits is permitted.

At 6 weeks, bony union is usually complete, all external protection can be discontinued, and progressive functional

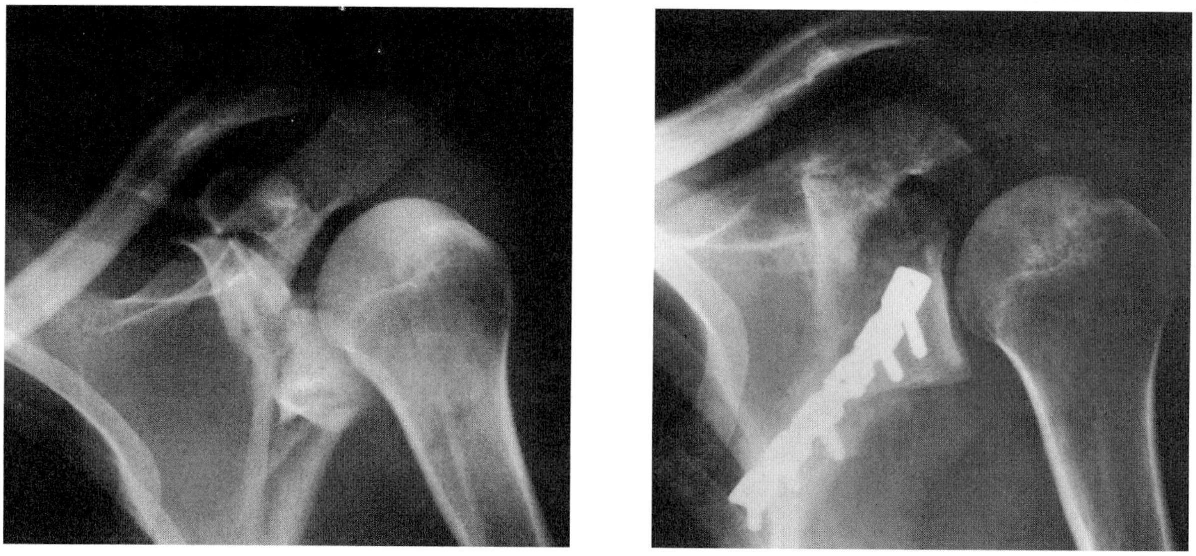

Fig. 7 Radiographs of an individual who sustained a Type II fracture of the glenoid neck. **Left,** Pre-operative AP radiograph showing significant angulatory displacement of the glenoid fragment. **Right,** A postoperative AP radiograph showing reduction and stabilization of the glenoid fragment.

use of the articulation is encouraged. Physiotherapy continues until range of motion and strength are maximized. The patient must be encouraged to continue to work diligently on the rehabilitation program because range of motion and strength can improve, and the patient does not achieve the end result for approximately 6 months to 1 year after injury.

The results of surgically managed fractures of the glenoid process depend on the specifics of the injury, the adequacy of the reduction, the quality of the fixation, and the rigor of the postoperative physiotherapy program. In a report of a 1984 study on 33 patients managed surgically for displaced intra-articular glenoid fractures, fractures of the glenoid rim associated with humeral head subluxation, and unstable fractures of the glenoid neck (6.5 years average follow-up), 79% had a good or excellent result.

The most significant complications associated with scapular fractures are those that result from accompanying injuries to adjacent and distant structures. Complications related to the scapular fractures themselves are relatively uncommon. Nonunion, although possible, is quite rare. Malunion can occur in a variety of forms depending on the particular fracture type. Malunion of scapular body fractures is generally well tolerated; however, painful scapulothoracic crepitus may occur. Fractures of the glenoid cavity may lead to symptomatic glenohumeral degenerative joint disease. Instability can occur following significantly displaced fractures of the glenoid neck (angulatory displacement) and fractures of the glenoid rim. Significantly displaced fractures of the glenoid neck (translational displacement) may give rise to glenohumeral dysfunction as a result of altered mechanics of the surrounding soft tissues.

Fractures of the Clavicle

Fractures of the clavicle are frequent; 85% involve the middle third, 10% the lateral third, and 5% the medial third of the clavicle. Most clavicular fractures are the result of direct trauma; however, a fall onto an outstretched arm can also be the mechanism of injury. Less than 3% of clavicle fractures have associated injuries.

With most middle third fractures, the medial segment is displaced superiorly and posteriorly by the sternocleidomastoid and trapezius muscles while the lateral fragment is displaced inferiorly and medially by the weight of the arm and the pectoralis major. Radiologic evaluation should include AP as well as cephalic and caudal tilt views to evaluate superoinferior and AP displacement, respectively. The vast majority of middle third fractures are treated nonsurgically with a figure-of-eight bandage, and a sling is worn during the initial 7 to 10 days to support the weight of the arm. Shortening and residual deformity usually result; however, in most cases this is painless and does not interfere with shoulder function. Indications for surgery include open fractures, severely displaced fractures (including those with impending skin compromise), and fractures with associated neurovascular injury/compromise. Internal fixation usually consists of either an intramedullary device or a plate and screws. Bone grafting should be considered for comminuted fractures. Ac-

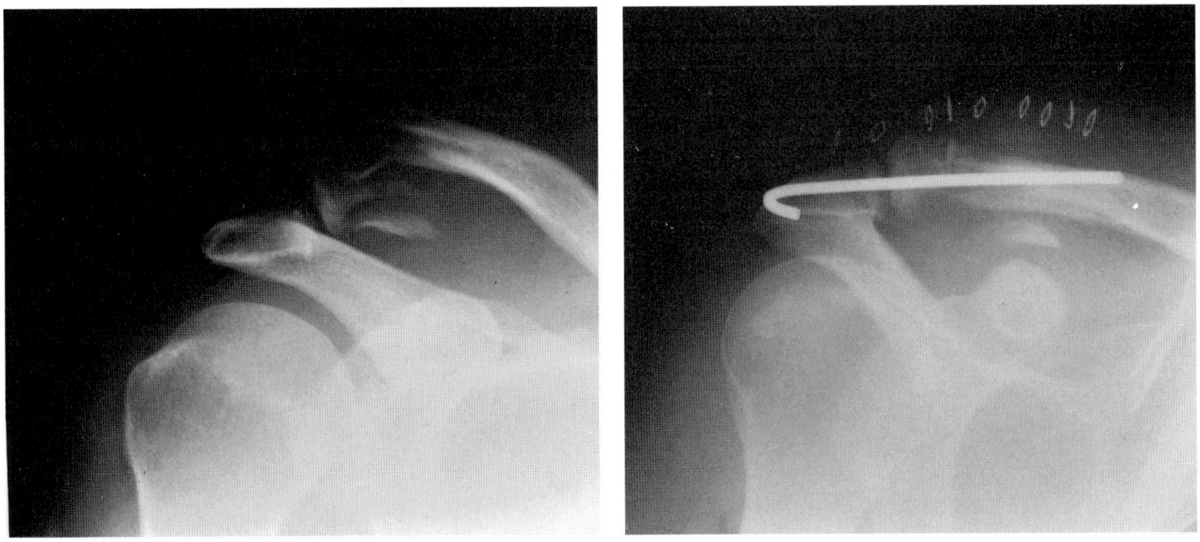

Fig. 8 Radiographs of the an individual who sustained a Type V fracture of the distal clavicle. **Left,** A pre-operative AP weightbearing radiograph of the involved area (note the major medial and lateral clavicular segments and the small inferior fragment to which the coracoclavicular ligaments are attached; note also the significant displacement at the fracture site). **Right,** Postoperative AP radiograph showing the major medial and lateral clavicular segments reduced and stabilized via an intra-medullary K-wire (note that the inferior intermediate fragment and the attached coracoclavicular ligaments are reapproximated to the distal clavicle).

cording to the report of a recent study on the use of a modified Hagie intramedullary pin in the treatment/stabilization of clavicular nonunions, union occurred in 95%. In addition, this technique was not associated with the significant complications that have been reported with other intramedullary devices used for the clavicle (K-wires, Steinmann pins). This technique would also seem to be applicable in the management of acute fractures that require surgical intervention.

Lateral third fractures are subclassified further. Type I injuries are minimally displaced because the coracoclavicular ligaments remain attached to the medial fragment. Type II (two variants) and type V fractures may be significantly displaced because the coracoclavicular ligaments are detached from the medial segments. In type IIA fractures, both the conoid and trapezoid ligaments remain attached to the distal fragment; in type IIB fractures, the conoid ligament is disrupted while the trapezoid ligament remains attached to the distal fragment; and in type V fractures, the conoid and trapezoid ligaments remain attached to a separate inferior cortical fragment. Type III fractures involve the articular surface of the lateral clavicle. Type IV injuries are epiphyseal separations in children. A weightbearing AP radiograph can be obtained to determine whether the coracoclavicular ligaments are functionally detached from the medial clavicular segment. AP and axillary radiographs are indicated to evaluate superoinferior and AP displacement, respectively. CT scanning is useful in determining whether the articular surface of the lateral clavicle has been involved and to what degree. Type I fractures are managed in the same manner as fractures of the middle third. Treatment of type II and type V fractures is controversial. The more displacement at the fracture site, the higher is the risk of nonunion and the greater is the indication for surgical reduction and internal stabilization. Intramedullary devices and coracoclavicular stabilization techniques have been described (Fig. 8). Type III fractures are generally managed nonsurgically. If a large fragment that results in a significant articular step off is present, however, ORIF may be indicated. If symptomatic degenerative joint disease occurs, a distal clavicle resection is the procedure of choice. In a recent study, 110 patients with fractures of the distal end of the clavicle (15-year average follow-up) were treated nonsurgically. Of the 73 type I fractures, 11% had persistent symptoms, 33% healed with deformity, four went on to nonunion, but none had severe disability. Of the 23 type II fractures, 22% went on to a nonunion, 17 were asymptomatic, and none were severely disabled. None of the 14 type III fractures required resection of the distal clavicle. Because none of the patients had severe residual disability, and eight of the ten nonunions were asymptomatic, the authors concluded that fractures of the lateral end of the clavicle do not require surgery. In another study, however, 43 patients with type II fractures were treated between 1965 and 1989; 20 were managed nonsurgically and 23 were managed surgically. The authors found a significant incidence of nonunion (30%), delayed union (45%), residual shoulder dysfunc-

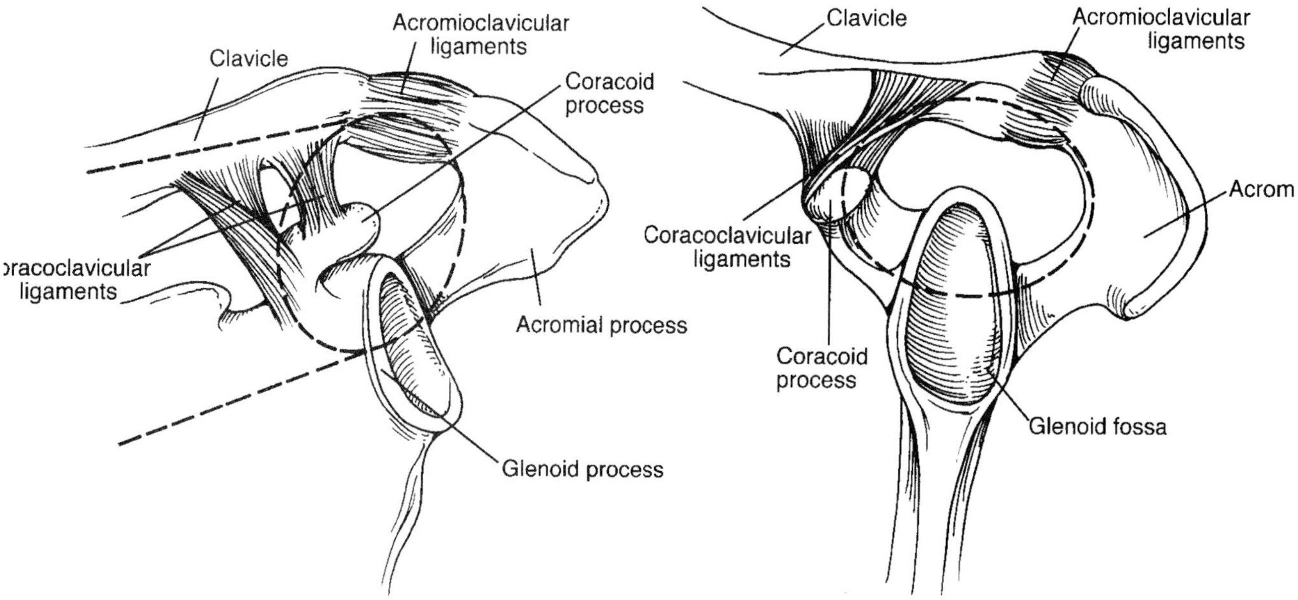

Fig. 9 Superior shoulder suspensory complex. **Left,** Anterioposterior view of the bone–soft-tissue ring and superior and inferior bone struts. **Right,** Lateral view of the bone–soft-tissue ring. (Reproduced with permission from Goss TP: Scapular fractures and dislocations: Diagnosis and treatment. *J Am Acad Orthop Surg* 1995;3:22–33.)

tion, and local complications in those fractures managed nonsurgically. They found ORIF gave superior results.

Fractures of the medial third of the clavicle are caused by high-energy direct trauma. Associated, even life-threatening, injuries, are not uncommon. Radiographic evaluation should include AP as well as cephalic and caudad tilt views; however, due to the complex bony anatomy in the area, CT scanning may be necessary to accurately detect and define these fractures. Treatment is nonsurgical and symptomatic.

Complications following clavicle fractures are uncommon and include nonunion, malunion, neurovascular sequelae, and postoperative degenerative disease of either the acromioclavicular or sternoclavicular joint. The incidence of nonunion has been reported to be 0.9% to 4.0%. Predisposing factors include inadequate immobilization, significant displacement, severity of trauma, soft-tissue interposition, refracture, and primary ORIF. If asymptomatic, no treatment is necessary. If symptomatic (pain, shoulder dysfunction, neurovascular compromise), ORIF (plating or intramedullary fixation) accompanied by bone grafting should be considered.

Malunion is common, although rarely symptomatic. Angulatory deformities are primarily a cosmetic issue, but significant shortening may lead to shoulder dysfunction. Neurovascular sequelae may be acute (secondary to fracture displacement) or delayed (secondary to compromise by exuberant fracture callus or a mobile nonunion). Post-traumatic arthritis can result from intra-articular fractures of either end of the clavicle. If sufficiently symptomatic, resection of the lateral or medial 1.5 cm may be necessary.

Double Disruptions of the Superior Shoulder Suspensory Complex

Double disruption of the superior shoulder suspensory complex (SSSC) is a concept that has been proposed to help the orthopaedist understand and unite a group of difficult-to-treat injuries (many of them involving fractures of the clavicle and scapula), which previously have been described in isolation (Fig. 9). The SSSC is a bone and soft-tissue ring at the end of a superior bony strut, the middle clavicle, and an inferior bony strut, the lateral scapular body. The ring is composed of the glenoid process, the coracoid process, the coracoclavicular ligaments, the distal clavicle, the acromioclavicular joint, and the acromial process. Single disruptions (eg, a type I fracture of the distal clavicle) are common, but because the overall integrity of the complex is maintained, displacement is minimal and nonsurgical treatment is sufficient. If, however, a double disruption occurs, the integrity of the complex is compromised and significant displacement may occur at either or both sites. This displacement, in turn, may have adverse healing and/or functional consequences. As a result, any injury to the SSSC should be evaluated carefully for the possible presence of a double disruption (CT scanning may be necessary). If it is present and displacement at one

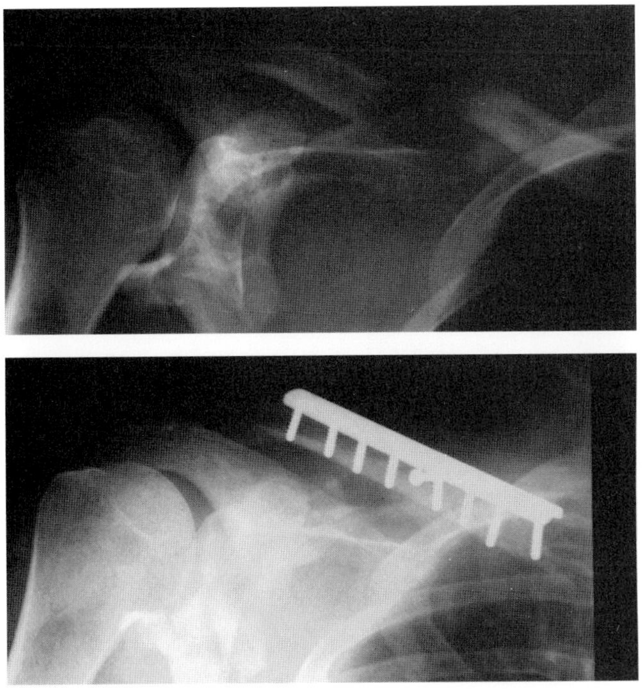

Fig. 10 Radiographs of an individual who sustained ipsilateral fractures of the glenoid neck and the middle third of the clavicle. **Top,** A preoperative AP radiograph showing the glenoid neck fracture and severe displacement at the clavicular fracture site. **Bottom,** A postoperative AP radiograph showing anatomic reduction and stabilization of the clavicle fracture as well as the persistently but acceptably displaced glenoid neck fracture.

or both injury sites is unacceptable, ORIF is indicated. Frequently, operative stabilization of one site will reduce and stabilize the other disruption indirectly and satisfactorily.

A combined fracture of the middle third clavicle and glenoid neck has been termed a floating shoulder. In isolation, each fracture is generally minimally displaced and managed nonsurgically. In combination, however, they constitute a double disruption of the SSSC; the clavicle fracture often allows the glenoid neck fracture to displace significantly, and the glenoid neck fracture frequently leads to unacceptable displacement at the clavicular fracture site. ORIF of the clavicular fracture has been recommended. The glenoid neck fracture is addressed if displacement remains unacceptable (Fig. 10). In one recently reported series in which 15 patients with such fractures were treated surgically (25-month average follow-up), 14 of the 15 fractures healed with a good or excellent functional result. Another series included nine patients (48.5-month average follow-up) with ipsilateral clavicle/glenoid neck fractures. Seven patients were treated surgically with plate fixation of the clavicle fracture and achieved an excellent result. Two patients were treated nonsurgically and were found to have decreased range of motion as well as drooping of the involved shoulder.

Scapulothoracic Dissociation

Scapulothoracic dissociation is a rare traumatic disruption of the scapulothoracic articulation, which is caused by a severe direct force over the shoulder accompanied by traction applied to the upper extremity. Although the skin remains intact, the scapula is torn away from the posterior chest wall prompting some to call this a "closed traumatic forequarter amputation." Any one of the three bones of the shoulder complex may be fractured and any of the three remaining articulations may be disrupted. Disruption of the subclavian (most frequent) or axillary vessels is common as well as complete or partial disruption of the brachial plexus. Damage to the soft-tissue support structures, especially those that run from the chest wall to the scapula or the chest wall to the humerus, may be severe.

Diagnosis is based on the presence of the following clinical findings: (1) a history of violent trauma; (2) massive soft-tissue swelling over the shoulder girdle; and (3) significant lateral displacement of the scapula seen on a nonrotated chest radiograph. A scapulothoracic dissociation is particularly likely if these findings are accompanied by a pulseless upper extremity indicative of a complete vascular disruption and a complete or partial neurologic deficit indicating injury to the brachial plexus. As with all rare injuries, awareness of the clinical entity is critical to making the correct diagnosis.

If the vascular integrity of the extremity is in question, an emergency arteriogram is performed followed by the appropriate surgical repair if necessary. A careful neurologic examination, including later electromyelography (EMG) testing if indicated, is necessary to assess the level and degree of injury. The prognosis for functional recovery in the face of a complete disruption/deficit is poor. Partial plexus injuries have a good prognosis; most individuals achieve complete recovery or regain functional use of the extremity. If portions of the plexus are intact, neurologic repair is a consideration. Late reconstructive efforts are guided/dictated by the degree of neurologic return. Care of the surrounding soft-tissue supportive structures that may be partially or completely disrupted has been nonsurgical.

Injury to the sternal-clavicular-acromial linkage (a disruption of the sternoclavicular or acromioclavicular (AC) joint or a fracture of the clavicle) is frequently if not invariably present in order for the scapula to displace posterolaterally. An associated clavicle fracture creates a very unstable anatomic situation—the clavicle fracture allows the scapula to displace severely and the unstable scapulothoracic articulation allows significant displacement to occur at the clavicular fracture site. Consequently, ORIF of the clavicular disruption (plating or tension band wiring) should be considered (Fig. 11). Similar reasoning would

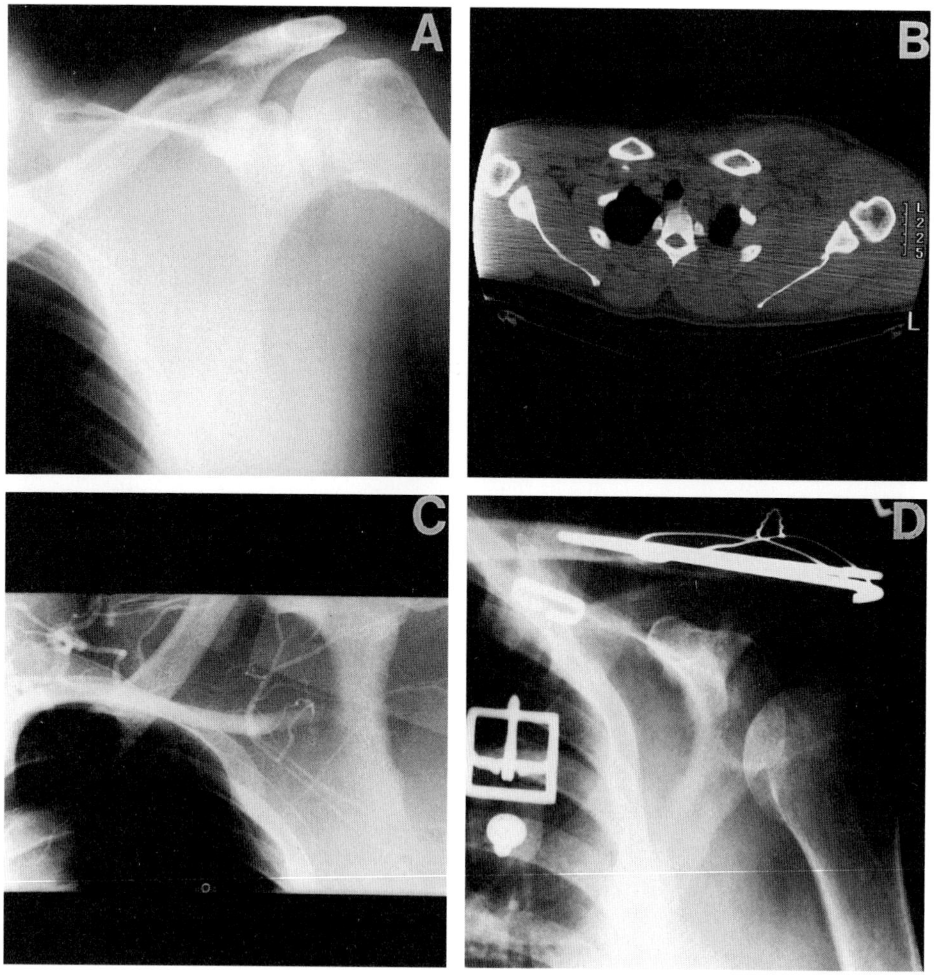

Fig. 11 Radiographs of a patient who sustained a left scapulothoracic dissociation. **A,** a pre-operative AP radiograph showing significant lateral displacement of the scapula and a significantly displaced fracture of the distal clavicle; **B,** a CT image showing significantly increased distance between the left scapula and the rib cage as compared to the opposite (uninjured) side; **C,** an arteriogram showing disruption of the subclavian artery; **D,** a postoperative AP radiograph showing reduction and stabilization of the distal clavicle (and the scapulothoracic articulation secondarily) using a tension band technique.

apply to scapulothoracic dissociations associated with a disruption of the AC joint. ORIF of a sternoclavicular disruption has less appeal due to the technical difficulty involved.

Humeral Shaft Fractures

Most fractures of the humeral shaft can be treated adequately by nonsurgical means, with healing often confirmed by 8 to 12 weeks. This injury makes up approximately 1% of all fractures and typically occurs as a result of direct violence, but fractures caused by indirect trauma, such as a fall on the elbow or even a violent muscle contraction, have been reported. Spontaneous humeral shaft fractures have occurred during a variety of throwing sports, including baseball pitching, javelin throwing, and handball, and several investigators have reported series of humeral fractures in arm wrestlers.

Numerous methods of nonsurgical treatment have been used including hanging casts, coaptation splints, shoulder spica casts, Velpeau immobilization, skeletal traction, and now, most commonly, functional bracing. The type and level of fracture, the patient's age and ability to comply, the degree of fragment displacement, and the presence of associated injuries influence the choice of treatment. Results of a comparative study of the nonsurgical treatment of these fractures in which functional cast bracing was used in 40 patients and coaptation splints in 25 demonstrated that the functional cast bracing group had a 2.5% nonunion rate, 8° of varus angulation with 50% of patients having less than 5° of varus, and that most patients exhibited complete restoration of shoulder and elbow motion at or soon after clinical evidence of union. These results were superior to those of the coaptation splinting group, which was found to have a 20% delayed union rate, an average of 12° varus angulation with only 16% less than 5°, and significant shoulder and elbow stiffness that required 3 to 12 months to resolve. Good functional results have been noted in the presence of residual coronal and sagittal plane

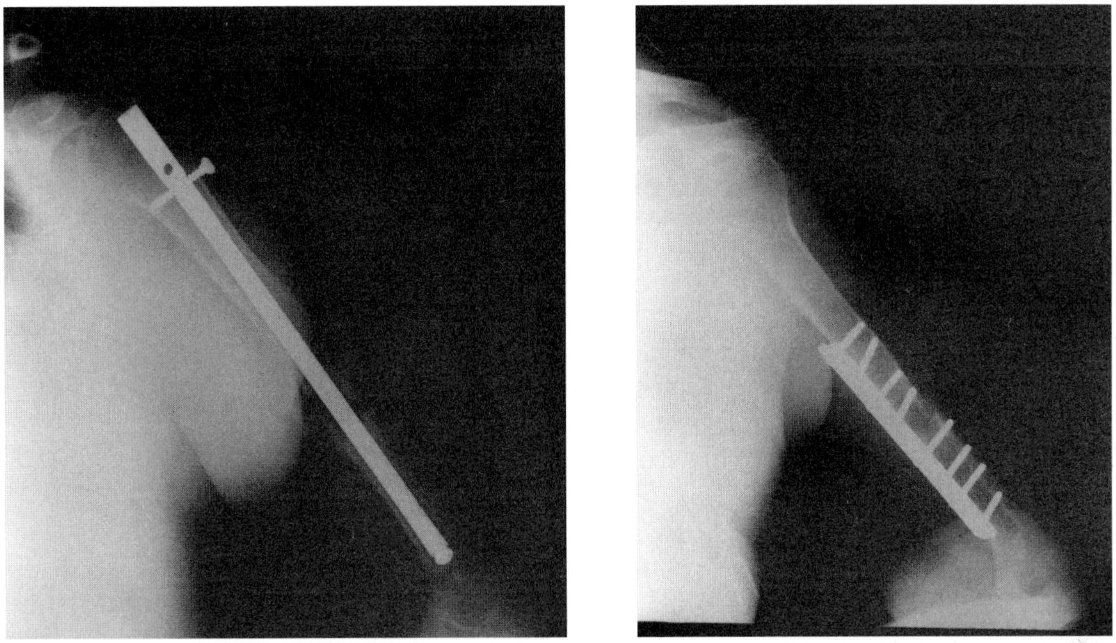

Fig. 12 **Left,** Nonunion of humeral shaft fracture treated with intramedullary nailing. Fracture was held distracted without rotatory stability. **Right,** Union was achieved after removal of the nail, followed by 4.5-mm dynamic compression plating with cancellous bone graft.

angulation of up to 30°. Functional bracing usually is instituted as soon as the patient is comfortable after initial splinting.

Indications for surgical intervention include segmental fractures, those with vascular involvement, multiply injured patients, floating elbow, open fractures, poor fracture alignment by closed methods, most pathologic fractures, bilateral humeral fractures, and patients who develop radial nerve palsies after closed reduction. Associated injuries remain important factors in management selection. ORIF in the form of compression plating is recommended in ipsilateral brachial plexus injuries. Operative stabilization, traction, and bracing were evaluated in 237 patients with humeral shaft fractures with varying degrees of associated injuries. Authors recommend operative intervention in the multiply-injured patient, but initial choice of treatment for moderately injured patients depended on the mobility of the patient. If the patient could be mobilized within 2 weeks, initial traction followed by bracing was preferable. In the singly injured, mobile patients, bracing was the optimum choice.

Various techniques of surgical intervention have been described, including plate and screw compression fixation, external fixation, and locked and unlocked intramedullary fixation via retrograde and antegrade approaches. One hundred twenty-seven patients with humeral shaft fractures were treated by ORIF using 4.5-mm dynamic compression plates. Complications included two transitory nerve palsies, two pseudarthroses, five fixation failures, and four infections. Despite this 10% complication rate, the authors reported 87.3% good to excellent results with full functional recovery.

Intramedullary fixation has gained popularity in the form of locked and unlocked rigid nails (with or without reaming) and stacked flexible Enders, Hackenthal, or Rush rods. Complications of antegrade nail fixation include rotator cuff injury and impingement of hardware, whereas retrograde insertion is associated with loss of elbow extension, heterotopic ossification, and distal nail migration. Criticism of flexible nails lies mainly with the less than optimum rotatory stability achieved and the associated incidence of nonunion. However, a report of 48 closed retrograde Hackenthal nail stabilizations demonstrated a 97% union rate at 1 year, with three occurrences of heterotopic ossification, one nonunion, and one delayed union. Removal of hardware was required in two cases due to migration, which may be avoided by proper impaction, bending of nail ends, and tight medullary fit. The authors recommended use of this technique for fractures below the flare of the proximal humeral metaphysis combined with splaying of nails within the head to improve rotatory stability.

Rigid intramedullary fixation combined with various locking techniques has been introduced mainly to improve rotatory and longitudinal stability, to prevent migration, and to allow crutch walking, although these techniques have met with some disfavor. Early results with the Seidel nail were promising. Most recent reports demonstrate high delayed and nonunion rates (up to 23%), complications up to 87% with significant technical difficulties that include nail protrusion due to proximal and distal locking flaws, intraoperative comminution associated with lateral pilot-hole placement, instrumentation failure, and canal underreaming leading to iatrogenic fracture (Fig. 12). Poor shoulder function was common. Decreased complication rates have been reported with modified 9-mm tibial nails inserted retrograde. Reaming remains controversial. Successful results have also been reported with modified Hansen-Street femoral nails inserted antegrade. External fixation continues to play a major role in open fractures with severe soft-tissue injury, infected nonunion, and in fractures with segmental bone loss.

Mechanical and biologic causes, including transverse fracture; inadequate immobilization; loss of vascularity; and fracture gap due to distraction, soft-tissue interposition, or bone loss, have been cited in the development of delayed unions and nonunions. The presence of osteopenia and obesity has also been implicated. Nonunion rates are reported as high as 15%. Rates of nonunion in those cases treated initially by ORIF appear to be decreasing according to recent reports whose authors cite strict attention to soft-tissue management and improved compression at the fracture site as responsible factors. Broad 4.5-mm dynamic compression plates are usually advised with eight cortices above and below the fracture.

Osteomyelitis is also a cause of delayed union and nonunion. Diagnosis is difficult based on plain radiographs, and hardware precludes the use of magnetic resonance imaging. Combined indium 111-labeled-leukocytes and technetium-99m methylene diphosphonate scintigraphy screening has recently been recommended for patients with delayed union or nonunion and a history of an open fracture, wound drainage, complication, infection, or radiographic findings suggestive of infection. These recommendations are based on the results of a series of 102 patients who underwent the above testing compared with results of open bone cultures of the delayed union or nonunion. False negatives were few, with a higher false-positive rate.

ORIF in the form of 4.5-mm broad dynamic compression plating supplemented with cancellous bone grafting remains the treatment of choice for nonunion of the humeral shaft. Intramedullary nailing and external fixation techniques have also been reported, but atrophic nonunions, fractures with radial nerve palsies, very proximal or distal nonunion sites, angular or rotational deformity, and need for implant removal may require exposure of the humerus, thereby facilitating the use of compression plating. Screw purchase in osteoporotic bone poses a formidable problem, but it may be enhanced with polymethylmethacrylate. Reconstruction of the humeral nonunion with an intramedullary fibular graft combined with compression plating has also been used with good results. Authors state that screw fixation was enhanced by passing the screws through the fibula as well as two humeral cortices (quadricortical) and that this fixation was as strong as polymethylmethacrylate augmentation and stronger than bicortical fixation in cadavers.

Injury to the radial nerve is associated with humeral shaft fractures in 2% to 17% of patients. It is most commonly seen both in spiral fractures of the distal humerus as described by Holstein and Lewis and in transverse midshaft fractures, especially when high-energy trauma is involved. Spontaneous recovery is seen in 76% of those injuries. Although most of these injuries tend to be neurapraxias, spiral distal third fractures have a higher incidence of nerve laceration and interposition between fragments. It is critical to identify these lesions prior to attempted closed reduction. Radial nerve palsies that develop after closed reduction and those associated with open fractures continue to be primary indications for early nerve exploration. In cases of progressive neurologic deficit or of deficits that do not improve clinically or electrophysiologically 3 to 4 months after treatment, exploration is often indicated.

Management of radial nerve palsies continues to be an area of research and controversy. Choice of early versus late exploration is based on degree of displacement, fracture site, degree of neurologic deficit, and whether or not the fracture is open. In a review of 12 patients who were treated surgically with delayed exploration for radial nerve lesions due to fractures, findings included three nerves entrapped in callus, four encased in perineural fibrosis, two partially lacerated (17%), and three completely lacerated (25%). Microsurgical reconstruction with interfascicular sural nerve grafting was performed in six, neurolyses in five, and tendon transfers in one, with 91% good to excellent results.

In a report of 14 cases of radial nerve palsies associated with open humeral shaft fractures that were treated by early exploration, either at the time of fracture debridement or delayed wound closure, nine (64%) patients had either nerve entrapment between fragments or laceration. There was an equal incidence of radial nerve lacerations or entrapments in grade I, II, and III open fractures. Epineural repair was performed with return of good motor function, but none regained radial sensibility. Based on the high incidence of laceration and entrapment between fragments, the authors recommend early nerve exploration in open fractures, with either repair or neurolysis in addition to skeletal fixation of the fracture.

Plate fixation of acute fractures with and without radial nerve injuries was performed in 44 consecutive patients. Of the 15 radial nerve palsies, 12 anatomically intact nerves were identified with three lacerations (20%). Radial nerve function returned in all 12 intact nerves and in one sutured nerve after plating, with two postoperative neurapraxias resolving in 3 weeks. Two lacerated nerves were left unrepaired. The authors recommended a posterior approach with the patient prone to provide access to the lower two thirds of the humerus for both plate fixation and radial nerve exploration.

Annotated Bibliography

Proximal Humerus Fractures

Cuomo F, Flatow EL, Maday MM, et al: Open reduction and internal fixation of two- and three-part displaced surgical neck fractures of the proximal humerus. *J Shoulder Elbow Surg* 1992;1:287–295.

Twenty-two patients with two- and three-part displaced surgical neck fractures were treated with open reduction and limited internal fixation with heavy nonabsorbable sutures incorporating the rotator cuff, tuberosities, and shaft. Humeral Ender nails were incorporated in a tension band fashion to increase rotatory and longitudinal stability. There were 82% good or excellent results, 14% satisfactory, and 5% unsatisfactory results reported. There were no cases of avascular necrosis or loss of fixation.

deLaat EA, Visser CP, Coene LN, et al: Nerve lesions in primary shoulder dislocations and humeral neck fractures: A prospective clinical and EMG study. *J Bone Joint Surg* 1994;76B:381–383.

Electrophysiologic evidence of nerve injuries was identified in 45% of 101 patients with primary shoulder dislocation or fracture of the humeral neck. Axillary, suprascapular, radial, and musculocutaneous nerves were most often involved. Authors stress early diagnosis to prevent lasting impairment of function.

Esser RD: Treatment of three- and four-part fractures of the proximal humerus with a modified cloverleaf plate. *J Orthop Trauma* 1994;8:15–22.

In 26 young patients who had three- and four-part fractures, open reduction and internal fixation utilizing a modified cloverleaf plate yielded good or excellent results in 24 patients, with no evidence of osteonecrosis. Plate malleability, the use of 4.0-mm rather than 6.5-mm screws in the head region, a low superior plate profile, and a youthful population with good bone stock were felt to be contributing factors to the successful results.

Flatow EL, Cuomo F, Maday MG, et al: Open reduction and internal fixation of two-part displaced fractures of the greater tuberosity of the proximal part of the humerus. *J Bone Joint Surg* 1991;73A:1213–1218.

Twelve patients with two-part greater tuberosity fractures treated with open reduction through a deltoid splitting approach, internal fixation with heavy nonabsorbable suture, and rotator cuff repair are reviewed. All fractures healed, with six excellent and six good results and average active forward elevation of 170°.

Hersche O, Gerber C: Iatrogenic displacement of fracture-dislocations of the shoulder: A report of seven cases. *J Bone Joint Surg* 1994;76B:30–33.

This retrospective report discusses seven cases in which open or closed reduction of a shoulder dislocation associated with fracture of the humeral neck led to displacement of the neck fracture. In three of the seven cases the neck fracture was unrecognized with biplanar views (scapular AP and lateral) reinforcing the need to obtain the axillary view.

Jaberg H, Warner JJ, Jakob RP: Percutaneous stabilization of unstable fractures of the humerus. *J Bone Joint Surg* 1992;74A:508–515.

Closed reduction and percutaneous pinning in 48 patients yielded good to excellent results in 70%, fair to poor results in 30%, loss of fixation in four, with complete avascular necrosis in two and subtotal avascular necrosis in eight. Authors suggest that three-part fractures with greater tuberosity displacement and four-part/head splitting fractures are better suited for open reduction and limited internal fixation and humeral head replacement, respectively.

Sidor ML, Zuckerman JD, Lyon T, et al: Classification of proximal humerus fractures: The contribution of the scapular lateral and axillary radiographs. *J Shoulder Elbow Surg* 1994;5:24–27.

Trauma series radiographs of 50 proximal humerus fractures were used to assess the relative contribution of the scapular lateral and axillary radiographs to fracture classification with the Neer four segment system. The authors report that when combined with the scapular anteroposterior radiograph, the axillary view contributes significantly more to fracture classification than the scapular lateral radiograph.

Sidor ML, Zuckerman JD, Lyon T, et al: The Neer classification system for proximal humeral fractures: An assessment of interobserver reliability and intraobserver reproducibility. *J Bone Joint Surg* 1993;75A:1745–1750.

The radiographs (trauma series) of 50 proximal humerus fractures were assessed by five different observers (shoulder specialist, orthopaedic traumatologist, skeletal radiologist and PGY-5 and PGY-2 orthopaedic residents). Pairwise comparisons showed a corrected intraobserver reliability coefficient of 0.48. Intraobserver reproducibility (two viewings 6 months apart) ranged from 0.50 to 0.83 and was best for the shoulder specialist.

Fractures of the Scapula

Goss TP: Fractures of the glenoid cavity. *J Bone Joint Surg* 1992;74A:299–305.

This article classifies fractures of the glenoid cavity, and mechanisms of injury are described. State-of-the-art guidelines regarding diagnosis, treatment (non-operative and operative), and postoperative management are detailed.

Goss TP: Fractures of the glenoid neck. *J Shoulder Elbow Surg* 1994;3:42–53.

This review article focuses on the evaluation and management of fractures of the glenoid neck, especially those that are significantly displaced. A classification scheme is proposed, and a review of the current literature is included.

Kavanaugh BF, Bradway JK, Cofield RH: Open reduction and internal fixation of displaced intra-articular fractures of the glenoid fossa. *J Bone Joint Surg* 1993;75A:479–484.

In this series, ten displaced intra-articular fractures of the glenoid fossa treated with open reduction and internal fixation (ORIF) at the Mayo Clinic between 1980 and 1989 are described. The authors found ORIF to be a "useful and safe technique for the treatment of selected displaced fractures of the glenoid fossa," which can "restore excellent function of the shoulder."

Zuckerman JD, Koval KJ, Cuomo F: Fractures of the scapula, in Heckman JD (ed): *Instructional Course*

Lectures 42. Rosemont, IL, American Academy of Orthopaedic Surgeons, 1993, pp 271–281.

This review chapter describes the various scapular fractures that may be encountered. Current diagnostic and therapeutic principles are detailed as well as results that can be expected and complications that may occur.

Fractures of the Clavicle

Boehme D, Curtis RJ Jr, DeHaan JT, et al: Non-union of fractures of the mid-shaft of the clavicle: Treatment with a modified Hagie intramedullary pin and autogenous bone-grafting. *J Bone Joint Surg* 1991;73A:1219–1226.

In this series, 21 patients with a symptomatic nonunion of the middle third of the clavicle underwent open reduction internal fixation with a modified Hagie intramedullary pin and autologous bone grafting (35 month average follow-up). Union occurred in 20 (95%) of the 21 individuals.

Double Disruptions of the Superior Shoulder Suspensory Complex

Goss TP: Double disruptions of the superior shoulder suspensory complex. *J Orthop Trauma* 1993;7:99–106.

This article introduces a biomechanical principle that underlies, unites, and allows understanding of several well-described but difficult-to-treat shoulder injuries, which have previously been described in isolation, as well as injuries that are rarely seen. Diagnostic and therapeutic principles are detailed, and several illustrative cases are described.

Humeral Shaft

Foster RJ, Swiontkowski MF, Bach AW, et al: Radial nerve palsy caused by open humeral shaft fractures. *J Hand Surg* 1993;18A:121–124.

In a series of 14 patients with radial nerve palsy caused by open humeral shaft fractures, 64% had a radial nerve that was either lacerated or interposed between fracture fragments equally distributed between grade I, II, and III open fractures. Authors recommend early nerve exploration and rigid internal fixation in patients with this combination of injuries.

Ingman AM, Waters DA: Locked intramedullary nailing of humeral shaft fractures: Implant design, surgical technique, and clinical results. *J Bone Joint Surg* 1994; 76B:23–29.

The authors report their experience with a modified Gross-Kemph 9-mm tibial intramedullary locked nail and a new technique of nailing in 41 patients. There was only one failure in a nail locked at only one end. Rehabilitation was faster with a retrograde approach.

Robinson CM, Bell KM, Court-Brown CM, et al: Locked nailing of humeral shaft fractures: Experience in Edinburgh over a two-year period. *J Bone Joint Surg* 1992;74B:558–562.

This retrospective review reports on 30 fractures treated with locked Seidel nailing. Technical difficulties and intraoperative and postoperative complications occurred in 87% of patients, which caused the authors to suggest considerable modifications to the nail and its insertion site.

Sharma VK, Jain AK, Gupta RK, et al: Non-operative treatment of fractures of the humeral shaft: A comparative study. *J Indian Med Assoc* 1991;89:157–160.

Forty patients with diaphyseal fractures treated by functional cast bracing were compared with 25 patients treated by coaptation splinting. Functional cast bracing yielded distinctly superior results, with minimal elbow/shoulder stiffness, average varus angulation of 8°, and 2.5% nonunion rates.

Classic Bibliography

Ada JR, Miller ME: Scapular fractures: Analysis of 113 cases. *Clin Orthop* 1991;269:174–180.

Ebraheim NA, An HS, Jackson WT, et al: Scapulothoracic dissociation. *J Bone Joint Surg* 1988; 70A:428–432.

Edwards DJ, Kavanagh TG, Flannery MC: Fractures of the distal clavicle: A case for fixation. *Injury* 1992;23: 44–46.

Hardegger FH, Simpson LA, Webber BG: The operative treatment of scapular fractures. *J Bone Joint Surg* 1984; 66B:725–731.

Herscovici D Jr, Fiennes AG, Allgower M, et al: The floating shoulder: Ipsilateral clavicle and scapular neck fractures. *J Bone Joint Surg* 1992;74B:362–364.

Leung KS, Lam TP: Open reduction and internal fixation of ipsilateral fractures of the scapular neck and clavicle. *J Bone Joint Surg* 1993;75A:1015–1018.

Leung KS, Lam TP, Poon KM: Operative treatment of displaced intra-articular glenoid fractures. *Injury* 1993; 24:324–328.

Nordqvist A, Petersson C: Fracture of the body, neck, or spine of the scapula: A long-term follow-up study. *Clin Orthop* 1992;283:139–144.

Nordqvist A, Petersson C, Redlund-Johnell I: The natural course of lateral clavicle fracture: 15 (11–21) year follow-up of 110 cases. *Acta Orthop Scand* 1993;64:87–91.

25

Shoulder: Instability

Instability is one of the most common disorders affecting the shoulder, particularly in younger, athletic patients. The glenohumeral joint is more frequently dislocated than any other major joint. The contributions of various structures to the stability of the glenohumeral joint and the way in which these structures may interact to stabilize the shoulder have been examined in recent biomechanical studies. Clinical studies have been focused on anatomic repairs, which aim at restoring stability without compromising motion or function. Techniques for arthroscopic repair of instability have been advanced, although recurrence rates of instability appear to be higher than after open repair in most series. The significance of superior labral pathology and the role of the biceps tendon as a glenohumeral stabilizer continue to be areas of uncertainty and controversy. Recent advances in these areas, as well as a consideration of instability involving the other articulations of the shoulder complex (ie, the acromioclavicular and sternoclavicular joints) will be covered in this section.

Glenohumeral Instability

Glenohumeral instability encompasses a spectrum of disorders of varying degree, direction, and etiology. The instability is classified according to the timing of diagnosis (acute versus chronic) and frequency of the event, the degree, the direction(s), the etiology of the first occurrence, and whether or not the individual can voluntarily produce the instability. Some investigators have stressed the importance of distinguishing traumatic unidirectional cases from those with atraumatic multidirectional instability. Those with atraumatic multidirectional instability typically manifest signs of generalized ligamentous laxity, which involve the contralateral shoulder, elbows, wrists, and metacarpophalangeal joints, in addition to shoulder instability in all three directions: anterior, posterior, and inferior. However, other surgeons have expressed concern that there is another subset of patients with an intermediate degree of instability, especially an inferior component. One group of authors has termed this group bidirectional (ie, anterior and inferior or posterior and inferior). Bidirectional instability may be seen more frequently in overhead athletes, because they subject the shoulder to repetitive microtrauma and develop instability on that basis. Patients also frequently present with a history suggestive of several etiologic factors for their shoulder instability. For example, a young swimmer with a great degree of inherent ligamentous laxity may not develop symptomatic instability until after swimming for several years (repetitive microtrauma) or until after a traumatic event, such as a motor vehicle accident. Such cases demonstrate that categories are not necessarily discrete, and that overlap between etiologic categories may exist in a clinical population. Determination of the direction of the instability, and in cases of instability in more than one direction, of the primary direction and of all lesser components of the instability, is essential in planning a successful strategy for treating the problem.

Finally, the issue of volition must be considered when deciding on treatment alternatives. When evaluating a patient with a voluntary component to the instability (usually, these are patients with predominantly posterior subluxation), the surgeon must determine whether this is merely positional (ie, occurs when the individual places the arm in a provocative position) or whether the individual actively subluxes the shoulder, either as a behavioral tic (muscular type) or in order to gain attention (signifying an underlying psychological disorder). Only the positional group will benefit from surgical reconstruction, and attempts at surgical repair in the last group will be very likely to fail.

Biomechanics of Glenohumeral Instability

The minimal bony constraint, which allows nearly a global range of motion for the shoulder, also predisposes it to instability. No single mechanism is responsible for stabilizing the glenohumeral joint. Rather, a number of factors influence glenohumeral stability, including the articular geometry, the mechanisms of surface adhesion and cohesion, atmospheric pressure, the muscles around the shoulder (particularly the rotator cuff muscles), and the static soft-tissue stabilizers (labrum and glenohumeral ligaments). Recent biomechanical studies have provided further insight into the function of each of the stabilizers and, more importantly, into how they may interact to stabilize the glenohumeral joint.

Data from stereophotogrammetric studies of the articular surfaces of the glenohumeral joint have demonstrated that the normal humeral head and glenoid articular surfaces are spherical with a high degree of conformity. The cartilage is thicker peripherally on the glenoid than in the center. The glenoid subchondral bone, however, is flatter than that of the humerus, giving an impression of nonconforming surfaces on plain radiographs. These findings of conforming spherical articular surfaces suggest that the articular geometry does play a role in providing stability, although the large differential in surface area between the larger humeral head and the smaller glenoid minimizes the overall effect of the conforming radii of curvature. Data from other studies have suggested that compression of the humeral head into the conforming glenoid cavity by the action of the rotator cuff muscles provides an important mechanism for stabilizing the shoulder. This mechanism of "concavity-compression" allowed the humeral head to resist tangential forces of up to 60% of the compressive load with the labrum intact in an in vitro study. Resection of the labrum reduced the effectiveness of this mechanism by approximately 20%. This mechanism is thought to be particularly important for providing stability in the mid-range of glenohumeral motion, when the capsular ligaments are lax.

The glenoid labrum has been regarded as an important structure in maintaining stability ever since Bankart described its detachment from the glenoid rim as the "essential lesion" in recurrent anterior instability. More recently, distinct morphologic differences have been found between the superior and anteroinferior regions. The superior labrum has a meniscal pattern with a roughly triangular cross section and a loose attachment to the glenoid. The anteroinferior portion is firmly attached to the glenoid rim and serves as a fibrous attachment site of the inferior glenohumeral ligament complex. In a recent cadaveric study, a simulated Bankart lesion resulted in an increase in anterior and inferior translation at all positions of elevation, but these increases were quite small (Fig. 1). The authors concluded that detachment of the anterior portion of the inferior glenohumeral ligament from the glenoid rim does not appear to be solely responsible for the increased glenohumeral translation that is necessary to produce an anterior dislocation of the shoulder. Permanent stretching or elongation of the inferior glenohumeral ligament may also be necessary for dislocation to occur. Other recent biomechanical studies have provided important information about the static or capsuloligamentous stabilizers. In the lower range of abduction, the superior and middle glenohumeral ligaments are the most important capsular structures that provide anterior stability.

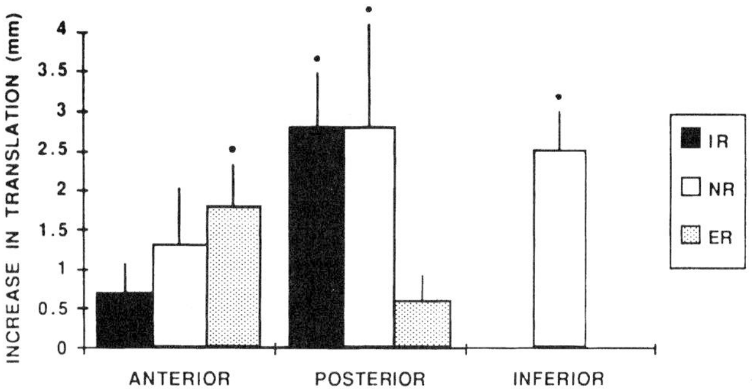

Fig. 1 The effect of a simulated anteroinferior labral attachment (Bankart lesion) on load-induced glenohumeral translations in cadaveric shoulders at 90° abduction. (Reproduced with permission from Speer KP, Deng X, Borrero S, et al: Biomechanical evaluation of a simulated Bankart lesion. *J Bone Joint Surg* 1994;76A:1819–1826.)

As the arm is placed into greater degrees of abduction and external rotation, the inferior glenohumeral ligament becomes the primary capsular restraint against anterior translations. Similarly, the primary restraint to inferior translation of the adducted shoulder is the superior glenohumeral ligament. With progressive abduction, the inferior glenohumeral ligament complex prevents inferior translations. These ligaments appear to act as checkreins to excessive translations of the humeral head when the extremes of motion are reached. Different regions of the capsule assume primacy as restraints, depending on the arm position, but the various regions appear to act in concert and share the tension required to stabilize the shoulder, particularly at the extremes of motion.

In another study, regional variations were found in structural and mechanical properties among the various regions of the inferior glenohumeral ligament. The superior band was consistently the thickest region, and thickness progressively decreased from anterosuperiorly to posteroinferiorly. Mechanical testing to failure demonstrated variation in strain to failure among the three regions, and strain at failure averaged 27%. In this study, capsular rupture (midsubstance failure) was seen almost as frequently as glenoid insertion failure as the mode of inferior glenohumeral ligament failure. Moreover, even in cases where the ligament failed at its glenoid insertion (a parallel with the clinical Bankart lesion), significant capsular stretching occurred prior to failure. This observation suggests that marked capsular stretching may occur, as well as labral detachment, in an event of traumatic anterior dislocation, and both of these elements may contribute to the resulting glenohumeral instability.

Finally, a number of recent studies have provided insight into how the various glenohumeral stabilizers may interact to provide joint stability. Several authors have recently reported that the rotator cuff tendons blend with the capsuloligamentous structures at their insertions. Contraction of the rotator cuff may create tension in these ligaments, thus "dynamizing" the ligaments. In another study, proprioceptive deficits were demonstrated in shoulders with anterior instability. These deficits were not found in shoulders that had undergone surgical reconstruction of the instability. Thus, the capsuloligamentous structures may provide afferent proprioceptive feedback to the muscles stabilizing the shoulder. When these structures become damaged and can no longer provide this afferent information, proprioceptive deficits occur, perhaps contributing further to recurrent episodes of instability. Surgical repair of the capsuloligamentous integrity appears to restore the proprioceptive properties.

Evaluation of Glenohumeral Instability

When standard radiographs are available to document a locked dislocation, the diagnosis of glenohumeral instability and the primary direction of the instability are straightforward. When these are not available or when the instability involves a transient subluxation, confirming the diagnosis is more difficult. In such cases, the history and physical examination are the most important diagnostic tools. The location of pain, by itself, is usually not sufficient to make the diagnosis of instability or to determine its direction. Although anterior shoulder pain in young athletes frequently is associated with anterior subluxation, it is also present in the syndrome of subacromial impingement. Moreover, patients with anterior instability may have pain that is predominantly posterior, perhaps due to overuse of the posterior rotator cuff or to synovitis of the glenohumeral joint. Placing the symptoms in the context of the arm position or the specific activity (or phase of activity) that causes the symptoms is usually more helpful in making the diagnosis. For example, in throwing athletes, knowing which phase of the throw elicits symptoms can assist in clarifying the predominant direction of the instability: usually, anterior instability is more symptomatic during late cocking, while posterior instability is more symptomatic during the follow-through. A sensation that the shoulder slips out, popping or clicking, and transient neurologic complaints ("a dead arm") when the arm is in provocative positions are other symptoms that are suggestive of glenohumeral instability.

On examination, the sulcus sign and provocative apprehension tests are helpful in diagnosing and characterizing an instability. The sulcus sign test is performed by pulling downward traction on the neutrally positioned arm and then with the arm at 90° of abduction. A dimple or gap between the humeral head and acromion appears in shoulders where there is an inferior component to the instability, as in bidirectional or multidirectional instability. However, it is important to recognize that a positive sulcus sign is not, by itself, sufficient for a diagnosis of instability. Two recent reports provided quantitative information on in vivo laxity of the glenohumeral joint and noted that not only is there marked variability in joint translations among normal shoulders, but also that there can be overlap in laxity between normal shoulders and those with clinical symptoms of instability. Thus, it is only when the excessive translations of the humeral head are symptomatic that clinical instability is said to be present.

The anterior apprehension test, performed by placing the arm in 90° of abduction with the elbow flexed to 90° and then progressively externally rotating and extending the arm with one hand and exerting an anteriorly directed force to the humeral head with the other, is quite useful in diagnosing anterior glenohumeral instability. The relocation test, in which the apprehension test is then repeated while stabilizing the humeral head with a posteriorly directed force over the anterior aspect of the joint, reportedly helps differentiate between anterior subluxation and subacromial impingement. In a recent report it was emphasized that this test did not distinguish well between these entities when a sensation of pain alone was considered. However, the accuracy of the test was greater than 80%, when only true apprehension (that is, a sense of an impending subluxation or dislocation) was considered. Finally, the provocative test for posterior instability consists of positioning the shoulder in 90° of flexion and combined adduction/internal rotation and then placing a posteriorly directed force on the humerus. A symptomatic subluxation or a sensation of impending subluxation will occur with this maneuver in those with posterior instability.

Radiographic evaluation of an acute traumatic shoulder injury consists of the trauma series, which includes a true anteroposterior (AP), a lateral scapular (Y-view), and an axillary view. The axillary view is particularly useful in diagnosing locked posterior fracture-dislocations, which unfortunately continue to be missed frequently on the initial emergency room evaluation. When the patient presents between episodes of dislocation or when the instability consists of subluxation, the radiographs may provide supporting evidence of the diagnosis of instability. The AP view in internal rotation may demonstrate the Hill-Sachs lesion that is frequently present after recurrent dislocations. The axillary and apical oblique views will best demonstrate glenoid rim fractures or erosions of the anterior glenoid. Other radiographic imaging techniques, such as double contrast computed tomographic (CT) arthrography and magnetic resonance imaging (MRI) can provide information about the structural integrity of the capsule and labrum and about capsular volume. However, these studies are significantly more costly than standard radiographs and should be used only when additional information is needed to confirm the diagnosis. The CT-arthrogram can add useful information in cases in which the standard radiographs demonstrate a fracture of the glenoid rim or suggest other bony abnormalities, such as excessive retroversion or hypoplasia of the glenoid. These studies may also add useful information about the status of the labrum after a failed instability repair.

In selected cases, where the diagnosis of glenohumeral instability is suspected but remains uncertain or the primary direction of the instability is unclear, an examination under anesthesia can assist in clarifying the diagnosis. This examination can be combined with an arthroscopic examination to provide additional information about the internal glenohumeral anatomy. Labral detachment and excessive capsular volume can be visualized directly, as well as fraying or abnormal wear on the anterior or posterior labrum.

Treatment of Anterior Glenohumeral Instability

Nonsurgical treatment of a primary anterior shoulder dislocation consists of a closed reduction, followed by a period of immobilization and activity restriction and then by a program of rehabilitative exercises. Although many surgeons employ immobilization for 3 to 6 weeks, the value of immobilization or of a particular length of time of immobilization has not been demonstrated. Shorter periods of immobilization are usually used for older patients or those who have had an episode of traumatic subluxation. The specific goals of nonsurgical treatment are to strengthen the muscular stabilizers of the shoulder (both the rotator cuff muscles and the scapular stabilizers), to gradually regain full motion, and to avoid provocative arm positions or activities during the early postinjury period.

The rate of recurrence after an anterior dislocation in young (less than 20 years old) athletically active patients is 90%, according to early reports. Several reports from the last decade have suggested that the overall rate of recurrence is probably lower (approximately 33%), although the youngest age group had a much higher rate (55% to 66%). In a recent prospective study, nonsurgical treatment was compared with arthroscopic suture repair for acute primary anterior dislocations of the shoulder in a population of military cadets. In this study, the group treated with immobilization for 4 weeks, followed by a supervised rehabilitation program before returning to full activity at 4 months, had a recurrence rate of instability of 80% (compared to 14% in the surgically treated group). Results of this study suggested a role for the use of surgical repair after the primary dislocation, in light of the high recurrence rate in this young, athletically active group.

Another recent study was on the treatment of 140 shoulders with subluxation (anterior, posterior, or multidirectional) using a specific program of muscle-strengthening exercises. With this program, 80% of patients with an atraumatic onset of instability had satisfactory results, compared with only 16% of those with traumatic subluxation. In each subgroup, patients who had posterior instability responded better than those with anterior instability. Results of this study, then, suggest differential benefits of nonsurgical treatment for patients with subluxation, based on the specific type of instability, and emphasize the importance of careful classification of the instability to predict the chances of success with an exercise program for a particular shoulder.

Anterior glenohumeral instability can be surgically repaired using open or arthroscopic methods. Many open surgical procedures have been described, and most of these have provided success in a high percentage (> 95%) of patients, when this is measured by recurrence of dislocation. However, as instability repairs are evaluated by stricter criteria, which emphasize motion and function (including the return to high-demand overhead sports activities), the limitations of some of the older, standard repairs, such as the Putti-Platt and Magnuson-Stack procedures, which tether the shoulder and limit external rotation, have become evident. The use of metal hardware, such as screws and staples, which can loosen and migrate into the joint, leading to degenerative arthritis, has also fallen into disfavor.

Increasingly, procedures that restore the normal glenohumeral anatomy and repair the capsular pathology (detachment from the insertion on the glenoid rim and/or excessive laxity of the capsular ligaments) have been used to treat recurrent anterior instability. A modified Bankart repair and a number of different capsulorrhaphy procedures (anterior inferior capsular shift, T-plasty modification of the Bankart repair, and the anterior capsulolabral reconstruction) have been shown to be effective in large series for stabilizing the shoulder and allowing a high level of unrestricted overhead function. The capsulorrhaphy procedures can be performed using either a lateral (humeral) or a medial capsular incision (Fig. 2). They allow a simultaneous repair of a detached anteroinferior labrum and a reduction in joint volume to restore effective function of the glenohumeral ligaments. The subscapularis is either split (to avoid detachment) or detached and repaired anatomically, but it is not shortened, thus allowing restoration of full motion. These repairs address inferior or multidirectional elements of the instability as well, if they are present, allowing the shoulder to be properly balanced. With these procedures, 75% to 80% of athletes are able to return to their sports at the same level of competition.

Arthroscopic stabilization has been performed over the past decade, using a number of different techniques. These techniques have included fixation with staples, sutures, suture anchors, and most recently, biodegradable tacks. The advantages of arthroscopic stabilization that have been cited include lower surgical morbidity, a smaller scar, and better postoperative motion (especially external rotation). However, in most reports, the recurrence of instability after arthroscopic stabilization has been significantly higher than after open repair. In one series of arthroscopic Bankart suture repairs, in which the rate of recurrence was 44%, the authors suggested that part of the reason for the high failure rate is the inability of the arthroscopic repair to address the plastic deformation that occurs in the glenohumeral ligament-labrum complex. One approach is to reserve the use of arthroscopic repair for cases of unidirectional anterior dislocation in which a Bankart lesion is found and in which there is no demonstrable inferior laxity. As a result of the variable success of arthroscopic stabilization procedures, the status of these procedures remains uncertain. Additional studies are needed to define specific indications and the preferred technique.

Failure after repair of instability usually involves one or more of the following: recurrent or persistent instability, stiffness, or the later development of glenohumeral osteoarthrosis. In a study on the management of a failed Bristow procedure in 40 shoulders, the primary etiology of failure was excessive laxity of the capsule in 80% and an untreated Bankart lesion in 20%. It was emphasized that, because of the extensive scarring in the area of the musculocutaneous and axillary nerves and the deficiency of the subscapularis, surgical treatment after a failed Bristow procedure was complex and difficult. Another retrospective study was of the management of patients with severe loss of external rotation after anterior capsulorrhaphy. Data from this study confirmed the findings in earlier reports, in which it was pointed out that an excessively tight anterior repair can result in posterior subluxation and the development of glenohumeral osteoarthrosis. In this situation, the performance of an anterior soft-tissue release for patients with 0° external rotation or less should be consid-

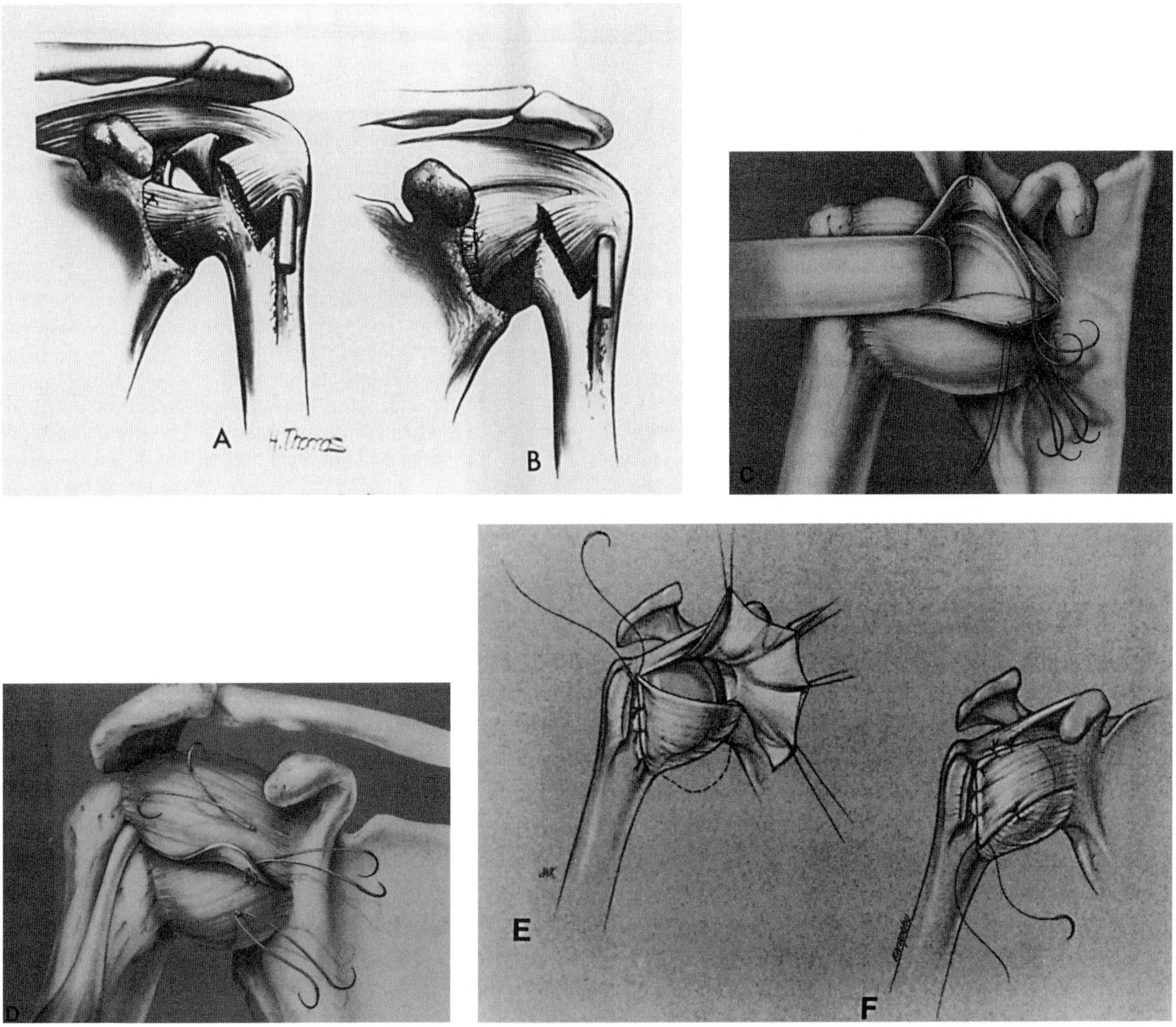

Fig. 2 Examples of capsulorrhaphy procedures for treating recurrent anterior glenohumeral instability. These procedures allow simultaneous repair of a detached labrum and a reduction in capsular volume, especially anteroinferiorly. Capsulorrhaphy may be performed either through a medial capsular incision [T-plasty capsulorrhaphy **(A, B)** (Reproduced with permission from Altchek DW, Warren RF, Skyhar MJ, et al: T-plasty modification of the Bankart procedure for multidirectional instability of the anterior and inferior types. *J Bone Joint Surg* 1991;73A:105–112.) and anterior capsulolabral reconstruction **(C, D)** (Reproduced with permission from Montgomery WH III, Jobe FW: Functional outcomes in athletes after modified anterior capsulolabral reconstruction. *Am J Sports Med* 1994;22:352–358.)] or a lateral capsular incision [anterior inferior capsular shift **(E, F)** (Reproduced with permission from Bigliani LU, Kurzweil PR, Schwartzbach CC, et al: Inferior capsular shift procedure for anterior-inferior shoulder instability in athletes. *Am J Sports Med* 1994;22:578–584.)].

ered. If severe osteoarthrosis has already developed, then total shoulder arthroplasty or humeral hemiarthroplasty should be considered.

Treatment of Posterior Instability

Locked posterior dislocations of the glenohumeral joint represent less than 5% of shoulder dislocations. They nearly always are manifested with an associated impression fracture of the anteromedial aspect of the humeral head. The patient presents with a prominent coracoid process anteriorly, a posterior shift to the axis of the arm, and an inability to externally rotate the arm. Obtaining an axillary radiograph will prevent missing the diagnosis. Due to the associated fracture and because locked dislocations behave differently from recurrent posterior subluxations, these injuries are classified with proximal humeral fractures, rather than with recurrent instability. Treatment options include closed reduction and immobilization with the arm in slight extension and external rotation (when the humeral defect is less than 20% of the articular surface), open reduction with transposition of the lesser tuberosity and the subscapularis tendon into the defect (when it is between 20% and 40% of the articular surface), and prosthetic hemiarthroplasty (when the defect exceeds 45% of the articular surface).

The treatment of recurrent posterior instability remains controversial. It is widely accepted that the initial treatment should be nonsurgical, consisting of a structured exercise program. However, there is no consensus on the surgical procedure of choice for those in whom conservative treatment has failed. Procedures that aim to provide bony stability have included the use of a posterior bone block to extend the posterior glenoid, an opening wedge osteotomy of the posterior glenoid (glenoplasty), and rotational osteotomy of the humerus. Soft-tissue repairs have included a posterior labral repair, a posterior capsular plication (reverse Putti-Platt repair), and posterior capsulorrhaphy. Unfortunately, few large series are available for evaluation of these different surgical repairs.

Increasingly, it has been recognized that many patients with instability that is predominantly posterior also have elements of inferior or multidirectional instability. This may account for the high failure rate following unidirectional posterior capsular plication in several series. Posterior capsulorrhaphy procedures that include a posteroinferior capsular dissection to reduce the capsular volume have had a higher degree of success (80% to 90%) in treating posterior instability. Because bony abnormalities appear to be quite uncommon in patients with posterior instability, posterior bone grafting is reserved for the few cases of posterior glenoid deficiency or for use in some revision procedures, when the soft tissues are particularly attenuated.

Treatment of Multidirectional Instability

The initial treatment of multidirectional instability is an extensive program of strengthening exercises for the rotator cuff and scapular muscles. However, when patients continue to have pain and disabling instability, surgical treatment should be considered. Unidirectional repairs are insufficient for treating this problem, because they do not address the inferior capsular redundancy that is the hallmark of this type of instability and may, in fact, create excessive tightness on the side repaired, leading to a fixed subluxation in the direction left unaddressed. The inferior capsular shift procedure, which allows reduction in volume on all sides of the joint while thickening or reinforcing the side of greatest instability, has been a satisfactory means for treating multidirectional instability. Recently, authors have reported success in greater than 90% with this repair. Moreover, there appears to be no deterioration of results at long-term follow-up.

Pathology of the Superior Labrum-Biceps Complex

Another area of recent interest concerns pathology involving the superior glenoid labrum and the origin of the long head of the biceps tendon at the superior labrum. Superior labral lesions were first noticed in young athletes who participated in overhead sports activities, such as throwing. It was postulated that this injury was due to repetitive traction of the biceps tendon on the labrum with repeated throwing motions. An injury to the superior labrum, which begins posteriorly and extends anteriorly to the region of the mid-glenoid notch, was described in another report. The authors coined the term "SLAP lesion" (superior labrum anterior and posterior) and identified the lesion in 27 patients via arthroscopy. The mechanism of injury is thought to be compression loading of the shoulder in a flexed and abducted position, resulting from a fall onto the outstretched arm. Typically, these patients present with shoulder pain, particularly with overhead activities, and with "clicking" or "popping" of the shoulder. On examination, pain is often elicited with resisted shoulder flexion with the elbow extended and the forearm supinated (biceps tension test). The compression rotation test, performed by placing a compression force on the humerus, with the shoulder abducted to 90° and the elbow flexed to 90°, and then rotating the arm, may catch the torn labrum. Radiographic studies, such as CT-arthrography and MRI, have not been useful in diagnosing SLAP lesions.

A classification system for SLAP lesions has been proposed, based on the anatomic configuration of the tear at arthroscopy (Fig. 3). In type I lesions, there is a frayed or degenerated appearance of the superior labrum, but its peripheral edge and the attachment of the biceps to the labrum are intact. In type II lesions, the superior labrum and attached biceps are separated from the glenoid at the usual peripheral attachment. Type III lesions consist of a bucket-handle tear in the superior labrum, with the central portion displaced into the joint, but the peripheral attachments of the labrum and biceps are intact. In type IV lesions, a bucket-handle tear is present and the biceps attachment is also compromised. Treatment is based on the type of lesion encountered, with the authors of the classification system recommending debridement for types I and III lesions, fixation back to the glenoid after debridement for type II lesions, and debridement with possible biceps tenodesis for type IV lesions.

There continues to be controversy concerning the appropriate treatment of superior labral pathology. The rationales for simple debridement include removing interposed damaged labrum that can catch in the joint, reducing inflammation by removing inflamed synovial and bursal tissue, and facilitating further rehabilitation efforts. Reported results, however, are mixed. For some early series, a high percentage of satisfactory results was reported

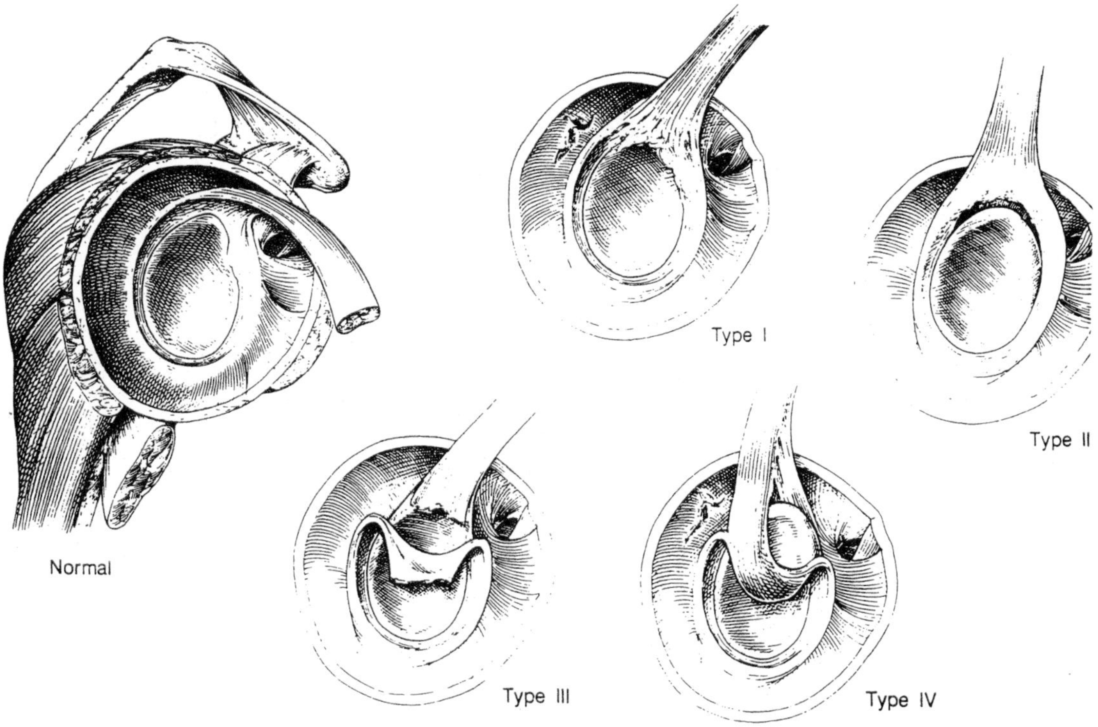

Fig. 3 Classification system for pathology of the superior labrum anterior and posterior lesions (SLAP lesions). (Reproduced with permission from Snyder SJ, Karzel RP, Del Pizzo W, et al: SLAP lesions of the shoulder. *Arthroscopy* 1990;6:274–279.)

when the lesion didn't extend to the anteroinferior quadrant, while for others, excellent short-term results were reported, but there was deterioration after 1 to 2 years. In several recent reports there was a high percentage of satisfactory results with arthroscopic repair of types II and IV SLAP lesions, although the average follow-up in these reports was less than 2 years.

The issue of whether or not these lesions of the superior labrum and long head of the biceps tendon are associated with subtle forms of glenohumeral instability remains unresolved. Data from a recent cadaver study suggested that the long head of the biceps contributes to anterior glenohumeral stability by increasing the shoulder's resistance to torsional forces when the arm is in the abducted, externally rotated position. It is suggested that detachment of the superior labral complex decreases the shoulder's resistance to torsion and places greater stress on the inferior glenohumeral ligament. Data from an earlier cadaver study had suggested that the long head of the biceps provides a stabilizing function against anterior and posterior translations in the hanging arm position. Authors of one clinical report on labral debridement found that many of these shoulders demonstrated instability on examination under anesthesia, while others found that glenohumeral ligament injury (especially to the superior or middle ligaments) was encountered in 58% of the shoulders with labral tears. Further biomechanical studies and longer-term follow-up in the clinical series of labral repair are needed to resolve these issues about the significance of the superior labrum-biceps complex as stabilizers and their possible role in subtle forms of glenohumeral instability.

Acromioclavicular Instability

The usual mechanism of acromioclavicular joint injuries involves a fall onto the point of the shoulder with the arm in an adducted position. The clavicle is generally maintained in its anatomic position by the sternoclavicular ligaments and the action of the trapezius muscle, while the scapula is driven in an inferior position and droops. These injuries are classified according to the degree of relative displacement of the distal clavicle and the amount of damage to the acromioclavicular capsular ligament, the coracoclavicular ligaments, and the fascia of the adjacent muscles (deltoid and trapezium).

Type I injury represents a sprain of the acromioclavicular ligament, and radiographs appear normal. Type II injury represents a tear of the acromioclavicular ligament and a sprain of the coracoclavicular ligaments. Radiographs demonstrate widening of the acromioclavicular joint, but no significant change in the coracoclavicular distance. Type III injury represents a tear of the acromioclavicular and coracoclavicular ligaments with dislocation of the joint. There is also damage to the fascia of the deltoid and trapezius overlying the distal clavicle. Radiographs demonstrate a coracoclavicular distance that is 25% to 100% greater than on the uninjured side. Type IV injury includes the damage described for a type III injury, but there is also more significant posterior displacement of the distal clavicle through the trapezius, and the skin may even be tented. Type V injury includes the damage described for a type III injury, but with a greater degree of displacement of the clavicle toward the base of the neck. The coracoacromial distance is 100% to 300% greater than on the uninjured side. Type VI injury, which is quite rare, is a subcoracoid or subacromial dislocation of the distal clavicle.

The treatment of acute types I and II acromioclavicular injuries is nonsurgical. Ice, analgesics, and the use of a sling for a short period are generally recommended, followed by gradual resumption of use, as symptoms decrease. The treatment of acute type III separations, however, remains controversial. Currently, the trend is toward nonsurgical treatment of most of these injuries. This treatment consists of accepting the deformity, using a sling for support and comfort in the early postinjury period, and then rehabilitating the shoulder with range-of-motion and strengthening exercises. Attempts at maintaining a reduction of the joint by means of straps or splints are presently not favored by most, because these instruments are often ineffective and can cause skin breakdown.

Over the past decade several investigators have compared the results of nonsurgical and surgical treatment of acute type III acromioclavicular injuries. Investigations included randomized, prospective studies, in which those treated nonsurgically had a shorter rehabilitation period, earlier return to work and sport, and fewer complications. Results of a recent study of patients treated nonsurgically for type III injuries indicated that strength and endurance levels of the injured shoulders were comparable to those of the uninjured side at follow-up. Discomfort levels were low, but increased with higher levels of activity. When the dominant shoulder is involved, particularly in young active patients or overhead laborers, surgical treatment is chosen by some surgeons for acute type III injuries. Also, acute surgical stabilization is routinely recommended for types IV, V, and VI injuries. In these injuries, there is greater damage to the deltotrapezial aponeurosis, leading to greater deformity and instability (Fig. 4).

Several methods of stabilization have been reported, including acromioclavicular joint fixation (with pins), coracoclavicular fixation (using a screw, wire, synthetic tape, or heavy suture material), and dynamic muscle transfer. Good results have been reported for use of a number of different techniques, although the trend appears to be toward the use of coracoclavicular fixation. In chronic cases, a transfer of the coracoacromial ligament and excision of the distal clavicle, in addition to some sort of coracoclavicular fixation, yields satisfactory results (stability) and avoids the development of degenerative arthritis.

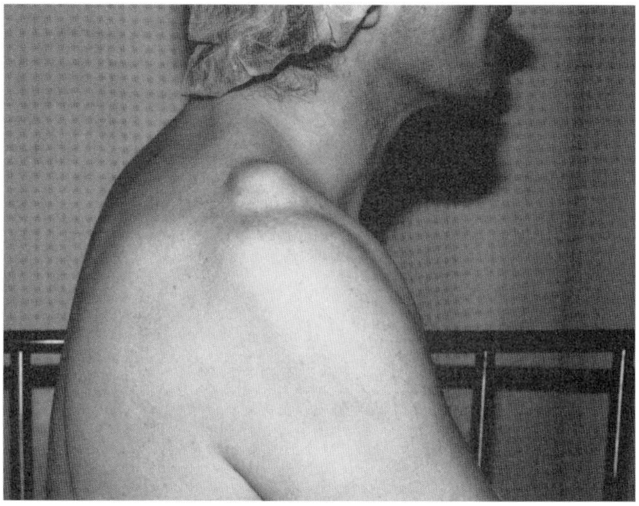

Fig. 4 Type IV acromioclavicular separation with the unstable distal clavicle displaced through the trapezius and tenting the skin.

Sternoclavicular Instability

Sternoclavicular dislocations are much less common than injuries to the acromioclavicular joint. These injuries occur with motor vehicle accidents and with violent sports activities. They can occur in either an anterior or posterior direction, with anterior dislocations seen with greater frequency. Greater attention has been paid in the literature to posterior dislocations, because they are more difficult to diagnose and may cause significant injury to the trachea, lungs, and great vessels. Patients with a posterior dislocation may present with hoarseness, dysphagia, dyspnea, or venous congestion of the neck and upper extremity. On physical examination, a posterior dislocation of the sternoclavicular joint can be difficult to diagnose, and these injuries can occasionally be mistaken for anterior dislocations. Anterior dislocations are more easily diagnosed by the prominence of the medial end of the clavicle. AP radiographs can be difficult to interpret; a 40° cephalic tilt view and tomograms can be helpful. CT is quite useful in these cases, clarifying the bony abnormalities as well as the relationship of the trachea, esophagus, and subclavian vessels to the bony structures. CT can also differentiate between a true dislocation and a displace physeal fracture of the medial end of the clavicle (pseudodislocation), which is seen in adolescents after trauma to the sternoclavicular joint (Fig. 5).

Anterior sternoclavicular dislocations are generally treated nonsurgically. Closed reduction frequently results

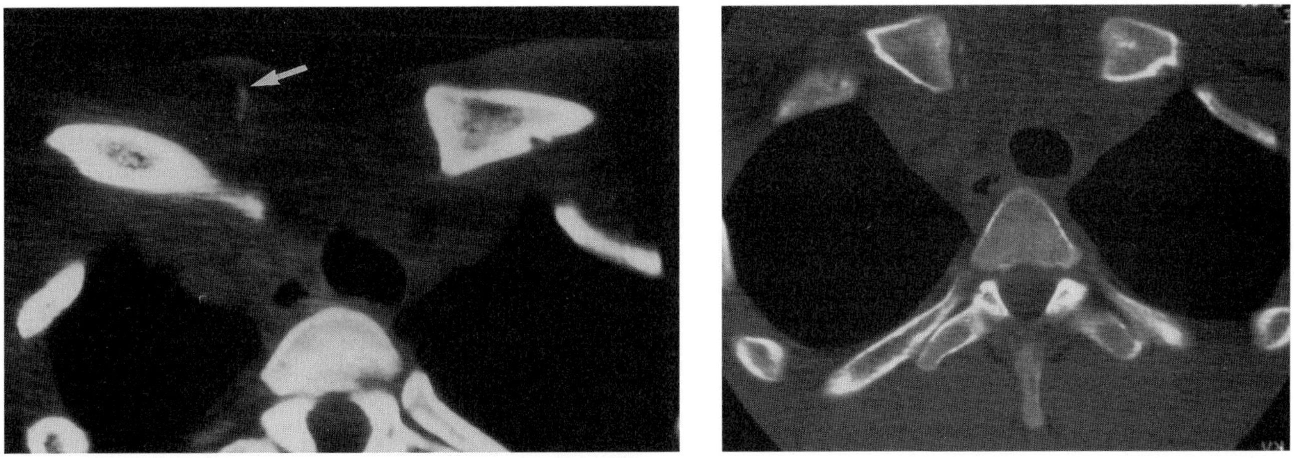

Fig. 5 A physeal fracture of the medial end of the clavicle with posterior displacement in a teenager, before (**left**) and after closed reduction (**right**). This injury can be mistaken for a posterior sternoclavicular dislocation clinically, but computed tomography is useful in establishing the diagnosis (arrow indicates epiphyseal fragment).

in failure, with an inability to maintain the unstable clavicle in the joint. Surgical treatment has been marked by high complication rates, with serious morbidity resulting from mediastinal or intracardiac migration of fixation pins. On the other hand, posterior sternoclavicular dislocations present peril to the mediastinal structures. Closed reduction is indicated. With the patient placed supine with a bolster between the scapulae, lateral traction is placed on the abducted and extended arm. Further traction anteriorly, with a sterile towel clip attached to the clavicle, may aid in difficult reductions. If closed reduction is unsuccessful, open reduction is undertaken. The reduction is usually stable in cases of posterior dislocation, and the arm is maintained in a figure-of-eight dressing or a sling for 4 to 6 weeks. Atraumatic or spontaneous subluxation or dislocation of the sternoclavicular joint is managed conservatively.

Annotated Bibliography

Glenohumeral Instability: Basic Science

Bigliani LU, Pollock RG, Soslowsky LJ, et al: Tensile properties of the inferior glenohumeral ligament. *J Orthop Res* 1992;10:187–197.

Structural and mechanical (tensile) properties of the three regions of the inferior glenohumeral ligament are reported in a cadaver study. The thickness of this ligament decreased significantly from its superior band (average, 2.8 mm) to its posterior axillary pouch (average, 1.7 mm). Ligament failures occurred both in the midsubstance (35%) and at the insertion sites (65%), although significant stretching occurred prior to failure, regardless of the ultimate failure mode.

Lippett SB, Vanderhooft JE, Harris SL, et al: Glenohumeral stability from concavity-compression: A quantitative analysis. *J Shoulder Elbow Surg* 1993;2:27–35.

Concavity-compression of the humeral head into the glenoid is an important mechanism for stabilizing the shoulder in the midrange of glenohumeral motion, where the capsular ligaments are lax. With an intact labrum, the humeral head resisted tangential forces of up to 60% of the compressive load; without the labrum, the effectiveness of this mechanism decreased by 20%.

Speer KP, Deng X, Borrero S, et al: Biomechanical evaluation of a simulated Bankart lesion. *J Bone Joint Surg* 1994;76A:1819–1826.

After simulation of a Bankart lesion in a cadaver model, mean joint translations increased by very small amounts (3.4-mm maximum, which occurred with inferior translations at 45° of elevation). Detachment of the anteroinferior labrum alone does not appear to be solely responsible for the increased glenohumeral translation that is necessary to produce an anterior dislocation of the shoulder.

Glenohumeral Instability: Clinical

Altchek DW, Warren RF, Skyhar MJ, et al: T-plasty modification of the Bankart procedure for multidirectional instability of the anterior and inferior types. *J Bone Joint Surg* 1991;73A:105–112.

The authors report on the results in 40 patients of a medially based capsulorrhaphy procedure, which allows combined repair of a Bankart lesion and the elimination of inferior laxity. A high percentage of patients (83%) returned to full sports activity, although throwers noted some decrease in velocity.

Arciero RA, Wheeler JH, Ryan JB, et al: Arthroscopic Bankart repair versus nonoperative treatment for acute, initial anterior shoulder dislocations. *Am J Sports Med* 1994;22:589–594.

This prospective study compared arthroscopic stabilization and nonsurgical treatment for acute primary traumatic shoulder dislocation in 36 military cadet-athletes. In the nonsurgical group, 80% developed recurrent instability and seven later required open repair, while in the arthroscopic group, only 14 % developed recurrence and only one required open repair.

Bigliani LU, Kurzweil PR, Schwartzbach CC, et al: Inferior capsular shift procedure for anterior-inferior shoulder instability in athletes. *Am J Sports Med* 1994;22:578–584.

Sixty-three patients (including 31 throwing athletes) with anteroinferior glenohumeral instability underwent a laterally based capsular shift procedure, combined with repair of a Bankart lesion when present (31%). Satisfactory results were achieved in 94%, and 92% returned to sports (75% at the same level). The rate of recurrence of instability was 3%.

Burkhead WZ Jr, Rockwood CA Jr: Treatment of instability of the shoulder with an exercise program. *J Bone Joint Surg* 1992;74A:890–896.

One hundred fifteen patients with glenohumeral subluxation were treated with a specific program of muscle-strengthening exercises. Those with a history of atraumatic instability responded favorably to treatment in 80% versus only 15% for those with traumatic subluxation.

Cooper RA, Brems JJ: The inferior capsular-shift procedure for multidirectional instability of the shoulder. *J Bone Joint Surg* 1992;74A:1516–1521.

Thirty-eight patients (43 shoulders) with disabling multidirectional instability were treated with an inferior capsular shift. Ninety-one percent had no recurrence of instability. Failures and recurrences of instability occurred early in the postoperative period, and results did not appear to deteriorate over time.

Grana WA, Buckley PD, Yates CK: Arthroscopic Bankart suture repair. *Am J Sports Med* 1993;21:348–353.

Twenty-seven patients were treated with arthroscopic Bankart suture repair for anterior glenohumeral instability. Twelve (44%) developed recurrent instability, and the authors recommend caution in the use of arthroscopic stabilization for the competitive athlete.

Green MR, Christensen KP: Arthroscopic versus open Bankart procedures: A comparison of early morbidity and complications. *Arthroscopy* 1993;9:371–374.

Thirty-eight patients with unidirectional anterior shoulder instability were treated with either an arthroscopic suture repair (n = 20) or an open modified Bankart repair (n = 18). Patients treated with the arthroscopic technique demonstrated a significant ($p < 0.001$) reduction in surgical time, estimated blood loss, postoperative narcotic use, postoperative fevers, duration of hospitalization, and work days missed compared to those treated with the open procedure.

Lephart SM, Warner JJP, Borsa PA, et al: Proprioception of the shoulder joint in healthy, unstable, and surgically repaired shoulders. *J Shoulder Elbow Surg* 1994;3:371–380.

Proprioceptive deficits were identified in the shoulders of patients with chronic anterior glenohumeral instability. Surgical stabilization appears to restore some of these proprioceptive properties, suggesting a proprioceptive role for the capsuloligamentous structures.

Lusardi DA, Wirth MA, Wurtz D, et al: Loss of external rotation following anterior capsulorrhaphy of the shoulder. *J Bone Joint Surg* 1993;75A:1185–1192.

Twenty shoulders with severe loss of external rotation after a previous anterior capsulorrhaphy were successfully managed with a release of the anterior soft tissues. In addition, nine shoulders with severe osteoarthritis underwent prosthetic arthroplasty. All shoulders had improvement in pain and range of motion (external rotation increased by an average of 45°).

Montgomery WH III, Jobe FW: Functional outcomes in athletes after modified anterior capsulolabral reconstruction. *Am J Sports Med* 1994;22:352–358.

Thirty-two consecutive athletes underwent anterior capsulolabral reconstruction with a horizontal capsulotomy and fixation with suture anchors. Ninety-seven percent good or excellent results were achieved, and 81% returned to the same sport at the same level of competition, including 9 of 13 (69%) baseball pitchers.

Superior Labral/Biceps Complex

Cordasco FA, Steinmann S, Flatow EL, et al: Arthroscopic treatment of glenoid labral tears. *Am J Sports Med* 1993;21:425–431.

This paper suggests that arthroscopic labral debridement may yield satisfactory short-term results, but the results deteriorate with time in a high percentage of cases.

Rodosky MW, Harner CD, Fu FH: The role of the long head of the biceps muscle and superior glenoid labrum in anterior stability of the shoulder. *Am J Sports Med* 1994; 22:121–130.

Data from a cadaveric shoulder model suggest that the long head of the biceps muscle contributes to torsional forces in the abducted, externally rotated position. With a superior labral detachment, peak torque and torsional rigidity was significantly reduced ($p < 0.01$).

Snyder SJ, Karzel RP, Del Pizzo W, et al: SLAP lesions of the shoulder. *Arthroscopy* 1990;6:274–279.

A classification system and methods for diagnosis and treatment are reviewed, based on arthroscopic findings in 27 shoulders with superior labral pathology. These lesions can be diagnosed best by arthroscopic means and may be treated successfully in a high percentage of patients using arthroscopic techniques.

Acromioclavicular Joint

Tibone J, Sellers R, Tonino P: Strength testing after third-degree acromioclavicular dislocations. *Am J Sports Med* 1992;20:328–331.

Strength testing at an average of 4.5 years after injury in 20 patients with a grade III acromioclavicular separation that was treated nonsurgically demonstrated no strength deficits for shoulder adduction, abduction, internal rotation, external rotation, flexion, or extension. Most grade III acromioclavicular dislocations should be treated conservatively.

Classic Bibliography

Allman FL Jr: Fractures and ligamentous injuries of the clavicle and its articulation. *J Bone Joint Surg* 1967;49A: 774–784.

Altchek DW, Warren RF, Wickiewicz TL, et al: Arthroscopic labral debridement: A three-year follow-up study. *Am J Sports Med* 1992;20:702–706.

Bankart ASB: The pathology and treatment of recurrent dislocations of the shoulder joint. *Br J Surg* 1938;26: 23–29.

Cooper DE, Arnoczky SP, O'Brien SJ, et al: Anatomy, histology and vascularity of the glenoid labrum: An anatomical study. *J Bone Joint Surg* 1992;74A:46–52.

Harryman DT II, Sidles JA, Harris SL, et al: Laxity of the normal glenohumeral joint: A quantitative in vivo assessment. *J Shoulder Elbow Surg* 1992;1:66–76.

Morgan CD, Bodenstab AB: Arthroscopic Bankart suture repair: Technique and early results. *Arthroscopy* 1987;3:111–122.

Neer CS II, Foster CR: Inferior capsular shift for involuntary inferior and multidirectional instability of the shoulder: A preliminary report. *J Bone Joint Surg* 1980; 62A:878–908.

Resch H, Golser K, Thoeni H, et al: Arthroscopic repair of superior glenoid labral detachment (the SLAP lesion). *J Shoulder Elbow Surg* 1993;2:147–155.

Rowe CR: Prognosis in dislocation of the shoulder. *J Bone Joint Surg* 1956;38A:957–977.

Soslowsky LJ, Flatow EL, Bigliani LU, et al: Articular geometry of the glenohumeral joint. *Clin Orthop* 1992; 285:181–190.

Thomas SC, Matsen FA III: An approach to the repair of avulsion of the glenohumeral ligaments in the management of traumatic anterior glenohumeral instability. *J Bone Joint Surg* 1989;71A:506–512.

Turkel SJ, Panio MW, Marshall JL, et al: Stabilizing mechanisms preventing anterior dislocation of the glenohumeral joint. *J Bone Joint Surg* 1981;63A: 1208–1217.

Warner JJ, Deng XH, Warren RF, et al: Static capsuloligamentous restraints to superior-inferior translation of the glenohumeral joint. *Am J Sports Med* 1992;20:675–685.

Wojtys EM, Nelson G: Conservative treatment of grade III acromioclavicular dislocations. *Clin Orthop* 1991;268: 112–119.

Young DC, Rockwood CA Jr: Complications of a failed Bristow procedure and their management. *J Bone Joint Surg* 1991;73A:969–981.

Zuckerman JD, Matsen FA III: Complications about the glenohumeral joint related to the use of screws and staples. *J Bone Joint Surg* 1984;66A:175–180.

26

Shoulder: Reconstruction

The armamentarium of treatment options is increasing as rapidly as understanding of pathologic conditions about the shoulder. Advances in diagnostic and therapeutic arthroscopy have expanded the orthopaedic surgeon's approach to rotator cuff disease, while other research has improved understanding of prosthetic design and technique. Clinical studies have provided a new perspective on some common, yet problematic disorders. Despite these advances, numerous questions pertaining to the management of massive rotator cuff tears, complications of prosthetic arthroplasty, and nerve lesions of the shoulder girdle still exist.

Muscular Function and Anatomy of the Glenohumeral Joint

The contribution of the deltoid and each of the rotator cuff muscles to elevation of the arm continues to remain a subject of debate. Data from studies in which selective blocks of the suprascapular and axillary nerves were used have suggested that the supraspinatus and middle deltoid contribute equally to measured torque in abduction. Selective block of the infraspinatus alone, however, has been reported to reduce abduction torque up to 45%, thus suggesting a role in arm elevation. The functional relationship of the deltoid and rotator cuff to humeral elevation was indirectly determined by calculation of changes in moment arms and measurement of muscular excursion in cadaveric specimens. In this way, both the infraspinatus and subscapularis were shown to contribute to abduction. Changes in rotation further affected the ability of either muscle to augment elevation in the scapular plane. Internal and external rotation enhanced the ability of the upper portions of the infraspinatus and subscapularis, respectively, to abduct the arm. The data help explain, in part, how a supraspinatus defect may not necessarily limit functional abduction of the arm.

Strength in external rotation and abduction can be effectively measured using isokinetic and isometric methods. Standardization of arm positions for strength testing in the scapular plane was found to be reliable and includes isometric strength of external rotation at 45° of abduction and 45° of internal rotation, isometric strength of abduction at 45° of abduction, and isokinetic strength of external rotation and abduction at 90° per second. Standard methods of testing can allow improved evaluation and comparison between results of treatment.

There now is a more detailed understanding of the gross and microscopic anatomy of the rotator cuff. The supraspinatus tendon is made up of five distinct layers and receives reinforcement by fibers extending from the coracohumeral ligament and adjacent tendons. Distribution of forces over an expanded area of the cuff could be expected to result from tension in any one musculotendinous unit.

Arthroscopy of the Shoulder

Arthroscopy of the shoulder has advanced from a purely diagnostic tool, and its use has led to new techniques and instrumentation for the treatment of both glenohumeral and subacromial problems. Orthopaedic surgeons have gained a clearer definition of shoulder pathology (impingement, labral injury, instability) through use of the arthroscope, and it has led to the development of techniques that address the pathology. Rehabilitation has been made easier.

The standard arthroscopic equipment used in the shoulder includes a 30° 4-mm arthroscope, video camera setup, graspers, biters, and shavers. One instrument that is particularly helpful in arthroscopy of the shoulder is the Wissinger rod for changing portals. There are basically two methods for positioning the patient: the lateral decubitus position in which the patient is positioned on the side with the arm abducted and 5 to 10 lbs of traction applied, and the beach chair position in which the patient is in a semisitting position with gravity as the only traction. Which of these methods is used depends on the surgeon's preference. Standard portals include anterior superior, posterior superior, and lateral subacromial. Posterior portal placement can be complicated by injury to axillary and suprascapular nerves, whereas the anterior portal can be complicated by cephalic vein, brachial plexus, or axillary artery injury. The use of pressurized fluid systems is mentioned with caution. Fluid extravasation into soft tissues can lead to increased postoperative pain or compartment syndrome. New fixation or anchoring techniques, laser usage, and office arthroscopy are being explored and show promise.

Rotator Cuff Disease

Etiology

It is generally accepted that rotator cuff disorders represent a spectrum of disease with a multifactorial etiology. Whether these disorders result from mechanical impingement or an intrinsic degenerative process requires further clarification.

The influence of various morphologic aspects of the coracoacromial arch has been evaluated in recent studies. The association of both acromion morphology and enthesopathy with rotator cuff disease is well established. Patients with an inferiorly projecting acromion or evidence of subacromial spurs are more likely to demonstrate impingement and associated lesions of the rotator cuff. Data from a recent study evaluating the anatomic characteristics of 200 scapulas revealed subacromial spurs and osteophyte formation in the anterior third of the acromion in 18% overall. Anatomic variations most closely associated with these lesions included a more horizontal lying acromion, an increased acromial length in the anteroposterior (AP) plane, and a decreased height of the coracoacromial arch. Although such factors have been suggested to play a role in the pathogenesis of impingement syndrome and rotator cuff disease in certain cases, standard acromioplasty may not adequately address these issues.

Mechanical forces about the coracoacromial arch, which are not fully understood, have also been implicated in rotator cuff disease. Biomechanical and geometric testing of the coracoacromial ligament has demonstrated that the lateral band (that portion of the ligament more likely to impinge on the tendinous cuff) was both shorter in length and smaller in cross-sectional area in shoulders with rotator cuff tears. Although histologically there were no structural differences in the ligament between normal shoulders and shoulders with rotator cuff tears, there was evidence of decreased mechanical properties in the latter. The reduction in mechanical integrity of the ligament was thought to reflect the multiple directional loads imposed on this structure in shoulders with rotator cuff tears. Data from an additional investigation in which scanning electron micrographs were used to evaluate rotator cuff deterioration in eight cadaveric shoulders demonstrated that observed degenerative changes were characteristic of alterations secondary to frictional and rubbing mechanisms. These observations support the contention that degenerative changes already present in the cuff, irrespective of etiology, can be aggravated by frictional or abrading type mechanisms.

Impingement Syndrome

Impingement syndrome is one of the most frequently diagnosed causes of pain about the shoulder. Appreciation of the pathoanatomy, etiology, and associated secondary findings remain important determinants for improved prognosis and successful treatment. Inadequate recognition of the primary source of symptoms, failure to adequately address associated pathology, and incomplete surgical decompression, in part, may help explain those cases refractory to accepted treatment strategies. Benefits of selective anesthetic injections into the glenohumeral joint, acromioclavicular joint, and subacromial space have been well documented in the literature and can aid in discriminating potential sources of pain.

A recent study highlighted a group of patients whose clinical picture was typical of impingement syndrome that had not responded to conservative treatment measures. Intraoperatively, these patients were found to have coexisting degenerative changes of the glenohumeral joint that were evident arthroscopically but had not been apparent on preoperative radiographs. Because such findings can alter prognosis, increased suspicion along with careful examination and both axillary and true scapular AP radiographs may aid in preoperative detection of these lesions.

Other potential sources of pain in some throwing athletes with painful arc syndrome include impingement of the deep surface of supraspinatus tendon on the posterosuperior glenoid rim. Arthroscopic confirmation of these findings with the arm in 90° to 150° of abduction and external rotation has been reported. Associated findings frequently found include degenerative lesions of the posterior superior labrum, corresponding osteochondral lesions of the humeral head, and partial tears of the rotator cuff. It has subsequently been suggested that abduction and external rotation of the arm can entrap a portion of the supraspinatus tendon between the humeral head and glenoid in susceptible individuals. Further investigation is necessary to better define this entity, clarify its pathoanatomy, and evaluate proposed treatment modalities.

Although open acromioplasty is a time-honored treatment for impingement syndrome, arthroscopic methods are associated with shorter hospital stays and faster achievement of maximal pain relief. Retrospective comparison of open and arthroscopic techniques for chronic impingement syndrome demonstrated no significant differences in mean postoperative shoulder scores at 1- to 5-year follow-up. Examination of postoperative radiographs, however, revealed the presence of subacromial calcifications in some individuals in the arthroscopic group, and these were associated with a worse result. Recent reports have generally confirmed that the results of arthroscopic acromioplasty are at least equivalent to those of open techniques. The benefits of shorter hospital stays and faster recovery have been consistently reported for arthroscopic acromioplasty and have led to the acceptance of this technique for the treatment of impingement syndrome in the absence of full-thickness rotator cuff tears.

The presence of residual acromion that extends beyond the anterior border of the clavicle has been emphasized as a potential cause of failed acromioplasty. Variations of Neer's technique that highlight the excision of the anterior acromion have demonstrated results comparable to previous series. Inadequate osseous resection can be readily assessed radiographically and may result in recurrent impingement and surgical failure (Fig. 1).

Rotator Cuff Tears

Imaging

Diagnostic imaging of rotator cuff disorders can be a useful adjunct to clinical examination when appropriately used in patients presenting with shoulder pain. Routine radiographs should include an AP view in the plane of the

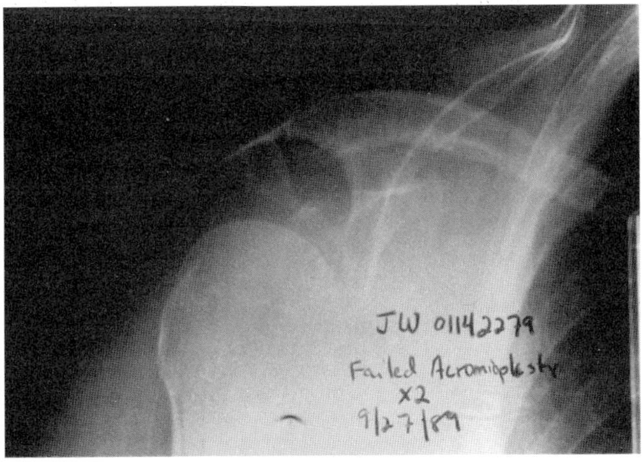

Fig. 1 Thirty degree caudal tilt view demonstrating a persistent subacromial spur after two failed attempts at acromioplasty.

scapula with the arm in internal and external rotation in addition to an axillary view. Additional images, such as the supraspinatus outlet view, can demonstrate acromial morphology, whereas an AP projection directed 30° caudally will often reveal subacromial spurs that are not entirely evident on conventional frontal views (Fig. 2). In one recent study, it was noted that of 100 subacromial spurs detected on the caudal tilt view, only 18 were demonstrable on the routine AP radiograph.

Results of ultrasonography depend largely on adequate technique and interpretive skills. In one retrospective study of 49 patients there was an accuracy of 84% in the detection of full-thickness rotator cuff tears with ultrasonography, in contrast to an accuracy of 94% with arthrography. The inability of ultrasound to reliably differentiate partial and small full-thickness tears was also noted.

Magnetic resonance imaging (MRI) has demonstrated a sensitivity and specificity of 100% and 95%, respectively, in the diagnosis of complete tears. Although it has the advantage of accurately depicting tear size and biceps pathology, MRI, like ultrasonography, presents difficulties in distinguishing partial and small full-thickness tears. In such instances, factors pertaining to technique, surface coil type, and interpretive skills become increasingly important. The effectiveness of MRI in determining defects of the rotator cuff in shoulders that previously underwent surgery has been evaluated. Complete tears were detected with an accuracy of 90%, although partial-thickness lesions were indistinguishable from repaired tendons.

Increasing dependence on MRI and inadequate correlation to clinical findings may contribute to improper diagnosis and treatment of patients presenting with shoulder pain. In a prospective study assessing MRI scans in 96 asymptomatic volunteers, complete and partial rotator cuff tears were demonstrated in 14% and 20%, respectively. Of individuals over 60 years of age, 54% were noted by MRI to have either a full or partial-thickness tear despite normal function and the absence of symptoms. The results highlight the dangers of basing surgical decisions on MRI scans alone. Additionally, they provide in vivo evidence that individuals with no history of shoulder complaints can have normal function regardless of the presence of a rotator cuff tear on MRI (Fig. 3).

Nonsurgical Management

The success of nonsurgical management—rest, local modalities, nonsteroidal anti-inflammatory drugs (NSAIDs), physical therapy, and judicious use of subacromial steroid injections—of rotator cuff disorders and impingement may vary from less than 50% to 90%. This wide range is

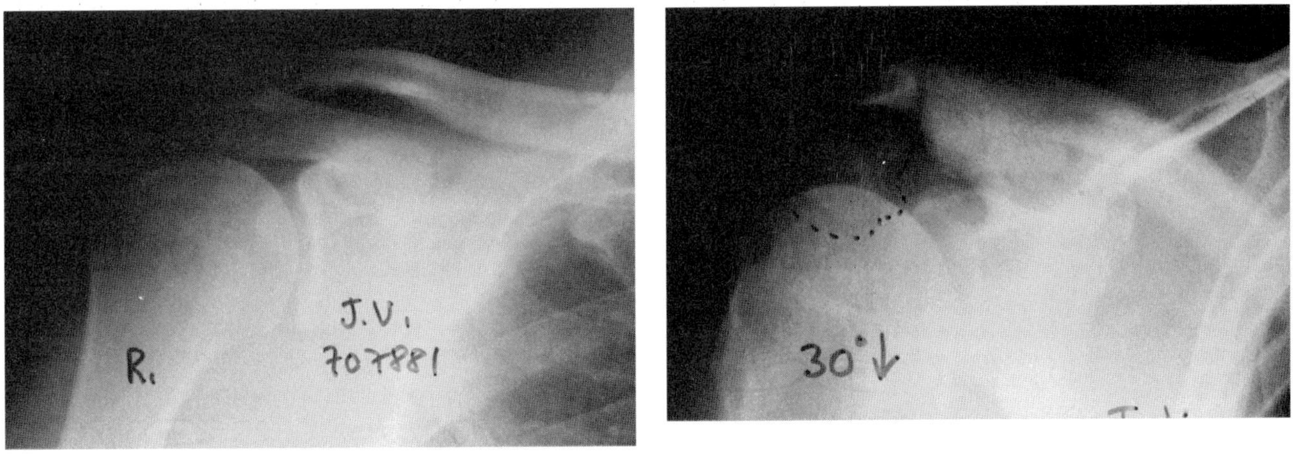

Fig. 2 Anteroposterior radiograph in the plane of the scapula **(left)** and 30° caudal tilt view **(right)** in a patient with impingement syndrome. A large anterior subacromial spur is apparent on the caudal tilt view **(outlined)** and obscured on the routine AP view.

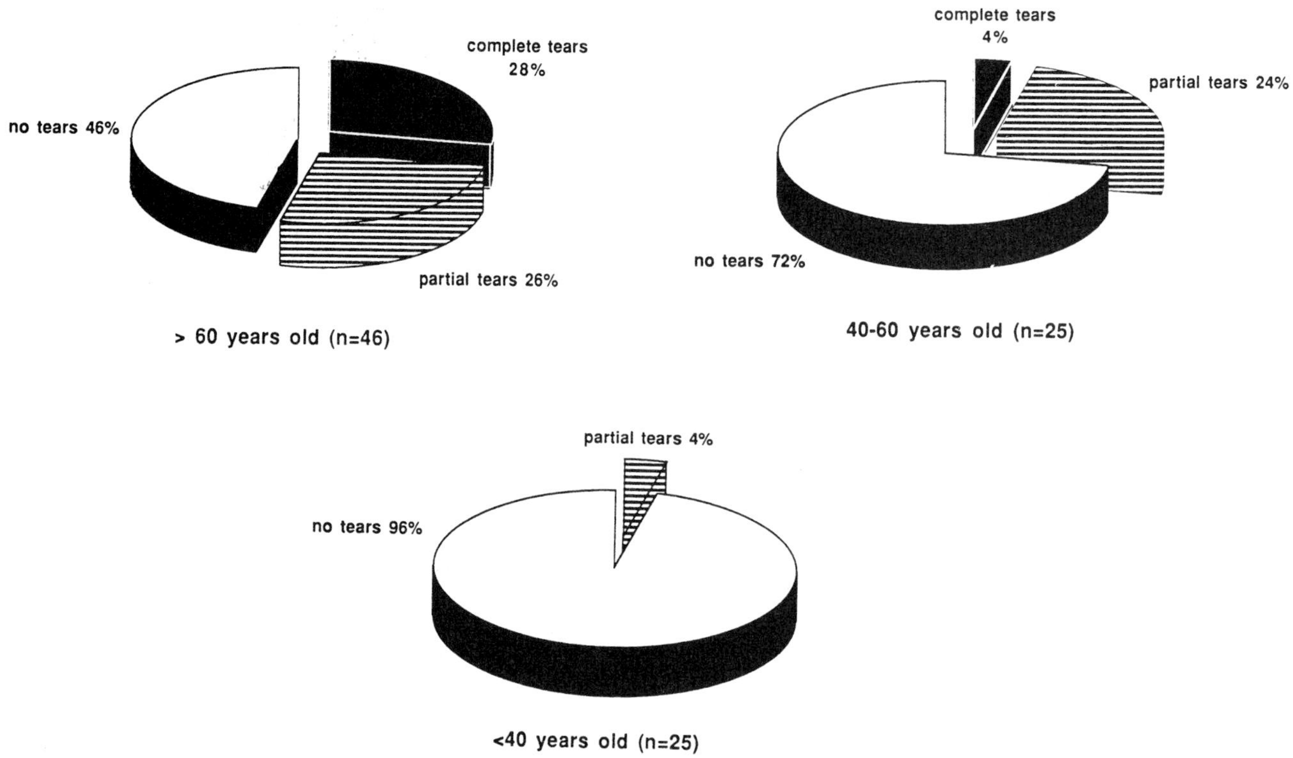

Fig. 3 Prevalence of MRI evident rotator cuff tears in asymptomatic volunteers over 60 years of age (**left**), 40 to 60 years (**right**), and under 40 years (**bottom**). (Adapted with permission from Sher JS, Uribe JW, Posada A, et al: Abnormal findings on magnetic resonance images of asymptomatic shoulders. *J Bone Joint Surg* 1995;77A:10–15.)

likely a reflection of the lack of uniformity in classification, indications, and treatment. The fact that many individuals can have rotator cuff tears with normal function and no discomfort while others may have disabling pain highlights the need for a better understanding of the precipitating factors responsible for symptoms. Furthermore, the multifactorial nature of rotator cuff disease makes it difficult to critically compare investigative studies and results of treatment. Although approximately 50% of individuals with symptomatic complete rotator cuff tears seem to achieve satisfactory results with conservative measures, in one retrospective study it was observed that patients evaluated beyond 6 years had worse results when compared to shorter follow-up evaluations. Duration of symptoms for less than 1 year and preservation of motion and strength prior to treatment were associated with improved shoulder scores; however, deterioration with time beyond 6 years was evident.

Surgical Management

Partial-Thickness Tears Optimal management of partial-thickness rotator cuff tears remains a subject of controversy. Arthroscopic debridement with or without acromioplasty has exhibited satisfactory results in 75% to 86% of individuals according to recent reports. Open excision and direct repair has also demonstrated comparable results in many patients. Although well-controlled studies are still lacking, excision and either side-to-side repair or suture into bone are generally recommended for partial tears involving greater than 50% of the tendon thickness in cases refractory to conservative treatment.

Full-Thickness Tears Rotator cuff repair is the mainstay of surgical treatment for symptomatic full-thickness lesions. Factors important in decision making include severity and duration of symptoms, functional limitations, patient demands and expectations, tear location, and tear size. Greater than 10-year follow-up of conventional open repair techniques has continued to demonstrate good results in small, medium, and many large sized tears. Optimal management of massive tears, however, remains a challenging problem.

Data from a recent prospective study comparing arthroscopic debridement and open repair in 45 patients with 1- to 4-cm rotator cuff tears demonstrated satisfactory pain relief and return of arm elevation in the two groups at 2- to 5-year follow-up. Although the open repair group had improved overall function and strength, patient satisfaction was similar. Arthroscopic debridement was recommended only in carefully selected individuals with limited demands, whose main goal was relief of pain. Similarly, data from a prospective study in 87 patients with chronic full-thickness rotator cuff tears of variable size demonstrated superior results in the open repair group. Shoulder scores in patients who had undergone debridement deteriorated with time and demonstrated no correlation with tear size, age, or preoperative activity level.

Other reports evaluating arthroscopic subacromial decompression and debridement in selected patients with complete cuff tears revealed satisfactory results in 90%, 50%, and 84% of individuals with small (0 to 2 cm), larger (2 to 4 cm) and massive (> 4 cm) tears, respectively, at 2- to 7-year follow-up. Although those patients with massive tears did not regain significant strength or motion, they did attain adequate pain relief and satisfaction, thereby achieving limited goal expectations. Individuals with larger, otherwise repairable tears, who had undergone debridement, did poorly when compared to historic controls.

Primary repair of full-thickness rotator cuff tears combined with acromioplasty offers the best opportunity for pain relief and return of strength and function. The management of unrepairable tendon defects, however, remains controversial. Surgical options include local tendon transposition (eg, subscapularis, teres minor) and distant tendon transfer (eg, latissimus dorsi, anterior deltoid, trapezius) as well as reconstruction with autografts, allografts, and synthetic materials. These techniques can be technically demanding and often yield unpredictable results. In carefully selected patients, acromioplasty combined with cuff debridement has been reported to yield satisfactory function and relief of symptoms. Further investigation is needed to better define the relative roles of each of these approaches to the management of unrepairable defects of the rotator cuff.

Arthroscopically assisted rotator cuff repair has had comparable results to open techniques in selected patients, although at shorter follow-up. Postoperative evaluation of 44 patients at an average of 4.2 years exhibited 84% good to excellent results with 88% patient satisfaction. Individuals with small and moderate tears had improved results over those with large and massive lesions. Reports of other investigations employing arthroscopic-assisted techniques indicated similar findings at an average follow-up of 4 years.

Multiple factors often contribute to failed rotator cuff surgery, which can consequently impose a surgical challenge. Evaluation of 31 patients undergoing repeat operations for unsuccessful cuff repairs revealed persistent subacromial impingement in 90% and the presence of a large or massive tear at the index operation in 97%. Factors associated with poor results after revision surgery were a previous lateral acromionectomy, deltoid detachment, and poor tissue quality (Fig. 4). Although sufficient pain relief was achieved in 81%, functional results were considerably less predictable.

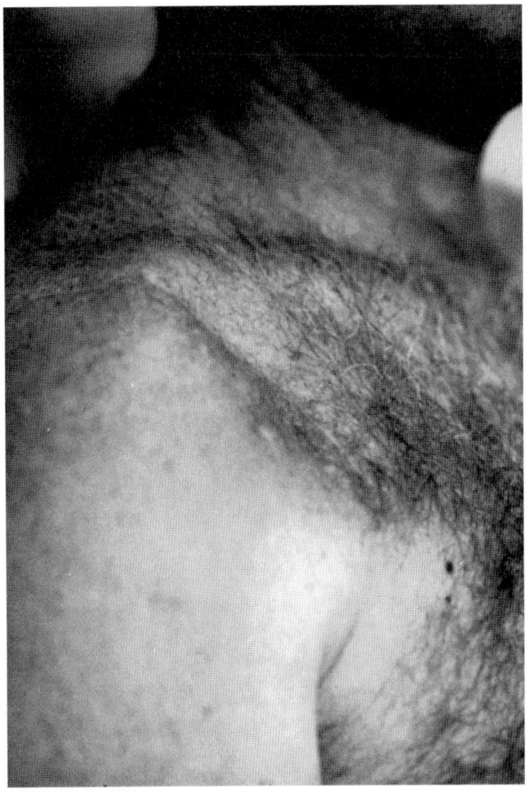

Fig. 4 Detachment of the anterior portion of the deltoid after open surgical repair of the rotator cuff.

Prosthetic Arthroplasty

Arthroplasty in the painful arthritic shoulder can accomplish satisfactory relief of symptoms and restoration of function in properly selected individuals. Patients with rheumatoid arthritis often present a diagnostic challenge because radiographic abnormalities do not always correlate with the source of pain. In a recent study, it was found that 55% of shoulders in rheumatoid patients demonstrated relief of symptoms after local anesthetic injection into the subacromial space or acromioclavicular joint despite advanced radiologic evidence of glenohumeral degeneration. Loss of sphericity of the humeral head, however, did positively correlate with pain generated from the glenohumeral joint. The results highlight the potential benefits of selective anesthetic injection in the evaluation of the rheumatoid patient with shoulder pain.

Design and Technique

Unconstrained prosthetic designs have demonstrated fewer complications and superior long-term results when compared to constrained components. In contrast to the situation in total hip arthroplasty, unconstrained total shoulder prostheses afford little joint stability and thus require sufficient rotator cuff integrity to limit humeral head excursion.

A recent study evaluated the effects of conformity and constraint of various prosthetic designs on translational force and frictional torque generated at the articular surface. The more conforming and constrained implants demonstrated greater forces with humeral head rotation and translation. Although the increase in measured articular forces may contribute to glenoid loosening in certain prostheses, objective data delineating the degree of stress and strain at the component interface remain absent in the literature. Such information can provide further insight into the mechanical factors contributing to loss of component fixation.

Effects of glenoid preparation on deformation and edge displacement of glenoid components have also been evaluated. Data from these studies demonstrated that reaming of the osseous surface so that it closely conformed to the back of the glenoid component helped stabilize the component against eccentric loads. Less conforming methods of bone preparation, such as hand burring or curetting of the glenoid, yielded greater displacement and deformation of the polyethylene socket.

Surgical considerations for proper reconstruction of the glenohumeral joint during arthroplasty include adequate soft-tissue release, repair of rotator cuff defects, proper sizing of components, and correct positioning of the implants. Observations of the anatomic relationships between the humeral head and glenoid in 140 shoulders were discussed in a recent report that highlighted the differential increase in radius of curvature of the glenoid relative to the humerus. Implications to prosthetic design and technique were emphasized, especially restoration of the lateral humeral offset for preservation of maximal deltoid and rotator cuff strength.

Press-fit stems that fill the medullary canal define the ultimate prosthetic head position more rigorously than loose-fitting or cemented stems. Geometric evaluation of the medullary canal axis with the orientation of the articular surface in cadaveric specimens demonstrated that changes in version of the press-fit stems had a minimal effect on the combined head and neck length. Accordingly, if influence on soft-tissue tension through changes in the humeral component version was minimal, undue compromise of the tuberosities and rotator cuff insertions could be avoided. Use of the tuberosity anatomy as an added reference for determination of proper version was emphasized rather than version selection based solely on the same degree of forearm rotation in every case.

Results

Results of hemiarthroplasty and total shoulder replacement using hybrid fixation techniques have generally been comparable to those of hip and knee arthroplasty. Satisfactory pain relief can be reliably achieved in 85% to 95% of patients, although functional results are more dependent on the integrity of the rotator cuff. A recent review of hemiarthroplasties in 18 shoulders with irreparable rotator cuff tears and severe glenohumeral arthritis was reported; satisfactory pain relief was achieved in 83% and functional improvement, although variable in degree, was present in all at 2- to 10-year follow-up.

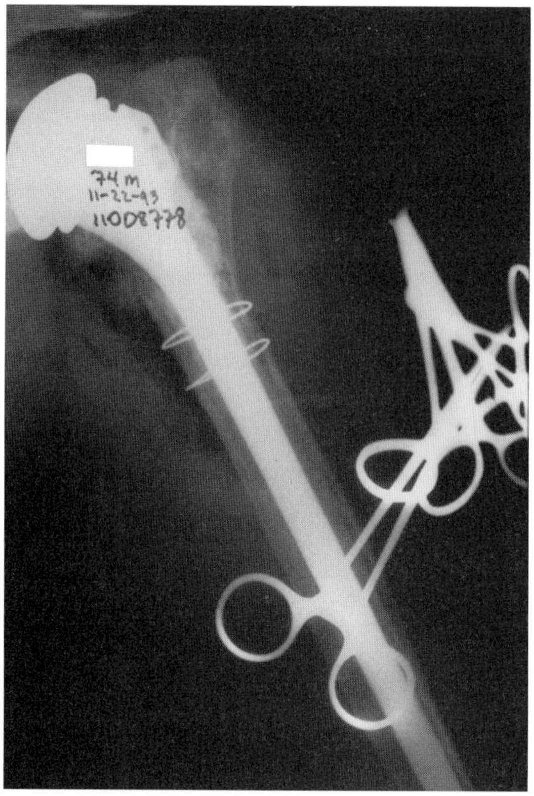

Fig. 5 Anteroposterior radiograph of a long-stem component placed after an intraoperative periprosthetic fracture which occurred during a revision procedure.

Complications

Intraoperative periprosthetic humeral fractures, while uncommon, are typically associated with overzealous insertion of reamers, broaches, and stems or aggressive manipulation of the arm during surgery. Risk of fracture is increased in osteopenic bone, and prompt recognition is vital to successful management. Intraoperative radiographs can help identify the extent of the fracture or rule out questionable injury in many cases. A recent report of three cases noted formation of a nonunion in all individuals in whom initial management was nonsurgical. Fracture healing was achieved after revision with a long-stem prosthesis or open reduction and internal fixation with bone grafting (Fig. 5).

Postoperative periprosthetic fractures of the humerus are an uncommon complication, which can lead to significant disability. Risk of fracture is also increased in osteopenic bone. A review of seven patients who had incurred a fracture and were initially treated nonsurgically revealed complications in all; complications included nonunion or a tardy radial nerve palsy. Surgical treatment resulted in ultimate healing at an average of 5 months, but incomplete pain relief and loss of motion were common sequelae. Nonsurgical management was associated with an increased likelihood of nonunion and injury to the radial nerve.

Instability after shoulder arthroplasty has been reported to range from 0% to 18% with unconstrained designs. Factors responsible for subluxation or dislocation typically include soft-tissue imbalance or component malposition. Subscapularis muscle rupture is responsible for most reported cases of anterior instability, and early recognition with repair remains critical to avoid permanent loss of function. However, posterior instability, although less frequent, was found to have a multifactorial etiology in a recent study (Fig. 6). Treatment of instability after total shoulder replacement can be difficult and was successfully achieved in ten patients with either soft-tissue reconstruction, prosthetic revision, or both.

Arthrodesis

Arthrodesis of the glenohumeral or scapulothoracic articulation is an infrequently performed procedure with limited indications. When it is achieved, limitation of humerothoracic motion can be expected. Typically, patients will have difficulty with activities at head level or behind the back, while functions at waist level are well tolerated. In a recent investigation using spatial electromagnetic sensors to evaluate residual motion in the unfused articulation, it was demonstrated that residual motion was similar to normal motion except for decreased external rotation and extension in scapulothoracic fusions and increased scapulothoracic internal rotation in glenohumeral fusions. However, functional limitation after either procedure was related most closely to activities that required extremes of internal rotation or elevation. These results further support those of previous investigations.

Various techniques have been described for glenohumeral arthrodesis that include the use of either internal or external fixation methods (Fig. 7). Analysis of 57 patients who had undergone fusion by one surgeon using single plate fixation without primary bone grafting revealed a 95% fusion rate. The three patients who had developed a nonunion ultimately healed after delayed bone grafting. Although successful fusion can be predictably achieved in the majority, a 14% complication rate was noted. Patients who had a brachial plexus injury and poor preoperative hand function or multidirectional instability refractory to previous stabilization procedures before undergoing fusion were most dissatisfied, had significant pain, and demonstrated the lowest cumulative activities of daily living scores at postoperative evaluation. Long-term follow-up in patients with scapulothoracic fusions for fascioscapulohumeral muscular dystrophy has continued to reveal improved function up to 21 years postoperatively.

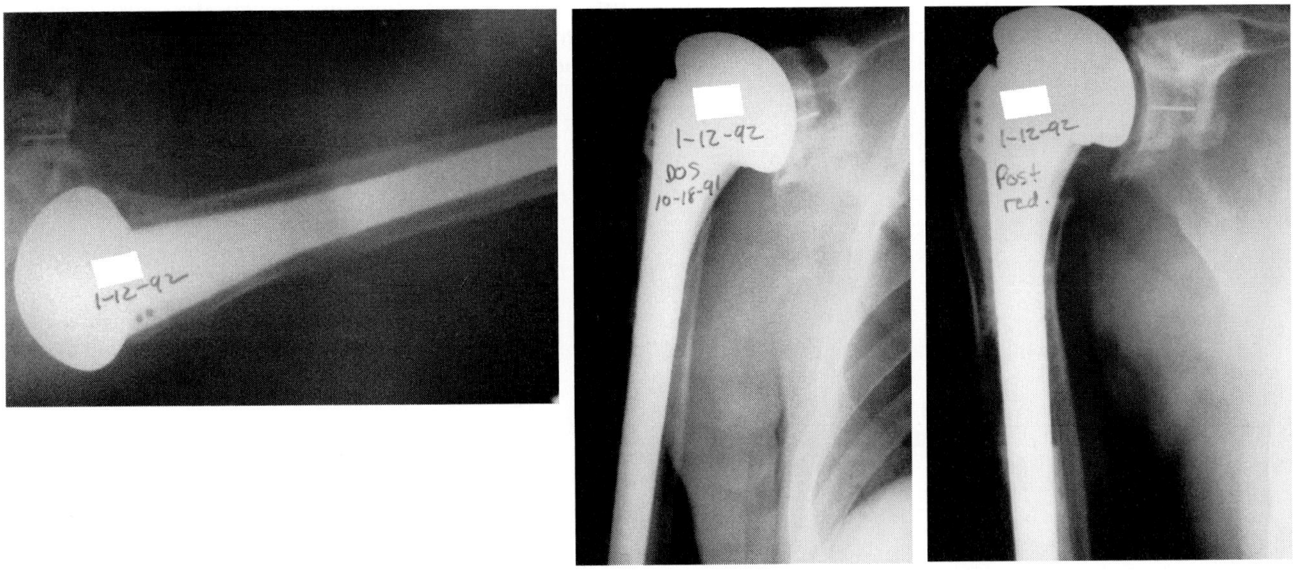

Fig. 6 Axillary (**left**) and AP (**center**) radiographs demonstrating a posterior dislocation after total shoulder replacement. Reduction was achieved after gentle closed manipulation (**right**).

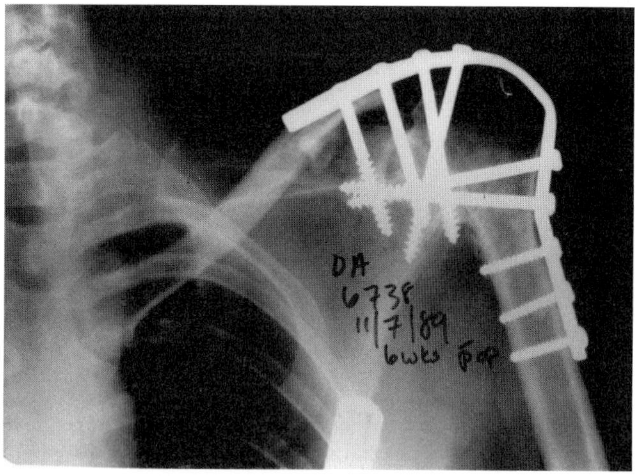

Fig. 7 Early postoperative radiograph of a glenohumeral arthrodesis using single plate internal fixation.

Frozen Shoulder

Frozen shoulder is an elusive disorder with a pathogenesis that is not fully understood. Although most patients can be effectively treated by nonsurgical means (a structured physical therapy program, NSAIDs), the duration of symptoms can be unpredictable and prolonged in many individuals. When patients do not respond to nonsurgical management, a manipulation under anesthesia should be considered as a method of improving motion. However, manipulation is generally required in only a small percentage of patients. Open soft-tissue release is only rarely used and is reserved for those who have not improved following manipulation or in whom manipulation poses an unacceptable risk of fracture. More recently, arthroscopic release techniques have been used with satisfactory results. However, the indications for this approach require further definition.

A review of 62 patients with idiopathic adhesive capsulitis revealed mild pain or residual stiffness in half of the subjects at an average follow-up of 7 years. Physical examination demonstrated restriction of motion in 60% and 18% when compared to calculated control values and the contralateral limb, respectively. Duration of symptoms ranged from 1 to 42 months, with an average of 12 months. Although a decrease in measured arcs of motion or a mild persistence of symptoms can often be found, they do not impose sufficient functional limitation to cause dissatisfaction in the majority of patients.

Long Thoracic Nerve Palsy

Injury to the long thoracic nerve is clinically manifested by the presence of shoulder pain, scapular winging, and difficulty in arm elevation (Fig. 8). Causes are multiple and include mechanical, toxic, and infectious etiologies. A review of 197 patients revealed that the majority of cases were secondary to either strenuous exertion or trauma and that the disorder was most common in young persons. Fifteen percent were of unknown etiology. Anatomic assessment of autopsy specimens has elucidated potential mechanisms of injury to this nerve as it courses inferiorly along the chest wall. Nerve compression as a result of anterior scapular motion or traction associated with posterior scapular movement were felt to be responsible, in part, for paralysis of the relatively unprotected nerve at the inferior angle of the scapula in susceptible individuals. It was suggested that asynchronous action of the periscapular muscles may predispose the nerve to injury through these mechanisms and that repeated scapular winging in patients with serratus muscle paralysis may be potentially harmful and delay recovery. It is hoped that additional studies will provide further insight into the possible etiologies of this disorder.

Although the majority of cases of isolated palsy of the long thoracic nerve resolve within 12 months, few patients fail to improve with expectant management. Surgery can be considered in those patients who continue to have symptoms refractory to conservative measures with no evidence of spontaneous recovery. Pectoralis major transfer to the inferior pole of the scapula has demonstrated consistently good results in most cases. A recent review of eight patients with scapular winging treated with pectoralis major transfer extended by a fascia lata graft revealed excellent results in all patients at an average follow-up of 2 years. Opinions differ as to the optimal time for surgery after the initial neurologic insult, however, it is generally recommended that surgery be delayed for at least 6 to 12 months. Consideration should be given to the mechanism of injury, residual symptoms, functional deficit, physical demands, and electrodiagnostic studies prior to contemplating surgical management.

Although nerve exploration and possible reconstruction might potentially be considered as an alternate surgical option, there is little evidence in the literature to support such procedures. Poor accessibility of the long thoracic nerve, extended time between the injury and ultimate anticipated return of nerve function, and the uncertain return of serratus activity can add significant morbidity and likely exceed the potential pitfalls of pectoralis major transfer.

Brachial Plexus Injury

Brachial plexus dysfunction may be secondary to a number of etiologies, some of which include traumatic, infectious, entrapment, and iatrogenic mechanisms. Commonly, it is a result of high-energy trauma creating a traction neuropathy as the head is forced laterally at the time of impact. The mechanism of injury, location, extent, and completeness of the impairment can be sufficiently de-

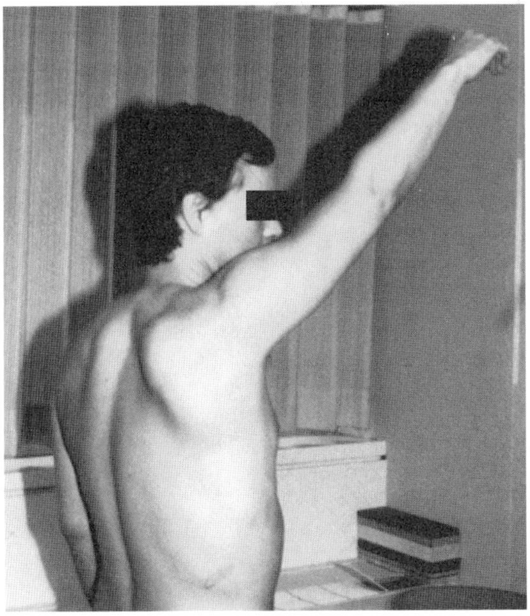

Fig. 8 Scapular winging in a patient with a serratus anterior nerve palsy.

termined in most cases after completion of a thorough history and neurologic evaluation supplemented with electrodiagnostic studies.

Prognosis in the adult typically correlates with the severity and the site of the lesion. High-velocity mechanisms, such as motorcycle accidents, are more likely to cause severe traction injuries with a less favorable outlook than lower-energy trauma, such as a simple fall or poor patient positioning during surgery. Other poor prognostic signs include the presence of Horner's syndrome, which is suggestive of a root avulsion. The immediate onset of severe and persistent pain may forecast a poor return of neurologic function. Moreover, age may be a consideration because elderly patients with significant neural disruption demonstrate a decreased potential for nerve recovery after surgical reconstruction. Multiple investigations have confirmed that, overall, supraclavicular and complete injuries carry a worse outlook than infraclavicular and incomplete lesions. Although lesions of the lower trunk of the brachial plexus are infrequent, the potential for recovery of intrinsic hand function is generally considered to be poor. Similarly, C5 and C6 disruption typically precludes recovery of good shoulder function with nerve reconstruction alone.

Examination will aid in the localization of the neurologic dysfunction and can offer information relevant to future management. A positive Tinel's sign over the supraclavicular fossa with radiating limb paresthesia is suggestive of at least one intact nerve root or postganglionic lesion that may have significance for potential reconstructive procedures. Manual muscle testing may note preservation of strength of the proximal musculature because the rhomboids and serratus anterior are innervated by root collaterals and their denervation can suggest a C5 and C5–C7 root avulsion, respectively.

Radiographs of the cervical spine and shoulder should be obtained and can be helpful in diagnosis. Scoliosis involving the cervical vertebrae or avulsion fractures of the transverse processes are associated with root avulsions. Lateral dislocation of the scapula reflects the severity of trauma and is also associated with significant damage to the plexus.

While many patients will incur less severe injuries and demonstrate either spontaneous neural recovery or minimal residual signs and symptoms, conservative treatment will typically be sufficient. Patients with more extensive neurologic injury who carry a poor prognosis may be considered reasonable candidates for surgical intervention. Selection of patients for surgery should include attention to signs of more extensive injury, which include high-velocity accidents, associated skeletal or regional trauma, and Horner's syndrome. Individuals with gunshot or blast wounds can be considered poor candidates for nerve grafting because the tissues are often devitalized, providing an insufficient bed for graft success. Spontaneous recovery of neural function within the first few weeks may reveal clues to the viability of intact neural pathways, but, short of exploration, offers little information as to the status of any persistently deficient pathways.

Multiple surgical options exist including neural repair, grafting, neurotization, neurolysis, tendon transfers, shoulder arthrodesis, and amputation. In general, most patients will not be agreeable to a shoulder arthrodesis, amputation, and prosthetic fitting when alternatives are available. Although reports indicate variable results for the surgical treatment of brachial plexus injuries, the lack of uniformity in classification, treatment, and assessment makes comparisons between studies less than ideal. Most experts would agree, however, that the earliest possible attempt at nerve reconstruction or repair affords the greatest potential for functional improvement. Furthermore, delay of exploration beyond 6 months may significantly decrease chances for surgical success. Some contend that the optimal time for surgery lies between the third and sixth weeks after the initial trauma.

As microsurgical techniques have continued to progress, so have the overall results of nerve repair and reconstruction. However, the degree of improvement remains limited and often unpredictable. In one review of 164 patients with traction injuries who underwent brachial plexus surgery, 55% of 58 patients with supraclavicular injuries demonstrated at least minimal improvement after either neurolysis, grafts, repairs, or neurotization. In contrast, 85% of 20 patients with infraclavicular injuries benefited to some extent from surgery. Just as variable degrees of functional improvement can be anticipated, the effect of surgery on pain continues to yield inconsistent results.

Intercostal neurotization of the musculocutaneous nerve with or without shoulder arthrodesis in an attempt to restore elbow flexion has been reported to yield moderate success in some limited series. In addition, nerve reconstruction offers the potential for restoration of distal sensation, albeit usually limited. Patients with isolated upper trunk disruption who have achieved limited success with peripheral nerve surgery and who possess good distal extremity function may benefit from an arthrodesis of the glenohumeral joint. Often, shoulder function can be improved provided there remains active control of at least some of the scapular muscles. The function of the trapezius and levator scapula are usually spared because they receive innervation from the spinal accessory nerve and anterior primary rami C3 and C4, respectively. Predictable fusion, functional improvement, reduction in pain, and correction of inferior humeral subluxation can generally be attained; however, the degree of functional gain appears to correlate with the preoperative functional status.

Annotated Bibliography

Basic Science

Clark JM, Harryman DT II: Tendons, ligaments, and capsule of the rotator cuff: Gross and microscopic anatomy. *J Bone Joint Surg* 1992;74A:713–725.

The gross and microscopic structure of the myotendinous rotator cuff was evaluated. The rotator cuff tendons were found to interdigitate and fuse, forming a common insertion on the humerus. Distinct layers of the tendon were defined histologically.

Collins D, Tencer A, Sidles J, et al: Edge displacement and deformation of glenoid components in response to eccentric loading: The effect of preparation of the glenoid bone. *J Bone Joint Surg* 1992;74A:501–507.

Effects of various methods of preparation of the osseous glenoid on edge displacement and deformation of a polyethylene glenoid component were evaluated in cadaveric specimens. Reaming revealed the least amount of displacement and deformation. Use of hand burrs and curettes resulted in a successive increase in measured parameters.

Iannotti JP, Gabriel JP, Schneck SL, et al: The normal glenohumeral relationships: An anatomical study of one hundred and forty shoulders. *J Bone Joint Surg* 1992;74A: 491–500.

Cadaveric and MRI analysis of 140 shoulders was performed to assess the normal anatomic relationships of the glenohumeral joint. It was noted that 85% of the humeral measurements fell within eight fixed combinations of the radius of curvature and thickness of the humeral head. Variability in dimensional parameters and its applications to prosthetic arthroplasty are discussed.

Kuhlman JR, Iannotti JP, Kelly MJ, et al: Isokinetic and isometric measurement of strength of external rotation and abduction of the shoulder. *J Bone Joint Surg* 1992; 74A:1320–1333.

Strength in abduction and external rotation in the plane of the scapula was measured using isometric and isokinetic methods in 39 volunteers. Reliability of testing at various arm positions was determined and results presented.

Otis JC, Jiang CC, Wickiewicz TL, et al: Changes in the moment arms of the rotator cuff and deltoid muscles with abduction and rotation. *J Bone Joint Surg* 1994;76A:667–676.

Changes in moment arms of the rotator cuff and deltoid with glenohumeral motion were evaluated in a cadaver model. The results demonstrated the potential capacity of both the infraspinatus and subscapularis muscles to contribute to arm elevation in the plane of the scapula.

Arthroscopy of the Shoulder

Field LD, Savoie FH III: Arthroscopic suture repair of superior labral detachment lesions of the shoulder. *Am J Sports Med* 1993;21:783–790.

Impingement Syndrome

Ellman H, Harris E, Kay SP: Early degenerative joint disease simulating impingement syndrome: Arthroscopic findings. *Arthroscopy* 1992;8:482–487.

Eighteen patients with a preoperative diagnosis of impingement syndrome, which was refractory to conservative management, were reviewed retrospectively. At the time of arthroscopic surgery they were found to have significant glenohumeral arthropathy that had not been evident radiographically.

Lazarus MD, Chansky HA, Misra S, et al: Comparison of open and arthroscopic subacromial decompression. *J Shoulder Elbow Surg* 1994;3:1–11.

Results of open and arthroscopic subacromial decompression were compared retrospectively in 68 patients. Mean postoperative shoulder scores were similar in the two groups; however, the arthroscopically treated patients had shorter hospital stays and more rapid achievement of maximal pain relief.

Rotator Cuff Disease

Etiology

Soslowsky LJ, An CH, Johnston SP, et al: Geometric and mechanical properties of the coracoacromial ligament and their relationship to rotator cuff disease. *Clin Orthop* 1994;304:10–17.

Geometric and mechanical analysis of the coracoacromial ligament in 20 specimens revealed decreased mechanical properties of this structure in shoulders with rotator cuff tears. The difference in findings when compared to cadavers with intact rotator cuffs was felt to reflect the multiple directional loads imposed on the ligament in shoulders with cuff defects.

Imaging

Owen RS, Iannotti JP, Kneeland JB, et al: Shoulder after surgery: MR imaging with surgical validation. *Radiology* 1993;186:443–447.

MRI scans in 31 patients obtained prior to repeat shoulder surgery were reviewed and compared with surgical findings. Detection of full-thickness cuff tears demonstrated an accuracy of 90%, while partial tears were indistinguishable from repaired tendons.

Paavolainen P, Ahovuo J: Ultrasonography and arthrography in the diagnosis of tears of the rotator cuff. *J Bone Joint Surg* 1994;76A:335–340.

The diagnostic performance of ultrasonography and arthrography in the detection of rotator cuff tears was reviewed retrospectively. Overall, ultrasound demonstrated an accuracy of 84% in the assessment of full-thickness tears, while arthrography revealed an accuracy of 94%.

Sher JS, Uribe JW, Posada A, et al: Abnormal MRI scans in shoulders of asymptomatic subjects. *J Bone Joint Surg* 1995;77A:1025.

MRI scans were obtained in 96 normal volunteers with no history of shoulder complaints or evidence of pathology on physical examination. The frequency of positive MRI findings increased with age. Complete and partial rotator cuff tears were evident in 14% and 20% of all individuals, respectively. Persons over 60 years had a 28% and 26% prevalence of complete and partial tears.

Treatment

Bigliani LU, Cordasco FA, McIlveen SJ, et al: Operative treatment of failed repairs of the rotator cuff. *J Bone Joint Surg* 1992;74A:1505–1515.

Review of 31 patients who underwent repeat operations for failed rotator cuff repairs revealed satisfactory overall results in 52%. Factors most commonly associated with failure of the index procedure included large or massive tears in 97% and persistent impingement in 90%.

Ellman H, Kay SP, Wirth M: Arthroscopic treatment of full-thickness rotator cuff tears: 2- to 7- year follow-up study. *Arthroscopy* 1993;9:195–200.

Arthroscopic debridement and subacromial decompression of full-thickness rotator cuff tears in 40 patients yielded satisfactory results in selected patients. Although adequate pain relief was attained in unrepairable cuff defects, restoration of lost strength and motion were not typically achieved.

Itoi E, Tabata S: Conservative treatment of rotator cuff tears. *Clin Orthop* 1992;275:165–173.

Fifty-four patients with full-thickness rotator cuff tears were treated nonsurgically and reviewed retrospectively at 1 to 9 years. Satisfactory results were achieved in 82% overall. Factors associated with worse results included duration of symptoms greater than 1 year and poor motion and strength prior to treatment.

Liu SH: Arthroscopically-assisted rotator-cuff repair. *J Bone Joint Surg* 1994;76B:592–595.

Full-thickness rotator cuff tears in 44 patients were repaired with arthroscopically assisted techniques and followed up for an average of 4 years. Satisfactory results were achieved in 84% overall. Individuals with massive tears (> 5 cm) were less likely to achieve a satisfactory outcome.

Montgomery TJ, Yerger B, Savoie FH III: Management of rotator cuff tears: A comparison of arthroscopic debridement and surgical repair. *J Shoulder Elbow Surg* 1994;3:70–78.

A prospective comparison of arthroscopic debridement versus open repair in 87 patients with chronic full-thickness rotator cuff tears demonstrated superior results in the surgical repair group at 2- to 5-year follow-up.

Prosthetic Arthroplasty

Arntz CT, Jackins S, Matsen FA III: Prosthetic replacement of the shoulder for the treatment of defects in the rotator cuff and the surface of the glenohumeral joint. *J Bone Joint Surg* 1993;75A:485–491.

A 2- to 10-year follow-up of hemiarthroplasties in 18 patients with preoperative massive rotator cuff tears and glenohumeral arthritis was performed. Satisfactory pain relief was achieved in 15 individuals, and a 43° average increase in active elevation was noted.

Ballmer FT, Sidles JA, Lippitt SB, et al: Humeral head prosthetic arthroplasty: Surgically relevant geometric considerations. *J Shoulder Elbow Surg* 1993;2:296–304.

Geometric evaluation of native and prosthetic humeral articular surfaces in relation to a surgically defined humeral reference was performed in ten cadavers. Results demonstrated a minimal effect on soft-tissue tension with changes in version of press-fit stems. Soft-tissue release and selection of head and neck size were identified as factors that give the surgeon greater control in restoring joint kinematics.

Bonutti PM, Hawkins RJ: Fracture of the humeral shaft associated with total replacement arthroplasty of the shoulder: A case report. *J Bone Joint Surg* 1992;74A: 617–618.

A case report and the authors' observations of intraoperative periprosthetic humeral fractures were presented.

Boyd AD Jr, Thornhill TS, Barnes CL: Fractures adjacent to humeral prostheses. *J Bone Joint Surg* 1992;74A:1498–1504.

Review of seven patients with postoperative periprosthetic humeral fractures revealed complications in all subsequent to injury. Five cases required surgical treatment after development of a nonunion.

Moeckel BH, Altchek DW, Warren RF, et al: Instability of the shoulder after arthroplasty. *J Bone Joint Surg* 1993;75A:492–497.

Experience and results of treatment in ten patients with glenohumeral instability after shoulder arthroplasty was presented.

Arthrodesis

Harryman DT III, Walker ED, Harris SL, et al: Residual motion and function after glenohumeral or scapulothoracic arthrodesis. *J Shoulder Elbow Surg* 1993;2:275–285.

Residual motion in the unfused articulation after either glenohumeral or scapulothoracic fusion using a three-dimensional electromagnetic apparatus was evaluated. The unfused articulation exhibited motion similar to normal except for decreased external rotation and extension in scapulothoracic fusions and increased scapulothoracic internal rotation in glenohumeral fusions. Humerothoracic motion was significantly decreased in all.

Richards RR, Beaton D, Hudson AR: Shoulder arthrodesis with plate fixation: Functional outcome analysis. *J Shoulder Elbow Surg* 1993;2:225–239.

Results of shoulder arthrodesis in 57 patients undergoing a single surgical technique by a single surgeon demonstrated successful fusion in 95% and an overall complication rate of 14%.

Frozen Shoulder

Shaffer B, Tibone JE, Kerlan RK: Frozen shoulder: A long-term follow-up. *J Bone Joint Surg* 1992;74A:738–746.

Two- to 11-year follow-up of 62 patients treated nonsurgically for idiopathic frozen shoulder revealed residual stiffness or pain in 50% and limitation of motion in 60% and 18% when compared to control values and the contralateral shoulder, respectively.

Long Thoracic Nerve Palsy

Post M: Pectoralis major transfer for winging of the scapula. *J Shoulder Elbow Surg* 1995;4:1–9.

Eight patients with irreversible isolated paralysis of the serratus anterior underwent a pectoralis major transfer extended with a fascia lata graft. Consistently good results were achieved, and the surgical technique is described.

Vastamäki M, Kauppila LI: Etiologic factors in isolated paralysis of the serratus anterior muscle: A report of 197 cases. *J Shoulder Elbow Surg* 1993;2:240–243.

Assessment of precipitating factors in 197 patients with isolated serratus anterior paralysis revealed strenuous exertion as a cause in 35%, trauma in 26%, infection in 5%, and an iatrogenic etiology in 7%.

Brachial Plexus

Phipps GJ, Hoffer MM: Latissimus dorsi and teres major transfer to rotator cuff for Erb's Palsy. *J Shoulder Elbow Surg* 1995;4:124–129.

Thirty-five patients with Erb's palsy were surgically managed with a transfer of the latissimus dorsi and teres major tendons. Active external rotation was restored in most cases and progressive deformity and dislocation was halted in all but three patients.

Classic Bibliography

Arthroplasty

Brenner BC, Ferlic DC, Clayton ML, et al: Survivorship of unconstrained total shoulder arthroplasty. *J Bone Joint Surg* 1989;71A:1289–1296.

Cofield RH: Total shoulder arthroplasty with the Neer prosthesis. *J Bone Joint Surg* 1984;66A:899–906.

Friedman RJ, Thornhill TS, Thomas WH, et al: Non-constrained total shoulder replacement in patients who have rheumatoid arthritis and class-IV function. *J Bone Joint Surg* 1989;71A:494–498.

Neer CS II, Watson KC, Stanton FJ: Recent experience in total shoulder replacement. *J Bone Joint Surg* 1982;64A: 319–337.

Basic Science

Gerber C, Schneeberger AG, Vinh TS: The arterial vascularization of the humeral head: An anatomical study. *J Bone Joint Surg* 1990;72A:1486–1494.

Harryman DT II, Sidles JA, Clark JM, et al: Translation of the humeral head on the glenoid with passive glenohumeral motion. *J Bone Joint Surg* 1990;72A: 1334–1343.

Howell SM, Imobersteg AM, Seger DH, et al: Clarification of the role of the supraspinatus muscle in shoulder function. *J Bone Joint Surg* 1986;68A:398–404.

Inman VT, Saunders JB, Abbott LC: Observations on the function of the shoulder joint. *J Bone Joint Surg* 1944;26: 1–30.

Lohr JF, Uhthoff HK: The microvascular pattern of the supraspinatus tendon. *Clin Orthop* 1990;254:35–38.

Rotator Cuff

Ellman H, Hanker G, Bayer M: Repair of the rotator cuff: End-result study of factors influencing reconstruction. *J Bone Joint Surg* 1986;68A:1136–1144.

Gartsman GM: Arthroscopic acromioplasty for lesions of the rotator cuff. *J Bone Joint Surg* 1990;72A:169–180.

Gerber C: Latissimus dorsi transfer for the treatment of irreparable tears of the rotator cuff. *Clin Orthop* 1992; 275:152–160.

Harryman DT II, Mack LA, Wang KY, et al: Repairs of the rotator cuff: Correlation of functional results with integrity of the cuff. *J Bone Joint Surg* 1991;73A:982–989.

Hawkins RJ, Misamore GW, Hobeika PE: Surgery for full-thickness rotator-cuff tears. *J Bone Joint Surg* 1985;67A:1349–1355.

Mudge MK, Wood VE, Frykman GK: Rotator cuff tears associated with os acromiale. *J Bone Joint Surg* 1984;66A: 427–429.

Neer CS II: Impingement lesions. *Clin Orthop* 1983;173: 70–77.

Neer CS II, Craig EV, Fukuda H: Cuff-tear arthropathy. *J Bone Joint Surg* 1983;65A:1232–1244.

Neviaser RJ, Neviaser TJ, Neviaser JS: Concurrent rupture of the rotator cuff and anterior dislocation of the shoulder in the older patient. *J Bone Joint Surg* 1988;70A: 1308–1311.

Ozaki J, Fujimoto S, Nakagawa Y, et al: Tears of the rotator cuff of the shoulder associated with pathological changes in the acromion: A study in cadavera. *J Bone Joint Surg* 1988;70A:1224–1230.

Imaging

Iannotti JP, Zlatkin MB, Esterhai JL, et al: Magnetic resonance imaging of the shoulder: Sensitivity, specificity, and predictive value. *J Bone Joint Surg* 1991;73A:17–29.

Arthrodesis

Cofield RH, Briggs BT: Glenohumeral arthrodesis: Operative and long-term functional results. *J Bone Joint Surg* 1979;61A:668–677.

Hawkins RJ, Neer CS II: A functional analysis of shoulder fusions. *Clin Orthop* 1987;223:65–76.

Frozen Shoulder

Ozaki J, Nakagawa Y, Sakurai G, et al: Recalcitrant chronic adhesive capsulitis of the shoulder: Role of contracture of the coracohumeral ligament and rotator interval in pathogenesis and treatment. *J Bone Joint Surg* 1989;71A:1511–1515.

Brachial Plexus

Leffert RD: Brachial-plexus injuries. *N Engl J Med* 1974; 291:1059–1067.

Narakas A: Surgical treatment of traction injuries of the brachial plexus. *Clin Orthop* 1978;133:71–90.

Rorabeck CH; Harris WR: Factors affecting the prognosis of brachial plexus injuries. *J Bone Joint Surg* 1981;63B: 404–407.

27

Elbow and Forearm: Pediatric Aspects

Congenital Anomalies and Acquired Disorders

Congenital Dislocation of the Radial Head

Congenital dislocation of the radial head usually is an isolated finding (Fig. 1). Bilaterality has been a criterion for the diagnosis of congenital dislocation of the radial head, and unilateral dislocation has been considered an acquired lesion. More recently, however, isolated unilateral congenital dislocation of the radial head has been reported in children. Arthrographic evaluation to differentiate congenital dislocation of the radial head from traumatic dislocation demonstrates that with congenital dislocation, the radial head is displaced from the capitellum but is covered by the capsule of the elbow joint, which also includes the humerocapitellar joint; in traumatic dislocation, the radial head is displaced from the capsule of the elbow joint and the lesion is extra-articular.

Limitation of motion, especially supination, of the involved elbow in congenital dislocation causes functional impairment. Radiographic signs that suggest congenital dislocation of the radial head include increased ulnar length in relation to the radius and a hypoplastic capitellum. Reduction attempts for isolated congenital dislocation are generally unsuccessful. Until additional information is available that refutes this experience, reduction of this congenital dislocation, either open or closed, is not recommended at any age.

If dislocation of the radial head is associated with acquired or congenital below-elbow deficiencies, the dislocation does not require specific surgical treatment and generally does not necessitate modification of any prosthesis. Radial head excision near skeletal maturity can improve elbow motion and decrease pain, but minor discomfort in the wrist may occur. Patient outcomes after this operation are generally quite satisfactory.

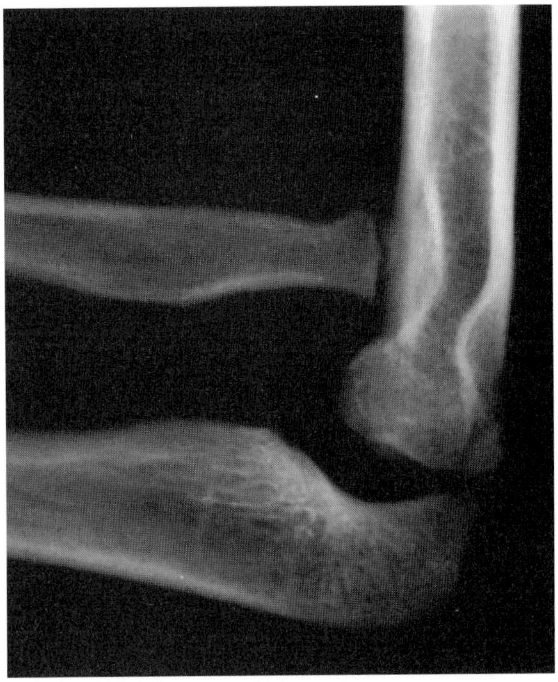

Fig. 1 Congenital anterior dislocation of the radial head.

Osteochondritis Dissecans of the Capitellum

Biomechanical considerations of the elbow suggest that differences in stiffness between the central radial head and the lateral capitellum increase the strain in the lateral capitellum. High valgus stress activities, such as pitching or throwing, localize this increased strain to the lateral capitellum and are a factor in the initiation of the osteochondritis dissecans lesion. In addition to adolescents who are throwing athletes, osteochondritis dissecans is seen commonly in young gymnasts who may show precocious signs of joint aging. Prognosis for continued high-level performance is poor once severe radiographic changes are seen.

Individuals with osteochondritis dissecans of the capitellum may have persistent symptoms of pain and permanent loss of elbow range of motion at long-term follow-up. These symptoms correlate with radiographic signs of degenerative joint disease in the lateral compartment of the elbow. Most elbow pain caused by overuse can be treated successfully with rest and activity modification. Surgery is indicated when loose bodies cause locking and catching of the elbow. The key to prevention is early recognition of overuse injury, rest, and activity modification.

Trauma

Supracondylar Fractures of the Humerus

Supracondylar humeral fractures are the most common pediatric elbow fracture and usually are caused by a fall on an outstretched hand. Normal ligamentous laxity allows the elbow to hyperextend, forcing the olecranon into the posterior humeral fossa. This concentrates forces along the weak metaphyseal bone of the distal humerus and most commonly results in a posteriorly displaced extension-type supracondylar humeral fracture. Flexion-type supracondylar injuries usually are caused by direct trauma to the elbow from a fall that displaces the supracondylar fragment anteriorly. Ninety-eight percent of supracondylar humeral fractures are extension-type injuries and 2% are flexion-type injuries.

Gartland's classification is the most frequently used and has been modified to include: type IA, nondisplaced fractures; type IB, medial impaction fractures; type IIA, fracture fragments with posterior angulation; type IIB, fracture fragments with malrotation with or without posterior angulation; type IIIA, complete posteromedial displacement; and type IIIB, complete posterolateral displacement. Complications of supracondylar fractures include Volkmann ischemia (fewer than 1%), nerve palsy (3% to 8%), vascular injury (2%), and cubitus varus (2% to 33%, depending on treatment; Fig. 2).

Treatment methods have consisted of traction, closed reduction and casting, closed reduction and percutaneous pinning, and open reduction and internal fixation (ORIF). Closed reduction and casting of displaced supracondylar humeral fractures has had an unacceptably high rate of poor results. To avoid loss of reduction, the elbow must be flexed to 120°, but flexing the elbow to 120° increases the chance of Volkmann ischemic contracture. Traction has been associated with an increased incidence of malunion, although it may be valuable if soft-tissue swelling is severe or the fracture is severely comminuted. Closed reduction and percutaneous pinning is the most frequently recommended treatment for displaced supracondylar humeral fractures. Stabilization is obtained with two lateral or crossed medial and lateral Kirschner wires (K-wires), and the arm is then extended to evaluate the reduction clinically and radiographically (Fig. 3). The elbow can be placed in 90° or less of flexion to allow for swelling and to prevent vascular compromise. Open reduction is indicated if an acceptable closed reduction cannot be obtained and for open supracondylar humeral fractures or fractures with vascular compromise. An anterior approach for posterior displaced fractures allows fracture reduction and vascular repair or vein grafting if necessary.

Type IA (nondisplaced) fractures should be treated with cast or splint immobilization, close observation, and follow-up evaluation of fracture alignment. Varus impacted type IB fractures require closed reduction and percutaneous pinning to recreate a normal carrying angle. Type II fractures usually require closed reduction and casting. If fracture stability is questionable or swelling is severe, the fracture should be stabilized after reduction with two lateral or crossed medial and lateral smooth K-wires. Type III fractures require closed reduction and pinning. Crossed K-wires have been shown to provide greater stability, but if the medial epicondyle cannot be adequately palpated or the location of the ulnar nerve is in question, a small medial incision can be made or two lateral K-wires are used. Open reduction of a supracondylar humerus fracture is indicated when closed reduction is not successful. An inadequate closed reduction is indicated by a change in Baumann's angle of more than 10° compared to the opposite elbow or a decrease in the carrying angle of approximately 15°. An anteromedial or anterolateral approach can be used, depending on the direction of displacement. When vascular insufficiency accompanies a supracondylar fracture, immediate closed or open reduction and K-wire stabilization is the treatment of choice. Arterial exploration is indicated if there is no distal limb perfusion after closed reduction and K-wire fixation; if there is any suggestion of decreased capillary refill, pallor, or increased compartment pressure; or if the pulse cannot be found by Doppler examination of an ischemic extremity. In a truly pulseless, pale, nonviable appearing extremity, a preoperative arteriogram is not needed before exploration and usually causes a delay in definitive treatment. Exploration is best performed through an anterior approach. The fracture can be reduced and pinned followed by exploration and repair or vein grafting of the arterial injury.

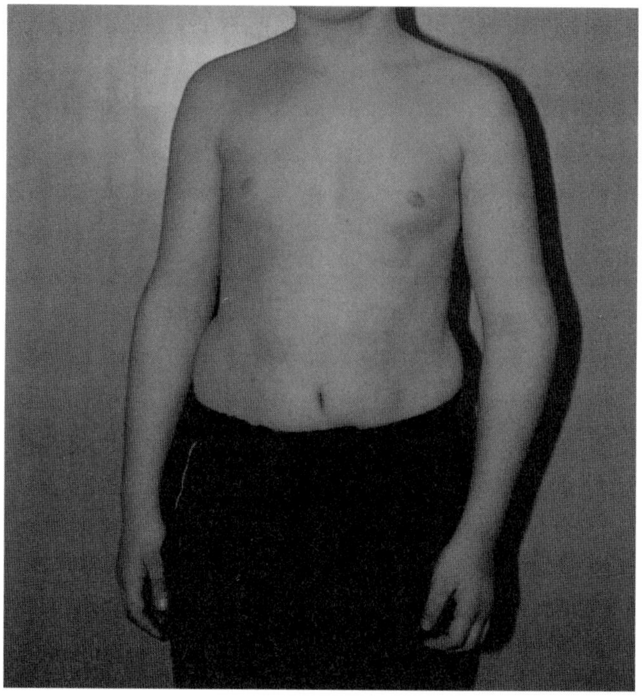

Fig. 2 Cubitus varus deformity after supracondylar humeral fracture.

Transphyseal Injuries

Transphyseal fractures through the distal humeral physis usually occur between birth and 4 years of age. Because the distal humerus is mostly cartilaginous at this age, accurate diagnosis is difficult. Transphyseal fractures usually are Salter-Harris type I or II injuries and are caused by a fall on an outstretched hand; child abuse also is a frequent cause. Transphyseal injuries should be differentiated from elbow dislocations and fractures of the lateral humeral

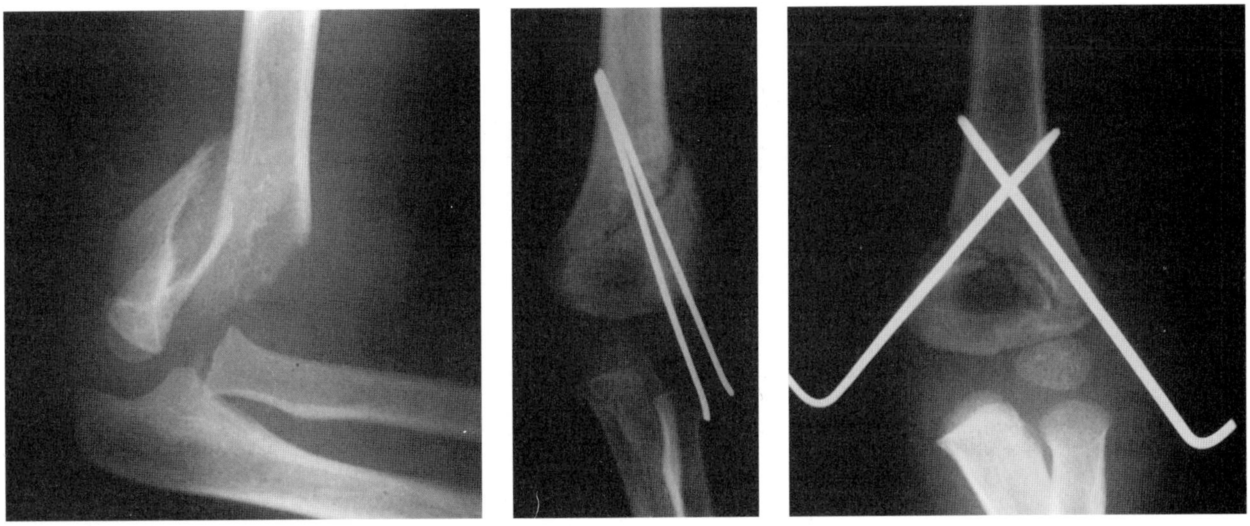

Fig. 3 **Left,** Supracondylar humeral fracture in a 6-year-old child. **Center,** Supracondylar humeral fracture after percutaneous lateral pin fixation. **Right,** Crossed pin fixation of supracondylar humeral fracture.

condyle. The normal location of the long axis of the radius through the center of the capitellum remains intact in a child with a transphyseal fracture, but is displaced lateral to the capitellum in a child with a posterolateral elbow dislocation and medial to the capitellum in a child with a lateral condylar fracture. If the diagnosis is questionable, an arthrogram can help determine the true fracture pattern. Magnetic resonance imaging (MRI) also is useful but because of the expense and the need for sedation, it should be used only if the diagnosis cannot be made by conventional methods.

Nondisplaced or minimally displaced transphyseal fractures are treated with closed reduction and splint or cast immobilization. Displaced transphyseal fractures are best treated by closed reduction and percutaneous pinning to avoid malunion.

Lateral Condylar Fractures of the Humerus

Fractures of the lateral humeral condyle account for approximately 15% of all elbow fractures in children and occur most often in children between the ages of 5 and 10 years. The most common mechanism of injury is a varus stress to an extended elbow with the forearm supinated. Lateral condylar fractures can be classified according to the amount of displacement and the integrity of the articular surface. A type I fracture has minimal (less than 2 mm) displacement with an intact articular surface; a type II fracture is displaced 2 to 4 mm, and the articular surface is disrupted (the condylar fragment may be moderately displaced in rotation), and a type III fracture is significantly rotated and completely displaced.

A lateral condylar fracture usually can be seen on standard anteroposterior (AP), lateral, and oblique radiographs of the elbow. If the diagnosis is uncertain or the stability of the fracture is questionable, gentle varus stress views may be obtained with the use of mild sedation. An arthrogram may determine the presence of an articular hinge, especially in type II fractures.

Treatment is based on the degree of fracture displacement and the presence or absence of an intact cartilage hinge. Nondisplaced fractures can be treated with 3 to 4 weeks of cast immobilization with the arm flexed 90° and the forearm supinated. Close follow-up is mandatory because late displacement may result in malunion or nonunion in 10% of type I fractures. Radiographs should be obtained regularly until the fracture has healed. This may require removing the cast and obtaining radiographs of the elbow in extension. If instability or displacement occur, percutaneous pinning or ORIF may be indicated. Type II fractures that are stable by stress examination and arthrography can be percutaneously pinned, but if the fracture fragments are rotated, ORIF should be performed through a lateral approach. Unstable type II and type III fractures are treated by ORIF. The posterior soft tissues of the lateral condyle should be left intact to decrease the risk of osteonecrosis of the fragment.

The most common complication after lateral condylar fractures is nonunion that results in progressive cubitus valgus deformity and tardy ulnar nerve palsy. The treatment of an established nonunion is controversial because of the risk of osteonecrosis of the capitellum and loss of elbow motion. If the distal fragment is in an acceptable position (minimally displaced and minimally rotated with separation of the fragments less than 1 cm), in situ bone grafting and internal fixation can be performed. The bone graft is placed between the metaphyseal portions of the proximal and distal fragments. Patients who develop tardy ulnar nerve palsy secondary to cubitus valgus deformity can be treated with anterior transposition of the ulnar nerve. The average time of onset of late ulnar neuropathy is approximately 22 years after injury.

Medial Epicondylar Fractures of the Humerus

Approximately 11% of injuries to the distal humerus in children involve the medial epicondyle. These injuries are most common between the ages of 9 and 14 years. Most often overpull of the forearm flexor tendon or a varus stress through the attachment of the ulnar collateral ligament causes an acute avulsion of the epicondyle. Cast immobilization generally produces good results in nondisplaced fractures. If the fracture occurs with dislocation of the elbow, the fragment may become entrapped in the joint and prevent reduction of the dislocation. Commonly cited indications for open reduction include: (1) rotation and displacement of more than 1 cm, (2) persistent entrapment of a fracture fragment in the joint after reduction of elbow dislocation, (3) ulnar nerve dysfunction, and (4) severe valgus instability.

Medial Condylar Fractures of the Humerus

Fractures of the medial humeral condyle are among the least common injuries of the elbow, accounting for fewer than 1%. Fractures with little or minimal displacement usually can be treated with cast immobilization; however, nonunion of the medial condyle has been reported after conservative treatment of these injuries. More severely displaced fractures (displacement of more than 2 mm) require ORIF. Early diagnosis, accurate reduction, and internal fixation are essential in both medial and lateral condyle fractures to avoid articular incongruity and functional disability, as in any Salter-Harris type III or IV fracture. Undiagnosed and untreated fractures may require supracondylar closing wedge valgus osteotomy to correct cubitus varus deformity.

Fractures of the Olecranon

Isolated olecranon fractures are rare in children. Nondisplaced fractures can be treated closed, but ORIF with tension band wiring are required for displaced fractures. Most authors recommend open reduction if displacement is more than 4 mm. Olecranon fractures in older children are more likely to be displaced than those in younger children. Growth abnormalities of the olecranon apophysis are uncommon after fracture, and most unsatisfactory results are because of loss of flexion and extension.

Vagaries of the physis of the proximal olecranon may be confused with a fracture. Identifying the normal sclerotic margins and the wider posterior portion of the physis will help distinguish a normal physis from a fracture.

Monteggia Fracture-Dislocations

All four types of Monteggia injuries described by Bado occur in children. Type I injuries (anterior dislocation of the radial head) are the most common, followed by type III injuries (lateral dislocation). Types II (posterior dislocation) and IV (anterior dislocation with fracture of both the radius and ulna) are rare. Several Monteggia equivalents also have been described, the most common of which is anterior dislocation of the elbow associated with an ulnar fracture and a radial neck fracture or separation of the proximal radial epiphysis. Another relatively frequent Monteggia equivalent is radial head dislocation (usually lateral) with an olecranon fracture.

Diagnosis of the Monteggia lesion can be difficult; misdiagnosis has been reported in up to one third of children with this injury. Often radiographs of the elbow are not obtained or subtle dislocation or subluxation of the radial head is not recognized on radiographs. On radiographs, the radial head should always point through the middle of the capitellum in any position, especially on the lateral view. This can be confirmed by drawing a straight line through the radial head; in any position this line should pass through the center of the capitellum.

Most Monteggia fractures in children can be treated by closed methods. Types I, III, and IV fractures should be immobilized for 6 weeks with the elbow in 100° of flexion and the forearm fully supinated; type II injuries are immobilized for 4 weeks with the elbow extended. Closed reduction may be unsuccessful because of interposition of the annular ligament or the capsule, and open reduction may be necessary. Surgical treatment may consist of closed reduction of the radial head and open reduction of the ulnar fracture, or open reduction of both the radial head and ulnar fracture with internal fixation of the ulna. In adolescents, the ulna can be fixed with a plate-and-screw device or an intramedullary rod; in younger children an intramedullary wire can be used. Percutaneous intramedullary rodding of the ulna also has been described. Regardless of the type of fixation, stripping of the soft tissues, including the periosteum, should be minimal. The length of the ulna should be maintained and angulation corrected to stabilize the radial head reduction.

Complications reported in association with Monteggia fractures and their equivalents include posterior and anterior interosseous nerve lesions, vascular compromise, compartment syndrome, malunion, and proximal radioulnar synostosis (Fig. 4). Radial nerve injury is most frequent after type III fractures. Most nerve injuries resolve within 3 to 6 months of injury. When the ulna is malunited, regardless of the amount of remodeling, osteotomy of the ulna usually is necessary to allow stable reduction of the radial head. In older children, an intramedullary pin or compression plate may be necessary to fix the osteotomy of the ulna. Internal fixation usually is not required in younger children.

According to recent reports, satisfactory reduction of the radial head may be obtained as late as 3 to 6 months or more after traumatic dislocation. This procedure generally requires osteotomy of the angulated ulna, followed by open reduction of the radial head, reconstruction of the annular ligament with fascia or other soft tissue, and stabi-

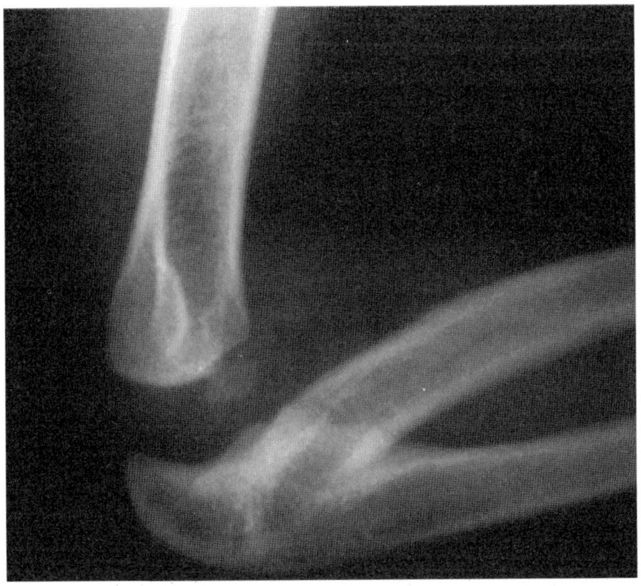

Fig. 4 Radioulnar synostosis and posterior dislocation of the radial head.

lization of the radial head in normal position against the capitellum.

Dislocations of the Elbow

Dislocation of the elbow in children is rare, accounting only for approximately 3% to 6% of all children's fractures and dislocations involving the elbow. In most large series of traumatic elbow dislocations, approximately half are reported to occur in persons younger than 20 years of age; the peak incidence is in adolescents between the ages of 13 and 14 years. Most pure dislocations are posterior, but they can occur anteriorly, medially, or laterally. Rarely, there is proximal radioulnar joint disruption (divergent dislocation) in either the AP or transverse plane.

Most elbow dislocations can be reduced closed. Reduction usually is stable, but the elbow should be immobilized for about 7 to 14 days. Open reduction is indicated when closed reduction cannot be obtained, when the dislocation is open, or because of associated displaced fractures, most commonly of the medial epicondyle, radial neck, or lateral condyle.

Neurovascular injuries and associated fractures are most frequent with posterior dislocations. The median nerve may be entrapped in the joint during closed reduction of the dislocation or may block closed reduction. Proximal median nerve deficit, limited passive elbow motion, and an associated medial epicondyle avulsion after reduction of a posterior elbow dislocation should arouse suspicion of nerve entrapment. Immediate surgical exploration and extraction of the nerve are indicated. Neurovascular status should be monitored for 12 to 24 hours after reduction to detect any late neurovascular compromise.

Arterial injuries that require surgical treatment usually are associated with open dislocations. Radiographs after reduction should be scrutinized for soft tissue or bony interposition in the joint space.

Chronic Recurrent Elbow Dislocation

Recurrent elbow dislocations in children are rare, and most occur in adolescents. Four primary underlying causes of recurrent dislocation of the elbow have been suggested in the literature: (1) a shallow trochlear notch that allows easy dislocation of the olecranon from the trochlea; (2) capsular laxity of the elbow, either medial, lateral, or combined; (3) intra-articular fractures that cause instability of the olecranon in the trochlea, either medial or lateral; and (4) congenital laxity of the medial and lateral ligaments about the elbow. Often the etiology consists of a combination of two or more of these conditions. The specific pathology should be determined by comparison AP and lateral radiographs, varus and valgus stress views, arthrography, fluoroscopy during surgery, or arthroscopy.

The need for surgical correction of symptomatic chronic dislocations is controversial, but elbow deformity, limited range of motion, chronic pain, and failed conservative treatment generally are agreed to be indications for surgical treatment. The surgical procedure should be selected to correct the specific pathology. A variety of procedures have been described for different pathologies; however, several authors have described posterolateral instability as the most common pathology and recommend soft-tissue repair and reconstruction on the lateral side of the elbow, reinforcement of this area, and reattachment of the lateral collateral ligament.

Radial Neck Fractures

Radial neck fractures in children usually are proximal metaphyseal fractures or physeal fractures, such as Salter-Harris type I or II injuries. The normal radial metaphysis is slightly angulated and, before the epiphysis ossifies, this angulation can be confused with a fracture. Ossification of this epiphysis usually begins around the age of 4 to 6 years.

The proximal radioulnar joint is a very exact and congruous joint. Any displacement or translation of the head and neck fracture fragment causes a decrease in rotation about the forearm. The usual mechanism of injury is a fall on an extended elbow with a valgus force applied to the forearm. Greenstick fractures of the olecranon and avulsions of the medial epicondyle often occur with radial neck fractures. Tenderness is localized laterally just distal to the elbow joint about the radial head. Pain is increased by rotation of the forearm rather than by elbow flexion and extension.

Before treatment, the parents must be informed that the child may lose forearm rotation regardless of the method of treatment. This is especially true if displacement of the radial head is severe. Displacement usually indicates significant soft-tissue injury, which usually accounts for the posttreatment stiffness. Most radial neck fractures can be treated nonsurgically. For fractures with less than 30° to 45° of angulation and less than 50% translation, posterior splint immobilization is recommended. Early protected motion is begun by 10 to 14 days. If the fracture fragments are angulated more than 45°, the fracture should be manipulated with the child under general anesthesia to obtain better alignment. In one method, the elbow is extended, a varus stress is applied to the forearm, and pressure is applied with the thumb directly against the radial head fragment. Others recommend manipulation with the elbow flexed and pressure applied over the radial head with the forearm forcibly pronated. Occasionally, a completely displaced fracture can be reduced by this flexion–pronation technique. Another technique is to wrap the forearm tightly with an elastic bandage, starting distally and progressing proximally up to the level of the radial head. This technique is moderately successful in fractures that have 30° to 60° of angulation and some translation. Fractures that remain angulated more than 60° or have significant residual translation require surgical intervention.

Percutaneous reduction can be performed by using a pin to manipulate the fracture fragment into a reduced position. If a percutaneous pin is used, it should be inserted as far laterally as possible with the forearm pronated as much as possible to avoid injury to the posterior interosseous branch of the radial nerve. Open reduction is indicated only if adequate reduction cannot be obtained by closed or percutaneous techniques. Open reduction should be performed as soon as possible to prevent the development of heterotopic bone formation or myositis ossificans.

The fracture is best approached laterally between the anconeus and extensor carpi ulnaris muscles. After reduction, interdigitation of the fracture fragments often provides adequate stability. If stability of the radial head fragment is questionable, it should be secured with two small oblique pins transfixing the radial head to the proximal radial metaphysis.

The fracture should be protected in a cast for at least 2 to 3 weeks, but early motion is essential to prevent stiffness. After cast removal at 2 to 3 weeks, active motion is begun in a posterior splint. If pin fixation is used, the pins are removed at 3 weeks and motion is begun.

Loss of motion is common after radial neck fractures, usually loss of pronation rather than supination. Radial head growth may be stimulated by the increased vascularity from injury, and this overgrowth may contribute to the loss of forearm motion. Overgrowth occurs in as many as 40% of children with radial neck fractures, but functional results usually are good.

Radial ulnar synostosis and myositis ossificans cause the most severe loss of motion and are probably the most serious complications that occur after this injury. They are more common after severely displaced fractures that are treated surgically. Delay in initial treatment also seems to increase the risk of these complications. Premature physeal closure can occur but generally does not cause significant shortening or affect function.

Fractures of the Forearm

Forearm fractures are common in children, and most, regardless of level, can be treated by closed techniques. Fractures of the distal third account for approximately 75% of forearm fractures. Most authors agree that after closed reduction, the arm should be placed in supination for proximal fractures, in neutral for fractures of the middle third, and in pronation for distal fractures. Although anatomic alignment is ideal, Price and associates believe that 40° of malrotation, 10° of angulation, complete displacement, and loss of radial angle can be accepted rather than resorting to open reduction in younger children. They recommend closed reduction as the treatment of choice for skeletally immature patients with diaphyseal fractures of the radius and ulna, and note that rotational alignment should be accurately restored, using the position of the radial tuberosity as a guide. Others recommend that, if initial closed reduction achieves apposition of more than 50%, repeated attempts at reduction should be avoided.

Radiographs should be obtained at 1 week and 2 weeks after closed reduction to detect any reangulation or displacement. Loss of acceptable alignment should be treated by remanipulation. Successful manipulation of nonphyseal fractures has been reported as late as 24 days after injury.

Open reduction generally is indicated for: (1) open fracture, (2) failed closed reduction in an older adolescent (10 years of age or older), (3) malalignment, and (4) irreducible fracture (because of soft-tissue interposition). If open reduction is indicated, internal fixation should be used to prevent nonunion or recurrence of malposition. Small compression plates, one-third tubular plates, intramedullary K-wires, and elastic intramedullary nails have all been used successfully for fixation.

Plastic deformation may occur in either the radius or ulna, most often in children between the ages of 2 and 15 years. In a review of reported series of plastic deformation of the forearm, the ulna was bowed in 83% of patients and the radius in 50%. In addition to the cosmetic deformity, bowing of one or both bones of the forearm may cause limitation of pronation and supination as the bowed bones encroach on the interosseous space. According to Sanders and Heckman, angulation of less than 20° in young children usually will remodel satisfactorily, but reduction should be considered in children older than 4 years or any child with a deformity of more than 20°, especially if it limits pronation and supination. They described a closed reduction technique reported to correct 85% of the angulation in plastic deformation. Others based their recommendations on the age of the patient and the severity of the deformity: in children older than 10 years of age, deformities of 15° or more should be manipulated and corrected; in children between 6 and 10 years of age, correction of deformities of 20° or more should be attempted; and in children 5 years of age and younger, remodeling most likely will restore correct anatomy and function of deformities of more than 20°. If reduction is attempted, parents should be informed that fracture of one or both bones may be necessary to obtain reduction. As a general rule, if the deformity is unsightly or the bowed bone seriously compromises pronation and supination, reduction should be done.

Cross union of the bones of the forearm is rare in children, but can limit function of the forearm because of limitation of pronation and supination. Several factors have been suggested as contributing to the development of cross union, including severe initial displacement, displacement after reduction, periosteal interposition, surgery, delayed surgery, remanipulation, excision of the radial head, and fractures of the radius and ulna at the same level. In a review of 10 cross unions in children, Vince and Miller concluded that the risk of cross union is increased by surgical trauma to the soft tissue between the radius and ulna and that excision of the radial head alone was a greater risk factor than open reduction alone. Although their results after excision of the cross union were not as good in children as in adults, they noted that delaying excision until the child is skeletally mature may preclude regaining full pronation and supination because of soft-tissue contractures.

Galeazzi Fracture-Dislocations

Galeazzi fracture-dislocations are rare in children, and disruption of the distal radioulnar joint is recognized in fewer than half of the initial injuries. Most of these fractures can be treated with closed reduction, but the distal radioulnar joint must be reduced with the forearm in supination, and the arm should be immobilized in a long arm cast for at least 6 weeks with the elbow in flexion and the forearm in supination. Rarely, adequate closed reduction cannot be obtained, and the distal radial fragment should be stabilized with a small compression plate before the forearm is placed in supination to reduce the distal radioulnar joint. The most serious complication of this injury is malunion, which can result in loss of supination and pronation.

Annotated Bibliography

Congenital Anomalies and Acquired Disorders

Agnew DK, Davis RJ: Congenital unilateral dislocation of the radial head. *J Pediatr Orthop* 1993;13:526–528.

Bilaterality has been a criterion for diagnosis of an isolated congenital dislocation of the radial head, with unilaterality regarded as an acquired lesion. This series confirms the existence of a unilateral congenital dislocation of the radial head.

Bauer M, Jonsson K, Josefsson PO, et al: Osteochondritis dissecans of the elbow: A long-term follow-up study. *Clin Orthop* 1992;284:156–160.

Impaired motion and pain on effort were the most common complaints. Radiographic signs of degenerative joint disease were present in more than half of the elbows and correlated with a reduced range of motion.

Campbell CC, Waters PM, Emans JB: Excision of the radial head for congenital dislocation. *J Bone Joint Surg* 1992;74A:726–733.

All patients were satisfied with the outcome of the operation. Excision of the radial head for congenital dislocation results in an increased range of motion and a decrease in pain in the elbow.

Cleary JE, Omer GE Jr: Congenital proximal radio-ulnar synostosis: Natural history and functional assessment. *J Bone Joint Surg* 1985;67A:539–545.

In a long-term review, the authors found no correlation between degree of deformity and functional status and concluded that surgical treatment is seldom indicated.

Maffulli N, Chan D, Aldridge MJ: Derangement of the articular surfaces of the elbow in young gymnasts. *J Pediatr Orthop* 1992;12:344–350.

There was a high incidence of osteochondrotic lesions, intra-articular loose bodies, and precocious signs of joint aging. The prognosis of elbow joint articular surface lesions in these athletes is not good.

Menio GJ, Wenner SM: Radial head dislocations in children with below-elbow deficiencies. *J Hand Surg* 1992;17A:891–895.

Two thirds of the children who have below-elbow deficiencies, congenital or acquired, have concomitant radial head dislocations. The dislocation does not require specific surgical treatment and rarely necessitates prosthetic modifications.

Miura T: Congenital dislocations of the radial head. *J Hand Surg* 1990;15:477–481.

The range of motion of the elbow and forearm is considerably limited and causes functional impairment, especially lack of supination. Increased ulnar length in relation to the radius and hypoplastic capitellum suggest that a dislocation is congenital.

Mizuno K, Usui Y, Kohyama K, et al: Familial congenital unilateral anterior dislocation of the radial head: Differentiation from traumatic dislocation by means of arthrography. A case report. *J Bone Joint Surg* 1991;73A: 1086–1090.

Arthrography of the elbow aids in diagnosis of congenital dislocation of the radial head by identifying the intra-articular location of the radial head.

Ruch DS, Poehling GG: Arthroscopic treatment of Panner's disease. *Clin Sports Med* 1991;10:629–636.

With the advent of arthroscopy, a diagnosis can be made and treatment with limited invasiveness instituted.

Schenck RC Jr, Athanasiou KA, Constantinides G, et al: A biomechanical analysis of articular cartilage of the human elbow and a potential relationship to osteochondritis dissecans. *Clin Orthop* 1994;299:305–312.

Significant differences exist in the mechanical properties and thickness of cartilage in the capitellum and radial head. The central section of the radial head is significantly stiffer than the lateral capitellum. The disparity in the mechanical properties of the central radial head and lateral capitellum increase strain in the lateral capitellum.

Elbow Trauma

Beaty JH, Donati NL: Recurrent dislocation of the elbow in a childen: Case report and review of the literature. *J Pediatr Orthop* 1991;11:392–396.

This is a report of successful treatment of an 8-year-old boy who had six dislocations in 2 years. Etiologies of recurrent elbow dislocation are discussed and emphasis is placed on aiming surgery at specific pathology.

Bernstein SM, McKeever P, Bernstein L: Percutaneous reduction of displaced radial neck fractures in children. *J Pediatr Orthop* 1993;13:85–88.

The authors describe the technique of percutaneous reduction of displaced radial neck fractures in children and report good results with the procedure.

Boyd DW, Aronson DD: Supracondylar fractures of the humerus: A prospective study of percutaneous pinning. *J Pediatr Orthop* 1992;12:789–794.

In this prospective study, there were good results when the Baumann angle was used as criteria for acceptable reduction. Acceptable results were obtained with the use of two lateral pins.

Camp J, Ishizue K, Gomez M, et al: Alteration of Baumann's angle by humeral position: Implications for treatment of supracondylar humerus fractures. *J Pediatr Orthop* 1993;13:521–525.

The authors recommend measurement of Baumann's angle on a true AP view with the humerus parallel to the radiographic plate and the x-ray beam perpendicular to the plate. This position is least sensitive to humeral rotation and easiest to reproduce.

Campbell CC, Waters PM, Emans JB, et al: Neurovascular injury and displacement in type III supracondylar humerus fractures. *J Pediatr Orthop* 1995;15:47–52.

In this report of neurovascular compromise in 29 (49%) of 59 children with type III fractures, the median nerve was most often injured with posterolateral displacement and all radial nerve injuries occurred with posteromedial displacement. The brachial artery injuries occurred most often (64%) with posterolateral displacement.

Cramer KE, Green NE, Devito DP: Incidence of anterior interosseous nerve palsy in supracondylar humerus fractures in children. *J Pediatr Orthop* 1993;13:502–505.

Of 101 children with supracondylar fractures, 15 had neural lesions, six of which were isolated anterior interosseous nerve palsies and four were injuries to the anterior interosseous nerve and another nerve. The authors caution that this injury may be overlooked.

Dias JJ, Johnson GV, Hoskinson J, et al: Management of severely displaced medial epicondyle fractures. *J Orthop Trauma* 1987;1:59–62.

The authors report good functional results after nonsurgical treatment of 20 severely displaced (mean 10 mm) medial epicondylar fractures with elbow dislocation.

D'souza S, Vaishya R, Klenerman L: Management of radial neck fractures in children: A retrospective analysis of one hundred patients. *J Pediatr Orthop* 1993;13: 232–238.

This is an analysis of a large series of radial neck fractures in children, with discussion of criteria for acceptable translation (< 5 mm) and angulation (< 45°) that can be treated nonsurgically.

Flynn JC: Nonunion of slightly displaced fractures of the lateral humeral condyle in children: An update. *J Pediatr Orthop* 1989;9:691–696.

The author recommends early stabilization and bone grafting in treatment of nonunion, the leading cause of which is inadequate initial treatment of the fracture.

Graves SC, Canale ST: Fractures of the olecranon in children: Long-term follow-up. *J Pediatr Orthop* 1993; 13:239–241.

Satisfactory results were reported in 93% of undisplaced fractures and 78% of displaced fractures in a series of 41 olecranon fractures. The most common cause of unsatisfactory results was loss of motion, but this did not prevent good function in most patients.

Kallio PE, Foster BK, Paterson DC: Difficult supracondylar elbow fractures in children: Analysis of percutaneous pinning technique. *J Pediatr Orthop* 1992; 12:11–15.

This is a report of acceptable results in a series of displaced supracondylar fractures treated with lateral divergent pins.

Marzo JM, d'Amato C, Strong M, et al: Usefulness and accuracy of arthrography in management of lateral humeral condyle fractures in children. *J Pediatr Orthop* 1990;10:317–321.

This is a communication of accuracy of arthrography and guidelines for its use.

Masada K, Kawai H, Kawabata H, et al: Osteosynthesis for old, established non-union of the lateral condyle of the humerus. *J Bone Joint Surg* 1990;72A:32–40.

The authors describe a technique of osteosynthesis, which is recommended only for nonunions in patients with severe pain or apprehension because of lateral instability.

Mehserle WL, Meehan PL: Treatment of the displaced supracondylar fracture of the humerus (type III) with closed reduction and percutaneous cross-pin fixation. *J Pediatr Orthop* 1991;11:705–711.

The authors report good results with crossed K-wire fixation of Type III supracondylar humerus fracutres. Baumann's angle and the lateral humeral capitellar angle were useful guides for assessing the adequacy of maintenance of fracture reduction.

Mintzer CM, Waters PM, Brown DJ, et al: Percutaneous pinning in the treatment of displaced lateral condyle fractures. *J Pediatr Orthop* 14:462–465.

The authors report good results with percutaneous pinning of lateral condylar fractures. This method is recommended for fractures that are displaced > 2mm and have a congruent joint surface by arthrogram.

Paradis G, Lavallee P, Gagnon N, et al: Supracondylar fractures of the humerus in children: Technique and results of crossed percutaneous K-wire fixation. *Clin Orthop* 1993;297:231–237.

The authors report good results after closed reduction and percutaneous pinning using crossed K-wire fixation.

Pirone AM, Graham HK, Krajbich JI: Management of displaced extension-type supracondylar fractures of the humerus in children. *J Bone Joint Surg* 1988;70A:641–650.

In a large series of displaced supracondylar fractures, there was a higher percentage of excellent results with closed reduction and percutaneous pinning than with other treatment methods.

Rodriguez-Merchan EC: Percutaneous reduction of displaced radial neck fractures in children. *J Trauma* 1994;37:812–814.

The authors correlate the degree of initial displacement with functional outcome in a series of displaced radial neck fractures.

Royce RO, Dutkowsky JP, Kasser JR, et al: Neurologic complications after K-wire fixation of supracondylar humerus fractures in children. *J Pediatr Orthop* 1991;11:191–194.

The authors report four neurologic complications in 143 children with K-wire fixation of supracondylar fractures. Two children had late ulnar neuropraxias; 1 ulnar nerve injury and 1 radial nerve injury were caused by direct trauma during wire insertion.

Shaw BA, Kasser JR, Emans JB, et al: Management of vascular injuries in displaced supracondylar humerus fractures without arteriography. *J Orthop Trauma* 1990; 4:25–29.

The authors report vascular impairment in 17 (12%) of 143 children with displaced supracondylar fractures. Rapid reduction and K-wire stabilization without arteriogram are recommended.

Forearm Trauma

Landfried MJ, Stenclik M, Susi JG: Variant of Galeazzi fracture-dislocation in children. *J Pediatr Orthop* 1991;11:332–335.

The authors describe a type of Galeazzi fracture-dislocation in which soft-tissue interposition blocks closed reduction.

Lascombes P, Prevot J, Ligier JN, et al: Elastic stable intramedullary nailing in forearm shaft fracture in children: 85 cases. *J Pediatr Orthop* 1990;10:167–171.

The authors report 92% excellent results with elastic stable intramedullary nailing. This technique is recommended for displaced fractures in children older than 10 years of age and in younger children in whom conservative treatment fails.

Price CT, Scott DS, Kurzner ME, et al: Malunited forearm fractures in children. *J Pediatr Orthop* 1990; 10:705–712.

This is a report of 39 children with malunions of the forearm, all of whom were satisfied with function and cosmetic appearance regardless of age, angulation, complete displacement, or loss of radial bow at the time of union. Closed reduction is recommended for diaphyseal forearm fractures in children.

Stoll TM, Willis RB, Paterson DC: Treatment of the missed Monteggia fracture in the child. *J Bone Joint Surg* 1992;74B:436–440.

The authors report eight missed Monteggia lesions, noting that reconstruction can be successfully obtained by open reduction or radial head and ulnar osteotomy in children up to 10 years of age and at least 4 years after injury.

28

Elbow and Forearm: Trauma

Adult Fractures and Dislocations

Olecranon Fractures

Olecranon fractures are among the most common elbow fractures. Most are caused by the tension of the triceps combined with a bending moment over the distal end of the trochlea. The tension and bending produce a transverse or oblique fracture, which frequently is associated with a compression fracture of the remaining intact distal portion of the olecranon fossa. Another frequent mechanism of fracture is direct trauma. Direct trauma produces complex comminuted fracture patterns, which may be associated with radial head fractures or dislocations and/or with fractures of the proximal radius and ulna. When the flexed elbow sustains high-energy trauma, olecranon fractures are frequently associated with open wounds, severely comminuted fracture patterns, and marked elbow instability. Finally, chronic stress overload can cause olecranon fractures in an adult or fracture through an unfused olecranon epiphysis in an adolescent. These stress fractures have been reported most commonly in throwing athletes, particularly baseball pitchers and javelin throwers.

There is no generally accepted classification of fractures of the olecranon. The factors that are used to define subgroups in the literature include the amount of displacement, the direction of the fracture line (transverse versus oblique), the presence or absence of articular comminution, the percent involvement of the olecranon, and the presence or absence of associated injuries, such as dislocations, coronoid fractures, or radial head fractures. These factors have been used to assist the surgeon in deciding between treatment alternatives and to prognosticate results.

The deforming force of the triceps usually produces fracture displacement and necessitates immobilization of the elbow in extension if manipulative reduction can be achieved. Nonsurgical treatment should be reserved for minimally displaced olecranon fractures that have little articular incongruity and enough soft-tissue stability to achieve union. Treatment should consist of a short period of protective immobilization with the elbow between 45° and 90° of flexion in a long arm splint or cast, followed by gentle mobilization and gradual return to function with fracture healing. Nondisplaced stress fractures of the olecranon have been reported to heal with nonsurgical treatments, such as activity modification or splinting.

Displaced fractures require surgery to prevent nonunion, eliminate articular incongruity, and restore the elbow extensor mechanism. Surgical repair consists of open reduction and internal fixation (ORIF) of the displaced olecranon or excision of the fractured proximal end of the olecranon process, with repair of the central triceps tendon to the remaining distal olecranon. Inadequate information exists in the literature to determine which fractures are most suitable for which technique. Generally favorable results have been reported with both.

Excision of the olecranon fracture fragments should be considered, particularly in cases with comminution or osteopenic bone, because internal fixation is more difficult and involves more complications in these cases. Although studies have shown little difference in strength between elbows treated by excision and those treated by internal fixation, excision is generally favored in elderly lower demand patients (Fig. 1).

The amount of the olecranon fractured may preclude surgical excision as the optimal treatment choice. Fracture fragments involving less than 60% of the olecranon can be safely excised without creating elbow instability. Treatment by excision of small proximal fragments is therefore ideal. Excision of up to 80% has been reported, but mechanical studies indicate that loss of this much of the olecranon could create elbow instability, and instability has been reported clinically with 60% excisions. Therefore, when greater than 60% is involved, excision should not be the primary treatment. Also, excision should be undertaken with caution if there is preexisting elbow instability or evidence of a coronoid fracture, both of which predispose to postoperative instability. When excision is chosen, the triceps should be repaired close to the articular surface of the residual ulna to decrease the chance of instability.

The generally excellent results reported for simple two-part fractures, whether transverse or oblique, make fixation the more attractive alternative for these fractures. A number of possible techniques are available, the most popular of which are longitudinal screw fixation, with or without a tension band wire; tension band wiring around two longitudinal Kirschner wires (K-wires); and plate fixation with a contoured one third tubular plate. Mechanical testing, used to compare the stability of simulated olecranon fractures fixed by these three methods, produced conflicting results. In more distal olecranon fractures, particularly those associated with anterior instability, plate fixation appears to be more stable and better suited than tension banding techniques to resist the deforming forces of the brachialis and the biceps. Good clinical results have been reported with all three methods. The major technical problems with any fixation technique are obtaining exact articular reduction, preventing redisplacement, and avoiding secondary problems relating to the hardware that require early removal. Data from one prospective study have dem-

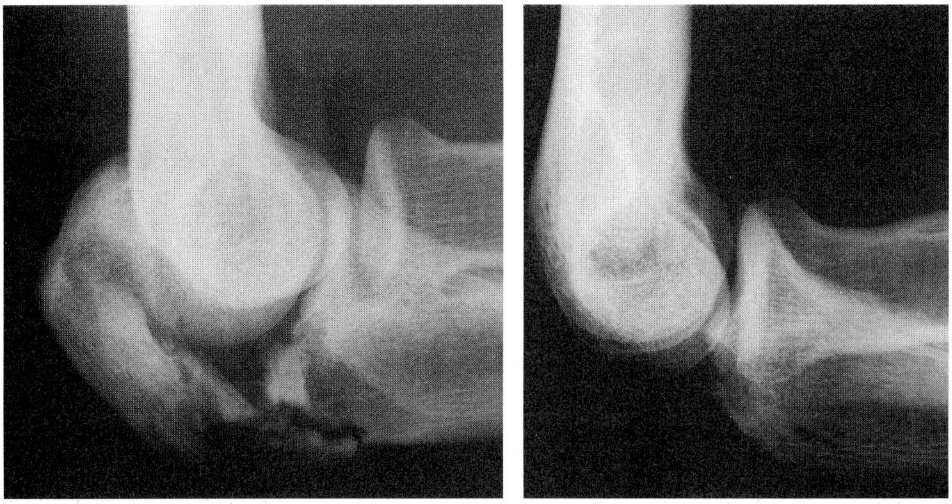

Fig. 1 **Left,** A lateral radiograph of a severely comminuted olecranon fracture involving approximately 60% of the olecranon surface. **Right,** Internal fixation was not possible. The proximal olecranon was excised and the triceps reattached through drill holes. Excising greater than this amount of the olecranon could lead to elbow instability.

onstrated better reductions, less loss of fixation, and fewer late problems in a group of elbows randomized to treatment with contoured one third tubular plates than in a group randomized to treatment with tension band wiring.

Most olecranon fractures heal, and the vast majority of patients recover a functional range of motion. Small losses of terminal extension are reported in greater than one half of cases. Pain is not a significant problem, and when it occurs it often relates to symptomatic hardware. Few long-term data exist on the incidence of arthrosis, but most arthritic changes that occur are reported as mild. Hardware complications are frequent in many series and include loss of fixation, which results in fracture displacement, or prominent protruded and symptomatic hardware, which requires removal. Attention to technical details of the chosen fixation technique is required to minimize the complications related to surgically implanted hardware.

Nonunion of the olecranon is uncommon (5% of cases). When it occurs, nonunion frequently causes pain and may be associated with instability and limitation of motion. Possible treatments include rehabilitation, arthroplasty, excision of the proximal fragment, and ORIF to obtain union. The majority of nonunions in symptomatic young patients with large proximal fragments unite when treated with ORIF with or without supplemental bone graft (Fig. 2). The combined data of two series demonstrated successful union in 20 of 21 cases surgically treated. Smaller proximal fragments can be treated with surgical excision and triceps repair. Elderly patients with associated arthrosis may be candidates for arthroplasty.

Coronoid Fractures

Coronoid fractures are frequently associated with elbow dislocations. Two percent to 10% of elbow dislocations have associated coronoid fractures, and in a recent series of coronoid fractures, one third had elbow dislocations. Displacement of the coronoid indicates avulsion of the brachialis muscle as well as some anterior capsule and the anterior bundle of the medial collateral ligament (MCL), especially if the fragment is large. In addition to the loss of these soft-tissue stabilizers, because the coronoid process itself can act as an anterior buttress, preventing posterior displacement of the elbow, elbow dislocations with coronoid fractures may be predisposed to increased instability of the elbow. Therefore, care should be taken to avoid recurrent dislocation in the first few weeks after dislocation. Coronoid fractures are one component of a complex spectrum of injuries that are frequently associated with acute elbow instability.

A recent study has subclassified coronoid fractures by the percent of involvement of the whole coronoid to determine the prognosis for recurrent instability as well as clinical outcome. Small avulsions of the tip of the coronoid (type 1) were found to have a good prognosis with treatment by only brief immobilization. Fractures involving 50% of the coronoid (type II) were sometimes associated with elbow instability, whereas fractures involving greater than 50% of the coronoid (type 3) were frequently found to be associated with elbow instability and had poor clinical outcomes. It was theorized that reduction and fixation of these large fragments would restore stability and improve patient outcome.

Capitellar Fractures

Fractures of the capitellum are rare, accounting for only 0.5% to 1% of all elbow injuries in the adult. The mechanism of injury has been debated, but it probably occurs by forces transmitted through the radial head from a fall on the outstretched hand. Radial head and capitellum fractures therefore have similar mechanisms, and both may be associated with ruptures of the MCL. Two types of capitellar fracture have been described. Type I fractures

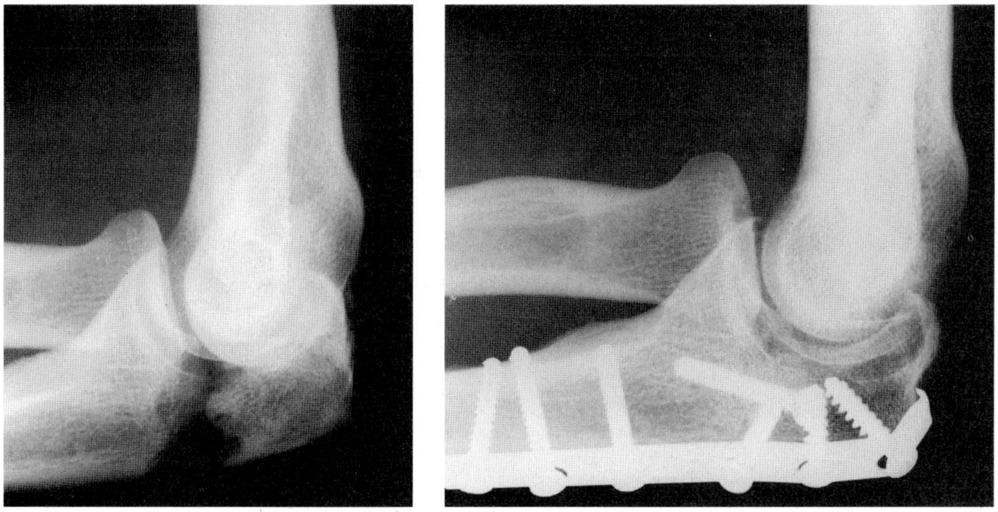

Fig. 2 Left, A lateral radiograph demonstrated a nonunion of the olecranon with a 1-cm gap 3 months after injury. The patient had had no previous treatment. **Right,** This lateral radiograph demonstrates that union was achieved after open reduction and fixation with a contoured one-third tubular plate and an interfragmentary screw.

(Hahn-Steinthal) constitute the majority of the capitellum, which is typically displaced anteriorly and superiorly. The type II fracture (Kocher-Lorenz) involves only a shell of the articular surface and a small amount of subchondral bone. Radiographic evaluation of the lateral compartment of the elbow is facilitated by obtaining a radial head–capitellum view, which is obtained by placing the elbow and the cassette in the lateral projection position and obliquing the tube 45° to the forearm. Tomograms may be necessary in some cases.

Nonsurgical management is indicated for nondisplaced fractures. Splinting in flexion for several weeks is required. For displaced fractures, excellent results have been reported after successful closed reduction. Problems with closed reduction include failure to obtain reduction, difficulties with accurate radiographic analysis of reduction, redisplacement, and the requirement for immobilization in marked flexion.

Two surgical approaches are ORIF or fragment removal. ORIF is most applicable to type 1 fractures in which the fragment is large (Fig. 3). A lateral approach is recommended, with detachment of the extensor origin if required for increased exposure. Fixation has been reported with K-wires, AO screws, or a Herbert screw. Care must be taken to avoid intra-articular hardware. Good results have been reported after fragment excision, and this is the least demanding technique. Excision is frequently necessary in type 2 fractures in which little subchondral bone exists to support internal fixation. If possible, excision should be avoided in cases with associated valgus instability of the elbow from an injury to the MCL.

Radial Head Fractures

Radial head fractures are common, accounting for approximately 20% of all elbow fractures. They typically occur from a fall on the outstretched hand with the forearm in pronation. Less common mechanisms are direct trauma and valgus loading. Radial head fractures may be associated with elbow dislocations.

Mason's classification is still the most commonly used in the literature. Type I fractures are nondisplaced, type II are marginal fractures with displacement, and type III are comminuted fractures involving the whole head of the radius. Some authors have used the designation of type III to refer to any comminuted fractures, even if the whole head of the radius is not involved; however, this does not fit with Mason's original description. The amount of involvement of the surface of the radial head and the number of millimeters of depression required to move from a type I to a type II fracture are not clear from the literature. This classification has been extended to include a type IV radial head fracture when there is an associated elbow dislocation.

Radial head fractures are frequently associated with soft-tissue injuries around the elbow and forearm. The presence of these soft-tissue injuries is important to diagnose because they influence the appropriate choice of treatment for the radial head fracture. Rupture of the MCL in association with a radial head fracture produces valgus instability, which is increased by radial head excision. Injury to the interosseous membrane of the forearm and the triangular fibrocartilage in the wrist produces axial instability of the forearm and subluxation of the distal radioulnar joint. The combination of a radial head fracture or dislocation and an acute distal radioulnar subluxation has been called the Essex-Lopresti injury. The more severe radial head fractures (types III and IV) have a higher chance of significant soft-tissue injury leading to elbow or forearm instability; therefore, there should be a higher index of suspicion when evaluating these fractures.

Controversy continues over the optimal treatment for

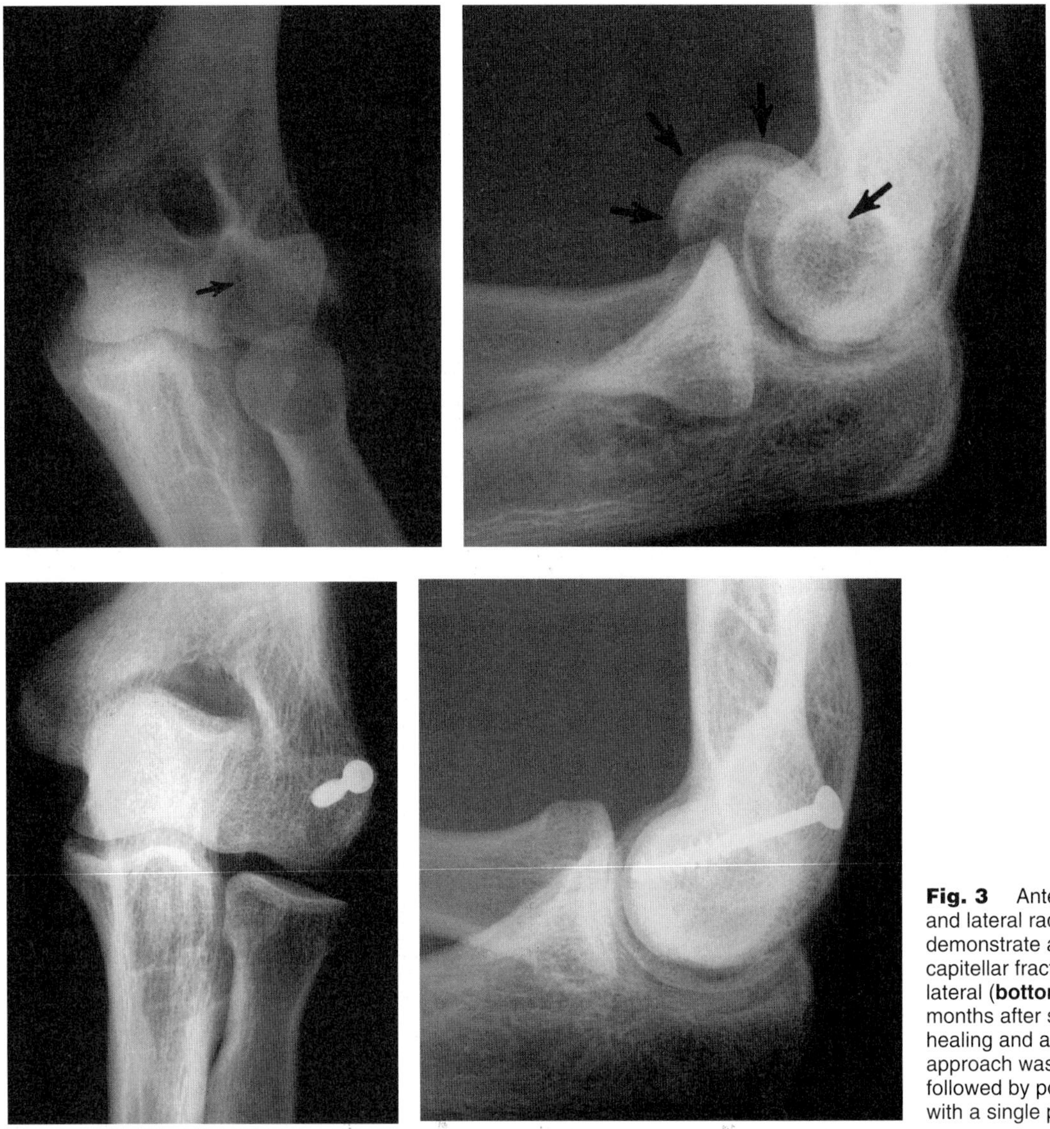

Fig. 3 Anteroposterior (AP) (**top left**) and lateral radiographs (**top right**) demonstrate a type I (Hahn-Steinthal) capitellar fracture. AP (**bottom left**) and lateral (**bottom right**) radiographs 2 months after surgery demonstrate healing and a congruous joint. A lateral approach was made to the elbow, followed by posterior to anterior fixation with a single partially threaded screw.

some types of radial head fractures. There is general agreement that nondisplaced or minimally displaced fractures (type I) should be treated nonsurgically with a brief period of splinting followed by early mobilization. Some authors have recommended aspiration and injection of the joint to enhance patient comfort. The results in the vast majority of cases are excellent, although nonunion and arthrofibrosis after these fractures have been reported.

Type II radial head fractures typically involve displacement of the anterolateral portion of the radial head, although other areas can be involved. The treatment options include conservative treatment similar to that described for type I fractures, excision of the depressed fragment, excision of the entire head, and ORIF. Good and excellent results have been reported for both conservative treatment and for ORIF. Acute excision for type II fractures is no longer recommended.

Conservative treatment of type II radial head fractures results in a satisfactory outcome in the majority of cases. Small losses of terminal extension and rotation may occur. For patients that develop pain or significant loss of motion, delayed excision of the radial head has been reported to decrease pain and increase function in 70% to 80% of cases.

Aspiration, injection with local anesthetic, and examination for a block to motion has been recommended to predict patients with type II fractures who will have poor outcomes after conservative treatment. However, the re-

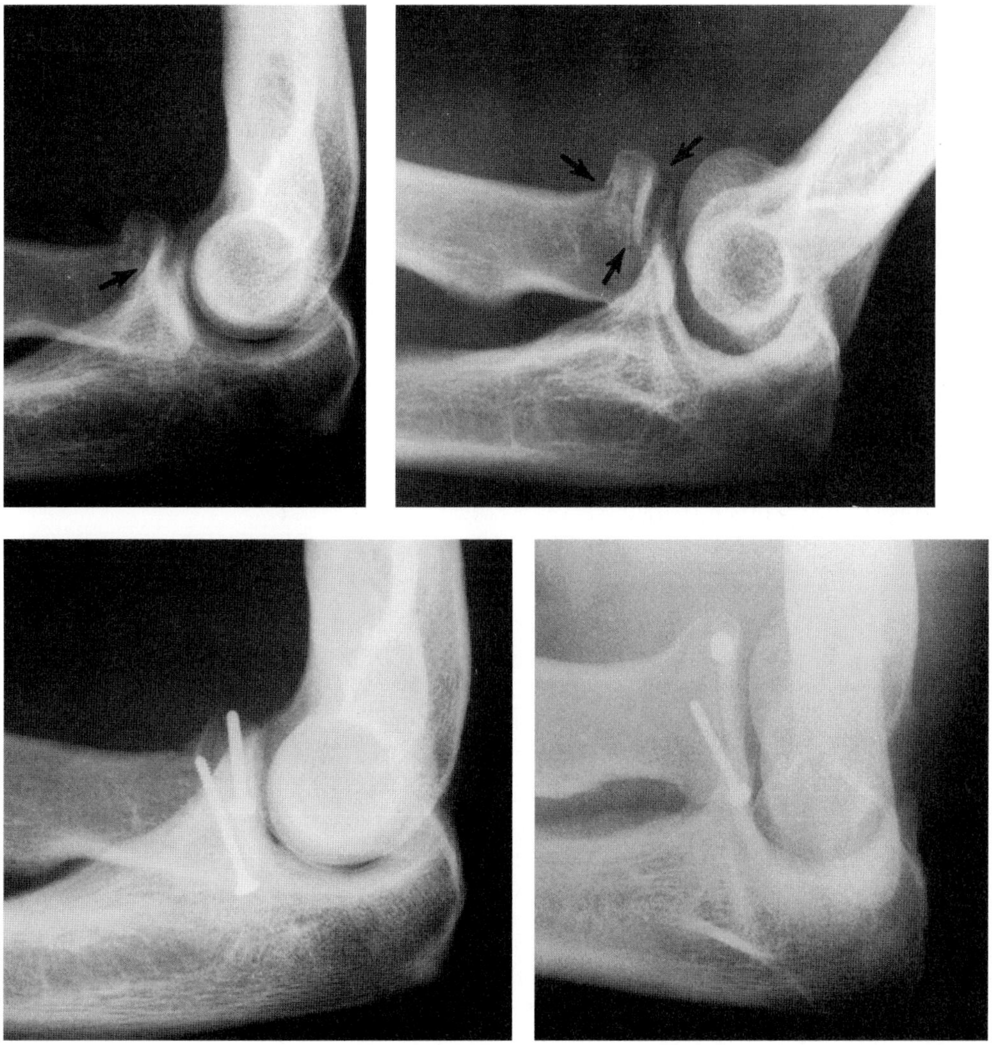

Fig. 4 Lateral (**top left**) and radial head view (**top right**) radiographs demonstrate a Mason type II radial head fracture with 4 mm of depression. Lateral (**bottom left**) and radial head view (**bottom right**) radiographs taken after open reduction and internal fixation with one 2.0-mm and one 1.5-mm screw.

sults of treatment based on this diagnostic approach have not been documented, and the amount of loss of motion on this examination that indicates more aggressive treatment is required is not known.

Treatment of all type II fractures by ORIF followed by early motion has an increasing number of advocates. This treatment has the advantage of preservation of the head and restoration of the articular surface. A high percentage of good and excellent results have been reported for a variety of fixation techniques, including Herbert screws, polyglycolide pins, and countersunk AO screws (2.0 or 1.5 mm) (Fig. 4). If only type II fractures with large marginal fractures are chosen, internal fixation can be accomplished without excessive technical difficulties and with predictably good results. Unfortunately, there are not enough data in the literature to determine the percentage of articular involvement and amount of depression that would most likely result in improved outcomes when reduced and stabilized.

In a retrospective review of two small groups of patients with type II fractures, better results were found after ORIF than after conservative treatment. Despite this report, both conservative treatment and ORIF for type II radial head fractures can still be supported by the literature.

Comminuted fractures of the entire radial head (type III) have commonly been treated by early surgical excision, and this is still the treatment of choice for most of these fractures. The optimal timing of excision has been an issue, but no new data have been reported. Many authors suggest that excision should be performed within 24 or 48 hours of injury to decrease the incidence of heterotopic bone formation. Other retrospective reviews of the long-term results of radial head excision have shown good results in cases where excision was performed within 1 week of injury. Finally, the results of delayed excision of the radial head from months to years after the injury have been shown to improve function and decrease pain in the majority of patients treated.

The results of radial head excision are favorable in the majority of elbows treated and do not deteriorate over time. Most patients lose 15° or less of rotation and have a small loss of strength in pronation and supination. Loss of the stability of the radiocapitellar joint typically leads to a small increase of the carrying angle at the elbow and an average of 2 mm of positive ulnar variance. Some patients have mild intermittent symptoms at the elbow, and a minority of patients develop pain at the wrist. These symptoms do not always correlate with the degree of proximal migration of the radius.

Despite these generally favorable results after acute radial head excision for type III fractures, a minority of patients develop significant problems. Those with associated elbow dislocations may have increased instability of the elbow, making it difficult to maintain reduction of the elbow. Those with evidence of acute injury to the distal radioulnar joint may develop wrist symptoms secondary to proximal migration of the radius. Either of these problems may be severe and difficult to manage. For these reasons, not all comminuted fractures should have early radial head excision as an isolated treatment. When there is associated valgus instability of the elbow, elbow dislocation (type IV fracture), or evidence of disruption of the distal radioulnar joint (Essex-Lopresti), preservation of the stability of the proximal radiocapitellar articulation may be necessary.

In cases in which fracture displacement is not severe, preservation of the fractured radial head through a nonsurgical approach combined with cast immobilization for 2 to 3 weeks may produce satisfactory results. Radiographs should be checked to confirm that redislocation does not occur in the cast. If symptoms warrant, delayed radial head excision can be performed.

If fracture comminution and displacement preclude conservative treatment and associated soft-tissue injuries increase the risk of instability following radial head excision, another strategy is necessary; although, no entirely satisfactory approach for this difficult combination has been documented in the literature. If possible, ORIF of the radial head is an attractive option. Unfortunately, for comminuted type III fractures, successful internal fixation is most difficult and has the least satisfactory results. Silicone replacement has been recommended but has also been criticized secondary to the lack of satisfactory mechanical properties of the implant, as well as to late fractures and silicone synovitis. Temporary use of a silicone prosthesis followed by removal after soft-tissue healing may be a satisfactory compromise, although the ability of this implant to even temporarily restore axial stability of the forearm has been questioned. Metallic implants, such as vitallium, have been used to replace the radial head and have better mechanical properties than silicone. Vitallium replacements have been reported to have clinically favorable results in one recent series of patients.

Regardless of which technique is chosen for the radial head, associated treatment may be required for repair of the MCL, brachialis avulsions, coronoid fractures, or the triangular fibrocartilage. Immobilization of the elbow, pinning of the distal radioulnar joint, or casting with the forearm in supination may be necessary in some of these complicated cases. The use of a hinged external fixator has been suggested, and may provide stability and motion while soft tissues heal. Results of this technique have not yet been reported.

Forearm Fractures

Diaphyseal fractures of the forearm frequently involve both bones, but can be of either the radius or the ulna, sparing the other bone. Isolated fractures of the radius should always be suspected of having distal radioulnar joint disruption (Galeazzi fracture dislocation). Isolated fractures of the ulna also may have associated joint subluxation or dislocation at the proximal radiocapitellar joint (Monteggia fracture dislocation). Unlike the radius, the ulna frequently sustains fractures from direct trauma (night stick fracture) without associated joint disruption.

Fractures of the forearm bones require accurate reduction to achieve excellent function. Forearm malunion has been studied in cadaveric models; its major effect is to produce a loss of forearm rotation. Each degree of rotational malunion produces a degree of rotational loss. Angular malunion of less than 10° produces little loss of rotation, but greater degrees of angular malunion produce increasingly significant decreases in rotation. One clinical study has demonstrated that even in plated fractures, if the radial bow was not restored, there was a loss of range of rotation and grip strength. The authors suggested that for optimal results, careful contouring of the plate and/or a slight obliquity of the plate across the radius is required to restore exact anatomy.

The need for an accurate reduction to obtain maximal motion has caused closed reduction and casting for forearm fractures to fall out of favor for all but isolated ulna fractures. Plating is the most common treatment for fractures of both bones of the forearm, isolated radial shaft fractures, and isolated ulna fractures not suitable for conservative treatment. Separate approaches should be used for each bone: the ulna is approached along the subcutaneous border, and the radius can be approached through a dorsal Thompson approach or a volar Henry approach. The traditional recommendation to use bone graft for cases with greater than one third comminution has been questioned because high healing rates have been obtained with less aggressive approaches. Small dynamic compression plates produce the best results for the majority of fractures. Postoperatively, protective splinting with early range of motion of the wrist and elbow allows relatively early return to function. Some authors have recommended casting in noncompliant patients. Casting is frequently required when proximal or distal joint disruption occurs in association with a fracture of one of the forearm bones. Ninety percent of the results have been reported as excellent or satisfactory. Patient follow-up commonly demonstrates a loss of less than 25% of forearm rotation and 10° of wrist or elbow motion.

These results of plating in closed fractures have led some authors to advocate immediate open reduction and plate fixation in open fractures of the forearm bones. Adequate data indicate that in conjunction with an excellent debridement, this technique produces good and excellent results and an acceptably low infection rate in types I, II, and IIIA open forearm fractures. The higher infection rate and poorer outcomes reported for immediate plate fixation of severe types IIIB and IIIC open forearm fractures may relate more to the injury than the fixation technique. Temporary periods of external fixation, followed by delayed plate fixation, may be a satisfactory alternative in the highest grade open injuries. Displaced low velocity gunshot fractures of the forearm appear to have better results when treated by open reduction and plate fixation than when treated by closed reduction and cast immobilization.

Refracture after plate removal is a complication of plate fixation of forearm fractures that has received considerable attention in the literature. Several studies have defined factors that increase the incidence of this complication. These are: the use of 4.5-mm plates, greater initial fracture displacement and comminution, early plate removal and/or the presence of fracture site radiolucency at the time of removal, and the failure to achieve adequate reduction and compression at the time of initial fixation. Many of the refractures have been within the first 6 weeks after plate removal, leading most authors to recommend a period of splinting or casting after removing the plates. However, some refractures have been reported beyond 6 weeks. In most series, there has been an association between refracture and early plate removal. If indicated, removal is not recommended until 15 to 24 months after fracture. It is not known whether newer types of plates (titanium), which theoretically reduce stress shielding, will decrease the incidence of refracture.

Attention to these details can significantly decrease the refracture rate that has been reported. However, to avoid this complication entirely, some authors recommend leaving forearm plates in situ. Studies on bone mineral density and forearm grip strength have demonstrated that these parameters are not affected by long-term in situ forearm plates. These studies support the philosophy of avoiding routine forearm plate removal.

Synostosis between the radius and the ulna is another complication of both bone forearm fractures. The incidence of this complication is increased in high-energy fractures and when comminuted fragments or long screws are left intruding into the interosseous space. Recent reports have indicated that, particularly for a midshaft synostosis, the results of surgical excision are good, with a low incidence of recurrence and a satisfactory return of forearm rotation. The use of low dose, postoperative radiation has been described to prevent recurrence of synostosis. It is generally recommended to wait at least 1 year for full maturation of the synostotic bone prior to excision. Resection of a proximal synostosis has less success; only one half of the patients benefited from this procedure in one series.

Isolated fractures of the shaft of the radius are often associated with disruption of the distal radioulnar joint (Galeazzi fracture dislocation), and the poor results of conservative treatment of this injury combination have been documented. The radius fracture is usually at the junction of the mid and distal thirds, but may be elsewhere in the shaft. It is typically dorsally angulated on the lateral radiograph and shortened on the anteroposterior radiograph. The best results have been reported after treatment by open reduction and plate fixation of the radial fracture. This treatment should be followed by intraoperative examination of the distal radioulnar joint clinically and radiographically. Some authors feel that if the joint is stable, splinting and early motion are all that are required postoperatively. Others have immobilized all of these fractures in supination. Any suspicion of instability of the distal radioulnar joint requires immobilization in a long arm cast in as much supination as is necessary to maintain reduction for 6 weeks. Some Galeazzi fractures are associated with an irreducible distal radioulnar joint or a soft incomplete reduction indicating entrapped soft tissues, such as the extensor carpi ulnaris tendon. Open reduction and removal of the entrapped tissue is required in these cases.

Unlike trauma to the radius, direct trauma to the ulna frequently produces a fracture without associated joint disruption. The majority of these ulnar nightstick fractures can be treated conservatively by casting or bracing. Data from a prospective study have shown that treatment with a short arm removable brace leads to better patient satisfaction and earlier return to work than treatment with a long arm cast. This study has confirmed the generally held impression that immobilizing the elbow is not necessary for repair of these fractures. The literature is not clear about which fractures are not amenable to simple bracing and require ORIF for optimal function. In one study, there were excellent results when less than 50% displacement of the ulnar shaft was used as a criteria for brace treatment. Whether greater degrees of displacement or angulation also achieve excellent results after conservative treatment is uncertain. In one study, fractures of the distal third of the ulna were found to be more problematic for functional brace treatment, particularly when they were displaced or angulated. The nonunion rate after conservative treatment is hard to determine from the literature.

Proximal ulna fractures extending into the olecranon should be treated with open reduction and plate fixation. These fractures require 3.5-mm compression plates, unlike isolated olecranon fractures, which need only one third tubular plates. Proximal ulnar fractures associated with radial head subluxation or dislocation (Monteggia) are best treated by open reduction and rigid internal fixation of the ulna, usually with plates and screws, and closed reduction of the radial head. If closed reduction of the radial head is not possible, then open reduction and removal of interposed soft tissues should be performed. If there is an associated radial head fracture, it may need to be addressed by internal fixation, prosthetic replacement, or excision. Most authors have recommended casting postoperatively, but if the ulna is anatomically reduced and the radial head is stable through a range of motion, protected early motion may be a safe alternative. The physician should be aware that there is up to a 20% incidence of posterior interosseous nerve palsy associated with Monteggia fracture dislocations.

Fractures of the Distal Humerus

Fractures of the distal humerus are uncommon, accounting for 1% or less of adult fractures. These fractures may involve either the medial or lateral condyle, but more commonly involve both condyles, usually with intra-articular extension. Complete fractures of the distal humerus without intra-articular extension occur in adults, but less commonly than in children. The major horizontal fracture line may be through the condyles (transcondylar) or above them (supracondylar). This complex set of injuries is produced by either axial load transmitted through the forearm to an extended elbow or direct trauma to the flexed elbow, each with variable degrees of associated abduction or adduction moments.

Knowledge of the local anatomy of the distal humerus is required to understand the injury patterns and to plan fixation. The distal humerus widens in the coronal plane but flattens in the sagittal plane to a narrow isthmus before expanding distally, forming medial and lateral columns. These two columns support the centrally positioned trochlea, which fits between the distal ends of the lateral and medial columns. The articular surface of the capitellum lies on the distal lateral column. The columns have a normal 40° anterior sagittal angulation and a 10° to 15° valgus angulation. The valgus angulation accounts for the carrying angle of the elbow. The coronoid and olecranon fossa lie between the two columns above the trochlea and are separated by a thin plate of bone.

The most common classification in the literature is that of Riseborough and Radin, which classifies distal humerus fractures into four types based on displacement, comminution, and the presence or absence of rotation of either the trochlea or capitellum. A more comprehensive anatomic classification, which has become increasingly popular, is that of Müller and associates, which divides fractures of the distal humerus into nonarticular type A fractures, partial articular type B fractures, and total articular type C fractures. Each of these are divided into three subtypes, which are again divided into three subtypes, making 27 separate types of distal humerus fractures.

As complex as the Müller classification is, further appreciation of the subtleties of the pathoanatomy are often required to plan accurate internal fixation. These subtleties include the location of the horizontal fracture line (high in the supracondylar region or low in the transcondylar region), the presence of separate fractures of the epicondyles, and comminution between the trochlear and capitellar fragments. Central comminution requires screw fixation without compression to maintain the width of the distal humerus. The fixation of a separate coronal fracture of the trochlea with a Herbert screw, in conjunction with internal fixation of the rest of the distal humerus, was described recently. This pattern was found to occur in the low transcondylar fracture types.

Single fractures of the humeral condyles are less common than fractures across both condyles, making up less than 5% of distal humerus fractures. If nondisplaced, they can be treated with simple splinting followed by early range of motion. When displaced, these fractures are best treated with ORIF with interfragmentary screws supported by a plate if necessary. The approach required may be medial, lateral, or posterior extensile, depending on the fracture. Isolated medial epicondylar fractures, if significantly displaced, can be fixed with a single screw, although some advocate nonoperative treatment of all epicondylar fractures, even when displaced.

Conservative treatment of supracondylar fractures has been reported. Simple splinting or casting is reserved for minimally displaced fractures, for those with comminution or osteopenia such that successful internal fixation and early motion are not possible, and for those patients in whom a major surgical approach is not feasible. Longitudinal skeletal traction followed by splinting or casting may decrease fracture displacement; however, the elderly patients that frequently sustain this type of fracture do not tolerate lateral arm traction well. Severe open fractures may require cross-joint external fixation.

Considerable data in the literature indicate that the majority of patients with displaced supracondylar or transcondylar fractures achieve optimal results when treated by early ORIF, usually through an extensile posterior approach. Although there have been improvements in approaches, surgical techniques, and internal fixation devices, these surgeries are technically demanding, and the results achieved depend on obtaining accurate reduction and sufficiently stable internal fixation to permit early motion without fracture displacement or hardware failure. When these goals are met, 70% to 90% good and excellent results have been reported. The average extension–flexion range obtained has been between 20° to 130°. Typically, there is no loss of rotation.

Despite these generally favorable results, complications have been reported in all series. Postoperative ulnar nerve palsy can affect patient outcome. Complications related to fixation of an olecranon osteotomy in one third of the cases in one series have been reported. Major fixation failures and nonunions are less common, but have occurred in up to 15% of cases.

These complications should cause the surgeon to be

cautious and to pursue all attempts to minimize their incidence. The patient's age, medical conditions, and postoperative expectations should be considered when choosing this surgery. The incidence of ulnar nerve palsy can be minimized by gentle technique and anterior subcutaneous transposition of the ulnar nerve at the end of the procedure. Problems with the olecranon osteotomy have caused some authors to recommend an extra-articular osteotomy or an extensile soft-tissue approach without olecranon osteotomy. These approaches make exposure of the distal aspect of the trochlea, where there is often comminution, more difficult.

Hardware failure and loss of fixation have stimulated studies on the optimum mechanical constructs for plate application. It is clear that two plates are mechanically stronger than any single column plate. To obtain two-plate fixation on low fractures, plates may need to be contoured very distally, sometimes incorporating the transcondylar screw as one of the distal plate screws. One third tubular plates have reportedly had a high failure rate, and they have generally been replaced by 3.5-mm pelvic reconstruction plates or even 3.5-mm dynamic compression plates. Different orientations of the two plates have been mechanically tested. The greater the spread between two plates, the greater the rigidity of fixation. Spread is increased by placing one or both plates on the medial or lateral side of the distal humerus rather than straight posterior. If the lateral plate is placed on the lateral side instead of straight posterior, a special contour is required because of the anterior angulation of the distal lateral column. Plate location should also be planned to obtain optimal screw purchase. When planning screw locations, the surgeon must be aware of the nonvisualized anterior articular surface on the lateral column.

Malunion and nonunion of supracondylar humerus fractures occur in a small percentage of cases. Data from a recent study have shown that healing of nonunions and restoration of articular congruity can be achieved in the majority of surgically treated patients. Extensile exposures, anterior and posterior capsulotomies, reconstruction of intra-articular pathology, and mobilization and neurolysis of the ulnar nerve are required. In some cases, three plates may be necessary. These major reconstructions of the distal humerus are indicated only in patients who are able to cooperate with the extensive postoperative protocols required. Total elbow replacement using a semiconstrained prosthesis for nonunion in older patients has also reportedly led to satisfactory results at an average 5-year follow-up.

Tendinopathies About the Elbow

Patients who have tendinitis in the region of the lateral or medial epicondyle of the elbow frequently present for treatment. These tendinopathies involve the wrist extensor group over the lateral epicondyle, and the wrist flexor–forearm pronator group over the medial epicondyle.

Most authors believe that the pathology is consistent with microscopic or macroscopic degeneration or tears in the extensor or flexor tendon origin. On the extensor side, the tendinous origin of the extensor carpi radialis brevis has been particularly implicated. Pathologic investigation shows fibroblastic proliferation, hyaline degeneration, and vascular invasion in the involved tendon origin. The process appears to be degenerative rather than inflammatory and indicates a failure of injury repair or degeneration in the tendon origin. Inflammatory cells are not frequently present.

A variety of nonsurgical treatment modalities have been described. Alterations of technique in sporting activities or changes in the workplace may lead to symptomatic improvement and cure. It has been shown that tennis players with lateral epicondylitis make greater use of their wrist extensors and pronators compared to tennis players without epicondylitis, indicating that stroke modification may be of benefit. Other modalities include the use of forearm bands to distribute the force away from the extensor origins, nonsteroidal anti-inflammatory medication, local steroid injections, and a variety of physical therapy and rehabilitative measures. These include rest, ice, and other local modalities, such as phonophoresis to decrease inflammation, followed by strengthening of the muscle tendon units involved.

Many surgical procedures have been described for tendinopathies about the elbow. Surgical options should be considered only for patients who have been recalcitrant to a variety of conservative modalities, because the majority of patients will improve without surgery. Many surgical procedures have been directed at the extensor origin, involving open or percutaneous release of the extensor tendons, or localized excision of the area of degenerated tendon. The success rate reported for the majority of these procedures is 80% or greater. It is not possible to determine a clear benefit of one technique over another, nor is it possible to know when conservative treatment should be abandoned in favor of surgical intervention. A recent report indicates that many patients continue to improve for years after surgical intervention.

A meta analysis has been attempted on the literature of both conservative and surgical treatments of lateral epicondylitis. Those conducting this analysis were not able to document evidence in the literature for the benefit of any treatment. The lack of knowledge of the natural evolution of the process and the placebo effect of treatments was emphasized.

Avulsion of the distal biceps tendon insertion is a relatively uncommon injury that typically occurs in the dominant extremity of men with an average age of 50 years. However, two recent reports document the occurrence of this lesion in young athletes. The average age of the patients reported in these series was 40 years, and nine of the 11 were weight lifters or body builders. One patient provided a 6-year history of anabolic steroid use and sustained bilateral avulsions.

The diagnosis of an acute, complete rupture is usually relatively straightforward. Other conditions may cause antecubital pain and swelling; these include brachialis injuries, partial biceps ruptures, gangliae, and inflammation of the bursa between the radial tuberosity and the biceps tendon. Two recent series have explored the role of magnetic resonance imaging (MRI) in evaluating patients with suspected injuries of the distal biceps tendon. Axial images were more valuable than sagittal images, and there was 100% agreement between MRI images and surgical findings in 15 cases that underwent surgical exploration in one of these two series.

Early reattachment of the avulsed tendon to the bicipital tuberosity using a modified two-incision technique remains the treatment of choice in this condition. Early reattachment provides normal or near normal strength and endurance in both flexion and supination. The two-incision technique reduces the risk of neurovascular injury, and if this method is modified by not exposing the ulna, the risk of heterotopic ossification and radioulnar synostosis appears to be minimal. The use of Mitek suture anchors has also been reported in a small series of four cases.

Annotated Bibliography

Olecranon, Coronoid and Radial Head Fractures

Morrey BF: Current concepts in the treatment of the fractures of the radial head, the olecranon, and the coronoid. *J Bone Joint Surg* 1995;77A:316–327.

In this current concepts review, Dr. Morrey provides a description of his methods of assessment and classification of injuries to the radial head, olecranon, and coronoid. He provides recommended treatment approaches and outcomes information in a succinct but comprehensive review.

Olecranon

Danziger MB, Healy WL: Operative treatment of olecranon nonunion. *J Orthop Trauma* 1992;6:290–293.

Five patients were treated for nonunion of the olecranon. Union was successfully achieved with improved function. A contoured dynamic compression plate was the fixation method of choice.

Hume MC, Wiss DA: Olecranon fractures: A clinical and radiographic comparison of tension band wiring and plate fixation. *Clin Orthop* 1992;285:229–235.

Forty-one patients were prospectively randomized for treatment by tension-band wiring around two longitudinal K-wires or plate fixation with a contoured one third tubular plate. Tension-band wiring achieved only 37% good clinical and 47% good radiographic results, compared with plate fixation, which achieved 63% good clinical and 86% good radiographic results.

Inhofe PD, Howard TC: The treatment of olecranon fractures by excision of fragments and repair of the extensor mechanism: Historical review and report of 12 fractures. *Orthopedics* 1993;16:1313–1317.

Twelve patients with olecranon fractures treated by excision of the proximal fragment were retrospectively reviewed. Up to 70% of the olecranon was excised. Eleven had good or excellent results. Excision was felt to have particular benefit for comminuted or osteopenic olecranons where internal fixation is most difficult.

Nuber GW, Diment MT: Olecranon stress fractures in throwers: A report of two cases and a review of the literature. *Clin Orthop* 1992;278:58–61.

The authors report two cases of olecranon stress fracture in throwing athletes, which healed with splinting and rest.

Papagelopoulos PJ, Morrey BF: Treatment of nonunion of olecranon fractures. *J Bone Joint Surg* 1994;76B:627–635.

The treatment of nonunion of the olecranon in 24 patients was retrospectively reviewed. Twenty nonunions were treated surgically; one with excision of the proximal olecranon, three with prosthetic replacement, and 16 with osteosynthesis. Sixteen patients achieved good or excellent results. Union was achieved in 15 of the 16 patients treated by osteosynthesis.

Coronoid Fractures

Regan W, Morrey B: Fractures of the coronoid process of the ulna. *J Bone Joint Surg* 1989;71A:1348–1354.

Thirty-five patients with fractures of the coronoid process were retrospectively reviewed and classified as type I, avulsion of the tip of the process; type II, 50% of the process or less; and type III, involvement of more than 50%. Twelve of the 35 were associated with elbow dislocations. According to an objective assessment, 92% of patients who had type I fractures, 73% who had type II, and 20% who had type III had satisfactory results. An aggressive approach to reduction and fixation of type III fractures was recommended.

Radial Head

Broberg MA, Morrey BF: Results of delayed excision of the radial head after fracture. *J Bone Joint Surg* 1986;68A:669–674.

Twenty-one patients who underwent delayed excision of a previously fractured radial head were retrospectively reviewed. The radial head was excised between 1 month and more than 20 years from injury. Seventy-seven percent had good or excellent results.

Coleman DA, Blair WF, Shurr D: Resection of the radial head for fracture of the radial head: Long-term follow-up of seventeen cases. *J Bone Joint Surg* 1987;69A:385–392.

Seventeen patients who had a fracture of the radial head that was not associated with a dislocation of the elbow and was treated by radial head excision were retrospectively reviewed at an average of 19.8 years after injury. These patients had an average loss of strength of pronation and supination of 5% and 11%, respectively. Compared to the opposite side, the ulnar variance was increased by an average of 2 mm, and the carrying angle increased by an average of 9°. Mild symptoms in the elbow were present in only a few patients. The results did not deteriorate with time.

Davidson PA, Moseley JB Jr, Tullos HS: Radial head fracture: A potentially complex injury. *Clin Orthop* 1993;297:224–230.

Fifty consecutive cases of radial head fracture were clinically examined and had valgus stress radiographs. The results demonstrated that the higher the Mason class of radial head fracture, the greater the chance of associated elbow instability.

Geel CW, Palmer AK: Radial head fractures and their effect on the distal radioulnar joint: A rationale for treatment. *Clin Orthop* 1992;275:79–84.

Nineteen patients treated with ORIF for radial head fractures were reviewed. Sixteen of the 19 patients had partial articular fractures; three had more complex fractures involving the whole head of the radius. Excellent results were obtained in 14 of the elbows; however, the follow-up was less than 12 months.

Khalfayan EE, Culp RW, Alexander AH: Mason type II radial head fractures: Operative versus nonoperative treatment. *J Orthop Trauma* 1992;6:283–289.

Ten cases of type II radial head fractures treated by ORIF were retrospectively compared to 16 cases treated closed. The results showed 90% good and excellent results in the surgically treated group and 44% good and excellent results in the conservatively treated group. This difference was statistically significant, even with the small group of patients studied.

King GJ, Evans DC, Kellam JF: Open reduction and internal fixation of radial head fractures. *J Orthop Trauma* 1991;5:21–28.

Fourteen elbows were followed up at an average of 32 months after ORIF for displaced fractures of the radial head. In the Mason type II fractures, 100% good or excellent results were reported. However, in the type III fractures, only 33% obtained good or excellent results.

Knight DJ, Rymaszewski LA, Amis AA, et al: Primary replacement of the fractured radial head with a metal prosthesis. *J Bone Joint Surg* 1993;75B:572–576.

In cadaveric specimens, a vitallium metallic radial head prosthesis came closer to restoring the normal mechanics of the radiocapitellar joint than a silicone implant. Clinically, 31 patients treated with this implant were reviewed with a mean follow-up of 4.5 years. Two implants had been removed for loosening, but there were no other complications secondary to the prosthesis, and its use was recommended in cases of severe radial head fracture with concomitant soft-tissue injuries.

Pelto K, Hirvensalo E, Böstman O, et al: Treatment of radial head fractures with absorbable polyglycolide pins: A study on the security of the fixation in 38 cases. *J Orthop Trauma* 1994;8:94–98.

Forty-three patients were treated for radial head fractures with absorbable polyglycolide pins. Excellent or good results were obtained in 36 of 38 patients (95%) available for follow-up. Unlike previous reports on polyglycolide implants, no adverse local soft-tissue reactions were noted in this series.

Trousdale RT, Amadio PC, Cooney WP, et al: Radioulnar dissociation: A review of twenty cases. *J Bone Joint Surg* 1992;74A:1486–1497.

Twenty patients with radioulnar dissociation, characterized by trauma to the lateral compartment of the elbow and instability of the distal radioulnar joint, were retrospectively reviewed. The results were unsatisfactory in 12 of 15 patients, in whom the two-level nature of the injury was not recognized initially. Radial head excision should be avoided if possible in cases with evidence of both proximal and distal injuries.

Vanderwilde RS, Morrey BF, Melberg MW, et al: Inflammatory arthritis after failure of silicone rubber replacement of the radial head. *J Bone Joint Surg* 1994; 76B:78–81.

A case is reported in which the inflammatory process secondary to long-term implantation of a silicone replacement for the radial head resulted in generalized cartilage degeneration in the elbow joint. This complication, along with others previously reported (fracture, dislocation, synovitis, lymphadenitis, and subchondral resorption), calls into question the long-term use of this implant for radial head replacement.

Forearm Fractures

Bruckner JD, Lichtman DM, Alexender AH: Complex dislocations of the distal radioulnar joint: Recognition and management. *Clin Orthop* 1992;275:90–103.

Eleven patients were identified who had fractures of the radius associated with dislocations of the distal radioulnar joint. After fixation of the radius, four of these were found to have complex dislocations defined as a failure to obtain closed reduction or a soft, incomplete reduction. The authors recommended exploration and removal of interposed soft tissues, such as the extensor carpi ulnaris tendon.

Duncan R, Geissler W, Freeland AE, et al: Immediate internal fixation of open fractures of the diaphysis of the forearm. *J Orthop Trauma* 1992;6:25–31.

Sixty-nine patients who sustained open fractures of one or both bones of the forearm were treated by irrigation, debridement, and immediate ORIF, followed by 48 to 72 hours of antibiotics. There were no infections in patients with grade I, grade II, or grade IIIA injuries, and 90% had satisfactory results. The four patients reviewed with grades IIIB and IIIC injuries had unsatisfactory results and developed infections.

Gebuhr P, Hölmich P, Orsnes T, et al: Isolated ulnar shaft fractures: Comparison of treatment by a functional brace and long-arm cast. *J Bone Joint Surg* 1992;74B:757–759.

This prospective randomized study allocated 39 patients with isolated fractures of the lower two thirds of the ulna to treatment by a long arm cast or a prefabricated functional brace. There were no nonunions in either treatment group. There was no significant difference in the time to healing; no fractures took longer than 20 weeks to heal. However, the patients treated with a brace were more satisfied with their treatment, had better wrist function, and returned to work earlier.

Lenihan MR, Brien WW, Gellman H, et al: Fractures of the forearm resulting from low-velocity gunshot wounds. *J Orthop Trauma* 1992;6:32–35.

The results of treatment of 37 extra-articular fractures of the forearm secondary to low-velocity gunshot wounds were reviewed. The results were poorest in patients with displaced fractures treated by cast immobilization, suggesting that ORIF should be the treatment of choice for displaced fractures.

Lindsey RW, Fenison AT, Doherty BJ, et al: Effects of retained diaphyseal plates on forearm bone density and grip strength. *J Orthop Trauma* 1994;8:462–467.

Bone mineral density and forearm grip strength were measured in 14 patients who had retained forearm plates. Two groups were analyzed; one between 2 and 5 years from fracture, and a second more than 5 years. In both groups, the forearm grip strength was less than in the opposite limb, but the difference was less in the group that was longer from treatment, and none of the differences were statistically significant. Bone mineral density was well preserved in both groups.

Ostermann PA, Ekkernkamp A, Henry SL, et al: Bracing of stable shaft fractures of the ulna. *J Orthop Trauma* 1994;8:245–248.

In a cadaveric experiment, it was found that displacement of less than 50% of the shaft of the ulna was stable through full pronation and full supination. In a clinical trial, 30 ulnar shaft fractures, meeting the criteria of not less than 50% displacement, were treated with a functional brace. The mean time to union was 7.3 weeks, with a range of 6 to 9 weeks. All fractures healed, and there was one delayed union.

Rosson JW, Petley GW, Shearer JR: Bone structure after removal of internal fixation plates. *J Bone Joint Surg* 1991;73B:65–67.

Fourteen patients were reviewed by single-photon absorptiometry after removal of internal fixation plates. No evidence of cortical atrophy was found in any patients who had the plates left for at least 21 months after the initial surgery.

Schemitsch EH, Richards RR: The effect of malunion on functional outcome after plate fixation of fractures of both bones of the forearm in adults. *J Bone Joint Surg* 1992;74A:1068–1078.

Fifty-five patients managed for both bones of the forearm fractures were followed for a mean of 6 years, and the results were assessed functionally and radiographically. The recovery of grip strength and the return of 80% of normal rotation of the forearm were found to be related to the restoration of a normal radial bow.

Fractures of the Distal Humerus

Figgie MP, Inglis AE, Mow CS, et al: Salvage of non-union of supracondylar fracture of the humerus by total elbow arthroplasty. *J Bone Joint Surg* 1989;71A:1058–1065.

Fourteen patients with nonunion of the distal humerus treated with total elbow arthroplasty were reviewed at an average of 5 years after reconstruction. The average postoperative elbow score was 84. There were three failures; one each secondary to dislocation, loosening of the humeral component, and deep infection.

Helfet DL, Hotchkiss RN: Internal fixation of the distal humerus: A biomechanical comparison of methods. *J Orthop Trauma* 1990;4:260–264.

Mechanical testing in a cadaveric model showed that two-plate constructs were significantly stronger in both rigidity and fatigue testing than cross-screws or a single posterior "Y" plate. Plates placed at 90° to each other posteriorly on the lateral column and medially on the medial column were recommended.

Helfet DL, Schmeling GJ: Bicondylar intraarticular fractures of the distal humerus in adults. *Clin Orthop* 1993;292:26–36.

A review of the literature on bicondylar intra-articular fractures of the distal humerus is presented, including classification, treatment options, indications for surgery, expected results, and complications.

Jupiter JB, Barnes KA, Goodman LJ, et al: Multiplane fracture of the distal humerus. *J Orthop Trauma* 1993;7:216–220.

Five patients had a coronal plane fracture of the trochlea in addition to the more common sagittal and horizontal plane fractures of the distal humerus. A Herbert screw was used to fix the trochlea before fixation of the rest of the distal humerus.

McKee M, Jupiter J, Toh CL, et al: Reconstruction after malunion and nonunion of intra-articular fractures of the distal humerus: Methods and results in 13 adults. *J Bone Joint Surg* 1994;76B:614–621.

The results of reconstruction of 13 patients with malunions and nonunions of intra-articular distal humeral fractures were reported with a mean follow-up of 25 months. Ten out of 13 patients obtained an average arc of motion of 97°, improved ulnar nerve function, and good or excellent clinical results.

Schemitsch EH, Tencer AF, Henley MB: Biomechanical evaluation of methods of internal fixation of the distal humerus. *J Orthop Trauma* 1994;8:468–475.

Five configurations of plating of cadaveric distal humeri were mechanically tested. Particularly in torsion, all two-plate constructs were stronger than an anatomically designed single lateral "J" buttress plate, even when augmented with a medial interfragmentary screw. When there was a gap, the lateral anatomic buttress plate, combined with a medial reconstruction plate, gave greater rigidity than either combination of two reconstruction plates placed at 90° to each other.

Tendinopathies About the Elbow

D'Alessandro DF, Shields CL, Tibone JE, et al: Repair of distal biceps tendon ruptures in athletes. *Am J Sports Med* 1993;21:114–119.

Visuri T, Lindholm H: Bilateral distal biceps tendon avulsions with use of anabolic steroids. *Med Sci Sports Exerc* 1994;26:941–944.

These two series combined report 11 cases of distal biceps tendon avulsion in young patients. All patients were very active and nine of the 11 were weight lifters or body builders. Surgical repair resulted in near normal supination strength and endurance and flexion strength and endurance. All repairs were done using a double incision technique. The importance of rehabilitation was emphasized.

Falchook FS, Zlatkin MB, Erbacher GE, et al: Rupture of the distal biceps tendon: Evaluation with MR imaging. *Radiology* 1994;190:659–663.

Fitzgerald SW, Curry DR, Erickson SJ, et al: Distal biceps tendon injury: MR imaging diagnosis. *Radiology* 1994;191:203–206.

These two reports document the value of MRI in evaluating patients with antecubital pain and suspected distal biceps tendon injuries. Correlation between surgical findings and MRI findings was high in those cases that underwent surgical exploration. The authors of these two studies conclude that MRI was helpful in evaluating distal biceps tendon injuries and in particular, in distinguishing complete ruptures from incomplete injuries and other conditions that mimic ruptures.

Labelle H, Guibert R, Joncas J, et al: Lack of scientific evidence for the treatment of lateral epicondylitis of the elbow: An attempted meta-analysis. *J Bone Joint Surg* 1992;74B:646–651.

A meta-analysis of the treatments for lateral epicondylitis was performed. Only 18 randomized controlled studies were identified. The mean score of these articles was low. The authors concluded that there was insufficient scientific evidence to support the current treatments for lateral epicondylitis.

Regan W, Wold LE, Coonrad R, et al: Microscopic histopathology of chronic refractory lateral epicondylitis. *Am J Sports Med* 1992;20:746–749.

The histopathologic features of 11 patients treated surgically for lateral epicondylitis were compared with those of 12 cadaveric specimens by a single pathologist. All 11 surgical specimens were interpreted as abnormal, and all 12 cadaveric specimens were interpreted as being histologically normal. The pathologic findings were vascular proliferation and hyaline degeneration. Histopathologically, the process was degenerative rather than inflammatory.

Verhaar J, Walenkamp G, Kester A, et al: Lateral extensor release for tennis elbow. *J Bone Joint Surg* 1993;75A:1034–1043.

This prospective study is a review of the results of 63 patients treated with an open extensor origin release for lateral epicondylitis. The results were shown to continue to improve out to 5 years after surgery. Seventy-six percent of patients had no pain or only slight pain 1 year from surgery; by 5 years this had increased to 92%.

29

Elbow: Reconstruction

In this past few years there have been significant advances in a number of areas relating to elbow reconstructive surgery. These advances have led to a better understanding of the indications for and contributions of imaging studies, the role of arthroscopy in the diagnosis and treatment of elbow disorders, applied biomechanics, prevention and treatment of elbow stiffness, correction of elbow instability, and the management of elbow arthritis, including total elbow arthroplasty (TEA).

Diagnostic Studies

As has been emphasized in the past, a careful history and physical examination combined with radiographs, including special views, yield adequate information to proceed with treatment in the vast majority, perhaps 90%, of cases. Lateral tomograms are indicated to assess osteophytes, impingement, osteoarthritis, and posttraumatic stiffness. Magnetic resonance imaging (MRI), although not routinely indicated, is useful to diagnose loose bodies, osteochondritis dissecans (OCD), tumors, and partial or complete ruptures of the distal biceps tendon insertion. Computed tomography (CT) arthrography can be used to assess the status of the articular cartilage in OCD and to confirm partial tears of the deep surface of the medial collateral ligament (MCL) as indicated by a "T-sign". Electrodiagnostic studies and bone scans are sometimes helpful. Although only a small percentage of patients presenting with elbow problems require diagnostic arthroscopy, this technique provides valuable information in about two thirds of the cases for which it is used.

Biomechanics and Kinematics

Although the elbow has often been thought of as a highly constrained articulation, it has been shown experimentally to behave as a loose, or sloppy, hinge with 3° to 5° of varus–valgus and rotational laxity. Modern unlinked (often called unconstrained) and linked (semiconstrained) TEAs recreate this loose hinge mechanism, which permits the soft tissues to absorb some of the forces and moments, protecting the prosthesis–cement–bone interface from them. The elbow is often misconceptually referred to as a nonweightbearing joint.

The axis of rotation of the elbow passes in a line through the lateral epicondyle to a point on the anterior inferior aspect of the medial epicondyle. This axis of rotation can be reproduced with a hinged external fixation device that can maintain elbow stability while permitting motion following surgery or trauma. This device has proven valuable in maintaining a functional arc of motion, which is from 30° to 130° of flexion. The functional arc of motion in rotation is from 50° pronation to 50° supination.

There are three primary constraints to elbow instability: an intact ulnohumeral articulation, the anterior band of the MCL (AMCL), and the ulnar part of the lateral collateral ligament (LCL), previously described as the lateral ulnar collateral ligament (LUCL). The AMCL is the primary constraint to valgus instability, and the radial head is of secondary importance. Replacement of the radial head with a silastic implant is inadequate when the AMCL is disrupted. The anterior capsule is an important constraint to instability only in full extension. On the lateral side, the ulnar part of the LCL is the primary constraint to posterolateral rotatory and varus instabilities. Finally, the coronoid process is a critical element in both valgus and posterolateral rotatory instability.

Functional Anatomy

The anatomy of the LCL complex is currently a topic of much discussion and interest, but also some confusion. The ulnar part of the LCL is the primary constraint to posterolateral rotatory instability, which is now thought to be a common mechanism of elbow subluxation and dislocation, especially those that are recurrent. This structure has occasionally been represented in schematic illustrations as a discrete band. However, it is only discrete at its insertion on the tubercle of the supinator crest of the ulna, where it can be palpated deep to the fascia covering the supinator and the extensor carpi ulnaris muscles by applying a varus or supination moment to the elbow (Fig. 1). At its origin on the lateral epicondyle and throughout the rest of its course it blends with the fibers of the lateral collateral/annular ligament complex from which it is indistinguishable.

Surgical Exposures

The posterior approach to the elbow has become the universal incision; in fact its utility and versatility led to the expression that "the front door to the elbow is at the back." It permits access to the ulnar nerve, the posterior elbow by posteromedial or posterolateral arthrotomies, and the anterior elbow via the deep portion of the Kocher approach. A posterior incision should not cross the tip of

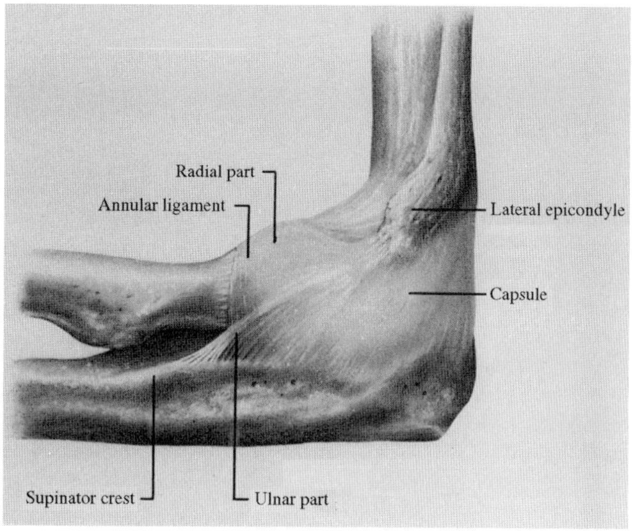

Fig. 1 The lateral collateral ligament is a capsuloligamentous complex consisting of an ulnar part, a radial part, and the annular ligament. The ulnar part has fibers that pass from the lateral epicondyle over the annular ligament (with which it blends) to insert on to the tubercle of the supinator crest on the ulna. It is distinct only near its insertion; further proximally it blends with the rest of the collateral ligament complex and the overlying common extensor tendon. It is the primary constraint to posterolateral rotatory instability of the elbow. The lateral collateral ligament complex is isometric at its origin on the lateral epicondyle. (Reproduced with permission from O'Driscoll SW, Horii E, Morrey BF, et al: Anatomy of the ulnar part of the lateral ligament of the elbow. *Clin Orthop* 1992;5:296–303.)

the olecranon; it should be slightly medial or slightly lateral. If there is a scar from a previous incision, it should almost always be used rather than making a new incision that might create a devascularized skin bridge. Careful dissection and handling of the ulnar nerve is important, and its blood supply must be preserved by avoiding skeletonizing the nerve. Access to the elbow joint can be accomplished using the Bryan-Morrey (Mayo) triceps-sparing approach by reflecting the triceps and anconeus as a flap. This approach is anatomic, versatile, and extensile, but requires careful technique and is occasionally complicated by triceps weakness. In certain cases, it is possible to leave the triceps attached to the olecranon and work on either side of it. This procedure greatly facilitates rehabilitation and prevents triceps weakness. In other cases, only the deep portion of the Kocher approach is needed. An olecranon osteotomy is used mainly for distal humeral fractures. Its main complication is the requirement for hardware removal, but it also has the potential for olecranon nonunion. The lateral Kocher approach is easy, quick, familiar to most, and extensile. It permits exposure of the entire joint, but not the ulnar nerve. The LCL traditionally has been divided longitudinally, but it can be left intact and the joint opened anterior and posterior to it. The latter modification to this approach should be considered whenever possible. The other approaches: anterior, medial, two-incision, and so forth each have more limited indications.

Arthroscopy

There has been an explosion of interest in elbow arthroscopy, which is now being performed by a rapidly increasing number of surgeons. Its role in the diagnosis and management of elbow problems has been partially established, but continues to evolve. Techniques such as capsular distension to displace the anterior neurovascular structures away from the instruments are well established.

Diagnostic Arthroscopy

Patients with suspected loose bodies can best be diagnosed with arthroscopy. The posterior compartment must be examined, because loose bodies may be missed there. Preoperative radiographs can be falsely negative in one fourth of patients with loose bodies, and the number of loose bodies present is often underestimated based on the preoperative radiographs. Those patients with pain and abnormal clinical or radiographic findings in whom the diagnosis remains obscure or unknown can usually be diagnosed by arthroscopy. Patients with snapping and idiopathic contractures of spontaneous onset usually have intra-articular pathology that can be identified with arthroscopy. Subtle degrees of valgus laxity due to partial tearing of the MCL from chronic valgus overload can be identified with the arthroscopic valgus stress test. It is performed by applying a valgus stress with the elbow flexed 70° while viewing the medial side of the ulnohumeral articulation from the anterolateral portal and observing for excessive opening. Patients who have pain but normal findings on examination and standard investigations typically remain undiagnosed after arthroscopy. Thus, diagnostic arthroscopy does not substitute for a careful history and physical examination or routine investigations. Diagnostic arthroscopy may assist in establishing a diagnosis in patients who present with snapping of the elbow or signs and symptoms consistent with cartilaginous loose bodies, posttraumatic arthritis, primary degenerative arthritis, dense soft-tissue adhesions (for example following radial head excision), ulnohumeral rotatory instability, and apparently spontaneous contractures. Patients with spontaneous onset of contracture typically are found to have a form of inflammatory arthritis.

Therapeutic Arthroscopy

The ideal indication for surgical arthroscopy is the removal of isolated loose bodies. However, patients with posttraumatic or primary degenerative arthritis associated with loose bodies do not benefit from simple loose body removal. The same is true for those with contractures. Not all loose bodies are detectable radiographically, and many patients have more than one loose body. Therefore, both anterior and posterior compartments should be examined. Other indications for surgical arthroscopy include debridement for OCD, debridement and localized synovectomy in

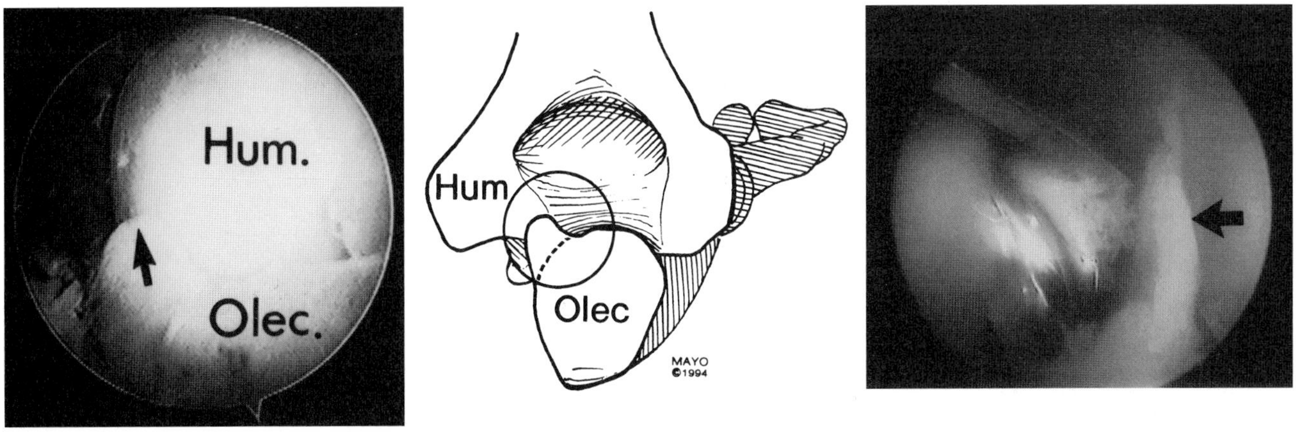

Fig. 2 Posteromedial osteophyte (arrrow) on the olecranon (Olec.) as seen in overhead throwing athletes from abutment of olecranon against the posterior humerus (Hum.). **Left,** The arrow indicates the posteromedial osteophyte. **Center,** The dotted line indicates the usual contour of the olecranon. (Reproduced with permission from the Mayo Foundation.) **Right,** The osteophytes can be removed with a burr, but this method often leaves cartilaginous projections (arrow). Attempts to remove these with the burr can damage the cartilage of the distal humerus. An effective way to remove them is with a small curved osteotome.

patients with posttraumatic arthritis, and removal of osteophytes from the olecranon and coronoid as well as from the olecranon and coronoid fossae in patients with early-stage primary degenerative arthritis (Fig. 2). Synovectomy is practical and efficacious for the management of inflammatory or septic arthritis, although it is technically highly demanding. The surgeon must be constantly aware of the fact that the neurovascular structures may be within 2 mm of the operating instruments in the anterior part of the elbow. Although the safety of arthroscopic synovectomy has not yet been clearly proven, the advantages over open synovectomy are readily apparent to those experienced with both techniques.

Arthroscopic capsular release for elbow stiffness (usually posttraumatic) is being performed in some centers (Fig. 3). Arthroscopy in stiff elbows is much more difficult than might be expected. Because the capsule is contracted and the intracapsular capacity is less than half that of normal elbows, the space available in which to work in the anterior elbow is reduced. Also, capsular compliance may be reduced to 14% of normal, indicating that the capsule is not as distensible either. Displacement of the anterior neurovascular structures away from the arthroscopic instruments by capsular distension may not be possible in stiff elbows. Also, nerves sometimes pass right through the thickened scar tissue surrounding the anterior capsule. Until this technique is proven safe, it should be considered experimental, and performed only by those individuals experienced with both open treatment of stiff elbows and elbow arthroscopy, because the risk of neurovascular injury may actually be higher in patients treated with arthroscopic capsular release. One recent report on arthroscopic release of simple elbow contractures included a permanent nerve injury.

Minor complications occur in 10% to 20% of patients and are usually not permanent. The prevalence of nerve injuries is not yet defined, but the number of anecdotal reports of cases is a serious concern. Substantial experience with arthroscopy in general and a thorough knowledge of normal and abnormal anatomy of the elbow are prerequisites to the safe and successful use of this procedure.

Elbow Instability

Recurrent Elbow Instability

Recurrent elbow instability is now better understood based on studies of the pathoanatomy, mechanism of injury, kinematics, and subsequent clinical experience. Elbow instability is a spectrum from subluxation to dislocation based on the extent of pathology (Fig. 4). In virtually all cases, the LCL complex is detached or attenuated. Damage to the ulnar part of the LCL is the essential lesion, because this structure normally prevents the ulna from rotating away from the humerus as occurs with recurrent elbow dislocation or subluxation. The MCL may or may not be intact. Posterolateral rotatory instability is being diagnosed with increasing frequency since its discovery, probably due to increased awareness of the condition.

Patients typically present with a history of recurrent painful clicking, snapping, clunking, or locking of the elbow, and careful interrogation reveals that this occurs in the extension half of the arc with the forearm in supination. A history of trauma (usually a dislocation but sometimes just a sprain) or surgery is usually present. Iatrogenic surgical causes include radial head excision and lateral release for tennis elbow (due to violation of the ulnar part

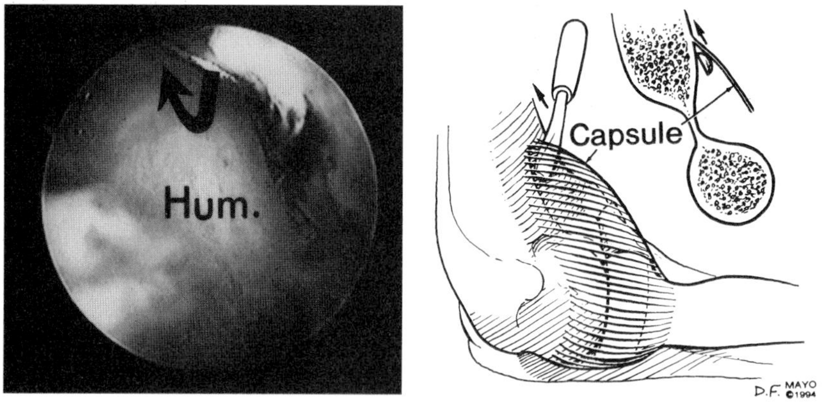

Fig. 3 The role of arthroscopy in release of posttraumatic capsular contractures is being explored. Various techniques are under consideration, including direct division of the capsule. There is usually excessive scarring, with distortion of the normal anatomy, which places the anterior neurovascular structures (especially the radial nerve) at risk. A safer technique being used by some is to release the contracted capsule and scar from the humerus (Hum.) with a sweeping motion from distal to proximal (arrow) using a blunt periosteal elevator. (Reproduced with permission from the Mayo Foundation.)

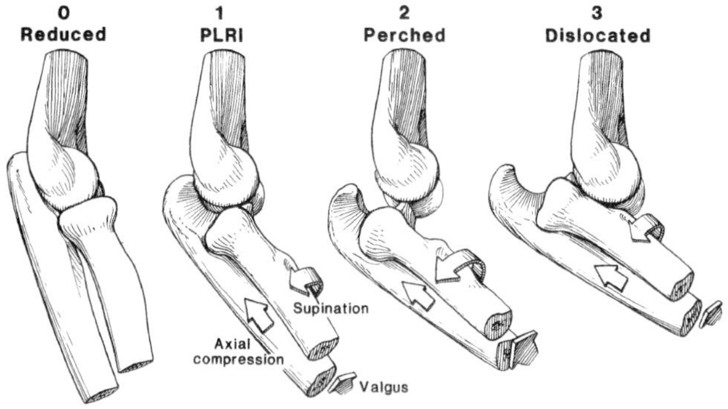

Fig. 4 Elbow instability is a spectrum from subluxation to dislocation, which can be thought of in three stages that correlate with the pathoanatomic stages of capsuloligamentous disruption and dictate treatment. PLRI refers to posterior lateral rotatory instability. The forces and moments responsible for displacements are illustrated by the arrows. (Reproduced with permission from O'Driscoll SW, Horii E, Morrey BF, et al: Anatomy of the ulnar part of the lateral ligament of the elbow. *Clin Orthop* 1992;5:296–303.)

of the LCL). Some patients with excessive soft-tissue laxity from long-term crutch walking or connective tissue disorders may also complain of such instability. The physical examination is typically unremarkable except for a positive lateral pivot shift apprehension test or posterolateral rotatory apprehension test (Fig. 5). With the patient in the supine position and the effected extremity overhead, the wrist and elbow are grasped in the same way as the ankle and knee when examining the leg. The forearm is supinated with a mild force at the wrist, and a valgus moment is applied to the elbow during flexion. This maneuver results in a typical apprehension response with reproduction of the patient's symptoms and a sense that the elbow is about to dislocate. The actual subluxation and the clunk that occurs with reduction can usually be reproduced with the patient under general anesthetic or, occasionally, after injecting local anesthetic into the elbow joint. The lateral pivot shift test performed in that manner results in subluxation of the radius and ulna off the humerus, which causes a prominence posterolaterally over the radial head and a dimple between the radial head and the capitellum (Fig. 5). As the elbow is flexed to approximately 40° to 60° or more, reduction of the ulna and radius together on the humerus occurs suddenly with a palpable visible clunk. A lateral stress radiograph taken prior to the clunk can help demonstrate the rotatory subluxation (Fig. 6).

Surgical correction is performed by reattaching the avulsed LCL or reconstructing it with a tendon graft such as that of the palmaris longus or the semitendinosus (Fig. 7). The current reconstruction technique involves isometric placement of the origin on the lateral epicondyle and fixation to bone at either end. When valgus instability is present, the MCL is also reconstructed. The surgeon must be cautious because what appears clinically to be valgus instability may actually be due to posterolateral rotatory instability. True valgus instability can be distinguished by testing for valgus laxity with the forearm fully pronated (to prevent the ulna subluxating off the humerus).

There appears to be no need for unusual, nonanatomic procedures for ligament reconstruction in recurrent or chronic instability. For example, transarticular pinning of the elbow for subluxation is no longer indicated. Immediate motion is possible, and stability has been maintained. The current approach in acutely injured elbows is to start immediate motion; those that are too unstable are reconstructed to permit such early motion. Clinical experience with aggressive ligament reconstruction in complex fracture dislocations of the elbow has been promising and supports these principles.

Chronic Elbow Dislocations

Chronic elbow dislocations are treated on similar principles. The additional factors of stiffness and joint surface damage are managed as indicated in the next section. The

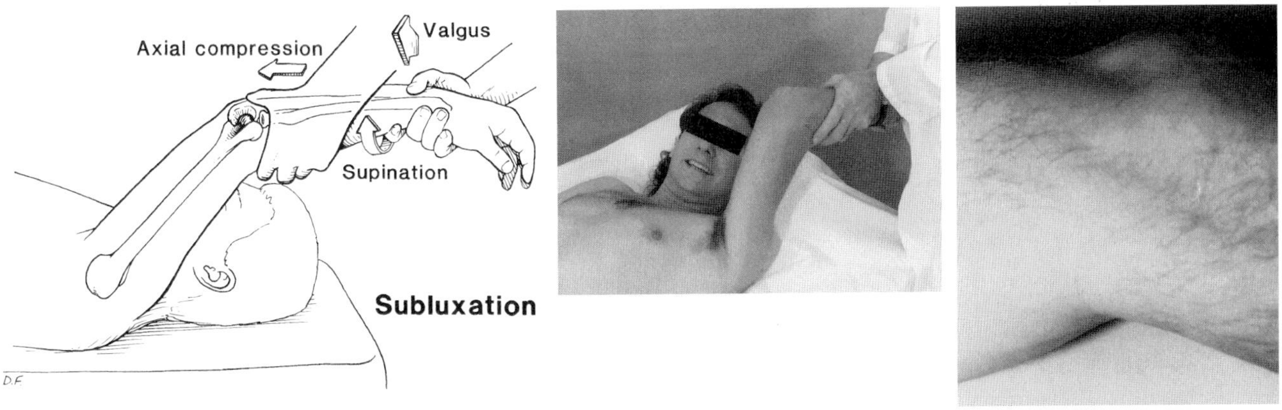

Fig. 5 **Left,** The lateral pivot shift test of the elbow for posterolateral rotatory instability is most easily performed with the arm in the overhead position. In this position the test is similiar to the examination of the lower extremity for anterior cruciate insufficiency of the knee. While flexing the elbow from the extended position, a combination of axial compression as well as valgus and suppination moments are applied to the elbow to cause it to subluxate. When the elbow is flexed past a certain position (typically 30° to 60° of flexion) the subluxation reduces with a palpable and visible clunk. (Reproduced with permission from O'Driscoll SW, Bell DF, Morrey BF: Posterolateral rotary instability of the elbow. *J Bone Joint Surg* 1991;73A:440–446.) **Center,** A patient with posterolateral rotatory instability of the elbow demonstrating a positive apprehension sign during the lateral pivot shift test. This is a highly sensitive sign and, in fact, the most important one in the awake patient because most patients are not able to relax adequately to permit subluxation of the elbow during the lateral pivot shift test. **Right,** A close up lateral view of the elbow with the arm in the same position as shown in the *center* (overhead, so that the head of the patient is to the left and the hand is to the right). Subluxation is marked by a prominence over the posterolateral aspect of the elbow and a dimple behind the radial head where the skin is "sucked into" the space between the ulna and the humerus as the elbow opens up. (Reproduced with permission from Frymoyer (ed): *Orthopaedic Knowledge Update 4.* Rosemont, IL, American Academy of Orthopaedic Surgeons, 1993, pp 335–352.)

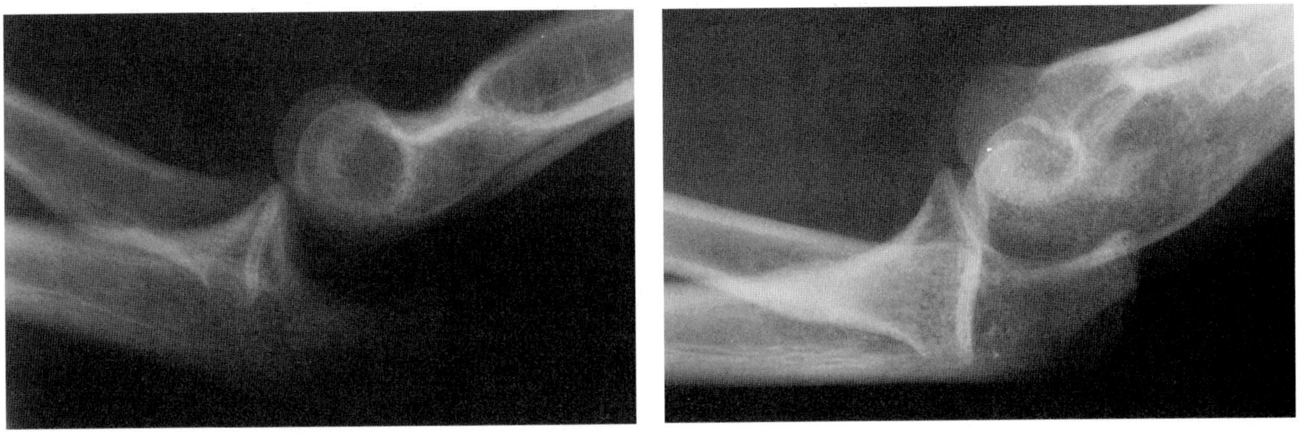

Fig. 6 **Left,** Lateral radiograph during the lateral pivot shift test showing posterolateral rotatory instability of the elbow, the features of which are ulnohumeral rotatory subluxation with the ulna supinating away from the humerus and creating a gap there. The radial head moves with the ulna so that the radiohumeral joint is also subluxated. **Right,** An oblique radiograph of the same elbow shows what is typically seen. The ulnohumeral subluxation is not as obvious because of overlying bone shadows, and the radial head appears to be subluxated posteriorly. This combination of features is responsible for this condition being mistakenly diagnosed as isolated posterior dislocation of the radial head when in fact the proximal radioulnar joint is reduced and the annular ligament is intact. (Reproduced with permission from Frymoyer JW (ed): *Orthopaedic Knowledge Update 4.* Rosemont, IL, American Academy of Orthopaedic Surgeons, 1993, pp 335–352.)

scar is excised, the joints resurfaced if destroyed, and the ligaments reconstructed. A hinged external fixation device is usually used to maintain stability while the soft tissues heal.

Valgus Instability The AMCL is the primary constraint to valgus instability, and the radial head is a secondary constraint. The radial head can be excised without significant valgus instability if the AMCL and the ulnohumeral

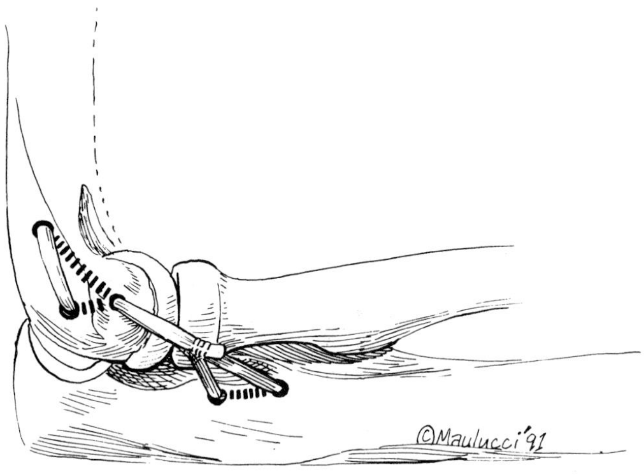

Fig. 7 Reconstruction of the ulnar part of the lateral collateral ligament (lateral ulnar collateral ligament) for the treatment of posterolateral rotatory instability of the elbow, is performed using the palmaris longus tendon graft attached to the ulna on either side of the tubercle of the supinator crest and to the humerus at the isometric point of origin on the lateral epicondyle (Reproduced with permission from Gino Maulucci, medical illustrator.)

articulation are intact. If the AMCL is not intact, every effort should be made to preserve the radial head and to repair or reconstruct the AMCL. Replacement of the radial head is not indicated following excision for a fracture unless there is medial collateral laxity and valgus instability or damage to the articulation (such as a coronoid fracture) that also compromises stability.

Chronic Valgus Overload Chronic valgus overload in throwers and overhead athletes can result in attenuation or detachment of the AMCL and is treated by reconstruction using a palmaris longus tendon graft. Ulnar nerve symptoms may be present, and if significant, are treated by ulnar nerve transposition at the time of surgery. Otherwise, the ulnar nerve is left in situ because routine transposition causes ulnar nerve complications in a small percentage of operations.

Chronic Posterior Dislocation of the Radial Head Isolated chronic posterior subluxation and dislocation of the radial head is classified into three types, according to the position of the anterior margin of the radial head: type I, above a horizontal line through the middle of the capitellum; type II, below a horizontal line through the middle of the capitellum; and type III, posterior to a vertical line through the middle of the capitellum. Type I is the most likely to go on to early painful degenerative changes, and type III least likely to. These outcomes are analogous to what occurs in developmental dysplasia of the hip when subluxated incongruent hips are compared to those with high posterior dislocations. Early radial head excision has not caused distal radioulnar problems. This is a very useful classification system that can be directly applied to clinical practices.

Stiffness and Ankylosis

The most common complication following elbow surgery or trauma is stiffness. The elbow also has a propensity for heterotopic ossification. The management of a stiff elbow can be thought of in terms of prevention, nonsurgical treatment, and surgical treatment. Soft-tissue contractures are prevented largely by early (preferably immediate) movement through a relatively full arc of motion. Soft-tissue contractures of less than 1 year duration can be treated with patient-adjusted static splints. These splints are also very helpful in preventing contractures in those patients who are slow to regain motion postoperatively. Using the principles of viscoelasticity, patient-adjusted static splints permit the contracted periarticular soft tissues to elongate by stress relaxation. This method is highly effective for regaining range of motion in the first 6 months following injury or surgery. Clinically important improvements can occur after 6 months, although the likelihood of such improvement occurring decreases up to a year following injury or surgery, after which time virtually no improvement can be expected. Physical therapy tends to be unsuccessful in the treatment of established contractures.

Patients who lack the functional arcs of motion (30° to 130° of flexion and 50° of pronation to 50° of supination) usually experience impairment of their activities of daily living (ADLs). The indications for surgery include impairment of function with limitation in the ADLs or other important activities that a patient may wish to pursue. The preoperative evaluation includes a careful history and physical examination, standard radiographs, and lateral tomograms. Contractures are classified as intrinsic (intra-articular adhesions, articular incongruity) or extrinsic (capsular contracture, heterotopic ossification, extra-articular malunion). Intrinsic contractures usually have extrinsic soft-tissue contractures.

Surgery is perhaps best performed through a posterolateral skin incision, which can then be used for any subsequent operations around the elbow. The deep portion of the approach is the modified lateral Kocher for extrinsic contractures. The traditional Kocher or the Bryan-Morrey approaches are preferred for intrinsic contractures. The selection of a surgical approach must take into consideration all necessary surgical steps, including access to the anterior and posterior aspects of the elbow as well as the requirement for anterior and posterior capsulectomies or removal of bone. A posterior approach is the most versatile and by raising flaps permits identification of the ulnar nerve and access to the entire joint. A lateral approach is highly versatile, although it sometimes requires a separate medial incision to ensure safety of the ulnar nerve. The anterior approach is indicated only in the presence of an isolated flexion contracture, with normal full flexion of the elbow and no evidence on the preoperative tomograms of bony abnormalities at the olecranon or in the olecranon fossa. This exposure is the most restricted, and therefore, its indications are limited. Its use in the presence of an extension contracture (loss of full flexion) is contraindicated, because it will not permit improvement in flexion and its use has been associated with loss of flexion. Flexion and extension contractures should be released at the same time if they are present.

The results of surgery are gratifying. When the principles outlined above have been adhered to, about 95% of patients can be expected to gain motion from surgery, about 90% to be within 10° of the functional arc of motion, and 80% to achieve a functional arc of motion. The preoperative severity of the contracture does not necessarily affect the final motion gained, although it does determine the complexity of the surgery required. More complex procedures, including distraction arthroplasty using fascia lata, have similar results because the complexity of the surgery is a function of the preoperative status and severity of the contracture. Distraction arthroplasty is highly demanding and requires significant experience. Many of these patients have had previous surgery and scarring around the elbow, which predisposes to soft-tissue problems and wound infection. There is a risk for significant neurovascular injury.

Radioulnar Synostosis

The best treatment for radioulnar synostosis is prevention. It can occur whenever subperiosteal stripping is performed and the radius and ulna are exposed through the same incision. Avoidance of such exposures and minimizing bone dust in the wound probably are helpful. Treatment of an acquired radioulnar synostosis depends to a certain extent on the level of the cross union, but overall a functional or nearly functional range of motion is achieved in approximately one half of the cases. Rarely is it possible to achieve a nearly full arc of pronation–supination, and this may be due to soft-tissue contracture.

Flail Elbow

The primary purpose of the elbow is to place the hand in space; therefore, a flail elbow typically results in significant functional impairment, although not necessarily pain. Bracing is not particularly successful. If the elbow is flail due to periarticular or intra-articular nonunions, treatment by open reduction, internal fixation, and bone grafting is appropriate if the patient is young. Recently, satisfactory results have been achieved with aggressive release of contractures and rigid internal fixation. However, in most cases there is extensive bone and soft-tissue loss. Fortunately, treatment by semiconstrained total elbow replacement (see below) is highly successful in restoring function and stability. In fact, the most gratifying results of elbow reconstruction are seen in these patients, who preoperatively have no or little use of the limb, and postoperatively frequently have normal or close to normal motion, strength, stability, and no pain.

Arthritis

Osteoarthritis

Primary osteoarthritis of the elbow, characteristic in its clinical and radiographic presentations, is a disorder almost exclusive to males. Men with a history of heavy use of the arm, weightlifters, and throwing athletes present in their third to eighth decades with mechanical impingement pain at the extremes of motion, classically in extension more than in flexion. Carrying anything, such as a briefcase, with the elbow extended is painful. Pain in the midarc of motion is present only in the late stage. A flexion contracture of approximately 30° is typical and may be associated with some loss of flexion as well. The typical finding is pain on forced extension or flexion. Radiographs show osteophytes on the olecranon and coronoid, osteophytes filling in the olecranon and coronoid fossae, and usually loose bodies, which may not be "loose" because they are often stuck in the synovium (Fig. 8). The radioulnar joint and, finally, the radiohumeral joint may become involved.

Treatment of primary degenerative arthritis is possible in the early stages by removal of the osteophytes from the olecranon and coronoid as well as from the olecranon fossa. Removal can be done by open or arthroscopic surgery. The open procedure is known as the Outerbridge-Kashiwagi (OK) or ulnohumeral arthroplasty. Improvement in pain and function occurs in approximately 90% of

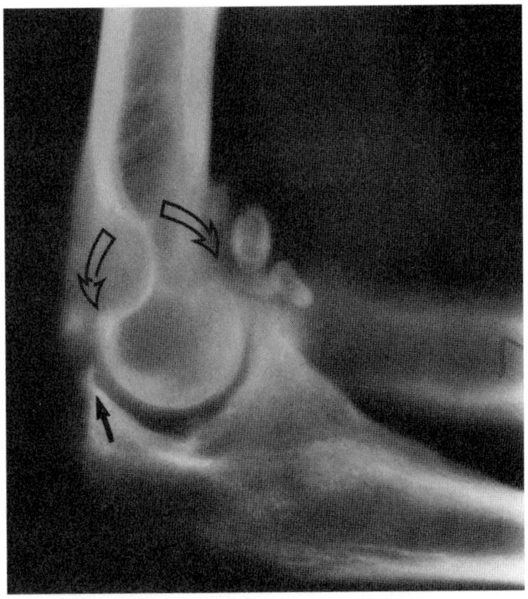

Fig. 8 Lateral tomogram showing the characteristic findings of osteoarthritis of the elbow with osteophytes on the tips of the olecranon (solid arrow) and coronoid as well as in the coronoid fossa and olecranon fossa (hollow arrows), as indicated by "filling in" of the fossae. Loose bodies can often be seen as well.

patients. Arthroscopic treatment is possible provided that both the osteophytes and the loose bodies are removed. Simple loose body removal alone does not improve these patients; the osteophytes must be excised. Removal of osteophytes from the coronoid fossa is more difficult than from the olecranon fossa. One approach is the arthroscopic equivalent of the OK arthroplasty, in which a fenestration is created in the distal humerus to permit removal of the anterior osteophytes and loose bodies.

A more extensive open debridement, the Tsuge operation, is designed to eliminate the oteophytes around the elbow and not just in the anterior and posterior impingement areas. Distraction interposition arthroplasty has been used more for posttraumatic than primary osteoarthritis.

Posttraumatic Arthritis

Posttraumatic arthritis can occur following different injuries, but is most common with distal humeral fractures that involve intra-articular comminution. Stiffness is common. Nonunions in this region usually result in a flail dysfunctional elbow. Treatment is dictated by the pathology, complaints, and age of the patient as discussed below.

Rheumatoid Arthritis

Rheumatoid arthritis, which affects the elbow less frequently than other joints, results in painful impairment of function. The severity of the disability is profoundly evidenced by patients who, after an extended period of disability, have one elbow replaced and then request surgery on the contralateral side within just a few months. After failure of appropriate medical treatment, surgical options considered include open or arthroscopic synovectomy and capsular releases, radial head excision, interposition or resection arthroplasty, and TEA. Selection of surgery and indications differ from one center to the next, and differ substantially between North America and Europe. In general, patients younger than 60 years are considered for synovectomy, while those older than 60 years are treated by TEA.

Synovectomy is typically thought of as useful in the earlier stages of arthritis, but there is controversy regarding its success in more advanced stages. There is a trend towards radioisotope injection because of its low morbidity, or arthroscopic synovectomy by those skilled with this technique. The advantage of radial head excision appears to be more for surgical exposure in open procedures than because of any beneficial effect. It may even hasten joint destruction by altering the biomechanics of the ulnohumeral joint.

Total Elbow Arthroplasty

The evolution of TEA has had similarities to that of total knee arthroplasty and is now considered highly reliable based on medium-term clinical results. There are two types of prosthetic joint designs in current use: unlinked (unconstrained) surface replacements (Fig. 9), and linked (semiconstrained) (Fig. 10). Fully constrained hinges are of historic interest and are not indicated.

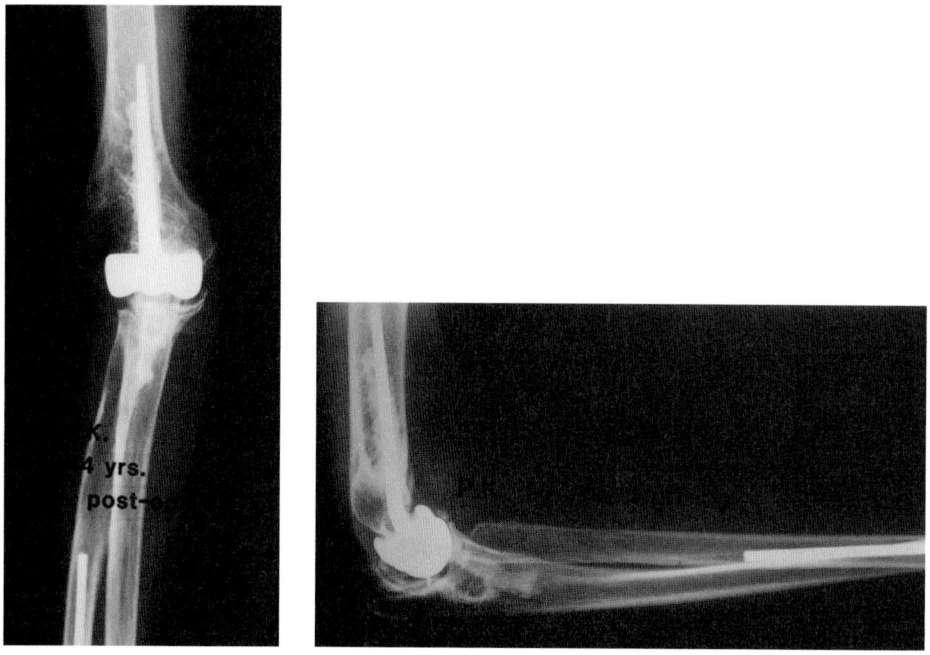

Fig. 9 Unlinked (nonconstrained) total elbow arthroplasty: Patients with adequate bone stock and soft tissues for stability can be treated with a nonconstrained arthroplasty, such as the capitellocondylar (Ewald) prosthesis. This is the oldest elbow prosthesis still in use and is reported by the originator to have excellent long-term results. (Reproduced with permission from Ewald FC, Simmons ED, Sullivan JA, et al: Capitellocondylar total elbow replacement in rheumatoid arthritis. *J Bone Joint Surg* 1993;75A:498–507.)

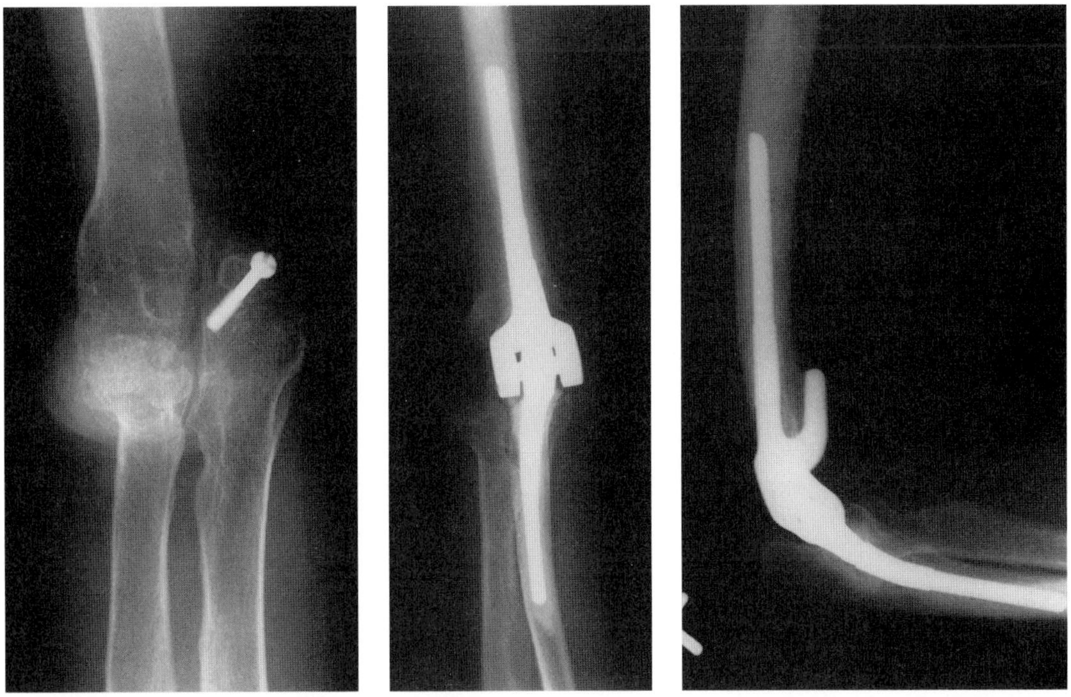

Fig. 10 Semiconstrained Total Elbow Arthroplasty (TEA): There are a number of types of semiconstrained implants available. Some use a snap-fit (which has the potential for uncoupling) while others are coupled with a loose-fitting bolt so they can not dislocate. These are necessary when bone loss is extensive, such as in the flail elbow (**left**). The Morrey-Coonrad TEA (**center and right**), has a porous-coated anterior flange under which a bone graft is placed to enhance fixation and resist the posterior forces and torsional moments on the humeral component. Incorporation of the bone graft and cortical remodeling is expected in 80% or more cases. This design has been proven to be highly versatile and clinically successful. (Reproduced with permission from Frymoyer JW (ed): *Orthopaedic Knowledge Update 4.* Rosemont, IL, American Academy of Orthopaedic Surgeons, 1993, pp 335–352.)

Indications

The indication for surgery, as for replacement of the hip, knee, or shoulder is to improve the quality of life by restoration of pain-free function (motion, stability, and strength) in a joint that is causing functional impairment. The commonest diagnosis for which TEA is performed is rheumatoid arthritis. Other indications include the treatment of supracondylar–intercondylar nonunions of the distal humerus, severely comminuted acute supracondylar–intercondylar fractures of the distal humerus in elderly patients with osteoporotic bone that cannot be reduced and fixed adequately, and flail elbow caused by posttraumatic loss of bone or structural integrity. The only absolute contraindication to TEA is active infection of the joint. Most would recommend reserving TEA for patients older than 60 years, although youth is not an absolute contraindication, just as it is not in the shoulder, knee, or hip. Loss or destruction of bone or soft tissue is not a contraindication to TEA, because these problems can be dealt with surgically. With appropriate implant selection, custom components are rarely required; such components usually are reserved for revisions or patients with juvenile rheumatoid arthritis.

In the presence of ipsilateral shoulder arthritis, the joint that is most disabling is generally operated on first. Bilateral TEAs in patients with rheumatoid arthritis can be performed simultaneously with results and morbidity comparable to those following unilateral TEA. The need for subsequent lower extremity surgery, which results in the requirement for walking aids, is not a contraindication for elbow replacement.

Biomechanics of Total Elbow Arthroplasty

As stated earlier, the elbow has been erroneously referred to as a nonweightbearing joint, even though the forces across it can exceed three times body weight. The principal forces and moments (posterior and rotational) about the humeral component of a TEA are largely responsible for loosening. The kinematics and biomechanics of several designs of TEA have been evaluated in the laboratory. The unlinked capitellocondylar design has little intrinsic constraint, relies on external forces for component stabilization, and behaves truly as a minimally constrained prosthesis. Adequate soft-tissue supports, which are properly balanced, are essential to prevent instability of this arthroplasty. The Morrey-Coonrad semiconstrained TEA has also been investigated and found to behave as a true semiconstrained joint. Simulated muscle loading stabilizes both types of prosthesis. The laxity permitted by these and other prostheses is greater than that of the normal elbow. This laxity should minimize the stress experienced by the bone–cement interface and may reduce the incidence of loosening.

Clinical Results

Pain relief after TEA is as dramatic and predictable as that found after total hip or knee replacement. At least 90% of patients are highly satisfied with pain relief. Functional improvement is also predictable following TEA. Extension strength remains relatively unchanged; this situation might be explained on the basis of surgical approach (detachment and reattachment of the triceps) and offset of the axis of rotation of the prosthesis. Excellent motion, close to the functional range, should be expected and is often possible, even in patients with complete ankylosis of the elbow. Gains in motion, especially extension, are usually greater with semiconstrained than minimally constrained prostheses. Use of the former permits complete release of contracted soft tissues and immediate unrestricted motion postoperatively; however, such soft-tissue release and unrestricted extension predispose to dislocation of surface replacement prostheses.

The incidence of instability (recurrent dislocation or subluxation) of nonconstrained elbow prostheses has decreased according to more recent reports, but still is in the range of 5% to 10%. Despite these problems, the minimally constrained TEA, such as the capitellocondylar, has been used with satisfactory long-term success for over 20 years. The inventor reported his results with 202 capitellocondylar prostheses after 2 to 15 years (mean: 6 years; Fig. 9). Pain relief and functional improvement were excellent, with patients scoring an average of 26 out of 100 points preoperatively and 91 out of 100 postoperatively on a 100-point rating scale. Repeated surgery was only required in 5% of the cases for loosening, dislocation, or infection. Also, it was the authors' impression that complications seen in earlier years had diminished. This report from the originator of the longest-used total elbow is extremely impressive and indicates that the results do not deteriorate much with time.

Dislocation can be eliminated with some semiconstrained designs. The concept is that the ulnar and humeral components are linked by a loose hinge, so that they cannot dislocate or subluxate (Fig. 10). Laxity built into the sloppy hinge permits some of the forces and moments applied across the elbow to be absorbed by the soft tissues around the elbow. The static (ligament) and dynamic (muscle) soft-tissue constraints thus theoretically take on the role that they play in a nonconstrained design and decrease the likelihood of loosening. There are a number of different semiconstrained designs, but all appear to be successful (although not all are permanently linked). They have been in use since 1976, and follow-ups averaging up to 9 years have been reported, with mechanical (nonseptic) loosening rates of less than 5%. The inventor of the most popular design reported a 95% Kaplan-Meier estimated survival at 7 years in 68 patients with rheumatoid arthritis treated by a Morrey-Coonrad TEA. There were no cases of mechanical loosening. Longer-term follow-up will determine whether or not the low incidence of loosening will continue to parallel that of the hip and knee. Problems that have been seen with some semiconstrained prostheses, such as uncoupling of the triaxial and disengagement of the axle pin in the Pritchard, have not been seen with the Morrey-Coonrad prosthesis. For these reasons, and because of the extreme versatility of this prosthesis, it is preferred by many.

The indications for minimally constrained surface replacement arthroplasties versus semiconstrained ones is not clear. At the present time, loss of bone or ligamentous integrity, ankylosis, and requirement for soft-tissue releases are indications for a semiconstrained prosthesis. The excellent clinical results with semiconstrained designs suggest that loosening might be no more common than with nonconstrained ones. The theoretical advantage of better preservation of bone stock with a resurfacing design is not necessarily true for elbows. Resurfacing designs require more resection of bone from the ulna and, in some designs, from the humerus than do certain semiconstrained ones. The theoretical advantages of a resurfacing design must be considered in light of the necessity for anatomic accuracy during insertion to avoid unbalanced eccentric forces and moments that can lead to instability and/or loosening.

Excisional Arthroplasty

Excisional arthroplasty remains an option, particularly following failed TEA. Its success (relatively pain-free, satisfactory range of active motion with reasonable stability) is more likely if the medial and lateral columns of the distal humerus remain present. If the elbow becomes flail or grossly unstable, it is usually nonfunctional.

Arthrodesis

Arthrodesis of the elbow is incompatible with satisfactory function because range of motion of the elbow is essential for use of the hand. It is almost never indicated as a primary procedure. Its indications are for intractable sepsis or situations in which there is no possibility of reconstruction by revision TEA. There might be an indication in a young man who performs heavy labor. Unfortunately, there is no single optimum position.

Annotated Bibliography

Boerboom AL, de Meyier HE, Verburg AD, et al: Arthrolysis for post-traumatic stiffness of the elbow. *Int Orthop* 1993;17:346–349.

In 12 patients who underwent arthrolysis of the elbow for posttraumatic stiffness, the arc of flexion–extension improved from 73° to 112°. Those operated on within a year of injury improved twice as much as those operated on after a longer period.

Bonutti PM, Windau JE, Ables BA, et al: Static progressive stretch to reestablish elbow range of motion. *Clin Orthop* 1994;303:128–34.

Twenty patients with elbow contractures who had limited success with other treatment modalities including surgery were treated for 1 to 3 months with patient-adjusted splints. Splints were worn for 30 minutes at a time, which allowed for stress relaxation of the contracted soft tissues. Motion increased an average of 31° (69%). No complications and no deterioration in range of motion were noted at 1-year follow-up.

Gallay SH, Richards RR, O'Driscoll SW: Intraarticular capacity and compliance of stiff and normal elbows. *Arthroscopy* 1993;9:9–13.

Elbow joint capacity and capsular compliance were measured in eight stiff and ten normal elbows of 11 patients. The capacity of the normal elbow joint was 14 ± 2 ml; that of the stiff elbow was 6 ± 3 ml. Capsular compliance of the stiff elbow was only 15% of normal, confirming that the capsule is structurally altered, not just contracted. Adequate capsular distension of the stiff elbow might not be possible, increasing the potential for neurovascular injury with use of anterior portals.

Hollister AM, Gellman H, Waters RL: The relationship of the interosseous membrane to the axis of rotation of the forearm. *Clin Orthop* 1994;298:272–276.

The relationship of the axis of rotation to the interosseous membrane was found in fresh cadaveric forearms to be constant and independent of elbow flexion or extension. The axis of rotation runs from the center of the radial head to the center of the distal ulna.

Jones GS, Savoie FH III: Arthroscopic capsular release of flexion contractures (arthrofibrosis) of the elbow. *Arthroscopy* 1993;9:277–283.

Twelve patients with flexion contractures of the elbow were managed by arthroscopic release of the proximal capsule and debridement of the olecranon fossa. Although all patients gained motion, there was one permanent injury to the posterior interosseous nerve.

King GJ, Itoi E, Niebur GL, et al: Motion and laxity of the capitellocondylar total elbow prosthesis. *J Bone Joint Surg* 1994;76A:1000–1008.

In 17 cadaveric elbows, the motion and laxity of the capitellocondylar unconstrained TEA were assessed with an electromagnetic tracking device and simulated muscle-loading. The axis of rotation of the TEAs averaged 2° of varus compared to the intact elbows. Maximum valgus–varus laxity of the TEA was 4° ± 2° greater than that of the normal elbow, indicating that it behaves as a minimally constrained prosthesis. Proper tracking of the components depends on appropriate positioning and soft-tissue tensioning.

Kraay MJ, Figgie MP, Inglis AE, et al: Primary semiconstrained total elbow arthroplasty: Survival analysis of 113 consecutive cases. *J Bone Joint Surg* 1994;76B:636–640.

A series of 113 semiconstrained TEAs in 95 patients with mixed diagnoses were analyzed for failure at a maximum follow-up of 99 months. The cumulative 5-year survival was 90% for inflammatory arthritis, versus 53% for posttraumatic arthritis or supracondylar nonunion.

Madsen F, Sojbjerg JO, Sneppen O: Late complications with the Pritchard Mark II elbow prosthesis. *J Shoulder Elbow Surg* 1994;3:17–23.

This paper presents disturbing longer-term results that show the predisposition of the axle pin to wear out and disengage, causing the prosthesis to uncouple and dislocate. A design change has been recommended and instituted.

Mahaisavariya B, Laupattarakasem W, Supachutikul A, et al: Late reduction of dislocated elbow: Need triceps be lengthened? *J Bone Joint Surg* 1993;75B:426–428.

The results in two groups of patients with late reduction of posterior elbow dislocations, one of which had lengthening of the triceps (36) and the other did not (34), were compared. The patients in the group without lengthening had better clinical results and significantly less postoperative flexion contracture ($p < 0.05$).

McAuliffe JA, Burkhalter WE, Ouellette EA, et al: Compression plate arthrodesis of the elbow. *J Bone Joint Surg* 1992;74B:300–304.

Union occurred in 14 of 15 patients in whom arthrodesis of the elbow was performed with an AO compression plate anteriorly or posteriorly. There remains no real optimum position for arthrodesis.

McKee M, Jupiter J, Toh CL, et al: Reconstruction after malunion and nonunion of intra-articular fractures of the distal humerus: Methods and results in 13 adults. *J Bone Joint Surg* 1994;76B:614–621.

Thirteen adults with painful, stiff, malunited and ununited intra-articular distal humeral fractures, including 9 with ulnar neuropathy, were treated by ulnar nerve neurolysis, anterior and posterior capsulectomy, osteotomy and open reduction where necessary, and stable internal fixation with or without bone grafting. All healed and noted improved function; the average arc of motion increased from 43° preoperatively to 97° postoperatively. Ulnar nerve function improved in all cases.

Morrey BF: Post-traumatic contracture of the elbow: Operative treatment, including distraction arthroplasty. *J Bone Joint Surg* 1990;72A:601–618.

Preoperative evaluation, surgical techniques, and postoperative rehabilitation for elbow contracture and ankylosis are described. Even for serious elbow derangements, a functional outcome is usually possible. The surgery is demanding with significant risk of complications, but patient satisfaction is high.

Morrey BF, Adams RA: Semiconstrained arthroplasty for the treatment of rheumatoid arthritis of the elbow. *J Bone Joint Surg* 1992;74A:479–490.

This paper reviews the results of 58 semiconstrained modified Coonrad TEAs for rheumatoid arthritis at an average follow-up of 4 years. Results were good or excellent in 90% of patients, with motion being greater than or equal to the functional arc of motion. Complications occurred in 22% but only 10% needed additional surgery. The Kaplan-Meier survivorship analysis revealed a 95% 7-year survival with no aseptic loosening.

Nestor BJ, O'Driscoll SW, Morrey BF: Ligamentous reconstruction for posterolateral rotatory instability of the elbow. *J Bone Joint Surg* 1992;74A:1235–1241.

Surgical reconstruction for recurrent dislocation of the elbow was performed by reconstructing the ulnar part of the LCL and plicating the attenuated lateral soft tissues. Success was over 90% in this small initial series of patients. Principles are outlined.

O'Driscoll SW: Elbow arthritis: Treatment options. *J Am Acad Orthop Surg* 1993;1:106–116.

This article reviews the current treatment options in the management of elbow arthritis.

O'Driscoll SW, An K-N, Korinek S, et al: Kinematics of semi-constrained total elbow arthroplasty. *J Bone Joint Surg* 1992;74B:297–299.

This biomechanical study in human cadaver elbows shows the Morrey-Coonrad semiconstrained elbow arthroplasty can mimic the normal kinematics of the elbow during simulated active motion with muscles loaded. Varus and valgus moments are absorbed, at least in part, by muscles about the elbow rather than transferred to the prosthesis–bone interface.

O'Driscoll SW, Bell DF, Morrey BF: Posterolateral rotatory instability of the elbow. *J Bone Joint Surg* 1991;73A:440–446.

The clinical and radiographic characteristics of this condition are described in detail, and this report is the first of a series that describe the anatomy, pathology, kinematics, surgical technique, and results of surgery for this condition.

O'Driscoll SW, Horii E, Morrey BF, et al: Anatomy of the ulnar part of the lateral collateral ligament of the elbow. *Clin Anat* 1992;5:296–303.

This anatomic study advances and corrects a misunderstanding about the anatomy of the LCL. The ulnar part of the LCL, also called the LUCL, originates isometrically on the lateral epicondyle as part of the LCL complex, passes over and blends with the annular ligament, and inserts on the ulna at the tubercle of the supinator crest just distal to the annular ligament. The LUCL is the primary constraint to posterolateral rotatory instability and is analogous to the anterior band of the MCL.

O'Driscoll SW, Morrey BF: Arthroscopy of the elbow: Diagnostic and therapeutic benefits and hazards. *J Bone Joint Surg* 1991;74A:84–94.

This article details the risks and benefits of arthroscopy of the elbow from an overall viewpoint and describes the diagnostic and therapeutic roles of this procedure.

O'Neill OR, Morrey BF, Tanaka S, et al: Compensatory motion in the upper extremity after elbow arthrodesis. *Clin Orthop* 1992;281:89–96.

Ten healthy male subjects were asked to complete a series of tasks that represented normal elbow function. They were then fitted with a custom adjustable brace that simulated elbow arthrodesis at 50°, 70°, 90°, and 110° flexion and asked to repeat the tasks. Significant impairment resulted because the adjacent shoulder and wrist joints cannot compensate.

Ogilvie-Harris DJ, Schemitsch E: Arthroscopy of the elbow for removal of loose bodies. *Arthroscopy* 1993;9:5–8.

Thirty-four patients with loose bodies in the elbow were treated arthroscopically. Overall, 89% of patients had significant improvement. There were two transient symptoms of numbness of the forearm but no permanent complications. Posterior portals should be used in all cases to avoid missing loose bodies.

Redden JF, Stanley D: Arthroscopic fenestration of the olecranon fossa in the treatment of osteoarthritis of the elbow. *Arthroscopy* 1993;9:14–16.

The authors describe their arthroscopic approach to the treatment of elbow osteoarthritis that permits debridement of the elbow joint together with the removal of intra-articular loose bodies. It is the arthroscopic equivalent of the open debridement procedure known as the Outerbridge-Kashiwagi arthroplasty.

Sakakibara H, Suzuki H, Momoi Y, et al: Elbow joint disorders in relation to vibration exposure and age in stone quarry workers. *Int Arch Occup Environ Health* 1993;65:9–12.

Elbow joint disorders were studied in 74 male stone quarry workers who operated vibrating chipping hammers and rock drills. Loss of motion and radiographic changes of osteoarthritis were significantly related to the duration of vibratory tool operation, even when the effect of age was taken into account.

Stinson LW Jr, Lennon R, Adams R, et al: The technique and efficacy of axillary catheter analgesia as an adjunct to distraction elbow arthroplasty: A prospective study. *J Shoulder Elbow Surg* 1993;2:182–189.

The use of an indwelling axillary catheter for continuous postoperative anesthesia has greatly improved the management of patients undergoing extensive elbow reconstructive surgery.

Timmerman LA, Schwartz ML, Andrews JR: Preoperative evaluation of the ulnar collateral ligament by magnetic resonance imaging and computed tomography arthrography: Evaluation in 25 baseball players with surgical confirmation. *Am J Sports Med* 1994;22:26–32.

A series of 25 baseball players with medial elbow pain were evaluated with CT arthrography, MRI, arthroscopy, and open exploration. Of the 25, 16 had an abnormal MCL. MRI and CT arthrography detected complete MCL tears accurately. A T-sign on CT arthrography indicated a partial undersurface tear of the MCL, which MRI was not sensitive in detecting.

Tsuge K, Mizuseki T: Debridement arthroplasty for advanced primary osteoarthritis of the elbow: Results of a new technique used for 29 elbows. *J Bone Joint Surg* 1994;76B:641–646.

At a mean of 64 months postoperatively, the average gain of range of motion was 34°, with good pain relief and improved grip in most patients. Two elbows required repeated surgery but there were no other serious complications.

Ward WG, Anderson TE: Elbow arthroscopy in a mostly athletic population. *J Hand Surg* 1993;18A:220–224.

Improvement in pain and function occurred in approximately 90% of 35 patients treated by arthroscopic removal of loose bodies and/or osteophytes of the elbow.

30

Wrist and Hand: Pediatric Aspects

Congenital Anomalies

Congenital deformities occur in approximately 6% to 7% of live births, with multiple anomalies in 1%. One in 626 live births has been estimated to have upper extremity anomalies, but only 10% of these patients have significant cosmetic or functional deficits. Of these congenital deformities, 1% to 2% are caused by chromosome abnormalities. A minor portion is secondary to defined genetic causes. In the majority of cases, the cause of the congenital malformation is unknown. The classification system adopted by the International Federation of Societies for Surgery of the Hand groups congenital deformities into seven categories: (1) failure of formation of parts; (2) failure of differentiation of parts; (3) duplication; (4) overgrowth; (5) undergrowth; (6) constriction band syndrome; and (7) generalized skeletal abnormalities.

In utero, the arm bud appears 26 days after fertilization and 24 hours before the appearance of the leg bud. Growth occurs in a proximal to distal fashion, and is guided by the apical ectodermal ridge, which induces the mesoderm to condense and differentiate. The upper limb anlage is initially continuous and extends to a hand paddle by day 31. The digital rays develop by day 36 with fissuring of the hand paddle, initially in the central rays, followed by the border digits. Mesenchymal differentiation also occurs in a proximal to distal fashion with chondrification, enchondral ossification, joint formation, and muscle and vascular development. Joint formation and digital separation require programmed cell death. The entire process is complete by 8 weeks postfertilization. Other major organ system development occurs simultaneously and accounts for the frequent association of cardiac, craniofacial, musculoskeletal, and renal anomalies with upper limb malformations.

Failure of Formation

Transverse Arrest Congenital amputations include amelia (absence of a limb), hemimelia (absence of the forearm and hand), acheiria (absence of the hand), adactylia (absence of digits), or aphalangia (absence of phalanges). The most common upper limb congenital amputation is a forearm level amputation (short below elbow) with an incidence of 1:20,000 live births. Upper arm amputations occur in 1:270,000 live births, and amputations related to constriction band syndrome occur in 1:15,000 live births. However, these are now considered a deformation caused by intrauterine amnionic bands and are not classified as a failure of formation.

The treatment options include observation, prosthetic fitting, and surgery. These children generally have minimal functional deficits. The cosmetic issues vary and need to be assessed on an individual basis. Early prosthetic fitting is routine for forearm level amputees when they are able to sit independently ("sit to fit"). This timing enables the child to develop spatial orientation with two limbs of equal length. The initial prosthesis is passive, with the introduction of a body-powered opening or closing terminal device at 2 to 3 years of age. Myoelectric prostheses are reserved for the adolescent or very functional body-powered prosthetic-using child. Unfortunately, long-term use of both body-powered and myoelectric prostheses is limited. The choice to discontinue use of the prosthesis most commonly occurs in adolescence. Surgery for the forearm level amputee is reserved for stump revision to improve cosmesis or prosthetic fitting.

For children with transverse deficiencies of the digits, surgical reconstruction is indicated to improve pinch and grasp. In the presence of sufficient soft-tissue pockets at the phalangeal level, nonvascularized toe phalanx transfers provide skeletal stability for pinch and grasp as well as the potential for growth of the transferred bone. Growth is most predictable if surgery is performed before 18 months of age. The periosteum and collateral ligaments of the toe phalanx should be preserved in order to enhance local revascularization and physeal preservation. In the older child with terminal digital deficiencies, surgical options include distraction lengthening, on-top plasty, intercalary bone graft, or microvascular toe transfer. Distraction lengthening requires meticulous pin care and patient cooperation to lessen the risk of complications. Lengthening is routinely performed at 1 mm/day with four 0.25-mm turns. When desired length is achieved, the external fixation device is left intact until skeletal consolidation occurs. The most common complications are pin tract infection and loosening. Intercalary bone grafting is performed with acute intraoperative skeletal lengthening. A Z- or transverse osteotomy is performed and external fixation is used intraoperatively to obtain desired length. Internal fixation with a neutralization plate stabilizes the bone graft. Five percent to 30% of initial skeletal length can be obtained using this method. On-top plasty grafts require sufficient soft-tissue coverage to lessen the risk of graft resorption. Pedicle flaps have been used for this purpose when there is insufficient local soft tissue. Microvascular toe transfer has been used for patients with monodactyly or adactyly to provide pinch. The concern is the presence of muscles, tendons, nerves, and blood vessels to provide blood supply, sensibility, and motor function to the transferred digit.

Constriction band syndrome has the most normal proximal anatomy when compared to other congenital terminal deficiencies. Vascular compromise of the transferred digit is uncommon. Postoperative malalignment and decreased mobility are common, and secondary procedures including osteotomies or tenolysis are often required to provide optimal pinch.

Phocomelia This intercalary segment deficiency is rare and is most often associated with craniofacial syndromes such as Roberts. There are three types: type I, the hand attaches directly to the trunk; type II, the forearm and hand attach directly to the trunk; and type III, the hand attaches directly to the humerus. These children become very facile and often use their feet for prehension. Treatment options include prosthetic fitting or limb lengthening with a vascularized fibula transfer or distraction osteoclasis. However, prosthetic use is often limited, and surgical lengthening is rarely indicated.

Radial Club Hand and Thumb Aplasia Radial dysplasia encompasses a broad spectrum of preaxial malformations that may involve the elbow, forearm, wrist, and thumb. The defects may be in isolation or be associated with cardiac (Holt-Oram), hematologic (Fanconi's anemia), musculoskeletal, or craniofacial (Nager's) syndromes. Radial dysplasia is usually a sporadic event, although it may be associated with chromosomal abnormalities (trisomy 18 or 21). Incidence ranges from 1:30,000 to 1:100,000 live births. It is bilateral in half of the cases. The degree of radial dysplasia ranges from complete absence of the radius and thumb to a minimally shortened radius. Classification is: (1) short radius with delayed distal physeal growth; (2) hypoplastic radius with delayed proximal and distal physeal growth; (3) partial absence of the radius; and (4) complete absence of the radius. Complete absence of the radius is the most common presentation and it is always associated with preaxial deficiencies of muscles, tendons, nerves, and blood vessels in addition to the obvious bone and joint defects. Associated hypoplasia or aplasia of the thumb is very common.

Treatment begins in the neonatal period with passive stretching exercises and corrective splints or casts. The goal is to correct the radial-sided contracture and allow passive placement of the hand on the distal aspect of the ulna. In infants with severe uncorrected deformities, distraction external fixators have been used to gradually correct the soft-tissue contracture over 6 to 12 weeks. When the soft tissues are flexible, then surgical radialization or centralization is performed if elbow range of motion is near normal. Generally, this occurs between 6 and 12 months of life. Surgical reconstruction includes centralization or radialization. Rebalancing of the tendons with transfer of the extensor carpi radialis or flexor carpi radialis to the ulnar carpus and reefing of the extensor carpi ulnaris lessens the risk of recurrence. Radial Z-plasties, ulnar excision of redundant skin, and ulnocarpal capsular reefing improve soft-tissue tension. Excision of the lunate is usually reserved for those deformities that are not otherwise correctable. Ulnar diaphyseal osteotomy is usually completed when the ulna is bowed more than 30°. It is extremely important that surgery not ablate the distal ulna physis or the forearm will become markedly shortened. In those situations, distraction osteoclasis to lengthen the forearm has been used in adolescence or adulthood. Often this requires a simultaneous wrist fusion. Complications with forearm distraction lengthening are nearly universal and include pin tract infections, neurovascular compromise, loss of digital motion and function, malalignment, poor bone healing, and refracture.

The majority of these children have hypoplasia or aplasia of their thumbs. Clinical findings include a contracted first web space, metacarpophalangeal (MCP) joint instability, thenar weakness, and interphalangeal (IP) joint stiffness or instability. Surgical treatment is indicated and should include first web space reconstruction with local flaps, opponensplasty with abductor digiti quinti or ring flexor digitorum superficialis tendon transfers, and MCP joint stabilization with ligament reconstruction or arthrodesis. Patients with aplasia and more severe forms of hypoplasia in which the basal joint is absent or unstable or the thumb has no motors (pouce flottant) are indicated for index finger pollicization. The surgical technique described by Buck-Gramko is most commonly used. Pollicization is preferred over microvascular toe transfer in this clinical setting and is generally performed between 6 and 18 months of age. The quality of the pollicized digit depends on the quality of the original index finger in terms of tendon function and joint motion.

Ulnar Club Hand Ulnar dysplasia is much less common than radial dysplasia. It is often sporadic but may be associated with other musculoskeletal defects (ulnar-fibular syndrome) or syndromes (Cornelia de Lange). Because the ulna stabilizes the elbow and the radius stabilizes the wrist, these patients predominately have elbow instability and dysfunction, whereas radial dysplasia patients have wrist instability and dysfunction. Classification is based on the degree of ulnar dysplasia: type I, hypoplasia of both proximal and distal ulna physis; type II, partial absence of ulna with radial bowing; type III, total absence of ulna; and type IV, total absence of ulna with radiohumeral synostosis. Type II is the most common.

Controversy exists regarding the ulnar anlage. In types II and III deformities, with progressive ulnar subluxation of the wrist, radial bowing, and proximal migration of the radial head, early resection of the ulnar anlage is indicated. Otherwise, resection is not indicated. Other surgical options include humeral or radial osteotomy to improve hand position and hand reconstruction to improve pinch. All are indicated if they improve function. Finally, in type II deformity with forearm instability and radial head dislocation, creation of a single bone forearm with resection of the radial head is indicated.

Cleft Hand/Symbrachydactyly Central defects of the hand have been described in the past as typical or atypical. Since 1992, the International Federation of Societies of Surgery of the Hand has classified typical cleft hands as cleft hands and atypical cleft hands as symbrachydactyly. Typical cleft hands occur in conjunction with cleft feet, have an autosomal dominant inheritance pattern, and are often associated with anomalies such as cleft lip/palate, congenital heart disease, and imperforate anus. This condition is generally bilateral and always includes partial or complete longitudinal deficiency of the middle ray. The adjacent digits are often syndactylized. Symbrachydactyly (atypical cleft hand) occurs sporadically, is not associated with other anomalies, and is unilateral. Multiple rays may be absent in the hand but the feet are normal.

Treatment of the typical cleft hand centers around closure of the cleft and reconstruction of the first web space. The thumb may be syndactylized partially or completely to the index finger. This adduction contracture needs to be corrected in conjunction with the cleft closure. Snow-Littler, Miura, and Ueba flaps involve transposition of the cleft skin to the first web space with simultaneous transposition of the index ray ulnarly. Associated fourth web space syndactylies are separated with z-plasties and skin grafts. There may be associated camptodactyly or clinodactyly of the adjacent digits requiring corrective splinting or surgery.

Symbrachydactyly reconstruction is more complex and individualized. With multiple absent digits, nonvascularized or microvascular toe transfers may be used to provide pinch function. Digital lengthening techniques are also frequently used.

Failure of Differentiation

Syndactyly Syndactyly is the most common congenital hand malformation. It may occur in isolation, be associated with other congenital hand anomalies (polydactyly, brachydactyly) or systemic malformations (Poland's, Apert's). It occurs in 1:2,000 live births and may be inherited in an autosomal dominant fashion. It is much more common in whites than blacks. It is classified as simple, involving skin only, or complex, involving skin, bones, and joints. The syndactyly may be incomplete, involving only part of the web space, or complete, involving the entire web space. Failure of the programmed cell death that allows for formation of the interdigital clefts causes this condition. The most common web space involved is the third, followed by the fourth, second, and first webs. It is bilateral in 50% of cases.

Treatment involves creation of a web space and separation of conjoined structures. There is always a need for skin graft in complete syndactylies. Local vascularized flaps, either dorsal rectangular or volar and dorsal triangular flaps, are used to reconstruct the web (Fig. 1). Skin graft, usually full thickness from the groin, is used to cover the sides of the digits. The eponychium often requires reconstruction because of conjoined nail plates. Local rota-

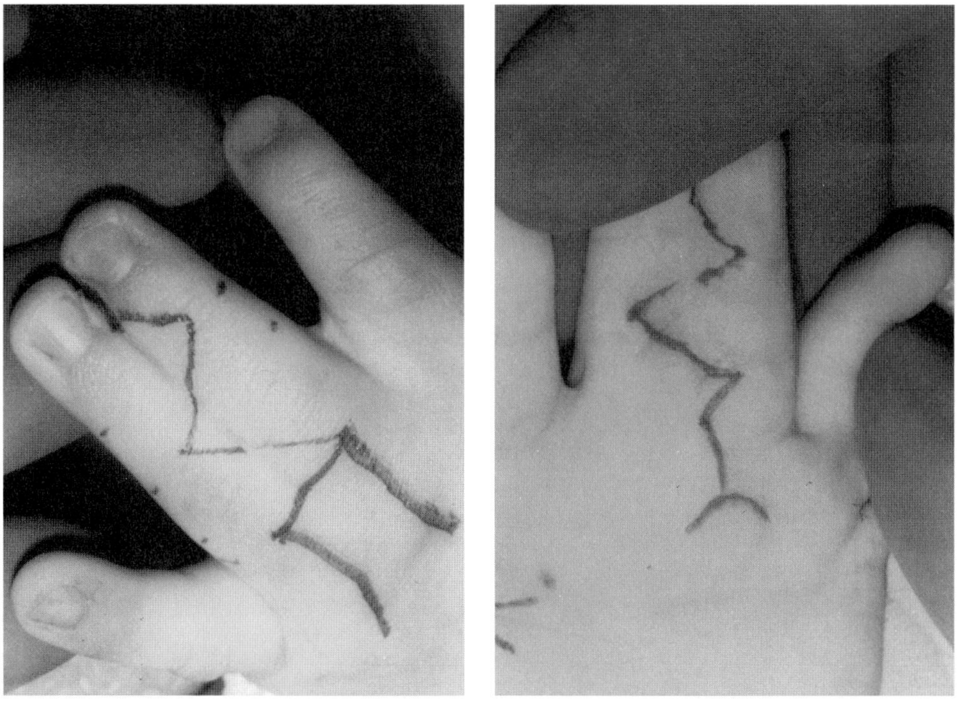

Fig. 1 Intraoperative photographs outlining skin flaps for release of a complete, simple syndactyly of the third web space. The dorsal rectangular flap provides vascularized skin for the reconstructed web space. The Z-plasties are mirror images. Full thickness skin graft will be needed dorsoulnarly and dorsoradially.

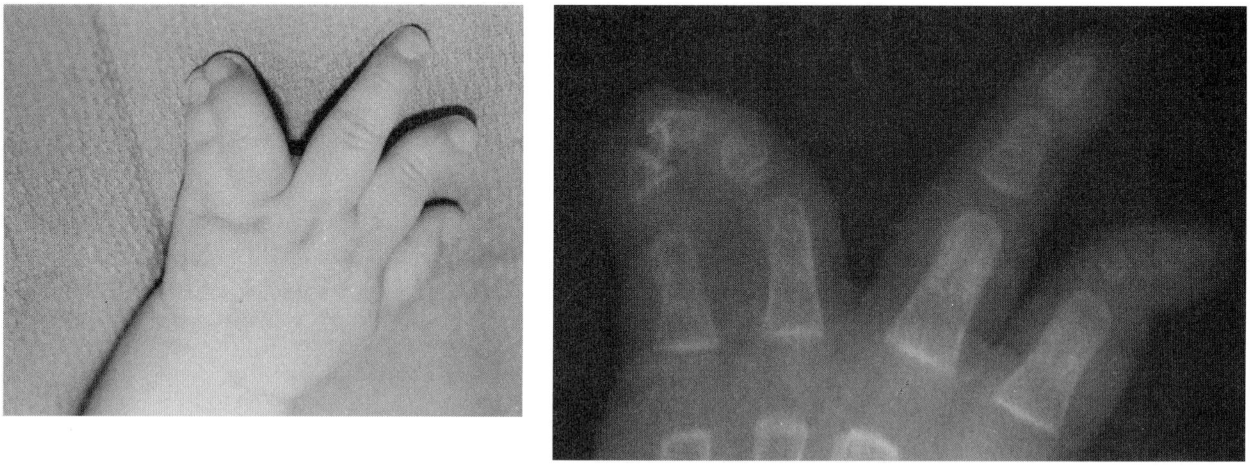

Fig. 2 Preoperative photograph (**left**) and radiograph (**right**) of a fourth web space complex syndactyly. The distal phalangeal synostosis between these digits of unequal length is causing progressive deformity. Surgical separation was performed at 4 months to lessen ring finger deformity.

tion flaps and composite skin grafts from the toe can be used to improve the contour and appearance of the nail area. Proximal dissection is limited by the digital artery bifurcation; the digital nerves do not limit dissection because the epineurium can be divided and the nerves separated.

The timing of surgery depends on the web space involved and the complexity of the deformity. Border digit syndactylies are between digits of unequal length and can cause growth deformity in the longer digit (Fig. 2). Release should be early (3 to 6 months of age) in these situations. Complex syndactylies are treated at 6 to 12 months of age. Simple, complete syndactylies between digits of similar length and incomplete syndactylies can be treated at any age before the child attends school. In all cases, the earlier the release, the higher the risk of recurrence of a mild syndactyly in the web space ("web creep"). Attempts at neonatal release have the highest risk of recurrence. In situations of multiple syndactylies (acrosyndactyly), each side of the involved digit should be released in a separate operation because of possible vascular compromise to the digit. The success of surgery depends on the degree of original deformity. Complex syndactylies may have residual limited range of motion or malalignment requiring further surgery. Simple syndactyly releases lead to normal function and pleasing cosmetic results, although skin graft is never the same as native skin in appearance. Attempts at tissue expansion have had too high a rate of complications to warrant its use.

Synostosis Synostosis occurs when conjoined structures fail to separate during development. This can lead to failure of formation of a joint (humeroulnar synostosis, symphalangism) or a fusion of normal bones (radioulnar synostosis, complex phalangeal syndactyly). The most common upper extremity synostosis is a proximal radioulnar synostosis. Treatment of this entity depends on functional impairment. A loss of forearm rotation can be compensated for by shoulder and wrist motion, except in situations of synostosis in extreme pronation. Attempts at resection of an osseous synostosis are rarely successful. The preferred treatment is derotation osteotomy through the synostosis, placing the forearm in neutral to 20° of pronation. Fixation with a longitudinal ulnar Kirschner wire (K-wire) and a transfixing K-wire is recommended because of the risk of postoperative compartment syndrome in up to 30% of patients. If a compartment syndrome develops, the transfixing K-wire can be removed to lessen the intracompartment pressure while the longitudinal K-wire maintains axial alignment.

Surgical attempts to reconstruct a joint in situations of joint synostosis have been disappointing in terms of maintaining the range of motion obtained intraoperatively. This is true even with the advent of distraction devices, such as the Ilizarov. If appropriate, corrective osteotomy to a more functional position is preferred.

Carpal coalition occurs between the lunate and triquetrium in up to 1.6% of the general population. It is most common in males and blacks. Coalitions of the capitate-hamate, trapezium-trapezoid, and pisiform-hamate also occur. Carpal coalitions may be familial and may exist with other syndromes (Holt-Oram, Turner's, arthrogryposis).

Camptodactyly Camptodactyly translates from Greek to mean "bent finger." These patients present with a flexion deformity of the proximal interphalangeal joint, most commonly in the small finger. It may manifest itself in infancy or in adolescence and can be associated with multiple other malformations. It is caused by an imbalance between the flexor and extensor mechanisms of the proximal interphalangeal (PIP) joint. Anatomic anomalies are frequent and include abnormal insertions of the lumbricals, flexor digitorum superficialis, or retinacular ligaments. Treatment is designed to restore normal flexor–extensor balance. In the infantile form, normal balance may be best achieved by progressive extension splinting. In the adolescent form, surgery is often indicated if splinting fails and the deformity is severe or progressive. Surgery is designed to correct the aberrant anatomy through release or transfer of abnormal origins or insertions. Unfortunately, the results of these procedures are often disappointing. If radiographs reveal bone and joint changes, corrective extension osteotomy is indicated rather than procedures designed to increase motion.

Clinodactyly Clinodactyly represents abnormal radial deviation in the middle phalanx or distal interphalangeal joint. It most often involves the small finger and is usually bilateral. Clinodactyly commonly occurs in otherwise normal children. It has an autosomal dominant inheritance, it is frequently associated with other syndromes (Down), and should alert the primary neonatal examiner to look for associated malformations or problems. Treatment is based on the degree of deformity. Most are mild and nonprogressive and, therefore, do not warrant surgical intervention. Progressive clinodactyly associated with a delta middle phalanx may require a closing-wedge or reverse-wedge osteotomy to improve alignment and function. Physeal bar resection and fat graft interposition have recently been reported to provide correction.

Duplication

Preaxial Polydactyly Thumb duplication may be a misnomer because it implies there are two normal thumbs; whereas, in reality, both are hypoplastic. In isolation, thumb duplication is usually a sporadic occurrence. It may be associated with genetic syndromes such as acrocephalopolysyndactyly or Robinow's. If associated with a triphalangeal thumb, it is autosomal dominant. The incidence of preaxial polydactyly is 0.08:100,000 live births. The Wassel classification system is most commonly used. This scheme is based on the number of bifid or duplicated phalanges and metacarpals. A duplicated proximal and distal phalanx is the most common type (type IV) (Fig. 3). Reconstruction involves excision of the more hypoplastic thumb, generally the radial one, and reconstruction of the remaining thumb. The extensor and flexor tendons are often eccentrically located and interconnected. They must be separated and centralized. Collateral ligaments must be preserved or reconstructed, and the thenar muscles are reattached to the base of the proximal phalanx of the retained thumb. Osteotomies are indicated to correct skeletal malalignment, and the bifid metacarpal head or proximal phalanx often seen in types IV and II must be narrowed. Occasionally surgical recombination of the distal phalanx and nail beds (Bilhaut-Clouquet procedure) in

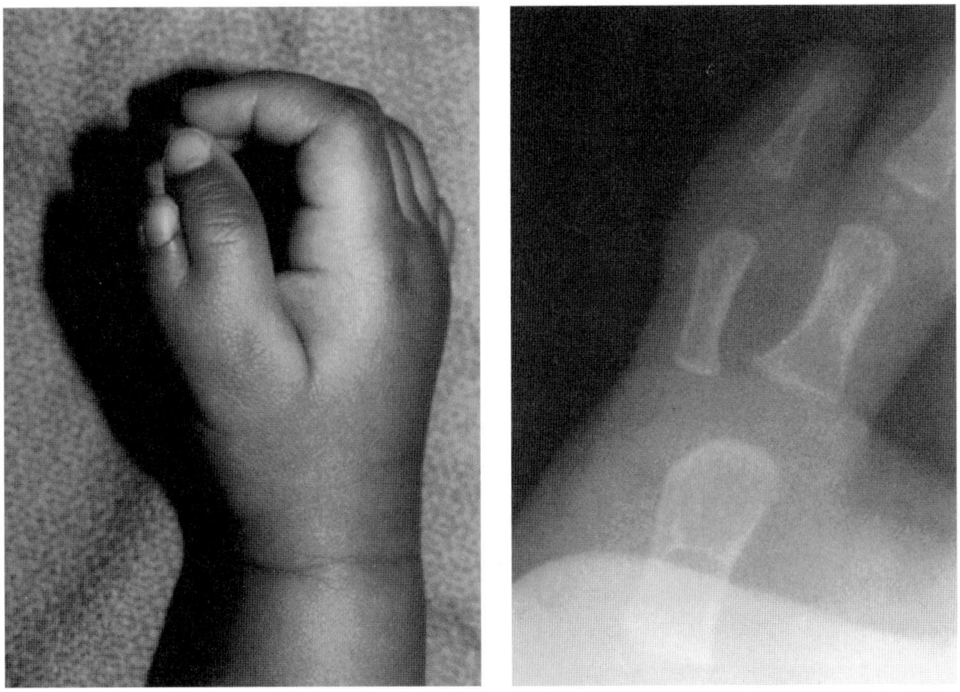

Fig. 3 Photograph (**left**) and radiograph (**right**) of a Wassel type IV thumb duplication. Surgical reconstruction involves excision of the radial-based digit including the radial aspect of the broad or bifid metacarpal head. The thenar muscles and metacarpophalangeal joint radial collateral ligament need to be transferred to the retained ulnar-based thumb.

types I and II is indicated but the results are generally disappointing because of persistent nail deformity and IP joint stiffness. Unlike postaxial polydactyly, thumb skin nubbins should never be ablated in the nursery with suture ligature because the thenar muscles attach to the radial polydactyly, and simple ablation will result in deformity and weakness of opposition.

The need for further surgery with growth may be as high as 40%; a Z-deformity of the proximal and distal phalanges is the most common problem. Adduction contracture of the first web space should be treated with 4-flap Z-plasty.

Postaxial Polydactyly Postaxial polydactyly is very common, with an incidence of 1:300 in blacks and 1:3,000 in whites. It has an autosomal dominant inheritance. It may be associated with other systemic anomalies (Ellis-van Creveld, Laurence-Moon, Bardet-Biedl syndromes). There are three types: type I, soft-tissue nubbin; type II, partial duplication including bone; type III, complete duplication including the metacarpal and phalanges. Most often, the primary care physician treats the skin nubbins with suture ligature amputation in the nursery. However, this treatment frequently leads to a residual mass at the base of the digit that many adults complain about. As a result, it may be better to excise the entire remnant, including its broad base, under local anesthesia. Duplications that include bone should be reconstructed in the operating room after the child is 6 months of age, when anesthesia is safer. Reconstruction of the tendons and ligaments follows the principles outlined in preaxial polydactyly.

Overgrowth

Fortunately for both the surgeon and the patient, macrodactyly is very uncommon. It is a very difficult problem to successfully reconstruct and the deformity is very disturbing cosmetically and socially to the patient. Macrodactyly is usually unilateral and predominately on the radial side of the hand. It most commonly affects the index finger. It more often involves multiple adjacent digits than an isolated finger, and it is often associated with neurofibromatosis of the median nerve. The differential diagnosis includes overgrowth caused by vascular or lymphatic malformations and hemihypertrophy.

Surgery is aimed at reducing the bulk of the digit. Soft-tissue resection is always a major component of treatment, but recurrent deformity is common. Epiphysiodesis and phalangeal reduction osteotomies designed to shorten and narrow the bone are commonly used. Amputation by ray resection may yield the best cosmetic and functional result in extreme cases. However, the patient and family should be forewarned that amputation may lead to accelerated growth of an adjacent digit. Most hand surgeons view this as the most difficult problem to deal with. The best results may come with very aggressive surgical interventions at an early age.

Undergrowth

Brachydactyly is a common malformation. In isolation, it has an autosomal dominant inheritance with variable penetrance. It is frequently associated with other syndromes (Turner's, Larsen's) or diseases (cretinism, sickle cell), especially with brachymetacarpia. Brachydactly most often involves the middle phalanx, especially in the small finger. It may occur in conjunction with symphalangism, camptodactyly, or clinodactyly. The presence of brachydactyly, especially brachymetacarpia, warrants systemic examination for associated malformations. Treatment options include digital lengthenings, bone grafting, microvascular transfer, or osteotomies for malalignment.

Thumb hypoplasia may cause a significant deficit in prehension and grasp. It may involve hypoplasia of the metacarpal (Cornelia de Lange's syndrome, diastrophic dwarfism) or phalanges (Rubinstein-Taybi, Apert's syndromes). It is most commonly associated with syndromes associated with radial ray deficiencies (Holt-Oram, Fanconi's). The most common presentation includes thenar muscle hypoplasia; metacarpal-phalangeal joint instability with ulnar collateral ligament deficiency; decreased first web space; interphalangeal joint instability or stiffness; and skeletal hypoplasia. These elements need to be reconstructed surgically by first web space 4-flap Z-plasty, opponensplasty, MCP joint collateral ligament reconstruction, or arthrodesis. More severe forms present with carpometacarpal (CMC) joint instability, multidirectional MCP joint instability, absent or deficient extrinsic motors, and severe skeletal hypoplasia. Recommended treatment for these patients is thumb ablation and index pollicization.

Constriction Band Syndrome

Constriction band syndrome is associated with acrosyndactyly and acral amputations. It is most likely a mechanical deformation related to early amnionic rupture with resultant oligohydramnios and amnionic bands. There is no inheritance pattern. It occurs in 1:15,000 live births. It is associated with other deformations in 50% of cases, the most common being clubfeet. There may be devastating cleft lip and facial deformations as a result of constricting amnionic bands. The ring finger is the most frequently affected. The constriction ring may lead to distal edema or cyanosis. In acrosyndactyly, there often are skin clefts that pass dorsal to volar indicating the embryonic formation of a web space before the amnionic rupture and subsequent deformation. Treatment involves excision of the constriction ring and staged Z-plasty reconstruction. This treatment frequently reduces the distal edema and cyanosis with minimal risk of recurrence. In the presence of acrosyndactyly, digits are separated with Z-plasties and skin graft.

Trigger Thumbs/Digits

Trigger thumb represents an abnormality of the flexor pollicis longus (FPL) and its tendon sheath at the A1 pulley.

There is a palpable nodular thickening ("Notta's node") of the FPL tendon at the A1 pulley, and the IP joint is usually fixed in flexion. In the past, trigger thumbs have been considered a congenital disorder. However, the vast majority are probably acquired in the first 2 years of life as evidenced by a recent prospective screening of neonates that failed to yield any trigger digits. Thirty percent of cases are bilateral. In infants younger than 9 months of age, 30% may go on to spontaneous resolution; in infants older than 1 year of age, less than 10% spontaneously resolve. Trigger digits are more often multiple and are frequently associated with syndromes (eg, Down). Surgical release of the A1 pulley and flexor tendon sheath restores normal IP joint motion. There have been no reported recurrences of trigger thumbs in infants or toddlers after surgical release. Recurrence does occur in trigger digit release.

Acquired Conditions

Cerebral Palsy

Wrist and hand involvement is common in cerebral palsy. These patients have limited hand function because wrist and finger flexor spasticity combined with weakness of wrist and digital extensors interferes with grasp, release, and pinch. Deficiencies of voluntary muscle control and sensibility also contribute to poor hand function. Patients with good voluntary muscle control, good sensibility, grade 5 muscle strength, and in-phase muscle activity by dynamic electromyography (EMG) are good candidates for surgical reconstruction and may expect an improvement in hand function after surgery. Patients with extreme spasticity, poor voluntary control, and limited sensibility often present with extreme wrist and finger flexion. Surgery in these patients may provide a more normal appearance, facilitate care of palmar skin, and assist caretakers responsible for assisting these patients with activities of daily living (ADL).

Poor release is usually secondary to flexor spasticity or contracture. Wrist and digital flexor lengthening can be performed by Z-lengthening, fractional lengthening, or flexor–pronator origin release. Flexor tendon sublimis-to-profundus lengthening will improve position but significantly weaken grasp and is not indicated in a patient with the potential for good hand function. If release is not improved by lengthening alone, then a transfer to the extensor digitorum communis may be indicated. Flexor carpi ulnaris or pronator teres transfers are most commonly used. Rarely, poor release is secondary to intrinsic tightness. Ulnar nerve block at the wrist will help determine if an ulnar motor neurectomy is indicated.

Thumb in palm deformity is common. Treatment should include release of contractures, augmentation of weak thumb extension and abduction, and stabilization of unstable MCP or IP joints. A four-flap Z-plasty of the first web space in conjunction with an adductor and first dorsal interosseous muscle release will improve passive abduction and lessen the effect of adductor spasticity. If the adductor pollicis is in phase by dynamic EMG, then release of only the transverse head with preservation of the oblique head may improve pinch postoperatively. Capsulodesis with the volar plate, fusion of the proximal phalanx epiphysis to the metacarpal head with physeal preservation in the skeletally immature, or arthrodesis in the skeletally mature all stabilize the hyperextensible MCP joint. The joint should be positioned in 20° to 30° of flexion. Transfer of the flexor carpi radialis, brachioradialis, or palmaris longus has been used to improve active thumb abduction and extension in conjunction with MCP joint stabilization.

Poor grasp is less common but secondary to wrist palmar flexion spasticity, weak wrist extension, and swan neck digital deformities. Improving active wrist extension will often increase grip strength. However, active digital extension in a neutral or extended wrist position is mandatory before a wrist dorsiflexion transfer is performed. Otherwise, tenodesis from a dorsiflexed wrist will prevent release because of digital flexion posturing. Flexor carpi ulnaris, brachioradialis, pronator teres, or extensor carpi ulnaris transfers all have been used successfully as wrist extensor transfers. Swan neck deformities are corrected by a volar PIP joint tenodesis with either a slip of the flexor digitorum superficialis tendon or the lateral band.

Juvenile Rheumatoid Arthritis

Chronic juvenile arthritis is rare. Hand and wrist involvement is most commonly secondary to polyarticular juvenile rheumatoid arthritis (JRA). It usually involves females older than 10 years of age and is usually seropositive. The IP, MCP, and radiocarpal joints are affected. The IP joints often have flexion contractures with associated synovitis. Boutonnière deformity is more common than swan neck deformity. The MCP joints are frequently radially deviated with associated ulnar deviation of the wrist. Spontaneous fusion of the intercarpal joints with subsequent carpal shortening is common. Loss of wrist extension occurs in approximately 25% of patients. The extensor tenosynovitis or wrist synovitis associated with decreased extension should not be mistaken for a dorsal wrist ganglion. Thumb CMC joint ankylosis was seen in 47% of one series of 100 patients with JRA. Growth acceleration with advanced ossification of the wrist occurs in early-onset JRA. Growth retardation occurs in long-standing or late onset JRA. The differential diagnosis of chronic juvenile arthritis includes hemophilia, multiple epiphyseal dysplasia, sickle cell disease, leukemia, child abuse, and infection. Physical therapy, splinting, and nonsteroidal anti-inflammatory medications are important to maintain joint mobility and hand function. Methotrexate treatment for a mean of 14 months led to remission of polyarticular JRA in 45% of children treated. Surgical tenosynovectomy is performed for triggering or impending tendon rupture. Wrist joint synovectomy rarely improves motion or function. PIP joint release may be indicated to improve position in severe flexion contractures.

Infections

Children, especially adolescents, are susceptible to the same hand infections as adults. The principles of treatment of infections secondary to animal bites, human bites, herpetic whitlow, and *Mycobacterium marinum* should be adhered to in children. Similarly, emergent drainage and appropriate antibiotic treatment for infections of the palmar and thenar spaces and compartments as well as the flexor tendon sheaths is also imperative in children.

Children who present with signs and symptoms consistent with a felon should be evaluated for the possibility of a distal phalangeal osteomyelitis. Initial radiographs will most likely be normal and it will be 5 to 10 days later before periosteal reaction or osteolysis appears. Therefore, emergent irrigation and debridement of the felon should include assessment of the distal phalanx for a periosteal abscess. Unilateral or bilateral axial incisions are used for drainage. The infecting organism is usually *Staphylococcus aureus.*

The differential diagnosis of a chronic paronchyia in a child includes psoriasis, candidiasis, herpes, or bacterial infection. Psoriasis is usually distinguished by nail pitting. The distinction between psoriasis and infection is important because treatment for psoriasis involves local steroid creams, which are clearly contraindicated in bacterial or fungal infections. Dermatologic consultation can be useful to assess for psoriasis as well as to perform a Tzanck test for possible herpes. Candidiasis will often have an associated diaper rash or oral involvement. Most of these children are not immunocompromised. Nail plate removal and incision and drainage is indicated only for true bacterial infections unresponsive to antibiotics.

Cellulitis in children may be the presenting manifestation of a deep-space infection, osteomyelitis, or septic arthritis, especially if there is significant soft-tissue swelling. If cellulitis is unresponsive to intravenous antibiotics, hand elevation, and immobilization, a deep-space infection should be aggressively sought. Fractures may also present with erythema and swelling that resembles infection. Finally, salmonellae osteomyelitis has been described in three of 11 cases of hand-foot syndrome in children with sickle-cell disease. The infection involves both the metaphysis and diaphysis. High fever, local tenderness and swelling, and elevated white cell or polymorphonuclear leukocyte counts were not helpful in distinguishing infection from infarction. Plain radiographs and bone scans were equivocal. Needle aspiration for culture and blood cultures should be obtained on sickle-cell patients presenting with dactylitis. Prophylactic antibiotics including *S aureus* and salmonella coverage should be initiated pending cultures.

The presence of a foreign body should also be suspected in a child with a hand infection. Plain radiographs are often negative. Ultrasound may be useful in defining the size and location of the foreign body prior to excision.

Burns

Scalding accounts for 85% of the burns sustained by children under the age of 3. At this age, most burns are caused by hot water; contact with hot objects such as heaters, irons, or stoves; or spills from cooking materials or liquids. If the burn is distributed in a stocking glove pattern without evidence of additional splash burns, child abuse should be suspected. Most of these children can be treated nonsurgically. Local wound care with nonadherent dressing changes and debridement of ruptured bullae is often all that is necessary acutely in this age group. Rapid reepithelialization occurs and skin grafts are often unnecessary. More extensive hand burns may need temporary pin fixation of the MCP joints in 70° to 90° of flexion with the IP joints in extension to prevent contractures. Elastomer and compressive gloves after acute healing can lessen scar formation. Skin grafting is reserved for more extensive third degree burns, especially in older children.

Older children and adolescents often suffer burns from experimentation with matches and gasoline. These hand burns may be associated with more extensive upper extremity or total body burns. Fluid resuscitation and care in a burn unit is necessary if the burns cover greater than 25% of the body. In that setting, more aggressive grafting, possible pedicle coverage, and escharotomies for vascular compromise are appropriate. Reconstructive surgery with Z-plasties for joint contractures and burn syndactylies are necessary if nonsurgical measures fail, if the contractures worsen with growth, or for more severe contractures.

Tumors

Benign soft-tissue tumors, such as joint ganglia, epidermal inclusion cysts, and cysts of tendon sheaths, are as common in children as they are in adults. Usually they are asymptomatic but the parents request evaluation because of concern regarding the potential malignancy of the mass. Observation of a ganglion is appropriate unless there is pain, limitation of motion or activities, or parental or physician concern regarding the diagnosis. Spontaneous resolution occurs more frequently in children than in adults. Aspiration and injection are difficult in the preadolescent. Surgery involves appropriate excision of the ganglion and its stalk.

Warts (verrucas) are common in children, usually asymptomatic unless traumatized, and often multiple. They are contagious and caused by a papova virus. Twenty-five percent resolve spontaneously in 6 months and all by 5 years. Repetitive cryotherapy is effective in two thirds of patients. Malignant hand tumors are rare in children. However, any firm, rapidly growing, painful mass, especially if in the palm, needs to be investigated thoroughly. Radiographic evaluation should include plain radiographs; hand magnetic resonance imaging (MRI) or computed tomography (CT) scans to assess soft-tissue and bony involvement; and bone scans, chest radiographs, and CT scans to stage for metastatic disease. Biopsy with both frozen and permanent sections should be staged separately from excision if malignancy is considered. Skin incisions need to allow for future resection without jeopardizing hand function. Single or multiple ray resections are most often performed for all hand malignancies, including Ewing's sarcoma, rhabdomyosarcoma, epithelioid sarcoma, and osteogenic sarcoma.

Trauma

Fractures

The hand is the most commonly injured body part in a child. Multiple series have indicated that the majority of fractures are physeal; that 80% to 90% can be treated closed; and that both growth disturbance and malunion are rare. The most common injury is a Salter-Harris II fracture of the small finger, and this occurs most commonly in the older child. In toddlers and young children, the most common injury is a distal phalanx fracture associated with a nail bed laceration or distal tip amputation from a crush injury.

Phalangeal Fractures Mallet fingers in a young child are secondary to physeal separation. Terminal tendon disruption is uncommon before adolescence because the extensor mechanism inserts into the epiphysis. These injuries may be associated with interposition of germinal matrix between the fracture fragments. Epiphyseal dislocation is rare but needs to be ruled out in a mallet finger, especially if the epiphysis is unossified. Treatment of the physeal separation includes open repair of the germinal matrix laceration and splinting of the distal phalanx in extension for 3 weeks. In a very young child, this may require a short arm cast. Chronic mallet fingers are rare in young children but may be successfully treated with surgery. Treatment of soft-tissue and bony mallets in the older child follows standard adult treatment. Distal interphalangeal (DIP) joint subluxation needs to reduced, but this can almost universally be done closed with splinting or by percutaneous pinning of the joint. Open reduction is rarely if ever indicated, even in the presence of a large fracture fragment. The complication of open reduction is subsequent loss of flexion.

Phalangeal neck fractures frequently occur and are associated with significant potential complications. Displacement of the fracture into extension and malrotation is common. The fragment is tethered by the collateral ligaments as it rotates dorsally up to 90°. The fracture is unstable and often will displace after closed reduction. Pin fixation is frequently necessary. In a young child, fixation may be accomplished with a single oblique pin. If open reduction is necessary, the collateral ligaments should not be dissected from the distal fragment. This maneuver significantly increases the risk of osteonecrosis. Frequently patients present late with an impending malunion because a satisfactory reduction was not achieved or maintained. Open reduction at this stage may increase the risk of osteonecrosis. On occasion, immature callus can be broken down by use of a percutaneous pin as a lever in the fracture site from the dorsum. This step allows for anatomic reduction and percutaneous pin fixation. Alternatively, the fracture should be allowed to heal, and a late subchondral fossa reconstruction should be performed if there is a bony block to flexion. An average of 90° of PIP joint flexion can be obtained with subchondral fossa reconstruction. Remodeling of this fracture is rare because of the significant distance from the physis but has been described in a single case report.

Intercondylar fractures in young children are often small osteochondral fractures. These have a high risk of nonunion, malunion, and osteonecrosis. This risk is particularly great in the middle phalanx if the injury is a crush injury that alters the local blood supply. In this situation, the fracture needs to be treated aggressively with open reduction while preserving the collateral ligament attachments to the fragment to lessen the risk of complication. However, this procedure does not guarantee a successful result. In the adolescent, treatment of intercondylar fractures is similar to that in adults. Anatomic reduction and pin fixation are necessary to restore the joint surface and to prevent loss of reduction that can occur with this unstable fracture. Generally this procedure can be performed closed, using distraction and a percutaneous towel clip to obtain reduction. Open reduction can be performed with a volar, midaxial, or dorsal approach. Early mobilization is important to prevent PIP joint stiffness.

Diaphyseal level phalangeal fractures are rare in a young child and more common in the teenager. The major issue with these fractures is malrotation, which may be most apparent with digital flexion (Fig. 4). Frequently children will not actively move their finger in the acute setting to allow for accurate assessment of digital rotation. However, passive wrist flexion and extension will cause enough digital motion to allow for an accurate assessment. If closed treatment is chosen, never immobilize a solitary finger but secure it to the adjacent digits to prevent subsequent loss of reduction. If the finger is malrotated and unstable, reduction with pin or screw stabilization is necessary.

Physeal fractures make up 30% to 70% of pediatric finger fractures. A Salter-Harris II fracture of the small finger is the most common. Closed reduction of the fractures is performed in MCP flexion to lessen the restraint of the more distal web space. The surgeon's thumb or a cylindrical object such as a pencil can be used. Postreduction stability is maintained by taping the digit loosely to the adjacent digit and applying a short arm mitten cast for 3 weeks. Less common type III physeal fractures require open reduction if there is greater than 2 mm of diastasis or articular step-off.

Metacarpal Fractures Boxer's fractures are common in adolescence. Closed reduction and cast immobilization with three-point fixation for 3 weeks is preferred for displaced fractures. Often these patients will not seek medical attention until there is significant healing. Fortunately, the

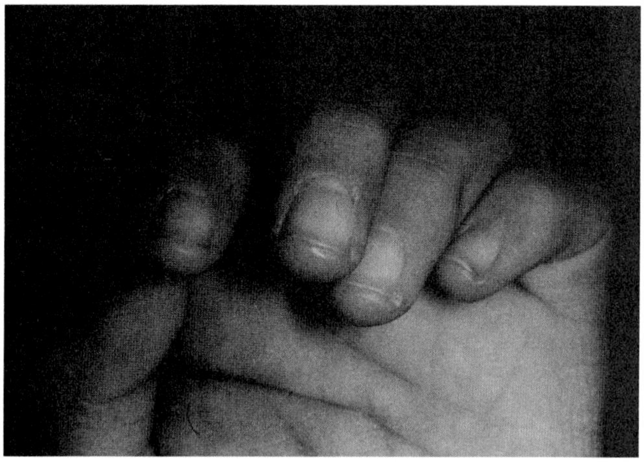

Fig. 4 Clinical photograph of digital malrotation that can be associated with phalangeal or metacarpal level fractures.

fracture is adjacent to the distal metacarpal physis, and the flexion malunion will remodel if there is sufficient growth remaining. Late open reduction carries the risk of physeal injury and should be avoided. Diaphyseal fractures of the fifth metacarpal have a higher risk of malunion that will not remodel. Closed reduction and percutaneous pinning to the adjacent metacarpals is the treatment of choice. Corrective osteotomy may be necessary in the severe, malunited diaphyseal fracture that fails to remodel a flexion deformity with growth.

The major issue with other diaphyseal metacarpal fractures, especially if there are multiple metacarpal fractures, is malrotation. Active digital motion or passive tenodesis of the wrist will allow the examiner to diagnose malrotation. Anatomic reduction and pin, screw, or plate fixation will correct the malrotation.

Thumb Fractures Two unique fractures of the thumb are Salter-Harris III fractures of the proximal phalanx and metacarpal base fractures. A type III physeal fracture of the thumb proximal phalanx is the equivalent of an adult ulnar collateral ligament disruption (Fig. 5). These fractures require open reduction and internal fixation to restore joint stability, and joint and physeal alignment. During surgical exposure, remember that the ulnar collateral ligament is intact so that after reflection of the adductor aponeurosis, the MCP joint may be exposed through the fracture site rather than by inadvertent incision of the ligament. Long-term results of anatomic open reductions are excellent.

Metaphyseal fractures at the base of the thumb metacarpal often displace. Immobilization and observation, even with displaced fractures, is appropriate because the malunited dorsal–radial prominence will remodel over the ensuing 6 to 12 months (Fig. 6). A displaced Bennet's fracture requires anatomic alignment of the intra-articular component and pin fixation of the thumb metacarpal to the adjacent second metacarpal and carpus.

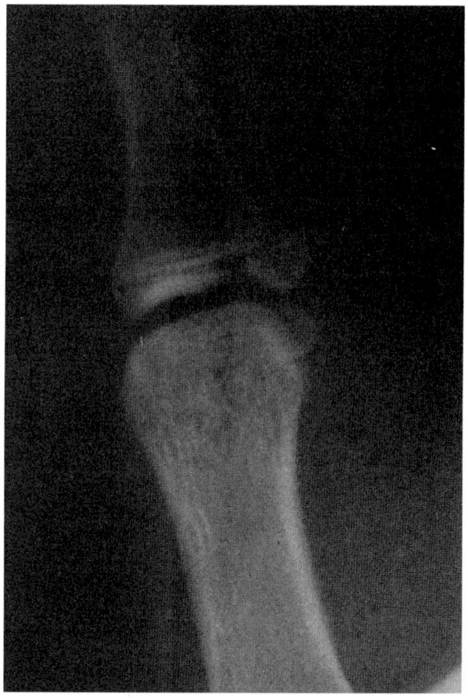

Fig. 5 Salter-Harris type III fracture of the ulnar proximal phalanx (thumb) that represents the equivalent of an ulnar collateral ligament injury in an adult. This fracture requires open reduction and internal fixation to restore the articular surface and ligamentous integrity.

Scaphoid Fractures Most scaphoid fractures in the skeletally immature patient are distal pole or avulsion fractures. These heal readily with thumb spica cast immobilization for 4 to 8 weeks without risk of nonunion or osteonecrosis. Waist fractures, however, carry the same risks of nonunion and osteonecrosis in the child as they do in an adult. Treatment of an established nonunion in a child should be with open reduction, bone grafting, and, potentially, internal fixation. Herbert screws have been used in children both with acute displaced waist fractures and with established nonunions. The issue of whether a bipartite scaphoid, even if bilateral, is congenital or post-traumatic is unresolved.

Radius and Ulna Fractures Of pediatric forearm fractures, 75% to 85% involve the distal radius. The majority of these fractures are metaphyseal and are associated with metaphyseal fractures of the ulna. Closed reduction and long arm cast immobilization has been the standard of treatment. Most recently, several studies indicate a high incidence of loss of reduction in these patients. Poor casting techniques, isolated radius fractures, associated displaced ulna fractures, and initial malangulation greater

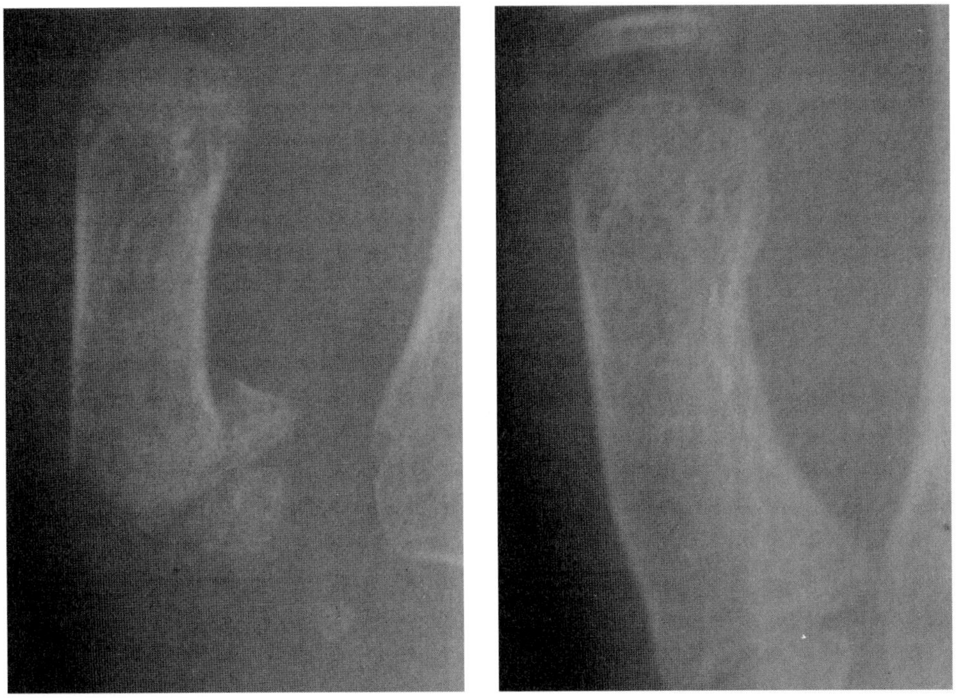

Fig. 6 Left, Base of thumb metacarpal fracture with significant displacement and angulation. **Right,** The fracture has remodeled to a near anatomic alignment in just 6 months.

than 30° have all been associated with loss of reduction. The rate of rereduction with closed treatment has been cited as high as 28%. A randomized, prospective study of isolated radius fractures (Galeazzi equivalent) indicated a 91% rate of rereduction with cast treatment versus no rereduction with percutaneous pin fixation. Malunited fractures will remodel in the flexion–extension plane and less so in the radial deviation–ulnar deviation plane. Rotational malunion will not remodel. Axis deviation, calculated from reference tables, may more accurately predict remodeling potential and outcome than malangulation alone.

Most distal radius physeal fractures are type II injuries in the adolescent. The incidence of associated nerve injuries was 8% in a prospective study. A recent retrospective series indicates that patients with symptoms or signs of median nerve injury at the time of presentation are best managed with percutaneous pin fixation rather than cast immobilization. This fixation reduces the risk of forearm compartment syndrome, acute carpal tunnel syndrome, and median neuropathy (Fig. 7). Patients whose fractures redisplace or who present 7 or more days after injury should not undergo rereduction in order to avoid iatrogenic physeal injury. If a malunion occurs but does not remodel with growth, a dorsal opening wedge osteotomy with bone graft and internal fixation can be performed when the patient is skeletally mature.

Galeazzi fractures do occur in children. Most commonly, there is an ulnar physeal fracture associated with a distal radius metaphyseal fracture. Late distal radioulnar joint instability is rare in this situation, but ulnar physeal arrest and ulnar shortening have been described. True ligamentous disruptions occur rarely and may lead to late instability, which usually presents as a volar dislocation of the ulna with forearm supination. Soft-tissue reconstruction with a portion of the fifth and sixth retinaculum and slip of the extensor carpi ulnaris tendon can stabilize the distal radioulnar joint. Any malunion causing instability should be corrected with an osteotomy.

Dislocations

Traumatic injuries to the joints in children are usually stable volar plate injuries with minimal Salter-Harris III physeal avulsions. Treatment should be brief immobilization for comfort followed by buddy taping until they are asymptomatic. This will prevent the PIP joint stiffness that can occur with prolonged immobilization. True interphalangeal dislocations are usually dorsal and occur more commonly at the PIP joint than the DIP joint. Closed reduction with distraction and dorsal to volar manipulation is generally successful. Rarely, a displaced epiphysis, flexor tendon, or interposed volar plate can block reduction and will require open reduction.

MCP dislocations of the thumb or index finger can be simple or complex. Complex dislocations are irreducible and have an interposed volar plate blocking closed reduction. Radiographs often reveal widening of the joint space as well as bayonet alignment of the proximal phalanx and metacarpal when the dislocation is complex. Open reduction can be performed through either a volar or dorsal ap-

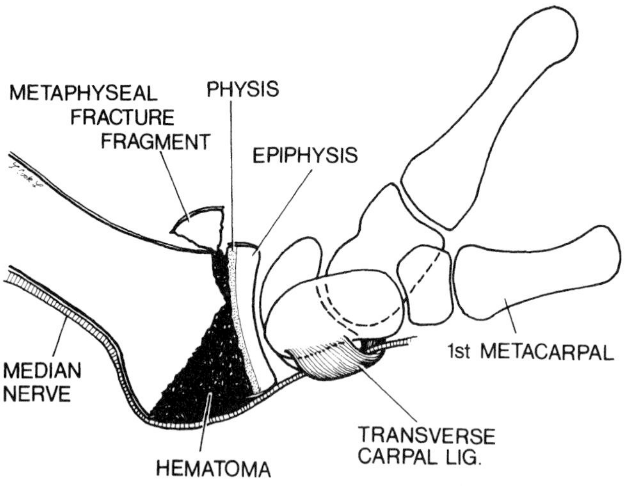

Fig. 7 Drawing depicts the possible etiology of median neuropathy with impingement of the nerve across the metaphysis and hematoma proximally and tethering by the transverse carpal ligament distally.

proach. Because the radial neurovascular bundle is tented just beneath the skin by the metacarpal head, extreme caution is necessary with the volar skin incision in order to prevent an iatrogenic nerve laceration. Regardless of approach, the volar plate must be incised and extracted from the joint to allow reduction and anatomic realignment of the flexor tendons, seasmoids, and collateral ligaments. Postoperative treatment includes early protected motion with buddy taping and extension block splinting. Chronic instability is rare, but limited MCP motion is not. The digital neurapraxia secondary to the dislocation will resolve in this age group.

Tendon Lacerations

The diagnosis, surgical care, and postoperative rehabilitation of flexor tendon injury may be more difficult in a child than an adult. This is especially true in the toddler and preschool age child, where patient cooperation is limited. Often observation of the digital cascade and digital excursion with wrist tenodesis serve as the basis for diagnosis (Fig. 8). If in doubt, explore the wound under anesthesia. Repair of tendon lacerations in zones I and II requires meticulous technique with fine sutures. In the infant, the core suture may be as fine as 6-0, and the epitenon suture an 8-0. Postoperative immobilization in a cast for 4 weeks is effective. There have been no differences in total active motion (TAM) between early mobilization protocols and cast immobilization for 4 weeks in the pediatric age group. The results of isolated profundus tendon lacerations in zone I averaged 90% to 94% of normal TAM. Isolated profundus lacerations in zone II averaged 71% to 78% of normal TAM. Combined superficialis and profundus lacerations in zone II averaged 72% TAM. However, if cast immobilization continued beyond 4 weeks, there was a significant decrease in TAM to 40% by 6 weeks. There was no difference in the results by age groups from 0 to 15 years of age. Associated nerve or palmar plate injuries slightly reduced the quality of the results. Tendon rupture following repair is rare. Two-stage reconstructions of unrecognized zone II lacerations in children have had poorer results than in adults, with a higher rate of complications and a mean TAM of only 140°. Results were better when postoperative care included supervised rehabilitation.

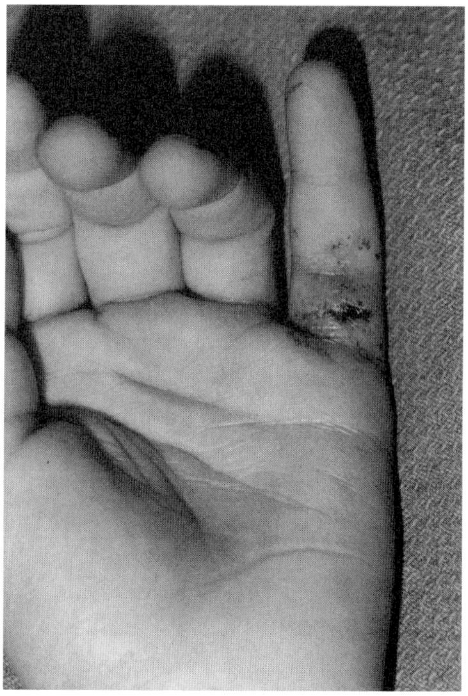

Fig. 8 Small volar proximal phalanx laceration with loss of small finger digital cascade indicative of a flexor tendon laceration.

Extensor tendon lacerations are treated the same way in a child as in an adult. Direct repair in the emergency room under sedation or in the operating room under general anesthesia is preferred. Cast immobilization in a protected position of wrist dorsiflexion and digital extension is continued for 4 weeks after repair. Results are excellent with primary repair. Associated fractures, dislocations, and flexor tendon injuries adversely affect the results.

Nerve Lacerations

Nerve lacerations should be suspected in any laceration that is deep across the path of a digital, median, or ulnar nerve. Because discriminatory sensibility does not develop until age 5 to 7 years, two point discrimination or fine light touch testing is often fruitless in younger children. If these tests are used, the examiner should always test the uninjured hand first to define accuracy. Pin prick testing may be painful and causes anxiety in a young child, making further examination impossible. An effective, nonthreatening method to assess cutaneous innervation is to soak the affected finger in saline for up to 20 minutes and to then examine for skin wrinkling. Absence of normal skin wrinkling following immersion indicates denervation. The motor examination in children may also be limited due to failure to understand instructions or anxiety. However, two easily understood maneuvers may provide important information about function of median and ulnar innervated muscles. The "good luck sign" (long finger crossed on index) requires an intact ulnar nerve and "snapping" the thumb and long finger requires an intact thenar motor nerve. Most children understand these maneuvers and are able to repeat them on request. If in doubt, explore the nerves under general anesthesia.

The results of microscopic epineural repair at digital, palmar, or wrist level in children are outstanding. The improved results in children compared to adults may be multifactorial: children have cerebral compliance that enables them to adjust to mixed peripheral signals; in the shorter limbs and digits of children, the distance from laceration to sensory end-organ is less; and the fascicular area in children may be as high as 80% compared with 60% in adults. For similar reasons, nerve grafting in late reconstruction has excellent results in children. In chronic, untreated nerve lacerations, there appears to be a decrease in digital length and girth. Finally, in failed ulnar or median nerve repairs at the forearm or wrist, tendon transfer reconstruction adheres to adult principles. However, this is rarely required.

Amputations

Fingertip amputations are very common in children. Incomplete amputations often involve the nail bed or germinal matrix and require meticulous closure with 6-0 chromic suture. Uncomplicated survival of the distal part is common with appropriate repair. Complete fingertip amputations can frequently be treated with nonadherent dressing changes. Local coverage with advancement flaps, skin grafts, composite grafts, or pedicle flaps is rarely necessary and should be reserved for significantly exposed bone. Because the physis of the distal phalanx is proximal to the level of injury, skeletal growth will continue and eventually compensate for any shortening that resulted from the injury in a toddler or preschool-age child. Longitudinal studies have found that nail deformity, digital foreshortening, and loss of sensibility are rare in children regardless of the method of treatment.

Treatment of more proximal, complete digital amputations with replantation in children as young as 1 year of age is now standard. In children, the indication for replantation is more liberal than in adults and includes multiple digit, thumb, midpalm, hand, and distal forearm amputations as well as single digit amputations in zones I and II. Crush amputations from doors, heavy objects, or bicycle chains have a peak incidence at age 5 years while sharp amputations occur more commonly in adolescents. Digital survival rates from replantation range from 69% to 89% in pediatric series. More favorable digital survival was seen

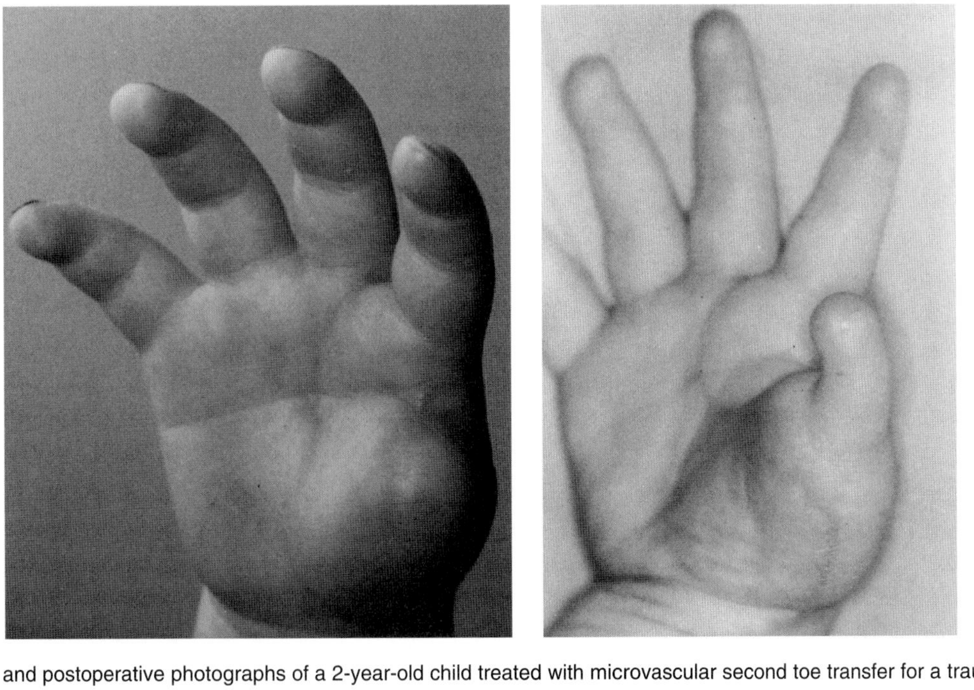

Fig. 9 Pre and postoperative photographs of a 2-year-old child treated with microvascular second toe transfer for a traumatic thumb amputation.

in sharp amputations, body weight greater than 11 kg, more than one vein repaired, bone shortening, interosseous wire fixation, and vein grafting of arteries and veins. Vessel size generally exceeds 0.8 mm in digital replants in children and is not a technical problem. Index and long finger replants have done better than small finger replants in children. A survival rate of 95% occurred in children if prompt reperfusion was seen after arterial repair, with at least one successful venous anastomosis compared with 0% survival if one or both of these were absent. Neural recovery rates far exceed those cited in adults, with return of two point discrimination less than 5 mm often present. Tenolysis may be necessary after tendon repair. Two-stage flexor tendon reconstruction in children has a higher rate of complications than in adults. Growth arrest or deformity is more common if there is a crush component to the amputation. Microvascular toe to thumb transfer is a very successful alternative to pollicization following a failed thumb replant in a young child (Fig. 9).

Annotated Bibliography

Congenital

Kruger L, Fishman S: Myoelectric and body-powered prosthesis. *J Pediatr Orthop* 1993;13:68–75.

Nationwide Shriner's Hospital experience with 120 pediatric below elbow amputees compares body-powered and myoelectric prosthetic use. Short-term preference was clearly for myoelectric prosthesis (78% versus 22%). However, only 44% used the myoelectric, 33% used the body-powered, and 23% were nonusers at 2-year follow-up.

Manske PR, Rotman MB, Dailey LA: Long-term functional results after pollicization for the congenitally deficient thumb. *J Hand Surg* 1992;17A:1064–1072.

Twenty-three patients underwent a comprehensive evaluation at an average of 8 years following surgery. Children with isolated thumb deficiencies had better results than those with associated conditions (eg, radial club hand), and age at time of surgery did not affect outcome.

Radocha RF, Netscher D, Kleinert HE: Toe phalangeal grafts in congenital hand anomalies. *J Hand Surg* 1993; 18A:833–841.

The authors report the Louisville experience with 72 nonvascularized toe phalanx transfers followed up for a mean of 42 months. Age at operation (< 12 months) and preservation of periosteum and ligamentous attachments were strongly associated with preservation of an open physis in the transferred bone and continued longitudinal growth.

Rodgers WB, Waters P: Incidence of trigger digits in newborns. *J Hand Surg* 1994;19A:364–368.

A prospective review of 1,046 newborn infants revealed no trigger digits. The article also reports a retrospective study of 89 trigger thumb and 11 trigger digit releases. Only seven of the children presented at less than 6 months of age and none less than 3 months of age. This study raises the possibility that trigger digits may be an acquired rather than congenital condition.

Acquired

Dado D, Angelats J: Management of burns of the hands in children. *Hand Clin* 1990;6:711–721.

This review article describes the scald or contact burns that occur in infants and toddlers as opposed to the burns from matches or gasoline that occur with adolescents. The authors outline treatment protocols for each type of burn.

Feinstein K, Poznanski AK: Evaluation of joint disease in the pediatric hand. *Hand Clin* 1991;7:167–182.

This review article describes the differential diagnosis of pediatric joint diseases in the hand to include JRA, leukemia, sickle cell disease, child abuse, and hypertrophic osteoarthropathy. It outlines methods of radiologic assessment to diagnose and monitor progress of these diseases.

Roth JH, O'Grady SE, Richards RS, et al: Functional outcome of upper limb tendon transfers performed in children with spastic hemiplegia. *J Hand Surg* 1993; 18B:299–303.

Seventeen patients treated by one surgeon are reviewed. At 2- to 6-year follow-up, total range of motion was unchanged but functional grading was improved by two grades and parental satisfaction was high.

Trauma

Fractures

De Boeck H, Jaeken R: Treatment of chronic mallet finger in children by tenodermodesis. *J Pediatr Orthop* 1992;12: 351–354.

Four children with chronic mallet fingers due to extensor tendon injury were treated successfully with tenodermodesis. No loss of motion or complications occurred.

Fischer MD, McElfresh EC: Physeal and periphyseal injuries of the hand: Patterns of injury and results of treatment. *Hand Clin* 1994;10:287–301.

The authors review a series of 1,048 finger fractures in patients less than 16 years of age. Fracture patterns are reviewed and recommendations provided with respect to assessment and treatment of these sometimes perilous injuries.

Gibbons CL, Woods D, Pailthorpe C, et al: The management of isolated distal radius fractures in children. *J Pediatr Orthop* 1994;14:207–210.

Twenty-three isolated distal radial metaphyseal fractures were prospectively randomized into cast treatment versus percutaneous pinning. There were no complications in the percutaneous pinning group; 91% of the cast immobilization group underwent further manipulation.

Letts M, Rowhani N: Galeazzi-equivalent injuries of the wrist in children. *J Pediatr Orthop* 1993;13:561–566.

Ten children with Galeazzi or Galeazzi-equivalent fractures are retrospectively reviewed. Galeazzi-equivalent fractures may include a fracture through the distal growth plate of the ulna and have a less favorable prognosis than standard Galeazzi fractures in this small series.

Waters PM, Kolettis GJ, Schwend R: Acute median neuropathy following physeal fractures of the distal radius. *J Pediatr Orthop* 1994;14:173–177.

This is a retrospective review of eight cases of median neuropathy after displaced distal radial physeal fractures. The authors outline a treatment protocol utilizing percutaneous pinning to lessen the risk of acute median neuropathy or forearm compartment syndrome associated with closed reduction and cast immobilization of these fractures.

Tendon

Amadio PC: Staged flexor tendon reconstruction in children. *Ann Chir Main Memb Super* 1992;11:194–199.

This is a retrospective review of 12 children with 14 staged flexor tendon reconstructions for zone II injuries. Mean total active motion was 140° (range: 90° to 210°). There were five infections and one tendon rupture.

O'Connell SJ, Moore MM, Strickland JW, et al: Results of zone I and zone II flexor tendon repairs in children. *J Hand Surg* 1994;19A:48–52.

This is a retrospective study of 78 children with 95 zone I or Zone II flexor tendon repairs. There was no difference in total active motion results from protocols for early motion versus cast immobilization for 4 weeks. There was no difference in age group between 0 and 15 years. There was significant loss of motion if immobilization continued beyond 4 weeks.

Microsurgery

Baker GL, Kleinert JM: Digit replantation in infants and young children: Determinants of survival. *Plast Reconstr Surg* 1994;94:139–145.

This is a retrospective review of 32 replantations in children under 34 months of age. Overall survival rate was 69%. Factors favorable to a successful outcome included body weight greater than 11 kg, vein grafting for arteries and veins, more than one vein repaired, and bone shortening. Prompt digital reperfusion and at least one successful vein anastomosis led to a success rate of 95%.

Barrios C, de Pablos J: Surgical management of nerve injuries of the upper extremity in children: A 15-year survey. *J Pediatr Orthop* 1991;11:641–645.

This is a retrospective review of 37 surgically treated nerve lesions in 33 children with greater than 2-year follow-up. There were 19 ulnar, 12 median, and six radial nerve injuries. All primary nerve repairs under age 10 years were normal. There was recovery to least an M4, S3 level with repairs delayed up to 1 year postinjury.

Devaraj VS, Kay SP, Batchelor AG, et al: Microvascular surgery in children. *Br J Plast Surg* 1991;44:276–280.

In this retrospective review of 43 microvascular procedures in 38 children with an average age of 5.4 years, overall vascular success rate was 93%.

Classic Bibliography

Congenital

Birch-Jensen A: *Congenital Deformities of the Upper Extremities.* Copenhagen, Ejnar Munksgaard, 1949.

Blauth W: Der hypoplastiche Daumer. *Arch Orth Un Fall Chir* 1967;62:225–246.

Broudy AS, Smith RJ: Deformities of the hand and wrist with ulnar deficiency. *J Hand Surg* 1979;4A:304–315.

Buck-Gramcko D: Pollicization of the index finger. *J Bone Joint Surg* 1971;53A:1605–1617.

Buck-Gramcko D: Radialization as a new treatment for radial club hand. *J Hand Surg* 1979;4A:304–315.

O'Rahilly R, Gardner E: The timing and sequence of events in the development of the limbs in the human embryo. *Anat Embryol* 1975;148:1–23.

Patterson TJ: Congenital ring-constructions. *Br J Plast Surg* 1961;14:1–31.

Wassel HD: The results of surgery for polydactyly of the thumb. *Clin Orthop* 1969;64:175–193.

Acquired

Dixon GL Jr, Moon NF: Rotational supracondylar fractures of the proximal phalanx in children. *Clin Orthop* 1972;83:151–156.

Hastings H II, Simmons BP: Hand fractures in children: A statistical analysis. *Clin Orthop* 1984;188:120–130.

Simmons BP, Peters TT: Subcondylar fossa reconstruction for malunion of fractures of the proximal phalanx in children. *J Hand Surg* 1987;12A:1079–1082.

31

Wrist and Hand: Trauma

Distal Radius Fractures

Distal radius fractures are common injuries usually sustained by elderly patients as a result of a fall and by younger patients as a result of high-energy trauma. The goals of treatment are to restore maximum function and to limit the development of posttraumatic arthritis. Accepted standards of treatment are the same as for other intra-articular and periarticular fractures and specify that the physician achieve and maintain a satisfactory reduction until healing occurs and then rehabilitate the wrist to restore motion and strength. Several descriptive classification schemes have been developed in an attempt to guide treatment and predict outcome. However, none of these systems is universally accepted or applied, and little information is available relative to their intra- or interobserver reliability.

Criteria for an acceptable reduction and the optimum techniques to achieve and maintain it are not clear for all fracture types in all age groups. Loss of the normal palmar tilt, decreased radial inclination, and radial shortening have all been implicated as causes of poor outcome, as has loss of articular congruity. In several recent clinical and laboratory studies, investigators have attempted to identify which of these factors is important in determining long-term outcomes following these injuries. The effect of residual dorsal tilt on range of motion and carpal alignment was investigated in 30 patients with extra-articular fractures. With increased dorsal tilt, range of wrist motion became more restricted and a dorsal intercalated segment instability (DISI) became apparent. Adverse effects were small when dorsal tilt was less than 10°. Residual deformity can also affect the distal radioulnar joint (DRUJ), leading in some cases to persistent pain and loss of forearm rotation. In a laboratory study, the effects of four common types of radial deformity on DRUJ mechanics were investigated. Radial shortening caused the greatest disturbance in kinematics and the most distortion of the triangular fibrocartilage. Decreased radial inclination and dorsal angulation caused intermediate changes, whereas dorsal displacement produced minimal changes. Radial deformity by itself did not produce DRUJ dislocation.

Long-term follow-up studies have been undertaken to identify the most important factors affecting outcome. Seventy-six patients were reviewed 27 to 36 years after conservative treatment for fractures of the distal radius as young adults. The authors attempted to correlate the clinical presentation at follow-up with radiographic parameters. Patients who had degenerative changes in the radiocarpal joint had more complaints than those who did not; however, this correlation was weak. Degenerative changes in the DRUJ were not associated with more complaints. As noted in earlier reports, radial shortening adversely affected the clinical outcome and was more often associated with radiographic degenerative changes in extra-articular fractures. In a subgroup analysis of patients with intra-articular fractures, the main factor related to the development of degenerative changes was found to be joint incongruity greater than 1 mm. Although there was a higher incidence of degenerative changes in the intra-articular fracture group compared to the extra-articular fracture group, there was no difference in clinical outcome between the groups. Findings were similar in another study of 42 patients who had sustained intra-articular fractures as young adults an average of 16 years prior to evaluation. Only six patients changed occupation as a result of the fracture, and only one fourth of the patients reported dysfunction, although more than half had visible residual deformity.

Despite these reasonably satisfactory long-term outcomes following closed reduction and cast treatment, surgical management is recommended for difficult fractures because it offers the potential to further minimize residual deformity and loss of function. In addition, surgical management is a more reliable method of reduction for significantly displaced intra-articular fractures and, thus, should decrease the risk of posttraumatic arthritis. In an attempt to provide the most appropriate care, management algorithms have been developed that adapt treatment to the functional requirements of the patient and the fracture pattern.

Selecting the most appropriate treatment depends on accurate delineation of the extent and displacement of the fracture. Dorsal or volar comminution, severe dorsal angulation at presentation, and incomplete reduction are signs of likely redisplacement and subsequent deformity following cast treatment. Although the ability to maintain a satisfactory reduction with cast treatment alone can often be predicted on the basis of the original radiograph, ancillary imaging studies such as tomograms and computed tomography (CT) scans are frequently required to more completely understand the fracture, especially if there are intra-articular extensions. In a study of 19 consecutive distal radius fractures, CT examinations were more sensitive than plain radiographs in identifying intra-articular involvement and resulted in a change in management in five patients. Intra-articular fractures deserve special attention; several studies have demonstrated a cor-

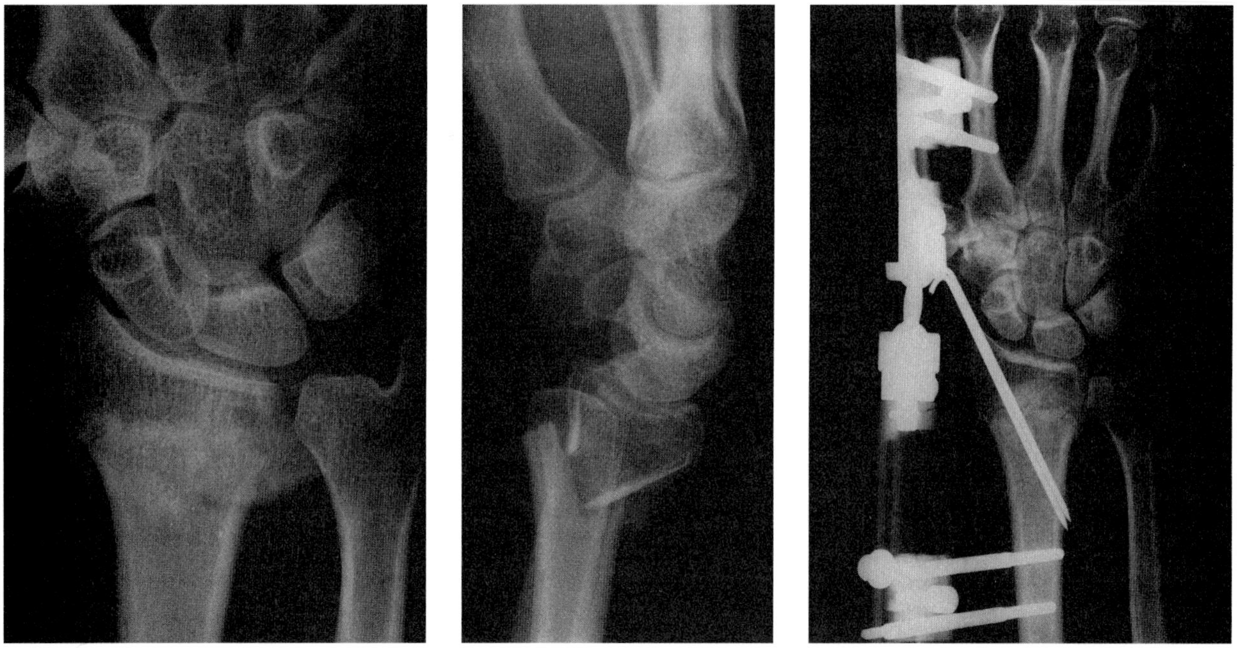

Fig. 1 **Left** and **center,** A distal radius fracture with significant extra-articular displacement, shortening, angulation, and dorsal comminution; the intra-articular fractures are minimally displaced. **Right,** Following reduction, the fracture was stabilized with Kirschner wires (K-wires) and external fixation. Bone graft was added through a limited dorsal exposure. The external fixator was removed at 4 weeks and the K-wires were removed at 6 weeks.

relation between final articular incongruency and the development of degenerative changes and a worse clinical outcome.

Several treatment alternatives to closed reduction and casting are available; these include closed reduction and external fixation, closed reduction and percutaneous pinning, and open reduction and internal fixation (ORIF) with or without bone grafting. Although anatomic reduction remains the goal, surgical techniques are evolving in an attempt to minimize postoperative stiffness, decrease surgical risks, and reduce the quantity of internal and external fixation hardware. Techniques such as intrafocal pinning, limited dorsal exposure with bone grafting, arthroscopic assisted reduction, and percutaneous pinning are attempts to achieve these goals (Fig. 1).

In a study of 26 patients with severe distal radius fractures treated by external fixation with distraction, outcome at 2 years was adversely affected in proportion to the amount and duration of distraction. Although a critical amount of distraction could not be defined, the authors recommended that external fixation be limited to less than 6 weeks if possible. Despite the adverse affects attributed to treatment, the patients in this series recovered 75% of their motion and grip strength.

A review of 100 cases of distal radius fracture treated by distraction and bone grafting with external fixation for 3 weeks followed by 3 weeks of functional bracing demonstrated excellent results at an average follow-up of 20 months. The indications included fractures with comminution, displacement, and intra-articular involvement. Ages of the patients ranged from 16 to 65 years; patients older than 65 years of age were excluded. Sixty of the fractures were Frykman type VII or VIII. Distraction with external fixation was used to achieve and maintain extra-articular reduction by ligamentotaxis. A 2-cm dorsal incision was then made over the fracture site, and iliac crest graft was pushed into the fracture. The contour of the carpal surface served as a mold to realign the articular surface. In about 10% of cases, packing the bone graft caused displacement of the palmar fragments, which required the addition of Kirschner wire (K-wire) fixation.

Intrafocal pinning was originally described in 1976 and has been widely used in Europe. Essentially a variation of percutaneous pinning, the technique consists of limited open placement of buttressing K-wires. The original indication was an unstable extra-articular fracture in a young adult; however, the indications have been extended to include elderly patients and intra-articular fractures with minimal displacement. Contraindications are significant intra-articular involvement, volar comminution, advanced osteopenia, and the inability to achieve a satisfactory reduction by closed manipulation prior to pinning. The current technique uses three 0.062-inch K-wires inserted through small incisions directly over the fracture between the first and second, the third and fourth, and the fourth and fifth dorsal wrist compartments. Pins are initially inserted directly into and parallel to the fracture and then directed 45° obliquely and proximally to engage the opposite cortex. This maneuver further reduces the fracture and provides a buttress for the distal fragment. Although no cast immobilization was used in the original description, a cast is now commonly used for 6 weeks. Several series from Europe have had good results using this method. A recent report from the United States of 23 patients claimed good and excellent radiographic results in 79% of patients younger than 65 years of age and in 60% of those older than 65. Seventy percent of patients younger than 65 years of age and 100% of those older than 65 years had a good or excellent clinical outcome. Thus, some loss of reduction occurred in the elderly, but it was well tolerated. The technique appears to offer many advantages for simple to moderately difficult fractures that cannot be managed by cast treatment alone.

ORIF using a wider exposure is indicated for comminuted intra-articular fractures and shear fractures, such as volar Barton's fractures. These types of fractures cannot be reduced by ligamentotaxis and are more unstable following reduction. Bone grafting, various types of hardware, and external fixation should be considered. The main objectives are to reduce the articular surface and to neutralize the forces that cause displacement during fracture healing. However, indiscriminate use of hardware will increase the risk of complications.

Scaphoid Fractures

Patients with pain and tenderness about the anatomic snuff box following trauma to the wrist should be suspected of having an acute scaphoid fracture. Initial radiographs should include at least a posteroanterior (PA), lateral, and PA in ulnar deviation. If these radiographs are normal, the patient should be immobilized in a thumb spica splint or cast and radiographs repeated in 7 to 10 days. If pain and tenderness persist, but standard radiographs remain negative, further investigation is indicated. In this clinical setting, it is imperative to determine whether or not the patient has sustained a fracture, because delays in recognition and treatment will increase the risk of an adverse outcome. Data from previous studies have demonstrated that a delay in treatment of 28 days from the time of fracture is associated with a 45% rate of nonunion compared to a 5% rate when treatment is begun within 28 days.

Several approaches have been used to evaluate suspected scaphoid fractures when initial plain radiographs are negative. The value of repeating plain radiographs was compared to that of using bone scans in a study of 78 patients with a clinically suspected scaphoid fracture. The sensitivity of radiographs decreased from 64% in the first day series to 30% in follow-up radiographs. The reliability among experienced radiologists was satisfactory for the initial radiographs, but poor for follow-up. These data imply that a first day series is meaningful, whereas repeated radiographs do not improve the diagnostic accuracy. Conversely, a bone scan was found to be 98% specific and 100% sensitive in these patients. A positive predictive value of 93% was calculated for the bone scan using CT scan and repeat plain radiographs to confirm fractures. The authors concluded that the best diagnostic approach for suspected scaphoid fractures is an initial radiographic series followed by a bone scan if the initial radiographs are negative. When this treatment strategy was used, there were no nonunions in a series of patients treated for suspected scaphoid fracture. These data, however, are in contrast to those in a previous report, which indicated that repeat radiographs are sufficiently reliable to provide appropriate care. The appropriate role of bone scans in the evaluation of patients with suspected scaphoid fractures remains unclear.

When radiographs reveal a scaphoid fracture, the physician should identify several radiographic features of the fracture that will assist in management decisions and influence prognosis. These features include the location and orientation of the fracture within the bone as well as the presence or absence of displacement. Fractures of the proximal third of the bone are associated with significantly higher rates of delayed union, nonunion, and osteonecrosis. Displaced fractures are considered unstable and are more likely to present problems with delayed union and nonunion than nondisplaced fractures. Generally acknowledged criteria for displacement or instability are 1 mm or more step off between the fracture fragments, a radiolunate angle of more than 15°, and an intrascaphoid angle of more than 25°. Some surgeons argue that any complete fracture through the body of the scaphoid should be considered an unstable fracture. This criterion has not been universally accepted. Additional imaging studies, such as CT scans or tomograms, should be obtained if the plain radiographs are inconclusive.

The indications for ORIF of acute scaphoid fractures include displaced or angulated fractures and fractures associated with perilunate fracture dislocations. Proximal pole fractures and fractures that are considered unstable due to fracture obliquity or comminution deserve consideration for internal fixation, although there are few data that document improved clinical outcomes following internal fixation of these particular fractures. K-wires and screws are most commonly used for fixation. K-wires are easier to insert but do not provide the stability of a properly placed bone screw. The fixation achieved by the different available screw designs has been compared in several biomechanical experiments; however, the minimum requirements for fixation in clinical applications are unknown. Although there are screws that provide better compression and rigidity than the Herbert Screw, its unique design and the reported satisfactory clinical results support continued use of this device.

Wrist Instabilities

Carpal instability refers to a malalignment of the carpal bones and is most commonly caused by a fracture or ligament injury. Patients typically complain of pain, weakness of grip, and a popping or catching sensation in the wrist. Despite a plethora of anatomic, biomechanical, and clinical studies, the definitions and classification of specific carpal instabilities continue to evolve, and the most appropriate diagnostic studies and treatment methods remain controversial. With the exception of carpal dislocations and fracture dislocations, the diagnosis of an acute ligamentous injury in the wrist requires a high index of suspicion, and in many cases, the identification of clinically important lesions may not be possible in early examinations.

An increasingly popular contemporary classification scheme groups carpal instabilities into two categories called dissociative and nondissociative. Dissociative instability is caused by an interosseous ligament tear, and the principal abnormal motion occurs between bones within a carpal row. Nondissociative instability is caused by a ligament tear in the radiocarpal or midcarpal joints, and there is normal motion within a row and abnormal motion between rows. The terms static instability and dynamic instability are used to differentiate between conditions that can be seen on standard PA and lateral radiographs of the wrist (static instability) and those that are seen only when the wrist is placed in nonstandard positions, such as extreme ulnar or radial deviation, or when stress is exerted by the examiner or the patient as in making a tight fist (dynamic instability).

DISI is the most commonly encountered form of carpal instability. Although several different ligament lesions have been implicated as the cause of DISI, the most common is an injury to the scapholunate interosseous ligament. Injury to this ligament uncouples (dissociates) the scaphoid and lunate; eventually, the lunate slips into dorsiflexion and the scaphoid rotates to a more vertical orientation, producing rotatory subluxation of the scaphoid and DISI. Early radiographic findings include a widened scapholunate gap that, if greater than 3 mm, is considered diagnostic of scapholunate dissociation. However, the reliability of gap measurements on standard wrist radiographs has been challenged. A slightly oblique projection of the scapholunate joint may create the impression of a smaller gap than is actually present. To improve diagnostic accuracy, the affected wrist should be compared to the contralateral wrist viewed in an identical projection. Alternatively, fluoroscopic spot films can be used to obtain an appropriate profile of the joint.

If plain radiographs or fluoroscopy are equivocal in a patient with a suspected scapholunate interosseous ligament tear, wrist arthrography can be used to evaluate the interosseous ligaments. The diagnostic accuracy of wrist arthrography has been evaluated in several studies. In one study, 20 consecutive patients with chronic wrist pain were evaluated by arthrography and arthroscopy, and 19 of 20 had an arthrotomy. Arthroscopy was found to be more specific than arthrography, particularly in identifying the location and severity of an interosseous ligament tear. However, the arthrogram technique used in this study did not routinely include all three compartments, ie, midcarpal, radiocarpal, and radioulnar injections. In those patients in whom a midcarpal injection was performed, there were no false negative or false positive arthrograms.

The clinical significance of ligament defects identified by either wrist arthrography or arthroscopy is an important issue that is very difficult to resolve. Communicating lesions are seen frequently in the asymptomatic contralateral wrist when arthrography is performed bilaterally. Data from recent biomechanical and histologic studies have shown that the most proximal portions of the scapholunate and lunotriquetral ligaments are membranous and provide little mechanical stability, whereas the dorsal and palmar portions are ligamentous structures that provide substantial stability to these joints. However, the dorsal and palmar portions are difficult to evaluate by either arthrography or arthroscopy, and asymptomatic defects in the membranous portion have been shown to occur with high frequency, especially with advancing age. Twenty-six patients with at least one symptom of a scapholunate ligament tear underwent arthroscopy to evaluate the significance of the tear. During arthroscopy, the wrist was manipulated in an attempt to visualize scapholunate instability. Approximately half of the patients had a visible tear; fewer than one third of these patients had associated findings of instability. The authors concluded that tears of the membranous portion of the scapholunate ligament can occur without an associated instability and that this type of tear is not the cause of occult wrist pain. However, the combination of a scapholunate tear and instability seen at arthroscopy does indicate a pathologic condition. Although this study offers a method to assess ligament tears and instability, the accuracy of that method has not been substantiated.

The primary goals for treatment of an acute scapholunate ligament tear associated with instability are anatomic reduction of the scapholunate joint and correction of any additional carpal malalignment. Currently, there is increased interest in direct primary repair of the scapholunate interosseous ligament. Internal fixation, usually with K-wires, is required to maintain the reduction. Although closed reduction and percutaneous pinning has been used, open reduction is usually required to achieve an accurate reduction, especially if the injury is more than several weeks old (Fig. 2). A review of 21 patients with scapholunate dissociations treated as early as 1 month after injury by direct repair with or without dorsal radioscaphoid capsulodesis demonstrated satisfactory results. It was concluded that sufficient dorsal and membranous ligamentous substance is usually available for repair, even in injuries that are several months old.

Perilunate dislocations and fracture dislocations represent an extreme example of acute carpal instability. They are caused by severe trauma that results in gross carpal malalignment with or without fractures. In a recent

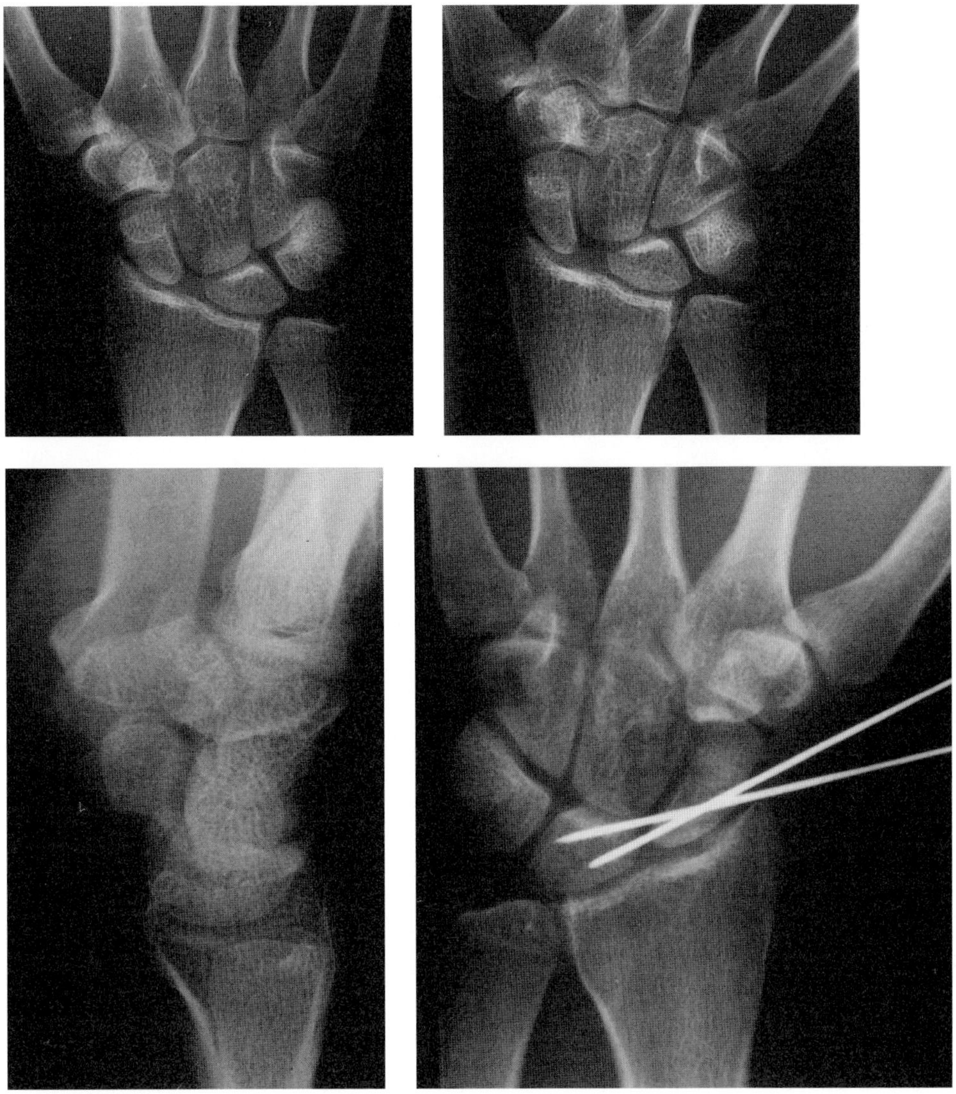

Fig. 2 **Top left,** A posteroanterior view of the wrist demonstrates scapholunate dissociation. **Top right,** The scapholunate gap is accentuated by ulnar deviation. **Bottom left,** The lateral view shows flexion of the scaphoid and extension of the lunate, typical of a dorsal intercalated segment instability. **Bottom right,** Treatment was by open reduction, direct ligament repair, and Kirschner-wire fixation for 10 weeks.

multicenter retrospective study of 165 patients with perilunate dislocations and fracture dislocations, outcomes were evaluated at an average follow-up of 6 years. In 25% of cases, the diagnosis was initially missed. Eight percent of the injuries were open. Factors that correlated with a poor outcome included open injuries and those in which the delay in treatment was greater than 1 week. There was no difference in the clinical outcome between perilunate dislocations and transscaphoid perilunate fracture dislocations. In closed injuries treated early, the incidence of malreduction was 71%, and the incidence of posttraumatic arthritis was 56%. In another study of 32 patients treated for lunate or perilunate dislocations, less residual carpal instability and a better clinical outcome were seen at an average follow-up of 5 years if the scapholunate ligament was repaired or reconstructed primarily than if the ligament was not repaired.

Phalangeal and Metacarpal Shaft Fractures

The vast majority of finger fractures can be successfully managed nonsurgically. The indications and the available techniques for surgical fixation are similar for phalangeal

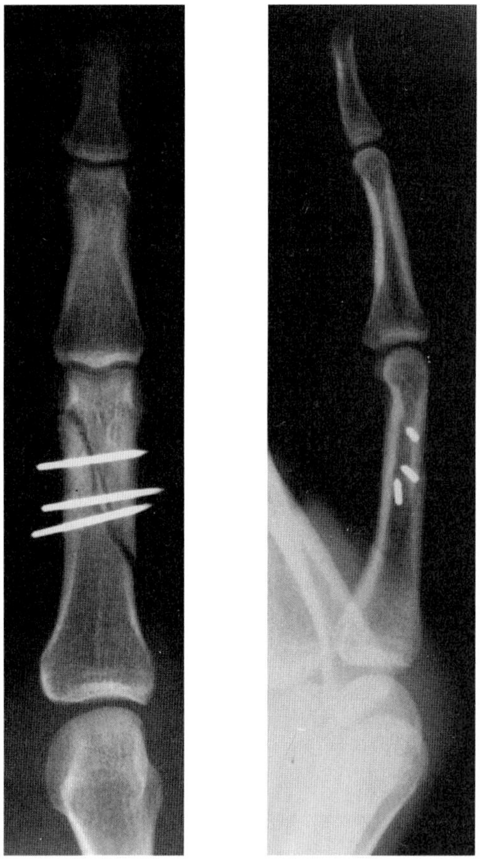

Fig. 3 A displaced spiral fracture of the proximal phalanx was treated by closed reduction and percutaneous Kirschner-wire fixation despite being 8 days after injury. The slight fracture gap due to hematoma did not impede healing. Early postoperative motion was initiated.

and metacarpal fractures. Fixation is indicated for: (1) an unstable fracture in which reduction cannot be maintained with closed techniques, (2) a fracture associated with significant soft-tissue injury when treatment of the soft-tissue injury may cause a loss of reduction, and (3) multiple fractures. Fracture patterns that indicate probable instability include displaced oblique and spiral fractures and comminuted fractures. The stability of transverse metacarpal and phalangeal fractures varies and commonly cannot be determined until closed reduction is attempted. Isolated fractures of the central metacarpals tend to be more stable, regardless of the fracture pattern, than fractures of the index and little finger metacarpals.

The criteria for satisfactory alignment vary among the phalanges and metacarpals. Sagittal plane angulation is not well tolerated in the index and long finger metacarpals, whereas up to 60° of angulation may be satisfactory in fifth metacarpal neck fractures. Small amounts of sagittal plane angulation in phalangeal fractures will disrupt digit balance and lead to deformity and dysfunction. Rotation and coronal plane angulation of both phalanges and metacarpals will cause digital overlap and are unacceptable.

Percutaneous fixation is best used when a satisfactory reduction can be achieved by closed means, but cannot be maintained by splints or casts. Available implants that can be inserted percutaneously include K-wires, absorbable pins, and screws (Fig. 3). When a closed reduction cannot be readily achieved, soft-tissue interposition is likely and surgical treatment is indicated. ORIF is considered when: (1) a closed reduction cannot be obtained, (2) percutaneous fixation cannot be achieved, or (3) a fracture is unstable as a result of segmental bone loss or comminution. When open reduction is performed, fixation must be sufficiently rigid to allow immediate range of motion, or the benefit of a well-reduced fracture will be outweighed by the additional scarring and stiffness caused by the surgical exposure. In a report on the outcomes of open hand fractures, the surgical dissection required for internal fixation had a negative effect on final finger motion. Based on these findings, the recommendation was to use the least invasive technique consistent with necessary stability.

Several alternatives to K-wires can be used in conjunction with open reduction. Intraosseous wiring, including the tension band technique, is an alternative that has been used successfully and remains popular for transverse fractures. Compression screws provide excellent fixation of long oblique and spiral fractures when the length of the fracture is at least twice the diameter of the bone. The fragment width should be three times the screw diameter to avoid iatrogenic fracture. An anatomic reduction and precise screw placement are required to achieve maximum stability. Plating is indicated for short oblique and unstable transverse metacarpal fractures and for metacarpal and phalangeal fractures that are unstable as a result of comminution or bone loss (Fig. 4). Plating is not as well tolerated in the phalanx because the hardware bulk can impede tendon function. Newer, low-profile screw and plate designs and application of the plate on the lateral aspect of the finger may reduce this problem, although the clinical efficacy of these implants is still unknown. Data from several laboratory and clinical studies have shown that adequate fixation can be obtained with a variety of techniques. Although several laboratory studies have demonstrated the mechanical superiority of plates and screws over K-wires, little information is available that compares the in vivo loads delivered to the fracture site during rehabilitation with the mechanical properties of each of these implant constructs.

External fixation of diaphyseal fractures is indicated for severely contaminated wounds, extensive comminution, and severe trauma in which further dissection will significantly compromise vascularity of the bone and soft tissues. A half-pin configuration is recommended for most frac-

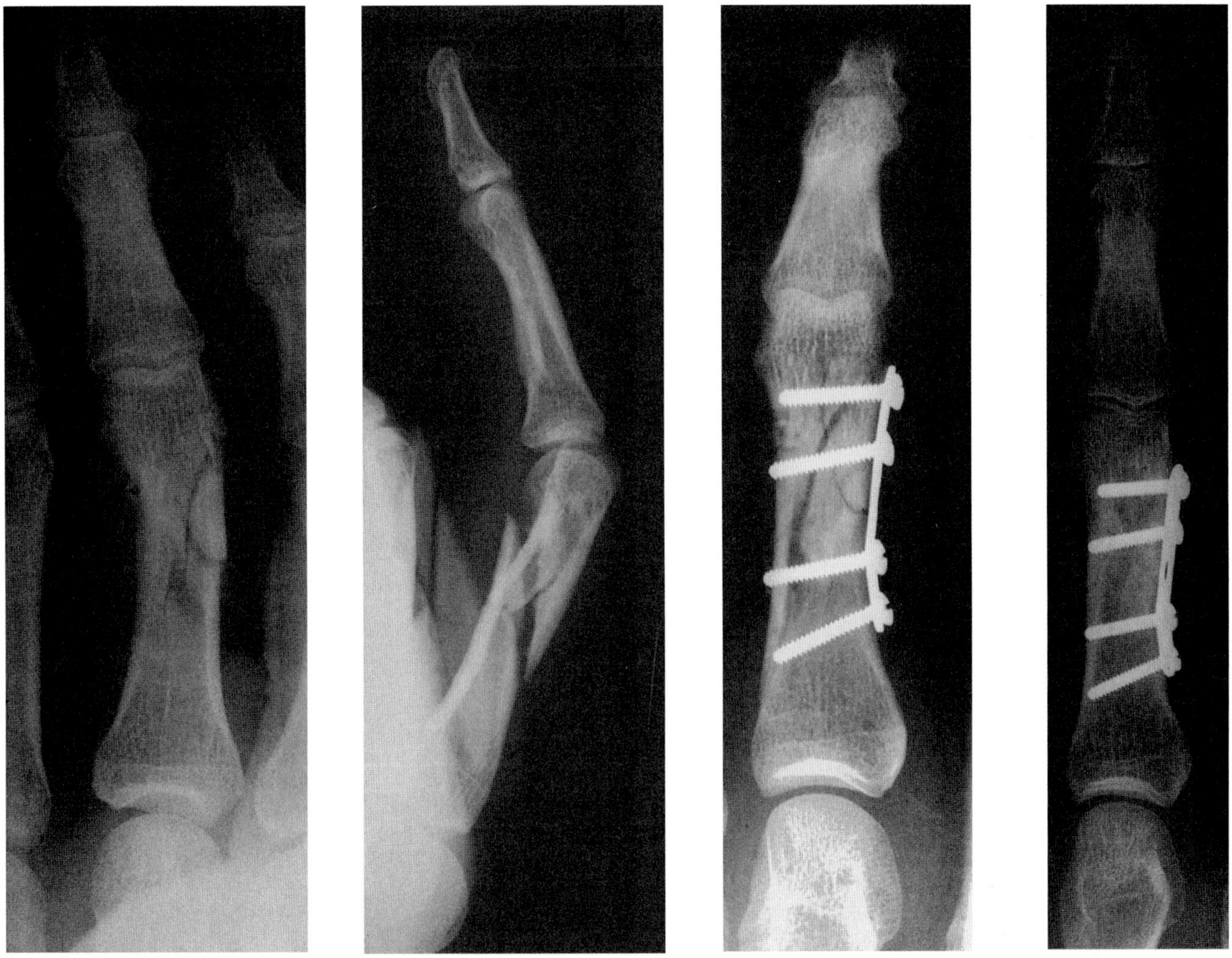

Fig. 4 **Left** and **left center,** A highly comminuted displaced fracture of the proximal phalanx. **Right center,** Plate fixation was required to gain fracture stability. **Right,** The fracture is shown to be well healed at 6 months; however, plate removal and extensor tenolysis was required to achieve maximum motion.

ture patterns. However, a full-pin configuration is considered when prolonged fixation is required, such as for fractures with severe bone loss that requires substantial grafting and for nonunion repairs with healing time that averaged 80 days in one series. Although external fixation offers advantages in these difficult wounds, even extensive trauma can be treated effectively by appropriate soft-tissue management and early internal fixation. A series of 64 metacarpal fractures from gunshot wounds were treated by internal fixation, bone grafting, and early range of motion exercises. All fractures united by 12 weeks, and there were no deep infections; metacarpophalangeal (MCP) joint motion averaged 65°, shortening averaged 1.4 mm, and angulation was less than 10°.

Proximal Interphalangeal Joint Fractures and Dislocations

A displaced transverse fracture through the neck of the proximal phalanx is difficult to manage because the small size of the metaphyseal fragment often precludes closed reduction, and the risk of joint stiffness is high. When a closed reduction is possible, it frequently requires extreme flexion of the joint to reduce and hold the fragment. If excessive flexion is required to hold a closed reduction, K-wires should be used to control the fracture and allow more appropriate positioning of the joint. Although motion will be restricted while the pins are in place, little functional loss will result if the pins are removed as soon as the

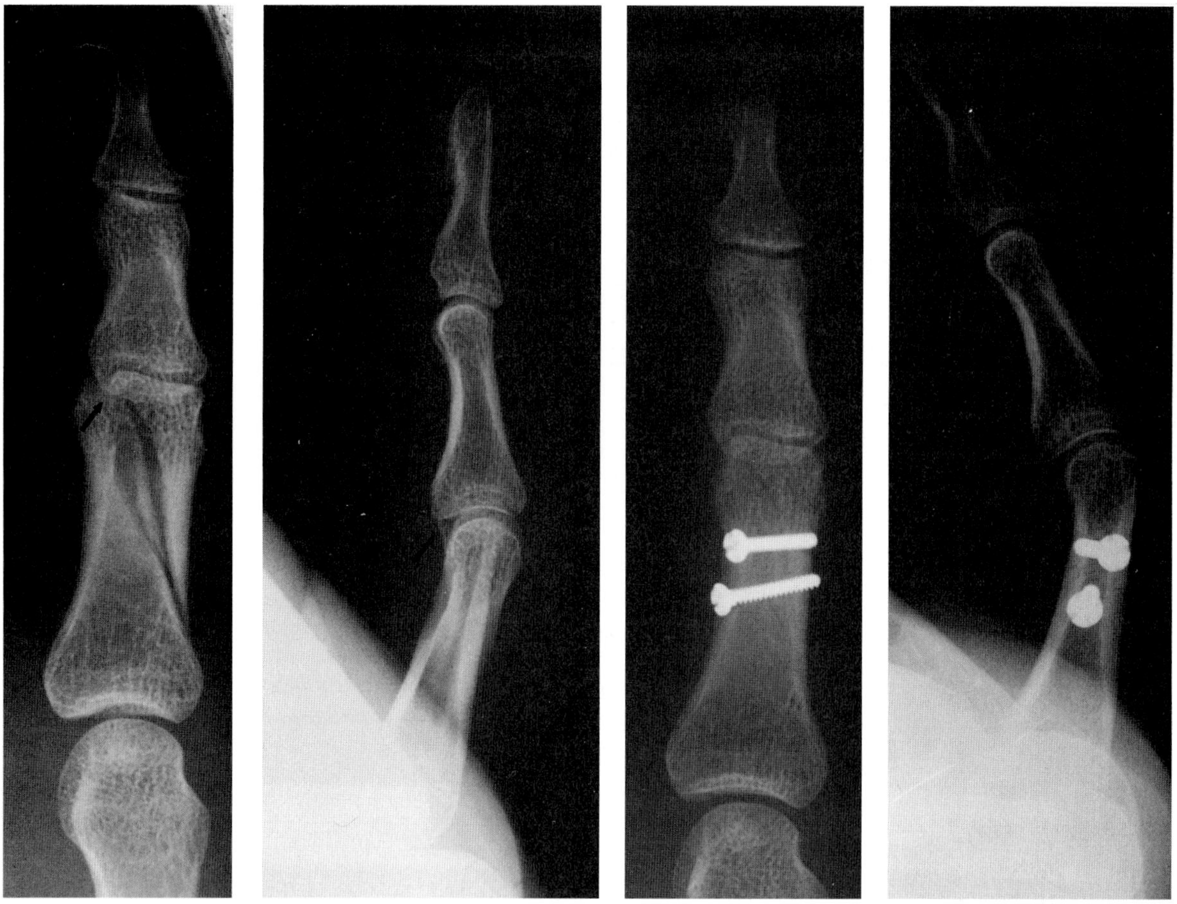

Fig. 5 **Left,** A spiral fracture of the proximal phalanx has shortened causing the distal spike (arrow) to protrude into the retrocondylar recess (arrow), which blocks proximal interphalangeal joint flexion. **Right,** The fracture was treated by open reduction and miniscrew lag fixation. Early motion was initiated.

fracture heals. Open reduction is the alternative; however, loss of final range of motion is frequent. Oblique and spiral fractures involving the distal diaphysis of the proximal phalanx can shorten causing a spike to protrude into the retrocondylar recess, which causes a mechanical block to proximal interphalangeal (PIP) joint flexion. Alignment will be normal clinically and on the PA radiograph; however, lateral and oblique radiographs will show the spike. An anatomic reduction is necessary to maintain motion (Fig. 5).

Unicondylar and bicondylar fractures of the proximal phalanx are unstable and require fixation to maintain joint congruency. In a review of 38 unicondylar fractures, four fracture patterns were identified: oblique volar, long sagittal, dorsal coronal, and volar coronal. The oblique volar pattern was the most common (58%). K-wire fixation resulted in the best final joint motion, however, in this retrospective study, the method of fixation was not randomized. Five of seven nondisplaced fractures treated by splinting and four of ten fractures treated by reduction and single K-wire fixation displaced. The authors recommended that multiple K-wires or miniscrew fixation be used to prevent displacement (Fig. 6). A short period of postoperative immobilization did not adversely affect final motion, although there was a trend toward diminished motion if mobilization was not initiated within 3 weeks.

Fractures involving the base of the middle phalanx result from either an avulsion of the collateral ligament or an axial compression injury. Large displaced avulsion fragments cause joint instability and incongruity and should be internally fixed. Compression injuries vary from nondisplaced, stable fractures involving a single plateau to highly comminuted pilon fractures characterized by depression of the central articular surface and displacement of the dorsal and volar articular fragments. Single-plateau fractures associated with joint angulation require elevation of the impacted fragment, possible bone grafting, and internal fixation. In a review of three different methods of

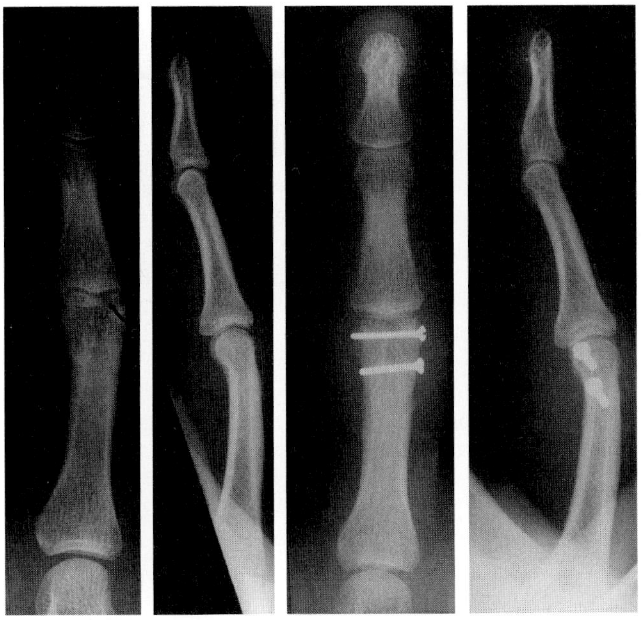

Fig. 6 **Left,** Fracture of the head of the proximal phalanx. The fracture pattern is an oblique volar type. The arrow points to the displacement and articular incongruity. **Right,** Treatment was by open reduction and miniscrew lag fixation. Early motion was initiated.

treatment for pilon fractures, skeletal traction produced better range of motion with fewer complications than splinting or ORIF.

Dorsal PIP dislocations with or without a small palmar plate avulsion fracture are usually stable after reduction and can be treated by buddy taping or static splinting in extension for a few days. A flexion contracture is the most common complication and is usually caused by prolonged immobilization in flexion. Splinting in extension reduces this complication; however, simple buddy taping results in an early return of motion and a low complication rate.

Treatment of dorsal PIP joint fracture-dislocations continues to evolve, with numerous treatment methods currently used. Recommended methods are based on the amount of articular surface involvement, because fractures involving approximately 40% or more of the base of the middle phalanx render the joint unstable. The primary objective of any method is to obtain and maintain a congruous reduction and preserve joint motion. Several methods have been designed to maintain the reduction while allowing early protected range of motion in an attempt to maximize final motion. Extension block splinting is the treatment of choice for injuries involving less than 30% of the articular surface that are stable following reduction. For more extensive injuries, the amount of comminution will affect treatment options. Repair by ORIF can be achieved only if the fracture fragments are large enough to be securely fixed. Extension block pinning is a new technique that is relatively simple and allows some early range of motion. The technique involves closed reduction by axial traction and PIP joint flexion followed by retrograde, percutaneous insertion of a K-wire into the distal, dorsal aspect of the head of the proximal phalanx to maintain joint reduction. The pin is also believed to eliminate the dorsal subluxing force of the central slip of the extensor tendon, however, active extension within the limit allowed by the pin is still afforded by the lateral bands. Gentle range of motion is initiated and the pin is removed at 4 to 6 weeks. Preliminary results with this method have been encouraging.

Palmar plate arthroplasty is advocated for acute injuries with extensive comminution and for chronic fracture dislocations. A review of 71 cases (22 acute fractures, 49 chronic cases) with a follow-up of 6 months to 4 years found that 87% of patients achieved a stable, pain-free range of motion from 5° to 95° within 2 months. Four patients had a flexion contracture of 10° to 35°, and five developed hyperextension, three of whom underwent successful revision of the palmar plate arthroplasty. A modification of the original technique was used, the collateral ligaments were preserved, and the palmar plate was freed from the accessory collateral ligaments and flexor sheath only in chronic cases.

Additional treatment alternatives include transarticular pin fixation, dynamic traction devices, and external fixation. Dynamic traction devices can produce good results in difficult articular fractures; however, application of these devices can be technically demanding. External fixation has been used for acute and late fracture dislocations, pilon and plateau fractures, and neutralization of internally fixed fractures. Several products designed specifically for external fixation of finger injuries are now commercially available, but clinical experience with these products is very limited.

Collateral Ligament Injuries of the Thumb Metacarpophalangeal Joint

Accurate assessment of injury severity is the key to providing appropriate initial care for patients with suspected injuries to the ulnar collateral ligament of the MCP joint of the thumb. Differentiation of incomplete from complete tears and complete nondisplaced from complete displaced tears is essential. Incomplete injuries and complete nondisplaced tears are treated nonsurgically with the expectation of an excellent functional result. Displaced tears are also known as a Stener lesion and require surgical repair. Several methods have been advocated to distinguish displaced from nondisplaced tears of the ulnar collateral ligament. These methods include palpation of the ligament proximal to the joint on clinical examination, arthrography, and magnetic resonance imaging (MRI). None of these methods is universally reliable or available. Functional bracing has been shown to be as efficacious as casting for the treatment of incomplete ulnar collateral ligament injuries and for protection following surgical repair.

To better define the technique and reliability of valgus stress testing in predicting a Stener lesion, a combined clinical and laboratory study was recently reported. The basis of this study is the observation that combined accessory and proper collateral ligament injuries are uniformly present when a Stener lesion exists. Conversely, an intact accessory collateral ligament appears to prevent ligament displacement. The study indicated that ligament displacement was probable (88% in the clinical series) when joint angulation during stress testing in extension was greater than 35°. The authors concluded that the presence of a palpable mass, which represents the ligament stump proximal to the adductor aponeuorosis, or lateral instability in extension exceeding 35° indicated that ligament disruption with displacement was likely and that surgery was indicated.

Numerous surgical techniques have been described to treat instability. Anatomic repair using one of several suture techniques is possible in most acute cases. Several commercial devices are also available to help attach the ligament stump to bone. In chronic cases, the ligament may be contracted and insufficient for repair. A review of 26 cases of ulnar collateral ligament reconstruction using a free tendon graft found that all patients had a stable joint with relief of pain and recovered 85% of their normal motion at an average follow-up of 4.5 years. This study contrasts with others in which restricted motion was seen after delayed reconstruction.

Radial collateral ligament injuries are less common than ulnar collateral ligament tears, and the site of injury within the ligament is more variable. In one study, 18 patients who had repairs of the radial collateral ligament were reviewed. Twelve patients who had repair delayed until 2 months after injury were compared to 6 patients who had immediate repair. The outcomes of the two groups did not differ significantly and 17 of 18 patients had a satisfactory result. Although the indications for late repair were instability and pain, the indications for early repair were not defined.

Metacarpal Base Fractures

Results of several studies have shown the importance of restoring axial length and continuity of the metacarpal shaft to the smaller medial fragment with its important anterior ligament attachment in Bennett's fractures. If ligament function is not reestablished through bony union, then painful subluxation and decreased pinch strength are more likely. Although accurate reduction of the articular surface has been advocated, there is clinical evidence that some incongruity is well tolerated long-term. In a study of 41 patients treated for Bennett's fractures, 21 of the 31 patients that were available for review had no symptoms, and the remaining ten had only slight pain at an average follow-up of 7 years. Fractures that healed with deformity of the articular surface had a higher incidence of radiographic degeneration. The authors concluded that late symptoms seemed to be less likely and less severe when the fracture healed in anatomic position. However, only six of ten patients with radiologic signs of arthritis had symptoms, and these were mild. Another study with a follow-up of nearly 10 years demonstrated similar findings with no correlation between articular incongruity of up to 3 mm and symptomatic arthritis. Based on these studies, the value of extraordinary techniques to achieve a perfect reduction is questionable. Union of the fracture and a stable joint appear to be most important. These objectives can be achieved by either direct fixation of the two fragments if the smaller anterior fragment is of sufficient size, or indirect fixation of the shaft to the trapezium or index metacarpal.

Fracture dislocations of the fifth carpometacarpal (CMC) joint are the ulnar side equivalent of the Bennett's fracture. The metacarpal is pulled dorsally and ulnarly by the extensor carpi ulnaris, with the exception of a fragment from the radial portion of the metacarpal base that is held reduced by the intermetacarpal ligaments. Closed reduction is often achieved easily with longitudinal traction and direct pressure; however, percutaneous K-wire fixation is recommended to prevent resubluxation. Although older studies indicate that articular incongruity is usually well tolerated, a recent report of 64 patients with an average follow-up of 4.3 years indicated that 38% of patients had intermittent dull pain, 49% had decreased grip, and 65% had radiographic arthritis. Review of radiographs revealed that although metacarpal subluxation was consistently corrected, articular alignment was improved in only 43% of fractures. Based on these results, accurate reduction of the joint surface was recommended. Combined fourth and fifth CMC fracture dislocations are often associated with comminuted dorsal hamate fractures or coronal fractures through the hamate (Fig. 7). These injuries are particularly unstable and require internal fixation. Open reduction is usually necessary to obtain an accurate reduction of the articular surfaces.

High Pressure Injection and Nail Gun Injuries

High pressure injection injuries of the hand frequently cause severe damage. Rates of amputation vary from 16% to 48%. The initial treating physician often does not recognize the significance of the injury, resulting in delayed treatment. Oil-based solvents (grease, paint, paint thinner) are particularly harmful.

The outcomes of 25 patients treated by an open wound technique were reviewed in a recent study. The surgical technique included wide exposure through zigzag incisions and debridement of devitalized tissue and injected material, with preservation of the neurovascular structures. The wound was irrigated with pulsed lavage and packed open. Surgery was repeated at 24 to 72 hours as necessary. These steps were followed by delayed wound closure or closure

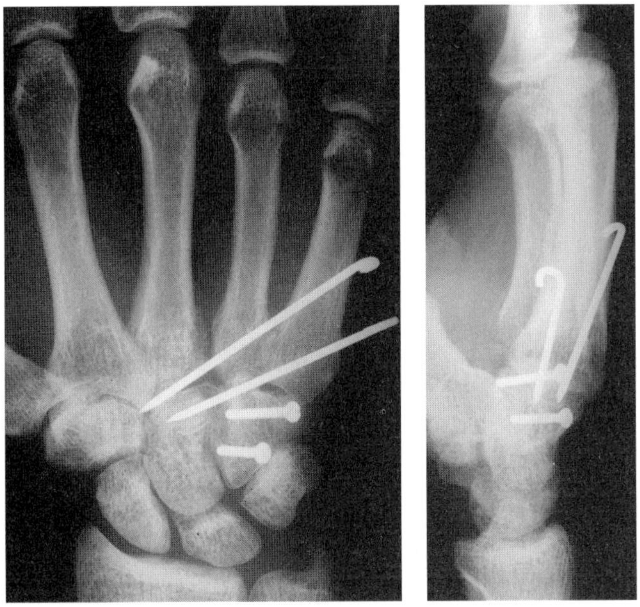

Fig. 7 A combined fourth and fifth carpometacarpal (CMC) fracture dislocation is associated with a coronal fracture through the hamate. This fracture pattern is unstable and requires open reduction and internal fixation. Two miniscrews fix the hamate fracture while temporary Kirschner-wires maintain reduction of the CMC joints.

by secondary intention. All patients received antibiotics, but none received steroids. Between debridements, whirlpools were used daily, and patients were started on intensive therapy emphasizing active range of motion. Four patients had amputations; however, these patients were seen 3 or more days after injury. Sixty-four percent had normal hand function and 84% of the hands and fingers were salvaged. These results are superior to those reported previously and were attributed to the surgical and rehabilitation techniques.

Nail guns are now routinely used in construction, and injuries to the hands are becoming more common. The nail is powered by an explosive charge of compressed air. Nails are manufactured with an adhesive coating and joined together into strips by copper wires. When the gun is fired, fragments of the wire form barbs that remain attached to the nail by the adhesive. These barbs considerably complicate removal by hooking soft tissues, including the neurovascular structures. Surgical exploration with nail removal under direct vision has been recommended to avoid further tissue damage. Because the barbs hook or point toward the head of the nail, an alternative method is to cut off the nail head and pull the nail out in the same direction as it entered (antegrade), thus avoiding soft-tissue entrapment by the barbs. The concept is the same as that used to remove a deeply penetrated fish hook.

Flexor Tendon Injuries

Primary repair of flexor tendon injuries and controlled postoperative mobilization remain the preferred treatment for flexor tendon lacerations, provided wound conditions are satisfactory. Several new suture techniques have been introduced in an effort to increase the strength of the repair sufficiently to allow early, active, controlled motion. Regardless of the suture technique used, experimental studies indicate that the number of suture strands crossing the repair site is the most important factor determining resistance to gap formation and the failure strength of the repair. Grasping and locking loops add little to repair strength and may actually contribute to gap formation by collapsing during tendon loading. Braided synthetic materials are popular choices for the core stitch because they make more secure knots, are stronger, and stretch less than monofilament sutures and are less brittle than stainless steel wire. The addition of a peripheral circumferential epitenon suture has been shown to increase repair strength, reduce gap formation, and improve healing. Several epitenon suture techniques that are stronger than a simple running suture have been described; however, the advantages of these modifications have not been demonstrated clinically.

A series of animal experiments have shown that passive motion improves the tensile strength, gliding surface, excursion, and vascularization in repaired flexor tendons. More importantly, the conclusions of numerous clinical reports indicate that controlled mobilization following repair improves clinical outcome. However, the optimum method of rehabilitation remains unclear. In one study, metal markers placed during surgery were used to compare tendon excursions between rehabilitation programs. The "four finger" method, which places all fingers, regardless of the presence of injury, into traction, produced markedly greater tendon excursion and joint motion compared to the standard rubber band traction protocol (Kleinert technique). The main disadvantages of the standard rubber-band traction method are the increased incidence of flexion contractures of the PIP joint and the often inadequate return of distal interphalangeal (DIP) motion. A program with a number of modifications, including a shorter dorsal splint that extended only to the level of the PIP joints and four finger traction, was used in a group of patients to decrease these problems. In addition, passive flexion was used to increase the range of motion achieved with traction alone, and the traction was intermittently removed. A volar splint was worn at night as needed to correct flexion contractures. Using this program, patients achieved 96% good or excellent and 4% fair results compared to 51% good or excellent, 40% fair, and 9% poor results using the standard protocol of a longer splint and traction to the injured finger(s) only.

The four finger method, the standard Kleinert method, and a modified Kleinert method that adds passive motion at the extremes of the traction range were compared in an additional study. The four finger method produced significantly greater PIP and DIP motion 4 weeks after surgery, with the improvements maintained throughout the remainder of the recovery. In an attempt to further improve outcome, early controlled active motion programs are gaining popularity. These programs are possible in part due to stronger suture techniques that can theoretically withstand the increased loads delivered to the repair site with active flexion. Although early clinical reports regarding these programs are encouraging, the results should be considered preliminary.

To evaluate the rate of recovery of motion following zone 2 tendon repair, a series of patients was examined at several time intervals during recovery. The PIP joints achieved 75% of their final motion by 4 weeks, 97% by 24 weeks, and 100% by 1 year after surgery. The DIP joints gained 44% of their final motion by 4 weeks, 63% by 12 weeks, 90% by 24 weeks, and 100% by 1 year. Fifty-eight percent of the total recovery occurred between 3 and 12 months. Those with poor results at 3 months had a greater rate of recovery after 3 months than those with an excellent result at 3 months. Based on these results, waiting 6 to 12 months is recommended before considering tenolysis following flexor tendon repair.

The best care of partial flexor tendon lacerations remains controversial. Although an unrepaired tendon may cause triggering or weaken and rupture, repair can cause adhesions with loss of motion. A series of patients with partial tendon lacerations ranging from 20% to 75% of the flexor tendon diameter were identified at surgery. Fourteen tendons were not repaired and eight were repaired. In the repair group, lacerations involving less than 50% of the tendon diameter were sutured with an epitenon suture only and those involving more than 50% were repaired with core suture (modified Kessler) and epitenon stitches. No triggering occurred in either group. Range of motion was better in the unrepaired group. Because most cases of triggering can be treated late with a good result, the primary indication for repair of a partial laceration is to prevent weakening and rupture. The authors concluded that a repair should be done only for lacerations involving more than 60% of the tendon. Authors of previous reports have made similar recommendations.

Repair of the flexor sheath in the finger remains controversial. Sheath closure, which is based primarily on theoretical advantages, may be attempted but extraordinary measures using tissue grafts are not justified because clinical studies have failed to show any benefit.

Extensor Tendon Injuries

Extensor tendon injuries are being given greater attention because of the increased recognition that not all lacerations respond well to traditional treatment. A retrospective study of 62 patients with 101 extensor tendon lacerations revealed that 60% of all fingers had an associated injury, such as a fracture, dislocation, joint capsule injury, or flexor tendon laceration. Results were good to excellent in 45% of fingers with combined injuries compared to 64% good to excellent results in fingers without associated injuries. Distal zone injuries (proximal phalanx to DIP joint) had a less favorable outcome than proximal zone injuries (forearm to MCP joint), and the average loss of flexion was greater than the average loss of extension.

After surgical repair, extensor tendon injuries have traditionally been managed by immobilization with the wrist in 40° of extension and the MCP joints in slight flexion for 3 to 4 weeks. Immobilization can result in extensor tendon adhesions, especially when the tendon injury is associated with other local tissue injuries. Improved results were reported for several studies in which a postoperative program of early, controlled passive motion by dynamic splinting, which is similar to programs used after flexor tendon repair, was used. Data from anatomic studies have shown that 27° to 41° of MCP joint flexion, depending on the finger, will produce 5 mm of extensor digitorum communis glide over the MCP joint, hand, and wrist. Although the clinical benefit of dynamic splinting has not been shown in a prospective study that compared dynamic to static splinting, the current trend is to use an early motion program, especially in cases that are more prone to adhesions, such as multiple extensor tendon injuries beneath the extensor retinaculum or those with injuries to adjacent tissues. The usefulness of dynamic splinting for extensor tendon injuries over the fingers is not apparent, and there are several probable difficulties with its application to these injuries. Dynamic splinting will most likely yield a good result in a cooperative patient with an injury at or proximal to the MCP joint and when a skilled hand therapist is available to fabricate the splint and to monitor progress. Traditional methods of immobilization are recommended for children and uncooperative adults.

Conservative management is appropriate for most closed mallet finger injuries. Surgical repair is not only unnecessary in most cases, but is probably contraindicated because splinting produces a satisfactory outcome. The exception may be those injuries with a fracture fragment involving greater than one third of the articular surface and associated with joint subluxation. Although an accurate reduction has been advocated to prevent joint deformity and subsequent arthritis, reduction and fixation of these fractures is challenging, and complications are frequent. In a study that included 45 surgically treated cases, 53% had a complication including nail deformity, joint incongruity, infection, loss of fixation, and joint angulation. However, treatment by splinting is not without complications; the most frequent problem is transient dorsal skin maceration and ulceration. In one study, a dorsal splint caused a higher rate of skin complications. Immobilization in hyperextension and dorsal external pressure should be avoided because they can exacerbate the relative hypovascularity in this region.

Closed acute boutonnière deformities without fixed contractures are treated by splinting the PIP joint in full extension and at the same time performing active and passive flexion exercises at the DIP joint to maintain the balance between the central slip and the lateral bands. If the patient has developed a PIP joint flexion contracture, treatment should begin with splinting or serial casting of the contracture until full passive extension is achieved. Active PIP joint extension is then assessed, and if it is inadequate, surgical treatment is indicated. Open lacerations over the PIP joint are likely to enter the joint; therefore, the first goal of treatment is to prevent infection. After wound and joint lavage, repair of the central slip and lateral bands is completed. Following repair, the PIP joint is splinted in extension for 5 to 6 weeks, and the patient does DIP joint flexion exercises.

Extensor tendon lacerations at the wrist level are under the retinaculum, which complicates repair and rehabilitation. Although some of the retinaculum can be excised for exposure and to prevent impingement at the repair site, a portion of the retinaculum should always be repaired or, preferably, preserved to prevent bowstringing.

Nerve Repair

The majority of acute nerve injuries can be repaired primarily. In a relatively clean wound, a primary repair using an end-to-end epineural or a group fascicular technique, depending on the internal topography of the nerve, is preferred. Matching fascicular orientation during repair is critical to prevent motor fibers from regenerating into sensory fibers and vice versa. In addition, accurate alignment of a pure sensory nerve will minimize incorrect localization of sensory recovery. Although it is usually not required for primary repair, awake stimulation is a useful technique to determine motor and sensory fascicular grouping in the proximal stump. Chemical staining of the nerve can also be useful; however, the technique is time-consuming and not widely available. Distally, it is not possible to use stimulation or staining, but surgical dissection aided by topography maps is useful. After the repair is completed, the digits and extremities should be put through a gentle range of motion to determine what motion is acceptable. Most repairs are protected in a splint for approximately 3 weeks.

Following nerve repair, range of motion of all affected joints must be maintained long-term to maximize potential motor recovery. Electrical stimulation of denervated muscle is controversial. However, early motor reeducation is beneficial after reinnervation begins. Later, reeducation emphasizes movements required for specific tasks and job activities. Aberrant sensory localization is common following nerve regeneration. Sensory reeducation will help the patient reinterpret the altered nerve impulses. As reinnervation progresses, the goals are to reeducate specific sensory perceptions and to improve localization. Later, reeducation focuses on improving task performance.

A review of 33 patients who had radial nerve repairs demonstrated useful results in 65% of patients. Nerve grafting was done in 21 cases and direct suturing in 12. Useful recovery was seen in only eight of the 21 grafted cases.

A review of 110 patients who had ulnar nerve repairs indicated that only 52% of the patients had useful recovery. Direct suturing was done in 34 cases and nerve grafting in 76 cases. The age of the patient, width of the nerve injury, delay to repair, and level of injury influenced results.

Intrinsic muscle recovery in 22 patients who had repairs of median and ulnar nerve transections at the wrist was examined clinically and with electromyography at an average follow-up of 5 years. Electrical activity was nearly always present despite the absence of clinically detectable function. Muscle power was clinically detectable when the maximum evoked muscle action potential reached 50% that of the contralateral side.

The outcomes of 15 patients who had combined median and ulnar nerve lacerations as well as multiple flexor tendon lacerations at the wrist were reviewed. The results of primary nerve repair were satisfactory; however, recovery of the median nerve was better than that of the ulnar nerve. Although wrist motion recovered well, recovery of finger flexion was often unsatisfactory. Poor finger motion was partially attributed to poor patient compliance in the rehabilitation program.

A long-held premise of proper nerve repair technique is that the repair should be completed free of tension, and when this is not possible, a graft should be used. A recent laboratory study in which a primate model was used challenged this approach. Axon regeneration after direct epineural repair under tension (15-mm gap) was compared to interfascicular nerve grafting via either standard grafting technique or a new technique using a collagen tube. Electrophysiologic measurements strongly favored direct nerve repair under tension, and histologic analysis demonstrated a similar tendency. The authors concluded that for modest defects, it is advantageous to accept modest tension with a direct repair rather than to use a nerve graft to achieve a tension-free repair.

Although numerous different biomaterials and tissues have been tried as a substitute for nerve autograft, none have reliably produced equivalent results, especially for long defects. The result of using autogenous vein grafts for 18 digital nerve defects were reported in a recent study. Excellent recovery occurred in only two digital nerves, good in nine, fair in five, and poor in two.

Replantation

Several factors influence the decision to replant an amputated part of the hand; however, the expected functional outcome from replantation should be one of the most important considerations. The anticipated final function should be equal to or better than function after an amputation revision or prosthesis. Factors that impact on functional outcome include the level of amputation, the mechanism of injury, ischemia time, and the age and health of the patient as well as the patient's potential for rehabilitation and occupational needs.

Replantation of the thumb should be attempted in almost all thumb amputations, including avulsion injuries. In multiple digit amputations, strong consideration should be given to replantation, especially of the least damaged digits. These digits can often be shifted to the most functional position of the hand or to the least damaged parts of the hand. Fingers replanted distal to the flexor superficialis insertion usually achieve satisfactory function. Replantation of a single digit proximal to the flexor superficialis insertion usually does not improve hand function and is rarely indicated. Replantation at the level of the palm, wrist, or distal forearm usually results in better function than would be achieved with a prosthesis. Higher levels of replantation can be complicated by muscle necrosis and infection, with significant systemic risk to the patient. Replantation of nearly all amputated parts should be considered in healthy children.

A study using multiple functional tests was done to compare the results of 25 patients who had thumb replantation with those of 18 patients who had revision amputation. Eighty percent of patients in both groups were able to perform activities of daily living 80% as well with the injured hand as with the uninjured hand. Grip strength averaged 84% of the opposite side in each group. Lateral pinch and work simulation assessments were better in the revision amputation group. Decreased sensibility was the leading complaint in both groups. Those patients with replanted thumbs that recovered good sensibility had better fine dexterity and the ability to hold certain objects. Most patients with an isolated thumb amputation distal to the MCP joint, regardless of treatment, resumed activities of daily living and their jobs. A clear advantage of either replantation or revision was not demonstrated in this study. These results should probably not be used to change the indications for thumb replantation, but they do emphasize the adaptability of most patients to an amputation.

The classification scheme most commonly used to guide treatment for ring avulsion injuries emphasizes the circulatory status of the finger at presentation. However, data from one study demonstrated that final functional outcome correlated more closely with the presence or absence of skeletal injury than with the amount of vascular damage. Prognosis was especially poor for ring avulsions with injury through the PIP joint. Thus, it appears that if the unique vascular problems caused by an avulsion injury can be managed by microvascular repair, the decision to save the digit should be based on criteria similar to those applied to amputations caused by other mechanisms.

Finger Tip Injuries

In finger tip amputations, the angle of injury has been used to guide treatment options. In dorsally angulated or transverse amputations, local finger flaps can be used. A wound with palmar angulation eliminates the possibility of using local flaps. A cross finger flap can be used in this case; however, the patient should be counseled concerning the resultant donor site scar. A thenar flap is an alternative, but should be used with caution in older patients because of the propensity for PIP joint stiffness. Allowing the wound to heal by secondary intention continues to be controversial. Some studies have shown that conservative treatment produces better results than skin grafting, shortening and closure, or flaps. However, some degree of a hook nail deformity will often occur with conservative management. A stable, satisfactory reduction of a tuft fracture is necessary to provide support for the nail bed. A K-wire or other internal fixation may be required to maintain stability. In children, the finger tip should be replaced, because even a composite amputation, including bone, nail bed, and pad distal to the level of the lunula, can be reattached as a composite graft.

Whether the nail should be removed in the presence of a subungual hematoma is controversial. The practice of removing the nail and repairing the nail bed when more than 50% of the nail is undermined by hematoma is supported by the good results reported using this technique. However, in another study, which was done to evaluate the treatment of subungual hematomas by drainage alone, the final result was not affected by the size of the hematoma or the presence of a tuft fracture.

In an acute nail bed injury with an avulsed nail, the nail bed should be repaired with fine chromic suture and the nail replaced as a stent. Larger fragments of avulsed nail bed should be carefully removed from the undersurface of the nail and replaced into the defects. Removal of smaller fragments from the nail will cause too much injury to the tissue; these fragments should be left in place and aligned when the nail is replaced. Good results were obtained in 29 and poor results in five of 34 digits treated by replacement of completely avulsed fragments of germinal or sterile matrix. There were only four cases of germinal matrix involvement, and half of these had a poor result. Ninety-one percent of cases with isolated sterile matrix grafting had a good result. In ten cases in which the fragments were replaced directly onto exposed bone, there were no nail deformities. It appears that no soft-tissue coverage of bone is needed to successfully graft sterile matrix.

Grafting acute nail bed defects in the sterile matrix has been advocated as a method to repair acute nail bed injuries complicated by loss of nail substance. This technique is most applicable when an unsalvageable digit is an available donor. Other alternatives include using a split-thickness sterile matrix graft from the uninjured portion of the same nail bed or a sterile matrix graft from the big toe, if the defect is large. Dermal and reversed dermal grafts have also been used, but the results appear to be less reliable. For germinal matrix defects, only full-thickness grafts of germinal matrix have the potential to produce nail growth. This type of reconstruction should be planned as a secondary procedure. In one study, 75 of 84 sterile matrix avulsions treated by split-thickness sterile matrix grafts had a good result. Nine cases resulted in some nail deformity, which was always within the injured region and not the adjacent donor region.

Annotated Bibliography

Distal Radius Fractures

Adams BD: Effects of radial deformity on distal radioulnar joint mechanics. *J Hand Surg* 1993;18A: 492–498.

Of four types of radial deformity tested in a laboratory study, radial shortening caused the greatest disturbance in DRUJ kinematics and the most distortion of the triangular fibrocartilage. Radial deformity alone did not cause dislocation of the DRUJ.

Greatting MD, Bishop AT: Intrafocal (Kapandji) pinning of unstable fractures of the distal radius. *Orthop Clin North Am* 1993;24:301–307.

Intrafocal pinning was used in 23 patients. Some loss of reduction was more common in patients older than 65 years of age. However, their clinical result was better than that of those younger than 65 years of age. Overall, the technique was satisfactory and appeared to offer advantages for simple to moderately difficult fractures.

Kaempffe FA, Wheeler DR, Peimer CA, et al: Severe fractures of the distal radius: Effect of amount and duration of external fixator distraction on outcome. *J Hand Surg* 1993;18A:33–41.

External fixation with distraction was shown to adversely affect outcome at 2 years in proportion to the amount and duration of distraction. However, a critical amount of distraction could not be defined.

Kazuki K, Kusunoki M, Yamada J, et al: Cineradiographic study of wrist motion after fracture of the distal radius. *J Hand Surg* 1993;18A:41–46.

The effect of residual dorsal tilt of the distal radius on wrist range of motion and carpal alignment was investigated in 30 patients with extra-articular fractures. Dorsal tilt greater than 10° was found to be associated with decreased range of motion and carpal malalignment.

Kopylov P, Johnell O, Redlund-Johnell I, et al: Fractures of the distal end of the radius in young adults: A 30-year follow-up. *J Hand Surg* 1993;18B:45–49.

Eighty-one percent of patients reported no difference between the injured and uninjured side, although they had significantly decreased wrist flexion and grip strength. The DRUJ of the fractured wrist did not demonstrate more pain or instability than the uninjured wrist, nor was there a difference in pronation–supination. Radiographs showed minor degenerative changes in the radiocarpal joint in 33% and in the DRUJ in 25%.

Leung KS, Shen WY, Tsang HK, et al: An effective treatment of comminuted fractures of the distal radius. *J Hand Surg* 1990;15A:11–17.

One hundred cases of comminuted fracture of the distal radius were treated by bone grafting and external fixation for 3 weeks followed by functional bracing. Additional K-wire fixation was used in some. The good results obtained using this method suggest that limited surgical exposure and fixation are adequate treatment for most patients.

Scaphoid Fractures

Tiel-Van Buul MM, Van Beek EJ, Borm JJ, et al: The value of radiographs and bone scintigraphy in suspected scaphoid fracture: A statistical analysis. *J Hand Surg* 1993;18B:403–406.

Repeat plain radiographs had a sensitivity of only 30% in detecting scaphoid fractures following an initial negative radiograph. Sensitivity and specificity of a bone scan was nearly 100%. A bone scan was the recommended diagnostic procedure for patients with suspected scaphoid fractures with an initial negative plain radiograph.

Wrist Instabilities

Dautel G, Goudot B, Merle M: Arthroscopic diagnosis of scapho-lunate instability in the absence of x-ray abnormalities. *J Hand Surg* 1993;18B:213–218.

Arthroscopy was combined with intraoperative wrist manipulation in order to identify scapholunate instability. Six of 26 scapholunate interosseous ligament tears identified during arthroscopy had no associated instability and were believed not to be the cause of wrist pain.

Herzberg G, Comtet JJ, Linscheid RL, et al: Perilunate dislocations and fracture-dislocations: A multicenter study. *J Hand Surg* 1993;18A:768–769.

In 166 cases reviewed, the diagnosis was initially missed in 25%. Open injuries and a delay in treatment of greater than 1 week were associated with a poor clinical outcome. Carpal alignment was better maintained following ORIF than after closed reduction and percutaneous pinning.

Lavernia CJ, Cohen MS, Taleisnik J: Treatment of scapholunate dissociation by ligamentous repair and capsulodesis. *J Hand Surg* 1992;17A:354–359.

Twenty-one patients with scapholunate dissociation were treated by ligament repair. Radioscaphoid capsulodesis was added in 14 patients. It was concluded that sufficient ligamentous substance is usually available for repair even in chronic injuries.

Phalangeal and Metacarpal Shaft Fractures

Gonzalez MH, McKay W, Hall RF Jr: Low velocity gunshot wounds of the metacarpal: Treatment by early stable fixation and bone grafting. *J Hand Surg* 1993;18A: 267–270.

Sixty-four metacarpal fractures due to gunshot wounds were treated by open reduction, bone grafting, internal fixation, and early motion. Final MCP joint motion averaged 65°. There was minimal shortening, and angulation averaged less than 10° in 63 fractures.

Hastings H II: Unstable metacarpal and phalangeal fracture treatment with screws and plates. *Clin Orthop* 1987;214:37–52.

Technical and clinical considerations in the treatment of metacarpal and phalangeal fractures by open reduction and internal fixation are reviewed.

Proximal Interphalangeal Joint Fractures and Dislocations

Durham-Smith G, McCarten GM: Volar plate arthroplasty for closed proximal interphalangeal joint injuries. *J Hand Surg* 1992;17B:422–428.

Seventy-one cases of volar plate arthroplasty were done using a technical modification of the original description. Eighty-seven percent of patients obtained a stable pain-free joint with an average range of motion of 5° to 95° within 2 months.

Viegas SF: Extension block pinning for proximal interphalangeal joint fracture dislocations: Preliminary report of a new technique. *J Hand Surg* 1992;17A: 896–901.

A new method of treatment for unstable dorsal fracture dislocations of the PIP joint uses a K-wire inserted into the head of the proximal phalanx to maintain reduction. Results are promising, although preliminary.

Weiss AP, Hastings H II: Distal Unicondylar fractures of the proximal phalanx. *J Hand Surg* 1993;18A:594–599.

The treatment of 38 distal unicondylar proximal phalanx fractures was retrospectively reviewed. Four types of fracture patterns were identified. The oblique volar pattern was the most common (58%). Multiple K-wires or miniscrew fixation was the most reliable. A short period of postoperative immobilization did not adversely affect final motion.

Collateral Ligament Injuries of the Thumb Metacarpophalangeal Joint

Durham JW, Kuhri S, Kim MH: Acute and late radial collateral ligament injuries of the thumb metacarpophalangeal joint. *J Hand Surg* 1993;18A:232–237.

The outcomes of acute and chronic repairs of the radial collateral ligament did not differ significantly. Seventeen of 18 patients had a satisfactory result. Although the indications for late repair were instability and pain, the indications for early repair were not defined.

Glickel SZ, Malerich M, Pearce SM, et al: Ligament replacement for chronic instability of the ulnar collateral ligament of the metacarpophalangeal joint of the thumb. *J Hand Surg* 1993;18A:930–941.

Excellent results were obtained in 24 of 26 patients with ligament reconstruction using a free tendon graft.

Heyman P, Gelberman RH, Duncan K, et al: Injuries of the ulnar collateral ligament of the thumb metacarpophalangeal joint: Biomechanical and prospective clinical studies on the usefulness of valgus stress testing. *Clin Orthop* 1993;292:165–171.

The valgus stress test for ulnar collateral ligament injuries was evaluated in a cadaver experiment and a clinical series. The key component of the test was stressing the joint in extension. Laxity greater than 35° indicated a probable Stener's lesion, which was confirmed in 88% of the patients in the clinical series.

Metacarpal Base Fractures

Kjaer-Petersen K, Jurik AG, Petersen LK: Intra-articular fractures at the base of the fifth metacarpal: A clinical and radiographical study of 64 cases. *J Hand Surg* 1992;17B: 144–147.

The results of 64 intra-articular fractures at the base of the fifth metacarpal were reviewed. Metacarpal subluxation was corrected; however, articular congruity was improved in only 53% of the fractures. Persistent symptoms were not uncommon, and 65% had radiographic arthritis at follow-up.

High Pressure Injection and Nail Gun Injuries

al-Qattan MM, Stranc MF: Nail gun injuries of the fingers: A safer method of nail removal. *J Hand Surg* 1993;18A:652–653.

An alternative technique for removal of a nail resulting from a nail gun injury is presented.

Pinto MR, Turkula-Pinto LD, Cooney WP, et al: High-pressure injection injuries of the hand: Review of 25 patients managed by open wound technique. *J Hand Surg* 1993;18A:125–130.

Twenty-five patients were treated by an open wound technique with debridement, drainage, open packing, and delayed closure. Eighty-four percent of the involved hands or fingers were salvaged and 64% had essentially normal hand function.

Flexor Tendon Injuries

Greenwald DP, Hong HZ, May JW Jr: Mechanical analysis of tendon suture techniques. *J Hand Surg* 1994;19A:641–647.

Seven different types of tendon repair were tested in a laboratory study in rabbits. A newer technique that includes four core suture strands crossing the repair site and criss-crossing within the tendon substance was stronger than more traditional suture techniques.

Karlander LE, Berggren M, Larsson M, et al: Improved results in zone 2 flexor tendon injuries with a modified technique of immediate controlled mobilization. *J Hand Surg* 1993;18B:26–30.

A rehabilitation program was used that included rubber-band traction to all four fingers, even if they are not injured. A dorsal splint extending only to the PIP joints decreased the incidence of PIP joint flexion contractures. The program achieved 96% good or excellent results compared to 51% good or excellent results using a more traditional protocol.

May EJ, Silfverskiold KL: Rate of recovery after flexor tendon repair in zone II: A prospective longitudinal study of 145 digits. *Scand J Plast Reconstr Surg* 1993;27:89–94.

The rate of recovery of PIP joint motion after flexor tendon repair was 75% of the final motion by 4 weeks and 97% by 24 weeks. The results indicate that there should be a waiting period of 6 to 12 months after flexor tendon repair before considering tenolysis.

McGeorge DD, Stilwell JH: Partial flexor tendon injuries: To repair or not. *J Hand Surg* 1992;17B:176–177.

Partial flexor tendon lacerations ranging from 20% to 75% were identified at surgery. Fourteen tendons were not repaired and eight tendons were repaired. No triggering occurred in either group. Range of motion was better in the group not repaired. It was concluded that a repair should be done only for lacerations greater than 60%.

Silfverskold KL, May EJ: Flexor tendon repair in zone II with a new suture technique and an early mobilization program combining passive and active flexion. *J Hand Surg* 1944;19A:53–60.

A new cross-stitch technique was used for flexion tendon repair in zone II in 55 digits. A rehabilitation program included passive and active motion. Two ruptures occurred. At 3 weeks postoperatively, DIP motion was 82% and PIP motion was 88% of the maximum possible.

Silfverskiold KL, May EJ, Tornvall A: Tendon excursions after flexor tendon repair in zone II: Results with a new controlled-motion program. *J Hand Surg* 1993;18A: 403–410.

Metal markers were placed in the tendon during surgery, and tendon excursion was measured during rehabilitation. The inclusion of four fingers in rubber-band traction increased FDP motion compared to a program with traction applied only to the injured digits.

Extensor Tendon Injuries

Browne EZ Jr, Ribik CA: Early dynamic splinting for extensor tendon injuries. *J Hand Surg* 1989;14A:72–76.

A dynamic splinting program was used following extensor tendon repairs. Motion was begun 2 to 5 days after repair and was continued for approximately 5 weeks. No ruptures occurred, and all patients recovered full flexion.

Newport ML, Blair WF, Steyers CM Jr: Long-term results of extensor tendon repair. *J Hand Surg* 1990;15A: 961–966.

In 101 extensor tendon lacerations, 60% of all fingers had an associated injury such as a fracture, dislocation, joint injury, or flexor tendon laceration. Combined injuries resulted in 45% good to excellent results compared to 64% good to excellent results in fingers without associated injuries.

Stern PJ, Kastrup JJ: Complications and prognosis of treatment of mallet finger. *J Hand Surg* 1988;13A: 329–334.

In 84 digits treated by splinting, there was a 45% complication rate; however, most complications were transient skin problems. There was a 53% complication rate in the surgically treated patients, with 76% of these complications still present at follow-up of 38 months.

Nerve Repair

Hentz VR, Rosen JM, Xiao SJ, et al: The nerve gap dilemma: A comparison of nerves repaired end to end under tension with nerve grafts in a primate model. *J Hand Surg* 1993;18A:417–425.

The concept of tension-free nerve repair was challenged in this study. It was concluded that for modest nerve defects, it is advantageous to accept modest tension with a direct repair rather than to use a graft to achieve a tension-free repair.

Hudson DA, de Jager LT: The spaghetti wrist: Simultaneous laceration of the median and ulnar nerves with flexor tendons at the wrist. *J Hand Surg* 1993;18B:171–173.

In 15 patients with combined median nerve, ulnar nerve, and flexor tendon lacerations at the wrist, results of primary nerve repair were satisfactory. However, recovery of the median nerve was better than that of the ulnar nerve.

Kallio PK, Vastamaki M, Solonen KA: The results of secondary microsurgical repair of the radial nerve in 33 patients. *J Hand Surg* 1993;18B:320–322.

A review of 33 radial nerve repairs demonstrated useful recovery in only 65% of patients. Nerve grafting was done in 21 cases and resulted in useful recovery in only eight of 21 cases.

Lester RL, Smith PJ, Mott G, et al: Intrinsic reinnervation-myth or reality? *J Hand Surg* 1993;18B: 454–460.

Intrinsic muscle recovery was studied at an average follow-up of 5 years in 22 patients who had repairs of the median and ulnar nerves at the wrist. Electrical activity was nearly always present despite the absence of clinically detectable function. Muscle power was detectable when electrical reinnervation reached 50% of the contralateral maximum evoked muscle action potential.

Tang JB, Gu YQ, Song YS: Repair of digital nerve defect with autogenous vein graft during flexor tendon surgery in zone 2. *J Hand Surg* 1993;18B:449–453.

Eighteen digital nerve defects identified during flexion tendon surgery in zone II were treated by interposition autogenous vein grafts. In defects over 2 cm, normal nerve slices were inserted inside the veins. Excellent recovery occurred in two nerves, good in nine, fair in five, and poor in two.

Vastamaki M, Kallio PK, Solonen KA: The results of secondary microsurgical repair of ulnar nerve injury. *J Hand Surg* 1993;18B:323–326.

In 110 patients who had ulnar nerve repairs, 52% recovered useful function. Patient age, width of nerve injury, delay to repair, and level of injury influenced results.

Replantation

Goldner RD, Howson MP, Nunley JA, et al: One hundred eleven thumb amputations: Replantation vs revision. *Microsurgery* 1990;11:243–250.

Multiple functional tests were used to compare the results of 25 patients who had thumb replantation with 18 patients who had revision amputation. Patients with replanted thumbs that recovered good sensibility had better fine dexterity and the ability to hold certain objects. Patients with an isolated thumb amputation distal to the MCP joint, regardless of treatment, resumed activities of daily living and their jobs.

Kay S, Werntz J, Wolff TW: Ring avulsion injuries: Classification and prognosis. *J Hand Surg* 1989;14A: 204–213.

Fifty-five cases of ring avulsion injuries were reviewed to determine how the extent of injury and the surgical treatment correlated with results. Injuries through the PIP joint had a poor prognosis, whereas through-bone amputations obtained satisfactory results.

Finger Tip Injuries

Shepard GH: Management of acute nail bed avulsions. *Hand Clin* 1990;6:39–56.

The treatment of nail bed injuries is reviewed. Replacement of avulsed nail bed is recommended, but when not available a sterile matrix graft can be done with a good result.

32

Wrist and Hand: Reconstruction

Carpal Tunnel Syndrome

Introduction/Epidemiology

Carpal tunnel syndrome (CTS) has now become one of the most frequently entertained musculoskeletal diagnoses, in part, because of public education and increasing awareness of the medical community. However, there also appears to be an increasing occurrence of CTS within a younger population. These patients have a history of performing repetitive tasks within a limited range of motion over prolonged periods of time. Along with CTS, the patients may present with complaints suggestive of multiple compressive neuropathies and multiple sites of musculotendinous irritation. This constellation of symptoms and physical findings has been lumped together under the ambiguous condition of "cumulative trauma disorders." That such a condition exists is controversial, especially with regard to its relationship as an etiologic source for CTS.

Sensory conduction of the median nerve has been used as an indicator to evaluate the relationship between CTS and age, gender, handedness, occupation, and clinical diagnosis. The study population was chosen at random, evaluated, and tested again 5 years later. The conclusions of the study were that slowing of sensory conduction and, by implication, the onset of CTS correlated more with age and hand dominance than any job-related factor. The investigators go on to state that there was no relationship between occupational hand use and CTS and that symptom-based diagnoses related to subjective pain were mercurial, rarely persisting for more than 5 years. Critics of this opinion are quick to point out that there was 33% attrition in the study population, which makes the statistical significance of the findings somewhat suspect, and that single-setting electrodiagnostic studies will miss dynamic CTS. Nevertheless, the study serves as a reminder that aging influences human tolerance of occupation-induced trauma.

The belief that there is a relationship between some occupations and the development of CTS is supported by an increasingly large number of international studies. Typical of these studies is one conducted by the California Department of Health Services, which evaluated CTS among grocery-store workers. The study was prompted by submission of an inordinately high number of CTS claims from employees of one particularly busy store. The investigators chose to measure forceful and repetitive wrist motion, identify a job classification scheme based on type of work tasks, and record the average time per week spent performing these tasks. A medical questionnaire and measurements of median sensory nerve conduction were used to measure CTS. Prevalence was 23% based on a sample of 56 participants drawn from a work force of 69 employees. Interestingly this is the same prevalence identified in the previously mentioned study. Rather then concluding that there was no correlation between occupation and CTS, the investigators demonstrated that there was a higher relative risk (95% confidence interval: 2.6 to 26.4) for a history of CTS-like symptoms among the high-exposure groups after adjustment for the potential confounders of age, sex, alcohol consumption, and high-risk medical history. In similar studies from Sweden, the prevalence of CTS in different occupational groups varied between 0.6% and 61%. The highest prevalence was noted for grinders, butchers, grocery-store workers, frozen food factory workers, platers, and workers with high-force, high-repetitive manual movements. At least 50% and as many as 90% of all of the CTS cases in these exposed populations were thought to be attributable to physical work load.

Diagnosis

The diagnosis should be based on sound historic facts, physical examination, and diagnostic findings. The history is that of pain and paresthesias along the palmar aspect of the radial digits, but not the palm; symptoms are usually worse at night and aggravated with prolonged wrist extension or flexion. In the past, the physical findings were usually an identifiable sensory deficit, thenar muscle atrophy in the severest cases, and symptom aggravation with easily performed maneuvers, such as Phalen's test. Because of heightened awareness, patients are presenting earlier in the course of the disease, their histories are prompted by the experience of others, and the cursory physical examination is usually normal, making accurate diagnosis dependent on provocative tests reinforced by adjunctive studies.

Phalen's sign, described as numbness and tingling in the median nerve distribution after sustained wrist flexion, has a reported sensitivity of 75% and specificity of 47% if the wrist position is held for more that 60 seconds. If this maneuver is combined with monofilament studies recorded prior to and 1 minute after wrist flexion, the sensitivity and specificity of the findings increases to 82% and 86% respectively. For the study to be considered positive, the monofilament sensibility must increase by one grade in thickness. Combined tests such as these are time consuming and require a well-trained and patient examiner. A combination of easily performed maneuvers may be just as useful. A sensitivity of 100% and a specificity of 97% have been reported after placing a sphygmomanometer about the wrist and inflating it to 150 mm Hg. Recapitulation of symptoms within 30 seconds of inflation is considered positive. The significance of this report is obscured by the failure of the authors to substantiate clinical findings with electrodiagnostic studies in a number of the cases. Nonetheless, pressure manipulation in combination with Phalen's maneuver and Tinel's sign certainly raises the suspicion that CTS is present. The diminution of two-point discrimination is a late finding consistent with long-standing nerve dysfunction and, like the presence of thenar atrophy, is being seen less frequently.

The remainder of the examination is directed towards identifying potential sites of proximal compression, particularly the cervical spine, thoracic outlet, elbow, and proximal forearm, and exploring the patient's history for contributing factors, such as endocrinopathies, collagen vascular diseases, dialysis, and acute and chronic trauma. The trauma history may be as obvious as an acute fracture or as subtle as the repetitive impact of crutches or wheelchairs.

CTS is said to be a clinical diagnosis that requires little investigation beyond a history and physical examination. Whether this represents cost-effective medicine or diagnostic arrogance remains unresolved. Arguably, adjunctive studies should be ordered for a reason. Radiographs are indicated for imaging the wrist if there is a history of trauma or long-standing inflammatory disease. If the examination raises suspicions, radiographs are used to help rule out distant compression points, such as a supracondylar process on the distal humerus or an accessory rib in the case of suspected thoracic outlet compression. Magnetic resonance imaging (MRI) and computed tomography (CT) scans are not routinely used because there currently is no evidence that either scan is a useful screening tool for CTS. The single most helpful adjunct remains electrodiagnostic testing.

Electrodiagnostic studies are not needed for diagnosis of most cases of CTS; they are most useful for identifying peripheral neuropathies and coexistent compression elsewhere in the extremity. With milder cases the findings may be subtle, underscoring the need for a consistent testing technique, preferably performed by the same electromyographer using the same equipment in the same setting. Each examiner should have established consistent norms, with values, including those for the ulnar nerve, compared bilaterally. The sensitivity of these studies increases from electromyograms (EMGs) and conduction velocities to distal latencies and ulnar–median nerve latency differences. EMGs are the most painful part of these studies and usually the least helpful. They require needle penetration for recording, and results are affected by needle depth and position. EMGs are rarely positive in the now typical case of early CTS, but remain useful when the history and examination suggest proximal median nerve entrapment, cervical radiculopathy, or peripheral neuropathy.

Conduction velocities measured along the length of the forearm and hand are helpful in identifying anomalous nerve communications, such as the Martin-Gruber anastomoses, but are not sensitive for the identification of mild CTS. Distal latency, the time in milliseconds required for an impulse to pass from the finger across the wrist or visa versa, is the most helpful study. Both motor and sensory distal latency can be recorded, but sensory latency is the more sensitive study. A distal sensory latency of greater than 3.5 ms is usually considered abnormal, although this may vary among examiners. An increase of 0.5 ms compared to the opposite wrist is also considered abnormal, but a significant difference may be masked by bilateral disease. In bilateral cases, it is helpful to compare the distal latency of the median and the ulnar nerve in the same hand. In a recent review of 56 normal patients, it was found that the distal latencies of the median and ulnar nerve differ by no more than 0.3 ms in many patients and no more than 0.5 ms in the great majority of patients. In the hands affected by CTS, the difference is usually greater than 0.3 ms. This subtle finding is particularly helpful in those cases where the distal latency is less than 3.5 ms (apparently normal), but the history and physical examination suggest otherwise.

Treatment

Treatment is predicated on history and physical examination. If there is a history of intermittent symptoms aggravated by a particular activity, conservative measures include wrist splinting, especially at night, and activity modification when possible. A review of systems and allergies will dictate whether or not nonsteroidal anti-inflammatory drugs (NSAIDs) and diuretics can be tolerated. NSAIDs are prescribed to reduce inflammation within the synovium of the carpal tunnel; but, based on intraoperative findings, their benefit may be no more than that of a mild analgesic. In a recent study, a synovial biopsy was submitted during carpal tunnel release (CTR) in 835 consecutive cases. Evidence of inflammation was seen in less than 5% of the specimens. The use of diuretics is also suspect because they are of little assistance unless there are notable fluid shifts. Steroid injections may offer temporary relief and serve as a prognostic tool. Those patients who have relief of symptoms after steroid injection, even if short lived, can anticipate the same relief with surgical intervention. However, poor results from injections do not necessarily presage poor results from surgery. Like all conservative measures, injections seem to be most helpful in those cases with the shortest interval between onset and presentation, normal sensibility, no atrophy, intermittent night symptoms, and positive electrodiagnostic studies limited to no more than 0.1 to 0.2 ms increases in distal latency.

Confounding the role of conservative management is a study from Japan in which 155 patients with electrodiagnostically confirmed CTS were followed up. Thirty-five percent of patients with idiopathic CTS had complete resolution of symptoms after 5 months without any specific treatment. These findings support the impression that in a number of cases, the symptoms reflect a transient stressful event that may resolve without specific treatment and that time should be allowed to pass before considering further intervention.

Surgery should be considered when other methods have failed. What constitutes failure depends on personal preference as well as clinical acumen. Most texts agree that 6 to 12 weeks of splinting and activity modification is prudent when the onset has been recent and the symptoms are transient. Most also agree that there is little reason to postpone intervention when there are constant complaints of numbness and weakness, decreased sensibility and atrophy, and prolonged distal latencies. The great majority of patients fall somewhere in between these two scenarios, and their care cannot be dictated by strict algorithms. Urgent intervention is necessary when carpal tunnel pressures are acutely elevated as a result of wrist fractures or dislocations, burns, or compartment syndromes.

In the last 5 years, the method for surgical treatment of CTS has undergone considerable modification, which was prompted in part by results of clinical and laboratory studies. The demonstrated elevation of the carpal tunnel pressure of patients with CTS, especially in the extremes of wrist flexion and extension, implies that the pressure leads not only to mechanical distortion but also to ischemia of the median nerve within the carpal tunnel. Releasing the pressure would resolve the ischemia, and symptoms should subside. Therefore, incising the transverse carpal ligament for the treatment of CTS may be the only treatment that is necessary or beneficial, even in the most severe cases. The benefit of incising the transverse carpal ligament in severe CTS versus release and epineurotomy was investigated in three prospective studies. In two studies open release and neurolysis was compared to open release alone; the third study used open release alone. In the first two studies, the end results for open release alone were as good as or better than the results of neurolysis. Results of the third study (open without neurolysis)—a resolution of pain in 90%, complete relief of numbness in 66%, and improved hand strength in 85%—reinforced these findings. If, as these data imply, the important aspect of surgical management of CTS is release of the transverse carpal ligament, then perhaps the procedure could be done through a limited incision with or without the assistance of an endoscope.

The role of endoscopic assisted CTR (ECTR) is controversial. There are at present over 20 reports representing several thousand ECTRs. The benefit of ECTR is reported to be decreased postoperative pain and an earlier return to gainful employment. For the most part, these studies are not randomized and surgery was done using a device designed by the author and subsidized by the medical instrumentation industry. One particular study in which CTR was compared to ECTR deserves note because it was a multicenter, randomized, prospective study, with the postoperative course documented by independent observers and because the report authors had no commercial connections. At the end of a 3-month observation period, both open and endoscopic techniques had high marks for relief of paresthesias and of hand pain. There was no significant difference in sensibility or strength. The ECTR group was shown to have a significant difference in scar tenderness: 39% compared to 64%. Four significant complications occurred in the ECTR study group. In another multicenter study, open CTR was compared to single portal ECTR. Although the study was poorly randomized and the follow-up was not blinded to the surgeons, the results reflect an advantage for ECTR for reduced pain and return to activities of daily living. It is interesting that in these and subsequent studies the return to work time was not affected by the method of release as much as by the insurance coverage. Patients undergoing the endoscopic technique with private insurance returned to work 2 weeks sooner than their open counterparts; whereas, patients with workers' compensation claims returned to work at the same time regardless of the technique.

Use of single and dual portal techniques in cadaveric models demonstrated or recapitulated potential problems with ECTR procedures. The most commonly encountered potential problem was incomplete transection of the transverse carpal ligament. The concern regarding incomplete transection may be overstated, the reported rate of repeated surgery for incomplete release after ECTR is the same as for open technique, less than 1%. Reported clinical complications have included complete transection of the median nerve and ulnar nerve, division of common and proper digital nerve branches, and complete or partial lacerations of the superficial palmar arch. Based on intraoperative findings in these complications and in the cadaver studies, it is recommended that ECTR instruments should always be passed within the synovial sheath of the carpal tunnel and directed along the axis of the ring finger, and that all incisions should be made with good visualization of the cutting instruments (Figs. 1 and 2). In the most recently reported series, performed by "experienced" surgeons, there have been no catastrophic complications; however, when a surgeon becomes "experienced" is not clear. There is a report of complete transection of the median nerve on case 59 of a 61-case series.

Detractors of endoscopic techniques are quick to point out that it is difficult to damage the median and ulnar nerves if these structures are protected while the transverse carpal ligament is divided under direct visualization. They also point out that carpal tunnel releases can be performed through incisions that avoid the base of the palm, thereby decreasing the potential for postoperative pain. Both a limited palmar and a double-incision technique have been proposed, with results that are similar to those of the best ECTR series. There are no randomized studies that compare limited incision and ECTR techniques (Fig. 3).

Results

Although the best surgical approach remains contested, these studies have brought up a number of helpful points. First, no matter what the technique or relationship to occupation, patient satisfaction at 6-months follow-up is uniformly high. Second, a good long-term clinical result can

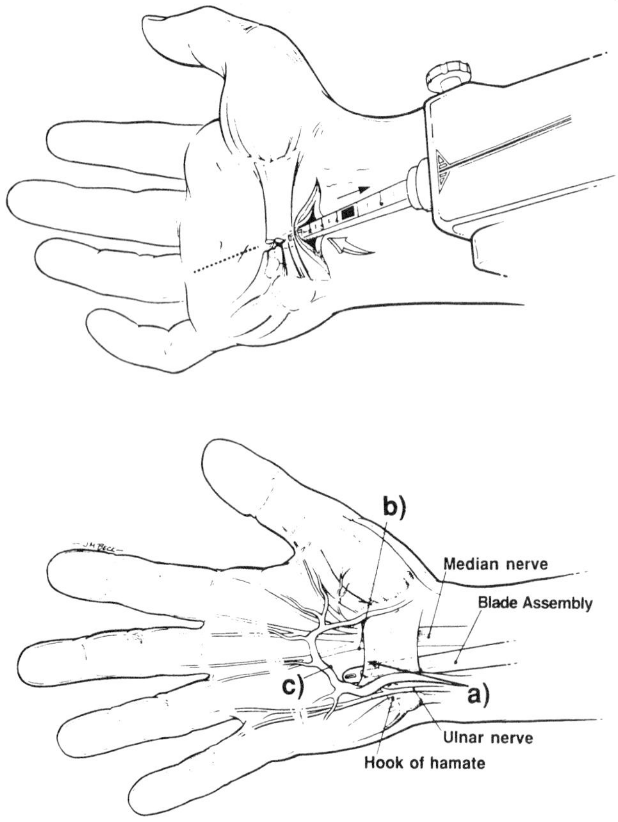

Fig. 1 This type of endoscope is introduced through a single wrist-level portal. A blade assembly located at the tip is trigger activated and is shown cutting the carpal ligament. Prior to blade elevation, the tip must be located in the "safe zone" in order to cut the distal edge of the carpal ligament while avoiding injury to the superficial vascular arch and the common digital nerves. The safe zone is defined by the ulnar half of the distal edge of the transverse carpal ligament (a), the ulnar border of the median nerve, ie, its common digital branch (b), and the ulnar proximal margin of the superficial palmar arch (c). (Reproduced with permission from Agee JM, McCarroll HR Jr, Tortosa RD, et al: Endoscopic release of the carpal tunnel: A randomized prospective multicenter study. *J Hand Surg* 1992;17A:987–995.)

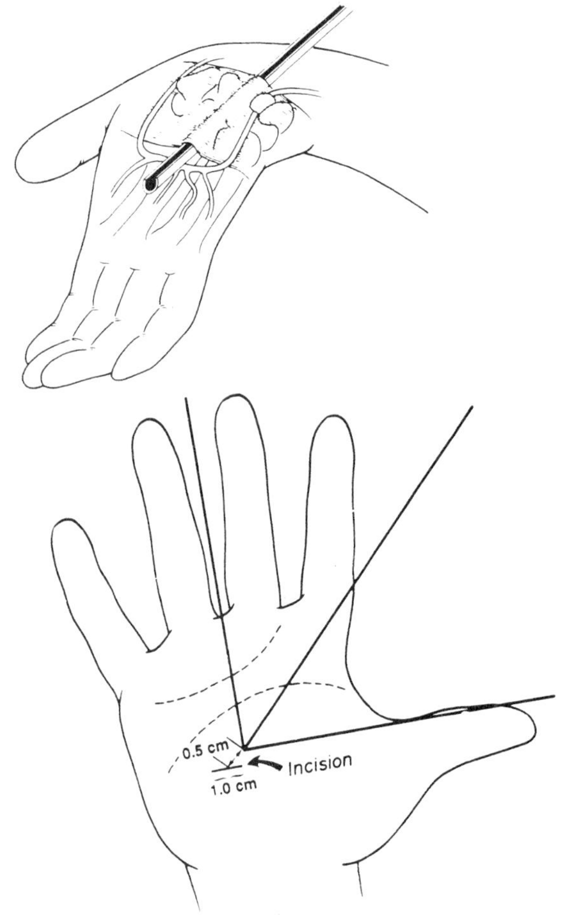

Fig. 2 The two-portal technique places a slotted cannula through the carpal tunnel that exits through the safe zone. The surface anatomy for the safe zone can be identified in two ways. The first, shown here, is described as being underneath a 1 cm transverse distal palmar skin incision along a line formed by the bisection of two lines drawn along a fully abducted thumb and the third web space. The incision is located 0.25 to 0.5 cm proximal to the junction of these lines. The second is described as a transverse incision based on the point of intersection between the long axis of the ring finger and Kaplan's cardinal line. (Reproduced with permission from Lee DH, Masear VR, Meyer RD, et al: Endoscopic carpal tunnel release: A cadaveric study. *J Hand Surg* 1992;17A:1003–1008.)

be anticipated in those cases in which symptomatic relief occurred within the first 24 hours postoperatively. Third, there is a relationship between certain occupations and the propensity to develop CTS, and this propensity is influenced by the general health of the patient. Therefore, health maintenance programs and measures taken to improve fitness may reduce an individual's risk of developing a CTS. Fourth, not every patient with CTS needs an operation; conservative measures are especially indicated in patients with transient symptoms or symptoms of recent onset. Fifth, an outcomes assessment tool for CTS has been introduced, which not only measures the objective findings of experienced clinicians but also takes into consideration the effect of the CTR on the patient's quality of life. Finally, no matter which technique is chosen to treat CTS, injury to either the median or the ulnar nerve as a result of that treatment is an unacceptable complication.

The outcomes assessment tool provides a global score to judge the benefit of various procedures. Preliminary findings, based on the tool's use for assessment of 104 patients, suggest that ECTR is better than a traditional long palmar incision. However, this study has several limitations: only seven of the 104 cases involved workers' compensation; the outcome is based on a single 3-month follow-up evaluation; a self-administered symptoms and

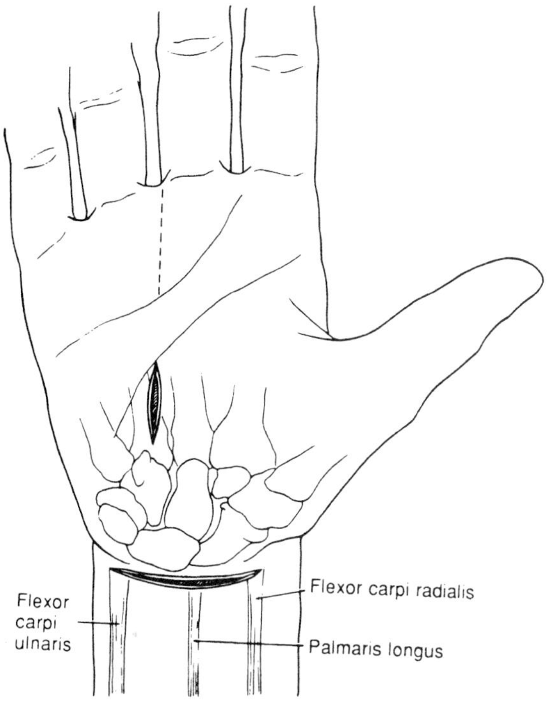

Fig. 3 The incisions proposed for minimal exposure carpal tunnel release. The proximal transverse incision is made just proximal to the wrist creases between the flexor carpi ulnaris and flexor carpi radialis tendons. The distal palmar incision is a longitudinal extension over the safe zone described in Figures 1 and 2. (Reproduced with permission from Wilson KM: Double incision open technique for carpal tunnel release: An alternative to endoscopic release. *J Hand Surg* 1994;19A:907–912.)

function questionnaire was not produced; a global cohort scheme was not developed outside of the cases presented; and the sample size is too small. All of these limitations are significant flaws in the development of a health outcome tool; nevertheless, this study presents an essential first step.

Wrist Salvage Procedures

A painless, stable, and mobile wrist is the desired goal of all wrist salvage procedures. The literature from the last 5 years demonstrates that these goals remain elusive. The wrist can be made stable and pain-free, but always at the cost of motion.

Wrist Arthrodesis

Rigid internal fixation with AO/ASIF plates and iliac crest bone graft has become an increasingly popular method for wrist arthrodesis in the treatment of traumatic, neurologic, and some inflammatory disorders. The fusion rate is between 93% and 100%, and complications, which until now have been described as minor, are usually related to prominent plates and screws. In a detailed look at 72 cases of wrist arthrodesis with AO plates, it was found that although the radiocarpal joint fused in all cases, there were 82 complications related to soft-tissue, bone, or unexplained pain. Early complications included wound problems (hematoma, excessive swelling, blisters, or partial dehiscence), limited metacarpophalangeal (MCP) joint motion, neurologic deficit (acute CTS or transient paresthesias), infection, and unexplained distal radioulnar joint pain. Complications related to the iliac crest donor site included hematoma and infection. Long-term or late complications were related to the fixation devices, pain at the distal radioulnar joint, unexplained pain, arthritis at the scaphotrapeziotrapezoid joint, MCP joint stiffness, and persistent neurologic deficits. Secondary procedures were required in 19 wrists, mostly to address problems related to the fixation devices, such as irritating or prominent hardware, or in the treatment of four fractures through the proximal most or distal most fixation screws. Despite an improved fusion rate, this technique has the same infection and complication rates as other techniques, and specific attention should be paid to the distal radioulnar joint and to problems related to the fixation device.

The AO Hand Study Group has introduced a specially designed fixation plate that addresses some of the problems noted above. The plate is precontoured to accommodate the dorsal recess of the carpus, places the wrist in neutral or 10° of extension, and is tapered distally. Proximal screws (3.5-mm) provide fixation to the radius and distal screws (2.7-mm) transfix the carpus and metacarpal (Fig. 4). It is recommended that the arthrodesis always include the radiocarpal, the scaphocapitate, and the third carpometacarpal articulations. Incorporation of the other intercarpal articulations and the second carpometacarpal articulation is optional. Cancellous bone graft is harvested from the distal radius, thereby avoiding the complications of distant donor sites.

In a study of wrist arthrodesis using plates and local bone graft, 18 of the 28 fusions were performed with the plate described above; 3.5-mm dynamic compression plates or 3.5-mm reconstruction plates were used for the other fusions. Immediate postoperative management included aggressive digit mobilization and edema control. All 28 wrist fusions were successful. Complications included one CTS that required release, one painful distal radioulnar joint palliated with steroid injection, and four cases of extensor tendonitis related to irritation from the prominent edge of 3.5-mm implants. The extensor tendonitis resolved in all four cases after implant removal.

Grip strength and the dexterity for activities of daily living were not significantly affected by the fusions. Shoulder, elbow, forearm, and digit motion were not affected. In a related article on comparison of wrist fusion with motion saving procedures, the same investigators reported no significant difference in the ability to perform rapid movements requiring manual dexterity in the course of activities of daily living. Activities requiring volar wrist flexion in

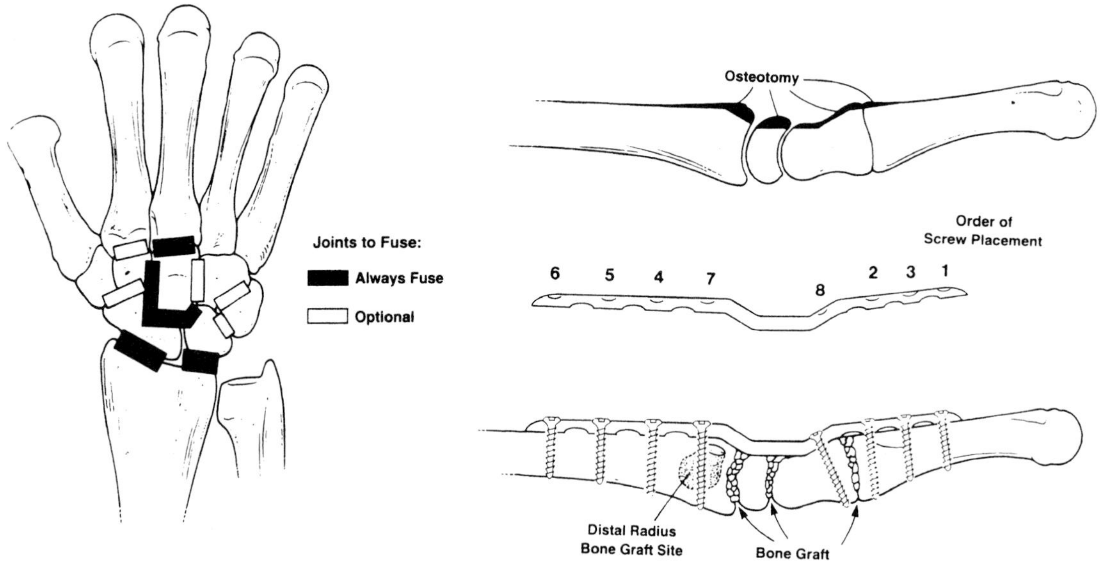

Fig. 4 Wrist arthrodesis with a contoured plate: The fusion always includes the joints marked with the dark boxes. The dorsal cortex is denuded to accommodate the plate and fixation is done in the order numbered. Bone graft, when necessary, is harvested from distal radius. A precontoured plate is now available with 3.5-mm screw holes proximally and 2.7-mm screw holes distally. (Reproduced with permission from Weiss AP, Hastings H II: Wrist arthrodesis for traumatic conditions: A study of plate and local bone graft application. *J Hand Surg* 1995;20A:50–56.)

which spatial limitation would not allow compensatory shoulder or elbow movement and activities requiring forceful pronation and supination combined with strong grasp were found to present difficulty in patients who had undergone total wrist fusion. For patients whose occupations require fine manual dexterity in tight spaces, wrist fusion might not be the most appropriate procedure. Unfortunately, motion sparing may not be appropriate either. These investigators found that there was no postoperative improvement in wrist motion after motion-sparing procedures. Thus, if the inability to perform a particular task or pursue a particular livelihood is related to limited motion, there are no procedures that will be appropriate. Finally, they noted that there was a 3 to 6 month learning curve to the patients' ability to perform specific activities postoperatively.

These authors conclude that wrist fusion is particularly attractive if the patient's preoperative motion is poor, arthritis is advanced, and the hand is to be used for heavy manual activity. Alternative motion-preserving procedures continue to have proponents.

Proximal Row Carpectomy

Proximal row carpectomy (PRC) is advocated in the treatment of Kienböck's disease, osteonecrosis of the scaphoid, scapholunate advanced collapse, perilunate dissociation, and arthrogryposis multiplex congenita. The durability of this procedure and its role in inflammatory arthritis were questioned in *Orthopaedic Knowledge Update 4.* Three studies provide further insight into the roll of PRC. In one multicenter study, 20 patients were evaluated a mean of 3.5 years after PRC; 14 were satisfied, noting decreased pain and increased strength despite a 15% decrease in motion, and six patients, three of whom had rheumatoid arthritis, continued to have moderate or severe pain. A second study of 18 wrists, nine with rheumatoid arthritis and nine with other various nonrheumatoid conditions, reinforces the dismal outlook for this procedure in patients with rheumatoid arthritis. All but two of the patients with rheumatoid arthritis failed because of persistent pain and imbalance. The third study assessed functional outcome, patient satisfaction, and radiographs of 23 wrists an average of 6 years following PRC. None of the patients had rheumatoid arthritis. Twenty patients were satisfied with the functional performance and pain relief. Wrist flexion–extension arc averaged 61% that of the opposite wrist, and grip strength averaged 79% of the opposite side. Radiocarpal arthritis developed in three wrists, but only one required arthrodesis for pain relief. Most importantly, the results did not decline at an average of 6 years after surgery.

PRC has been compared to other procedures in the treatment of scapholunate advanced collapse (SLAC). In a study of 24 wrists treated for symptomatic SLAC arthritis, treatment consisted of either PRC or limited wrist fusion (LWF) combined with scaphoid excision. Satisfactory pain relief, grip strength, and functional performance were observed in all but three patients in the PRC group. Differences in subjective and objective results between PRC and LWF were not statistically significant except for greater flexion–extension with PRC (77°) than with LWF (52°). A review of the Mayo Clinic experience with different reconstructive procedures for SLAC wrist, which involve the scaphoradial joint (stage II) or the capitolunate joint (stage III), indicated that six of 51 motion-sparing cases required later total wrist fusion. Scaphoid excision and four-corner arthrodesis reliably diminished wrist pain in patients with stage III SLAC wrist while maintaining a 54° flexion–extension arc. Stage II SLAC wrists were successfully treated with LWF, radioscaphoid arthrodesis, or PRC. Of the three procedures, PRC best preserved wrist mobility, with a flexion–extension arc of 71°. The advice drawn from both studies is that a stage-dependent surgical approach to the symptomatic SLAC wrist is appropriate. For wrists without capitolunate arthritis, PRC avoids the technical demands, lengthy postoperative immobilization, and risk of nonunion associated with LWF, but for stage III disease (capitolunate arthritis), pain relief may be unsatisfactory, and LWF is therefore recommended.

Other Motion-Sparing Procedures

Intercarpal Fusion The results and potential complications of limited intercarpal fusions were reviewed in *Orthopaedic Knowledge Update 4;* these procedures will generally provide 50% to 60% of motion, 50% to 80% grip strength, lead to relief of symptoms in 50% to 60% of patients, and have complication rates as high as 52%. In a 44-month follow-up of 100 limited wrist fusions combined with scaphoid excision for the treatment of SLAC wrist, strength and motion were similar to previously reported data. Contrary to the results noted in the studies of PRC versus LWF, there was only a 3% nonunion rate and complications occurred in less than 10% of patients. The majority of employed patients returned to their original jobs. The most common problem was dorsal impingement of the capitate and radius (12%), which was felt to be technique-related and avoidable by careful capitolunate alignment. This complication was treated surgically by excision of the dorsal margin of the radius and the abutting portion of the capitate. None of the 100 cases required arthrodesis despite the fact that 15 patients had pain at rest or with some activities of daily living.

Scaphocapitolunate arthrodesis is an alternative procedure to scaphoid excision in early SLAC, scapholunate dissociation, and Kienböck's disease. Twenty-one patients with either chronic incompetence of the scapholunate ligament or a scaphoid nonunion were followed an average of 28 months after scaphocapitolunate arthrodesis. Pain was significantly reduced in 80% of the patients, and the only major complication was an infection. Sixteen of 20 patients were able to return to work. The surgical procedure was done through a dorsal approach, with the use of autogenous bone grafting and Kirschner wire fixation. The average flexion–extension arc was 65°. Radiographic examination at final follow-up showed mild degenerative changes at the radiocarpal joint in two patients. Although the length of follow-up in this study is relatively short, these results are promising, and the procedure deserves consideration as an alternative to scaphotrapeziotrapezoid fusion for the treatment of scapholunate instability or recalcitrant scaphoid nonunion with minimal scaphoid fossa–radial styloid arthritis.

Radiocarpal Fusion Radiocarpal fusion (RCF) has been described for treatment of the rheumatoid wrist. Two studies accounting for 47 patients have been used to determine the efficacy of RCF in patients with wrist disorders other than rheumatoid arthritis. The most frequent indication was posttraumatic changes secondary to distal radius fracture (41 cases). Less frequent indications were Kienböck's disease, localized arthritis secondary to sepsis, and acute comminuted fracture of the distal radius. The average arc of wrist flexion and extension was between 48° and 52°. Grip strength was between 70% to 80% of that of the uninvolved hand. Pain relief was achieved in all patients who had no evidence of midcarpal arthritis at the time of surgery. The presence of midcarpal arthritis, however slight, was associated with uniform failure and is now considered a contraindication to RCF. In one study, all 11 patients returned to their previous employment. In the second study, seven patients went on to wrist fusion and their work status was not reported, 18 patients returned to their original employment, five did not return to work because of wrist problems, and six either retired or changed jobs for reasons other than their wrist.

Total Wrist Arthroplasty The indications for total wrist arthroplasty remain unchanged. The procedure is limited to low demand patients with intact wrist extensor tendons and adequate distal radius and metaphyseal bone stock. The ideal candidate is the patient with rheumatoid arthritis who leads a sedentary life and avoids the heaviest activities of daily living. Silicone spacers are the most frequently used implants. A 6.5-year study of 33 cases reveals that patients were satisfied and pain relieved in 63%. Implants fractured in 52%, and revision was required in 30%. Radiographic changes consistent with particulate synovitis were seen in 30%. Prosthetic settling, bony resorption, or implant fracture was seen in more than 70% of the patients at 58 months and 100% of patients at 70 months.

Wrist replacements with rigidly fixed metal-backed plastic components have now been reported with more than 8 years follow-up. In one series of 18 patients followed for 103 months, the 14 patients with rheumatoid arthritis had 30% loosening of components but continued to function well. Three of four patients with degenerative joint disease failed. These optimistic results are comparable to those of a previous study in which a different implant was used in the same patient population.

Distal Radioulnar Joint The Sauve-Kapandji procedure first described in 1936 has received considerable attention for the treatment of chronic instability or impingement problems about the distal radioulnar joint (DRUJ). It is believed that preservation of the head of the ulna minimizes the potential for some of the complications that can follow its excision. Retention of the head of the ulna secures a more normal transmission of loads across the wrist, maintains full support for the carpus, and preserves the normal contour of the wrist. Recent reports have better defined the role of this procedure. Radioulnar joint pain subsided in all of 37 cases, including 13 with rheumatoid arthritis and 17 with posttraumatic arthritis, ulnar instability, or ulnar impingement. In seven cases, proximal ulnar instability was associated with variable disability and was considered a potential problem. Patients with rheumatoid arthritis fared better than their posttraumatic counterparts. The instability of the proximal ulna after a Sauve-Kapandji procedure was also investigated (Fig. 5). Radiographic examination of 15 forearms revealed an unstable proximal ulnar stump and radioulnar convergence similar to that associated with the Darrach resection. The conclusion derived from both these studies is that the Sauve-Kapandji procedure can preserve ulnar support of the wrist and is believed to yield more satisfactory results than the Darrach resection in the rheumatoid wrist. However, its use for the treatment of nonrheumatoid DRUJ disorders, especially subluxed or dislocated DRUJs, is not recommended.

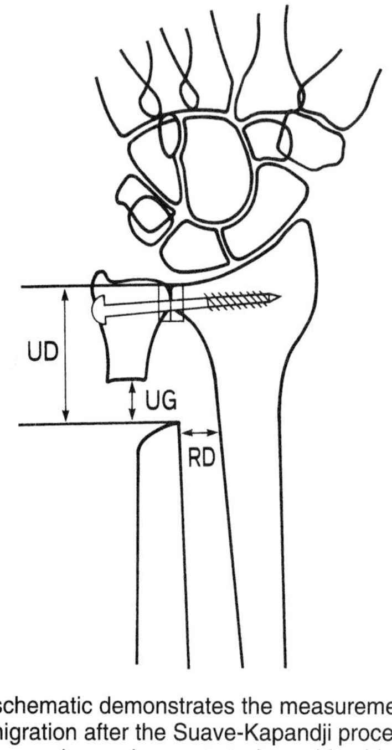

Fig. 5 This schematic demonstrates the measurements used to assess ulnar migration after the Suave-Kapandji procedure. RD, the radioulnar distance always demonstrated considerable narrowing. (Reproduced with permission from Nakamura R, Tsunoda K, Watanabe K, et al: The Sauve-Kapandji procedure for chronic dislocation of the distal radio-ulnar joint with destruction of the articular surface. *J Hand Surg* 1992;17B:127–132.)

A particularly vexing problem is the management of the dorsally subluxed or dislocated DRUJ. Various authorities hold opposite opinions regarding the effect of motion on the volar and dorsal distal radioulnar ligaments (DRUL) during pronation and supination. The opinions are so varied that the exact opposite techniques have been recommended for reconstruction. One novel experiment has shed some light on this controversial subject. The displacement of the volar and dorsal DRUL during pronation and supination was measured with a Hall-effect transducer. The investigators found that displacement increases in the dorsal DRUL during pronation and in the palmar DRUL during supination. These findings prompted the authors to consider reinforcing the dorsal capsule with a tendon weave for the treatment of ulnar dorsal DRUJ instability (Fig. 6). In a series of 14 patients treated for dynamic ulnar dorsal DRUJ instability, 12 had complete pain relief. An average of 8° of supination was lost while the remainder of wrist and forearm motion was preserved. Grip strength improved 76%, and no patients changed avocations or occupation.

Ulnar impaction, triangular cartilage tears, or the combination of both have been treated with hemiresection interposition arthroplasty, Darrach resections, and ulnar shortening osteotomies. A limited resection osteotomy has been introduced in which a "wafer" of the distal ulna is removed while preserving the ulnar styloid and the sigmoid notch articulation (Fig. 7). The dorsal DRUL is reinforced with retinaculum. Two reports with a total of 28 patients indicated that with the wafer resection, a full pain-free range of motion was obtained in 70%; the remaining 30% had mild pain with strenuous exercise. The operation resulted in improvement in all of these patients, but in some cases the improvement occurred slowly over 6 months. Prospective randomized trials are needed to compare the clinical effectiveness of this relatively complex intra-articular procedure with that of simpler extra-articular procedures, such as ulnar shortening osteotomy.

Scaphoid Nonunion

The authors of three recent articles debate the premise that scaphoid nonunion has a uniformly bad prognosis. Two articles are based on clinical acumen and the third questions the epidemiologic process by which present assumptions were made. In the first study, the investigators identified 25 patients (30 wrists) that had radiographic evidence of SLAC; there was no pain in 22 wrists and mild pain in eight. The pathology was discovered while examining the hand for other complaints. When these patients were reevaluated 2 years later, 20 wrists were totally free of symptoms and there was occasional pain in 10, especially with increased activity. The investigators caution against treating the pain-free but arthritic wrist. In a second study, 33 patients were reviewed 10 to 17 years after the diagnosis

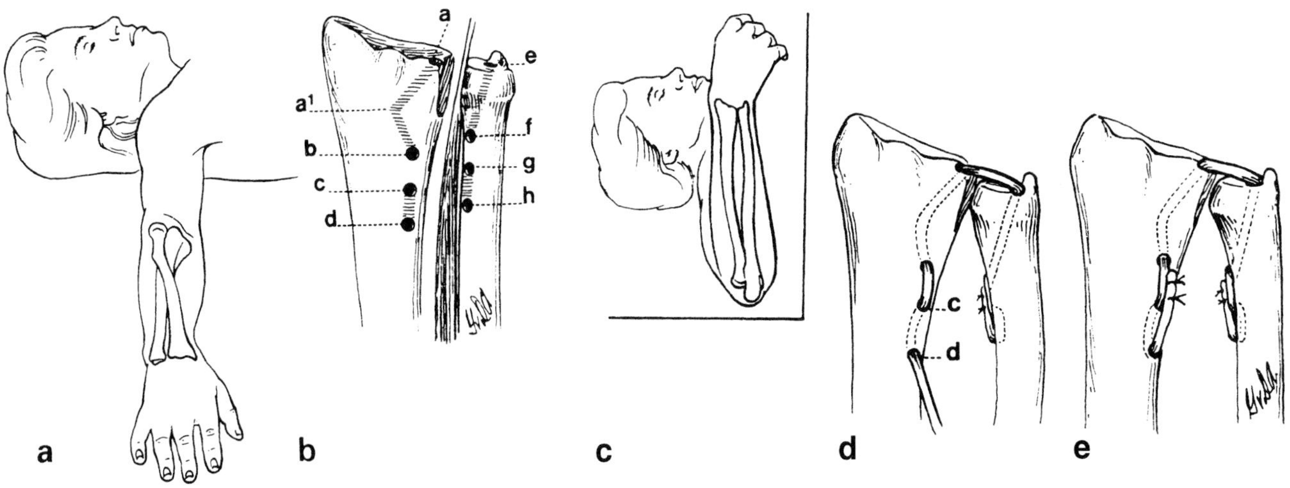

Fig. 6 A proposed reconstruction for dorsal capsule insufficiency of the distal radioulnar joint. Drill holes for a tendon weave are passed through the distal radius and ulna while the forearm is in pronation (a & b). The elbow is flexed and the forearm supinated while the repair is pulled tightly (c, d, & e). (Reproduced with permission from Scheker LR, Belliappa PP, Acosta R, et al: Reconstruction of the dorsal ligament of the triangular fibrocartilage complex. *J Hand Surg* 1994;19B:310–318.)

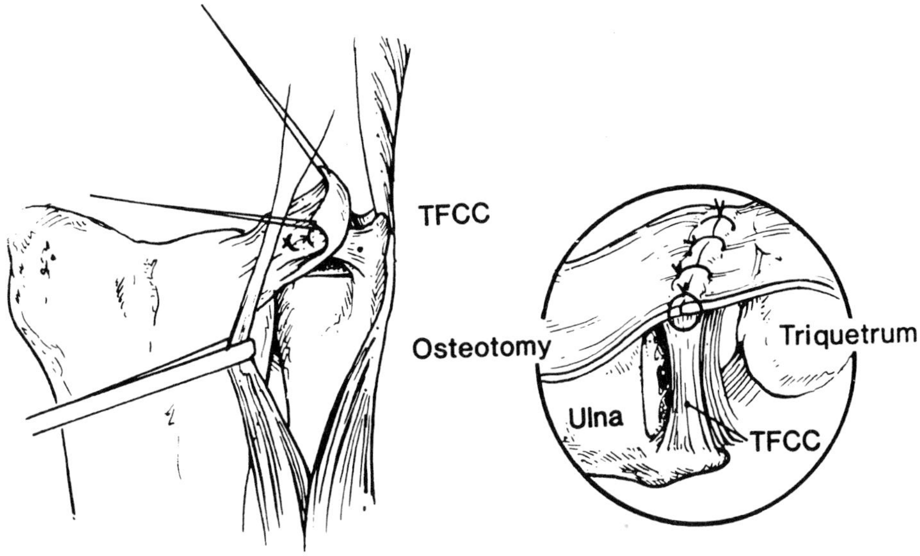

Fig. 7 The "wafer" procedure for impingement of the distal ulna is performed through a dorsal approach. The retinaculum of the fifth dorsal compartment is elevated from ulnar to radial, left intact at the septum between the forth and fifth compartments, and used to reconstruct the dorsal capsule of the distal radioulnar joint after resection of a 3- to 4-mm wafer of distal ulna. TFCC is the triangular fibrocartilage complex. (Reproduced with permission from Feldon P, Terrono AL, Belsky MR: The "wafer" procedure: Partial distal ulnar resection. *Clin Orthop* 1992;275:124–129.)

of scaphoid nonunion was established. Radiographs revealed a 100% incidence of progressive radiocarpal osteoarthritis. Five of the wrists were pain free. These investigators concluded that although in some patients the radiographic evidence of arthritis and clinical findings do not correlate, freedom from pain was not a reliable prognostic indicator. They recommend surgical treatment of the pseudarthrosis with the exception being well-established arthrosis, in which case treatment is tailored to patient demands and symptoms.

The authors of the third article critically evaluated those studies on the natural history of scaphoid nonunion from the viewpoint of the epidemiologist. Using six standard methodologic criteria for the performance of a valid natural history study, they determined that no study satisfied all criteria. Moreover, none developed the single most important method of a valid natural history study, an inception cohort. In the example of a scaphoid fracture, an inception cohort would be either patients with a new nonunion followed into the future or patients whose nonunion has run its entire course. In each study, the direction of the bias was identifiable and the natural history of scaphoid nonunion was distorted to make the outcome more severe than if methodologic problems had not been present. The authors concluded that the natural history of scaphoid nonunion is not as severe as has been reported in the literature, but the magnitude of the difference is not yet known. Their article demonstrates that clinical conclusions drawn from uncontrolled case series may be erroneous.

Trapeziometacarpal Joint

The trapeziometacarpal joint is the most commonly identified site for surgical treatment of osteoarthritis in the upper extremity and provides an excellent avenue for investigating the biology and pathophysiology of degenerative joint disease. In a study of 47 cadaver thumbs, Pelligrini and associates confirmed that the deep palmar or beak ligament is the cornerstone to translational stability of the thumb metacarpal on the trapezium. There was a direct correlation between the status of the articular surfaces and the integrity of the beak ligament. Degeneration was always associated with attrition of the beak ligament and occurred only in the palmar contact areas. In advanced arthritis, the palmar region demonstrated the greatest effect of stress, whereas the dorsal joint surfaces exhibited nonprogressive chondromalacia.

In two other studies by this same group, the surface ultrastructure of hyaline cartilage and the biochemical properties of the hyaline cartilage from four distinct quadrants in normal and osteoarthritic thumb trapeziometacarpal joints were analyzed. Scanning electron microscopy revealed that the earliest changes were observed in the tangential surface lamina and occurred in areas of chondromalacia in the palmar contact area of the joint. Progressive disruption of this superficial fibrillar layer of the articular cartilage was followed by disorganization of the underlying chondrocytes and matrix. Disruption of the protective surface lamina of trapeziometacarpal articular cartilage occurs in a geographic pattern corresponding to joint contact areas and regions of selective biochemical decomposition of proteoglycan matrix. Chondromalacic surfaces in the palmar contact areas of arthritic specimens were characterized by preferential loss of glycosaminoglycan, an increasing chondroitin sulfate/keratin sulfate ratio, and a retention of collagen. In contrast, articular cartilage from the dorsal portion of arthritic joints biochemically resembled that from adjacent normal specimens. These findings suggest an interdependent relationship between mechanical factors (attrition of the beak ligament) and biochemical matrix degradation in production of the cartilage lesion of trapeziometacarpal osteoarthritis. Therefore, it is necessary to address the palmar beak ligament in reconstruction of the arthritic trapeziometacarpal joint, the common denominator of all recently described thumb basal joint arthroplasty procedures.

Bony Deformity of Digits

Finger deformities, malalignment, and joint incongruity limit hand function because of pain and interference with hand closure. The uniformly dismal long-term results of interphalangeal (IP) joint replacement has prompted a closer look at the best methods for and consequences of small-joint arthrodesis. Crossed Kirschner pins, interfragmentary wire and longitudinal Kirschner pin, and a Herbert screw are used most frequently for fusion of the thumb IP joint and distal IP (DIP) joint. Each of these methods was used in a study of 181 terminal joint fusions. The union rate was 90% and was not affected by technique. Major complications, including nonunion, malunion, deep infection, and osteomyelitis, occurred in 20% of the cases. Minor complications, including dorsal skin necrosis, cold intolerance, proximal IP (PIP) joint stiffness, parasthesias, superficial wound infection, and prominent hardware, occurred in 16% of the joints fused. In a review of 290 tension band fusions of the thumb MCP joint and PIP joint, the union rate was 93%. Complications included ten superficial infections and three fusions that were malrotated. Late hardware removal was required in 25 fusions. The conclusion drawn from these two extensive studies is that the essential components to successful arthrodesis are appropriate preparation of the joint surfaces, careful positioning, and coaptation of the bone ends. Without these components, regardless of fixation technique, a pseudarthrosis is likely.

Metacarpophalangeal Joint Arthroplasty

Silicone implant arthroplasty remains the treatment of choice for reconstruction of dislocated MCP joints in patients with rheumatoid arthritis. This procedure reduces pain, corrects deformity, and improves function. Recent intermediate term (6 to 8 years) follow-up studies document that patients regain a functional arc of motion that undergoes little deterioration over time. Although PIP joint motion tends to improve in the first 2 years after MCP joint arthroplasty, motion in this joint deteriorates by 6 to 8 years after surgery.

Osteotomy

The best location for osteotomy of proximal phalangeal malunions remains controversial. Osteotomy at the malunion site has the greatest potential for correction of the deformity, but places the adjacent flexor and extensor tendons at risk for injury and subsequent loss of motion. Creating a compensatory deformity in the proximal metacarpal has been advocated as a way to avoid these problems. This latter technique has been reported to be satisfactory in a number of small series, none of which report the degree of preoperative deformity or postoperative correction. Critics of this procedure point out that although metacarpal rotational osteotomy may correct the apparent finger malrotation, there remains rotational malalignment in complete digital flexion. In addition, the digit assumes an S-shaped appearance in full extension, which reflects two diametrically opposed angular deformities—the traumatic deformity and the correctional osteotomy—separated by a distance of 3 to 4 cm. Complete correction of a malunion can be done only by addressing the malunion site.

The benefit of a step cut osteotomy was demonstrated in 16 proximal phalanx malunions. Increased postoperative motion was reported in most patients, although several patients lost up to 15° of extension. The largest series, 36 malunions corrected at the site of deformity, comes from the AO center in Switzerland. All 36 were corrected and maintained with plate and screw fixation; 86% of patients had satisfactory digital function. The poor results were related to chronic periarticular injury. Data from a more recent series reinforces these findings. Full correction of the preoperative deformity was achieved in nine patients, bony union was 100%, and no loss of preoperative range of motion was observed in eight patients. The ninth patient underwent correctional osteotomy and joint arthrodesis.

Amputation

Severe chronic bony deformities of the finger force the patient and physician to choose between multiple reconstructive procedures or amputation. The impact of digit amputations on the well-being of patients has been discussed in the report of a study of 120 patients who underwent amputation of at least one of the four ulnar fingers. None of the patients had attempted replantation because of injury severity. At an average of 12 years after injury, 80% of the patients assessed their condition as good or fair; those patients sustaining single digit amputation were the best. The authors felt that their observations bring into question the benefit of digit replantation when only one of the ulnar fingers has been amputated. Although the benefit of single digit replantation may be questionable for adult border digits, especially if the amputation is proximal to the flexor digitorum superficialis (FDS) insertion, amputation of a central digit presents a unique problem.

With a central digit amputation, the hand becomes increasingly more unsightly and clumsy as the level of amputation approaches the MCP joint. The accepted management of this problem is ray resection. There are four components to central resection: removal of the metacarpal, bony realignment, neuroma prevention, and preservation of web space. With ring-finger ray amputation, the fourth metacarpal is disarticulated and the mobility of the fifth carpometacarpal joint is used to close the gap. The mobility of the fourth and fifth carpometacarpal joints can be used when the long finger ray is amputated, but as the gap is closed the position and shape of the carpal articulations force the digits to rotate. Malrotation is prevented by allowing for a larger gap between the index and ring finger or transposing the index finger into the long finger position. Problems with index to long finger transposition include prolonged immobilization, nonunion, malunion, and inordinate loss of strength. These problems can be circumvented with the use of rigid fixation. Painful neuromas are prevented by placing the nerve ends dorsally in the substance of the interosseus muscles or suturing the ends together. Web space is best preserved by retaining the skin from either the radial or ulnar aspect of the amputated proximal phalanx and insetting the entire web space into the adjacent digit. In a series of ten patients treated with these methods, motion was preserved or improved after removal of the dysfunctional digit. Eighty percent of pinch and grip strength was retained in acutely injured patients. Strength improved postoperatively in patients with chronic problems but only to 50% that of the uninjured hand.

Tendon Problems

Boutonnière Deformity

The magnitudes of the extensor forces generated across the PIP joint by a variety of commonly used reconstructive procedures for the treatment of boutonnière deformities were measured in a laboratory study. Results showed that each method produced adequate extensor forces and restored full PIP joint extension. These data suggest that the preoperative condition of the finger and postoperative care are more important than any particular type of repair. For example, there is a remarkable difference between the results of boutonnière repairs for rheumatoid arthritis and repairs for chronic trauma. In a study of 19 fingers with rheumatoid boutonnière deformity, initial postoperative gains deteriorated with time. The results were unpredictable and disappointing. Patients with rheumatoid arthritis should be forewarned that within a year of reconstruction, a substantial extensor lag will still exist and some flexion will be lost. Based on this experience, the authors recommend PIP joint fusion in the face of severe extensor deficits and rigid deformities for the treatment of boutonnière deformity in patients with rheumatoid arthritis.

Trauma-related deformities do better, but the outcome of reconstruction remains directly proportional to the state of the PIP joint and the presence of a full pain-free passive range of motion. In one study, in which a modified Matev technique was used (Fig. 8), the 14 patients with a complete passive range of motion preoperatively had an average of 14° to 96° of active motion at the PIP joint and 9° to 59° of motion at the DIP joint postoperatively. However, the six patients with contractures had an average of 21° to 80° of active motion at the PIP and 13° to 41° of motion at the DIP joint. Given that all of the reconstruction techniques have the same potential for generating PIP extension, the Matev technique is attractive because it uses local tissue and addresses the lateral bands, the PIP joint, and the DIP joint. Mallet deformity occasionally results

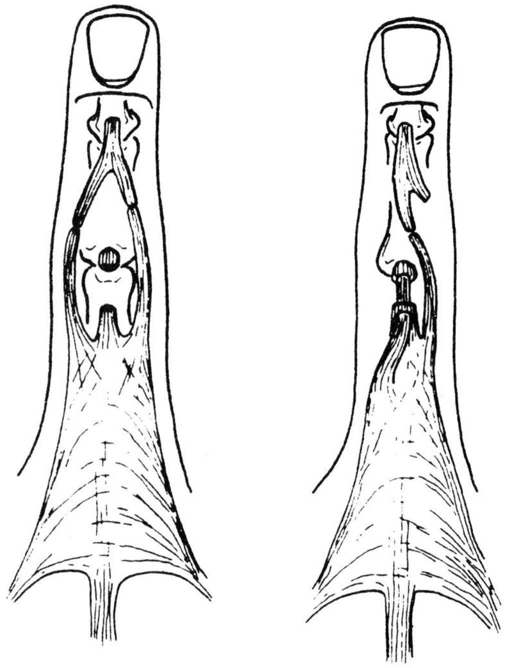

Fig. 8 Modified Matev reconstruction for boutonnière deformity. The lateral bands are step cut; the shorter proximal band is passed through the central tendon and sutured to the central slip stump. The longer lateral band is sutured to the terminal tendon.(Reproduced with permission from Terrill RQ, Groves RJ: Correction of the severe nonrheumatoid chronic boutonnière deformity with a modified Matev procedure. *J Hand Surg* 1992;17A:874–880.)

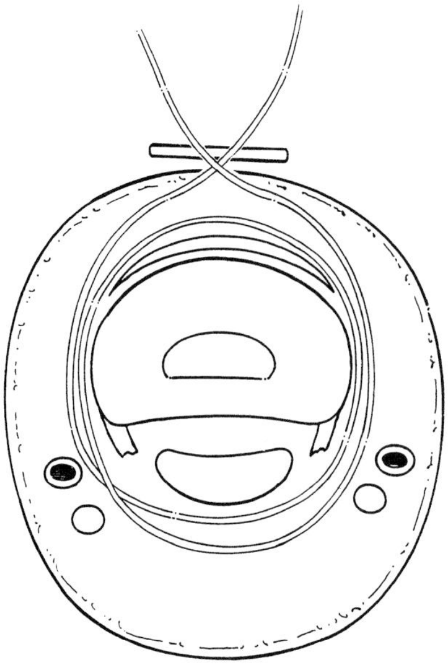

Fig. 9 Flexor tendon pulley reconstruction with a double wrap secured through dorsally placed button. (Reproduced with permission from Foucher G, Lenoble E, Ben-Youssef K, et al: A post-operative regime after digital flexor tenolysis: A series of 72 patients. *J Hand Surg* 1993;18B:35–40.)

from the Matev technique but usually resolves with 6 to 12 weeks of DIP joint extension splinting.

Flexor Tendon Tenolysis

The timing of tenolysis after flexor tendon repair depends on the maturity of the wound, skeletal stability, the patient's perception of disability related to limited motion, and failure to demonstrate improvement over time. In a series of 145 zone II flexor tendon repairs followed up prospectively, it was noted that a mean of 37% of the final DIP joint range of motion and 9% of the final PIP joint range of motion was recovered between 3 months and 1 year postoperatively. The results indicate that it is worth waiting 6 or 12 months before considering tenolysis; this period of time is considerably longer than is stated in most texts. The timing for tenolysis in children has recently been addressed. In a group of 26 patients between 1 and 16 years old at the time of tenolysis, those older than 11 years did much better than their younger counterparts.

In a report of flexor tenolysis in 78 fingers, two technical aspects were emphasized: stout pulley reconstruction, with a double circumferential wrap anchored over a button (Fig. 9), and immediate postoperative immobilization, with the finger in the flexed position. The procedure uses two incisions: a volar zig-zag (Bruner) incision along the digit for removal of adhesions and a palm or distal forearm incision to pull on tendons and test the adequacy of the release. The incisions are closed from distal to proximal making sure that the digit is pulled into flexion prior to wound closure. Two days postoperatively the digit is anesthetized and the IP joints are gently pulled into extension while the wrist and MCP joints remain flexed. Active flexion is initiated, and the wrist and MCP joint are gradually brought into extension over the next 3 weeks. At follow-up there was no improvement in four digits, and nine were actually made worse. In the remaining patients, the average improvement of total active motion in fingers was from 135° before surgery to 203° after, and in thumbs, from 65° to 115°. These results of a procedure performed by a skilled surgeon should emphasize that flexor tenolysis is an onerous task. Although there is great potential for improving function, there are also considerable risks.

Tenosynovitis

Cadaver studies and surgical biopsies of the A1 flexor tendon pulley have helped elucidate the possible mechanism and pathophysiology of trigger digits. The number of chondrocytes and adjacent extracellular matrix found within the A1 pulley of a triggering digit is significantly increased, which suggests that the process is characterized by fibrocartilage metaplasia. Whether this metaplasia is the cause of or is caused by the triggering is not yet clear.

Based on data from a number of large series, the most effective approach to this problem is injection. The success rate of a single injection is reported to be between 35% and 84%, with the success rate of three or more injections being 77% to 88%. If injections fail, the A1 pulley can be released surgically with an anticipated success rate of 98%. The procedures can be performed with local anesthetic infiltration and tourniquet control, using either a longitudinal or oblique incision.

Alternatively, a percutaneous method of release has been reported to be successful in all but three of 35 triggering digits. The technique consists of infiltrating the skin overlying the MCP joint with lidocaine and inserting a 19-gauge needle into the flexor sheath of the extended finger. The needle is centered over the metacarpal at all times and pierces the skin perpendicular to the point of triggering. The location of the needle within the sheath is confirmed by having the patient flex the digit slightly and observing the movement of the needle. The needle is then withdrawn 1 or 2 mm and rotated so that the bevels are in line with the digit. The needle is moved to and fro along the digit, cutting the A1 pulley in its course. Cadaver studies have demonstrated that the digital nerves of the thumb and the radial digital nerve of the index finger may be at risk for injury with this technique, and the authors are wary of using this method for these digits. With this caveat, the technique proved to be simple, safe, and cost effective in the management of this common problem.

Percutaneous techniques similar to that noted for trigger fingers would not be applicable to the treatment of de Quervain's disease. Cadaver dissection reveals that one or more terminal branches of the superficial branch of the radial nerve cross the area of dissection directly beneath the typical transverse incision for De Quervain's release. No matter how a needle was inserted, wiggling it to and fro would place these branches at risk for injury. As with trigger fingers, it appears that the first line of treatment for de Quervain's disease is conservative management with injection, splinting, or both injection and splinting. One study found that injection alone was more effective than splints alone or splinting combined with injection. Overall, 43 of 93 wrists responded to conservative management. Of the 50 wrists that failed conservative management, 45 were treated surgically. Twenty-two of the surgically treated wrists had a septum within the first compartment; this number is 14% higher than would be anticipated from cadaver studies. The finding of an increased incidence of a septum within the first dorsal compartment of patients with de Quervain's disease supports the argument that patients with septa are more prone to persistent symptoms or recurrent symptoms with conservative management.

Kienböck's Disease

The etiology, natural history, and most effective treatment methods for Kienböck's disease remain elusive. The stage of disease and ulnar variance remain the two most important variables that guide selection of treatment alternatives. Recent clinical and laboratory reports continue to support the use of extra-articular procedures, such as radius shortening osteotomy in patients with no evidence of carpal collapse or intercarpal degenerative changes (Lichman's stages I to IIIA) and negative ulnar variance. Several in vitro studies have shown that extra-articular procedures effectively reduce lunate compressive stress and strain and do not have a deleterious effect on carpal kinematics. In one recent clinical series, average grip strength increased 44% and range of motion 17% following radius shortening osteotomy. A radioscaphoid angle of 60° or more indicated that carpal collapse was significant and that an unfavorable outcome was likely. Patients with both lunate collapse and carpal collapse (Lichman's stage IIIB) may be more appropriately indicated for intra-articular procedures, such as limited arthrodeses or PRC regardless of ulnar variance. Limited arthrodeses, such as scaphoid-trapezoid-trapezium and scaphoid-capitate effectively unload the lunate but they also increase radioscaphoid contact pressures, and they have a deleterious effect on carpal kinematics as well.

Alternatives to radius shortening osteotomy, including angular and displacement osteotomies, have also been developed because of concern over the possible deleterious effects of radius shortening on ulnocarpal and DRUJ relationships, especially in patients with neutral or ulnar positive variance. The long-term clinical efficacy of these procedures is uncertain. Capitate shortening osteotomy combined with capitate-hamate arthrodesis may be indicated in patients with stages I to IIIA disease and neutral or positive ulnar variance. Lunate revascularization procedures are also under investigation.

Arthroscopy and Arthrography

Recent studies have demonstrated a poor correlation between patients' symptoms, physical findings, and findings on arthrogram. A review of three-compartment wrist arthrograms completed in 82 patients revealed a low correlation between noncommunicating defects in the capsule, triangular fibrocartilage (TFC), and interosseous ligaments seen on the arthrogram with the location of the patient's pain. In another study, these authors also demonstrated a lack of correlation between complete communications and the location of the patient's pain. Even more revealing was a study that reviewed the findings of bilateral wrist arthrograms completed in 56 patients with unilateral symptoms. In this study, 88% of radial TFC injuries, 59% of lunotriquetral, and 57% of scapholunate defects were bilateral. These studies indicate that the results of an arthrogram should be interpreted with extreme caution and must be considered in the context of the information obtained from a careful history and physical examination as well as other ancillary studies.

The role of wrist arthroscopy in the evaluation and treatment of patients with wrist pain continues to evolve.

Reported applications include resection of partial TFC tears; debridement of degenerative lesions of TFC, articular surface, and interosseous ligaments; and arthroscopically assisted reduction and pinning of intra-articular distal radius fractures, scaphoid fractures, and acute carpal instabilities. The long-term efficacy of many of these techniques remains unclear. Arthroscopy appears to have a more valuable role as a diagnostic technique. Several studies have documented the efficacy of arthroscopy in establishing a diagnosis of chondral defect, TFC tear, and partial or complete ligament tears. Twenty patients with chronic wrist pain underwent arthrography and arthroscopy in one series. Nineteen of the 20 also underwent arthrotomy. The authors concluded that arthroscopy was a more valuable technique for determining the size, location, and extent of ligament and TFC injuries in the wrist, and that arthroscopy may also assist the physician in planning surgical approaches to the wrist. As with arthrography, the findings at arthroscopy must be carefully interpreted in the context of the patient's clinical presentation, in order to ensure that the abnormalities noted provide a reasonable and likely explanation for the patient's pain.

Diagnostic and therapeutic wrist arthroscopy has a lower associated morbidity than wrist arthrotomy. Nevertheless, tendons, cutaneous nerves, and arteries are at risk from this procedure. An anatomic study of arthroscopic portals confirmed that the 3–4, 4–5, midcarpal, and distal radioulnar portals were relatively safe entry sites. The 1–2, 6R, and 6U portals place the radial artery, the superficial radial nerve, and dorsal cutaneous branches of the ulnar nerve at risk for injury because they may be located within a few millimeters of these structures. The authors emphasize the importance of careful technique when developing portals in wrist arthroscopy and recommended longitudinal incisions through skin only, followed by blunt dissection to the level of the capsule.

Annotated Bibliography

Epidemiology

Futami T, Kobayashi A, Wakabayshi N, et al: Natural history of the carpal tunnel syndrome. *J Jpn Soc Surg Hand* 1992;9:128–130.

Adults with CTS from all age groups and all occupations reported resolution of symptoms within 5 months in 54 of 155 patients. No specific treatment was initiated. This study emphasizes that a period of observation is prudent in the treatment of idiopathic CTS.

Hagberg M, Morgenstern H, Kelsh M: Impact of occupations and job tasks on the prevalence of carpal tunnel syndrome. *Scand J Work Environ Health* 1992; 18:337–345.

On the basis of epidemiologic and other evidence, it was concluded that exposure to physical work load factors, such as repetitive and forceful gripping, is probably a major risk factor for CTS in several types of worker populations.

Nathan PA, Keniston RC, Myers LD, et al: Longitudinal study of median nerve sensory conduction in industry: Relationship to age, gender, hand dominance, occupational hand use, and clinical diagnosis. *J Hand Surg* 1992;17A:850–857.

Sensory conduction of the median nerve was measured at 5-year intervals in an attempt to determine the relationship between age, gender, hand dominance, occupational hand use, and clinical diagnosis. In this report, age and hand dominance were more important than any job-related factor in the prediction of sensory conduction slowing after 5 years.

Osorio AM, Ames RG, Jones J, et al: Carpal tunnel syndrome among grocery store workers. *Am J Ind Med* 1994;25:229–245.

Alerted by a cluster of patients with CTS, the authors explored the relationship between forceful and repetitive wrist motion and CTS. Patients in higher-exposure jobs were more prone to complain of carpal tunnel like symptoms.

Diagnosis

Jablecki CK, Andary MT, So YT, et al: Literature review of the usefulness of nerve conduction studies and electromyography for the evaluation of patients with carpal tunnel syndrome: AAEM Quality Assurance Committee. *Muscle Nerve* 1993;16:1392–1414.

This article reviewed the medical literature through May of 1991 to determine the sensitivity and specificity of nerve conduction studies (NCS) and EMG in the diagnosis of CTS. The authors concluded that median sensory and motor nerve conduction studies are valid and reproducible with a high degree of sensitivity and specificity. This article serves as a ready bibliography for anyone interested in the electrodiagnostic literature relative to CTS.

Koris M, Gelberman RH, Duncan K, et al: Carpal tunnel syndrome: Evaluation of a quantitative provocational diagnostic test. *Clin Orthop* 1990;251:157–161.

Combining wrist flexion with Semmes-Weinstein monofilament measurement is recommended as the most accurate and sensitive quantitative clinical test for median nerve compression.

Redmond MD, Rivner MH: False positive electrodiagnostic tests in carpal tunnel syndrome. *Muscle Nerve* 1988;11:511–518.

This study concludes that certain reported criteria for CTS are abnormal in a high percentage of normal subjects, thereby making them of limited diagnostic value. Of all the criteria studied, it appeared that the comparison of the median to ulnar sensory latency across the carpal tunnel is most helpful.

Williams TM, Mackinnon SE, Novak CB, et al: Verification of the pressure provocative test in carpal tunnel syndrome. *Ann Plast Surg* 1992;29:8–11.

Three provocative tests (pressure, Phalen's test, and Tinel's sign) were studied. Sensitivity was 100% for the pressure provocative test, 88% for Phalen's, and 67% for Tinel's sign. The pressure-provocative test is performed by placing a pneumatic tourniquet about the distal forearm-wrist and inflating the cuff to 150 mm Hg. The study is considered positive if paresthesias occur within 30 s of inflation.

Treatment

Agee JM, McCarroll HR Jr, Tortosa RD, et al: Endoscopic release of the carpal tunnel: A randomized prospective multicenter study. *J Hand Surg* 1992;17A: 987–995.

A single portal endoscopic device was used to perform CTR in 122 patients from 10 different centers. The patients were said to be randomized and followed prospectively; however, the randomization is questionable. The results were quite favorable for ECTR. The median time for return to work was about 3 weeks less than that for the control group.

Brown RA, Gelberman RH, Seiler JG III, et al: Carpal tunnel release: A prospective, randomized assessment of open and endoscopic methods. *J Bone Joint Surg* 1993;75A:1265–1275.

In a prospective randomized trial a classic palmar incision was compared with two-portal carpal ECTRs. Both methods resulted in a high level of pain relief and resolution of paresthesias. Four complications occurred in the ECTR group.

Foulkes GD, Atkinson RE, Beuchel C, et al: Outcome following epineurotomy in carpal tunnel syndrome: A prospective, randomized clinical trial. *J Hand Surg* 1994; 19A:539–547.

Thirty-six wrists in 33 patients were prospectively randomized into epineurotomy and nonepineurotomy treatment groups. The addition of an adjunctive epineurotomy, although safe, offered no clinical benefit in the surgical treatment of CTS in this series.

Kerr CD, Gittins ME, Sybert DR: Endoscopic versus open carpal tunnel release: Clinical results. *Arthroscopy* 1994;10:266–269.

In this large series ECTR was found to be safe. No surgical complications were noted. Patients undergoing the endoscopic technique with private insurance returned to work 15.6 days sooner than their open counterparts. Patients with workers' compensation claims returned to work at the same time regardless of the technique used.

Murphy RX Jr, Jennings JF, Wukich DK: Major neurovascular complications of endoscopic carpal tunnel release. *J Hand Surg* 1994;19A:114–118.

This paper reports a case of transection of the median nerve and a pseudo aneurysm of the superficial palmar arch following single-portal ECTR.

Nolan WB III, Alkaitis D, Glickel SZ, et al: Results of treatment of severe carpal tunnel syndrome. *J Hand Surg* 1992;17A:1020–1023.

The results of this retrospective study indicate that carpal tunnel decompression is of benefit to patients with severe CTS.

Alternative Surgical Treatment

Bromley GS: Minimal-incision open carpal tunnel decompression. *J Hand Surg* 1994;19A:119–120.

Wilson KM: Double incision open technique for carpal tunnel release: An alternative to endoscopic release. *J Hand Surg* 1994;19A:907–912.

These two papers describe using a small palmar incision alone (Bromley) or combined with a transverse wrist crease incision (Wilson) for CTR.

Cadaver Studies

Lee DH, Masear VR, Meyer RD, et al: Endoscopic carpal tunnel release: A cadaveric study. *J Hand Surg* 1992;17A: 1003–1008.

Rotman MB, Manske PR: Anatomic relationships of an endoscopic carpal tunnel device to surrounding structures. *J Hand Surg* 1993;18A:442–450.

Anatomic relationships of an endoscopic carpal tunnel device to surrounding soft-tissue structures along the ring finger and the long-ring interspace axis were investigated using adult cadaver hands. The anatomic observations indicate the greater safety of using the ring finger axis for ECTR.

Seiler JG III, Barnes K, Gelberman RH, et al: Endoscopic carpal tunnel release: An anatomic study of the two-incision method in human cadavers. *J Hand Surg* 1992; 17A:996–1002.

A cadaver study was designed to determine the relationship of neurovascular structures to the sites of portal placement and transverse carpal ligament division during two-portal ECTR. An extrasynovial approach previously recommended by Chow was compared to a modified technique in which the proximal incision was made in a more distal location and a distally based ligamentous flap was created. This modified (intrasynovial) approach was found to be potentially safer and is now the approach recommended by most surgeons who perform ECTR.

Results

Clarke AM, Stanley D: Prediction of the outcome 24 hours after carpal tunnel decompression. *J Hand Surg* 1993;18B:180–181.

Results of a prospective study demonstrated that in all cases where there was symptomatic relief of pain and paresthesias within the first 24 hours postoperatively, a good or excellent outcome could be anticipated.

Katz JN, Gelberman RH, Wright EA, et al: A preliminary scoring system for assessing the outcome of carpal tunnel release. *J Hand Surg* 1994;19A:531–538.

A global score was created in which outcomes were selected and weighted according to their independent association with patient satisfaction with the results of surgery.

Kerr CD, Sybert DR, Albarracin NS: An analysis of the flexor synovium in idiopathic carpal tunnel syndrome: Report of 625 cases. *J Hand Surg* 1992;17A:1028–1030.

Synovial tissue was analyzed from the wrists of 835 consecutive patients undergoing surgery for idiopathic CTS. The authors conclude that tenosynovitis is not a part of the pathophysiologic process in chronic idiopathic CTS.

Weiss AP, Sachar K, Gendreau M: Conservative management of carpal tunnel syndrome: A reexamination of steroid injection and splinting. *J Hand Surg* 1994;19A: 410–415.

Seventy-six hands in 57 patients with mild CTS were treated with steroid injection and splinting and followed up for an average of 11 months. Young women (< 40 years old) were the least likely to have resolution of CTS symptoms when treated conservatively.

Wrist Arthrodesis

Lee DH, Carroll RE: Wrist arthrodesis: A combined intramedullary pin and autogenous iliac crest bone graft technique. *J Hand Surg* 1994;19A:733–740.

Forty-six wrist arthrodeses in 36 patients were performed using an autogenous iliac crest bone graft, with an intramedullary Steinman pin placed within the distal radial and third metacarpal shafts, and an obliquely-placed Kirschner wire across the second metacarpal base into the radius. This patient populations all had low demands on the wrist fusion related to congenital anomolies or collagen vascular disease in the majority of cases. The technique should be kept in mind for the treatment of patients with limited bone stock.

Weiss AP, Hastings H II: Wrist arthrodesis for traumatic conditions: A study of plate and local bone graft application. *J Hand Surg* 1995;20A:50–56.

Wrist fusions were performed with contoured AO/ASIF plates and local bone graft. A solid arthrodesis was obtained in all 28 cases. Complications included late extensor tenosynovitis treated with plate removal in four cases, one acute CTS treated with decompression, and one painful DRUJ treated with steroid injection.

Zachary SV, Stern PJ: Complications following AO/ASIF wrist arthrodesis. *J Hand Surg* 1995;20A:339–344.

This candid review of 71 patients treated with AO/ASIF 3.5-mm DC plates divided complications into short and long term. There were no nonunions. All told, there were 82 complications, 63 of which resolved.

Proximal Row Carpectomy

Culp RW, McGuigan FX, Turner MA, et al: Proximal row carpectomy: A multicenter study. *J Hand Surg* 1993;18A: 19–25.

Twenty patients underwent PRC. The procedure failed in all three patients with rheumatoid arthritis. Better results were seen in patients with mild preoperative arthritic changes.

Krakauer JD, Bishop AT, Cooney WP: Surgical treatment of scapholunate advanced collapse. *J Hand Surg* 1994; 19A:751–759.

This study reports the outcomes of six different reconstructive procedures in 55 patients for stage II and stage III SLAC wrist. Scaphoid excision and four-corner arthrodesis reliably diminished wrist pain in patients with stage III SLAC wrist and maintained useful wrist motion. Stage II SLAC wrist was successfully treated with radioscaphoid arthrodesis, PRC, or four-corner fusion. PRC preserved the most wrist mobility.

Tomaino MM, Delsignore J, Burton RI: Long-term results following proximal row carpectomy. *J Hand Surg* 1994;19A:694–703.

The majority of patients experienced satisfactory pain relief, functional wrist motion, and effective grip strength following PRC. The study, which has the longest follow-up of any, noted that the results did not decline at an average of 6 years after surgery.

Other Motion Sparing Wrist Procedures

Ashmead D IV, Watson HK, Damon C, et al: Scapholunate advanced collapse wrist salvage. *J Hand Surg* 1994;19A:741–750.

This is a report on 100 of 160 SLAC wrist procedures done between 1977 and 1990 and followed up for average of 44 months. The extension/flexion arc averaged 72°, there was excellent functional status and a high rate of patient satisfaction. Complications were three nonunions, 13 cases of dorsal impingement between the capitate and radius with wrist extension, and seven cases of particulate synovitis. Inherent to all retrospective studies is the failure to provide follow-up of all the cases treated by these authors, which in this report is 37% of their experience.

Bach AW, Almquist EE, Newman DM: Proximal row fusion as a solution for radiocarpal arthritis. *J Hand Surg* 1991;16A:424–431.

Thirty-six patients treated by radius-scaphoid-lunate arthrodesis for posttraumatic radiocarpal arthritis were studied. Seven patients required revision to complete wrist fusion because of pain. Arthritic changes in the midcarpal joint had been noted in these patients at the time of the limited fusion. The remainder did well, retaining about 45° of flexion–extension.

Bosco JA III, Bynum DK, Bowers WH: Long-term outcome of Volz total wrist arthroplasties. *J Arthroplasty* 1994;9:25–31.

The outcomes of 18 consecutive Volz total wrist arthroplasties were followed up for an average of 8.6 years. Overall, the long-term outcome of total wrist arthroplasty was favorable in patients with rheumatoid arthritis and poor in patients with degenerative joint disease.

Figgie MP, Ranawat CS, Inglis AE, et al: Trispherical total wrist arthroplasty in rheumatoid arthritis. *J Hand Surg* 1990;15A:217–223.

Thirty-four patients, with 35 trispherical total wrist arthroplasties for treatment of rheumatoid arthritis are reviewed. The results are especially promising for those patients with intact extensor tendons before surgery.

Fortin PT, Louis DS: Long-term follow-up of scaphoid-trapezium-trapezoid arthrodesis. *J Hand Surg* 1993;18A: 675–681.

A series of 19 consecutive patients who underwent scaphoid-trapezium-trapezoid arthrodesis for chronic scapholunate instability or isolated arthrosis was reviewed. The authors conclude that fusion without reduction of the scaphoid to a normal orientation was predictive of a poor result, but normal scaphoid positioning did not preclude development of arthrosis. Development of a painful degenerative thumb carpometacarpal joint may occur as an isolated phenomenon after scaphoid-trapezium-trapezoid arthrodesis.

Jolly SL, Ferlic DC, Clayton ML, et al: Swanson silicone arthroplasty of the wrist in rheumatoid arthritis: A long-term follow-up. *J Hand Surg* 1992;17A:142–149.

Twenty-three Swanson silicone rubber implants in patients with stage III or stage IV rheumatoid arthritis were reviewed at an average of 72 months after surgery. Survivorship analysis demonstrated 42% survival at 77 months.

Rotman MB, Manske PR, Pruitt DL, et al: Scaphocapitolunate arthrodesis. *J Hand Surg* 1993; 18A:26–33.

Since 1985, scaphocapitolunate arthrodesis has been performed on 21 patients. Pain was significantly reduced in 80% of the patients. Sixteen of 20 patients were able to return to work.

Distal Radioulnar Joint

Acosta R, Hnat W, Scheker LR: Distal radio-ulnar ligament motion during supination and pronation. *J Hand Surg* 1993;18B:502–505.

Using a Hall-effect displacement transducer during pronation and supination it was noted that the dorsal DRUL undergoes relative displacement during pronation, while the palmar DRUL undergoes relative displacement during supination.

Linscheid RL: Biomechanics of the distal radioulnar joint. *Clin Orthop* 1992;275:46–55.

This article presents a point of view opposite to that of Acosta and associates.

Nakamura R, Tsunoda K, Watanabe K, et al: The Sauve-Kapandji procedure for chronic dislocation of the distal radio-ulnar joint with destruction of the articular surface. *J Hand Surg* 1992;17B:127–132.

This paper investigated the role of Sauve-Kapandji procedure for nonrheumatoid patients with chronic DRUJ injuries. The clinical results were favorable. However, radiographic examination revealed an unstable proximal ulnar stump and radioulnar convergence in all patients.

Scheker LR, Belliappa PP, Acosta R, et al: Reconstruction of the dorsal ligament of the triangular fibrocartilage complex. *J Hand Surg* 1994;19B:310–318.

These authors proposed that DRUJ instability is secondary to dorsal DRUL rupture or attenuation and presented a reconstruction using a tendon graft weaved through the dorsal DRUL and anchored into the radius and ulna.

Taleisnik J: The Sauve-Kapandji procedure. *Clin Orthop* 1992;275:110–123.

This paper presents the author's experience using this procedure for rheumatoid arthritis, osteoarthrosis, and posttraumatic changes of the DRUJ. The Sauve-Kapandji procedure is probably contraindicated in the treatment of unstable or dislocated distal radioulnar joint.

Vincent KA, Szabo RM, Agee JM: The Sauve-Kapandji procedure for reconstruction of the rheumatoid distal radioulnar joint. *J Hand Surg* 1993;18A:978–983.

This procedure seems most suited for rheumatoid arthritis.

Scaphoid Nonunion: Natural History

Kerluke L, McCabe SJ: Nonunion of the scaphoid: A critical analysis of recent natural history studies. *J Hand Surg* 1993;18A:1–3.

This article is essential reading. It points out the epidemiologic flaws in previously published studies regarding the fate of scaphoid nonunion.

Lindstrom G, Nystrom A: Natural history of scaphoid non-union, with special reference to "asymptomatic" cases. *J Hand Surg* 1992;17B:697–700.

Thirty-three patients with nonunion of the carpal scaphoid were diagnosed by radiographic examination 2 to 37 years following the original trauma. Radiographs revealed a 100% incidence of progressive radiocarpal osteoarthritis.

Trapeziometacarpal Joint

Pellegrini VD Jr: Osteoarthritis of the trapeziometacarpal joint: The pathophysiology of articular cartilage degeneration. I: Anatomy and pathology of the aging joint. *J Hand Surg* 1991;16A:967–974.

Pellegrini VD Jr, Smith RL, Ku CW: Pathobiology of articular cartilage in trapeziometacarpal osteoarthritis: I. Regional biochemical analysis. *J Hand Surg* 1994;19A: 70–78.

Pellegrini VD Jr, Smith RL, Ku CW: Pathobiology of articular cartilage in trapeziometacarpal osteoarthritis: II. Surface ultrastructure by scanning electron microscopy. *J Hand Surg* 1994;19A:79–85.

These three studies provide incredible insight into this common problem. The conclusions drawn from these articles is that there is an interdependent relationship between mechanically-induced abrasive surface wear and biochemical matrix degradation in the production of the cartilage lesion of trapeziometacarpal osteoarthritis and that the cornerstone to stability is the palmar beak ligament.

Bony Deformity of Digits

Hanel DP, Lederman ES: Index transposition after resection of the long finger ray. *J Hand Surg* 1993; 18A:271–277.

Ten patients underwent index-to-long-finger ray transposition for repair after resection of the long finger ray. The authors reconstructed the hand by taking advantage of rigid fixation, web space preservation, and neuroma reduction with end-to-end suturing of the digital nerve stumps. There were no nonunions. Postoperative motion was equal or better than preoperatively. The same was true for grip strength.

Stern PJ, Fulton DB: Distal interphalangeal joint arthrodesis: An analysis of complications. *J Hand Surg* 1992;17A:1139–1145.

One hundred eighty-one arthrodeses of the DIP joints or thumb IP joints were noted to have major complications in 20% of the fusions and minor complications in 16% of the joints fused.

Stern PJ, Gates NT, Jones TB: Tension band arthrodesis of small joints in the hand. *J Hand Surg* 1993;18A:194–197.

There is no larger series of the MCP and PIP joint arthrodeses than the 290 tension bands reported here. With a 3% nonunion rate and minimal complications, the authors suggest that tension band arthrodesis should be the treatment of choice for fusion of the MCP and PIP joints.

van-der-Lei B, de-Jonge J, Robinson PH, et al: Correction osteotomies of phalanges and metacarpals for rotational and angular malunion: A long-term follow-up and a review of the literature. *J Trauma* 1993;35:902–908.

This series reinforces the findings of an older Swiss series of in situ correctional osteotomies for the treatment of rotational and angular malunion. Full correction of the preoperative deformity was achieved in 13 of the 15 patients, bony union in 100%, and all but one patient maintained or improved preoperative motion.

Tendon Problems

Boutonnière Reconstruction

Kiefhaber TR, Strickland JW: Soft tissue reconstruction for rheumatoid swan-neck and boutonniere deformities: Long-term results. *J Hand Surg* 1993;18A:984–989.

Nineteen fingers with rheumatoid boutonnière deformity were treated with central slip reconstruction. The results were unpredictable, with only modest improvement in the PIP extension, which deteriorated over time. The authors now recommend arthrodesis for most severe rheumatoid boutonnière deformities. The results of soft-tissue procedures for swan neck deformities were more promising but even these deteriorated with time.

Klasson SC, Adams BD: Biomechanical evaluation of chronic boutonniere reconstructions. *J Hand Surg* 1992;17A:868–874.

The magnitudes of the extensor forces generated across the PIP joint by four popular boutonnière deformity reconstructions was measured.

Smith PJ, Ross DA: The central slip tenodesis test for early diagnosis of potential boutonnière deformities. *J Hand Surg* 1994;19B:88–90.

The early diagnosis of closed central slip disruption is difficult. The authors describe an examination technique that assists in making the diagnosis.

Terrill RQ, Groves RJ: Correction of the severe nonrheumatoid chronic boutonniere deformity with a modified Matev procedure. *J Hand Surg* 1992;17A:874–880.

Chronic nonrheumatoid deformities were treated with a modification of the Matev procedure. Those with near normal preoperative range of motion did the best with 85% good or satisfactory results compared to 67% good or satisfactory results in fingers with contracture.

Tenolysis

Birnie RH, Idler RS: Flexor tenolysis in children. *J Hand Surg* 1995;20A:254–257.

Twenty-nine digits in 26 children underwent flexor tendon tenolysis. Children younger than 11-years-old did poorly obtaining only fair or poor results, whereas older children obtained mostly good or excellent results.

Foucher G, Lenoble E, Ben-Youssef K, et al: A post-operative regime after digital flexor tenolysis: A series of 72 patients. *J Hand Surg* 1993;18B:35–40.

Two technical modifications were introduced: reconstruction of a robust pulley and initial immobilization with the tendon in a flexed position. When therapy is started, the digit is coaxed into extension breaking the early adhesions.

Tendonitis

Auerbach DM, Collins ED, Kunkle KL, et al: The radial sensory nerve: An anatomic study. *Clin Orthop* 1994; 308:241–249.

The superficial branch of the radial nerve has an average of 5.8 branches crossing the wrist joint. The message here is that there are no uniquely safe incisions about this region whether longitudinal or transverse, and cautious dissection is warranted in this region.

Eastwood DM, Gupta KJ, Johnson DP: Percutaneous release of the trigger finger: An office procedure. *J Hand Surg* 1992;17A:114–117.

Pope DF, Wolfe SW: Safety and efficacy of percutaneous trigger finger release. *J Hand Surg* 1995;20A:280–283.

These two articles deal with a new technique for percutaneous release of the trigger finger using a 19- or 21-gauge hypodermic needle to release the A1 pulley. The results matched other series of open treatment.

Weiss AP, Akelman E, Tabatabai M: Treatment of de Quervain's disease. *J Hand Surg* 1994;19A:595–598.

These authors discuss the efficacy of steroid injection, steroid injection and splinting, and splinting alone for the treatment of de Quervain's disease. The authors recommend the use of a mixed steroid/lidocaine injection alone as the initial treatment of choice in this condition.

Arthroscopy/Arthrography

Abrams RA, Petersen, M, Botte MJ: Arthroscopic portals of the wrist: An anatomic study. *J Hand Surg* 1994;19A: 940–944.

Twenty-three cadaver specimens were dissected for the purpose of studying periportal anatomy. The authors indicate that the 3–4, 4–5, midcarpal, and DRUJ portals are relatively safe. However, the 1–2, 6R, and 6U portals were perilously close to the radial artery, superficial radial nerve, and the dorsal cutaneous branches of the ulnar nerve.

Cantor RM, Stern PJ, Wyrick JD, et al: The relevance of ligament tears or perforations in the diagnosis of wrist pain: An arthrographic study. *J Hand Surg* 1994;19A: 945–953.

Fifty-six consecutive patients with unilateral wrist pain underwent bilateral wrist arthrograms. In patients with ligament defects on the symptomatic side, 88% of the patients with radial TFC defects, 59% with lunotriquetral defects, and 57% with scapholunate defects had identical defects on the contralateral side.

Cooney WP: Evaluation of chronic wrist pain by arthrography, arthroscopy, and arthrotomy. *J Hand Surg* 1993;18A:815–822.

Twenty consecutive patients with confirmed wrist injuries and chronic wrist pain underwent arthrography and arthroscopy. Nineteen underwent arthrotomy. The author concluded that wrist arthroscopy was more accurate in localizing wrist injuries and was a more valuable technique in determining the location, size, and extent of ligament injuries within the wrist.

Metz VM, Mann FA, Gilula LA: Lack of correlation between site of wrist pain and location of noncommunicating defects shown by three-compartment wrist arthrography. *AJR Am J Roentgenol* 1993;160: 1239–1243.

Three compartment wrist arthrograms were completed in 82 patients with wrist pain. Noncommunicating defects of the capsule and incomplete defects of interosseous ligaments and the TFC were identified in 65 patients. The authors found no statistically significant correlation between these defects and the patients' symptoms. Age did not affect this correlation.

Kienböck's Disease

Coe MR, Trumble TE: Biomechanical comparison of methods used to treat Kienböck's disease. *Hand Clin* 1993;9:417–429.

This is a concise but comprehensive review of the available experimental data related to joint leveling procedures and intercarpal arthrodeses.

Condit DP, Idler RS, Fischer TJ, et al: Preoperative factors and outcome after lunate decompression for Kienböck's disease. *J Hand Surg* 1993;18A:691–696.

Twenty-three patients with Kienböck's disease underwent either radius shortening osteotomy (14) or scaphoid-trapezium-trapezoid (STT) fusion (nine) and were followed for a minimum of two years. A radioscaphoid angle greater than 60° precluded a good outcome in both groups.

Classic Bibliography

Bilos ZJ, Chamberland D: Distal ulnar head shortening for treatment of triangular fibrocartilage complex tears with ulna positive variance. *J Hand Surg* 1991;16A:1115–1119.

Feldon P, Terrono AL, Belsky MR: Wafer distal ulna resection for triangular fibrocartilage tears and/or ulna impaction syndrome. *J Hand Surg* 1992;17A:731–737.

Gelberman RH, Pfeffer GB, Galbraith RT, et al: Results of treatment of severe carpal-tunnel syndrome without internal neurolysis of the median nerve. *J Bone Joint Surg* 1987;69A:896–903.

Pichora DR, Meyer R, Masear VR: Rotational step-cut osteotomy for treatment of metacarpal and phalangeal malunion. *J Hand Surg* 1991;16A:551–555.

Richards RS, Roth JH: Simultaneous proximal row carpectomy and radius to distal carpal row arthrodesis: *J Hand Surg* 1994;19A:728–732.

IV

Lower Extremity

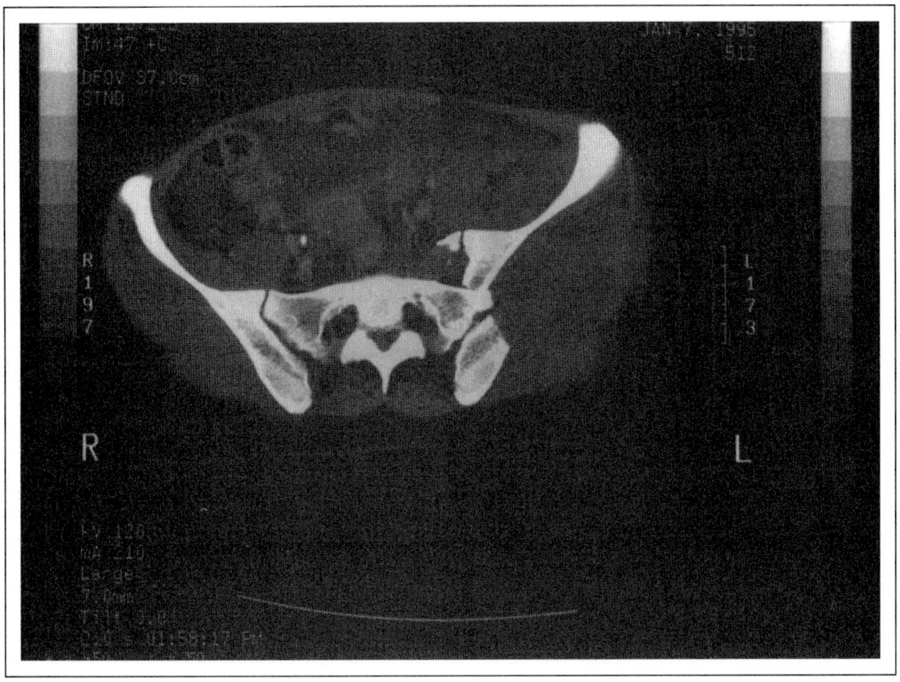

33

Hip, Pelvis, and Femur: Pediatric Aspects

Congenital Disorders

Developmental Dysplasia of the Hip

Developmental dysplasia of the hip (DDH) encompasses a wide range of disorders, including teratologic dislocation (severe, high-riding, occurring early in fetal life), neonatal hip instability, subluxation, dislocation, and acetabular dysplasia. All can be bilateral, and are found more frequently on the left side when unilateral. Causes can be both genetic and environmental; risk factors include family history, sex (female), intrauterine position (breech), and birth weight. DDH may be associated with a number of musculoskeletal anomalies, including torticollis, congenital knee hyperextension or subluxation, and foot deformities.

Diagnosis Clinical examination of the newborn is the best method for detection of DDH. Prospective neonatal screening has proven very successful, but no series has detected 100% of the abnormal hips. Three tests (abduction, Barlow's test, and the Ortolani test) are useful. Inguinal skin folds extending posteriorly to the level of the anus, while not specific, are suggestive of dislocation.

Radiographs usually are of little help in a child younger than 3 months of age, although sometimes they can be clearly abnormal. Ultrasound is very sensitive, but it is expensive and requires a knowledgeable operator. False positives are especially common in children younger than 6 weeks of age, and many hips that appear unstable will ultimately be normal without any treatment. Ultrasound may be helpful in high-risk infants (positive family history, breech) older than 6 weeks of age, in children who have an inconclusive clinical examination, and to confirm reduction of the hip in a Pavlik harness.

Treatment The goal is to obtain gentle, atraumatic concentric reduction, confirm it, and maintain it by flexion and abduction positioning until capsular laxity resolves and the hip is stable. If dysplasia of the acetabulum is present, stable positioning should be maintained until radiographic or ultrasonic demonstration of significant resolution. Treatment depends on age at detection: most neonates can be treated with a Pavlik harness; children under walking age, with closed reduction; those above walking age, with open reduction; and those over 18 to 24 months, with open reduction and pelvic or femoral osteotomy.

The most common method for achieving reduction in infants is the Pavlik harness, which allows successful spontaneous reduction of dislocated hips within 2 weeks in 75% to 90% of patients. Subluxatable hips and hips with a positive Ortolani test are most likely to respond favorably to Pavlik harness treatment; failures are more frequent in bilateral cases, Ortolani negative dislocations, and infants older than 2 to 3 months of age.

The Pavlik harness must be properly applied. The chest strap should cross the nipples, and the anterior foot straps should not allow extension beyond 90° to 100° of flexion; conversely, too much flexion can cause reversible femoral neuropathy. The posterior straps should not be too tight (which can cause osteonecrosis), but should limit adduction to 0°. Pavlik treatment is most successful before 7 weeks of age, but may effect reduction up to 3 to 6 months of age.

If brace treatment does not effect a concentric reduction after 3 to 4 weeks of proper use, or if the child is over 6 to 9 months of age, alternative treatment (closed or open reduction) should be considered. It is unwise to persist with unsuccessful bracing because it can cause posterior acetabular deformation that makes future treatment more difficult. At the present time, the value of traction is controversial. Skin traction can be carried out safely at home if the family is cooperative and able to supervise the child. Lightweight frames of polyvinyl chloride pipe can be adapted to home use, and are well-described in the literature.

Closed reduction is done under general anesthesia. The hip must be stable in a safe position, with flexion and abduction of 45° to 60°. If the adductor muscle is tight, percutaneous tenotomy can be performed, but excessive abduction should be avoided. Arthrograms are helpful to evaluate reduction and stability. Computed tomography (CT) may help to confirm reduction after the child is placed in a spica cast. The spica cast is changed every 6 weeks under anesthesia until the joint is stable (usually 12 to 16 weeks), and the child may be placed in an abduction brace for an additional 3 to 6 months at night only.

The upper age limit for closed reduction is determined by pathology, not age, but children older than 12 to 18 months usually require open reduction. Open reduction can be performed through an anterolateral (modified Smith-Peterson), medial (Ferguson), or anteromedial approach (Weinstein and Ponseti). The choice of approach varies with surgical training and experience; a Smith Peterson approach, modified by use of a transverse inguinal incision and without stripping of the abductors from the pelvis, allows excellent visualization of pathology.

Pelvic or femoral osteotomy can be performed at the time of reduction if necessary to stabilize the reduction or to correct acetabular dysplasia. If open reduction requires excessive force (compression) and femoral shortening is appropriate, femoral varus or derotation can be achieved simultaneously. If the reduction is unstable (especially in a child older than 18 months of age), combining reduction with pelvic or femoral osteotomy, or both, is wise, because remodeling may not correct significant acetabular dysplasia.

Isolated femoral osteotomies are useful for management of residual acetabular dysplasia after successful reduction of the hip only in children younger than 4 years of age. Between ages 4 and 8 years, acetabular response to femoral osteotomy is variable. Beyond 8 years of age, there is no role for isolated femoral osteotomy as treatment for residual acetabular dysplasia. In general, pelvic osteotomy (either Salter or Pemberton) is the procedure of choice for resolution of residual acetabular dysplasia in the management of DDH. Children with an enlarged acetabulum may benefit from an osteotomy that reduces the capacity of the acetabulum while rendering its superior roof more horizontal (Pemberton acetabuloplasty).

The treatment of asymptomatic radiographic dysplasia and early degenerative changes in adolescents and young adults is controversial. Most surgeons avoid major reconstructive procedures based on radiographic changes alone, in the absence of pain, but reconstructive osteotomies have been recommended to postpone symptomatic degeneration. Reconstruction or salvage procedures may be indicated for painful residual dysplasia. With adequate joint space, aggressive acetabular reorientation (Ganz, Wagner, Steel, Eppright), sometimes combined with femoral osteotomy, can improve joint mechanics and relieve pain. If complex reorientation to a concentric hip is impossible, a true salvage procedure, such as Chiari osteotomy or acetabular shelf (Staheli), can reduce pain and improve bone stock for later total joint arthroplasty. Trendelenberg limp after these procedures can be improved by distal and lateral tranfer of the greater trochanter.

Osteonecrosis (ON) may complicate any stage of DDH treatment. It may be mild, transient (radiographic only), and of little acute importance, although late growth arrest is possible. More frequently, ON leads to joint collapse and deformity as well as failure of proximal femoral physeal growth. A combination of collapse and residual subluxation should be treated by continued abduction bracing or pelvic osteotomy, despite the fact that results of osteotomy are compromised by the presence of ON. Leg-length inequality can be managed by contralateral femoral epiphysiodesis at the appropriate age; if a limp is present at that time, distal and lateral transfer of the trochanter is carried out under the same anesthetic.

Congenital Coxa Vara

Congenital coxa vara, an anomaly of the proximal femur, is characterized by a decreased neck-shaft angle and the presence of a femoral neck defect, typically a triangular fragment of bone located at the inferior metaphyseal—physeal junction. Unilateral involvement is more common than bilateral involvement and the sex ratio is equal. Patients typically present with a Trendelenburg, waddling gait and increased lumbar lordosis; pain rarely is present.

The neck-shaft angle on radiographs is decreased; however, it is often difficult to measure this angle. Because of the unreliability of the neck-shaft angle, the Hilgenreiner-epiphyseal (HE) angle was defined (Fig. 1). Several recent reports recommend valgus osteotomy (Fig. 2) for hips with an HE angle of $> 60°$; hips with an angle of $< 45°$ generally correct spontaneously. Hips with an HE angle between 60° and 45° should be observed closely because they can worsen easily. At the first sign of worsening, osteotomy should be performed. The surgical goal should be to obtain an HE angle of $\leq 35°$ or a neck shaft angle of $\geq 140°$, with overcorrection to try to prevent recurrent deformity. The femoral retroversion that is always present should be corrected at the same time. The most important facet in treatment is removing the shear stress from the abnormal physeal area. Correction is maintained better in children older than 5 years of age than in younger children. Because the proximal femoral physis frequently fuses after successful surgery, follow-up for leg length discrepancy is appropriate.

Bladder and Cloacal Exstrophy

Bladder exstrophy is an abnormality of the lower genitourinary tract that occurs in one of 10,000 to 25,000 live births. Cloacal exstrophy is an even rarer, more severe abnormality that involves both the lower genitourinary tract and the hindgut. The pubic diastasis associated with these exstrophies often requires bilateral pelvic osteotomy to

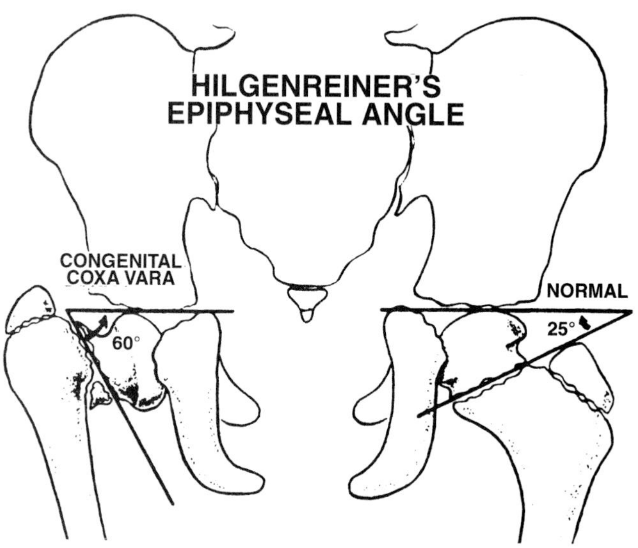

Fig. 1 Determination of the Hilgenreiner-epiphyseal angle, using Hilgenreiner's line as the horizontal axis and a line through the defect adjacent to the metaphysis axis. (Reproduced with permission from Weinstein JN, Kuo KN, Millar EA: Congenital coxa vara: A retrospective review. *J Pediatr Orthop* 1984;4:70–77.)

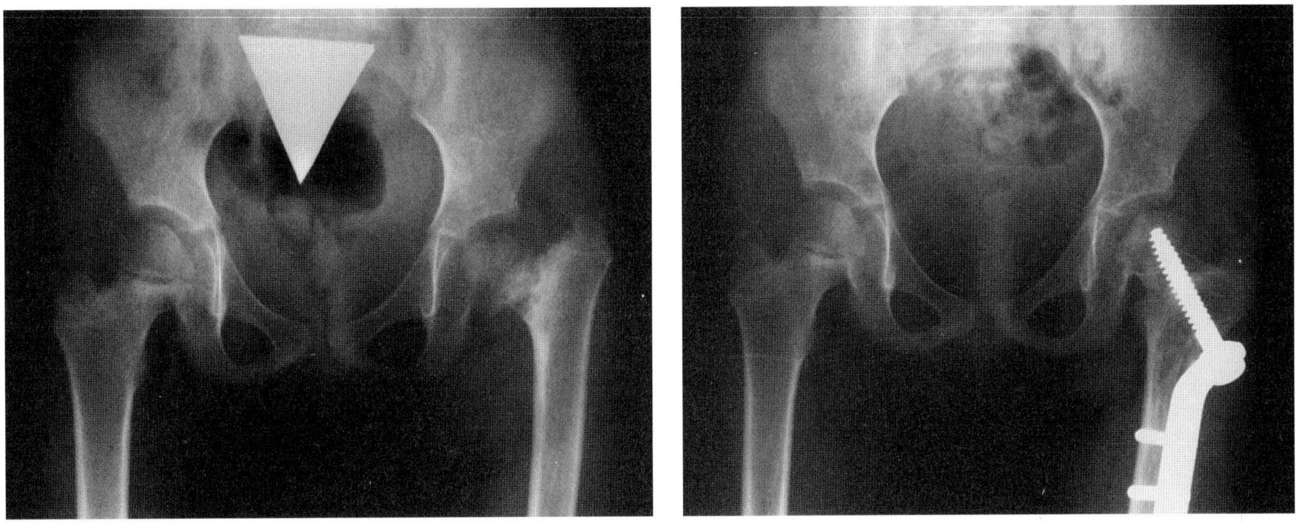

Fig. 2 **Left,** Congenital coxa vara in a 5-year-old child. **Right,** After valgus subtrochanteric osteotomy with compression-screw fixation.

ease closure. These osteotomies traditionally have been performed posteriorly, just lateral and parallel to the sacroiliac joint from the superior ilium into the sciatic notch, but the use of newer methods of osteotomy has been described. These include superior pubic ramomotomy, innominate osteotomy (the standard Salter, modified by an internal rotation maneuver, pin fixation, and without a wedge bone graft), and, most recently, an oblique osteotomy that is equidistant between the posterior and Salter osteotomies.

All children should have spinal radiographs to ensure that no coexistent spinal deformities are present. Those with cloacal exstrophy have a 100% incidence of spina bifida, often associated with a lipomeningocele and lower extremity paralysis, and frequently have foot deformities and hip dysplasia, which need orthopaedic care.

Congenital Femoral Anomalies

Congenital femoral anomalies usually involve the proximal femur and are classified into those with and without an osseous defect. This spectrum includes proximal femoral focal deficiency (PFFD), developmental coxa vara, and congenital short femur.

Proximal Femoral Focal Deficiency PFFD is characterized by shortening of the femur and a defect in the proximal femur, which is either unossified cartilage or a true discontinuity. Several different classifications exist, but the most widely used is that of Aitken (Fig. 3). In type A, there is initially a gap between the proximal and distal femur, but it is ossified eventually (by maturity). The femur is short with varus of the neck and subtrochanteric region. In type B, the gap fails to unite, and the acetabulum and femoral head are hypoplastic. In type C, the femoral head is absent or hypoplastic, and the acetabulum is markedly dysplastic; the distal femur migrates progressively proximally. In type D, both the acetabulum and femoral head are absent, and the distal femur consists of little more than the condyles.

The etiology of this condition is unknown. Because the foot is often involved as well, it may be a multifocal teratogenic process. The only known teratogen is thalidomide. On physical examination, the affected proximal femur of the limb is flexed, abducted, and externally rotated. Fifteen percent of patients have bilateral involvement, and over 50% have anomalies distal to the femur, especially paraxial fibular hemimelia, absence of lateral rays of the foot, and tarsal coalition.

Radiographic features vary with age. Portions of the proximal cartilage anlage ossify late, especially in types A and B. The presence of an acetabulum usually indicates that a cartilaginous femoral head also is present. Magnetic resonance imaging (MRI) may help better define what is present. MRI also has delineated the soft-tissue anatomy. Virtually all of the muscles are present. The sartorius is hypertrophied and may contribute to the flexed-abducted externally rotated position of the limb. The obturator externus is also enlarged and may function as a depressor of the femur. Several other muscles, especially the hip adductors and abductors, form a cuff to stabilize the proximal femur and probably contribute to the surprising stability of the dysplastic shaft fragment.

Treatment must correct as many as possible of the four functional defects in PFFD: (1) major limb length inequality (if unilateral); (2) pelvic–femoral instability; (3) malrotation of the lower extremity, including hip flexion-abduction-external rotation and knee flexion contracture; and (4) proximal hip muscle weakness.

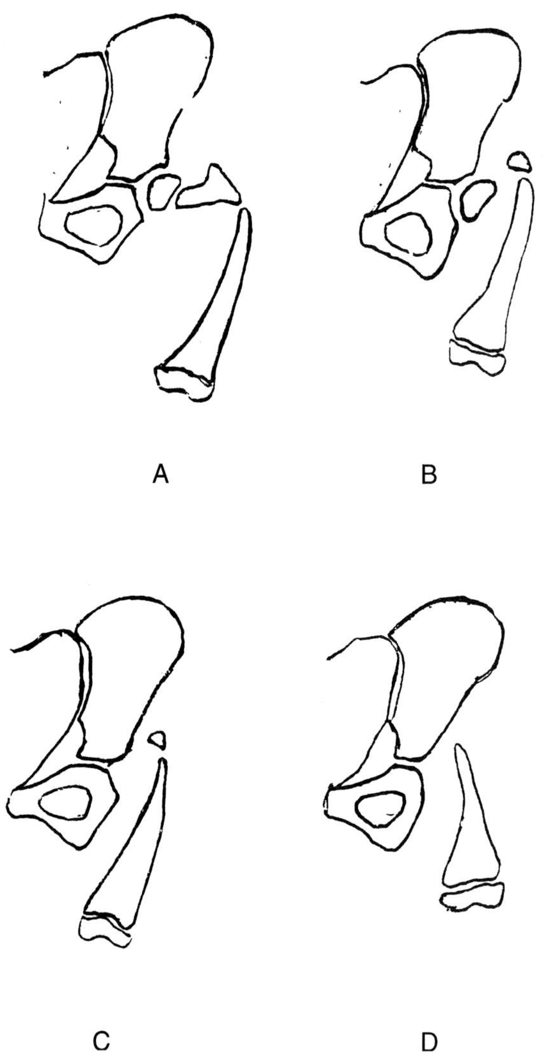

Fig. 3 Aitken classification.

For most patients with unilateral PFFD, treatment is geared toward fitting a prosthesis. A proximal femoral valgus osteotomy is needed to decrease coxa vara in type A and to secure union in type B. This procedure is followed by knee fusion and a rotationplasty or a Syme or Boyd amputation, depending upon the length of the limb, structure of the foot, and patient preference. The Syme or Boyd amputation allows fitting as an above-knee amputee, while the rotationplasty allows fitting as a below-knee amputee. Recent studies have shown that rotationplasty leads to a more normal quality of gait and decreased oxygen consumption during gait, with no measurable decrease in self-image. Types C and D PFFD may be treated with Syme amputation and prosthesis. In selected patients, pelvic–femoral fusion is performed to gain hip stability to allow for rotationplasty, with the true knee functioning as a hip.

Patients with bilateral PFFD usually are most functional without any prosthesis. When desired to increase height, however, extension prostheses may be constructed to wear fitted below the shoe, with the ankle at knee level.

Congenital Short Femur This term is used when shortening of the femur is the predominant limb anomaly and there is no major femoral defect or angulation. Many authors believe it is part of a spectrum with PFFD, but the treatment implications are different. Usually, the shortening is 5 to 10 cm at maturity. There is no known inheritance pattern. Physical findings include bowing of the femoral shaft in the direction of flexion-abduction-external rotation. The femoral head and neck may be slightly small. The knee often has anteroposterior (AP) laxity, which is indicated on radiographs by flattening of the intercondylar notch. The leg itself also may be slightly short, and there is a lower incidence of fibular deficiency compared to classic PFFD.

Radiographically, the growth inhibition is proportionate throughout development. Many patients with the condition are best treated with limb lengthening, depending on the status of the ipsilateral hip, knee, and foot. Lengthening done proximally has less risk of knee stiffness, but some surgeons believe that the regenerate bone formed is not as abundant as in a normal femur. Knee subluxation is a frequent complication, which is due to the cruciate laxity present in many of these patients.

Acquired Disorders

Transient Synovitis of the Hip

Transient synovitis is a benign, self-limited condition of unknown etiology, manifested by hip or knee pain, restiction of motion, and a limp. The challenge is to differentiate this condition from septic hip and Perthes disease. The child's temperature, sedimentation rate, and leukocyte count are helpful, but if there is any doubt, aspiration of the joint is indicated to rule out septic arthritis.

Radiographs are normal in transient synovitis; the capsular sign has been proven to be unreliable. Ultrasound (to demonstrate effusion) and clinical examination may be sufficient to make the diagnosis. Bone scan and MRI have not proven useful for diagnosis, and routine follow-up radiographs are unnecessary if the child remains asymptomatic after recovery from synovitis. There is no proof that transient synovitis leads to Perthes disease, although early Perthes disease can masquerade as synovitis. Only 2% of children with transient synovitis are diagnosed with Perthes disease, and these should eventually be detectable clinically and radiographically.

Septic Arthritis

Septic arthritis of the hip is a surgical emergency. A high index of suspicion is important, because in early stages it may mimic transient synovitis. Usually, sedimentation rate, leukocyte count, and temperature are elevated, but all may be normal early in the course of the disease. Neonates are particularly prone to sepsis without clinical signs or fever. Radiographs may show loss of normal soft-tissue planes around the hip. Ultrasound can suggest effusion, but there are false negatives in 25%. Bone scan may be abnormal, but is nonspecific, and false negatives can occur; it is usually unwise to delay definitive treatment while awaiting isotope studies.

Although blood cultures may be positive, definitive diagnosis is made by aspiration of the hip. If synovial fluid is not obtained, arthrographic confirmation of needle position is required. Aspirated fluid should be sent for culture, cell count, and Gram stain, and if the fluid is abnormal (white blood cell count > 50,000/mm^3), immediate surgical drainage is indicated. Appropriate empiric antibiotics are started as soon as the abnormal aspirate is obtained and are changed according to culture results. *Staphylococcus aureus* is the most common pathogen, but *Streptococcus* and gram-negative organisms are common, particularly in the newborn.

Most experts prefer drainage from an anterior approach, performed through a transverse-oblique inguinal incision. It is unnecessary to split the iliac apophysis; separation between tensor fascia lata and sartorius and reflection of the rectus femoris medially will expose the capsule. An anterior capsular window should be excised, and a drain may be used for 24 to 48 hours. Because osteomyelitis of the femoral neck can mimic septic hip, some surgeons drill the neck, but this probably is unnecessary in an infant because spontaneous decompression has already occured if the joint is septic, especially in a child younger than 18 to 24 months of age. A posterior exposure can be used, but the risk of injury to the retinacular vessels is significant, and the dissection should not extend distally on the femoral neck. Spica cast immobilization for 2 to 3 weeks is necessary in unstable septic hips following drainage. Hips drained by the anterior approach often are not unstable, allowing early motion, which is beneficial to articular cartilage.

Late sequelae of septic hip include subluxation, dislocation, ON, joint narrowing, acetabular dysplasia, coxa vara, resorption of the proximal femur, growth arrest (proximal or distal), and degenerative arthritis. Even slight motion usually is clinically preferable to arthrodesis.

Legg-Calvé-Perthes Disease

This disorder is still poorly understood, in etiology and treatment, with controversies about all aspects. Although a metabolic basis for the disorder has been suggested, to date none has been definitely found. There is a tendency toward higher thyroid levels with more epiphyseal involvement, and the levels are not influenced by stage of disease or mode of treatment in longitudinal studies. Some parallels with attention deficit hyperactivity disorder (ADHD) have been described recently. One third of children with Perthes have abnormal psychological profiles in impulsivity and hyperactivity, which are also associated with ADHD. Certain epidemiologic characteristics of Perthes (sex ratio, socioeconomic status, and geographic location) are also similar to those of ADHD, thus suggesting a correlation between the two disorders.

The "standard" in describing magnitude of epiphyseal involvement has been the Catterall classification. The shortcoming of any classification system is that further collapse and deformity may occur with disease progression, necessitating reclassification. The newer lateral pillar classification (Fig. 4) has been used recently, and studies have shown that it is more reliable in both interobserver reliability and in predicting the final outcome.

The treatment of Perthes remains controversial. A general consensus is that for patients younger than 6 years of age, the recommended treatment is alleviation of symptoms by home traction, nonsteroidal anti-inflammatory medications, and decreased activity; there is no definitive evidence that any treatment alters outcome in this group of patients. For children 6 to 8 years of age, the bone age becomes important. For those with a bone age ≤ 6 years and lateral pillar A and B severity (generally, Catterall I and II), the outcome does not appear to be altered by treatment. For those with a bone age of more than 6 years and lateral pillar B involvement, the outcomes appear to be improved by "containment." As of this writing, there is no evidence that any particular containment method (bracing, pelvic or femoral osteotomy) is superior. The effects of treatment are inconclusive for those with lateral pillar C involvement (generally, Catterall III and IV) and a chronological age of 6 to 8 years, regardless of bone age. Most children have lateral pillar B or C involvement when their chronological age is ≥ 9 years. Orthotic management in children of this age is difficult, and surgical management by innominate osteotomy often is the treatment of choice. The overall long-term effect of containment on these few patients is not yet clearly determined, but those with moderate involvement may have good results.

Generally, once reossification has started the potential for further femoral head deformity is minimal, although new information suggests that some hips become progressively flatter after onset of reossification. This phenomenon is more likely to occur in older patients, in those with more severe lateral pillar classification, and in those who have a prolonged reossification phase. Recent studies have suggested improved sphericity and congruency after shelf acetabuloplasty in older children.

Slipped Capital Femoral Epiphysis

The etiology of slipped capital femoral epiphysis (SCFE), although presumed to be idiopathic, may actually be a subtle endocrinopathy. Although screening of all children with SCFE may not be cost effective, the orthopaedist should have a high index of suspicion for hypothyroidism in children younger than 10 to 12 years of age with SCFE. SCFE is bilateral in 20% to 40% of children without endo-

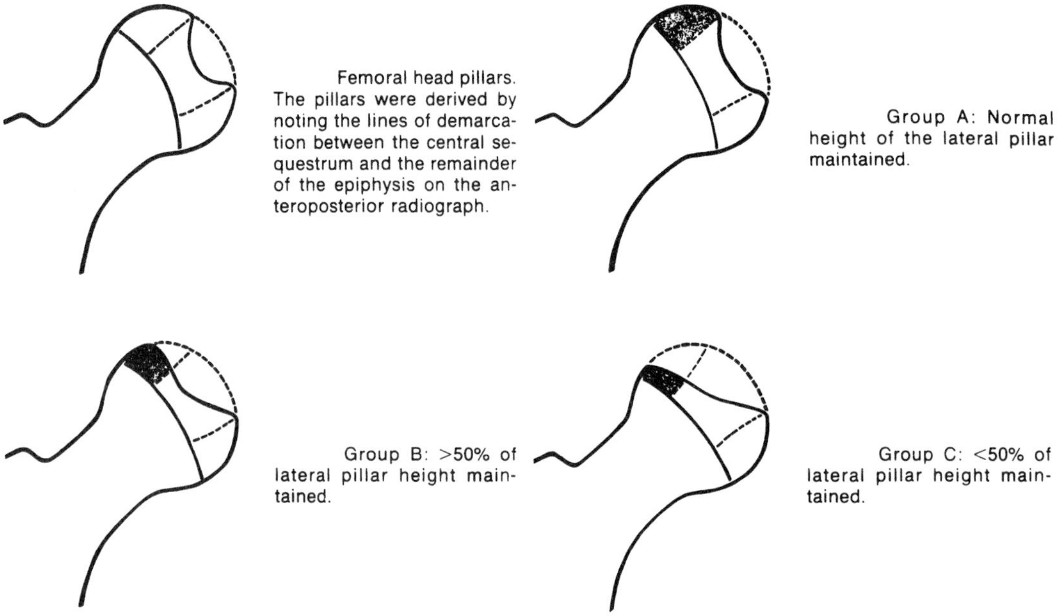

Fig. 4 The lateral pillar classification. (Reproduced with permission from Herring JA, Neustadt JB, Williams JJ, et al: The lateral pillar classification of Legg-Calvé-Perthes' disease. *J Pediatr Orthop* 1992;12:143–150.)

crine disorders, half of whom present with bilateral involvement. The other half develop contralateral SCFE later, usually within the first 18 months after the first SCFE. Frequent follow-up for the first 2 years after the diagnosis of a unilateral SCFE is recommended to prevent a delay in the diagnosis of a second SCFE.

Traditionally, the classification of SCFE has been acute (symptoms < 3 weeks), chronic (symptoms > 3 weeks), and acute/chronic (long-term pain with a recent increase in severity). A new classification system for acute SCFE has been proposed: unstable slips are those in which weightbearing is not possible, with or without crutches, and stable slips are those in which weightbearing is possible, with or without crutches. The unstable slips have a much poorer prognosis, with a very high chance of ON. In a recent study, the timing of internal fixation and the presence or absence of reduction in unstable, acute slips did not seem to have any relation to the development of ON, although this remains controversial. The development of ON, although devastating, often can be treated expectantly. Most children will reach adulthood before needing reconstructive procedures, which often can be delayed for 30 years after the development of ON.

Multiple pinning in situ, the mainstay of treatment for many years, has now mostly been replaced by fixation with a single screw (Fig. 5). This screw is larger than a Steinmann pin, usually 6 to 7 mm in diameter, and it can be inserted through a small skin incision using a triangulation technique (Fig. 6). The ideal placement of the screw is in the center of the epiphysis in both AP and lateral projections. The central single screw minimizes the chance of inadvertent, persistent pin penetration into the joint, thereby decreasing the risk of chondrolysis.

Realignment osteotomy can be done at the level of the femoral neck and physis (cuneiform osteotomy), the base of the neck, or the subtrochanteric level (Southwick osteotomy), but these operations are technically demanding and should be performed only by an experienced pediatric hip surgeon. Cuneiform osteotomy is anatomically the most sound, but carries the highest risk of ON; basilar neck osteotomy is less risky regarding ON; and subtrochanteric osteotomy carries a negligible risk of ON but does have an increased risk of chondrolysis. Because of these risks, osteotomies generally are reserved for moderate to severe cases of SCFE. Two recent reports of osteotomy (one cuneiform, one basilar neck) had excellent results, with the ON occurring only in acute (unstable) SCFEs.

Traumatic Disorders

Pelvic Fractures

Fractures of the pelvis in children are uncommon, and open reduction and internal fixation (ORIF) are rarely indicated. Severe soft-tissue injuries that often occur in conjunction with pelvic fractures may require emergency treatment. Abdominal injuries occur in 1% of patients with isolated pubic fractures, in 15% of those with iliac or sacral fractures, and in 60% of those with multiple frac-

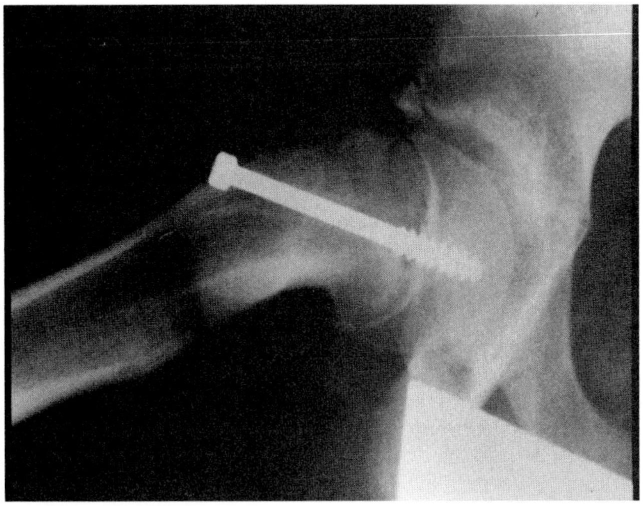

Fig. 5 Stable slipped capital femoral epiphysis after in situ fixation with single cannulated screw.

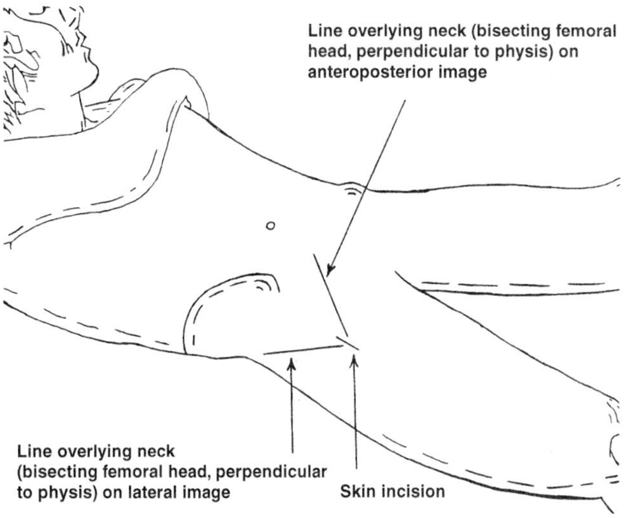

Fig. 6 Diagram of the landmarks used to mark the skin incision for in-situ insertion of a single cannulated screw in the treatment of a slipped capital femoral epiphysis. (Reproduced with permission from Aronson DD, Carlson WE: Slipped capital femoral epiphysis: A prospective study of fixation with a single screw. *J Bone Joint Surg* 1992;74A:810–819.)

tures of the pelvic ring. In children with associated visceral injuries, mortality ranges from 9% to 19%. Volume replacement is essential for hemodynamic stabilization, and the use of an external fixator, selected embolectomy, or ORIF may make this easier.

Because of the remodeling potential in children, long-term results of conservative treatment usually are satisfactory. Despite radiographic evidence of pelvic deformities after conservative treatment, excellent functional results have been noted. Treatment guidelines for pelvic fractures are not the same for children as for adults, and surgery (external or internal fixation) should be used only when conventional methods have been exhausted or in older adolescents approaching skeletal maturity.

Avulsion fractures of the pelvis occur most often in adolescent athletes. Surgical treatment of these fractures is rarely, if ever, indicated. Results appear to be the same after conservative treatment as after ORIF, regardless of the amount of displacement. In some children, displaced ischial avulsion injuries may result in excessive callus, myositis ossificans, and nonunion, but rarely cause impairment.

Acetabular fracture-dislocations in children differ from those in adults because damage to the triradiate cartilage may cause growth arrest and development of a shallow dysplastic acetabulum. Because injury to the triradiate cartilage is easily overlooked on initial radiographs, a CT scan may help to determine the extent of acetabular involvement and femoral head stability.

Salter-Harris type I or II injuries of the triradiate cartilage have favorable prognoses for continued normal acetabular growth. Salter-Harris types IV and V crushing injuries have poor prognoses because of premature closure of the triradiate cartilage resulting from formation of a medial osseous bridge. In young children, especially those under the age of 10 years, abnormal acetabular growth with premature closure of the triradiate cartilage may result in a dysplastic acetabulum that requires surgical treatment.

Hip Fractures

Hip fractures in children differ from those in adults because in children (1) epiphyseal separation may occur, (2) the blood supply of the femoral head is more vulnerable, (3) a higher incidence of ON has been noted, and (4) nondisplaced fractures, if treated with screw fixation across the physis, may result in premature physeal closure. Displaced fractures of the hip in children should be treated by closed reduction, if possible, and internal fixation with cannulated hip screws to avoid coxa vara deformity and nonunion. Internal fixation varies from smooth pins in infants to cannulated screws in adolescents. Spica cast supplementation is necessary in addition to internal fixation for hip fractures in children. Reports suggest that the occurrence of ON is related to the type of fracture and amount of displacement. Data from recent studies confirm that the frequency of ON in children with displaced femoral neck fractures ranges from 47% to 87.5%, depending on the type of fracture.

Hip Dislocations

Minor trauma may cause the hip to dislocate in a young child, and recurrent dislocations can occur because of cartilaginous pliability and ligamentous laxity syndromes. Of-

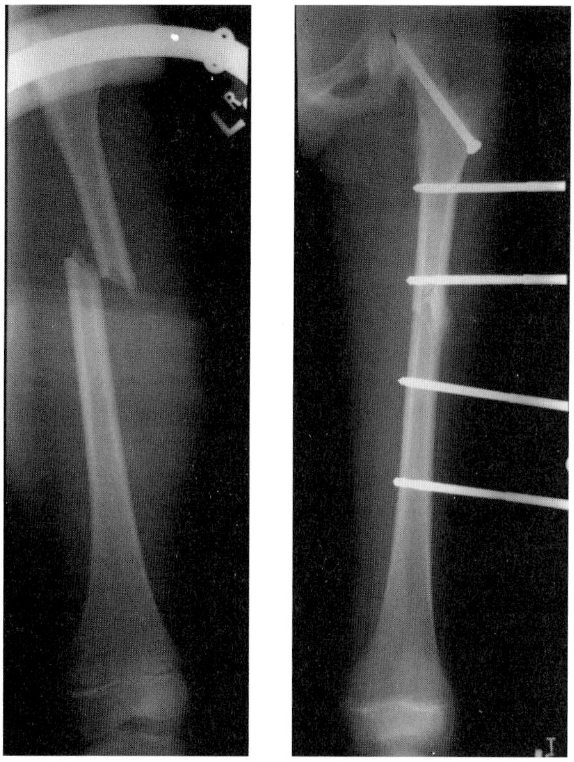

Fig. 7 **Left,** Ipsilateral femoral shaft and neck fractures in a 7-year-old child. **Right,** After external fixation of the femoral shaft fracture and cannulated screw fixation of the femoral neck fracture.

ten a less than concentric reduction is obtained because of interposition of capsular labrum or osseous cartilaginous fragments, and open reduction and removal of the fragment are necessary. Radiographs of both hips should be made after closed reduction to carefully compare the width of the joint spaces. CT may reveal entrapped soft tissues or osseocartilaginous fragments. The ON rate after hip dislocation seems to be the same for children as for adults (8% to 10%).

Femoral Shaft Fractures

Thirty percent of femoral shaft fractures in children younger than 4 years of age are caused by child abuse; 70% are abuse-related in children younger than 1 year of age. Abuse should be suspected if any of the following are present: an unreasonable history, inappropriate delay in coming to the hospital, previous history of abuse, evidence of other fractures in various stages of healing, multiple acute fractures, and characteristic fracture patterns of abuse (epiphyseal corner fractures and twisting spiral fractures).

Recommendations for treatment of femoral fractures vary depending on the age of a child. In children from infancy to 6 to 8 years, immediate spica casting or traction followed by spica casting is recommended. In children between the ages of 6 and 12 years, external fixation or traction, followed by spica casting and occasionally fixation with flexible reamed intramedullary nails is appropriate. In children older than 12 years or in those with polytrauma or head injuries, intramedullary rod fixation can be used.

If immediate spica casting is used, meticulous attention

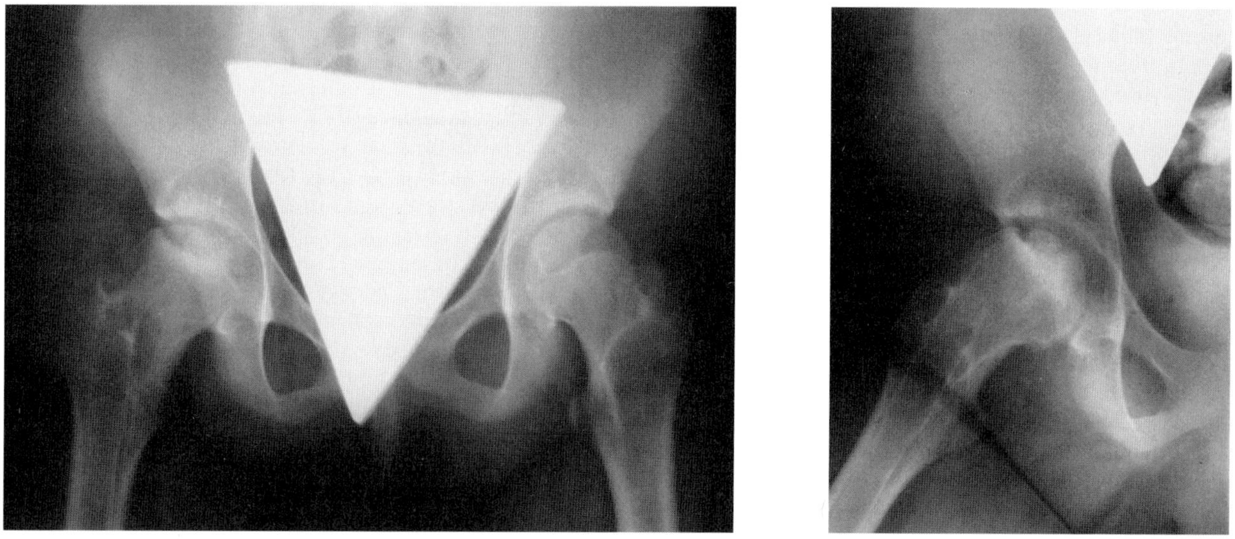

Fig. 8 Segmental avascular necrosis of the femoral head in a 13-year-old girl whose femoral fracture was nailed at 11 years and 6 months of age. (Reproduced with permission from Beaty JH, Austin SM, Warner WC, et al: Interlocking intramedullary nailing of femoral shaft fractures in adolescents: Preliminary results and complications. *J Pediatr Orthop* 1994;14:178–183.)

should be given to control of angulation and shortening. Fractures treated with skeletal traction followed by spica casting generally heal satisfactorily. If alignment and length are maintained, mild rotation usually corrects with growth. External fixators have been used successfully for femoral fractures in children between the ages of 4 and 12 years with polytrauma or head injuries (Fig. 7). The fixators generally are left in place until fracture healing occurs. Flexible Ender rods also have been used to avoid the proximal and distal femoral physes in children between the ages of 6 and 10 years for whom traction was not feasible because of head injury or polytrauma. Few complications have been noted with flexible intramedullary nailing, and a high rate of union has been demonstrated. Recently, ON after locked intramedullary nailing of the femur in adolescents has been reported (Fig. 8). Plate fixation also has been recommended for children with severe head injuries or polytrauma. Because of the possibility of plate failure, supplemental bone graft or spica casting may be used for fractures with medial cortex comminution.

Newton and Mubarak analyzed the financial aspects of femoral shaft treatment in children and adolescents, including both hospital and physician charges (orthopaedists, radiologists, and anesthesiologists). The lowest cost was for the early spica casting ($5,494) and the highest for skeletal traction followed by spica casting and for intramedullary rodding ($21,093 and $21,359, respectively).

Annotated Bibliography

Developmental Dysplasia of the Hip

Ando M, Gotoh E: Significance of inguinal folds for diagnosis of congenital dislocation of the hip in infants aged three to four months. *J Pediatr Orthop* 1990;10:331–334.

In 2,111 infants screened, abnormal inguinal folds were present in all patients with complete dislocation and in some with subluxation. Abnormal inguinal folds are asymmetric or, if symmetric, extend posteriorly beyond the anus.

Atar D, Lehman WB, Tenenbaum Y, et al: Pavlik harness versus Frejka splint in treatment of developmental dysplasia of the hip: Bicenter study. *J Pediatr Orthop* 1993;13:311–313.

Of 84 hips, 90% were successfully treated at one institution with Pavlik harness, with 7% ON rate (mostly type I). At another institution, 88% of 48 hips were successfully treated with a modified Frejka splint with an ON rate of 6% (type I). Guidelines are included.

Faciszewski T, Kiefer GN, Coleman SS: Pemberton osteotomy for residual acetabular dysplasia in children who have congenital dislocation of the hip. *J Bone Joint Surg* 1993;75A:643–649.

Of 52 hips with residual acetabular dysplasia treated by Pemberton osteotomy, 42 developed normal radiographic appearance at an average follow-up of 10 years. ON prior to surgery made results unpredictable.

Fish DN, Herzenberg JE, Hensinger RN: Current practice in use of prereduction traction for congenital dislocation of the hip. *J Pediatr Orthop* 1991;11:149–153.

A survey of members of the Pediatric Orthopaedic Society of North America revealed 95% of respondents used traction at least sometimes for treatment of DDH. Most common use was in children 12 to 18 months old; 28% rarely or never used it for children younger than 6 months; 31% used home traction. Use of preliminary traction is controversial.

Jones GT, Schoenecker PL, Dias LS: Developmental hip dysplasia potentiated by inappropriate use of the Pavlik harness. *J Pediatr Orthop* 1992;12:722–726.

Prolonged use of Pavlik harness (> 8 weeks) without reduction leads to changes that ultimately reduce success of closed reduction. Of 28 hips "overtreated," 17 required open reduction, with dysplasia of posterolateral acetabulum found. Authors recommend no more than 4 weeks harness use unless concentric reduction can be radiographically confirmed.

Kahle WK, Anderson MB, Alpert J, et al: The value of preliminary traction in the treatment of congenital dislocation of the hip. *J Bone Joint Surg* 1990;72A: 1043–1047.

Forty-seven hips were treated by closed or open reduction without the use of preliminary traction and were immobilized with the hip in marked flexion and slight abduction. The ON rate was 4% at 2-year minimum follow-up. Authors do not recommend traction for children younger than 2 years of age.

Mankey MG, Arntz CT, Staheli LT: Open reduction through a medial approach for congenital dislocation of the hip. *J Bone Joint Surg* 1993;75A:1334–1345.

In 66 hips treated by medial approach open reduction, the ON rate was 11%, and 33% had residual acetabular dysplasia requiring surgery. One re-dislocation and two subluxations required remanipulation. The authors believe the procedure is direct, cosmetic, and successful, and is a good alternative for children younger than 2 years of age.

Mubarak SJ, Beck LR, Sutherland D: Home traction in the management of congenital dislocation of the hip. *J Pediatr Orthop* 1986;6:721–723.

The article contains a practical description of the use of home traction and describes an inexpensive traction frame.

Tredwell SJ: Economic evaluation of neonatal screening for congenital dislocation of the hip. *J Pediatr Orthop* 1990;10:327–330.

Formal, routine screening of all infants at large children's hospitals in British Columbia was found to save considerable money in treatment costs. Screening was done (at no charge) by orthopaedic surgeons and a registered nurse.

Tucci JJ, Kumar SJ, Guille JT, et al: Late acetabular dysplasia following early successful Pavlik harness treatment of conjenital dislocation of the hip. *J Pediatr Orthop* 1991;11:502–505.

After Pavlik harness treatment of 74 hips, all were radiographically normal at 5-year follow-up. However, at average follow-up of 12 years, 17% had radiographic acetabular dysplasia (mild), suggesting the need for continued follow-up.

Viere RG, Birch JG, Herring JA, et al: Use of the Pavlik harness in congenital dislocation of the hip: An analysis of failures of treatment. *J Bone Joint Surg* 1990;72A:238–244.

Analysis of reasons for failure of Pavlik harness treatment in 25 patients revealed statistically significant risk factors: absent Ortolani sign, bilaterality, and age > 7 weeks. Of the 30 failures, 17 ultimately required open reduction.

Congenital Coxa Vara

Desai SS, Johnson LO: Long-term results of valgus osteotomy for congenital coxa vara. *Clin Orthop* 1993;294:204–210.

In this review of 20 hips treated by valgus subtrochanteric osteotomy, satisfactory results were obtained when the postoperative head-shaft angle was ≥ 130° and the Hilgenreiner-epiphyseal angle was ≤ 35°.

Weinstein HN, Kuo KN, Millar EA: Congenital coxa vara: A retrospective review. *J Pediatr Orthop* 1984;4:70–77.

This review of 22 patients introduced the concept of the Hilgenreiner-epiphyseal angle. Surgery is indicated when the angle is > 60°, and those < 45° generally correct spontaneously. Angles between 45° and 60° should be observed closely.

Bladder and Cloacal Exstrophy

Greene WB, Dias LS, Lindseth RE, et al: Musculoskeletal problems in association with cloacal exstrophy. *J Bone Joint Surg* 1991;73A:551–560.

In this study of 13 patients with cloacal exstrophy, all had spina bifida and lipomeningocele, with lower extremity paralysis in 11. Spinal deformities (congenital scoliosis and kyphosis, noncongenital scoliosis), foot deformities (calcaneus and equinovarus), and hip dysplasia also were common. A tethered cord was common.

Loder RT, Dayioglu MM: Association of congenital vertebral malformations with bladder and cloacal exstrophy. *J Pediatr Orthop* 1990;10:389–393.

This review of 33 patients with bladder and cloacal exstrophy noted a 33% incidence of congenital vertebral malformations. Entire spinal radiographs are recommended in these patients.

McKenna PH, Khoury AE, McLorie GA, et al: Iliac osteotomy: A model to compare the options in bladder and cloacal exstrophy reconstruction. *J Urol* 1994;151:182–187.

Using both an experimental model and early clinical experience, these authors found that an anterior midiliac diagonal osteotomy provided the best correction of the deformed ilia and resulted in the best pelvic symmetry.

Perovic S, Brdar R, Scepanovic D: Bladder exstrophy and anterior pelvic osteotomy. *Br J Urol* 1992;70:678–682.

These authors used superior pubic ramus osteotomy in 36 children for reconstruction of the pelvic ring during closure of bladder exstrophy. At 3.5 years follow-up, only 8 (22%) had recurrence of pubic diastasis.

Schmidt AH, Keenen TL, Tank ES, et al: Pelvic osteotomy for bladder exstrophy. *J Pediatr Orthop* 1993;13:214–219.

In this series, superior pubic ramomotomy (15 patients) had results equal to posterior iliac osteotomy (10 patients). Posterior iliac osteotomy has a longer time in surgery and requires postoperative immobilization, whereas pubic ramus osteotomy decreases the time in surgery without requiring postoperative immobilization.

Sponseller PD, Gearhart JP, Jeffs RD: Anterior innominate osteotomies for failure or late closure of bladder exstrophy. *J Urol* 1991;146:137–140.

These authors report their experience with 12 older patients undergoing either late closure or secondary reconstructions. They believe that this technique allows for excellent closure of the pubic diastasis.

Proximal Focal Femoral Deficiency

Boden SD, Fallon MD, Davidson R, et al: Proximal femoral focal deficiency: Evidence for a defect in proliferation and maturation of chondrocytes. *J Bone Joint Surg* 1989;71A:1119–1129.

A fetal specimen of mild PFFD was studied, showing altered chondrocyte proliferation.

Pirani S, Beauchamp RD, Li D, et al: Soft tissue anatomy of proximal femoral focal deficiency. *J Pediatr Orthop* 1991;11:563–570.

Magnetic resonance imaging studies show all muscles to be present but small, forming a soft-tissue cuff that stabilizes proximal femur and prevents pistoning.

Steel HH, Lin PS, Betz RR, et al: Iliofemoral fusion for proximal femoral focal deficiency. *J Bone Joint Surg* 1987;69A:837–843.

This procedure, used in unilateral type C or D PFFD, can improve femoropelvic stability in selected patients.

Congenital Short Femur

Grill F, Dungl P: Lengthening for congenital short femur: Results of different methods. *J Bone Joint Surg* 1991;73B:439–447.

Proximal diaphyseal corticotomy in this condition heals less well than in a normal femur.

Renzi-Brivio L, Lavini F, de Bastiani G: Lengthening in the congenital short femur. *Clin Orthop* 1990;250:112–116.

Multiple complications were seen but the end result was usually satisfactory.

Transient Synovitis

Bickerstaff DR, Neal LM, Booth AJ, et al: Ultrasound examination of the irritable hip. *J Bone Joint Surg* 1990; 72B:549–553.

In a study of 111 patients with irritable hip, effusion was present in 71% on sonography but only 15% by radiography. Because early Perthes is managed clinically, authors suggest sonography only rather than radiography in initial evaluation of uncomplicated irritable hip. This study again demonstrates the lack of radiographic criteria for diagnosing effusion of the hip.

Brown I: A study of the "capsular" shadow in disorders the hip in children. *J Bone Joint Surg* 1975;57B:175–179.

The commonly described radiographic finding of capsular swelling was demonstrated to be the product of lateral rotation and abduction. Dissection confirmed the presence of a normal plane of tissue that produces the sign. The finding appears to be an artifact.

Royle SG: Investigation of the irritable hip. *J Pediatr Orthop* 1992;12:396–397.

Radiographs of hips with synovitis have low diagnostic yield, but will detect Perthes disease. Scintigraphy is unlikely to be abnormal if sonogram is normal. Author recommends routine radiograph and sonogram without radionuclide studies.

Terjesen T, Osthus P: Ultrasound in the diagnosis and follow-up of transient synovitis of the hip. *J Pediatr Orthop* 1991;11:608–613.

Because only 2% of patients with clinical acute synovitis ultimately develop Perthes disease, authors suggest diagnosis and follow-up of uncomplicated cases by ultrasound. Anterior ultrasound with a difference of 2.0 mm or more in distance between anterior femoral neck and joint capsule (ACD difference) between sides indicates effusion.

Septic Arthritis

Betz RR, Cooperman DR, Wopperer JM, et al: Late sequelae of septic arthritis of the hip in infancy and childhood. *J Pediatr Orthop* 1990;10:365–372.

Multicenter follow-up and examination revealed few patients with pain or activity restriction, but many with radiographic abnormalities (absent or deformed head, premature fusion of physis, dysplasia or dislocation, unstable segments). Many had abductor lurches and length discrepancy. Older children had stiff hips, many of which were fused. Preservation of even slight motion was better than surgical fusion; reconstructive surgery may worsen long-term result.

Legg-Calvé-Perthes Disease

Herring JA: The treatment of Legg-Calvé-Perthes disease: A critical review of the literature. *J Bone Joint Surg* 1994;76A:448–458.

This thorough and critical review of the literature concludes that children less than 6 years of age need little active treatment. Those who are 6 to 8 years, lateral pillar B, and have a bone age more than 6 years appear to improve with containment treatment. Those ≥ 9 years of age usually need surgical treatment.

Herring JA, Williams JJ, Neustadt JN, et al: Evolution of femoral head deformity during the healing phase of Legg-Calvé-Perthes disease. *J Pediatr Orthop* 1993;13:41–45.

After the onset of reossification, 15 of 136 hips became progressively flatter. Progressive flattening was more likely in older children, those with more severe lateral pillar involvement, and those with prolonged reossification.

Hoffinger SA, Henderson RC, Renner JB, et al: Magnetic resonance evaluation of "metaphyseal" changes in Legg-Calvé-Perthes disease. *J Pediatr Orthop* 1993;13:602–606.

On the basis of MRI studies, metaphyseal changes are mostly physeal and epiphyseal irregularities; metaphyseal changes are much less common than previously thought. These data confirm an earlier cadaver study that showed that epiphyseal changes can appear to be metaphyseal on plain radiographs.

Kruse RW, Guille JT, Bowen JR: Shelf arthroplasty in patients who have Legg-Calvé-Perthes disease: A study of long-term results. *J Bone Joint Surg* 1991;73A:1338–1347.

Shelf arthroplasty at a long-term follow-up of 19 years showed an increased sphericity, center-edge angle, and Iowa hip score compared to those who were managed nonsurgically.

Loder RT, Schwartz EM, Hensinger RN: Behavioral characteristics of children with Legg-Calvé-Perthes disease. *J Pediatr Orthop* 1993;13:598–601.

In 24 children with Perthes, one third had abnormally high psychological profiles associated with attention deficit hyperactivity disorder (ADHD, impulsivity, hyperactivity). Certain epidemiologic characteristics of Perthes and ADHD are also similar.

Neidel J, Boddenberg B, Zander D, et al: Thyroid function in Legg-Calvé-Perthes disease: Cross-sectional and longitudinal study. *J Pediatr Orthop* 1993;13:592–597.

In this series of 59 children with Perthes disease, free T4 and T3 concentrations were increased by 16% and 10%, respectively, supporting the fact that systemic abnormalities exist in Perthes. These hormonal changes were evident at the time of diagnosis of Perthes.

Ritterbusch JF, Shantharam SS, Gelinas C: Comparison of lateral pillar classification and Catterall classification of Legg-Calvé-Perthes disease. *J Pediatr Orthop* 1993;13: 200–202.

In this review of 71 hips, the lateral pillar classification was a better predictor of Stulberg outcome than the Catterall classification. The interobserver reliability of the lateral pillar classification was also better than that of the Catterall classification.

Willett K, Hudson I, Catterall A: Lateral shelf acetabuloplasty: An operation for older children with Perthes' disease. *J Pediatr Orthop* 1992;12:563–568.

Lateral shelf acetabuloplasty was performed in 20 children over 8 years of age. Compared to 14 children who received no treatment, those with the shelf acetabuloplasty had significantly fewer subluxations and an increase in the number of congruent hips.

Slipped Capital Femoral Epiphysis

Abraham E, Garst J, Barmada R: Treatment of moderate to severe slipped capital femoral epiphysis with extracapsular base-of-neck osteotomy. *J Pediatr Orthop* 1993;13:294–302.

In this series of 36 hips with moderate to severe slips, 90% had good or excellent results after basilar neck osteotomy at an average follow-up of 9 years; none had ON.

Aronson DD, Carlson WE: Slipped capital femoral epiphysis: A prospective study of fixation with a single screw. *J Bone Joint Surg* 1992;74A:810–819.

Fifty-four of 58 hips treated with a single central screw had excellent or good results at a 3-year follow-up, further supporting this method of treatment.

Canale ST, Azar F, Young J, et al: Subtrochanteric fracture after fixation of slipped capital femoral epiphysis: A complication of unused drill holes. *J Pediatr Orthop* 1994;14:623–626.

Subtrochanteric fracture of the femur after in situ fixation of SCFE occurred in only 1.4% of patients over a 10-year period. However, the incidence of this complication is likely to rise with increased use of the technique. All four subtrochanteric fractures occurred through unused drill holes, and avoiding extraneous screw holes seems to be the best preventative measure. Once subtrochanteric fracture occurs, immediate open reduction and internal fixation with a compression hip screw device is the recommended treatment.

Fish JB: Cuneiform osteotomy of the femoral neck in the treatment of slipped capital femoral epiphysis: A follow-up note. *J Bone Joint Surg* 1994;76A:46–59.

Sixty-six hips were treated by cuneiform osteotomy for SCFE more than 30°; ON developed in three hips, all of which were acute-on-chronic slips.

Karol LA, Doane RM, Cornicelli SF, et al: Single versus double screw fixation for treatment of slipped capital femoral epiphysis: A biomechanical analysis. *J Pediatr Orthop* 1992;12:741–745.

Using a calf model of an acute slip, there was only a 33% increase in stiffness when two cannulated screws were used instead of one to fix the epiphysis. The stiffness of double or single screw fixation did not approximate that of the intact physis.

Krahn TH, Canale ST, Beaty JH, et al: Long-term follow-up of patients with avascular necrosis after treatment of slipped capital femoral epiphysis. *J Pediatr Orthop* 1993; 13:154–158.

The natural history of children with ON after an SCFE is one of gradual degenerative changes for which reconstructive surgery most often can be delayed until adulthood.

Lindaman LM, Canale ST, Beaty JH, et al: A fluoroscopic technique for determining the incision site for percutaneous fixation of slipped capital femoral epiphysis. *J Pediatr Orthop* 1991;11:397–401.

A fluoroscopic technique, and its geometric basis, used to determine the incision site for percutaneous fixation of SCFE is described.

Loder RT, Aronson DD, Greenfield ML: The epidemiology of bilateral slipped capital femoral epiphysis: A study of children in Michigan. *J Bone Joint Surg* 1993;75A:1141–1147.

The prevalence of bilaterality was 37% in this series; obese children were younger at the time of diagnosis. The presentation was simultaneous in 50%. Of the remaining children who had sequential slips, 88% were diagnosed within 18 months after the first slip. Frequent follow-up is thus recommended for the first 2 years after the diagnosis of a unilateral slip.

Loder RT, Richards BS, Shapiro PS, et al: Acute slipped capital femoral epiphysis: The importance of physeal stability. *J Bone Joint Surg* 1993;75A:1134–1140.

Fifty-five hips with an acute slip (less than 3 weeks of symptoms) were classified as stable (able to bear weight with or without crutches) or unstable (unable to bear weight, even with crutches). Satisfactory results were seen in 96% of the stable and 47% of the unstable hips; the poor results were largely due to the development of ON.

Meier MC, Meyer LC, Ferguson RL: Treatment of slipped capital femoral epiphysis with a spica cast. *J Bone Joint Surg* 1992;74A:1522–1529.

Three months of spica cast immobilization had an 83% complication rate. The complications were pressure sores, slip progression, and chondrolysis (53% incidence of chondrolysis). This high complication rate has led these authors to abandon this method of treatment.

Ward WT, Stefko J, Wood KB, et al: Fixation with a single screw for slipped capital femoral epiphysis. *J Bone Joint Surg* 1992;74A:799–809.

In 29 slips, a single central screw provided adequate fixation and promoted premature physeal closure without any chondrolysis or ON.

Wells D, King JD, Roe TF, et al: Review of slipped capital femoral epiphysis associated with endocrine disease. *J Pediatr Orthop* 1993;13:610–614.

Because hypothyroidism can be easily missed, these authors recommend screening all children with SCFE. Any child with an endocrine deficiency and unilateral SCFE should have the other hip prophylactically stabilized.

Pelvic and Hip Fractures in Children

Bond SJ, Gotschall CS, Eichelberger MR: Predictors of abdominal injury in children with pelvic fracture. *J Trauma* 1991;31:1169–1173.

Location of pelvic fractures in children was strongly associated with the probability of abdominal injury: 80% with multiple pelvic fractures had concomitant abdominal or genitourinary injury compared with 33% with fracture of the ilium or pelvic ring and 6% with isolated pubic rami fractures. The probability of abdominal injury given physiologic stability was less than 1% for isolated pubic fractures, 15% for iliac or sacral fractures, and 60% for multiple fractures of the pelvic ring.

Bucholz RW, Ezaki M, Ogden JA: Injury to the acetabular triradiate physeal cartilage. *J Bone Joint Surg* 1982;64A: 600–609.

Injury to the triradiate cartilage in nine patients was described. Salter-Harris type I or II injuries had favorable prognoses for continued normal acetabular growth. Salter-Harris type IV crush injuries had poor prognoses with premature closure of the triradiate physis secondary to formation of a medial osseous bridge. This was especially true in younger children who developed a shallow acetabulum.

Davison BL, Weinstein SL: Hip fractures in children: A long-term follow-up study. *J Pediatr Orthop* 1992;12: 355–358.

Nine (47%) of 19 children with hip fractures developed ON; seven required surgical treatment.

Forlin E, Guille JT, Kumar SJ, et al: Transepiphyseal fractures of the neck of the femur in very young children. *J Pediatr Orthop* 1992;12:164–168.

Five very young patients (8 to 26 months of age) were treated with closed reduction of transepiphyseal fractures. Four healed with deformities, but in two the varus deformity corrected with growth. The authors recommend spica casting without reduction in young children, with later correction of coxa vara by osteotomy if necessary.

Hughes LO, Beaty JH: Current concepts review: Fractures of the head and neck of the femur in children. *J Bone Joint Surg* 1994;76A:283–292.

Anatomy, classification, treatment guidelines, decision-making, and complications are discussed.

Nierenberg G, Volpin G, Bialik V, et al: Pelvic fractures in children: A follow-up in 20 children treated conservatively. *J Pediatr Orthop* 1993;1:140.

Twenty children treated mainly with skin traction and bed rest had excellent or good functional results, despite radiographic evidence of pelvic deformity. Guidelines for treating children with pelvic fractures differ from those for adults, and internal or external fixation should be used only as a last resort when conventional means have been exhausted.

Sundar M, Carty H: Avulsion fractures of the pelvis in children: A report of 32 fractures and their outcome. *Skel Radiol* 1994;23:85–90.

Avulsion injuries of the apopohysis of the pelvis are generally regarded as trivial injuries, but may result in disabilities that persist into adult life. Of 32 patients, ten reported limited sporting abilities and six had persistent symptoms, most often those with ischial avulsion injuries.

Femoral Shaft Fractures

Aronson J, Tursky EA: External fixation of femur fractures in children. *J Pediatr Orthop* 1992;12:157–163.

Forty-four femoral fractures were treated with external fixators, which were left in place for an average of 70 days. Femoral overgrowth averaged 5.8 mm. The authors recommended external fixation as an alternative to casting for the treatment of isolated femoral fractures in children aged 4 to 12 years.

Beaty JH, Austin SM, Warner WC, et al: Interlocking intramedullary nailing of femoral-shaft fractures in adolescents: Preliminary results and complications. *J Pediatr Orthop* 1994;14:178–183.

Of 31 adolescents (10 to 15 years of age) in whom locked intramedullary nails were used for fixation of femoral shaft fractures, one developed ON. All fractures united. Locked intramedullary nailing seems to be a reasonable alternative for femoral shaft fractures in older adolescents and in younger patients with polytrauma.

Evanoff M, Strong ML, MacIntosh R: External fixation maintained until fracture consolidation in the skeletally immature. *J Pediatr Orthop* 1993;13:98–101.

Twenty-five femoral fractures in skeletally immature patients were treated with external fixation. All fractures consolidated with fixators in place and most patients regained preoperative joint motion. Eighty-four percent of the fractures lost no position in the fixator. The authors recommend external fixation for all femoral fractures in children between the ages of 3 and 13 years.

Hansen TB: Fractures of the femoral shaft in children treated with an AO-compression plate: Report of 12 cases followed until adulthood. *Acta Orthop Scand* 1992;63:50–52.

AO compression plates were used for fixation of 13 femoral shaft fractures in 12 children. All fractures healed without angulation or rotation with a mean overgrowth of 7 mm. All patients had unrestricted motion of the hip and knee.

Heinrich SD, Drvaric DM, Darr K, et al: The operative stabilization of pediatric diaphyseal femur fractures with flexible intramedullary nails: A prospective analysis. *J Pediatr Orthop* 1994;14:501–507.

Flexible intramedullary nails were used in 77 patients, 68% of whom had equal leg lengths and 8% of whom had minimal rotational malalignment of 8°. The authors recommend flexible intramedullary rods for selected pediatric diaphyseal fractures in patients 6 to 10 years of age with polytrauma or head injury.

Kasser JR: Femur fractures in children, in Eilert RE (ed): *Instructional Course Lectures XLI.* Park Ridge, IL, American Academy of Orthopaedic Surgeons, 1992, pp 403–408.

In children younger than 4 years of age, 30% of femoral fractures are caused by child abuse, and in children younger than 1 year of age, 70% of femoral fractures are abuse-related. Abuse should be suspected if (1) there is an unreasonable history or delay in coming to the hospital, (2) there is a previous history of abuse or fractures in various stages of healing, and (3) multiple acute fractures or characteristic fracture patterns of abuse are apparent.

Newton PO, Mubarak SJ: Financial aspects of femoral shaft fracture treatment in children and adolescents. *J Pediatr Orthop* 1994;14:508–512.

Analysis of the financial aspects of femoral shaft fracture treatment, including hospital and physician charges, revealed that the lowest cost was for the early spica casting ($5,494) and the highest for skeletal traction and intramedullary rodding ($21,093 and $21,359, respectively).

Probe R, Lindsey RW, Hadley NA, et al: Refracture of adolescent femoral shaft fractures: A complication of external fixation. A report of two cases. *J Pediatr Orthop* 1993;13:102–105.

Refractures occurred after frame removal in two adolescent patients treated with external fixation. The authors believe that refracture is a clinical expression of the detrimental effects of prolonged rigidity imposed by the external fixator.

Strong ML, Wong-Chung J, Babikian G, et al: Rotational remodeling of malrotated femoral fractures: A model in the rabbit. *J Pediatr Orthop* 1992;12:173–176.

Mid-shaft femoral osteotomies were performed on 16 rabbits, the limbs were internally rotated, and external fixators were applied and left in place until the osteotomies healed. An average of 55% of rotational remodeling occurred spontaneously. This study supports the clinical experience that few patients with mildly malrotated fractures of long bones have complaints as adults.

Wallace ME, Hoffman EB: Remodelling of angular deformity after femoral shaft fractures in children. *J Bone Joint Surg* 1992;74B:765–769.

Twenty-eight children with unilateral middle third femoral fractures had angular deformities ranging from 10° to 26°. The average correction was 85% of the initial deformity; 74% occurred at the physis and 26% at the fracture site.

Ward WT, Levy J, Kaye A: Compression plating for child and adolescent femur fractures. *J Pediatr Orthop* 1992; 12:626–632.

AO compression plate fixation was used for femoral fractures in children and adolescents. All fractures healed without angulation or rotation. The authors noted, however, that stress fracture may occur through the screw holes during the first few months after plate removal.

Classic Bibliography

Gabuzda GM, Renshaw TS: Current concepts review: Reduction of congenital dislocation of the hip. *J Bone Joint Surg* 1992;74A:624–631.

Harcke HT, Kumar SJ: Current concepts review: The role of ultrasound in the diagnosis and management of congenital dislocation and dysplasia of the hip. *J Bone Joint Surg* 1991;73A:622–628.

34

Pelvis and Acetabulum: Trauma

Pelvic Fractures

Pelvic fractures continue to challenge the orthopaedic surgeon. In most cases, these fractures result from low-energy injuries and are managed conservatively. However, unstable pelvic ring disruptions caused by severe trauma may result in life-threatening hemorrhage, sepsis syndrome, and long-term problems with pain and disability (Fig. 1).

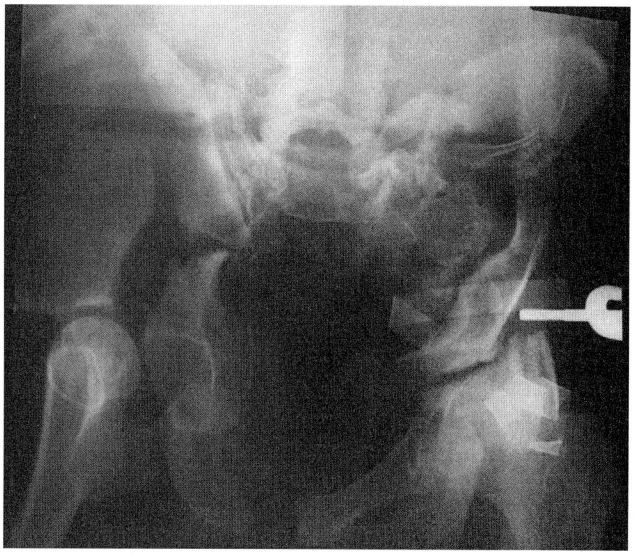

Fig. 1 This patient was crushed by a concrete wall. His severe pelvic ring disruption produced uncontrollable torential hemorrhage. Note the sacral displacement.

Evaluation of Injury

The patient with an unstable pelvic ring disruption, who is awake and communicative, complains of severe pelvic pain. Patients with genitourinary tract disruptions may complain of the inability to urinate. The physical examination proceeds simultaneously with resuscitation and treatment, especially in instances of hemodynamic instability. Observation of the pelvic soft-tissue envelope identifies lacerations and closed degloving injuries. Anterior pelvic and perineal open wounds are identified and covered with sterile compressive dressings. In male patients, the scrotal contents are palpated to rule out testicular displacements, and the penile urethral meatus is inspected for blood. Absence of blood at the meatus does not rule out urethral injury, especially if the patient is evaluated within 1 hour of the traumatic event. Female patients are examined bimanually, and the external genitalia are inspected for lacerations. Traumatic lacerations may involve the urethra, vagina, and bladder in these patients. Vaginal speculum evaluations are difficult but necessary, and are best performed in the operating room with the patient under general anesthesia. The lithotomy position is not used in order to avoid further pelvic displacements and potential clot disruption. Vaginal bleeding may be due to menstruation, laceration, or both. Vaginal lacerations are thoroughly debrided and managed open.

The mechanical integrity of the pelvis is often difficult to assess manually. A single manual pelvic stress evaluation performed using fluoroscopy by an experienced member of the resuscitation team is preferable. Repetitive stressing of the unstable pelvic ring may disrupt clots, thereby increasing bony bleeding. A rectal examination reveals prostatic displacements, mucosal abnormalities, and the presence of bleeding. Evaluation of the posterior pelvis is performed using spine "log-rolling" techniques. Inspection for lacerations and hematoma formation, as well as palpation, is important in these patients. Small posterior lacerations may be missed, especially in the gluteal folds, unless a careful examination is performed.

In responsive patients, lower extremity and perineal neurologic examinations are carefully detailed. All neurologic abnormalities are noted prior to reduction maneuvers. Repeat neurologic assessments are performed after manipulations, including the application of traction. Excessive traction may cause (or worsen) ipsilateral lower extremity neurologic dysfunction. Peripheral pulses are also carefully assessed.

Radiographic examinations of the unstable pelvic fracture begin with a good quality screening anteroposterior (AP) plain radiograph. Obvious fractures and asymmetries are identified. The stability of pelvic fractures is determined by many factors other than the pattern of bony injury and the associated soft-tissue injury. The displacement that occurs at the time of injury may be far greater than might be expected from the admission radiograph.

In patients with pelvic ring disruptions, pelvic inlet and outlet images are obtained after the AP radiograph. The pelvic inlet radiograph demonstrates AP deformities, especially symphysis pubis disruptions and sacroiliac joint dislocations. Posterior or anterior translation of the injured hemipelvis is best seen on the inlet view. The pelvic outlet image identifies flexion deformities and cephalad migration of the injured hemipelvis. Discrepancies between the iliac crests and ischial tuberosities on each side alert the physician to injuries. Cephalad displacements of the hemipelvis are seen as iliac and ischial height differences. Hemipelvic flexion deformities are noted when the iliac heights coincide, yet the ischial tuberosities are at different levels (Fig. 2).

True lateral sacral plain radiographs identify displaced transverse sacral fractures and demonstrate the sacral alar slope. Fractures involving the greater sciatic notch are visible on the true lateral sacral image. Judet oblique radiographs are obtained in those patients with acetabular fractures as a part of the pelvic disruption. These oblique images are also useful when displaced iliac fractures are present (Fig. 3).

Special radiographic evaluations of the genitourinary tract are obtained in those patients with hematuria, urethral meatal blood, difficulty or the inability to urinate, and/or the inability to easily insert a urinary catheter. These tests are performed by the consultant urologist and radiologist and include the (pericatheter) retrograde urethrogram and cystogram.

Pelvic computed tomography (CT) is used to gain further information about the pelvic ring disruption. These pelvic CT scans can be obtained in conjunction with an abdominal scan. Five-millimeter contiguous slices using a large field of view and bone reformation algorithms are advocated. In patients with complex and displaced sacral fractures, a direct coronal CT scan is also obtained by orienting the CT gantry parallel to the upper sacral segment. Routine pelvic CT scanning often identifies occult posterior pelvic ring injuries. For example, an air density within the sacroiliac joint on CT scan may represent a nondisplaced injury to the sacroiliac joint. Other, more severe, displacements are better identified on the CT scan (Fig. 4).

Classification

Numerous classification schemes exist for pelvic ring disruptions. An ideal system would describe the injured anatomic zone and the displacement (deformity) patterns, guide treatment, and predict outcomes. No such ideal system for pelvic classification exists for several reasons. These injuries are unusual outside of the trauma-center setting, making any scheme difficult to recall accurately, and combination injuries frustrate any classification scheme. Also, associated injuries other than those to the pelvis alone have significant impact on patient outcomes. Most physicians use the Tile classification, which is based on simplistic load applications and resultant deformities (Table 1).

Treatment

Resuscitation/Hemorrhage Effective resuscitation starts immediately. Airway management is imperative. Definitive resuscitation is based on simultaneous evaluation and treatment by a team of physicians who specialize in resuscitation. Hypovolemia is addressed immediately. Major

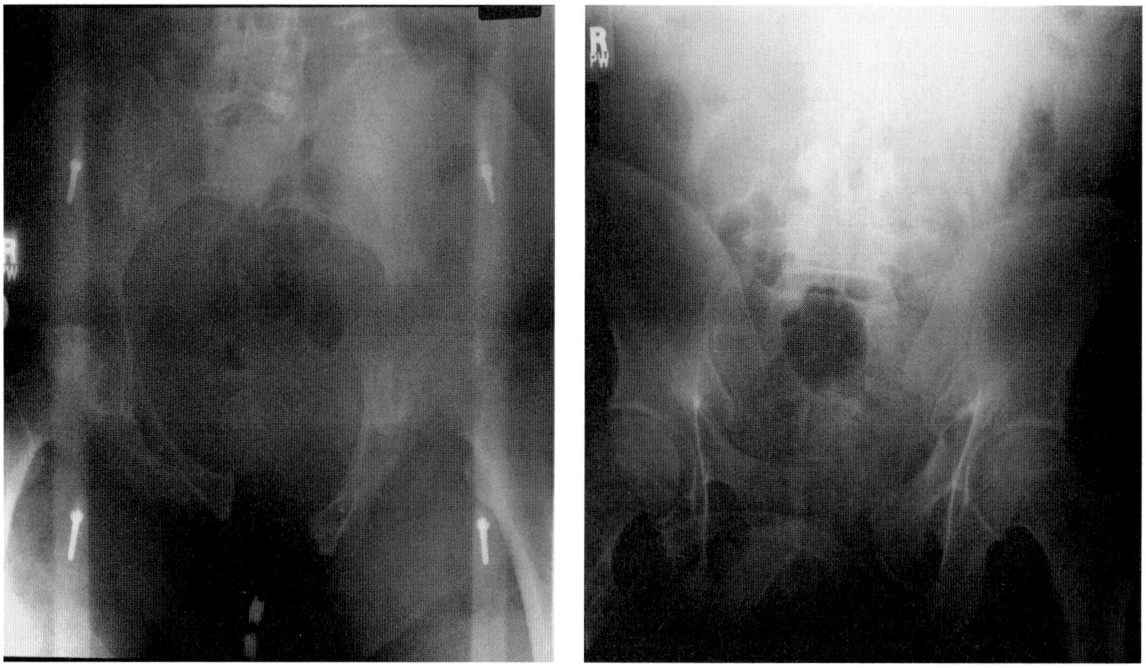

Fig. 2 Left, The pelvic inlet image identifies anterior and posterior pelvic distraction/compression deformities, as well as anterior/posterior displacements of the injured hemipelvis. **Right,** The pelvic outlet radiograph demonstrates cephalad/caudad displacements (vertical shear) of the injured hemipelvis. The upper sacral foramina are best seen on the outlet image. Hemipelvic rotation (flexion/extension) is identified on the outlet radiograph when the iliac crests are level and the ischial tuberosities are not.

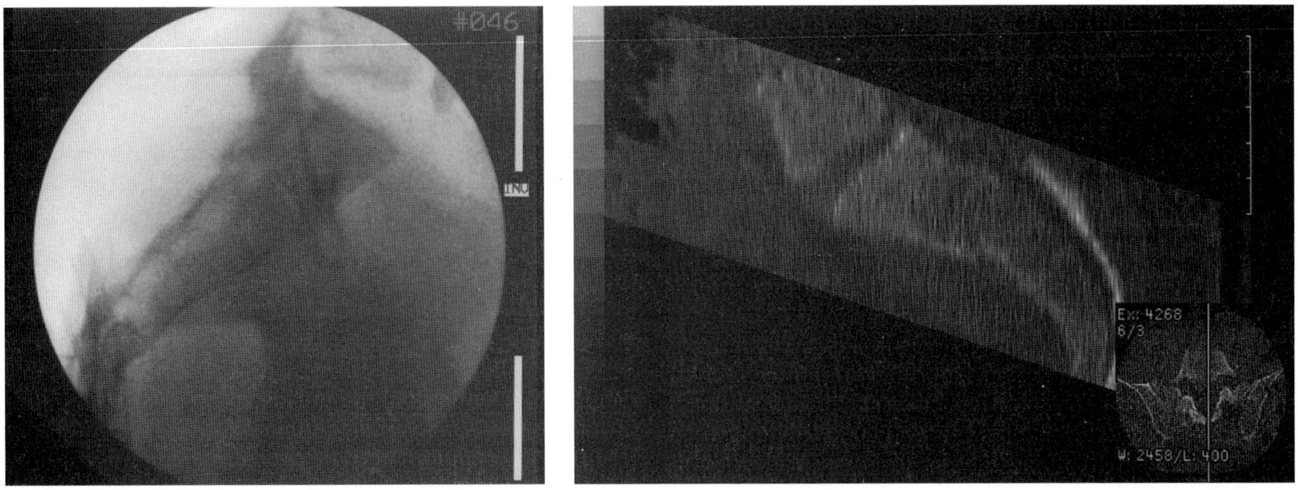

Fig. 3 **Left,** The true sacral lateral radiograph identifies the sacral alar slope indirectly. **Right,** Sagittal CT reconstruction of the sacrum demonstrates horizontal (transverse) sacral fractures. Judet oblique images are needed to classify acetabular fractures. The iliac oblique view is helpful to demonstrate iliac fractures and their displacement patterns.

blood volume losses occur in five areas: (1) intrathoracic, (2) intraperitoneal, (3) retroperitoneal, (4) external, and/or (5) intravascular (coagulopathy). External sources are usually obvious and controllable with direct pressure. The other four are not so obvious and are evaluated using mini-laparotomy, plain radiographs, CT scans, and coagulation screening tests. Volume replacement is instituted using warmed fluids through large vascular catheters. The patient is kept warm using heat lamps and by avoiding repetitive and prolonged exposures.

Hemorrhage should be viewed as a preventable cause of death. Bleeding in pelvic fractures occurs from exposed bone fracture surfaces, venous plexus disruptions, and arterial sources. Because of the spherical configuration of the pelvis, pelvic volume increases in proportion to the fourth power of its radius. The retroperitoneal space can accommodate up to 4 liters of blood before tamponade occurs. Fractures with posterior instability may have a blood product requirement three times higher than those without instability.

The patient at highest risk is one who has a posterior pelvic disruption with a major thoracic, abdominal, or head injury. These multiple injuries can be associated with up to 50% mortality, which increases directly with age. A direct correlation between injury severity scale rating and mortality rate has also been demonstrated.

External Treatment In situations of hemodynamic instability at the accident scene, all potential bleeding sources are addressed. Several techniques are available to temporarily stabilize the pelvis. Military antishock trousers (MAST) are pneumatic counterpressure suits and have been advocated as a prehospital stabilization option in a civilian setting since 1973. Some of the problems encountered with MAST have included (1) inability to perform groin cutdowns for vascular access; (2) difficulty performing abdominal, rectal, and pelvic examinations; (3) difficulty in evaluating complex groin wounds; (4) resultant compartmental syndromes of the lower extremities; (5) restricted ventilation; (6) accelerated lactic acidosis; (7) potential irreversible cardiac collapse if the MAST are rapidly deflated; (8) prolonged prehospital transport for application of MAST; and (9) potential diaphragmatic herniation of abdominal organs into the thorax. Other simpler external devices used to control the pelvic volume temporarily include vacuum beanbags and sheets lashed circumferentially about the pelvis.

Percutaneous Fixation The current management of pelvic fractures is aimed at immediate stabilization to control hemorrhage with delayed definitive fixation to prevent malunion. Ideally, these two treatment strategies occur simultaneously. Early surgical stabilization of the disrupted pelvic ring improves patient care. Urgent restoration of the stable spherical pelvic anatomy provides a tamponade effect, thereby decreasing hemorrhage. Transfusion requirements are reduced as is the duration of shock. Pelvic stability allows the patient to be upright and mobile. Pulmonary care is facilitated, the need for narcotic analgesic medications is diminished, and nursing care is facilitated.

Pelvic stability can be achieved using temporary external devices or with definitive internal fixation. External fixation frames are advocated as resuscitation aids to provide rapid pelvic stability. These frames serve a temporary function in limiting further pelvic expansion, thereby decreasing hemorrhage, and in facilitating patient transport to centers familiar with severe pelvic ring trauma for definitive care. Even large, complex pelvic external fixation

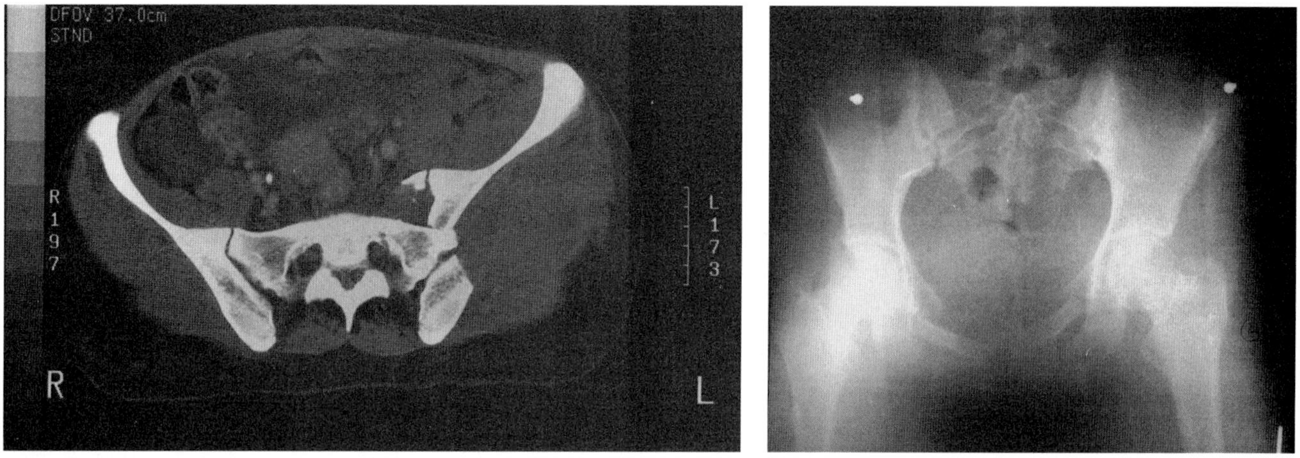

Fig. 4 This patient has a severely displaced fracture-dislocation of the left SI joint. The pelvic CT scan **(left)** readily identifies this injury which is poorly seen on the AP pelvis radiograph **(right).**

Table 1. Classification of pelvic fractures

Classification	Description
Type A	Stable
A_1	Avulsion, ring spared
A_2	Nondisplaced, involving ring
A_3	Transverse sacral/coccygeal, ring spared
Type B	Rotationally unstable
B_1 Stage 1	Open book distraction injury anteriorly (symphysis pubis or rami) with no posterior injury
Stage 2	Same as Stage 1 with unilateral, incomplete posterior disruption
Stage 3	Same as Stage 1 with bilateral, incomplete posterior disruptions
B_2	Lateral compression injury to the ipsilateral anterior and posterior hemipelvis
B_3	Lateral compression injury with bilateral anterior pelvic ring injuries and unilateral posterior disruption
Type C	Rotationally and vertically unstable
C_1	Complete hemipelvic instability due to anterior and unilateral posterior pelvis disruptions
C_2	Same as C_1 but with bilateral posterior complete instabilities
C_3	Any pelvic ring fracture/dislocation with an associated acetabular fracture

frames are mechanically inferior to most internal fixation devices. Complex frames may not permit active transfer from bed to chair and may restrict independent partial weightbearing unless supplementary posterior fixation is used. Combination anterior–posterior frame constructs using through and through pins have been described for use in special cases. Complications involved with the use of pelvic external fixation for definitive care include loss of reduction, with resultant pain and deformity, and pin-track infections.

Pin placement into the ilium is difficult, especially in obese patients or in those with significantly displaced fractures. The surgeon anticipates the amount of deformity so the skin stab incisions for pin insertion will not be extensive. The pelvic outlet image using the C-arm fluoroscopy unit guides accurate pin placement between the tables of the ilium at the gluteus medius pillar expansion. Large incisions for pin placement may complicate subsequent surgical procedures, especially if open treatment is delayed to the point of wound colonization or infection. Simple uniplanar resuscitation frame constructs are advocated. The connecting bars are positioned to allow hip flexion of at least 90° so the patient can sit. When properly positioned, these low-profile frame constructs do not obstruct abdominal and genitourinary access. Early supplementation with or conversion of these simple frames to definitive internal fixation is advocated.

Standard anterior external fixation frames poorly control the posterior pelvis. The pelvic resuscitation clamp was recently introduced to rapidly stabilize posterior pelvic ring disruptions. Pins attached to this C-shaped clamp are inserted percutaneously into the posterior ilium. The clamp is advocated as a temporary resuscitation device to diminish the pelvic volume and improve posterior pelvic stability. Early clinical results are promising when the pins are accurately inserted. Pin placement is facilitated by fluoroscopic imaging. Overcompression is avoided in transforaminal sacral fractures (Fig. 5).

Percutaneous fixation techniques in which iliosacral screws are used after closed reductions of the posterior pelvis have also proven beneficial by providing stability while lowering infection and blood loss rates. Insertion of these screws is possible due to the improved quality of intraoperative fluoroscopic imaging. Accurate visualization of the posterior pelvis aids implant placement.

Open Fixation Open reduction and internal fixation (ORIF) of the displaced pelvic disruption has become

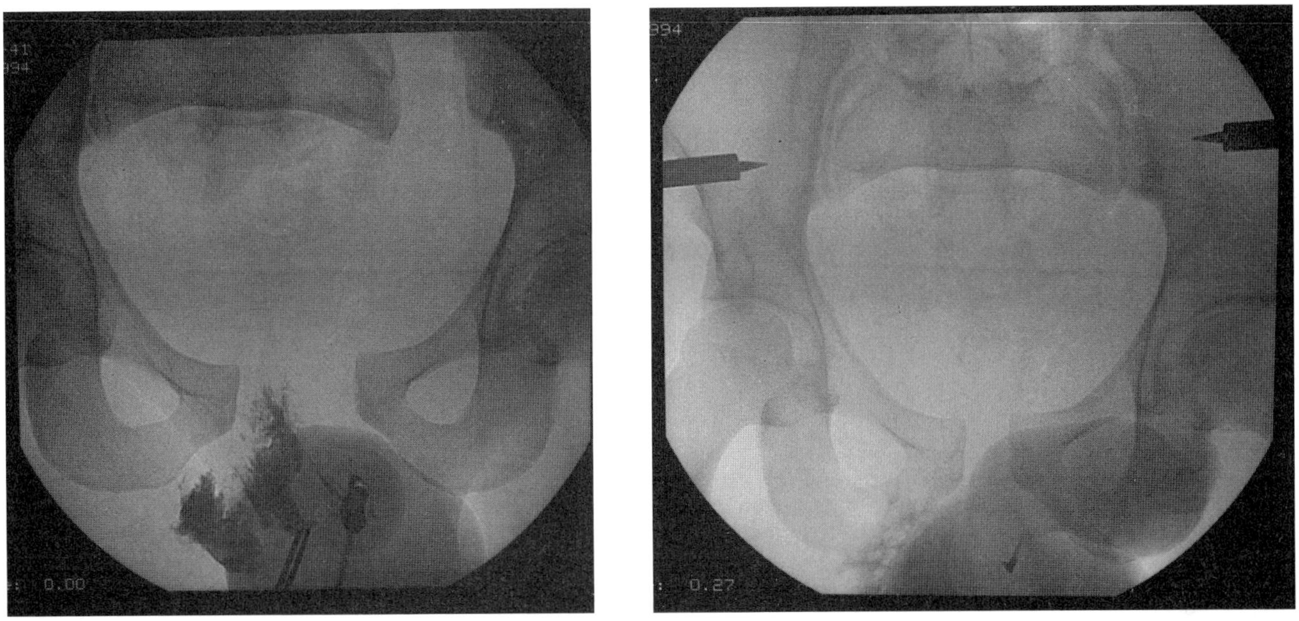

Fig. 5 The antishock clamp provides posterior pelvic stability for certain injuries. This hemodynamically unstable patient was crushed sustaining a complete symphysis pubis dislocation and left sided sacroiliac joint dislocation **(left).** The antishock clamp was applied in the angiography suite using fluoroscopic imaging. The reduction is noted **(right).**

more accepted as clinical experience and certain technologies have improved. The superiority of internal over external pelvic fixation is supported by several recent biomechanical evaluations. In one study, it was demonstrated that internal fixation of each disruption within the ring improves the overall pelvic stability. This information indicates that all components of the unstable pelvic ring injury should be stabilized whenever possible in order to improve stability.

ORIF of the anterior pelvis may be possible acutely as a part of the resuscitation efforts, especially when an exploratory laparotomy is performed. Symphysis pubis dislocations are reduced and plated either using the inferior extension of the midline laparotomy wound or through a separate Pfannenstiel incision. When possible, the pelvic reduction and fixation are performed before the laparotomy to diminish potential bleeding. The Pfannenstiel incision is also preferred in those patients with bladder and/or urethral disruptions, especially when primary genitourinary repairs are performed.

Controversy still exists over the ideal anterior pelvic implant, especially in patients with significant posterior pelvic instabilities that further stress the anterior fixations. Simple two-hole plates maintain some of the symphyseal inherent mobility. Pelvic reconstruction plates are also recommended by some authors. Two plates oriented at right angles to each other have been shown to be biomechanically more rigid than a single plate, but they require more extensive soft-tissue stripping and have increased potential for blood loss.

Although isolated pubic ramus fractures are usually treated conservatively, in those patients with instability, internal fixation is accomplished using either plates or medullary screws. Unstable pubic ramus fractures that are lateral to the iliopectineal eminence usually require an ilioinguinal exposure for reduction and plate fixation. Alternatively, a medullary screw can be used to stabilize superior pubic ramus fractures in certain patients. The ilioinguinal exposure is avoided in such cases. The use of retrograde medullary ramus screws is biomechanically equivalent to standard plating techniques.

Acetabular fractures may be noticed in association with pelvic ring disruptions. Pelvic stability is given first priority in patients with hemodynamic instability. The acetabular fracture may complicate resuscitative fixation, especially if the iliac crest is destabilized as a part of the acetabular fracture. In these cases, routine pelvic external fixation frames are not possible, and alternative strategies are used. In stable patients, the acetabular fracture is prioritized. After the acetabular fracture is anatomically reduced and fixed, the pelvic ring instabilities are stabilized. Reduction of the acetabular fracture may be complicated by displaced fractures or dislocations of the pelvic ring; therefore, these injuries may require simultaneous attention (Fig. 6).

Because of the subcutaneous location of the ilium, certain fractures may be associated with open skin wounds or severe local contusions. Iliac fractures displaced through the greater sciatic notch may injure the gluteal neurovascular complex and produce hemodynamic instability. Preoperative angiographic embolization is indicated in such

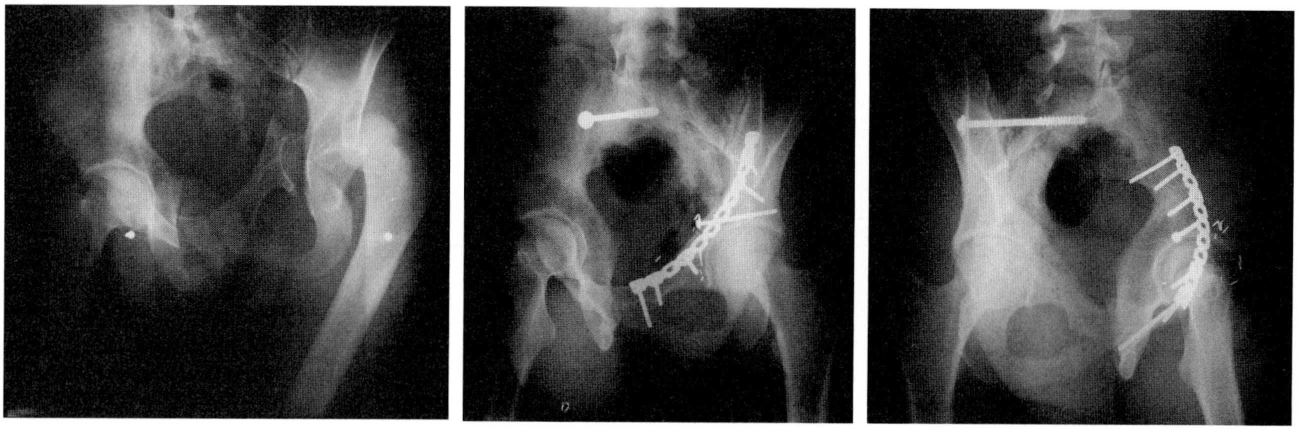

Fig. 6 Left, This patient sustained a left posterior hip dislocation and anterior column acetabular fracture. Right-sided pubic rami fractures and an anterior sacroiliac joint dislocation were also present. The hip dislocation was reduced closed in the emergency ward using intravenous sedation. **Center,** On the day following the accident, the acetabulum was reduced and stabilized using an ilioinguinal exposure. **Right,** The SI joint was reduced using an anterior pelvic compressor (femoral distractor) and stabilized with a percutaneously inserted iliosacral lag screw.

cases. Most iliac fractures occur in association with anterior pelvic fractures or dislocations. External fixation is not advocated for iliac fractures. Open reduction is performed using an intrapelvic iliac exposure or the open wound. Reduction of the iliac fracture is facilitated by simultaneous reduction of the anterior pelvic injury. Stable fixation is provided using lag screws between the iliac tables, supplemented with plate fixation. Fixation of the associated anterior pelvic injury improves overall stability (Fig. 7).

Disruptions of the sacroiliac joint occur in stages. There can be pure ligamentous injuries or fracture-dislocations. Complete ligamentous sacroiliac dislocations occur when all of the constraining tissues are interrupted at the time of injury. Associated lumbosacral plexopathies of variable severity are not uncommon in these complete dislocations, and local vascular structures may also be affected. These neural and vascular injuries can be caused by stretch or laceration. Incomplete sacroiliac joint dislocations usually result from a less violent transfer of energy and imply an anterior disruption only. Associated neural and vascular injuries are consequently less frequent. The sacroiliac joint disruptions can also be combination injuries, involving both fracture and dislocation. The sacrum cannot be ignored in instances of sacroiliac disruptions, because combination injuries of the posterior pelvic ring are common, especially with high-energy loading. In other cases, in which the sacroiliac joint ligaments yield while the interosseus ligaments remain intact and tether the posterior ilium, an avulsion fracture of the posterior ilium known as a "crescent" fracture is produced. These injuries reflect posterior pelvic ring instability that is similar to a complete sacroiliac joint dislocation. Conversely, sacral alar impaction fractures from lateral pelvic compression loads may mimic a sacroiliac joint dislocation radiographically, although the ligaments remain intact.

Complete sacroiliac joint dislocations are best treated with ORIF. Both anterior and posterior exposures have been advocated. The anterior iliac exposure provides direct visualization of the articular surfaces of the sacroiliac joint. Both plate fixation and iliosacral lag screw fixation have been recommended. The fifth lumbar nerve root may be injured by excessive medical retraction along the sacral ala. The lateral femoral cutaneous nerve may also be injured in this exposure. Posterior surgical approaches to the sacroiliac joint are associated with higher infection rates. The joint surfaces may also be difficult to visualize. The treatment of incomplete sacroiliac joint disruptions is controversial. Most authors advocate closed management.

Displaced sacral fractures usually occur through the neural foramina. Bone debris may impinge on the sacral nerve roots and produce neurologic abnormalities. Open reduction of sacral fractures is accomplished using a posterior exposure. The nerve roots are decompressed. Accurate open reduction and stable internal fixation are difficult to achieve, but when accomplished should protect the neural structures and allows healing. Various implants, including transiliac sacral bars, tension band plates, iliosacral screws, and combinations, are advocated. Direct sacral plating techniques have been advocated at some European centers. The treatment of transverse sacral fractures remains controversial (Table 2).

Patients with spinal cord injuries and pelvic fractures demand special attention. In these patients, the pelvic ring is exposed to abnormal forces during simple activities, such as sitting, because normal muscle forces are not available to counteract gravitational stresses. Even initially nondisplaced fractures may demonstrate instability and

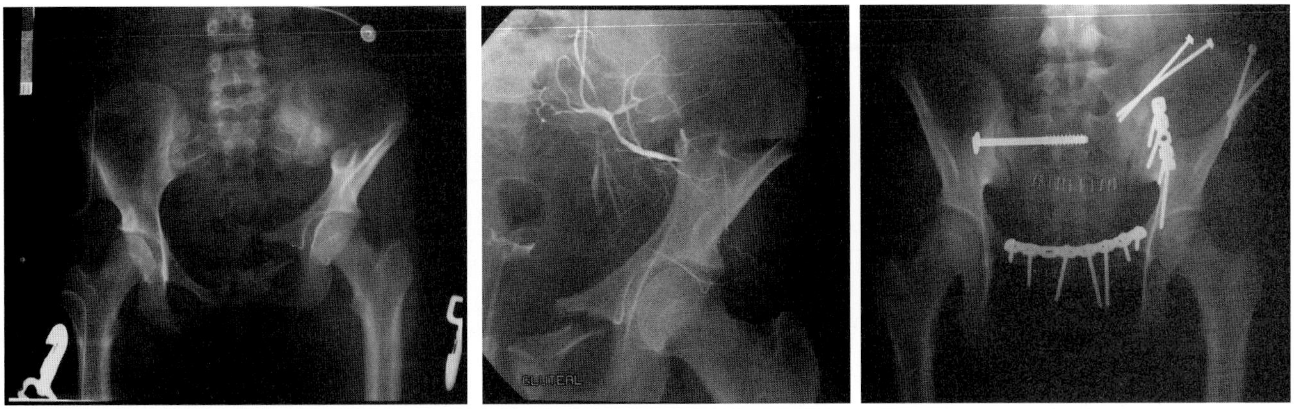

Fig. 7 **Left,** This patient jumped from a third floor window and sustained pelvic ring injuries including bilateral pubic rami fractures, a left iliac fracture, and a right incomplete sacroiliac disruption. She was hemodynamically stable after fluid resuscitation. **Center,** Because of the iliac fracture displacement through the greater sciatic notch, a pelvic arteriogram was performed and an avulsion of the superior gluteal artery was noted. The artery was embolized. **Right,** The day of injury, the patient was reduced and stabilized using simultaneous right percutaneous, left iliac, and anterior Pfannenstiel approaches.

Table 2. **Classification of sacral fractures**

Classification	Description
Zone I	Extraforaminal alar fractures
Zone II	Transforaminal fractures
Zone III	Fractures involving the central sacral canal

deformity because of these unusual load applications. These deformities are often quite severe and cause sitting imbalance, skin breakdown, and late spasticity due to pain. Orthopaedic surgeons should be aware of these potential problems when treating spinal-cord injured patients with pelvic fractures. Close radiographic follow-up or early rigid fixation using simple techniques is advocated.

Angiography Angiographic evaluation and embolization are used in those patients who demonstrate hemodynamic instability despite pelvic stabilization, adequate volume replacement, and no other source of ongoing bleeding. Certain fracture patterns, such as unstable iliac fractures displaced through the greater sciatic notch, are not amenable to external fixation and have a high incidence of associated vascular injuries. In these instances, arteriography becomes the primary therapeutic intervention.

Acetabular Fractures

A fracture of the acetabulum is often the result of a high-energy force indirectly transmitted to the acetabulum through the lower limb. The injury pattern and the associated injuries determine the method and urgency of treatment. The pattern of an acetabular fracture depends on the position of the femoral head at the time of impact, the magnitude and direction of the provocative force, and the quality of the underlying bone. Injuries frequently associated with a fracture of the acetabulum in a multiply injured patient include a sciatic nerve palsy, a bowel or bladder disruption, or a thoracic injury. Often unrecognized is a blunt shearing injury of the soft tissue adjacent to the acetabulum or the greater trochanter, termed a Morel-Lavalle lesion. This soft-tissue injury may separate the subcutaneous fat from the deep fascia, leading to a partial necrosis of the subcutaneous fat. Surgical excision of the devascularized subcutaneous tissue or the avoidance of surgical incisions through this area is recommended in order to avoid postoperative wound complications.

Classification

A fracture of the acetabulum is identified on anteroposterior (AP) and 45° Judet oblique radiographs of the pelvis (obturator oblique and iliac oblique). The fracture is further delineated using computed tomography (CT) at 3-mm intervals. A CT scan enables visualization of the quadrilateral surface, the acetabular dome, loose intra-articular fragments, and marginal impaction of the femoral head or acetabulum. A three-dimensional (3-D) reconstruction provides an overall view of the pelvis and a spatial relationship of the fracture fragments. However, the image summation that occurs in the 3-D reconstruction may lead to an underestimate or overestimate of certain acetabular fracture lines.

The classification of acetabular fractures, originally described by Letournel and Judet, is based on acetabular anatomy and describes ten fracture patterns. Each pattern is based on an analysis of the anterior and posterior columns, the anterior and posterior walls, the dome, and the teardrop of the acetabulum. Five are simple fracture patterns involving a posterior wall, a posterior column, an anterior wall, or an anterior column. The fifth simple pattern is a transverse fracture that can be designated as transtectal, infratectal, or juxtatectal depending on where the fracture line traverses the acetabulum. The five complex fractures have at least two fracture planes present in the acetabulum. These patterns include a combined posterior column and posterior wall fracture, a transverse fracture with a posterior wall component, an anterior column fracture with a posterior hemitransverse component, a T-shaped fracture, and a both column fracture. In a both column fracture, no articular segment remains intact, and only a small portion of the iliac wing remains attached to the sacrum. A spur sign is pathognomonic radiographically and represents the inferior tip of the fractured ilium seen lateral to the medially displaced acetabular fragments. This spur sign is best visualized on the obturator oblique radiograph.

Surgical Treatment

Emergent intervention is necessary if a hip dislocation or a femoral head subluxation is associated with an acetabular fracture. Ideally, the closed reduction of the femoral head into the acetabulum should avoid damage to the articular surfaces and should be performed with muscle relaxation using intravenous sedation in the emergency department or general anesthesia with fluoroscopy in the operating room. Temporary skeletal leg traction is used to maintain the reduction and prevent vascular insult to the femoral head or further cartilage damage. Laterally directed traction through a trochanteric screw is rarely indicated. Other indications for urgent surgical reduction of the acetabulum include the entrapment of large bony fragments within the joint following a closed reduction of the femoral head (Fig. 8), an open acetabular fracture to facilitate soft-tissue management, or a postreduction complete sciatic nerve palsy.

In nonemergent cases, the acetabular fracture pattern is analyzed using plain radiographs and CT imaging. Most authors recommend a displacement of the articular weight-bearing surface of >3 mm, marginal impaction of the acetabular articular cartilage, or a loss of acetabular congruency as indications for open reduction and internal fixation (ORIF). In addition, the roof arc measurement on plain radiographs or CT scan has been correlated with the need for acetabular ORIF. The roof arc angle is the angle formed between a line drawn from the fracture to the geometric center of the reduced femoral head subtended by a vertical line drawn to the geometric center of the reduced femoral head. A roof arc angle of less than 45° on plain radiographs (AP and Judet views) indicates a disruption of the superior acetabular dome and is a relative indication for ORIF. Certain fractures, such as a posterior wall or a both column fracture, are not amenable to the roof arc measurement. Relative contraindications to surgical fixation of the acetabulum include severe systemic illness, extreme osteoporosis, and systemic or local infection. Moreover, the physiologic age of the patient is more important than the chronologic age when considering acetabular fracture surgery.

The major surgical goal in acetabular surgery is to combine fracture rigidity with the anatomic restoration of the articular surface. Successful anatomic reduction often depends on use of the operative exposure appropriate for the fracture pattern. Fractures involving one column or wall (posterior wall, anterior wall, posterior column, anterior column, and posterior column/wall) can be stabilized through a single posterior Kocher-Langenbeck exposure or an anterior ilioinguinal exposure. A two-column fracture (transverse, transverse/posterior wall, anterior column/posterior hemitransverse, T, and both column) may require a single, an extensile (extended iliofemoral or triradiate), or a two-incision approach (Kocher-Langenbeck and ilioinguinal) depending on numerous variables. The Kocher-Langenbeck and the ilioinguinal approaches are nonextensile, enabling visualization of the posterior and the anterior columns, respectively. Both of these approaches provide acetabular exposure without detachment of the abductors from the ilium or the greater trochanter of the femur. In addition, the ilioinguinal approach allows for direct exposure of the entire inner aspect of the ilium from the sacroiliac joint to the pubic symphysis including the quadrilateral surface. The Kocher-Langenbeck approach is directed posteriorly and exposes the posterior column and wall from the greater sciatic notch to the upper ischium.

The extended iliofemoral and the triradiate approaches are considered extensile and expose both columns of the acetabulum through one incision. These two exposures provide good visualization of the acetabulum and facilitate the reduction of the articular surface, especially in fractures more than 14 days old. The extensile approaches, however, do not expose the anterior column medial to the iliopectineal eminence owing to the location of the external iliac vessels. Moreover, the extended iliofemoral and triradiate approaches have been associated with skin flap and muscle necrosis, abductor muscle weakness, and a higher incidence of symptomatic heterotopic ossification. Some authors recommend that patients requiring an extended iliofemoral approach have a preoperative angiogram to assure that the superior gluteal artery is patent. A relative contraindication to the use of an extended iliofemoral approach is an occlusion of the superior gluteal artery because the ascending branch of the lateral femoral circumflex vessel is ligated routinely during the surgical approach. It has been shown that the circumflex vessel is the collateral source of blood to the hip abductor musculature.

The combined surgical approach affords access to both acetabular columns and provides adequate visualization without excessive devascularization of bone fragments. In addition, associated injuries to the femoral head, the ipsilateral sacroiliac joint, and the symphysis pubis can be assessed through the anterior approach (Fig. 9). Staged anterior and posterior approaches have been recommended by some authors. However, the first procedure may lead to malalignment with rigid fixation, precluding proper reduction during the second operation.

The methods and instrumentation (specialized bone

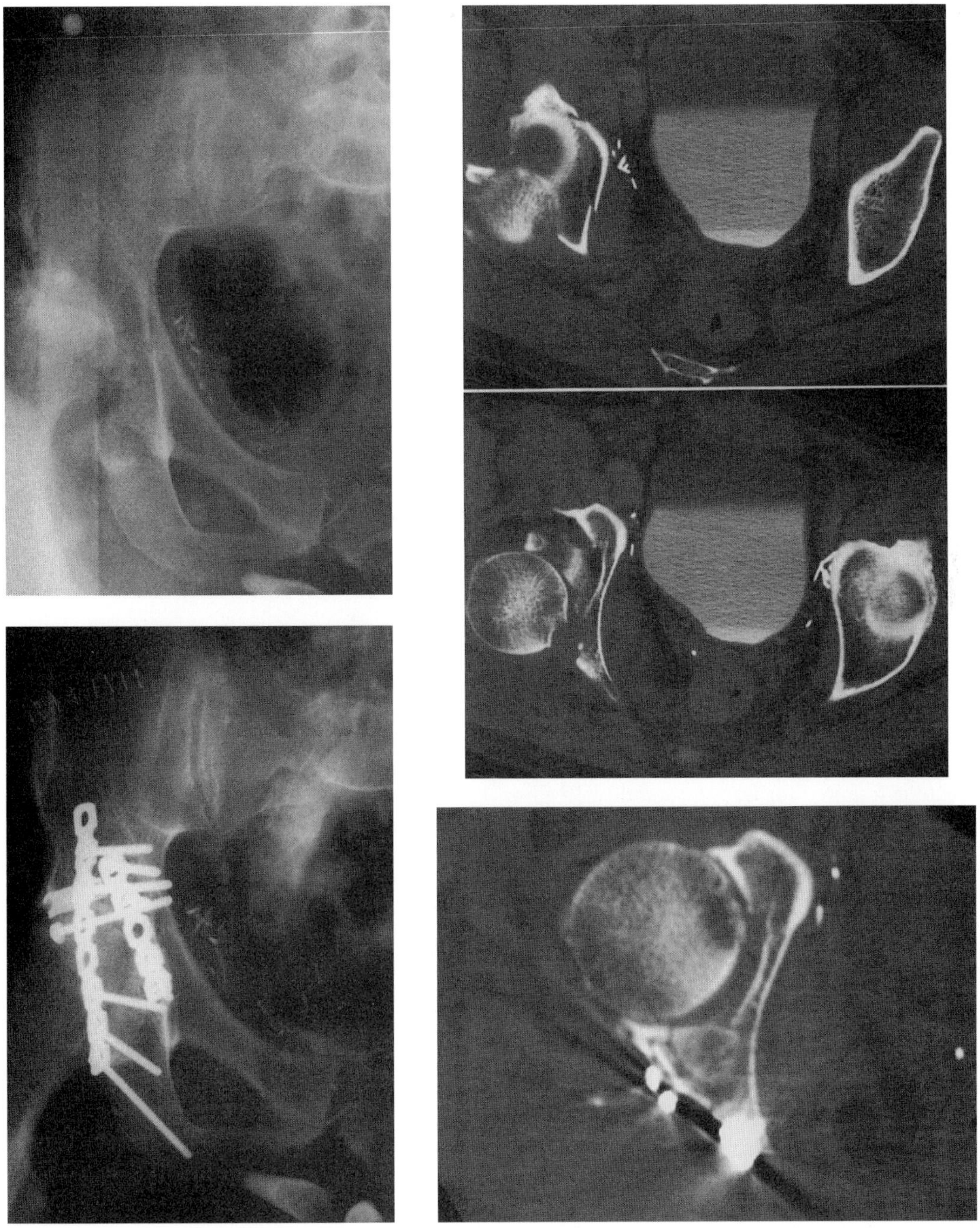

Fig. 8 Top left, Anteroposterior radiograph of a fracture-dislocation of the acetabulum in a 61-year-old male following a motor vehicle accident. The posterior wall is extremely comminuted and the femoral head is subluxed. **Top right,** Emergent computed tomography (CT) scan demonstrates several large fragments of the posterior wall lodged in the acetabulum. **Bottom left,** Postoperative radiograph of the acetabulum following the emergent open reduction and internal fixation of the acetabulum. **Bottom right,** Postoperative CT scan confirms the reduction of the femoral head and the satisfactory position of the acetabular screws.

clamps, reduction tools, and implants) used to reduce and stabilize an acetabular fracture are well described. Certain fracture patterns, specifically the posterior wall, require an additional comment. The posterior wall fracture is frequently associated with fracture comminution and soft-tissue disruption of the capsule. Because loss of fixation results in chronic instability, the initial fixation is critical. Cadaveric studies have shown that fractures of the superior one third portion of the posterior wall are most unstable and, if left untreated, result in subluxation or dislo-

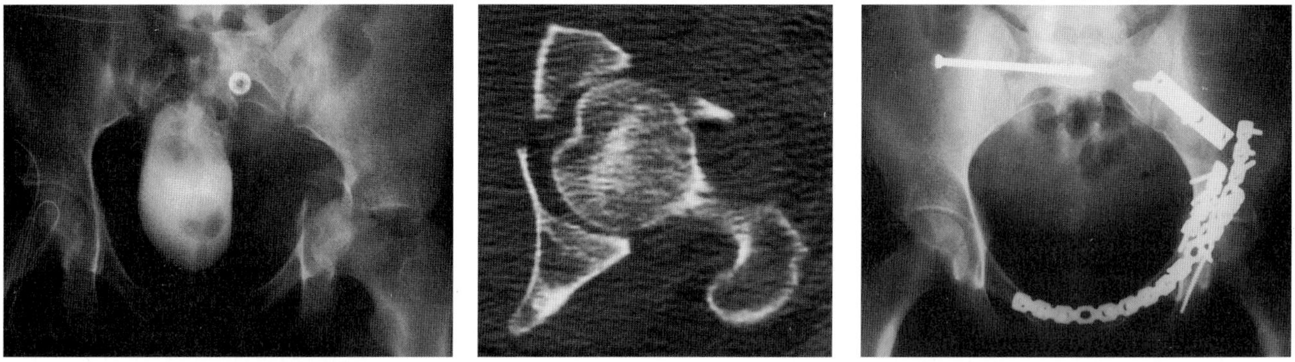

Fig. 9 **Left,** Anteroposterior radiograph of a T type fracture of the acetabulum in a 25-year-old female following a motorcycle accident. The femoral head has displaced the anterior and posterior columns of the acetabulum, and there is a displacement of the symphysis pubis and the sacroiliac joints. **Center,** The computed tomography scan confirms the acetabular displacement and demonstrates joint incongruency. **Right,** Postoperative radiograph of the pelvis following open reduction and internal fixation of the acetabulum using a combined anterior ilioinguinal and posterior Kocher-Langenbeck exposure. Surgical stabilization is also achieved of the symphysis pubis and the ipsilateral sacroiliac joint using the ilioinguinal portion of the combined incision.

cation of the femoral head. Fractures of the lower one third of the posterior wall are relatively stable and may not require surgical fixation unless fragments of bone are incarcerated in the joint. Cadaveric studies have also demonstrated that fixation with a buttress reconstruction plate is stronger than fixation with lag screws alone. For vertically comminuted fractures extending towards the margin of the posterior wall, a spring plate combined with a reconstruction plate is required for fracture stability. In this technique, a two- or three-hole, one-third tubular plate is modified. The end hole of the plate is cut intraoperatively, leaving two sharp prongs, which are bent 90° to the plate. By sliding the plate beneath and perpendicular to the contoured buttress reconstruction plate, a spring effect is produced over the thin section of acetabular wall. The hooked portion of the plate (prongs) provides bone support of the acetabulum where screws would violate the joint or be too large for the size of the fracture fragment. The hook should not engage the acetabular labrum.

Perioperative antibiotics are administered prior to the surgical procedure and maintained for 48 hours. Closed suction drainage is used postoperatively. Touch-down weightbearing is allowed at postoperative day 3 and continued for 12 weeks. If a posterior approach is required and there has been a significant disruption of the posterior capsule and the external rotators, then a limitation of hip flexion to 60° is maintained for 6 weeks to allow for soft-tissue healing.

Late Reconstruction of Acetabular Fractures

Surgical reconstruction of an acetabular fracture 3 weeks or more after injury requires special considerations. The ability to achieve a successful reduction is made difficult by the formation of callus between bone fragments, the absence of acute fracture planes, and a nonsupple soft-tissue envelope. Furthermore, as the fracture remodels, the muscle attachments to the individual bone fragments shorten. The incongruent acetabulum leads to permanent changes in the acetabular and femoral head cartilage.

An extensile approach is usually required for the delayed reconstruction of an acetabular fracture. However, the functional outcome is generally worse than with earlier treatment, despite an anatomic reduction, because of cartilage necrosis and posttraumatic arthritis. Certain fracture patterns with extensive displacement of the posterior column or wall (transverse, T, and posterior wall) are associated with a lower rate of achieving an anatomic reduction and a higher incidence of osteonecrosis and posttraumatic arthritis.

Results/Outcome

Previous clinical studies have shown that patient outcome is better with an anatomic reduction of the acetabulum than with a residual deformity of greater than 3 mm. In one study, 11% of 56 patients with an anatomic reduction of the acetabulum required a total hip arthroplasty at 2 years. In addition, 20% to 23% of patients developed femoral head osteonecrosis during the same period. Surprisingly, 83% of patients with a poor clinical result had a reduction with less than 3 mm of residual displacement. Therefore, important factors other than the adequacy of reduction include the presence of a dislocation at the time of injury, postoperative Brooker class III or IV heterotopic ossification, and patient age under 40 years. Additional studies have shown that postoperative subluxation of the femoral head or a failure to maintain a concentric reduction alters force transmission properties and accelerates posttraumatic degenerative arthritis of the acetabular cartilage.

A nonextensile approach to the acetabulum, combined with an anatomic reduction, may improve long-term outcome. Moreover, iatrogenic injury of the skin flap, devascularization of the abductor musculature, and severe heterotopic ossification are less likely with a nonextensile approach than with an extensile incision.

The quantitative strength of the hip musculature decreases 27% after ORIF of acetabular fractures. The greatest loss of strength occurs in the abductor musculature (50%), followed by the adductor musculature (28%). The severity of the strength deficit appears to be influenced by fracture pattern and surgical approach. Patients requiring a Kocher-Langenbeck approach had a greater loss of hip abductor strength if a transverse fracture was present compared to a posterior wall fracture. Other factors that diminish strength include fracture comminution, marginal impaction of the acetabular weightbearing dome, cartilage necrosis, and incongruency of the acetabular surface.

A relatively common problem associated with acetabular fracture is local soft-tissue injury, including local wounds, abrasions, and a closed degloving injury. With a closed degloving injury, the subcutaneous tissue is torn away from the underlying fascia creating a significant cavity, which contains hematoma and liquefied fat. This occurs as a result of the severe blunt trauma required to produce an acetabular fracture. When this lesion is present over the greater trochanter, it is known as a Morel-Lavalle lesion. These areas must be drained and debrided prior to or at surgery to decrease the chance of infection.

The functional outcome and complication rate in obese patients has been described. Several reports have noted a higher surgical complication rate in comparison to the nonobese patient with an acetabular fracture. Reported problems include wound dehiscence, septic arthritis, and loss of fixation.

An adverse functional outcome can be related to screws directed into the acetabulum causing accelerated acetabular deterioration. A recently described technique of auscultation using an esophageal transducer has been helpful in avoiding this complication. In addition, an acetabular danger zone, based on a cadaveric model, has been defined to avoid the intraoperative complication of acetabular screw penetration. This region was along the posterior column at the midacetabular level. Screws inserted 2 cm and 3 cm medial to the posterior acetabular labrum and angled medially at 45° and 15°, respectively, did not violate the acetabulum. Intraoperative fluoroscopy is useful in avoiding misdirected screws.

Complications

Inherent to all surgical procedures are the immediate postoperative complications of infection and thromboembolism. The risk of a wound infection can be minimized with appropriate soft-tissue management, the avoidance of large devascularized flaps, and perioperative antibiotics. The potential for thromboembolism can be decreased with the use of pneumatic compression stockings and anticoagulation. Preoperative and postoperative venous duplex ultrasonography is advocated, and in patients with positive findings, caval filters should be placed to reduce the risk of pulmonary embolism. In addition, caval filter prophylaxis has been recommended for patients undergoing acetabular surgery with two or more of the following risk factors: advanced age, delayed surgery, anticoagulation contraindications, prolonged immobilization, malignancy, obesity, intracranial or spinal hemorrhage, and a history of deep vein thrombosis or pulmonary embolism.

The rate of injury to the sciatic nerve secondary to the acetabular trauma is reported to be approximately 20%, with the rate of iatrogenic injury being another 5%. In one series, a satisfactory functional outcome was documented after a mean follow-up of 27 months in 13 of 14 patients who had sciatic nerve injuries associated with displaced acetabular fractures. However, residual neurologic sequelae were common, and patients with severe peroneal nerve injury did not recover good function. The likelihood of intraoperative sciatic neurapraxis, most common with posterior approaches, can be diminished by careful leg positioning, avoidance of improper retractor positioning, and somatosensory-evoked potential monitoring.

Traumatic and iatrogenic injuries of the superior gluteal artery are major causes of postoperative abductor flap necrosis and muscle weakness. In recent cadaveric angiographic studies, no evidence was found of circulation in the abductor muscles of limbs with occluded superior gluteal arteries that underwent an extended iliofemoral exposure. This was not the case in cadavers in which the combined ilioinguinal and Kocher-Langenbeck approach was used. The ilioinguinal approach is associated with thrombosis of the femoral artery, injury to the lateral femoral cutaneous nerve, and vascular bleeding in patients with a corona mortise. The corona mortise is an aberrant vascular conduit that connects the external iliac or the inferior epigastric artery with the obturator vascular system.

The reported incidence of heterotopic ossification after an acetabular fracture ranges from 20% to 100%, and because it leads to functional disability, recent studies have focused on preventing this complication. Several investigators have recommended a 6-week postoperative course of indomethacin to reduce the overall incidence of heterotopic bone formation, especially in patients with craniocerebral trauma and in those who require an extensile surgical approach. In addition, low dose targeted irradiation alone or combined with indomethacin has been effective in the prevention of heterotopic bone formation.

Annotated Bibliography

Pelvic Fractures

Albert MJ, Miller ME, MacNaughton M, et al: Posterior pelvic fixation using a transiliac 4.5-mm reconstruction plate: A clinical and biomechanical study. *J Orthop Trauma* 1993;7:226–232.

This combined study advocates posterior transiliac tension band plate fixation. The surgical exposures are outlined. Both infection and complication rates were low. Mechanical evaluations demonstrated comparable stability with sacral bars.

Duwelius PJ, Van Allen M, Bray TJ, et al: Computed tomography-guided fixation of unstable posterior pelvic ring disruptions. *J Orthop Trauma* 1992;6:420–426.

In this clinical series, iliosacral and transiliac screws were inserted to stabilize posterior pelvic disruptions. The screws were inserted using CT guidance with the patients in either the lateral or prone position. Reductions were obtained prior to screw insertion using skeletal traction and/or anterior external fixation. This iliosacral screw insertion technique may be indicated for nondisplaced posterior pelvic ring disruptions.

Ganz R, Krushell RJ, Jakob RP, et al: The antishock pelvic clamp. *Clin Orthop* 1991;267:71–78.

The pelvic antishock clamp is introduced. The technique of application is illustrated.

Gruen GS, Leit ME, Gruen RJ, et al: The acute management of hemodynamically unstable multiple trauma patients with pelvic ring fractures. *J Trauma* 1994;36:706–713.

Aggressive resuscitation of these patients included early internal pelvic fixation. Uncontrolled hemorrhage from the pelvic injury and/or surgery was not encountered. Anterior and posterior internal fixation of the pelvis after anatomic reduction provided stability while avoiding the complications of external fixation.

Koury HI, Peschiera JL, Welling RE: Selective use of pelvic roentgenograms in blunt trauma patients. *J Trauma* 1993;34:236–237.

This series concludes that alert, oriented, and reliable patients involved in blunt trauma do not need routine pelvic radiographs if the physical findings are negative.

Pohlemann T, Angst M, Schneider E, et al: Fixation of transforaminal sacrum fractures: A biomechanical study. *J Orthop Trauma* 1993;7:107–117.

A new technique of plate fixation of unstable sacral fractures is shown to be comparable to standard fixation techniques.

Pohlemann T, Bosch U, Gansslen A, et al: The Hannover experience in management of pelvic fractures. *Clin Orthop* 1994;305:69–80.

This series advocates accurate reduction and stable fixation of unstable pelvic ring injuries. An aggressive management protocol is outlined according to a strict timetable.

Simonian PT, Routt ML Jr, Harrington RM, et al: Biomechanical simulation of the anteroposterior compression injury of the pelvis: An understanding of instability and fixation. *Clin Orthop* 1994;309:245–256.

Internal fixation constructs of pelvic ring disruptions were evaluated in this biomechanical study. The most rigid overall pelvic fixation was achieved when both the symphyseal and sacroiliac disruptions were internally stabilized. Sacroiliac joint fixation using either an iliosacral lag screw or two anterior plates was comparable.

Simonian PT, Routt MLC Jr, Harrington RM, et al: Box plate fixation of the symphysis pubis: Biomechanical evaluation of a new technique. *J Orthop Trauma* 1994;8: 483–489.

This biomechanical study evaluates a new technique of symphyseal fixation. The box plate construct was more rigid than other routine forms of symphyseal fixation.

Simonian PT, Routt MLC Jr, Harrington RM, et al: Internal fixation of the unstable anterior pelvic ring: A biomechanical comparison of standard plating techniques and the retrograde medullary superior pubic ramus screw. *J Orthop Trauma* 1994;8:476–482.

This biomechanical study compared the retrograde medullary superior pubic ramus screw to standard plate fixation for pubic ramus fractures. Both techniques provided equivalent stability.

Acetabular Fractures

Dickinson WH, Duwelius PJ, Colville MR: Muscle strength testing following surgery for acetabular fractures. *J Orthop Trauma* 1993;7:39–46.

The overall muscle strength deficit was 27% following acetabular open reduction and internal fixation with the abductor musculature accounting for a 50% loss of strength. Factors that contributed to an unsatisfactory outcome included comminution of the weightbearing dome, marginal impaction of the acetabulum, and posterior acetabular exposures.

Fassler PR, Swiontkowski MF, Kilroy AW, et al: Injury of the sciatic nerve associated with acetabular fracture. *J Bone Joint Surg* 1993;75A:1157–1166.

A sciatic nerve injury was associated with the fracture in 11 patients and was iatrogenic in three patients. Intraoperatively, six of eight patients with a hemorrhagic contusion of the epineurium had a poor recovery of the peroneal division. Clinically, the peroneal division of the sciatic nerve was injured in all 14 patients and had a limited recovery if the injury was severe. However, in patients with an injury of the peroneal and tibial division, the prognosis for recovery of the tibial division was good.

Helfet DL, Schmeling GJ: Somatosensory evoked potential monitoring in the surgical treatment of acute, displaced acetabular fractures: Results of a prospective study. *Clin Orthop* 1994;301:213–220.

In a prospective review of 103 patients, the sciatic nerve (tibial and peroneal division) was traumatically injured in ten patients (10%) and the peroneal division in 18 (18%). Postoperatively, 5% of the patients had a peroneal division injury. In all five patients, the fracture pattern had significant posterior column or wall displacement.

Juliano PJ, Bosse MJ, Edwards KJ: The superior gluteal artery in complex acetabular procedures: A cadaveric angiographic study. *J Bone Joint Surg* 1994;76A:244–248.

The results of this cadaveric study demonstrated that with the extensile approaches, there was no evidence of vascular circulation in the abductor musculature when the superior gluteal artery was occluded. However, abductor muscle vascularization was intact after a combined ilioinguinal and Kocher-Langenbeck approach even when the superior gluteal artery was occluded. The authors concluded that the circulation to the abductor musculature depends on the superior gluteal pedicle. Ligation of the ascending branch of the lateral femoral circumflex artery during development of the abductor muscle flap eliminates the major collateral circulation.

Moed BR, Karges DE: Prophylactic indomethacin for the prevention of heterotopic ossification after acetabular fracture surgery in high-risk patients. *J Orthop Trauma* 1994;8:34–39.

In this study, 19 patients who did not receive indomethacin were compared to 16 matched patients who received indomethacin following acetabular surgery. The indomethacin-treated group had a 6% incidence of Brooker class III/IV heterotopic ossification compared to a 53% incidence in the untreated group. The authors recommend a 6-week postoperative course of indomethacin.

Olson SA, Matta JM: The computerized tomography subchondral arc: A new method of assessing acetabular articular continuity after fracture (A preliminary report). *J Orthop Trauma* 1993;7:402–413.

The criteria for the nonsurgical management of acetabular fractures included: (1) an intact articular surface along the superior 10 mm of the acetabulum on CT; (2) femoral head congruency with the superior acetabulum on plain radiographs without traction; (3) a minimum of 50% of the posterior wall remaining intact at the most involved level as determined by CT. Of those fractures meeting the nonoperative CT criteria, 82% had a good or excellent result at 1 year using the modified d'Aubigne scoring system.

Schmidt CC, Gruen GS: Nonextensile surgical approaches for two-column acetabular fractures. *J Bone Joint Surg* 1993;75B:556–561.

Twenty-one two-column fractures of the acetabulum were surgically managed through a single or a combined nonextensile approach. A reduction to within 3 mm was achieved in 18 patients (86%) without osteotomy of the greater trochanter. The average Harris Hip Score was 81. Skin and abductor muscle necrosis, which has been reported as a complication of extensile approaches, did not occur in this series.

Classic Bibliography

Pelvic Fractures

Ben-Menachem Y, Coldwell DM, Young JW, et al: Hemorrhage associated with pelvic fractures: Causes, diagnosis, and emergent management. *Am J Roentgenol* 1991;157:1005–1014.

Browner BD, Cole JD, Graham JM, et al: Delayed posterior internal fixation of unstable pelvic fractures. *J Trauma* 1987;27:998–1006.

Bucholz RW: The pathological anatomy of Malgaigne fracture-dislocations of the pelvis. *J Bone Joint Surg* 1981;63A:400–404.

Burgess AR, Eastridge BJ, Young JW, et al: Pelvic ring disruptions: Effective classification system and treatment protocols. *J Trauma* 1990;30:848–856.

Dahners LE, Jacobs RR, Jayaraman G, et al: A study of external skeletal fixation systems for unstable pelvic fractures. *J Trauma* 1984:27:876–881.

Dalal SA, Burgess AR, Siegel JH, et al: Pelvic fracture in multiple trauma: Classification by mechanism is key to pattern of organ injury, resuscitative requirements, and outcome. *J Trauma* 1989;29:981–1002.

Denis F, Davis S, Comfort T: Sacral fractures: An important problem. Retrospective analysis of 236 cases. *Clin Orthop* 1988;227:67–81.

Failinger MS, McGanity PL: Unstable fractures of the pelvic ring. *J Bone Joint Surg* 1992;74A:781–791.

Henderson RC: The long-term results of nonoperatively treated major pelvic disruptions. *J Orthop Trauma* 1989; 3:41–47.

Huittinen VM, Slatis P: Nerve injury in double vertical pelvic fractures. *Acta Chir Scand* 1972;138:571–575.

Kellam JF, McMurtry RY, Paley D, et al: The unstable pelvic fracture: Operative treatment. *Orthop Clin North Am* 1987;18:25–41.

Kraemer W, Hearn T, Tile M, et al: The effect of thread length and location on extraction strengths of iliosacral lag screws. *Injury* 1994;25:5–9.

Lange RH, Hansen ST Jr: Pelvic ring disruptions with symphysis pubis diastasis: Indications, techniques, and limitations of anterior internal fixation. *Clin Orthop* 1985;201:130–137.

Latenser BA, Gentilello LM, Tarver AA, et al: Improved outcome with early fixation of skeletally unstable pelvic fractures. *J Trauma* 1991;31:28–31.

Matta JM, Saucedo T: Internal fixation of pelvic ring fractures. *Clin Orthop* 1989;242:38–97.

Peltier LF: Complications associated with fractures of the pelvis. *J Bone Joint Surg* 1965;47A:1060–1069.

Pennal GF, Tile M, Waddell JP, et al: Pelvic disruption: Assessment and classification. *Clin Orthop* 1980;151: 12–21.

Simpson LA, Waddell JP, Leighton RK, et al: Anterior approach and stabilization of the disrupted sacriliac joint. *J Trauma* 1087;27:1332–1339.

Slatis P, HuittinenVM: Double vertical fractures of the pelvis: A report on 163 patients. *Acta Chir Scand* 1972; 138:799–807.

Stocks GW, Gabel GT, Noble PC, et al: Anterior and posterior internal fixation of vertical shear fractures of the pelvis. *J Orthop Res* 1991;9:237–245.

Tile M: Pelvic ring fractures: Should they be fixed? *J Bone Joint Surg* 1988;70B:1–12.

Acetabular Fractures

Baumgaertner MR, Wegner D, Booke J: SSEP monitoring during pelvic and acetabular fracture surgery. *J Orthop Trauma* 1994;8:127–133.

Bosse MJ: Posterior acetabular wall fractures: A technique for screw placement. *J Orthop Trauma* 1991;5:167–172.

Brueton RN: A review of 40 acetabular fractures: The importance of early surgery. *Injury* 1993;24:171–174.

Daum WJ, Scarborough MT, Gordon W Jr, et al: Heterotopic ossification and other perioperative complications of acetabular fractures. *J Orthop Trauma* 1992;6:427–432.

Ebraheim NA, Waldrop J, Yeasting RA, et al: Danger zone of the acetabulum. *J Orthop Trauma* 1992;6:146–151.

Heeg M, Klasen HJ, Visser JD: Operative treatment for acetabular fractures. *J Bone Joint Surg* 1990;72B:383–386.

Heeg M, Otter N, Klasen HJ: Anterior column fractures of the acetabulum. *J Bone Joint Surg* 1992;74B:554–557.

Helfet DL, Borrelli J Jr, DiPasquale T, et al: Stabilization of acetabular fractures in elderly patients. *J Bone Joint Surg* 1992;74A:753–765.

Helfet DL, Hissa EA, Sergay S, et al: Somatosensory evoked potential monitoring in the surgical management of acute acetabular fractures. *J Orthop Trauma* 1991;5: 161–166.

Kaempffe FA, Bone LB, Border JR: Open reduction and internal fixation of acetabular fractures: Heterotopic ossification and other complications of treatment. *J Orthop Trauma* 1991;5:439–445.

Kebaish AS, Roy A, Rennie W: Displaced acetabular fractures: Long-term follow-up. *J Trauma* 1991;31: 1539–1542.

Letournel E: The treatment of acetabular fractures through the ilioinguinal approach. *Clin Orthop* 1993; 292:62–76.

Martinez CR, Di Pasquale TG, Helfet DL, et al: Evaluation of acetabular fractures with two- and three-dimensional CT. *Radiographics* 1992;12:227–242.

McLaren AC: Prophylaxis with indomethacin for heterotopic bone after open reduction of fractures of the acetabulum. *J Bone Joint Surg* 1990;72A:245–247.

Oransky M, Sanguinetti C: Surgical treatment of displaced acetabular fractures: Results of 50 consecutive cases. *J Orthop Trauma* 1993;7:28–32.

Probe R, Reeve R, Lindsey RW: Femoral artery thrombosis after open reduction of an acetabular fracture. *Clin Orthop* 1992;283:258–260.

Roffi RP, Matta JM: Unrecognized posterior dislocation of the hip associated with transverse and T-type fractures of the acetabulum. *J Orthop Trauma* 1993;7:23–27.

Routt ML Jr, Swiontkowski MF: Operative treatment of complex acetabular fractures: Combined anterior and posterior exposures during the same procedure. *J Bone Joint Surg* 1990;72A:897–904.

Schopfer A, Willett K, Powell J, et al: Cerclage wiring in internal fixation of acetabular fractures. *J Orthop Trauma* 1993;7:236–241.

Tornkvist H, Schatzker J: Acetabular fractures in the elderly: An easily missed diagnosis. *J Orthop Trauma* 1993;7:233–235.

Vrahas M, Gordon RG, Mears DC, et al: Intraoperative somatosensory evoked potential monitoring of pelvic and acetabular fractures. *J Orthop Trauma* 1992;6:50–58.

Webb LX, Rush PT, Fuller SB, et al: Greenfield filter prophylaxis of pulmonary embolism in patients undergoing surgery for acetabular fracture. *J Orthop Trauma* 1992;6:139–145.

Wright R, Barrett K, Christie MJ, et al: Acetabular fractures: Long-term follow-up of open reduction and internal fixation. *J Orthop Trauma* 1994;8:397–403.

35

Hip: Trauma

Trauma to the hip, particularly hip fractures in the elderly, continues to be a medical, social, and economic challenge. An increasing number of hip fractures occur each year in an older and frailer population. Technical improvements in fracture fixation and prosthetic replacement have decreased the incidence of postoperative complications. However, continued improvements are necessary to improve functional outcome. This chapter will discuss hip dislocations, risk factors associated with hip fractures, and the treatment principles of femoral neck, intertrochanteric, and subtrochanteric fractures.

Hip Dislocations

Hip dislocations are usually the result of high-energy trauma. Severe associated injuries are common and include craniofacial, chest, abdominal, and other musculoskeletal trauma. It is essential to obtain radiographs of the pelvis and entire femur to identify the most commonly associated musculoskeletal injuries. Hip dislocations are divided into anterior and posterior types. Each will be discussed separately. Treatment for patients with a hip dislocation includes (1) careful evaluation to detect associated injuries; (2) immediate gentle closed or, if necessary, open reduction followed by assessment of hip stability; and (3) careful radiographic evaluation, including computed tomography (CT) scan, for congruency of reduction and to identify any associated femoral head or acetabular fracture.

If a concentric, stable reduction is obtained, the patient should be mobilized with protected weightbearing for 4 to 6 weeks. If the reduction is concentric but unstable, without associated fracture, the extremity should be placed in traction for 4 to 6 weeks until soft-tissue healing occurs. A nonconcentric reduction, resulting from either intra-articular osteochondral fragments, interposed soft tissue, or malreduction of associated fracture, necessitates open reduction and joint exploration. Treatment of associated femoral head or acetabular fractures depends upon the size and location of the fragments and the stability of the reduction.

Femoral artery and nerve injuries are very uncommon and are associated with anterior dislocations. Sciatic nerve injuries occur in approximately 10% of posterior dislocations. Osteonecrosis can occur up to 5 years after injury; the risk of osteonecrosis increases with time delay of more than 6 to 12 hours between injury and reduction. It is generally accepted that simple dislocations have an excellent long-term prognosis if reduced within 6 hours of injury. Authors of a recent study, however, reported poor long-term clinical outcome, particularly after posterior dislocation, in a series of hip dislocations without fracture followed for greater than 2 years.

Anterior Dislocations

Anterior dislocations are rare (10% to 18% of all hip dislocations) and can be classified as either superior or inferior. Anterior hip dislocations result from abduction and external rotation; superior dislocations occur in extension, and the far more common inferior dislocations in flexion. Closed reduction can be accomplished by traction followed by extension and internal rotation.

Associated femoral head fractures occur in 22% to 77% of cases and are classified as either transchondral or indentation types. Transchondral fractures that result in nonconcentric reduction require open reduction and either excision or internal fixation, depending on the fragment size and location. Indentation fractures, typically located on the superior femoral head, require no specific treatment, but fracture location has significant prognostic implications.

Ten percent of anterior dislocations develop osteonecrosis. Risk factors include a time delay from injury to reduction and repeated reduction attempts. The risk factors for posttraumatic degenerative arthritis include transchondral fracture, indentation fracture greater than 4 mm in depth, and osteonecrosis.

Posterior Dislocations

Posterior dislocations account for up to 90% of all hip dislocations and are classified based on the presence or absence of associated acetabular and/or femoral head fracture. Posterior dislocations result from an axial force applied to the flexed knee. If the hip is in a neutral or adducted position, a simple dislocation occurs; if the hip is abducted, a posterior acetabular rim fracture-dislocation results. Closed reduction involves traction on the adducted and flexed hip. Postreduction radiographs and computed tomography (CT) scan should be evaluated carefully for concentricity of reduction, intra-articular fragments, and associated fractures. If closed reduction under general anesthesia is unsuccessful or nonconcentric, an open reduction should be performed.

Hip stability must be assessed following either closed or open reduction. CT can be used to help determine stability after reduction of posterior wall fracture-dislocations. Stability is inversely related to the size of the posterior acetabular fragment; data from cadaveric CT studies have indicated that fragments involving $<$ 20% to 25% of the acetabular wall do not affect hip stability whereas those involving > 40% to 50% result in instability. The status of the posterior capsule may determine stability for fragments of transitional size. The acetabular depression fracture is a rotated, impacted, osteocartilaginous fragment of the posteromedial acetabulum that occurs as a result of a posterior fracture-dislocation. This fracture, with a reported 23% incidence using CT evaluation, should be elevated and bone grafted.

Osteonecrosis of the femoral head occurs in 10% of simple posterior dislocations and in over 50% of fracture-dislocations. The risk of osteonecrosis is related to the severity of the injury, time delay to reduction (> 6 to 12 hours), and repeated closed reduction attempts. The risk factors for posttraumatic degenerative arthritis include higher energy initial injury, presence of a nonconcentric reduction, time delay between injury and reduction, and the development of osteonecrosis.

Posterior Dislocations with Femoral Head Fracture

Approximately 10% of posterior dislocations have associated fractures of the femoral head or neck. These fractures have been further categorized by Pipkin into four types: type I, fracture of the femoral head caudad to the fovea; type II, fracture of the femoral head cephalad to the fovea, type III, type I or II plus femoral neck fracture; and type IV, type I, II, or III plus fracture of the acetabular rim. Femoral head fractures result from an axial force applied to the flexed knee with the hip adducted and flexed less than 50°.

Identification and sizing of the femoral head fragment are difficult with standard radiographs; CT scanning can provide this important information (Fig. 1). A CT-directed pelvic oblique radiograph has recently been described and found to be an accurate determinant of fracture displacement and joint congruity. This radiograph can be used postoperatively to monitor fracture healing. A gentle closed reduction should be attempted for Pipkin types I, II, and IV; type III injuries require open reduction. Postreduction radiographs, including CT scans, should be evaluated for concentricity and reduction of the femoral head fragment.

An unsuccessful or nonconcentric closed reduction (including under general anesthesia) mandates an open reduction. Pipkin types I and II fractures generally require open reduction from an anterior approach and internal fixation with well-recessed cancellous or Herbert screws. Authors of a recent study comparing the efficacy of an anterior versus posterior approach for Pipkin types I and II fractures reported improved fracture visualization and fixation with the anterior approach. Type III fractures in young active patients should be treated with open reduction and internal fixation of the femoral neck fracture, followed by internal fixation of the femoral head fracture. In the elderly or low functional demand patient, prosthetic replacement is indicated. Treatment of type IV injuries depends on the stability and concentricity of the reduction. If the reduction is unstable or nonconcentric, open reduction with fixation of the femoral head and posterior acetabular fracture is indicated.

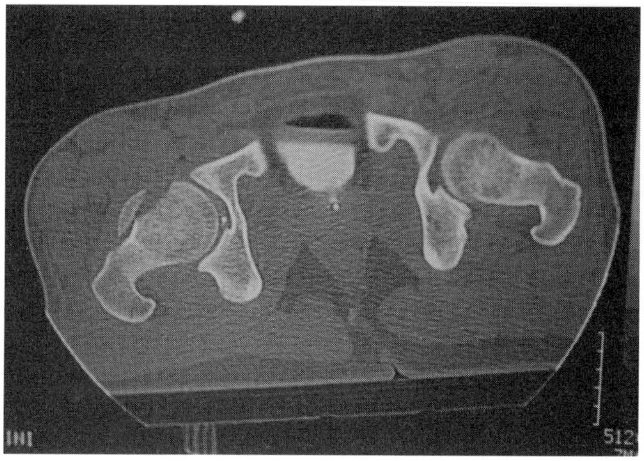

Fig. 1 Computed tomography scan of a Pipkin I right femoral head fracture.

Posterior hip dislocations with associated femoral head fractures are at high risk for developing osteonecrosis and posttraumatic degenerative arthritis. The prognosis for these injuries varies. Pipkin types I and II are reported to have the same prognosis as a simple dislocation. Pipkin type IV injuries have the same prognosis as posterior fracture-dislocations without a femoral head fracture. Pipkin type III injuries have a poor prognosis.

Hip Fractures

General Considerations

Risk Factors The incidence of hip fracture increases with increasing age, doubling for each decade beyond 50 years of age. Females are more commonly affected by a ratio of 2 to 3 to 1. The incidence in white women is 2 to 3 times higher than that reported for black and hispanic women. Additional risk factors include urban dwelling, excessive alcohol and caffeine intake, physical inactivity, previous hip fracture, use of psychotropic medication (hypnotics-anxiolytics, tricyclic antidepressants, and antipsychotics), and senile dementia. In general, osteoporosis should not be considered the cause of hip fractures in the elderly, but rather a potential contributing factor along with the other risk factors described. Osteomalacia has not been shown to be a risk factor for hip fractures. The hip axis length (the distance from the greater trochanter to the inner pelvic brim) has been demonstrated to be predictive of hip fracture independent of patient age and bone mineral density in elderly women. Coxarthrosis of the ipsilateral hip is rarely associated with an intracapsular femoral neck fracture, whereas intertrochanteric fractures do occur in the presence of degenerative changes.

Approximately 90% of hip fractures in the elderly result from a simple fall. Fall characteristics (ie, protective responses) and body habitus have been implicated as factors influencing the risk of hip fracture after a fall. Recent work has suggested that use of external hip protectors may decrease the risk of hip fracture in the elderly. Age-related changes in neuromuscular function may increase the likelihood that a fall will result in a hip fracture. These changes include decreased speed of ambulation, which makes it more likely that the point of impact from a fall will be near the hip, and decreased reaction time, which limits the potential for a protective response.

Mortality The current overall mortality rate in elderly patients 1 year following hip fracture ranges from 14% to 36%. There is general agreement that the highest mortality risk occurs within the first 4 to 6 months following fracture. After 1 year, the mortality rate approaches that for age- and sex-matched controls. Factors associated with increased mortality include advanced age, poorly controlled systemic disease, male sex, institutionalized living, psychiatric illness, and surgical treatment before medical stabilization. There is no agreement as to whether fracture type or type of surgical procedure are risk factors for increased mortality.

The influence of nutrition on the mortality and morbidity of hip fracture patients is well documented. Serum albumin level has been found to closely correlate with mortality. A recent study has reported the value of lymphocyte counts as a prognostic indicator of survival following femoral neck fracture.

Treatment Nonsurgical management is appropriate only in selected nonambulators who experience minimal discomfort from the injury. These patients, however, should be rapidly mobilized to avoid the complications of prolonged recumbency. It is important to evaluate and correct all comorbid medical conditions in the elderly hip fracture patient prior to surgery. Although most hip fracture patients can undergo surgery within 24 hours of injury, longer delays to stabilize medical problems have not been shown to increase morbidity or mortality. Surgical treatment of medically unstable patients, however, significantly increases the mortality risk. Several studies have evaluated the efficacy of preoperative skin traction in both femoral neck and intertrochanteric hip fracture patients. No benefit in pain control was found between patients treated with skin traction and those whose injured leg was placed on a pillow. Anesthetic choice (regional versus general) has not been shown to significantly affect the incidence of postoperative confusion or mortality in elderly hip fracture patients.

Postoperative management should be directed at early patient mobilization. The ability to ambulate within 2 weeks following surgery has been shown to correlate with living at home 1 year after surgery. Because nonweightbearing and partial weightbearing are difficult for elderly patients and there are no reported negative effects of full weightbearing after either internal fixation or prosthetic replacement, most geriatric hip fracture patients should be allowed to bear weight as tolerated.

Imaging Studies The vast majority of hip fractures can be identified on standard radiographs. However, occult hip fractures require additional imaging studies. It may require 2 to 3 days for bone scintigraphy to become positive in the elderly patient with a hip fracture. Magnetic resonance imaging (MRI) has been shown to be at least as accurate as bone scanning in the assessment of occult fractures of the hip and can be performed within 24 hours of injury (Fig. 2). However, MRI within 48 hours of fracture does not appear to be useful for assessing femoral head viability/vascularity or predicting the development of osteonecrosis or healing complications.

Hip Fractures in Young Adults Hip fractures in young adults are the result of high-energy trauma. It is essential to carefully evaluate these patients for head, neck, chest, abdominal, and other long bone or pelvic injuries. Immediate stabilization of orthopaedic injuries in these frequently multiply injured patients is essential. Specific attention must be given to the treatment of the hip fracture to minimize the risk of complications. In all cases, femoral neck fractures in younger patients (below the age of 50) should be treated as an emergency to decrease the incidence of osteonecrosis.

Functional Recovery

Evaluation of functional recovery following hip fracture has become increasingly important as it is realized that

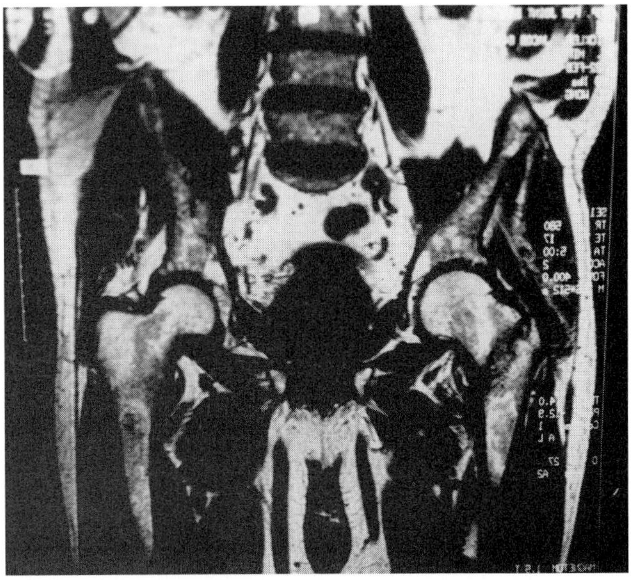

Fig. 2 Magnetic resonance imaging study of a left intertrochanteric hip fracture. This fracture was not apparent on plain radiographs.

treatment success is measured by those patients who are able to regain their prefracture level of function. Forty percent to 60% of geriatric hip fracture patients are able to return directly home after hospitalization. Factors predictive of a hospital to home discharge are younger age, prefracture and early postfracture independent ambulation and ability to perform activities of daily living (ADLs), and the presence of another person at home. Forty percent to 60% of patients will regain their prefracture ambulatory status within 1 year after fracture. The factors associated with regaining prefracture ambulatory status include younger age, male sex, and the absence of preexisting dementia. In addition, the use of a multidisciplinary team to treat geriatric hip fracture patients has been shown to improve outcomes.

Pathologic Fractures

The proximal femur is a common site for metastatic lesions, which result in pathologic fractures or impending fractures. The indications for stabilization of impending fractures include a lesion more than 2.5 cm in diameter or destruction of 50% or more of the cortex of a long bone. Patients treated prophylactically for impending fractures have less surgical mortality, fewer complications, fewer stabilization failures, and more successful rehabilitation than those undergoing surgery for pathologic fractures. In addition, stabilization of an impending fracture is easier and spares the patient the pain and disability associated with fracture. Life expectancy has been used as an indication for surgical treatment. Some have recommended at least a 90-day life expectancy, and others have utilized 30 days. Although there is no universal agreement, surgical treatment of impending and pathologic fractures is indicated in patients whose quality of life will be enhanced, regardless of the anticipated life expectancy. Surgical management provides pain relief and allows better patient mobilization.

Preoperative evaluation and preparation of the patient must be meticulous because these patients are often quite debilitated. Particular attention should be given to serum calcium levels, because hypercalcemia is commonly encountered. Metastatic lesions that are radiosensitive should undergo radiotherapy preoperatively or immediately after stabilization of the fracture. Radiotherapy has not been shown to decrease soft-tissue healing, but does interfere with incorporation of bone graft. Methylmethacrylate is an important adjunct for stabilization of these fractures. It is used to fill defects that remain after tumor removal and for implant fixation. Surgical management usually consists of internal fixation using adjunctive methylmethacrylate or prosthetic replacement. The choice depends on location and size of the lesion and sensitivity to radiotherapy.

Femoral Neck Fractures

The Garden classification of femoral neck fractures is used most commonly in the literature. However, there is difficulty in differentiating the four types of fractures as shown by studies of interobserver reliability. Therefore, it may be more accurate to classify femoral neck fractures as nondisplaced (Garden types I and II) or displaced (Garden types III and IV). Nondisplaced femoral neck fractures (Garden types I and II) should be internally stabilized using multiple lag screws or pins placed in parallel (Fig. 3). There has been no consensus as to the optimal number of pins, although most authors report successful use of three or four pins or screws for both nondisplaced and displaced fractures. Nonunion and osteonecrosis are uncommon complications following nondisplaced fracture, with nonunion occurring in less than 5% of cases and osteonecrosis in less than 10%.

Treatment of displaced femoral neck fractures remains controversial. Most authors advocate closed or open reduction and internal fixation in younger active patients, and primary prosthetic replacement in older, less active patients. There is general agreement that when internal fixation is chosen, achieving anatomic reduction is probably the most important factor in avoiding healing complications. An acceptable reduction may have up to 15° of valgus angulation and less than 10° of anterior or posterior angulation. Prompt reduction of displaced fractures has been advocated, but has not been shown consistently to decrease the incidence of nonunion or osteonecrosis. If a closed reduction is not acceptable, open reduction is required. Multiple lag screws or pins placed in parallel are most commonly used for internal fixation of displaced fractures. Nonunion and osteonecrosis continue to be problems following displaced femoral neck fracture. The incidence of nonunion has ranged from 10% to 30% and

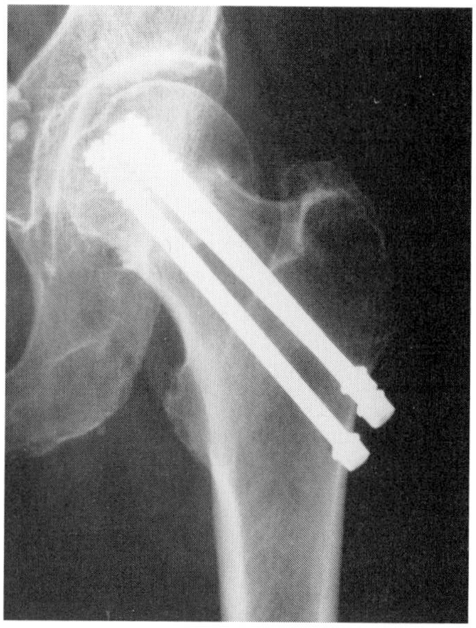

Fig. 3 Impacted femoral neck fracture stabilized with three cannulated cancellous screws.

for osteonecrosis, from 15% to 33%. Capsular distension with increased intracapsular pressure has been implicated as a possible cause of posttraumatic osteonecrosis. However, the clinical usefulness of immediate joint aspiration following femoral neck fracture is unclear. The need for additional surgery following internal fixation of displaced fractures has been variable. Approximately 33% of patients with osteonecrosis will require additional surgery; approximately 75% of patients with nonunion or early fixation failure will require additional surgery.

Prosthetic replacement should be used for the treatment of displaced femoral neck fractures in older and less active patients. Progressive acetabular erosion has been found to be a problem in some series of cemented unipolar hemiarthroplasties; the factors that have best correlated with the severity of acetabular erosion are patient activity level and duration of follow-up. The bipolar prosthesis (a prosthesis with an inner bearing) was designed to decrease the incidence of acetabular erosion (Fig. 4). Although many authors have reported superior results with use of bipolar prostheses compared to unipolar designs, controversy remains regarding the indications for use of the bipolar prosthesis as well as the amount of motion that occurs at its outer and inner surfaces.

The results of primary cemented total hip replacement after femoral neck fracture have been disappointing. At an average follow-up of 56 months, 18 of 37 patients (49%) younger than 70 years of age who had a primary total hip replacement after femoral neck fracture had undergone or were waiting revision surgery. Four more (11%) had definitive radiologic signs of loosening. Activity level correlated with early failure. The results of secondary total hip replacement after failed internal fixation of a femoral neck fracture are reported to be comparable to those obtained after primary arthroplasty for femoral neck fracture.

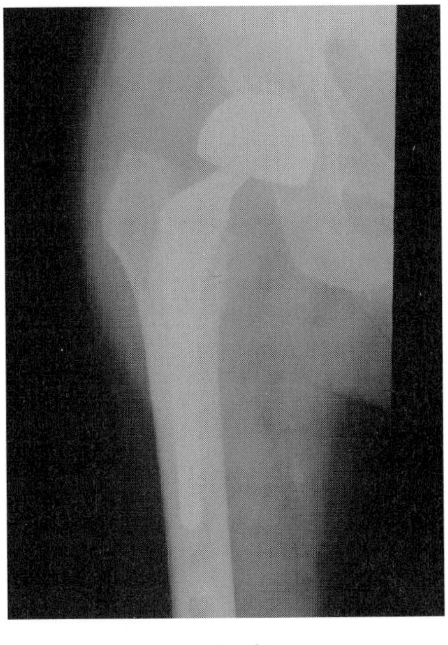

Fig. 4 A cemented bipolar prosthesis.

Young Adults

A femoral neck fracture in a young person is an orthopaedic emergency that requires prompt evaluation and definitive management. Nondisplaced fractures should be stabilized with multiple lag screws or pins. Care should be taken to avoid any loss of reduction during the surgical procedure. Nonunion and osteonecrosis are very uncommon following nondisplaced fractures, except in cases where the fracture was not identified initially. Successful treatment of displaced fractures is related to achieving anatomic reduction and stable internal fixation as soon as possible after the injury. A gentle, closed reduction should be attempted. If the reduction is unacceptable, an open reduction should be performed followed by multiple lag screw or pin fixation. When the principles of prompt anatomic reduction and internal fixation are followed, the incidence of nonunion should be less than 10% and osteonecrosis 20% to 33%.

Special Problems

Neurologically impaired patients include those with Parkinson's disease, previous stroke, and severe dementia. For patients with Parkinson's disease who sustain a femoral neck fracture, both internal fixation and prosthetic replacement have been recommended. The choice of treatment in these patients should be based on patient age, fracture type, and severity of disease. All of these patients require meticulous medical and nursing care to avoid complications. If prosthetic replacement is chosen, correction of a hip adduction contracture by tenotomy and an anterior surgical approach should be considered. Both measures may decrease the risk of dislocation. Patients with a previous stroke are at increased risk for hip fractures, primarily because of residual balance and gait problems and osteoporosis of the paretic limb. Treatment approach depends on fracture type and functional status. When the fracture occurs within 1 week of the stroke, poor functional recovery can be anticipated. If prosthetic replacement is chosen, hip contractures may require tenotomy, and an anterior approach may be preferred. Institutionalized patients with severe dementia present a particular challenge. In-hospital mortality has been reported as high as 50%. Nondisplaced fractures should be treated by internal fixation. Prosthetic replacement for displaced fractures should be performed through an anterior approach to decrease the risk of dislocation and infection from wound contamination in incontinent patients. For nonambulatory patients with severe dementia who do not experience significant discomfort from the injury, nonsurgical management with early bed to chair mobilization should be considered.

Femoral neck fractures in patients with rheumatoid arthritis are associated with an increased incidence of complications. In general, nondisplaced fractures can be successfully treated by internal fixation. Prosthetic replacement is generally recommended for displaced femoral neck fractures. If significant acetabular degeneration is present, total hip arthroplasty is indicated. Femoral neck fractures are very uncommon in patients with underlying osteoarthritis of the hip. When they do occur, total hip arthroplasty is preferred.

Patients with chronic renal disease or hyperparathyroidism who have femoral neck fractures (nondisplaced and displaced) are at increased risk for complications of internal fixation because of associated metabolic bone disease. In these patients, cemented primary prosthetic replacement is recommended.

Femoral neck fractures in patients with Paget disease should be carefully evaluated because of the potential for preexisting acetabular degeneration and deformity of the proximal femur. Nondisplaced fractures can be treated with internal fixation. For displaced fractures, prosthetic replacement is preferred. If there were prefracture symptoms of hip pain in the presence of acetabular degeneration, total hip arthroplasty is preferred; if acetabular degeneration is not present, cemented hemiarthroplasty may be performed. Deformity of the proximal femur and the tendency for excessive bleeding are technical difficulties often encountered.

Femoral neck fractures that occur as a result of metastatic disease require prosthetic replacement. With involvement of the entire proximal femur, a calcar or proximal femoral replacement may be necessary. For patients with acetabular involvement, a cemented acetabular component should be used. If acetabular involvement is extensive, portions of the ilium may have to be reconstructed using methylmethacrylate, wire mesh, and specialized acetabular components. Before performing prosthetic replacement for pathologic fractures of the proximal femur, it is important to identify any metastatic lesions that may be present in the femoral shaft. This will decrease the risk of intraoperative fracture or shaft perforation.

Intertrochanteric Fractures

Intertrochanteric fractures occur with approximately the same frequency as femoral neck fractures in patients with similar demographic characteristics. The most important aspect of fracture classification is determination of stability. Stability is provided by the presence of an intact posteromedial cortical buttress. Unstable fracture patterns include those with loss of the posteromedial buttress, intertrochanteric fractures with subtrochanteric extension, and reverse obliquity fractures.

Sliding Hip Screw

The sliding hip screw is the implant of choice for the treatment of both stable and unstable intertrochanteric fractures (Fig. 5). Sliding hip screw sideplate angles are available in 5° increments from 130° to 150°. The 135° plate is utilized most commonly; this angle is easier to insert in the desired central position of the femoral head and neck than higher angle devices. In addition, the insertion point is in metaphyseal bone, which produces less of a stress riser than the diaphyseal insertion point required for the 150° plate. Clinical studies have not shown a significant difference in the amount of sliding and impaction between these two plate angles.

The most important aspect of sliding hip screw insertion is secure placement of the screw within the proximal fragment. This requires insertion of the screw to within 1 cm of the subchondral bone. A central position within the femoral head and neck is recommended most commonly. If a central position is not possible, a posteroinferior position is preferred. Anterosuperior positions should be avoided because the bone is weakest in this area, thereby increasing the likelihood of superior screw cut out.

The necessity of a medial displacement osteotomy with use of the sliding hip screw remains controversial. Because the sliding hip screw allows controlled fracture collapse, unstable fractures anatomically reduced can be expected to impact into a stable pattern that is often medially displaced. This collapse usually results in less shortening of the extremity than a formal medial displacement osteotomy. In recent clinical studies comparing medial displacement to anatomic reduction for unstable fractures, no advantage of medial displacement over anatomic reduction was found.

Use of the sliding hip screw for intertrochanteric fractures is associated with a 4% to 12% incidence of loss of fixation. This most commonly occurs in unstable fractures

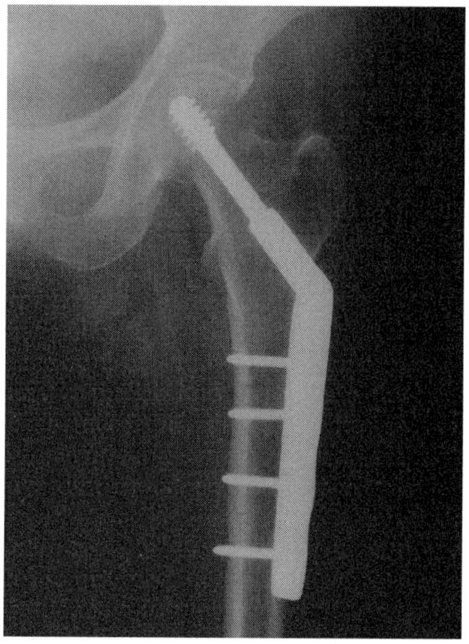

Fig. 5 An anteroposterior radiograph of a stable intertrochanteric fracture stabilized with a sliding hip screw. The screw is positioned in the center of the femoral head and neck, within 1 cm of the joint.

with severe osteopenia. Most fixation failures can be attributed to technical problems that involve poor fracture reduction and screw placement. Although the sliding hip screw allows postoperative fracture impaction, it is essential to obtain an impacted reduction at the time of surgery. This procedure avoids excessive collapse postoperatively that may exceed the sliding capacity of the device. If screw sliding brings the screw threads in contact with the plate barrel, additional impaction will not be possible and the device becomes the biomechanical equivalent of a rigid nail–plate.

Methylmethacrylate has been advocated as adjunctive fixation in extremely osteoporotic, unstable fractures treated with a sliding hip screw. Currently, however, its routine use with sliding hip screw fixation for nonpathologic fractures is not recommended.

Intramedullary Devices

The results of Ender nailing for intertrochanteric fractures have been variable and, in general, disappointing. Complication rates have ranged from 16% to 71%, with the most common being varus deformity, knee pain caused by distal migration of the nails, and external rotation deformity. Early repeated surgery has been required in up to 19% of cases. The highest complication rates were reported when these devices were used for unstable fractures.

The Gamma nail is an intramedullary nail/sliding hip screw device that has been used for the treatment of intertrochanteric hip fractures (Fig. 6). Its theoretical advantages are both technical (limited exposure, closed insertion, reduced operating room time, decreased blood loss) and mechanical (shorter lever arm and bending moment on the device due to its intramedullary design) compared to the sliding hip screw. However, most studies comparing the Gamma nail to a sliding hip screw have found no differences with respect to time in surgery, duration of hospital stay, infection rate or wound complications, implant failure, screw cut out, or screw sliding. However, patients treated with the Gamma nail were at increased risk of femoral shaft fracture at the distal nail tip and the insertion sites of the distal locking bolts. The Gamma nail may be best used in the treatment of comminuted intertrochanteric fractures with subtrochanteric extension, reverse obliquity fractures, and high subtrochanteric fractures.

A biomechanical evaluation of the Gamma nail in an experimentally created stable and unstable intertrochanteric fracture model was recently reported. The Gamma nail was shown to transmit decreasing load to the calcar with decreasing fracture stability. Virtually no strain on the bone was seen in four-part fractures with the posteromedial fragment removed. Insertion of the distal locking screws did not change the pattern of proximal femoral strain.

Prosthetic Replacement

Prosthetic replacement for intertrochanteric fractures has been used successfully to treat postoperative loss of fixation when repeat open reduction and internal fixation was not possible or desirable. A calcar replacement prosthesis is necessary because of the level of the fracture. Primary prosthetic replacement for comminuted, unstable fractures has also been used successfully in a limited number of patients. The disadvantages include a larger and more extensive surgical procedure and the potential for dislocation. The indications for the use of prosthetic replacement in the treatment of acute intertrochanteric fractures have not been defined; it does not appear to offer any advantages over a properly inserted sliding hip screw. However, prosthetic replacement may be indicated in patients with preexisting hip arthritis, pathologic fractures, or failed internal fixation.

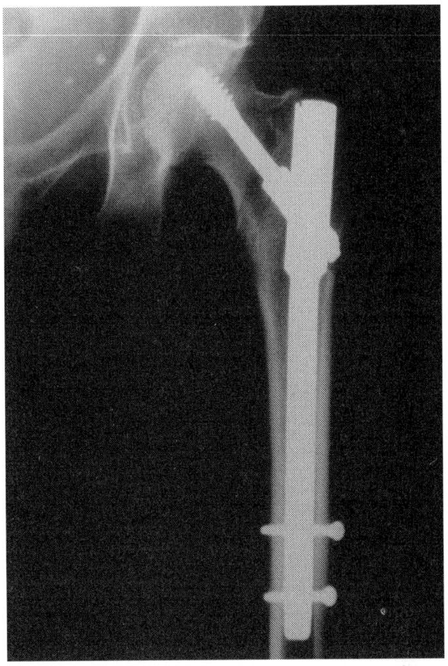

Fig. 6 Stabilization of an intertrochanteric fracture with an intramedullary hip screw.

Subtrochanteric Fractures

Subtrochanteric fractures account for approximately 15% of all proximal femur fractures. These fractures start at or below the lesser trochanter and involve the proximal femoral shaft. They are generally seen in three groups of patients: (1) young patients who are involved in high-energy trauma; (2) older patients with weakened bone whose fracture occurs as a result of a minor fall; and (3) older patients with pathologic or impending pathologic fractures from metastatic disease. The subtrochanteric area experiences some of the highest biomechanical stresses in the body. The medial and posteromedial cortex is a site of high compressive forces, while the lateral cortex experiences high tensile stresses. This stress distribution has important implications in fracture fixation and healing.

Various classification systems have been proposed, but as yet, none has been universally accepted. As in intertrochanteric fractures, fracture stability is based on the presence or absence of a posteromedial buttress. In stable fractures, medial and posteromedial cortical support is intact or can be reestablished. In unstable fractures, comminution results in loss of medial cortical continuity. These fractures are at highest risk for healing complications and implant failure.

The interlocking reconstruction nail is the implant of choice for subtrochanteric femur fractures (Fig. 7). Essentially all nonpathologic subtrochanteric fractures can be stabilized with interlocking nails, regardless of the fracture pattern or degree of comminution. Favorable mechanical characteristics of interlocking nails have eliminated the requirement of surgically reconstituting the medial femoral cortex. High rates of union with both first and second generation interlocking nails have been reported in large series of subtrochanteric femur fractures.

The sliding hip screw has also been used, particularly in low-energy subtrochanteric fractures in the elderly; a 95% rate of union was reported for one series. For this device to function optimally, the sliding component of the device must cross the fracture site. Therefore, subtrochanteric-intertrochanteric fractures are most suitable for use of a sliding hip screw. More distal fractures can be stabilized using a 95° fixed angle device: the condylar blade plate or screw. These devices provide improved fixation of the proximal fragment and act as a lateral tension band if the medial cortex is intact. The condylar screw is technically easier to insert than the blade plate; similar results with use of either device for the treatment of subtrochanteric fractures have been reported for recent series. Complication rates up to 20% have been reported after use of these 95° implants; complications usually are related to an inability to restore the medial femoral cortex. The surgeon may be able to minimize the risk of complications through use of indirect reduction techniques. If significant medial cortical comminution or soft-tissue stripping is present, bone grafting should be performed.

Postoperative management depends on the fracture pattern and the method of fixation. For subtrochanteric-intertrochanteric fractures treated with a sliding hip screw that allows fracture impaction, early weightbearing can be allowed. Stable fractures treated with intramedullary devices can also be treated with early weightbearing. Fractures with medial or segmental comminution must be protected, regardless of the device used, for at least 6 to 8 weeks until early healing is evident.

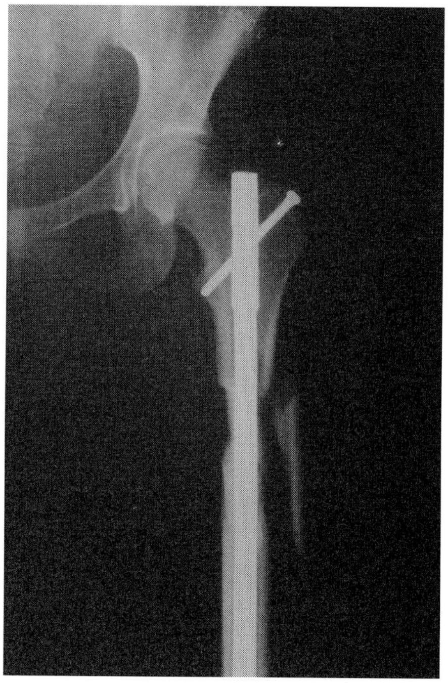

Fig. 7 Subtrochanteric femur fracture stabilized with an interlocked intramedullary nail.

Pathologic fractures and impending pathologic fractures in the subtrochanteric region have been treated successfully using interlocking nails, both with and without adjunctive methylmethacrylate. These devices provide the benefits of proximal fixation and an intramedullary rod that can bridge more distal lesions.

Annotated Bibliography

Hip Dislocation

Dreinhofer KE, Schwarzkopf SR, Haas NP, et al: Isolated traumatic dislocation of the hip: Long-term results in 50 patients. *J Bone Joint Surg* 1994;76B:6–12.

Fifty hip dislocations without fracture (12 anterior, 38 posterior) were retrospectively reviewed; 37 had a closed reduction within 3 hours of injury. No statistically significant difference in results was found between dislocations reduced in less than 1 hour and those that had a delay of 1 to 6 hours. The important factors affecting long-term prognosis were the direction of dislocation and the overall severity of injury.

Moed BR, Maxey JW: Evaluation of fractures of the femoral head using the CT-directed pelvic oblique radiograph. *Clin Orthop* 1993;296:161–167.

Ten patients with femoral head fractures were evaluated using conventional radiographs, CT scan, and a CT-directed pelvic oblique radiograph. The CT-directed pelvic oblique radiograph was found to be the most accurate determinant of the extent of fracture displacement and joint congruity. In addition, similar radiographs, reproducible from one examination to the next, could be used to assess progression of fracture healing.

Hip Fractures

Lauritzen JB, Petersen MM, Lund B: Effect of external hip protectors on hip fractures. *Lancet* 1993;341:11–13.

Ten of 28 wards in a nursing home were randomized to receive external hip protectors. Over an 11-month period, there were eight hip and 15 nonhip fractures in the hip protector group and 31 hip and 27 nonhip fractures in the control group. None of the eight residents in the intervention group who had a hip fracture was wearing the device at the time of fracture. The authors concluded that external hip protectors can be used to prevent hip fractures in nursing home residents.

Needoff M, Radford P, Langstaff R: Preoperative traction for hip fractures in the elderly: A clinical trial. *Injury* 1993;24:317–318.

Sixty-seven mentally competent patients who suffered a femoral neck fracture were randomly assigned to receive either 2.5 kg preoperative skin traction or no traction. Using pain assessment scales and records of analgesic consumption, there was found to be little difference between the two groups. The authors concluded that preoperative skin traction offers no benefits in pain control for the patient who suffers a femoral neck fracture and, therefore, should not be used routinely.

Rizzo PF, Gould ES, Lyden JP, et al: Diagnosis of occult fractures about the hip: Magnetic resonance imaging compared with bone-scanning. *J Bone Joint Surg* 1993; 75A:395–401.

MRI and bone scanning were performed in 62 patients in whom a fracture about the hip was clinically suspected, but not radiographically evident. MRI was performed within 24 hours of hospital admission; bone scanning was performed within 72 hours of hospital admission. MRI was as accurate as bone scanning in the detection of occult hip fractures.

Functional Recovery

Koval KJ, Skovron ML, Aharonoff GB, et al: Ambulatory ability after hip fracture: A prospective study in geriatric patients. *Clin Orthop* 1995;310:150–159.

Of 336 community dwelling, ambulatory, geriatric hip fracture patients followed up prospectively to determine ambulatory ability at 1-year minimum follow-up, 137 (40.8%) maintained their prefracture ambulatory ability, and 134 (39.9%) remained either community or household ambulators but became more dependent on assistive devices. Factors predictive of a patient regaining preinjury level of ambulation were age less than 85 years, poorer prefracture ambulatory ability, ASA rating of operative risk 1 or 2, and intertrochanteric fracture.

Ogilvie-Harris DJ, Botsford DJ, Hawker RW: Elderly patients with hip fractures: Improved outcome with the use of care maps with high-quality medical and nursing protocols. *J Orthop Trauma* 1993;7:428–437.

A prospective cohort study was performed on 106 elderly hip fracture patients. Fifty-one had standard nursing and medical treatment and 55 had a more intensive and standardized protocol involving both medical and nursing personnel. Patients in the study group had a statistically better outcome at 6-month follow-up and statistically fewer postoperative complications.

Thorngren KG, Ceder L, Svensson K: Predicting results of rehabilitation after hip fracture: A ten-year follow-up study. *Clin Orthop* 1993;287:76–81.

One hundred and three consecutive home dwelling hip fracture patients older than 50 years were followed for 10 years postfracture. The three most important variables for hospital to home discharge were the ability to walk 2 weeks after surgery, living with someone, and general good health. The most important positive variable for continuing to live at home was an active prefracture lifestyle; the most persistent negative variable was older age.

Femoral Neck Fractures

Broeng L, Bergholdt-Hansen L, Sperling K, et al: Postoperative Tc-scintimetry in femoral neck fracture. A prospective study of 46 cases. *Acta Orthop Scand* 1994;65: 171–174.

A prospective study was performed on 46 patients who had an internally stabilized femoral neck fracture (eight nondisplaced, 38 displaced). Healing complications, defined as loss of reduction or segmental collapse, were associated with decreased uptake in early (1 to 3 weeks) and 2-month scintimetry, but the specificity was only 50%. With normal or increased uptake, uncomplicated fracture healing was predictable with 90% to 100% sensitivity.

Intertrochanteric Fractures

Aune AK, Ekeland A, Odegaard B, et al: Gamma nail vs compression screw for trochanteric femoral fractures: 15 reoperations in a prospective, randomized study of 378 patients. *Acta Orthop Scand* 1994;65:127–130.

Three hundred seventy-eight intertrochanteric and subtrochanteric hip fractures were prospectively randomized to treatment with either a Gamma nail (177) or sliding hip screw (201). At a median follow-up of 17 months, 15 patients needed reoperation: 13 treated with a Gamma nail and two with a sliding hip screw. Ten patients, all stabilized with a Gamma nail, had suffered a femoral shaft fracture, either along the nail or at its distal tip.

Blair B, Koval KJ, Kummer F, et al: Basicervical fractures of the proximal femur: A biomechanical study of 3 internal fixation techniques. *Clin Orthop* 1994;306:256–263.

A biomechanical cadaver study was performed to compare the stability and ultimate strength of three standard fixation techniques used for the treatment of basicervical hip fractures: (1) three parallel 6.5-mm cannulated cancellous screws; (2) a 135° sliding hip screw with a four-hole side plate; and (3) a 135° sliding hip screw with a four-hole side plate and an additional 6.5-mm cannulated cancellous screw placed proximal and parallel to the sliding screw. The group instrumented with the multiple cancellous screws had a significantly lower ultimate axial load to failure than either sliding hip screw group.

Desjardins AL, Roy A, Paiement G, et al: Unstable intertrochanteric fracture of the femur: A prospective randomised study comparing anatomical reduction and medial displacement osteotomy. *J Bone Joint Surg* 1993; 75B:445–447.

A prospective randomized study was performed on 127 consecutive patients who had an unstable intertrochanteric hip fracture, to compare the results of anatomic reduction to medial displacement osteotomy. At an average follow-up of 11 months, no difference was found in walking ability or incidence of fixation failure. However, time in surgery and blood loss were significantly higher in the osteotomy group.

Gehrchen PM, Nielsen JO, Olesen B: Poor reproducibility of Evans' classification of the trochanteric fracture: Assessment of 4 observers in 52 cases. *Acta Orthop Scand* 1993;64:71–72.

Radiographs of 52 consecutive intertrochanteric hip fractures were assessed by four observers using the Evans' classification. Only 23 of 52 radiographs were classified identically by all four observers. When assessing only stability, the four observers agreed in only 34 of 52 cases.

Subtrochanteric Fractures

Mullaji AB, Thomas TL: Low-energy subtrochanteric fractures in elderly patients: Results of fixation with the sliding screw plate. *J Trauma* 1993;34:56–61.

Thirty-one patients older than age 70 years who suffered a low energy subtrochanteric hip fracture were internally stabilized using a sliding hip screw. Of patients alive at 6-month follow-up, 91% had successful union.

Classic Bibliography

Hip Dislocations and Fractures

Cummings SR, Phillips SL, Wheat ME, et al: Recovery of function after hip fracture: The role of social supports. *J Am Geriatr Soc* 1988;36:801–806.

Kenzora JE, McCarthy RE, Lowell JD, et al: Hip fracture mortality: Relation to age, treatment, preoperative illness, time of surgery and complications. *Clin Orthop* 1984;186: 45–56.

Magaziner J, Simonsick EM, Kashner TM, et al: Predictors of functional recovery one year following hospital discharge for hip fracture: A prospective study. *J Gerontol* 1990;45:M101–M107.

Patterson BM, Cornell CN, Carbone B, et al: Protein depletion and metabolic stress in elderly patients who have a fracture of the hip. *J Bone Joint Surg* 1992;74A:251–260.

Swiontkowski MF, Thorpe M, Seiler JG, et al: Operative management of displaced femoral head fractures: Case-matched comparison of anterior versus posterior approaches for Pipkin I and Pipkin II fractures. *J Orthop Trauma* 1992;6:437–442.

Zuckerman JD, Sakales SR, Fabian DR, et al: Hip fractures in geriatric patients: Results of an interdisciplinary hospital care group. *Clin Orthop* 1992;274:213–225.

Femoral Neck Fractures

Garden RS: Malreduction and avascular necrosis in subcapital fractures of the femur. *J Bone Joint Surg* 1971;53B:183–197.

Pearse MF, Bande S, O'Dwyer KJ, et al: The Exeter bipolar prosthesis in the active elderly patient: The results at 7 years. *Intern Orthop* 1992;16:344–348.

Scheck M: The significance of posterior comminution in femoral neck fractures. *Clin Orthop* 1980;152:138–142.

Intertrochanteric Fractures

Chang WS, Zuckerman JD, Kummer FJ, et al: Biomechanical evaluation of anatomic reduction versus medial displacement osteotomy in unstable intertrochanteric fractures. *Clin Orthop* 1987;225:141–146.

Dimon JH, Hughston JC: Unstable intertrochanteric fractures of the hip. *J Bone Joint Surg* 1967;49A:440–450.

Hopkins CT, Nugent JT, Dimon JH III: Medial displacement osteotomy for unstable intertrochanteric fractures: Twenty years later. *Clin Orthop* 1989;245:169–172.

Kyle RF, Gustilo RB, Premer RF: Analysis of six hundred and twenty-two intertrochanteric hip fractures. *J Bone Joint Surg* 1979;61A:216–221.

Leung KS, So WS, Shen WY, et al: Gamma nails and dynamic hip screws for pertrochanteric fractures: A randomised prospective study in elderly patients. *J Bone Joint Surg* 1992;74B:345–351.

Meislin RJ, Zuckerman JD, Kummer FJ, et al: A biochemical analysis of the sliding hip screw: The question of plate angle. *J Orthop Trauma* 1990;4:130–136.

Rosenblum SF, Zuckerman JD, Kummer FJ, et al: A biomechanical evaluation of the Gamma nail. *J Bone Joint Surg* 1992;74B:352–357.

Subtrochanteric Fractures

Ovadia DN, Chess JL: Intraoperative and postoperative subtrochanteric fracture of the femur associated with removal of the Zickel nail. *J Bone Joint Surg* 1988;70A: 239–243.

Winquist RA, Hansen ST Jr, Clawson DK: Closed intramedullary nailing of femoral fractures: A report of five hundred and twenty cases. *J Bone Joint Surg* 1984; 66A:529–539.

Wiss DA, Brien WW: Subtrochanteric fractures of the femur: Results of treatment by interlocking nailing. *Clin Orthop* 1992;283:231–236.

36

Hip and Pelvis: Reconstruction

Evaluation of the Hip

Clinical Assessment

All hips should be carefully checked for range of motion in flexion–extension, abduction–adduction, and internal and external rotation, with motion-associated pain noted. Loss of internal rotation is often the first demonstrable abnormality on physical examination of the arthritic patient. In later stages, fixed flexion or adduction contracture is common and should be noted.

One of the most frequent causes of patient dissatisfaction after hip surgery is unexpected change in limb length, particularly lengthening after total hip replacement arthroplasty or shortening after varus osteotomy. Leg lengths should be measured from both the umbilicus and the anterior–superior iliac spine to each medial malleolus. Accurate clinical measurements require compensation for ipsilateral contractures by placing the opposite limb in a comparable position. When significant discrepancies exist between true and apparent leg length measurements, quantitative scanograms can be obtained. Scanograms are also helpful when the position of the anterior–superior iliac spine has been altered by prior surgery or trauma. Functional leg length inequality can be documented by placing blocks under the shorter limb until the pelvis is level or the tendency of the knees to bend is equalized.

Abductor strength should be evaluated with the patient lying on the opposite side and elevating the examined limb. Although subtle weakness may manifest itself as a limp only after prolonged muscular activity, significant weakness results in a constant limp and is not necessarily associated with discomfort. The major causes of limp include pain, leg length inequality, and abductor weakness. It is not uncommon for more than one to be present in the same hip.

During examination of the hip, maneuvers or positions that either produce or relieve pain, or provoke clicking or snapping, provide potentially important clinical information. For instance, the regular demonstration of a click or pain with combined flexion, adduction, and internal rotation or in extension and simultaneous external rotation may strongly suggest a torn labrum. Presence of pain with abduction may signify impingement, either due to osteophytes or to a high-riding greater trochanter. Conversely, relief of pain in flexion or abduction or adduction can be used to identify a so-called "position of comfort" in prospective osteotomy candidates. Active strength of the limb in straight leg raising should be noted.

Sensory and motor integrity of the femoral and sciatic nerves should be documented before any hip procedure and rechecked as soon as possible after surgery. The presence of pulses in the foot should be documented in the same way.

Radiographic Assessment

Routine plain radiographs of the hip should include an anteroposterior (AP) radiograph of the pelvis, as well as AP and lateral views of the involved side. In dysplastic hips, the false profile radiograph is extremely useful. It is an oblique of the pelvis and true lateral of the upper femur taken in the standing position, and it allows better visualization of anterior coverage of the femoral head than any other plain radiographic view. Also in dysplasia, an AP radiograph in abduction and internal rotation is useful in screening patients for rotational pelvic osteotomy. Acceptable candidates for the procedure should demonstrate good centering of the femoral head and congruent opposing surfaces on this view (Fig. 1). AP views of the involved hip in abduction and adduction help to identify positions of increased or decreased impingement and congruency; both are useful parameters in selecting patients for osteotomy procedures. AP views of the hip should be centered over the hip and include enough of the upper femur to plan surgery.

Plain arthrography of the hip is seldom used in adult hip evaluations. In experienced hands, it can be useful in screening for tears of the acetabular labrum. Fluoroscopically controlled diagnostic injection of the hip joint with a short acting anesthetic agent can help separate pain of articular origin from pain with other causes.

Computed tomography (CT) scans may be useful to assess for loose bodies and incongruities of the joint surfaces when plain films are inconclusive. A CT scan may be necessary if three-dimensional (3-D) reconstruction is needed. An arthrogram combined with the CT is occasionally effective in allowing visualization of a torn or detached acetabular labrum. A CT scan can also be used to quantify anteversion and to quantify parameters of axial rotation, ie, distal femoral, upper tibial, and ankle rotation in the same limb.

Alternatives to Total Hip Arthroplasty

Arthrodesis

Arthrodesis is indicated in severe posttraumatic and postinfectious unilateral arthritis in young, otherwise healthy patients and in cases of severe, premature developmental arthropathies. Active infection, whether bacterial or from

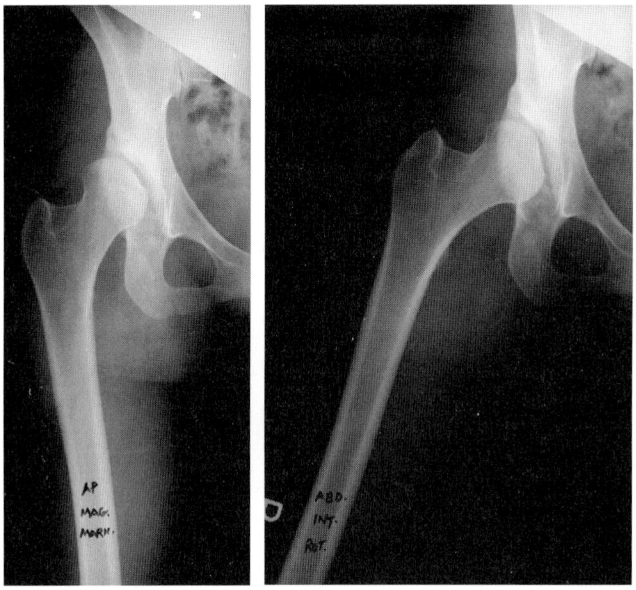

Fig. 1 **Left,** Anteroposterior (AP) radiograph of high-grade dysplasia with minimal arthritic deterioration. Radiographic appearance indicates an additional radiograph in AP internal rotation to verify centering of the hip. **Right,** Abduction internal rotation AP radiograph confirms suitability for rotational osteotomy.

other microorganisms, is a contraindication. Less frequent indications include end-stage failed arthroplasties and pelvic sarcoma resections. Unilateral arthrodesis has been shown to increase oxygen consumption in normal gait by 32%. Successful rehabilitation from arthrodesis permits return to full-time employment, including heavy labor that does not involve running. Nonunions (22% to 47%) were a major problem prior to the introduction of rigid, stable internal fixation. Although the classic Cobra plate technique included transiliac osteotomy and detachment of the abductors from the greater trochanter, these aspects of the original technique are no longer routinely used because transiliac osteotomy complicates acetabular cup placement in future total hip surgery, and preservation of abductor function is important for future conversion to total hip arthroplasty (THA). The Cobra plate can be used without transiliac osteotomy by performing trochanteric osteotomy and reattaching the greater trochanter over the plate. Successful use of other techniques, including multiple transarticular bolts, multiple compression screws, and transarticular hip nails, has been reported. Nonunion rates with the Cobra plate are very low (0% to 8%) according to several major reports.

The preferred position for a fused hip is 20° to 25° of flexion, neutral adduction, and neutral rotation. Up to 5° of adduction and 15° of external rotation can be tolerated. Deliberate abduction and internal rotation are to be avoided. Less than 20° of flexion makes sitting too difficult, and greater than 25° of flexion compromises walking and creates excessive apparent limb shortening as well as excessive lumbar lordosis.

In general, normal low back and ipsilateral knee function are considered prerequisites for patient selection. However, in one series, 49% of patients reported improvement in low back symptoms 4 to 5 years after surgery. After successful arthrodesis, over 20 years of good function can be anticipated in the majority of patients. Several excellent long-term reviews with 20- to 30-year follow-up have documented high patient satisfaction (comparable in men and women) with regard to pain relief, ability to work, and sexual function.

Every arthrodesis should be performed with anticipation of a need for eventual conversion to THA. The best indication for conversion of hip fusion to THA is severe low back pain. Thirty years after arthrodesis approximately 60% of patients have significant low back symptoms. Unfortunately high failure rates (20% to 33%) have been reported within 7 years of conversion of a surgically arthrodesed hip to THA. However, conversion of a spontaneously arthrodesed hip to THA has a natural history comparable to primary THA with regard to failure rate and complication rate. The high failure rates appear to apply only to surgically created fusions.

Ipsilateral knee arthritis, which occurs in approximately 50% of patients 30 years after fusion, can be treated with total knee replacement arthroplasty (TKA) independent of takedown of the hip fusion. If takedown and TKA are both deemed necessary, the hip surgery should precede the knee surgery. This order permits both flexion of the hips and better control of knee alignment. Range of motion of THAs after arthrodesis averaged 70° to 87° in several large series, with regard to total arc of motion in the flexion plane.

Hip Arthroscopy

Current indications for hip arthroscopy include suspected acetabular labral tears, loose bodies, and infection. In a series of 59 patients who had no prior surgery; had pain, click, or locking; and were unresponsive to prior treatment for up to 2 years, 35 (59%) had labral tears, which were most often anterior in location, and 29 (39%) had intra-articular loose bodies. Other findings included degenerative arthritis in 18 (30%) and a chondral defect on either the acetabular or femoral side in 16 (27%).

There was very poor correlation between imaging studies (magnetic resonance imaging, CT, and arthrogram-CT) and surgical findings. Only two of the 35 patients with arthroscopically proven labral tears had imaging studies (arthrograms) that suggested a tear. Magnetic resonance imaging (MRI) did not detect a single labral tear. Imaging studies were better for loose bodies, detecting them in 10 of 23 cases (43%). CT and MRI did not detect any nonossified loose bodies. Chondral defects found in 16 patients, usually in association with the labral tear or degenerative arthritis, were not detected by any imaging study.

In patients with arthroscopically proven labral tears,

there was a much stronger correlation with history and physical examination findings than with imaging studies; 90% of patients reported an intermittently painful click, 70% giving way, and 57% locking episodes. Similarly, patients with loose bodies had an 87% correlation with locking episodes reported during preoperative history. Overall, for 76% of the patients, no radiographic test contributed to a definitive preoperative diagnosis. These results should decrease reliance on MRI and CT as definitive diagnostic modalities.

In another report, arthroscopy of the hip was successfully used to drain and debride septic hips in four cases with results equivalent to open arthrotomy, but with much lower morbidity.

Osteotomies

Pelvic Osteotomies Osteotomies can be grouped into two categories: reconstructive and salvage. Reconstructive osteotomies correct significant architectural abnormalities associated with minimal clinical symptoms and no radiographic evidence of secondary arthritis. A result lasting decades is possible, and the need for THA may be permanently eliminated.

A salvage osteotomy is done for similar architectural abnormalities, but is associated with significant symptoms and radiographic evidence of arthritic deterioration (joint space narrowing, osteophytes, cysts, and femoral head deformity). The goals and expectations are more limited: reduction in pain, maintenance of or modest improvement in function, and postponement of THA for a finite but important period of time.

Over the last 3 to 5 years, a strong shift towards pelvic osteotomies in the treatment of adults with the sequelae of developmental dysplasia has resulted from long-term European success and the evolution of techniques that permit multidirectional correction combined with medial displacement of the hip center. There are no data from controlled, prospective studies in which adult patients with or without surgical treatment for dysplasia are compared. Thus, the decision to recommend major osteotomy surgery for an adult who is just beginning to have symptoms is a difficult one.

When surgery is necessary, rotational osteotomy of the acetabulum, rather than intertrochanteric osteotomy of the upper femur, should be performed whenever possible for the management of moderate to high-grade dysplasia. As a general rule, these procedures should be reserved for cases in which the center edge angle of Wiberg is less than 10°. When concomitant valgus of the femoral neck shaft angle is greater than 145°, adjunctive varus or varus extension osteotomy of the femur should also be considered.

For rotational pelvic osteotomies, a congruent, mobile hip with minimal or no degenerative changes is preferable. Where mild subluxation is present in addition to the dysplasia, centering of the femoral head into the socket on the abduction and internal rotation view is an important radiographic selection criterion for candidates. Until the advent of the false profile view (Fig. 2), the magnitude of anterior coverage deficiency was not appreciated, except at the time of surgery.

Among the pelvic osteotomies, the periacetabular osteotomy developed in the mid 1980s appears to offer the most advantages, preserving the integrity of the posterior column by isolating the acetabulum and its surrounding bone from the ilium, ischium, and pubis. Both rotational correction in three dimensions and medial displacement are possible, providing an advantage that sets this operation apart from the classic dome and other rotational osteotomies. The operation requires careful study and preoperative preparation and is technically challenging. Significant vascular and nerve injuries, as well as intra-articular fracture, can occur and must be avoided. Because of the free mobility of the fragment, overcorrection is as frequent a problem as undercorrection. Furthermore, retroversion or anteversion of the acetabulum can occur and must be carefully avoided by using intraoperative radiographs.

Recent data indicate that approximately 20% of patients require some form of major subsequent reconstructive procedure within 5 years of the index osteotomy, with results corresponding to the status of the joint at the time of surgery; patients who have moderate to severe arthrosis at the time of osteotomy have a much higher short-term failure rate. Patients with minimal evidence of joint space loss or arthrosis do much better during the first 5-year follow-up interval. The triple innominate osteotomy is associated with fewer intraoperative or perioperative complications than the periacetabular osteotomy. This relative safety factor is offset by several disadvantages, including complete transection of the ilium, greater resistance to movement of the fragment, and longer healing time.

Salvage Osteotomy The Chiari osteotomy, as a salvage procedure, still has a role in subluxing painful hips that do not satisfy criteria for rotational reconstructive osteotomy. The Chiari osteotomy is a type of shelf arthroplasty. Displacement of the fragment anteriorly, as well as laterally, is desirable. Because the true width of the ilium narrows dramatically proximal to the immediate subchondral region of the acetabulum, the bone cut should be as close to the joint capsule as possible. When the femoral head is subluxed proximally, very little bone actually is available for coverage. Degenerative arthritis is common after Chiari osteotomy. Many of the long-term follow-up reports in the literature are based on the use of Chiari osteotomy in skeletally immature patients for whom rotational reconstructive procedures would now be performed instead. The authors of one review of 500 Chiari osteotomies have suggested that the procedure be abandoned whenever reconstructive rotational osteotomy is possible. Approximately 50% of their cases involved combining valgus upper femoral osteotomy with the Chiari osteotomy; the combined procedure resulted in a significant improvement in long-term results.

The Chiari osteotomy makes the acetabular portion of

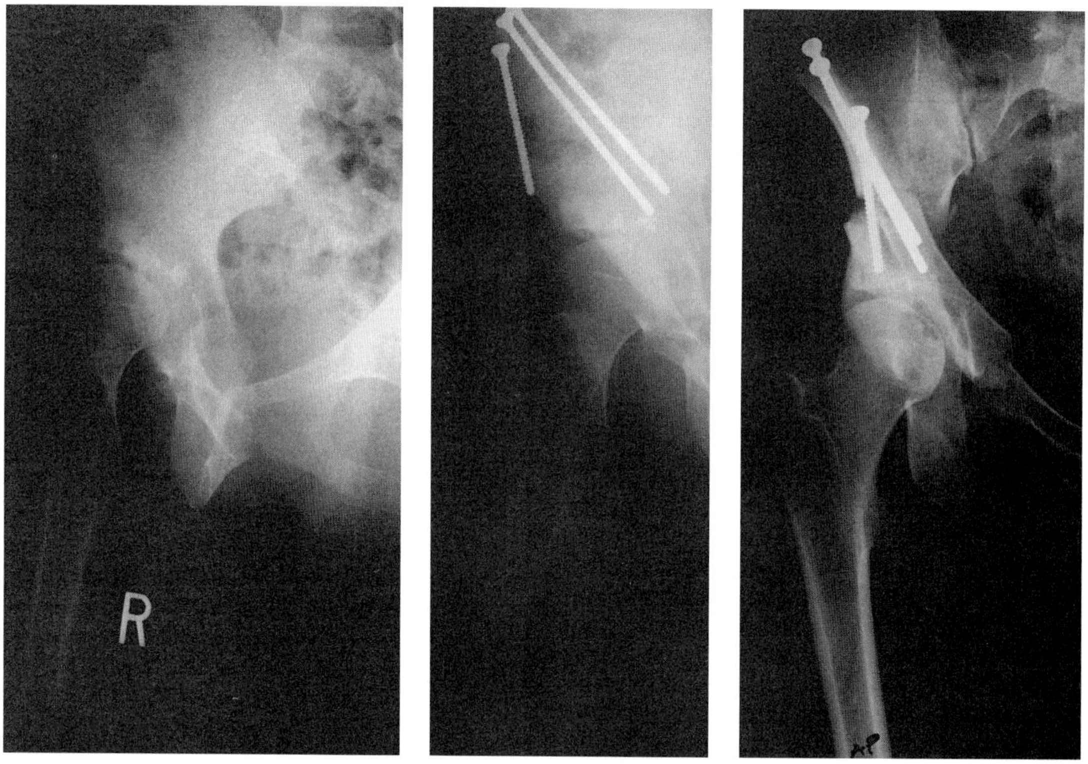

Fig. 2 **Left,** The false profile radiograph of Lesquene demonstrates deficiency of acetabular converage anteriorly; it is similar to the iliac oblique radiograph for assessment of pelvic fractures. The false profile represents a true lateral of the femur and an oblique of the pelvis. **Center,** Enhancement of anterior coverage after rotational periacetabular osteotomy. **Right,** Anteroposterior (AP) projection after periacetabular rotational osteotomy.

THA much more difficult. Widening of the medial-lateral dimension encourages overreaming of the more critical anterior and posterior walls. This problem is not true of rotational pelvic osteotomies, which actually facilitate conversion to THA. A common consequence of Chiari osteotomy is abductor weakness and limping. The factors responsible for the limp include the surgical stripping of the rectus and gluteal muscles from the lateral ilium wall, lateral translation to the abductor origin, verticalization of the abductor lever arm vector, and shortening of the muscle mass. Minimal surgical dissection and careful repair are important at the time of original surgery. In an otherwise satisfactory result, trochanteric lateral and distal transfer is indicated as a secondary procedure.

Femoral Osteotomies The ability to reverse a hip flexion contracture, to correct rotational imbalance, and to lengthen or shorten an extremity are particular assets of the femoral osteotomy, which cannot be duplicated as well or as easily during pelvic osteotomy. In general, the recovery time is 4 to 6 months before return to work at moderately demanding occupations. Return to work, with the use of two crutches, is possible within 5 to 6 weeks after surgery. Good mobility of the hip (at least 60° in the flexion arc), absence of osteopenia, and young age are favorable selection factors.

Valgus Intertrochanteric Osteotomy Valgus osteotomy repositions the proximal fragment as if the extremity were placed in adduction, positioning the distal fragment as if it were abducted at the osteotomy site. Valgus combined with extension in the sagittal plane is equivalent to extension of the distal fragment on the proximal fragment at the osteotomy site. Indications in osteoarthritis include dysplasia with mushroom cap deformity of the femoral head associated with at least 15° of passive adduction, improved radiographic appearance in adduction, and a favorable position of comfort test. Comfort in adduction refers to a patient's subjective response to passive adduction of the extremity during examination while lying supine on an examination table. It is further tested by having the patient stand with the ipsilateral foot adducted over the midline and placed lateral to the opposite foot. The patient is asked to stand and to walk in this position. This information should favorably correlate with the appearance of the plain AP radiograph in adduction and the morphology of the patient's problem. As an example, in a patient with post Perthes hinged abduction, passive abduction should provoke discomfort and meet resistance. Conversely, passive adduction should be well tolerated, or preferred, and the radiograph in adduction should show improvement, compared to the neutral AP view and the view in abduction.

Other indications for valgus osteotomy include nonunion of the femoral neck, acquired varus deformity, certain cases of osteonecrosis, and hinged abduction impingement as a sequela of Perthes disease. Valgus osteotomies inherently lengthen the femur. This lengthening can be offset by appropriate wedge resection; however, even full wedge resection is often insufficient to prevent unintended lengthening, and an addition block resection may be necessary.

Varus Intertrochanteric Osteotomy Varus is equivalent to abduction of the extremity at the hip level, or adduction of the distal fragment at the osteotomy level. Indications include coxa valga subluxans or high valgus neck shaft angle in a patient who has dysplasia associated with a round, congruent femoral head, at least 15° of passive abduction, improved radiographic appearance in abduction, and a favorable position of comfort test in abduction. Other indications include certain cases of osteonecrosis and idiopathic osteoarthritis. Varus inherently shortens. Open-hinged techniques can reduce shortening to an absolute minimum when necessary but may prolong healing time. Severe shortening can occur when full wedges are resected. Varus of greater than 20° is rarely indicated.

In one report of over 2,000 angulation intertrochanteric osteotomies, one third of the patients had enduring good results, one third had satisfactory outcome, and one third were failures, most of which occurred in the first 2 to 3 years after surgery. Results for a number of series of angulation osteotomies for arthritis secondary to dysplasia have been reported with good or excellent outcomes in more than 80% of patients at 10 years. In concentric arthritis without evidence of dysplasia osteotomy is less effective, but good results are reported at 5 years in the majority of patients who have had simple medial displacement osteotomies. Most of these patients have had conversion to THA by 8 to 10 years postoperatively. Osteotomy complicates future total hip stem insertion when displacements greater than 5 mm have occurred. This correlates with a higher incidence of intraoperative fracture. Careful preplanning of the osteosynthesis by superimposing THA templates may help to minimize this.

Femoral Neck Nonunion Biomechanical consequences of the valgus osteotomy include reduction of the shear forces at the nonunion site, with concomitant enhancement of compressive forces. In one report, 50 patients under the age of 70 who were treated by valgus intertrochanteric osteotomy for nonunion demonstrated a rate of conversion to total hip of 14% at an average of 7.1 years postoperatively. The average Harris score in the remaining patients was 91. Clinical results in patients with known osteonecrosis prior to the osteotomy were equivalent to those with bone scan proven head viability. It was concluded that osteonecrosis without collapse is not a contraindication to osteotomy in the physiologically young with femoral neck fracture nonunion. In the physiologically elderly, prosthetic replacement is indicated. If the ipsilateral leg is short, the inherent lengthening effect of valgus osteotomy can help to make up the difference. When the leg lengths are equal, full wedge resection is advisable to avoid lengthening.

Osteonecrosis

Although the precipitating etiologies for the onset of osteonecrosis of bone may vary, they share a final common pathway. This pathway often culminates clinically with the onset of joint pain, radiographic evidence of subchondral sclerosis or collapse, and eventual progression to severe degenerative joint disease.

Mechanism

Four basic mechanisms are implicated in the disruption of blood flow to bone to the degree necessary to produce osteonecrosis. These include mechanical disruption, (eg, displaced femoral neck fracture), external pressure on or damage to a vessel wall (eg, Gaucher's disease or radiation therapy), arterial thrombosis or embolism (eg, sickle-cell crisis), and venous or outflow occlusion (eg, septic osteonecrosis).

Etiology

The relationship between the inciting event and the onset of osteonecrosis is clear in some cases, such as vascular disruption from a femoral neck fracture or arterial thrombosis from sickled blood cells. However, the inciting event for idiopathic osteonecrosis, in general, and to some extent other nontraumatic etiologies (eg, alcohol intoxication and systemic lupus erythematosus) are poorly defined. Several theories have been proposed and differ largely based upon the model studied. Venous compression has been implicated in dysbaric osteonecrosis, pregnancy, and thrombophlebitis. Embolic causes largely revolve around arterial fat embolism and subsequent infarction. Sources of extraosseous emboli include corticosteroid use, Cushing's disease, and ethanol consumption. Intraosseous fat embolism, in addition to directly obstructing blood flow, is hypothesized to mediate vascular occlusion through an intermediary pathway of focal intravascular coagulation. An ischemic threshold, which results in deficient local clearance of procoagulants, especially tissue thromboplastin, is felt to be reached. Subsequent vascular stasis, hypercoagulability, and endothelial damage lead eventually to intravascular coagulation.

Some authors have hypothesized that osteonecrosis is the end result of a gradual continuum of bone disorders that begins with osteoarthrosis and finally results in osteonecrosis. This progression to osteonecrosis depends on the degree of intraosseous loading of embolic fat. As the concentration of fat increases, procoagulants fail to be cleared, resulting in intravascular coagulation and osteonecrosis. Other factors have been implicated, including prostaglandin release, vasoactive amines, and altered platelet function. Conditions that directly damage vessel walls may increase arterial susceptibility to or indirectly promote intravascular coagulation by exposing sequestered vessel-wall proteins. It has been hypothesized that traumatic osteonecrosis results from a single high dose–short duration shower of fat emboli, and that nontraumatic osteonecrosis occurs as a result of repeated exposure to low-dose embolic showers over a longer duration. Early diagnosis, with the subsequent administration of fibrolytic agents or anticoagulants, may play a role in the future treatment of this disorder.

Thirty-five years ago, the incidence of nontraumatic osteonecrosis was quite low. The reasons for the dramatic rise in the number of patients with nontraumatic osteonecrosis are not fully understood. In most reported osteonecrosis series, idiopathic osteonecrosis is the most common, followed either by alcohol-related or corticosteroid-induced osteonecrosis. The threshold of alcohol ingestion reported to be associated with osteonecrosis is the equivalent of 400 cc or more per week of 100% ethyl alcohol, resulting in a cumulative lifetime dose of 150 liters. Large incremental and cumulative doses of steroids have been correlated with an increasingly proportional risk of developing osteonecrosis in humans who have lupus erythematosus. Laboratory rabbits exposed to corticosteroids developed hyperlipemia, fatty livers, and varying degrees of osteolytic osteonecrosis.

The epidemiology of the risk of developing osteonecrosis from brief exposure to therapeutic corticosteroids is not well understood. The potential risk appears great enough to justify caution in prescribing systemic corticosteroids when reasonable alternatives exist. There is no known risk of osteonecrosis attributable to single or repetitive trigger-point or intra-articular injections.

Among traumatic causes of osteonecrosis, fracture of the femoral neck is associated with a 15% to 30% risk of osteonecrosis, and dislocation of the hip with a 10% to 15% risk. Other nontraumatic causes of osteonecrosis include hemoglobinopathies, ionizing radiation, and dysbarism. Some investigators also have found underlying, otherwise asymptomatic coagulopathies to be associated with osteonecrosis.

Diagnosis

The reparative process influences the density and strength of bone via altered osteoblastic and osteoclastic activity. This activity results in a perimeter zone of sclerosis (the necrotic sector) and subsequent subchondral collapse, which often is preceded by a precollapse appearance on plain radiographs of a crescent-shaped chondral lucency (crescent sign).

In the early stages of osteonecrosis, plain radiographs are often normal. MRI is the best single imaging study to establish the diagnosis, with reported specificity of 98%. Once the diagnosis has been established, plain radiographs are usually sufficient to follow the subsequent course of the condition. In addition to AP and lateral views, the tangential views of Schneider help to visualize the anterior and posterior aspects of the head (Fig. 3). The Steinberg classification (Table 1) improves on the original system of Ficat and Arlet (Table 2) by incorporating both MRI information and data on the size of the lesion.

Management

The natural history of osteonecrosis is linked to the size of the necrotic sector. Very small (less than 15% of the femoral head) lesions may resolve without any formal treatment. Conversely, very large lesions (greater than 50% of the femoral head) progress to collapse and arthrosis in greater than 85% of cases and are not well treated by any method other than THA. In nontraumatic osteonecrosis, the incidence of bilaterality is 50% to 80%. Verification of the status of the opposite hip is another strong indication for MRI as part of the evaluation of osteonecrosis. A number of historic reviews of the natural progression of os-

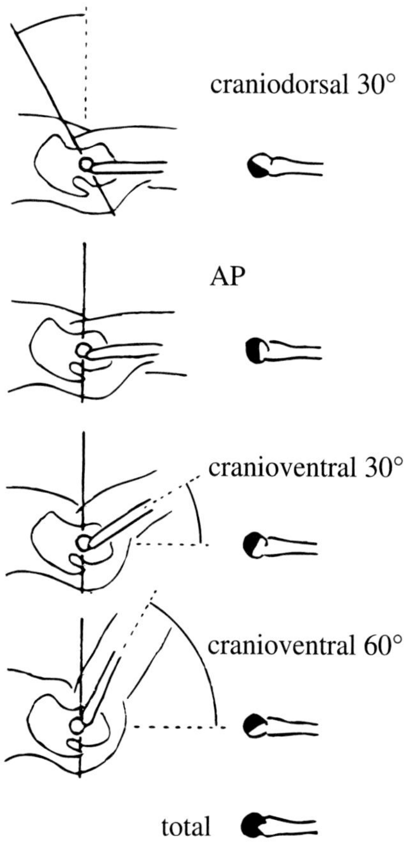

Fig. 3 Tangential views according to Schneider. These four views permit interpretation of a relatively large area of the femoral head circumference.

teonecrosis in nonsurgically managed cases, treated with crutches and partial or nonweightbearing ambulation, document an 85% to 92% risk of progression. In one series of 55 such hips, 84% required subsequent THA, usually within 3 years of diagnosis. Even in the most favorable stages (Ficat stage I and II), 69% required THA. This information was reviewed and published prior to the recognition of the influence of the size of the lesion on outcome and prior to the advent of MRI.

Table 1. Radiographic evaluation and staging of the hip in avascular necrosis of the femoral head

Stage	Characteristics
0	Normal radiograph; normal bone scan
I	Normal radiograph; abnormal bone scan
II	Sclerosis and/or cyst formation in femoral head
	A. Mild (< 20%)
	B. Moderate (20% to 40%)
	C. Severe (> 40%)
III	Subchondral collapse (crescent sign) without flattening
	A. Mild (< 15%)
	B. Moderate (15% to 30%)
	C. Severe (> 30%)
IV	Flattening of head without joint narrowing or acetabular involvement
	A. Mild (< 15% of surface and < 2 mm of depression)
	B. Moderate (15% to 30% of surface or 2 to 4 mm of depression)
	C. Severe (> 30% of surface or > 4 mm of depression)
V	Flattening of head with joint narrowing and/or acetabular involvement
	A. Mild, B. Moderate, C. Severe } determined as above plus estimate of acetabular involvement
VI	Advanced degenerative changes

(Reproduced with permission from Steinberg ME: Early results in the treatment of avascular necrosis of the femoral head with electrical stimulation. *Orthop Clin North Am* 1984;15:153–175.)

At least 14 methods of treatment other than THA have been espoused over the last 25 years, including autogenous grafting via arthrotomy and dislocation (the so-called trap door procedure), frozen segmental allograft, fresh cadaver osteocartilaginous allograft, femoral head devascularization, core decompression, rotational osteotomy, angulation osteotomy, vascularized pedicle graft, free microvascular fibular grafts, internal or external electric bone stimulation, nonvascularized strut graft, and combinations of the above. Clearly, such a litany exposes the lack of data documenting the reliability of any one procedure.

Core Decompression

One of the few prospective studies in the field compared core decompression with nonsurgical management in 55 patients. With minimum 2-year follow-up, the failure rate was 80% in the nonsurgical group and 30% in the core decompression group.

Long-term follow-up of a series of 101 patients, demonstrated 70% radiographic progression and 40% conversion to THA between 8 and 18 years after initial core decompression. In this series, there was a strong correlation between the Ficat stage at the time of core decompression and the percentage ultimately requiring THA during the follow-up period: I (4%); II (39%); and III (59%).

In a series of 350 patients treated by multiple cores through one lateral cortical window and adjunctive bone grafting, with 2- to 12-year follow-up of 300 of the patients, there was a 35% rate of conversion to THA. For stages I and II lesions, there was a strong correlation between size of lesion and outcome. Only 7% of hips with lesions involving less than 15% of the head required THA. Because there was no concurrent, nonsurgical control group among the small lesion patients, it is not known if the outcome represented effectiveness of the treatment

Table 2. Radiologic classification of ischemic necrosis of the femoral head

Clinical Data	Simple Necrosis		Necrosis Complicated by Collapse	
	Stage I	Stage II	Stage III	Stage IV
Joint line	Normal	Normal	Normal	Narrowed
Femoral head contour	Normal	Normal	Flattened subchondral infraction collapse	Collapsed
Trabeculae	Normal or very slight osteoporosis	Osteoporosis, mixed sclerosis/porosis	Sequestrum formation	Destruction of superior pole
Diagnosis				
By radiograph	Impossible	Probable	Certain	Very difficult to distinguish among arthrosis, flammatory arthritis, and necrosis
By functional exploration of bone	Hemodynamic, probable; histopathologic, certain	Hemodynamic, probable; histopathologic, certain	Confirmation	Hemodynamic insufficient; combined biopsy necessary

(Adapted with permission from Ficat RP, Arlet J: Necrosis of the femoral head, in Hungerford DS (ed): *Ischemia and Necrosis of Bone.* Baltimore, MD, Williams & Wilkins, 1980.)

method or if these hips might have done well without treatment. Historic control hips were chosen on the basis of Ficat classification alone, and not with regard to size of lesion. Therefore, use of historic controls is not helpful in sorting out this particular question.

In 10 reports involving 393 cumulative hips treated nonsurgically, the conversion rate to THA was approximately 70%. Five studies of a total of 354 hips treated using core decompression yielded an average rate of conversion to THA of 20%.

Electric Stimulation

The use of pulsed electromagnetic fields for the treatment of osteonecrosis has been studied extensively over the past 10 years. A report on the survival of hips in populations matched for prognostic variables indicated that, overall, 65% of hips were preserved with electric stimulation and 52% with core decompression. Electric stimulation and core decompression were equally effective in Ficat stages I and II hips. In stage III hips, electric stimulation was two times as effective as core decompression in reducing the need for THA. There have been no studies of electric stimulation with concurrent controls. Although promising, this method has not yet been approved by the FDA for the treatment of osteonecrosis.

Vascularized Fibular Graft

With the evolution of microvascular free-tissue transplantation in the 1970s, the classic fibular strut graft technique of Bonfiglio was modified to include its venous and arterial vascular pedicle. This approach is heroic, complex, and costly. It is accompanied by significant donor site morbidity. In a report of 425 free-fibular grafts between 1979 and 1992, 103 with more than 5-year follow-up, there was a 21% conversion rate to THA at 5 years. Results were best in patients with no sector collapse prior to surgery. Unfortunately, the reported results do not break down outcomes versus lesion size at the time of treatment, but only on the basis of Steinberg classification.

Further data will be necessary to demonstrate effectiveness in large-sized, precollapsed lesions. The effectiveness of this procedure may in large part be due to the core decompression that is a component of it. The rate of conversion to THA after free-vascularized graft is identical to the 20% figure for the combined core decompression series reported earlier in this chapter.

Endoprosthesis

Bipolar arthroplasty for osteonecrosis has a high failure rate. One author reported a 7% revision rate, 20% groin pain rate, and only 48% good or excellent evaluations of 31 hips at an average of 4.6 years. The histology of articular cartilage on the acetabular side of the hip joint at the time of THA for osteonecrosis has been studied in patients with radiographically normal appearing acetabulae. In 40 of 41 samples, gross abnormalities of the cartilage were noted. There currently is little support in the literature for the use of bipolar arthroplasties for osteonecrosis.

Total Hip Arthroplasty

Because most patients with osteoarthritis are relatively young, compared to the total hip population as a whole, a considerable portion of the difficulties associated with THA in this patient population can be reasonably attributed to their age at the time of surgery. One report of 28 THAs for osteonecrosis documented a 37% failure rate with minimum 5-year follow-up. Another series reported a 50% failure in osteonecrosis patients at 10 years. In 25 sickle cell patients with osteonecrosis, a revision rate of 40%, a complication rate of 49%, and an infection rate of 20% was reported. One author compared the outcomes of 64 osteonecrotic hips and 615 osteoarthritic total hips done during the same period of time and found comparable rates of complications and revisions, with a minimum follow-up of 3 years. Until developments of technology and techniques permit consistently good results for THA in young patients, the failure rate for THA in osteonecrosis patients is likely to remain high.

Osteotomy

Rotational osteotomy of 180° at the intertrochanteric level was devised and performed for osteonecrosis in the 1970s. The success rate reported for this extensive procedure was no better than that for angulation osteotomy, and the approach was abandoned. The Sugioka osteotomy, using a different technique, was associated with favorable initial reports. There were numerous reports, however, of disappointing results. Several independent Japanese investigators reported results of the Sugioka osteotomy that linked outcome to a small size lesion at the time of surgery. When the necrotic sector involved more than 50% of the femoral head, results were consistently poor.

Angulation osteotomies are effective in small to medium size lesions, but for an intermediate period of time only. Initial results are favorable, with approximately 60% to 75% good to excellent at 3 to 5 years. All authors have reported dramatic deterioration in the success rate over time, with approximately 40% to 50% of hips surviving 7 to 10 years. Osteotomy is useful in a small subset of patients in whom involvement is focal and occupies less than 50% of the femoral head. The size criteria are equally applicable to rotational and angulation osteotomies. Many types of intertrochanteric osteotomies have been espoused without the emergence of any clearly superior approach.

In general, for superolateral lesions with collapse of the femoral head at the lateral aspect of the femoral head, valgus or flexion valgus is indicated. Alternatively, when the superolateral segment of the femoral head is not involved and the lesion is more central, varus or flexion varus is preferable. Approximately one third of the patients who undergo osteotomy for osteonecrosis can be expected to gain 10 years or more before conversion to THA.

Total Hip Arthroplasty

Demographics

Over 123,000 THAs per year are currently carried out in the United States, at an estimated total cost in excess of $2.5 billion per year. Because individuals over the age of 65 years account for around two thirds of all hip replacements, the aging of the population will accentuate the trend toward increased utilization in the future. Age-specific incidence rates peak at 306 THAs per 100,000 men 65 to 74 years of age and 421 per 100,000 women 75 to 84 years of age.

Hip implants may be subjected to prolonged usage even in more elderly patient groups. In one recent Scandinavian study of patients with cemented THA, the long-term life expectancy was better than the average values for the general population, with 78% surviving an additional 10 years after 65 years of age.

A major factor in the increasingly widespread application of THA has been the tremendous benefits most patients derive from the procedure. In a recent, carefully performed prospective study of primary THA, this benefit was quantitated using quality-adjusted-life-year measurements. The majority of the derived benefits were evident by 3 months postsurgery, and included marked improvements in physical function, social interaction, and overall health. This study provides much needed and timely objective quantification of the cost effectiveness of THA.

Ironically, it has been the tremendous effectiveness of hip arthroplasty that has fueled not only the increasing use of the procedure but also the high level of interest in finding ways to solve or prevent the very real problems that still occur in some cases. Some of the recent failed efforts at innovation in THA have been attributed to the frequent combination of incompatible design goals and clinical tolerance of a trial-and-error culture that tended to bypass adequate testing.

Significant changes have occurred over the past decade in the costs associated with THA. In a study of actual costs (not charges) associated with primary THA at a Boston hospital, actual costs rose 46.5% between 1981 and 1990. Adjusted for inflation, this translates into a real increase of only 1.9% during the decade under study. Costs associated with the implant grew 212% during the same period (a real increase after inflation of 117%). The implant accounted for 24% of the total costs in 1990 versus 11% in 1981. Whereas overall hospital costs were controlled by decreased consumption of other resources, mainly because of shorter hospital stays, this study clearly shows where future cost containment efforts will need to be directed as institutions and providers come under increased fiscal pressures.

Cement Fixation

Controversy regarding the optimal mode of implant fixation for acetabular and femoral components in selected patient populations continues. Additionally, particulate wear problems are increasingly seen as an important cause of implant failure, and subsequently, prevention of particulate wear-related osteolysis has increasingly come to influence the discussion regarding choice of implant fixation method.

First-Generation Cemented Methods Long-term follow-up studies, some with 20-year data, on the outcome of the Charnley implants and methods document the overall durability of this approach, especially in older patients (Table 3). Failure rates tend to be linear over the first two decades and average around 1% or less per year, with greater than 80% implant survivorship at 15 to 20 years postimplantation reported by several groups. Cemented acetabular fixation was less durable than femoral fixation, with higher cup revision rates observed. Acetabular component linear wear averaged about 0.1 mm/year with the Charnley system.

Poor acetabular bone quality can adversely influence the longevity of these implants. A pattern of early loosening in cemented sockets has been correlated with deficient bone stock. In a series of 680 hips, early loosening (before 10 years) was associated with deficient acetabular bone as seen in previous developmental dysplasia of the hip, acetabular fracture, or protrusio. Late loosening (after 10 years) occurred in 56% of those with more than 2 mm of linear wear, inferring a biologic process for late loosening.

Proper anatomic socket positioning may not always be possible in acetabular deformities. Reasonable results have been reported long-term for proximally placed sockets. In a clinical study of cemented sockets placed proximally, 16% radiographic loosening occurred in those without any associated lateralization of the hip center, and only one cup was revised at 11 years average follow-up.

Retrieval studies of failed and well-functioning hip prostheses have added considerably to understanding of this operation. In a series of successful asymptomatic THAs retrieved at autopsy up to 17.5 years postsurgery, host bone was still in direct contact with the cement in the vast majority of patients, and an intervening fibrous membrane was rarely seen. A dense neocortex or shell of bone around the cement has been described. This bone is connected to the original cortex by trabecular struts and is associated with porosis and thinning of the original cortex. The cement–bone interface has been observed to remain intact despite occasional areas of implant–cement interface debonding. Postmortem histologic correlation has shown that for the majority of thin radiolucent lines frequently observed radiographically at the femoral cement–bone interface in well-fixed stems, the cement is intimately opposed to the bone. In these instances, the radiolucent line is due to the endosteal and cortex remodeling described above rather than to a fibrous membrane. When a fibrous membrane does occur, the density of histiocytes correlates with the membrane thickness, density of polyethylene particles, and time after implantation. On the acetabular side of the joint, radiolucent lines correlate more reliably with fibrous membrane formation, which is believed to be particulate induced.

Table 3. Results of first-generation cement methods

Location, Date	Hips (final)	Age at Surgery (range in years)	Follow-up (range in years)	Survivorship*	Revision Rate	Radiographically Loose	Comment*
Iowa, 1993	330 (98)	65 (29–86)	20 (20–22)	80% ± 8%	15%, 10% cup, 3% stem	22% cup, 7% stem	single surgeon
Minnesota, 1994	333 (112)	65 yrs	20 yrs minimum	84%	16%	17%	linear rate of failure
Wrightington, 1993	1,324 (193)	47 (23–68) for the 193 final	21 (18–26)		7% cup, 6% stem		
Denmark, 1994	241 (103)	?	17.6 (15–20.6)	89.3%, 20 yrs	8.30%	5% cup, 30% stem	
Wrightington, 1993	218 (166)	under 40	16 (10–24)	75%, 20 yrs OA: 51%; RA: 96%	16% cup, 14% stem		OA worse than RA
Iowa, 1994	89 (58)	under 50	18 (16–22)	68% ± 14% at 22 yrs	13% cup, 2% stem	50% cup, 8% stem	single surgeon

*OA is osteoarthritis, RA is rheumatoid arthritis

One risk factor associated with higher failure rates is young age at the time of arthroplasty. In one long-term review, the probability of revision at 20 years was 27% for those younger than 59 years of age at time of arthroplasty, 13% for those 59 to 65 years, 7.5% for those 65 to 70 years, and 12% for patients age 70 years or older when operated on.

Other factors shown to increase the risk of failure include increased weight, male sex, high activity level, and diagnoses of osteoarthritis or osteonecrosis versus rheumatoid arthritis. The increased failure rates associated with these risk factors (many of which may occur concurrently) were first noted after earlier shorter-term studies of first generation methods, and served as a major stimulus for the development of alternative devices and fixation methods.

Second-Generation Cemented Methods The use of a femoral canal plug and retrograde filling of the femur with a cement gun constitute minimum criteria for "improved" or second-generation methods, to which some also added pulsatile lavage for cleaning the bone interstices before cement insertion. Initial 5-year reports from three different institutions where these methods were used were superior to first-generation results from both these and other centers (Table 4). Longer term (8 to 14 years postimplantation) follow-up continues to be excellent, even in young patients, with regard to revision and loosening rates on the femoral side. This is in contrast to the acetabular side, on which fixation has been no more durable than with first-generation cemented methods.

Third-Generation Cemented Methods A more heterogeneous third generation of cemented methods comprises all the above second-generation methods plus pressurization of the cement after insertion, surface changes to the implant to attempt to improve implant–cement bonding, and some form of cement porosity reduction (via vacuum mixing or centrifugation). Both centrifugation and vacuum mixing of bone cement have been shown to produce significant reductions in porosity, with subsequent improvements in mechanical characteristics, including fatigue strength.

Surface enhancements have included roughening or textured treatments to stems or metal-backed cups and precoating of the implant with cement during manufacture to achieve the strongest possible cement bond to the implant. Proof of the relative clinical effectiveness of the addition of these various methods to generally accepted second-generation techniques awaits long-term follow-up study and validation. The same is true of even more recent changes, such as the use of spacers to try to ensure the uniformity of the cement mantle. This concept has been adopted because of the clinical and radiographic studies in which results were improved when the femoral cement mantle in the proximal medial region was no less than 2 mm and no more than 5 mm in thickness (Fig. 4). In one series, a thin cement mantle at the medial diaphysis (Gruen zone 5) was observed to contribute to mechanical failure of the stem, a problem often associated with valgus stem positioning. However, another study documented the adverse effect of varus stem position on stem-loosening rates. Although these data support the desirability of providing for reliable, reproducible neutral stem alignment with controlled cement thickness, the exact benefit derived from the several currently used systems for centralizing stems remains to be established.

Isolation of the several potentially significant factors that may affect prosthetic longevity may be difficult given the usual clinical setting in which several variables that may have different effects undergo simultaneous change or are uncontrolled. Examples of potentially confounding covariables include use of modular femoral heads, metal-backing of cups, use of elevated rim acetabular inserts, and changes in the quality, preparation, and manufacturing of the polyethylene. Many of these variables have been introduced or undergone change in parallel with introduction of third-generation cement methods, complicating the study of these issues. Nevertheless, reported results over the first decade after cemented THA using second-generation methods are successful enough that it seems reasonable that the proponents of alternative fixation tech-

Table 4. Results of second generation cement methods

Location, Date	Hips (final)	Age at Surgery (range in years)	Follow-up (range in years)	Revision Rate	Radiographically Loose or Redone
Boston, 1990	105	57.4 (20–84)	11.2 (10–12.7)	4.9% cup, 1.9% stem	42% cup, 2.9% stem
Boston, 1992	50	under 50	12 (10–14.8)	22% cup, 0% stem	44% cup, 2% stem
Iowa, 1994	42	under 50	11 (10–15)	24% cup, 5% stem	36% cup, 17% stem

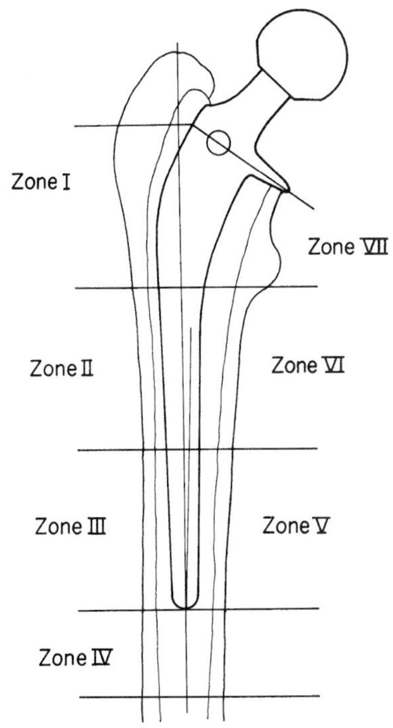

Fig. 4 This stylized drawing of an anteroposterior view of the proximal femur with hip stem in place demonstrates the subdivisions of the periprosthetic bone into the Gruen zones used to classify the location of periprosthetic interface and bone changes noted on radiographs. A similar convention can be applied to the lateral projection.

niques or implant designs bear the burden of proving significant advantage before widespread usage is encouraged.

Cemented Metal-Backed Versus All Polyethylene Cups
Data have been reported by one group of investigators regarding a single implant system in which a titanium cemented stem with 28-mm head, and either a cemented metal-backed cup or an all polyethylene socket was used. Wear, loosening, and revision rates were compared. In the metal-backed group, linear wear was greater (0.11 versus 0.08 mm/year), and volumetric wear was increased (66.2 versus 48.2 mm^3/year). In an earlier report by the same group, metal-backed cups also showed increased rates of radiolucency (39% versus 23%), loosening (4% versus 2%), and revision (6% versus 2%). All these differences were statistically significant. If adverse effects of similar magnitude are confirmed for other designs, these data would strongly support the abandonment of metal-backed cemented acetabular cups in favor of all-polyethylene ones.

Cementless Fixation
As clinical experience was obtained with cementless implants, new concerns surfaced—thigh pain and localized bone loss (osteolysis) quite similar to that seen in cases of loosened cemented implants. Cementless implant design developments have included use of hydroxyapatite coatings on smooth, textured, and even porous surfaces; increased stem modularity to attempt to improve implant fit and reduce implant stiffness on the femoral side; and use of custom designs to try to optimize the match of the implant to the patient's anatomy.

Extensively Porous-Coated Stems In a review of the results of 166 THAs performed with the extensively coated version of the AML stem, the rate of femoral revision for aseptic loosening at 6 to 13 years follow-up was 0.6%, with another 1.8% radiographically unstable, but not revised. Revision for all other indications such as dislocation, infection, marked polyethylene wear of the cup, and focal osteolysis (believed to be due to the polyethylene wear observed) totaled 15%. Cup wear and osteolysis was the cause of revision four to five times more often than component loosening (5.3% of overall series versus 1.2%). This difference may be related, at least in part, to the routine use of 32-mm heads.

The stability of fixation achieved with extensive coating of the stem has been confirmed by postmortem retrieval studies of instrumented specimens subjected to simulated physiologic loads and histologic analysis. Maximum relative motion at the porous coating–bone interface was only 40 μm when ingrowth was present histologically.

However, concerns regarding stress shielding and the potential for significant bone loss due to remodeling continue to limit the widespread use of this implant. In a review by the originator of this device, radiographic assessment showed that 14% of patients had moderate bone loss and 4% had severe bone density decrease. Greater bone loss was observed radiographically in association with apparent bone ingrowth and use of larger diameter (and thus stiffer) femoral stems. Significant variation in the actual quantity of remodeling, ranging from a 7% to a 78% decrease in bone mineral, was found in cadaveric retrieval studies. A separate determination, using dual-energy x-ray absorptiometry analysis of paired femora, confirmed similar variability in bone density decrease due to periprosthetic remodeling. Greater bone loss has been observed in hips with preexistent or contralateral osteoporosis of the proximal femur. This association may be aggravated by the endosteal enlargement, commonly seen in osteoporotic patients, which, when present, necessitates the use of larger, stiffer stems. Although thigh pain was noted in 14% of patients in an early series, this finding correlated with implant sizing errors or mismatch and dropped to 1.2% with improved fitting of the stem to the femoral canal once a larger inventory of implant sizes became available.

Proximally Porous-Coated Stems Initial results following implantation of proximally porous-coated femoral components were encouraging (Table 5). With experience and longer follow-up, revision rates have risen, many of the initial designs have been modified or abandoned by their developers, and understanding of the causes of loosening and the associated bone loss often seen with both cemented and cementless systems has increased. Because a plethora of uncemented designs was introduced in the United States, implanted in large numbers, and then redesigned and modified, usually before long-term outcomes were known, it becomes necessary to look for general trends or observations common to multiple designs, recognizing that some of the problems noted may be design specific. In addition, many of these femoral devices were inserted in combination with equally novel uncemented porous acetabular designs. In some instances, the performance of these cups may have impacted overall success rates for many of these arthroplasties.

Soon after the widespread introduction of proximally porous-coated stems in the United States, questions surfaced regarding thigh pain, which seemed to occur more often and with greater severity than seemed the case with earlier cemented systems. Reported rates varied depending on implant design and the criteria used to designate thigh pain. Although overall reported rates of thigh pain ranged up to 16%, some of these patients had minimal transient symptoms and were not adversely effected. Others (a much smaller percentage) had limiting pain, with symptoms severe enough to prompt revision surgery in some cases.

Although there were early concerns that significant thigh pain represented lack of bone ingrowth and stable fixation, it has become clear that some proximally porous-coated stems may both subside and show periprosthetic lucency and demarcation circumferentially, but still function well. It has also been found at revision that some patients with severe thigh pain may have excellent bone ingrowth of the proximally coated stem. Thus, thigh pain following porous-coated femoral component insertion may be caused by several different processes, including stress concentration at the stem tip, undersizing of the stem, stem motion (loosening), progressive osteolysis without loosening, and infection, or it may have a muscular origin.

Bone ingrowth does not ensure long-term success because later failure of the bone fixing the implant is possible. A recent histologic study of five proximally porous-coated stems revised for subsidence and loosening showed bone ingrowth in each, ranging from 4% to 44% of the pore spaces available for ingrowth. Each of the patients in this series had delayed onset of pain (at least 1 year postsurgery), and each tended to be active, heavy, or both, which suggests late fatigue fracture of the bony trabeculae that initially fixed the implant.

Cementless Press-Fit Nonporous Stems Several nonporous cementless femoral stem designs have been explored.

Table 5. Porous ingrowth femoral stem results

Center, Year	Design*	No. of Hips	Follow-up (years)	Revision: Stem Loosening	Radiograph: Stem Loosening	Thigh Pain
Arlington, VA, 1987	AML	307	2–5			14%
Arlington, VA, 1994	AML	166	6–13, avg 9.5	0.6%	1.8%	1.2% (better fit)
Washington, DC, 1988	PCA	50	2			16%
Newcastle, UK, 1994	PCA	241	2–9, avg 5	2%		
Seoul, Korea, 1993	PCA	116	6–7.5			
Washington, DC, 1993	PCA	100	5–7	1%	5%	15%–26% during first 5 yrs
Chapel Hill, NC, 1992	Harris-Galante	100	2–5, avg 37 mos	1%	0%	
Chicago, IL, 1992	Harris-Galante	121	3–6.2	3.3%	9% loose, 8% stable + tip lysis	
Toronto, Canada 1994	S-ROM	48	2–6	0%	0%	6.3%

*AML (DePuy, Warsaw, IN); PCA (Howmedica, Rutherford, NJ); Harris-Galante (Zimmer, Warsaw, IN); and S-Rom (Joint Medical Products, Johnson & Johnson, Raynham, MA).

Early experience in the United States was somewhat disappointing, with relatively high failure rates noted. There has been continued interest in devices of this type in Europe in the recent past, particularly with the addition of roughened surfaces to titanium devices designed to encourage intimate bone contact with the device. At present, the relative advantages, disadvantages, and proper clinical role for these implants remains uncertain.

Porous-Coated Acetabular Components Results with uncemented porous-coated acetabular components have been encouraging. If excessive polyethylene wear can be avoided, these devices may offer a more durable fixation solution than cement for some patients. One of the more successful early porous-ingrowth cup designs used titanium wire mesh fixed to the metal shell of the cup for fixation. Porous ingrowth has been reliably achieved with this design, as evidenced by clinical radiographic results and quantitative histology of autopsy retrievals of well-functioning arthroplasties. Ten of 11 such retrievals showed an average volume fraction of bone ingrowth of 12.1%, with more bone seen around screw holes through which screws were inserted. However, metal debris within histiocytes has been observed adjacent to screw holes in retrievals of this same design, with the amount present appearing to increase as a function of time since implantation. The significance of this observation is uncertain.

The variability in amount of ingrowth achieved has been confirmed in another retrieval study of well-functioning porous-coated cups. In one report, all nine cups showed bone ingrowth, but this ranged from 3% to 84%. When radiographic appearance was correlated with the histologic picture, it was found that radiographs underestimated the presence and extent of gap areas and overestimated the occurrence of bone apposition.

Intermediate term clinical results have also been encouraging. In a series of 83 consecutive primary arthroplasties in which line to line acetabular reaming of the same diameter as the cup was used, there was no radiographic loosening and there were no cup revisions because of loosening after a minimum 5-year follow-up. However, two revisions were required because of failure of the polyethylene liner locking mechanism. New, thin radiolucencies, not present initially after surgery, were observed in 59% of cases at 2 years, but these were less than 1 mm wide and incomplete or discontinuous. Further observation of these radiolucencies will be needed to assess their significance, but these results compare favorably to those reported with cemented methods.

In a prospective, randomized study of migration, no significant difference was found between Charnley and uncemented Harris-Galante cups inserted in patients undergoing bilateral THAs.

This same cup has been used in a press-fit fashion without screws, relying on slight underreaming of the prepared acetabular cavity, with equally excellent results and no loosening or revisions at 5-year follow-up. This approach has the advantage of avoiding the potential vascular risks involved with screw fixation that penetrates the inner cortex of the pelvis.

Initial contact between the metal shell and bone may be improved in some designs by underreaming. A comparison of initial contact with three designs—hemispheric, hemispheric with spikes, and threaded hemispheric—showed gaps and less than complete contact with all three despite 1-mm underreaming in all. Contact seemed to be limited by asymmetric reaming and incomplete seating due to areas of dense bone from the subchondral plate and spikes or threads when present. Excessive underreaming of the acetabulum risks fracture of the acetabular rim. In a recent cadaver study, 4 mm or more of underreaming resulted in a fracture risk of at least 40%.

The intermediate-term follow-up results for the PCA cup compare less favorably, mainly due to excessive polyethylene wear and secondary osteolysis rates. The PCA hip, which had a porous-coated chrome-cobalt acetabular component with peripheral pegs, also had a 32-mm femoral head. The polyethylene insert used was thinner than that which would have been used with a smaller head size. The routine use of these larger diameter heads probably has had an adverse effect on the acetabular wear and osteolysis rates in most reported series. One recent report of the minimum 6-year follow-up on a series of PCA hips indicated a 3% cup revision rate. The most ominous finding in this study was a high incidence of excessive wear (5 to 11 mm of thinning) noted in 17%. Osteolysis was visible radiographically in 33% of the hips, suggesting the longer-term revision rate will be high.

Another report on the PCA implant system revealed an 11% acetabular failure rate at an average 5-year follow-up (range 2 to 9 years). Twenty of the 26 acetabular failures were associated with excessive polyethylene wear and local osteolysis. Survivorship analysis with recommendation for revision as the failure endpoint was 91% at 6 years, 73% at 7 years, and 57% at 8 years, reinforcing the need for ongoing long-term follow-up of these patients.

A recent review has documented the occurrence and features of severe pelvic osteolysis associated with well-fixed and well-functioning porous-coated uncemented acetabular cups. All 15 cups in this series had polyethylene inserts 10 mm or less in thickness, and 12 were 8 mm thick or less. The osteolysis was not detected on radiographs despite regular follow-up films until over 5 years after surgery on average (range 53 to 84 months). Because 12 of 15 had hip scores over 90 despite what was, in some, extensive bone damage, these results show that regular ongoing long-term radiographic review of all such joints is important.

Threaded Acetabular Components Recent reports on the intermediate-term results of two different threaded nonporous titanium acetabular designs have been disappointing. One study showed only an 85% cup survivorship at 4 years for primary surgery and 52% survivorship in revision cases. A recent review of a different threaded titanium cup at 5 to 9 years follow-up revealed that 31% of the primary cups had been revised or were pending revision due to loosening and migration. Both groups of authors have abandoned the use of this design.

Hydroxyapatite-Coated Femoral and Acetabular Components There has been a great deal of recent interest in hydroxyapatite (HA), tricalcium phosphate (TCP), and other ceramic materials that are potentially resorbable and to which bone may bond directly. In a multicenter series of over 400 proximally HA-coated titanium stems, the 320 hips with 2-year follow-up had a Harris hip score of 95, and the 142 hips followed up 3 years, a score of 96. The mechanical loosening rate was 0.46%. A recent update of 206 hips from this same series at a minimum 5-year follow-up showed continued excellent radiographic results on the femoral side with no subsidence and only one case of endosteal osteolysis.

Cadaver retrieval and histologic analysis of five hips with satisfactorily functioning, pain-free HA-coated stems in place 5 to 25 months at the time of death has been reported. The histologic features were of a mechanically stable implant with remodeling at the implant-bone interface and bone apposition to the implant of 32% to 78% of the available surface.

The results for HA-coated acetabular components have been less favorable than the stem results. In a comparison of 129 HA-coated cups and 121 porous-coated cups, all inserted with identical HA-coated stems, the mechanical failure rate was 10.1% for the HA-coated cups compared to 3.3% for the porous-coated cups at minimum 5-year follow-up.

Total Hip Arthroplasty Complications

Pain

When diagnosing painful THA, the orthopaedist must consider etiologies that are extrinsic to the hip. These etiologies include spinal pathology or vascular claudication. Intrinsic hip pain can result from loosening, tumor, stress fracture, infection, and bursitis. A multitude of clinical tests can be used to differentiate extrinsic and intrinsic causes. The value of these methods is discussed below. Algorithms for evaluation of painful cemented and cementless devices are presented to provide guidance (Fig. 5).

Value of Plain Radiographs Vertical cup migration as measured on standard radiographs can predict late aseptic loosening. For both cementless and cemented hips, a threshold migration of 1.2 mm per year during the first 2 years after implantation indicated that hips were likely to fail. This measurement had a specificity of 86% and a sensitivity of 78%.

Role of Aspiration Hip aspiration has been reported to be a cost-effective and accurate method of evaluating potential hip infections. The sensitivity of hip aspiration has been reported at between 60% and 70%, with false negatives reported between 12% and 36%. A series of 147 aspirations had a high sensitivity (92.8%) and specificity (91.7%) with a negative predictive value of 99.2%, but only a 54.2% positive predictive value. Preoperative joint aspiration in 72 joint replacements (knee and hip) had a sensitivity of 67% and specificity of 96%. Compared to erythro-

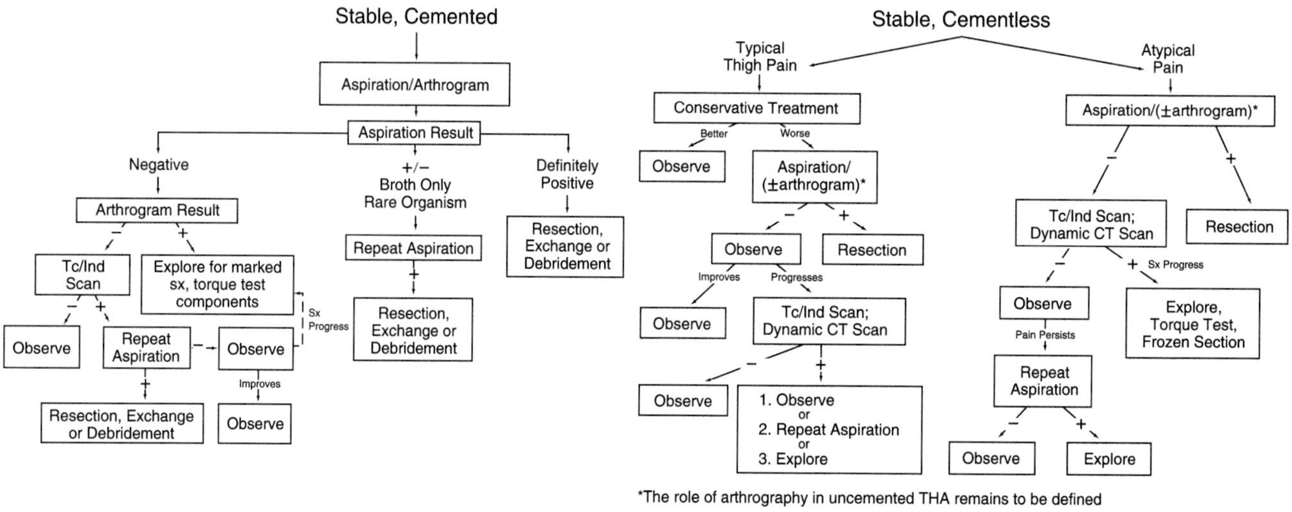

Fig. 5 Algorithms for painful cemented (**left**) and cementless (**right**) hips that appear stable radiographically.

cyte sedimentation rate, plain radiographs, and three-phase bone imaging, the aspiration was considered to be the most useful single test in the workup of the painful joint arthroplasty.

In a series of 143 hip aspirations, there was 100% specificity and 79% sensitivity. The sensitivity was increased to 91% by including criteria of joint fluid leucocytosis higher than 10,000/mm^3, presence of an arthrographic fistula, or organism isolation in joint fluid or rinsing fluid. In a study of 270 hip aspirations, a 13% false positive and 6% false negative rate were reported. On the basis of cost-effectiveness, it was recommended that the selection of patients to undergo preoperative aspiration should be based on a history that is suspicious of infection (early postoperative component loosening, painful arthroplasty, a distant infectious site) or radiographic findings of aggressive nonfocal osteolysis, focal lysis, or periostitis. It is not necessary to aspirate every THA prior to revision.

Osteolysis

Osteolysis, rather than fixation, has become the major concern in implant longevity. Osteolysis (originally termed "cement disease") results from the biologic reaction to particles—polymethylmethacrylate (PMMA) debris in the form of unpolymerized polymer or mechanical fragments and metal and polyethylene particles.

In cemented THA, debonding of the cement from the metal allows PMMA debris to interact with surrounding bone (Fig. 6). In a study of cement debonding, particulate PMMA was detected in eight of the 25 cases with available histology. This local fragmentation of PMMA can be the stimulus for local osteolysis. In a study of four cases of lysis (without looseness) in cemented stems, each case was associated with a cement mantle defect.

The earliest report of aggressive granulomatous lesions in cementless prostheses appeared in 1990. The etiology appeared to be polyethylene debris. The membranes surrounding loosened cementless implants contained both polyethylene and metal fragments. The use of a cementless prosthesis does not always rule out osteolysis. Sixteen cases of lysis were found in 474 stable cementless femoral components (Fig. 7); none showed subsidence or position change. Three of the 16 were firmly fixed. The periprosthetic membrane also demonstrated particulate polyethylene and metal debris.

The Mechanical Behavior of Debris Indirect evidence exists for an effective joint space around the prosthesis. The finding of particulate debris, for example polyethylene, at a distance from the articulation (in areas of linear or lytic osteolysis) demonstrates a communication of the joint with distant areas (Fig. 8). The space between the stem (or cement) and bone appears to be a conduit for transfer of joint debris. Free particles are found in joint fluid, in fibrin exudates on the surface of the joint capsule, and at the implant–bone interface. Within tissues, the particles are usually incorporated by histiocytes.

Stems with noncircumferential ingrowth surfaces may allow for easier migration of particles by allowing migration of debris along the smooth portion of the stem (Fig. 7). Stems without circumferential ingrowth surfaces have been reported to have an 8% rate of distal lysis without loosening at 5 years. Of those stems showing this distal lysis, 12% need revision due to the extent of lysis.

Peripheral-fit acetabular prostheses have not been found to protect against osteolysis of the pelvis. In a study of cementless sockets with "rim fit," communicating areas of pelvic lysis, with peripheral rim osteolytic defects allowing migration of particulate debris, were found at the time of socket revision. Even well-fixed cemented sockets may not effectively seal the pathway of particulate polyethylene into pelvic bone (Fig. 8).

Migration of particles to distant sites along lymphatic pathways has been found. Microscopic examination of pelvic lymph nodes from patients with cobalt-chrome and titanium implants show ipsilateral "metastasis" of metal and polyethylene particles.

Particle Type, Load, Size, and Osteolysis A study of tissues from implant retrievals and revisions evaluated the relationship between the amount of particulate polyethylene debris and the number of macrophages (tissue histiocytes) in the periprosthetic membrane, finding the concentration of particles proportional the degree of inflammatory response and bone resorption.

Cell culture studies of macrophages obtained from membranes about loose prostheses yield important insight into macrophage behavior in response to cement particles. Cement particles less than 12 μm in diameter are phagocytized by the macrophage. The phagocytes respond by increasing production of tumor necrosis factor (TNF), a bone-resorbing mediator. Larger particles avoid phagocytosis and do not stimulate release of TNF.

Human cell culture study demonstrates stimulation of monocytes by PMMA particles to produce specific bone-resorbing mediators: interleukin 1 (IL-1), TNF, and prostaglandin E_2 (PGE_2). Cell culture work has also demonstrated that metal particles are capable of monocyte stimulation and subsequent PGE_2 release. Membranes from implants with a polyethylene articulation produce higher levels of collagenase and IL-1, but PGE_2 tends to be constant regardless of the type of particle (polyethylene, cobalt-chrome, or titanium). Although many investigators have implicated polyethylene as the major contributor to the particle reaction, metal particles may also play a role in the osteolytic response. Metal deposits have been documented in 75% of osteolytic lesions; however, their relation to bone loss has not been demonstrated. Data from animal studies demonstrate a varied response to the two common metals used in THA: cobalt-chromium and tivanium (titanium, aluminum, vanadium). Although cobalt-chrome particles are very toxic to macrophages compared with same-sized tivanium particles, tivanium induces the release of higher levels of mediators of bone-resorbing

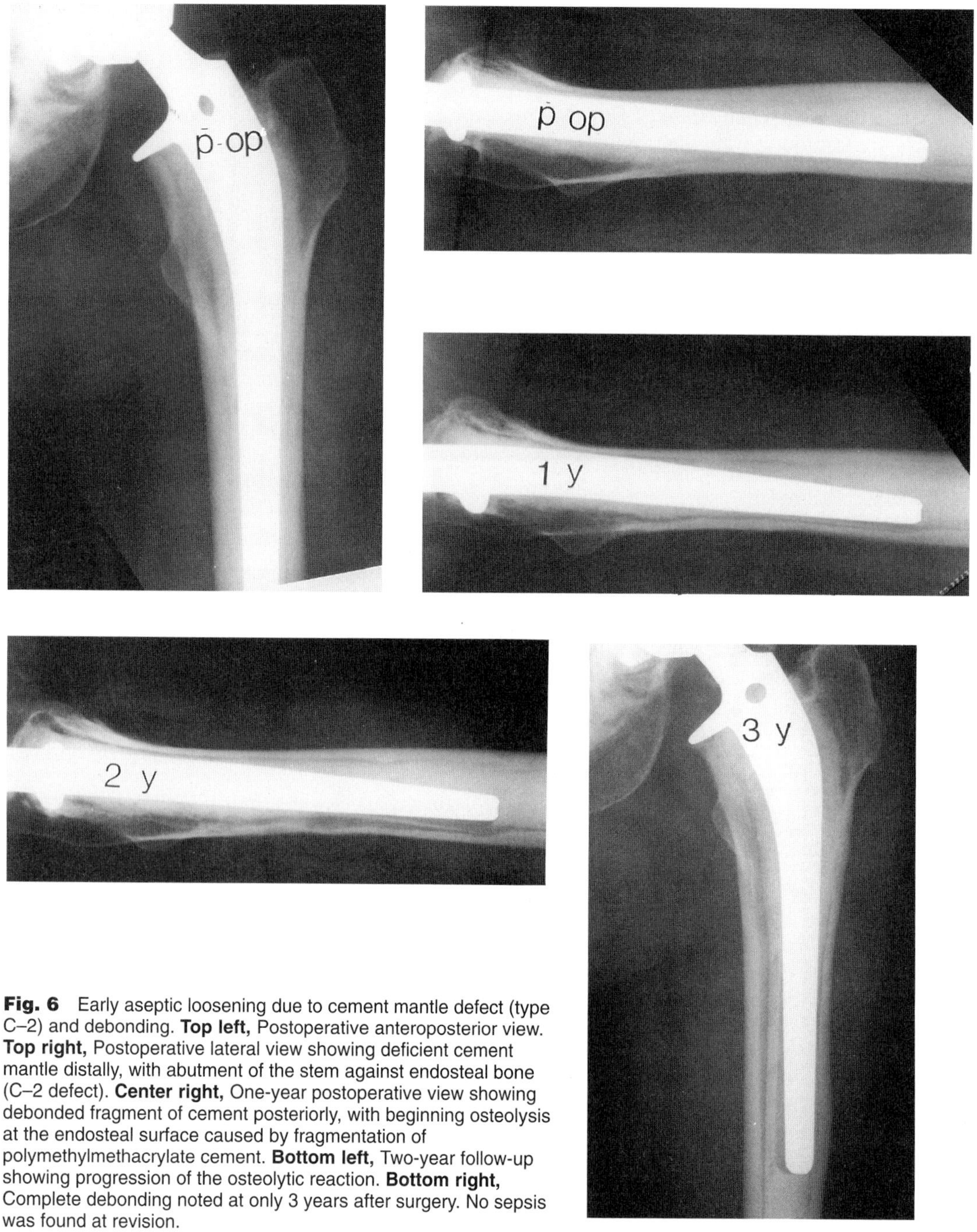

Fig. 6 Early aseptic loosening due to cement mantle defect (type C–2) and debonding. **Top left,** Postoperative anteroposterior view. **Top right,** Postoperative lateral view showing deficient cement mantle distally, with abutment of the stem against endosteal bone (C–2 defect). **Center right,** One-year postoperative view showing debonded fragment of cement posteriorly, with beginning osteolysis at the endosteal surface caused by fragmentation of polymethylmethacrylate cement. **Bottom left,** Two-year follow-up showing progression of the osteolytic reaction. **Bottom right,** Complete debonding noted at only 3 years after surgery. No sepsis was found at revision.

agents over a wide range of concentrations. However, analysis of membranes retrieved from about cobalt-chrome and titanium implants shows no difference in biochemical findings. Autopsy retrieval studies of HA-coated femoral stems indicate that ceramic particles may act as a stimulus of osteoclastic activity adjacent to the component.

Wear: Sources and Types of Debris Material Because polyethylene has been implicated as the major source for particle debris, emphasis has been directed at reducing wear. In metal–polymer bearings, the softer polymer is much more prone to wear than the metal and more likely to be found in surrounding tissues. However, polyethylene

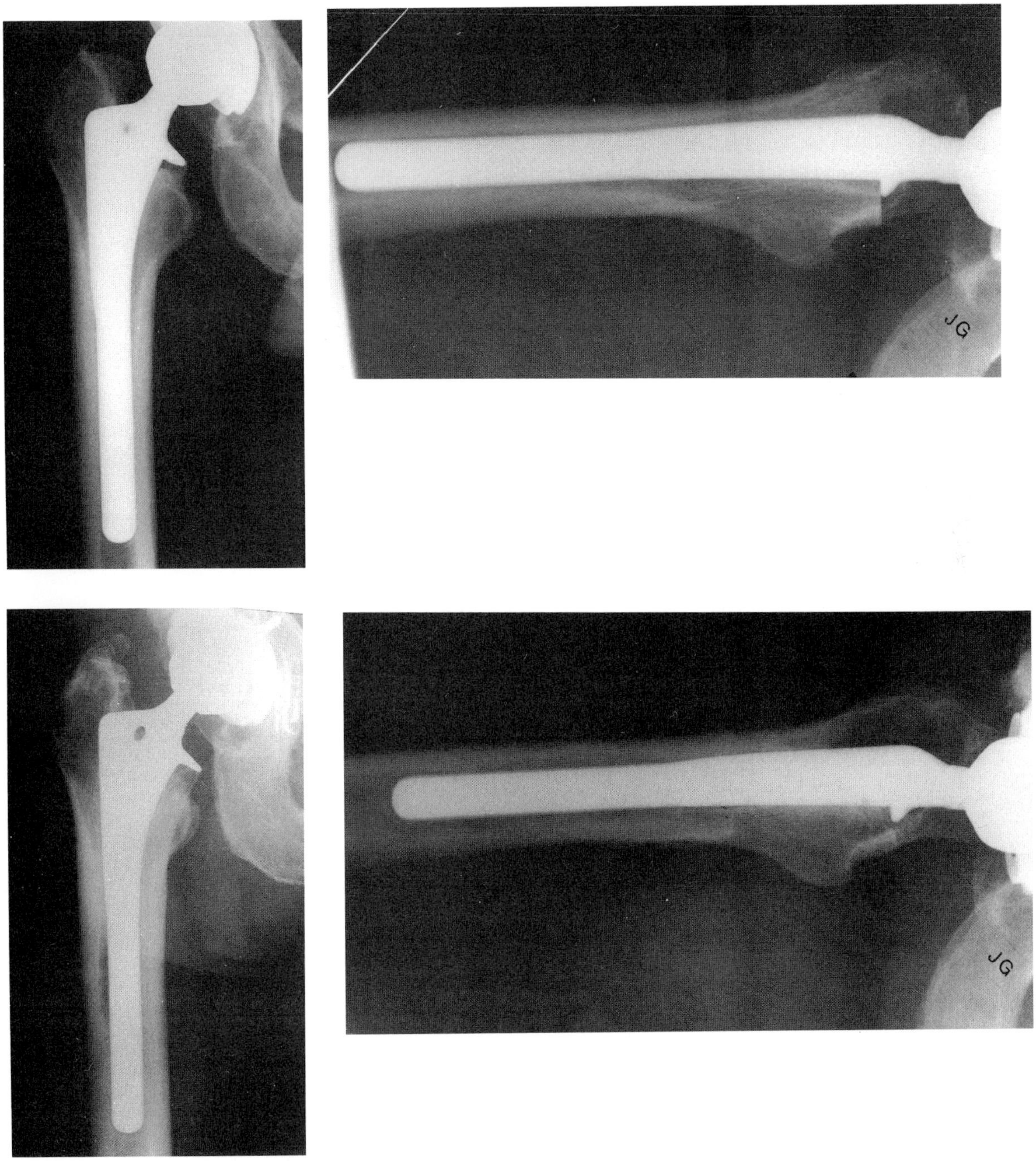

Fig. 7 Osteolysis without looseness of a cementless femoral component with noncircumferential proximal ingrowth pads. **Top left,** Early postoperative anteroposterior view. **Top right,** Postoperative lateral view. **Bottom left,** Distal femoral lysis 3 years later in zone II and zone I, with large greater trochanter lesion caused by polyethylene debris. **Bottom right,** Lateral view at 3 years showing extensive distal osteolysis and better distinguished greater trochanter lesion. The stem was not loose at repeated surgery and was treated by currettement and bone-graft, which have stopped the progression 5 years later.

is not directly cytotoxic, and it is the cellular processing of the polyethylene particles that leads to osteolysis.

Volumetric wear rates increase proportionately with increase in femoral head diameter. Measurements of polyethylene wear by radiographic technique closely correlate with actual wear of retrievals, although linear radiographic measurements tend to underestimate the true wear.

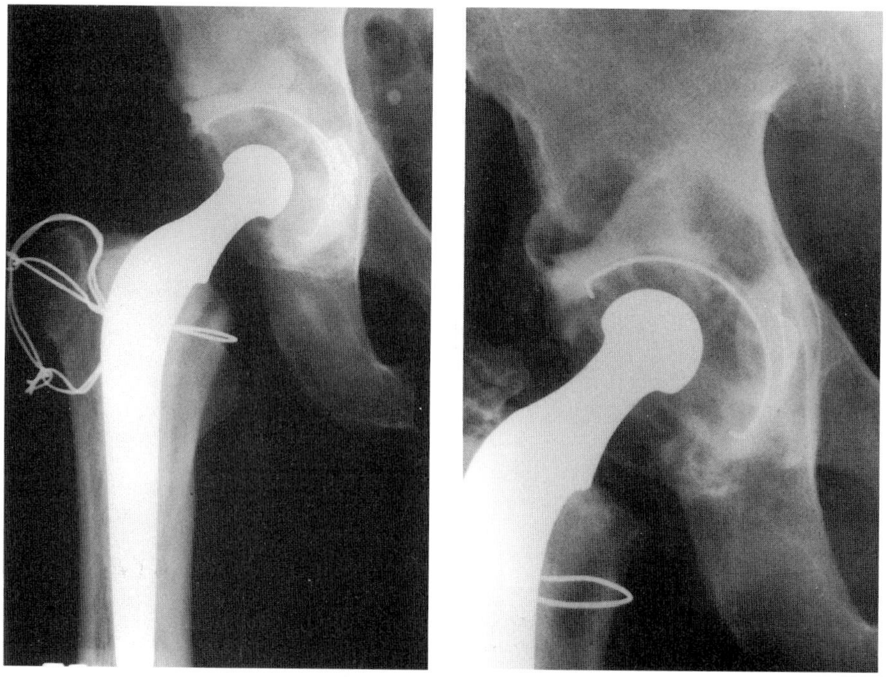

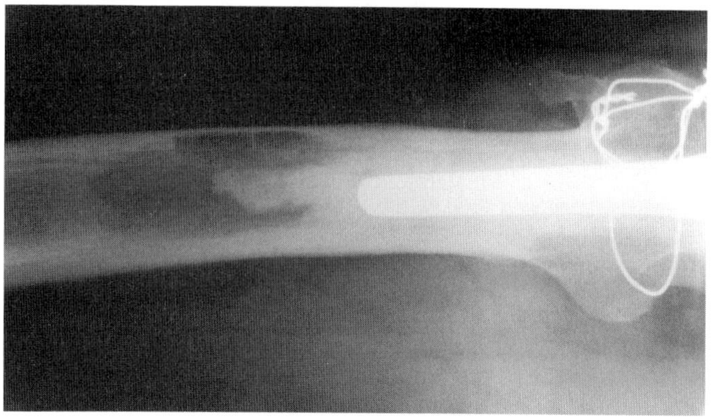

Fig. 8 Osteolysis without looseness of a cemented THA caused by polyethylene wear. **Top left,** Early postoperative view. **Top right,** Extensive polyethylene wear with severe periacetabular lysis 17 years later. **Bottom,** Extensive distal femoral lysis, without looseness, subsequently revised. All components were found to be firmly fixed; no debonding was noted. It demonstrates the concept of an effective joint space via polyethylene particles transmitted around a rigid cement mantle.

Wear rates in Charnley design sockets have been reported to vary by a factor of 100. Possible correlations to patient weight, activity, time of implantation, femoral head surface finish, polyethylene-batch variation, and sterilization technique have not been conclusive.

A spectrum of interrelated, complex macro and microtribologic factors exists that governs wear and friction of THAs. These factors include surface shape; contact stress; surface velocity; surface energy; roughness and adhesion; transfer films; oxidative wear; microabrasion from hard oxides and other larger three-body wear debris, such as bone cement and porous metal; lubrication and protein effects; and the mechanical properties of the bearing materials.

Few clinical data exist to demonstrate any advantage to alternative bearing materials. Wide variation exists in reports on wear of ceramic on ceramic, cobalt-chrome on cobalt-chrome, and ceramic on polyethylene bearings. Although a clinical report demonstrated ceramic on polyethylene to wear less than cobalt-chrome by a factor of 2.5, wear simulator data have not demonstrated any wear advantage of ceramic over cobalt-chrome as a bearing material.

Fretting and Corrosion Fretting occurs as a result of relative motion causing wear between two materials, and it has been documented at the back surfaces of polyethylene liners, at the junction of acetabular shell and screws, and at Morse taper junctions. A retrieval study of titanium prostheses showed screw-hole metal debris, which increased during the duration of the implant. Metal tapers are an additional source for metal debris as a result of mechanical fretting and corrosion and occur in similar and dissimilar metal junctions. Corrosive attack at the grain boundaries of the taper appears to be an important factor in Morse taper failure.

The Nature of Lysis Membranes The interface membrane found about aseptic loosened cemented implants contains a number of cells, including macrophages (60% to 80%), fibroblasts (15% to 30%), and T-lymphocytes (5%). Cytokines implicated in the inflammatory reaction against particulate debris of THA include: IL-1, IL-1-B, platelet derived growth factor, PGE_2, and TNF. Collagenase, IL-1, and PGE_2 have all been obtained from the membrane of loose prostheses. Macrophages, foreign-body giant cells, and osteoclasts arise from the monocyte-macrophage cell line and share many properties. However, osteoclasts resorb bone by a different mechanism. Mediators (eg, PGE_2) can stimulate bone resorption and are released by both macrophages and foreign body giant cells.

Progression of Lysis Osteolysis about both cemented and cementless femoral stems tends to be progressive. In stable femoral stems with noncircumferential porous coating, lysis appears earlier than about cemented stems, and it may progress more rapidly. When lysis develops about stable noncemented femoral stems, it frequently occurs in less than 3 years. The size of the lytic lesion increases progressively with time. When lysis develops about well-fixed cemented stems, the majority of cases develop 6 years after implantation.

Treating Osteolysis Because lysis is progressive in most cases, careful follow-up is essential and early intervention may be appropriate. Osteolysis as detected by radiographs is generally underestimated, particularly in the acetabulum. The periacetabular and femoral lesions are frequently asymptomatic, despite large areas of bone involvement. This observation emphasizes the importance of regular radiographic follow-up for early detection of osteolysis. Recurrence of osteolysis ("lysis after lysis") after a recemented revision is slight. Recurrence is reported in only 6.9% after a 5-year minimum follow-up (avg: 8.5 years).

Heterotopic Ossification

Heterotopic ossification (HO) arises from noncirculating connective-tissue cells with fibroblastic features. The reported rate of radiographic HO following "hip procedures" is between 8% and 90% and depends on the sex, bilaterality, preoperative nonsteroidal anti-inflammatory medication use, and age (over 60 years). Males have about twice the prevalence (42% versus 21%). Usually only the severe grades of HO (Brooker grades III or IV) are symptomatic, and the incidence of symptomatic HO after THA ranges from 1% to 33%.

A retrospective review of 637 THAs demonstrated that previous HO is a significant risk factor (82% chance of contralateral side developing HO). Revision surgery increased the severity from one to four Brooker classes in 50% of cases. Male sex and cemented THA were found to be significant risks by multivariate analysis.

A comparison study of 66 THAs found no difference between cemented and cementless fixation in HO formation. Although trochanteric osteotomy increased the risk (80%), there were no differences in anterolateral and posterior approaches. A comparison study of 65 primary hybrids with cementless primary THAs showed a significant increase in the number of high grade HOs (Brooker grades III or IV) and the subsequent need for repeated surgery (6%) in the cementless group. Factors such as the type of prosthesis, cement, preoperative range of motion, or the surgical approach have not been clearly proven as risk factors. At highest risk for HO are males with high grade HO (grade III) after the initial arthroplasty (73% association of second side with grade III after the first). These males are therefore candidates for prophylaxis.

Both nonsteroidal anti-inflammatory drugs (NSAIDs) and radiation therapy are effective preventative agents. Indomethacin, ibuprofen, diclofenac, and aspirin have all been shown to inhibit formation of HO in animal and human studies. In a prospective trial, 6 weeks of indomethacin after surgery reduced the HO incidence in a group of 100 patients. Side effects occurred in 20%, but most completed 4 weeks of treatment. A retrospective comparison of groups with or without aspirin during their hospital course showed an HO (grade III or IV) incidence of 3% with aspirin, and 48% without.

Naproxen at a dosage of 250 mg three times a day for 4 weeks was found to reduce the overall incidence of HO (48% versus 14%) in a study of 53 patients undergoing THA. In a double blind, prospective, randomized study, diclofenac twice a day for 6 weeks was effective in reducing overall HO from 55% to 15% and eliminating severe degrees of HO.

Higher risk patients may require irradiation at higher doses to prevent HO. New HO developed in 58% of a series of 33 patients treated with single fraction 700 cGy radiation therapy; those with three or more risk factors had a high rate of recurrence. The treatment should take place within 3 days of surgery with shielding of cementless implants or trochanteric osteotomies. In a randomized study, 141 hips at high risk to develop HO were treated postoperatively with either low-dose (five exposures of 200 cGy each) or high-dose (ten exposures at 200 cGy or 5 at 350 cGy) irradiation. The high dose was more effective. NSAIDs lowered the failure rate in both low- and high-dose groups. The only effective treatment for established HO is surgical excision.

Stress Shielding

Stress shielding of bone represents an adaptive remodeling of bone to altered stress and is found in both cemented and cementless arthroplasties. Cancellous bone is one tenth to one fiftieth as stiff as cortical bone, and cortical bone is one tenth as stiff as cobalt-chrome. Titanium has an elastic modulus about half that of cobalt-chrome. Large modulus mismatches between the femoral stem and proximal femur can lead to stress redistribution in the bone. Reduction in the stresses of the calcar region by as much as 70% have been measured after metal stem insertion. A reduction in the elastic modulus of the stem increases the bone stresses in the calcar region, but also increases cement stresses in the case of the cemented stem. Larger diameter cementless femoral stems (especially if bone ingrown) lead to increased stress shielding. Larger stem diameters lead to higher rigidity (axial rigidity increases directly with cross-sectional area or square of the stem diameter; flexural rigidity increases with the moment of inertia or fourth power of the stem diameter). In a clinical series of extensively coated, cobalt-chrome stems, two thirds of the more pronounced stress-shielded femora occurred with stem diameters greater than 15 mm (five to 10 times the flexural rigidity of smaller diameter stems). Risk factors for stress shielding include age, sex, preexisting osteopenia, extent of porous coating, and diameter and stiffness of the stem. In the canine model, stem stiffness is a major factor in the bone remodeling response of the proximal femur. The remodeling process, as detected by retrieval or absorptiometry, can be quite profound at times, particularly in cases of extensively porous-coated femoral prostheses (Fig. 9).

Dual energy x-ray absorptiometry is an accurate and reproducible method for measuring bone mineral density (BMD). In a study of 72 femoral prostheses, a small but progressive decrease in BMD continued for 5 to 7 years after implantation. A study of the natural history of stress shielding demonstrated a 40% bone loss proximally, and 28% bone loss distally at 3 years, but at later follow-up (between 7 and 14 years), 40% proximal and 49% distal loss were measured. The greatest decrease in BMD (34%) occurred in the proximal 1 cm of the medial femoral cortex, around stiffer, more extensively coated porous implants. Although stress shielding is also characteristic of cemented stems, the effect does not appear to be adverse in long-term retrieval studies. Osteoporosis occurring in the bone surrounding the cement mantle appears to be a reorientation of the endosteal trabeculae. As the endosteal bone expands and the cortical bone thins, the trabeculae reorient, connecting the neocortex against the cement with the endosteal cortex. The implant remains mechanically fixed to the neocortex.

Infections

Overall, the incidence of sepsis is approximately 1% over the lifetime of the prosthesis. An analysis of 2,651 THA cases identified diabetes, failed fracture osteosynthesis, a breakdown of sterility during surgery, postoperative urinary tract infection, and an unhealed wound at discharge as perioperative risk factors for deep sepsis. Most deep infections of total joint implants are thought to result from airborne contaminants. About half of THA sepsis is thought to arise at the time of operation. A comparison of prophylaxis given for 1 day (cefuroxime) compared with cefazolin given for 3 days found no difference in the infection rate in a prospective double blind study of 1,354 total

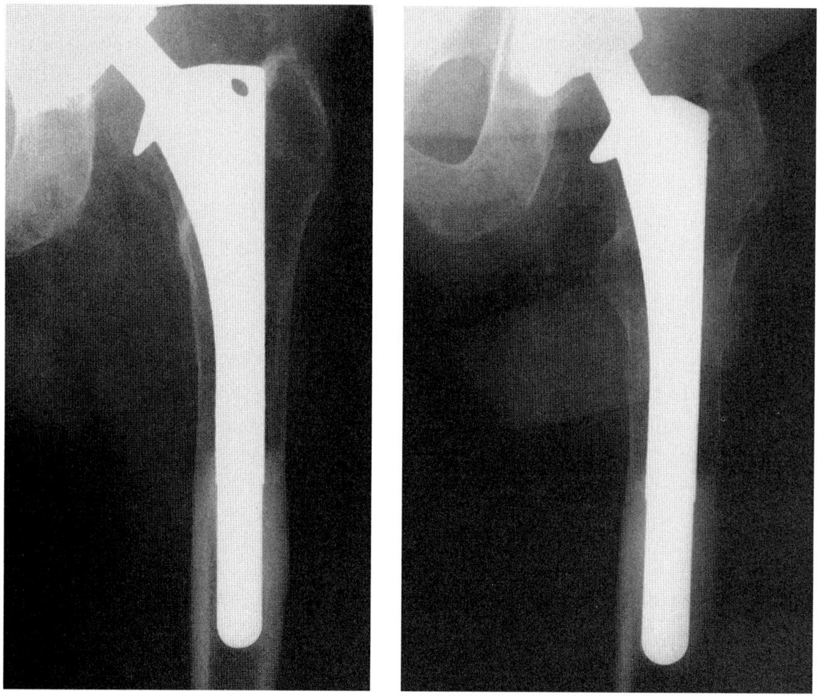

Fig. 9 Spontaneous fracture through weakened bone caused by stress shielding from an extensively coated cementless stem. **Left,** Advanced proximal stress shielding with distal cortical hypertrophy in a bone-ingrown stem. **Right,** Fracture and buckling noted in the lateral cortex and trochanter with remainder of distal stem well fixed.

joint patients. In a large multicenter study, there was a 50% reduction in infection with the use of ultra clean air, and an additional 50% reduction with the use of body-exhaust suits. Ultraviolet light is bactericidal and has been effective in disinfecting operating theater air.

Isotope Scans for Sepsis The results of technetium Tc 99m nanocolloid scintigraphy in 21 prosthetic infections were at least equivalent to those of indium In 111 leucocyte scintigraphy. The sensitivity was 94%, the specificity 84%, and the accuracy 87% (versus 75%, 90%, and 85%, respectively, for the leucocyte scintigraphy). Additional advantages were shorter examination time, less complexity, and better radiation dosimetry.

In a study comparing 43 arthroplasty patients undergoing scans using leukocytes labeled with technetium Tc 99m or indium In 111, diagnostic value of the two tests was similar in detecting prosthetic infection. Data from a comparison study of the effectiveness of plain radiographs, bone scans, and hip aspiration in 54 painful arthroplasties indicated that bone scanning was useful only when radiography was inconclusive. There is no concensus about the relative merit of one type of radionuclide scan versus another in the evaluation of the painful THA.

Intraoperative Frozen Section Intraoperative diagnosis of infection by the use of frozen tissue section has been considered unreliable according to results of several studies. The key to better sensitivity with frozen section technique may be appropriate deep sampling of periprosthetic tissue, microscopic scanning under low power to seek the maximally inflamed tissue, averaging 10 (at 400×) high-power fields to interpret the cell counts, and lowering the criteria established by Mirra from 5 cells per field to 1 to 5 cells (polymorphonuclear leucocytes, lymphocytes, and plasma cells in nonrheumatoid patients). These techniques have been reported to improve the sensitivity of intraoperative frozen section for diagnosis of infection to 90% and accuracy to 95%.

Dental Prophylaxis A review of the case reports of dental sepsis leading to joint infection by hematogenous spread has shown that actual confirmation of the oral pathogen and correlation with blood culture are rare. Although there is clear evidence that THA infection can result from dental manipulation, there is disagreement on the use of prophylactic antibiotics based on risk-benefit analysis. Some authors advocate prophylaxis only for those at high risk for prolonged bacteremia, namely patients with diabetes mellitus and rheumatoid arthritis and the immunosuppressed patient. Most dental manipulations leading to bacteremia are due to streptococcus. The transient bacteremia is detectable within 5 minutes after the procedure and persists for 10 to 30 minutes. Although the majority of orthopaedic surgeons surveyed recommend predental antibacterial prophylaxis (93%), a substantial number (41%) believe the practice lacks foundation or is of minor importance.

The American Heart Association standard prophylaxis recommendation is for amoxicillin, 3 g orally 1 hour before the procedure, and then 1.5 g 6 hours after the initial dose. They recommend the following standard regimen for patients allergic to penicillin: erythromycin ethyl succinate, 800 mg, or erythromycin stearate, 1 g, orally 2 hours before the procedure, then half the dose 6 hours after the initial dose; or clindamycin, 300 mg orally 1 hour before the procedure, and 150 mg 6 hours after the initial dose. For patients at high risk but allergic to amoxicillin, ampicillin, and penicillin, the recommendation is for vancomycin, 1 g intravenously over 1 hour, starting 1 hour before the procedure. No repeat dose is necessary.

Management of the Infected THA Surgical management of deep prosthetic infections has been successful with both single-stage revision (surgical debridement and immediate reimplantation followed by systemic antibiotic administration) and two-stage revision (surgical debridement, with or without placement of an antibiotic spacer, administration of systemic antibiotics, and prosthetic reimplantation at a later date). The addition of antibiotics to the cement can improve the salvage rate of both one- and two-stage reimplantations.

A two-staged treatment is the most successful method of eradicating infection from a THA. Two-staged reconstruction has recently been reported to be successful in eradicating infection in 84% to 97% of cases (Table 6). The two-stage method is generally considered a safer technique (lower recurrence), particularly when the infection is caused by a more virulent organism. Evidence has shown an increased risk for recurrence if a more virulent organism is treated with antibiotics for less than 28 days. Factors that increase the risk of recurrence include multiple previous surgeries, host compromise and malnutrition, extensive infection, highly virulent organism, and inadequate debridement.

The use of antibiotic beads placed in the deep wound at the time of resection has not conclusively improved results. A prospective multicenter randomized study of prosthetic infections showed no difference when treated by either debridement plus gentamicin PMMA beads or debridement and a conventional systemic antibiotic therapy.

The use of an antibiotic-impregnated spacer placed at the time of the initial debridement in a two-stage reconstruction has been reported to provide high local concentrations of antibiotic while allowing maintenance of soft-tissue tension and leg length to facilitate later reconstruction. The use of a gentamicin-impregnated spacer had 80% success in a small series of two-stage reconstructions. Only two of the five cases were ambulatory with the spacer. In a study of 15 cases using an antibiotic spacer prosthesis, it permitted 93% ambulatory status.

A two-stage technique of debridement and creation of a spacer prosthesis (autoclaved femoral component surrounded with high dose, 24 cc of tobramycin powder per 40 g pack of cement) and a polyethylene cemented socket in 14 THAs was followed 2 weeks later by reimplantation

Table 6. Success rates for one and two stage revisions

Year of Study	Cases	Success (%) One-stage	Success (%) Two-stage
1981	583	77	
1986	102	91	
1987	37	93	
1988	78	76	
1992	243	78	
1989	82		87
1992	86		87
1994	37		84*
1994	32		91

*Plus one additional debridement

of a conventional prosthesis with antibiotic cement. After 6 weeks of systemic antibiotics followed by 6 months of oral antibiotics, 96% success rate in eradication of the infections was reported. A high rate of dislocation (35%) in the revised hips was the primary cause of patient dissatisfaction. Data from a minimum 2-year study of 46 patients using a two-stage procedure with a temporary spacer of antibiotic-coated metal and a polyethylene socket indicated treatment was successful in controlling infection in 93.5% of cases.

A retrospective review of 46 infected THAs treated with two-stage resection and 6 weeks of systemic antibiotics showed a 91% success in 32 hips that were suitable for reimplantation. Minimum follow-up was 2 years. Fourteen hips were not reimplanted because of inadequate bone stock, poor soft-tissue quality, or antibiotic resistance of the infecting organism.

A retrospective review of 37 infected THAs treated by three-stage reimplantation (resection with debridement, redebridement at 1 week, and reimplantation at 4 weeks) showed a success rate of 84%. This report emphasized an aggressive surgical approach to management while shortening the interval of reimplantation to 4 weeks.

Dislocation

One goal of THA is to create adequate mechanical offset and soft-tissue tension to provide a stable reconstruction. Dislocation varies from 1% to 10% and studies have associated it most consistently with additional surgery. Diagnosis, age, and head size have never been clearly shown to be associated risks. The approach to the hip affects the dislocation rate, with (generally) higher risk of posterior dislocation with a posterior approach. Posterior dislocation is the most common direction of instability reported and represents 60% to 90% of dislocations.

Forty percent to 70% of dislocations occur in the first month after surgery. The chance of recurrent dislocation is less in those whose first dislocation is in the first postoperative month and higher in those who dislocate 3 months after surgery. Less than 1% of patients first dislocate after 5 years; most of these are women (3:1 ratio). Successful treatment has been reported in 63% to 83% of chronic dislocators following 6 to 12 weeks of immobilization. Thus, about one third of dislocations will recur despite treatment with appropriate immobilization.

When additional surgery for recurrent dislocation is undertaken, reorientation of the components only will be required in 40% of cases. Socket orientation may be the most important variable in hip dislocation. The use of modular devices may prove to be of substantial benefit in this situation. When the cause is known and corrected, success is about 70%. When the specific cause for instability is not clearly identified, or the only procedure performed is removal of the impingement, the success rate drops to under 50%. If the cause is unknown, and simple trochanteric advancement is done, the success is about 75% overall and 84% if trochanteric union occurs. Trochanteric nonunion and migration can increase the risk of dislocation two to six times. A series of 21 patients with recurrent dislocation without component malposition were treated with trochanteric osteotomy and distal advancement alone with a success rate of 81%.

The use of an elevated rim liner to improve stability of a hip appears dependent on the cause of instability, the orientation of the shell and liner, and the elevated rim liner geometry. The primary use for an elevated rim liner is to change the orientation of a malpositioned metal shell without having to revise the shell. The use of a wall-socket design may be important when considering use of a 22-mm diameter socket with a posterior approach. In a comparative study of a 22-mm simple hemispherical design and a 22-mm high posterior wall Charnley cup, the dislocation rate was statistically higher with the hemispherical design when surgery was performed with a posterior approach.

Periprosthetic Fractures

Periprosthetic fractures of the proximal femur can be classified according to the AAOS Committee on the Hip, based on both fracture location and pattern (Fig. 10). The classification of Duncan and Masri (Fig. 11, Table 7) is based on fracture location, fixation of the stem, and the quality of the bone. Complications associated with periprosthetic fractures include malunion, nonunion, and late loosening of the femoral component. The AAOS types IV and V are difficult fractures to manage closed because of the high chance of malalignment and malunion. Types III, IV, and V are associated with higher rates of late femoral loosening.

Fractures associated with a rigidly fixed femoral component can be managed by open or closed means. A plate or allograft strut is usually helpful in buttressing the fracture that is fixed with screws, and/or cerclage wires or cables. Combination plates that allow screw and/or cable fixation can be quite beneficial in these fractures. When the bone stock is inadequate for plate fixation, the femoral cement mantle is violated, or a canal-filling cementless device is present, an extracortical allograft and fixation may be

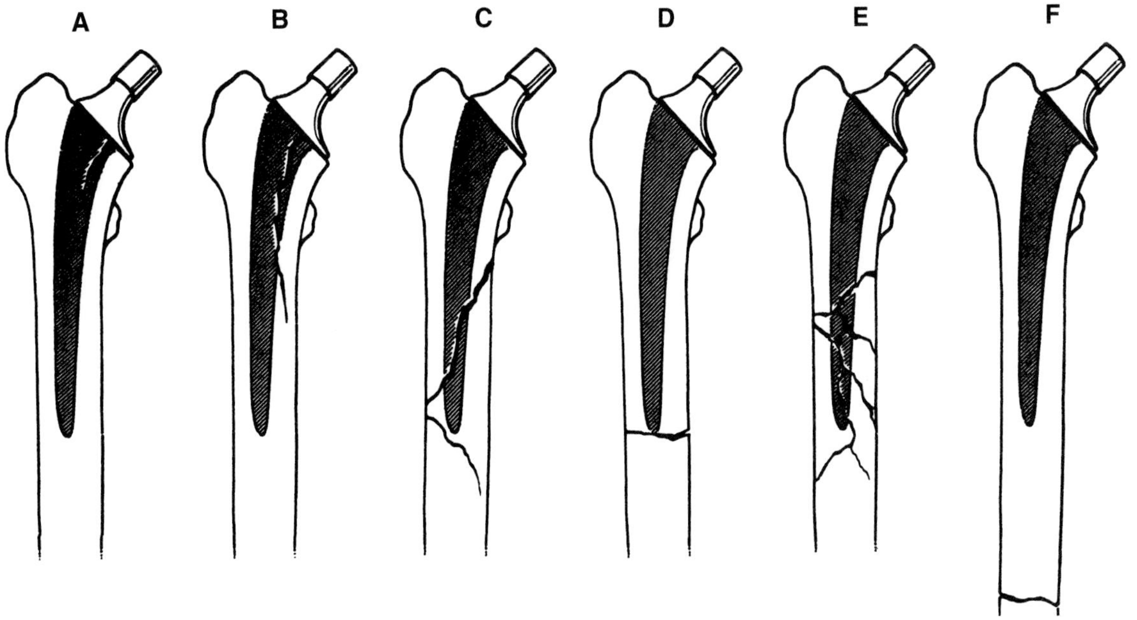

Fig. 10 Classification of femoral fractures associated with total hip arthroplasty based on location and pattern of fracture. Type 1 (not shown), located proximal to intertrochanteric line, commonly occurs preoperatively and does not alter the treatment of total hip arthroplasty. **A,** Type II, level 1 is vertical or spiral fracture (split) that does not pass the lower margin of the lesser trochanter. **B,** Type III, level 2 is vertical split or spiral fracture that extends to or beyond the lower margin of the lesser trochanter but does not pass the junction of middle and lower third of femoral stem. **C,** Type IV, level 2 includes area of femoral stem tip; IVA is spiral, and IVB is transverse, **D. E,** Type V, level 3 extends distal to stem with comminution. **F,** Type VI, level 3 fracture line is located distal to prothesis. (Courtesy of the American Academy of Orthopaedic Surgeons Committee on the Hip.)

used. Postoperative management must follow the principles of standard fracture management, with protective casting or bracing and restricted weightbearing.

Fractures associated with an existing loose femoral component are generally best treated by revision to provide stable fixation and early mobilization of the patient. At the time of revision, restoration of the cortical tube is achieved through fixation of the fracture around a trial stem using cerclage and/or plate fixation. Conceivably, both cementless and cemented femoral components may be used in the reconstruction if they are long enough to provide stability of the distal fracture fragment. Use of cement in conjunction with fractures of the femoral shaft is successful as long as the cement does not interfere with the apposition of the bone fragments. In a series of ten patients, compression plating for femur fractures at 2-year follow-up was reported to have a 90% union rate. Cemented revision long-stem fixation of periprosthetic fractures provides immediate rigid fixation that is advantageous in the postoperative rehabilitation of the patient. If the prosthesis is loose and the bone stock is inadequate due to osteoporosis, osteolysis, or severe comminution, revision with a proximal femoral replacement may be indicated. In the younger individual, proximal allograft replacement may be a better choice.

Femoral Component Revision Arthroplasty

The tremendous diversity of pathology and the wide range of difficulty encountered during revision THA results in a situation in which no one method can perform ideally in all instances. The challenge is to identify the optimal device and technique for a particular patient based on the bone loss, quality of residual soft tissues, and anticipated demands that will be placed on the reconstruction. Soft-tissue compromise, associated femoral periprosthetic fractures, and presence or absence of prior infection are only a few of the additional factors that may have a significant impact on outcome. Each patient's unique circumstances at the time of reconstruction must be carefully considered in order to optimize the final result.

Removal of the Failed Femoral Component

The mode of prior implant failure may affect revision difficulty and the quality of the remaining bone. Although the use of large superalloy stems of titanium or chrome-cobalt instead of small stainless steel stems has markedly reduced the incidence of stem fracture, rare cases of failure have been reported at the junction of some modular femoral heads with the implant neck (Fig. 12). This situation usually results in the need to remove an otherwise well-

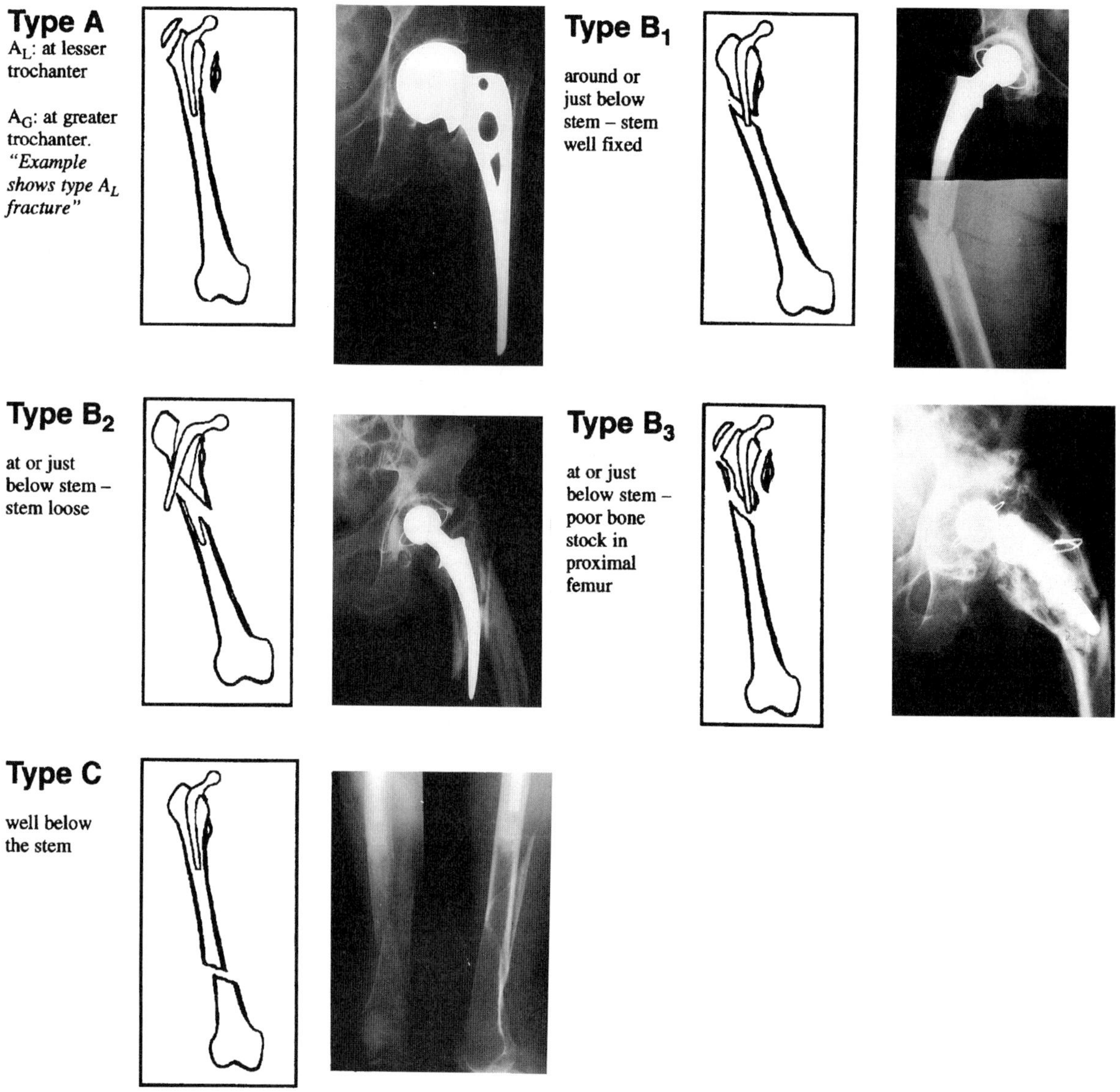

Fig. 11 Duncan and Masri classification system for fractures of the femur after total hip arthroplasty. (Reproduced with permission from Duncan CP, Masri BA: Fractures of the femur after hip replacement, in Jackson DW (ed): *Instructional Course Lectures 44.* Rosemont, IL, American Academy of Orthopaedic Surgeons, 1995, pp 293–304.)

fixed stem. Other failure modes seen with stems that are often solidly fixed and difficult to extract are recurrent dislocation, localized osteolysis, and some infection.

Bone Loss

The most widely accepted classification system is that proposed by the American Academy of Orthopaedic Surgeons Committee on the Hip, which uses the designation of cavitary, segmental, and combined defects to describe the type of bone loss present in any of the three specified zones used in this system (Table 8). Defect classification can facilitate the study of patients following reconstruction and allows treatment guidelines to be offered specific to the type and location of bone loss encountered. In general, traditional cemented and porous-coated implant systems have experienced poorer results in the face of greater

Table 7. Proposed classification of fractures of the femur following total hip arthroplasty

Type	Location	Subtype
A	Trochanteric region	A_G: Greater trochanter A_L: Lesser trochanter
B	Around or just distal to the stem	B_1: Prosthesis stable B_2: Prosthesis unstable B_3: Bone stock inadequate
C	Well below the stem	

(Reproduced with permission from Duncan CP, Masri BA: Fractures of the femur after hip replacement, in Jackson DW (ed): *Instructional Course Lectures 44.* Rosemont, IL, American Academy of Orthopaedic Surgeons, 1995, pp 293–304.)

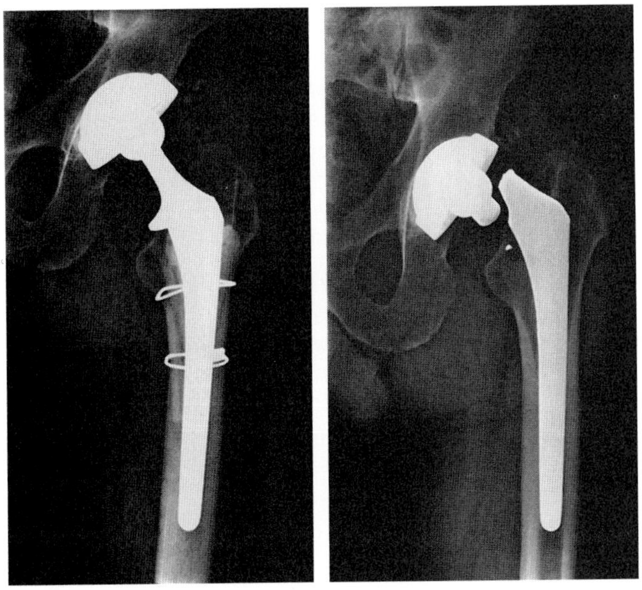

Fig. 12 Fatigue fracture of modular head of a well-fixed porous ingrowth femoral component.

degrees of bone loss, leading some to recommend increasingly distal fixation as proximal bone damage increases.

Femoral Reconstruction

Bone Grafting Although prosthetic replacement of lost femoral bone stock with large segment replacement stems (originally developed for tumor surgery) is possible, high rates of dislocation, infection, and subsequent stem loosening have been noted, with an overall survivorship of 73% at 11 years postsurgery in one reported series. This procedure is best reserved for salvage of massive bone loss in elderly or low-demand patients. Thus, restoration of lost bone with bone grafting is a frequent adjunct to femoral revision surgery.

Cancellous Morcellized Bone Graft Smaller cavitary defects, which remain between uncemented stems and host

Table 8. American Academy of Orthopaedic Surgeons Committee on the Hip classification of femoral defects in total hip arthroplasty

Defect Type	Description
1	Segmental
2	Cavitary
3	Combined (segmental and cavitary)
4	Malalignment
5	Femoral stenosis
6	Femoral discontinuity

bone, can be filled effectively with cancellous graft. Some degree of radiographic incorporation is frequently observed. However, if larger cavitary defects are present and the impacted cancellous bone is used to contribute to stability of a proximally porous-coated implant, increasing rates of subsidence and revision are encountered. In cemented revision surgery, use of cancellous graft densely packed in to the deficient cavitary proximal femur in combination with a tapered femoral component has been described by Ling as detailed below. Cancellous bone graft is a frequent adjunct to solid allograft struts or large segment allografts when these are needed for more extensive bone deficiencies.

Onlay Cortical Strut Allograft Recent reports have documented the efficacy of onlay strut allografts in restoring segmental defects in the proximal femur. A review of 174 patients undergoing strut grafting in combination with a cementless proximally coated calcar replacement stem during revision hip surgery showed that graft union was observed in 98% of cases. Similar high union rates have been recently reported for cortical struts used in combination with an extensively coated stem. The combination of distal stem fixation and proximal bone struts was radiographically observed to successfully restore lost femoral bone stock. Small segments of bone, measuring 1 to 2 cm, used in the medial calcar area have shown a high rate of subsequent resorption, which is most ikely related to rapid revascularization.

Large Segment Allografts When massive bone deficiency is present, replacement of the entire proximal femur with a large segment allograft allows restoration of anatomic relationships and provides potential sites for bony healing of the distal host to the graft and of the trochanter or other proximal bone fragments to the outside of the graft (Fig. 13). The resulting allograft prosthetic composite usually involves a long stem extending distally into the host bone. Stem fixation to the graft should be with cement, and the use of antibiotic-impregnated cement may have value in protecting the allograft from subsequent infection. Distal stem fixation is frequently uncemented, but the use of cement may be necessary if the extent or quality of the distal bone remaining is poor.

Proponents of this method cite rapid return to weightbearing, physiologic loading of the distal femur, and reconstruction of proximal bone stock as advantages of the method. Disadvantages include dislocation rates of 17% to 55%, nonunion rates of 19% to 25%, and infection rates of 6% to 8%. These problems have led many authors who are experienced with this method to suggest its use be reserved for those massive defects not amenable to other reconstructive methods. Use of alternative techniques such as onlay strut grafting of remnant host bone whenever possible is suggested.

Cemented Femoral Fixation Following Revision

First-Generation Cement Methods Repeat revision rates from several centers have ranged up to 6% by 4.5 years with radiographic evidence of loosening in as many as 44%. With longer follow-up, ongoing deterioration of results has been observed both radiographically and by clinical criteria. In one report of 210 cemented revision stems with 10 years average follow-up, 64% of the stems were either loose or had been revised.

Second-Generation Cement Methods Improvement in both clinical and radiographic results in cemented revisions can be achieved using these methods. In one series of 43 cases followed up for an average of 6.2 years, definite or probable radiographic loosening was present in 11% and repeat revision for aseptic loosening had been required in only one hip (2%). Later follow-up of this same group of patients revealed that the re-revision rate had increased to 10.5% by 11.7 years after surgery with another 10.5% radiographically loose. In a separate study of 42 hip replacements in patients who were younger than 50 years old at surgery, femoral revision was needed in 5% and another 12% were radiographically loose at an average of 11 years follow-up. Thus, a revision rate of 0.5% to 1% per year over the first decade has been reported with second-generation cemented methods on the femoral side. This rate represents a significant improvement over the failure rates observed with earlier cement techniques. When the bony bed precludes significant cement interdigitation, it is reasonable to expect a reduction in fixation durability over time. The relative value in revision surgery of more recent so-called third-generation cement methods, including the use of spacers and stem centralizers, cement porosity reduction, and stem surface enhancements, remains to be established with long-term follow-up studies, but may allow some improvement in results observed with second-generation techniques.

Uncemented Femoral Revision

Proximally Porous-Coated Stems Although initial short-term reports of proximally porous-coated femoral components for revision surgery were encouraging, subsequent experience has led to abandonment of first-generation proximally coated implants in most revision cases. Initial reports of the proximally-coated Harris-Galante prosthe-

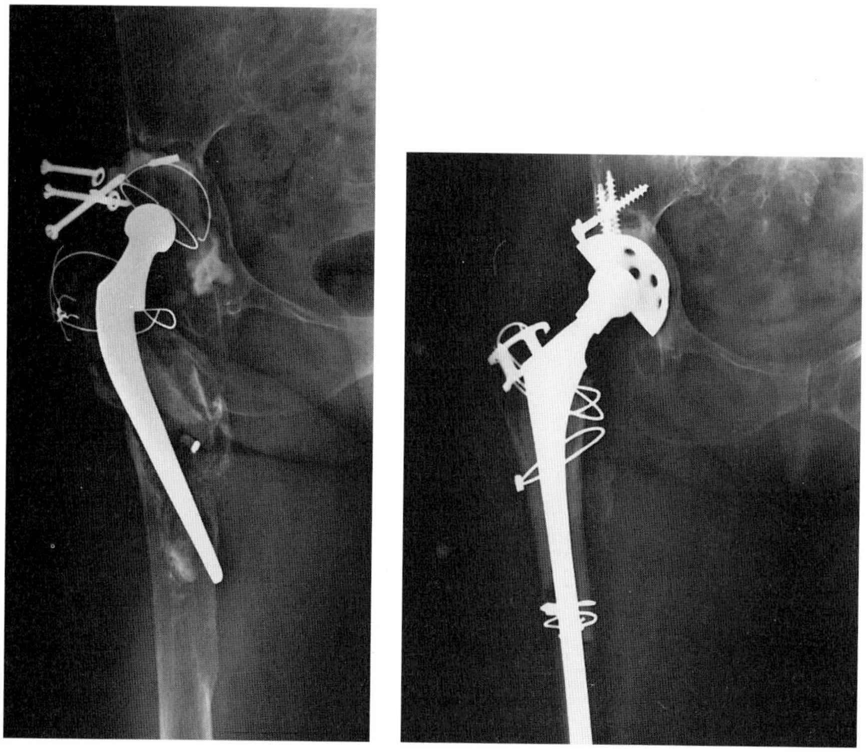

Fig. 13 Allograft prosthetic composite for reconstruction of massive osteolysis and periprosthetic fracture of the proximal femur.

sis for revision surgery in 28 cases revealed a re-revision rate of 20% at 5.5 years follow-up and a subsidence rate of 45%. Design modifications, including long-curved smooth stems and increases in proximal bulk with wedge-shaped geometries designed to facilitate proximal loadbearing were also followed by disappointing results, marked by significant rates of subsidence, radiographic loosening, and re-revision. Rates of intraoperative fracture increased significantly due to efforts at achieving a tight fit and maximum filling of sclerotic, damaged proximal femur (Fig. 14).

In a recent report of 69 femoral component revisions using an uncemented curved long-stem metaphyseal filling, proximally coated cobalt device (Osteonics Omnifit Long Stem), no clear-cut advantage was demonstrated by the addition of a longer stem to a tapered proximal geometry designed to maximize fit and fill of the proximal femur. With a mean follow-up of 3 years, repeat revision had been required in 9%, intraoperative fractures were noted in 46%, and significant rates of subsidence were observed. At 5 years, 82% of the entire series were free of revision or moderate pain, compared to only 58% of those with an intraoperative femoral fracture. These data clearly document an adverse effect on outcome from this complication.

A recent report of 375 consecutive revisions using six different proximally porous-coated implant designs (both long and short stem) showed that none of the devices performed in satisfactory fashion over the first 5 years postrevision. The revision rate for the overall series was 20%. Twenty-four percent of patients had moderate to severe pain and 29% mild pain. Forty percent of the devices were radiographically loose and an additional 17% possibly loose. Twenty-six percent of the cases in this series were associated with intraoperative fracture. Increased subsidence and decreased survivorship was noted when more severe bone loss was present.

Extensively Porous-Coated Stems Diaphyseal fixation using extensively coated long stems has been shown in recent reports to provide durable fixation for 10 years, with success rates equal to or exceeding those reported with other methods (Fig. 15). A recent report of 81 cases with 5- to 13-year follow-up documented 90% stem survivorship at 9 years. Radiographic loosening was noted in 11% and repeat revision was required in 10%, with five of the eight revisions in patients in whom the stem was undersized. In another review of 297 uncemented femoral revisions using an extensively coated implant that were followed up for 5.1 years, the aseptic loosening rate was 2% and an additional 1% of patients had radiographic loosening, but had not yet been revised. Potential tradeoffs with such a design include the potential for significant difficulty if the implant needed removal, and concerns about the long-term effects of proximal stress shielding. However, in the revision setting in which proximal bone has already been severely compromised, the only effective method of achieving stable noncemented implant fixation may be by distal diaphyseal fixation, which can then be combined with bone grafting to reconstitute the proximal femur. Not all patients are ideally suited for this type of implant. Fem-

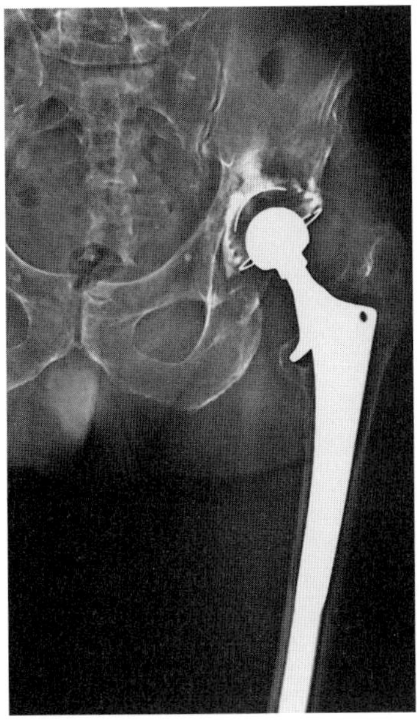

Fig. 14 Painful subsidence of an uncemented proximally porous-coated long-stem revision stem.

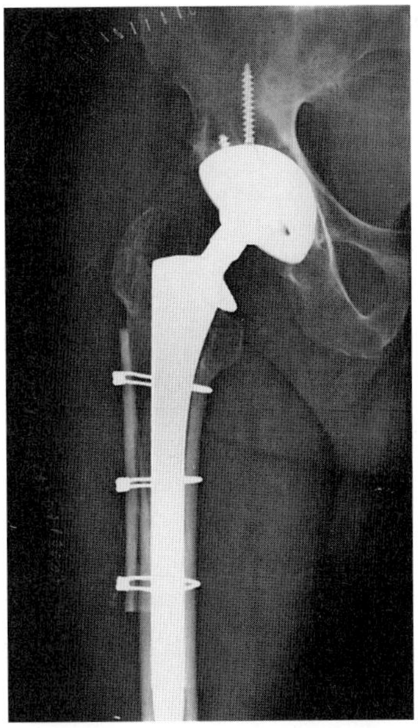

Fig. 15 Extensively coated revision femoral component placed with endosteal cancellous graft and onlay cortical strut grafts to restore proximal femoral bone stock.

oral canals with excessively large diameters may require placement of stems 18 mm or larger and risk increased rates of thigh pain due to presence of such a large stiff implant, while increasing the risks of proximal stress shielding.

Certain key points relating to the use of extensively porous-coated implants for revision surgery bear emphasis. First, complete cement removal is essential because residual plaques of cement can cause eccentric reaming, deviation of the implant at the time of impaction, and femoral fracture. The quality of canal fit has been correlated with subsequent outcome in several series. Diaphyseal fit over an area of 5 cm is recommended, and because many femoral canals are larger in the AP dimension than in the medial lateral plane, some overreaming in the medial lateral direction is often needed.

Intrafemoral Impaction Cancellous Allografting and Cement: The Ling Technique

Recent reports describe a method of femoral reconstruction in which compressed morcellized cancellous allograft is placed into the endosteal aspect of the femur, which is then further compacted with a series of tamps and trials prior to placement of a cemented, collarless, polished femoral stem within an envelope made up entirely of allograft cancellous chips (Fig. 16). In 68 femoral revisions followed up for 30 months, no repeat revisions have been required and significant improvement in function and pain scores was maintained over the follow-up period. Some slight subsidence of the polished stem within the cement mantle was noted in over 50% of the hips in this series. In a more recent report of 37 patients followed up for 2 to 5 years, subsidence of the stem within the cement was again noted in just over half. Subsidence of the cement within the surrounding bony envelope occurred in 11%. Grafts were judged to have incorporated in 77% of the hips at 2 years, and the initial results were encouraging.

The impaction cancellous allograft method appears promising, especially as a method for reconstructing cavitary deficiencies of the metaphysis and upper diaphysis. The long-term durability of this reconstructive method is uncertain, however, and the actual degree to which the bone graft incorporates and achieves viability and, therefore, potential value for subsequent revision surgery or long-term implant support is also unknown at the present.

Acetabular Revision

Bone Defects

Bone defects are broadly classified into contained and noncontained defects. Contained defects are pockets that are closed against the surface of the acetabular implant. Noncontained defects are segmental deficiencies of bone that allow the prosthetic hemispheric surface to contact or communicate with the surrounding soft tissues. The AAOS classification of acetabular deficiencies attempts to incorporate these concepts into anatomic location and

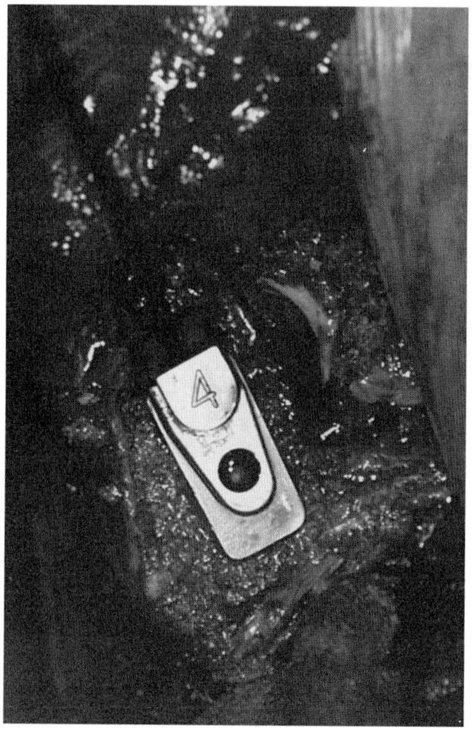

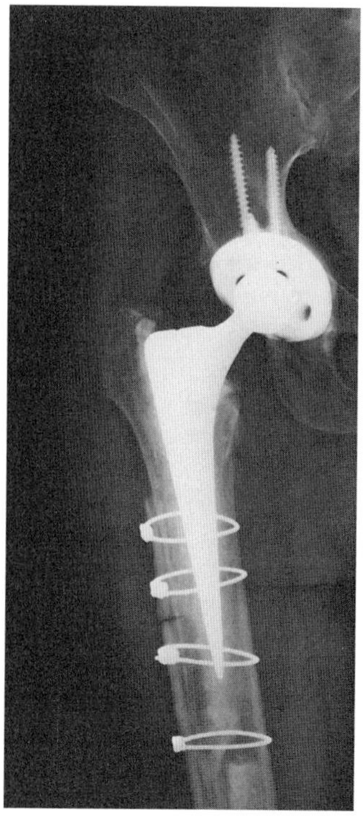

Fig. 16 Example of impaction and cancellous bone grafting of the proximal femur and placement of a cemented stem within the column of allograft chips. Onlay cortical strut allografting was used to prevent concentration of stress at the stem tip and reconstruct a segmental defect of the proximal femur as well.

combinations. This classification uses the terms segmental and cavitary to correspond to noncontained and contained defects, respectively. Type I deficiencies are segmental and divided into rim and medial wall locations. Type II are cavitary deficiencies divided into location (superior, anterior, posterior, and medial). Type III are combinations of segmental and cavitary defects. In addition, type IV deficiency is designated for pelvic discontinuity, and type V as arthrodesis. Major segmental deficiencies (type I) or combinations may require structural allograft reconstruction in order to provide component stability. In cases of type I medial deficiency, allograft reconstruction is technically difficult, and these cases are proven to be well managed by peripheral rim-fit sockets (ie, the support of the socket is obtained by oversizing the socket to the existing bony rim diameter). Type IV pelvic discontinuity defects usually require additional fixation across the discontinuity with the use of plate and screw fixation.

Joint Center Restoration

Restoration of the normal joint center is one of several goals in revision arthroplasty. This goal may be difficult to achieve in cases of proximal cup migration with associated bone deficiency and can require oblong sockets or allografts. Mechanical studies of sockets placed nonanatomically with the center lateral (20 mm), proximal (20 mm), and posterior (10 mm) indicate they have significantly higher stresses, with implications for fixation longevity. The cementing of sockets proximal to the anatomic center but without lateralization has been reported with acceptable 11-year results. This method may also be applicable to cementless sockets, but long-term data are not yet available.

It is generally agreed that the use of structural allografts is not preferable to the choice of a high cementless socket location without graft, although long-term data for cementless high sockets are not available. The use of an oblong socket allows fixation with a porous-coated device in contact with host bone (type II reconstruction), thereby eliminating the need for structural allograft (type III reconstruction) while restoring the joint center. However, no intermediate or long-term data exist to support this technique.

Methods of Reconstruction

Bipolar Reconstruction The bipolar acetabular component has not shown satisfactory performance in revision acetabular cases. The use of morcellized allograft with a bipolar device in severe cavitary acetabular defects is not structurally sound, and it should be considered only as a salvage procedure for the elderly or infirm patient. In an early follow-up study of 81 revision hips treated with a bipolar device, there was more than 50% bone graft resorption and migration, with a 13.3% revision rate at less than 3 years. At a minimum 5-year follow-up, satisfactory clinical results were reported in 58%.

In a study of 18 patients, only 22% showed radiographic improvement of the acetabular bone stock with this technique. Less than 40% had satisfactory clinical outcomes. The only other potential indication for the use of this device may be in instability of the hip reconstruction (lack of hip abductors) in the presence of sufficient acetabular bone stock.

Porous, Fixed Component Intermediate results for porous-coated, fixed, hemispheric sockets are remarkably good if the cases requiring structural supporting bone grafts are excluded. At 3 to 6 years' follow-up, a series of 138 revision sockets of a hemispheric, titanium mesh-coated design fixed with screws had a combined revision or migration rate of 5%. If only the aseptic cases were considered, no components migrated or were revised. This technique as reported has the best results for an acetabular revision series with any type of fixation at this length follow-up. In a study of porous acetabular components from a larger series of 166 hip revisions with an average follow-up of 4.4, there was 95% stable fixation with none revised.

Threaded Socket Threaded ring sockets have demonstrated substantial (12%) early failure rates in primary cases, with even worse results in revision cases (39%). At an intermediate follow-up of 62 months (range: 27 to 108), 31% of 52 primaries, and 62% of 16 revisions failed. When combined with structural allograft, a series of 32 threaded rings failed in 44% of cases at less than 4 years' follow-up. This technique has generally been abandoned.

Cemented Socket The poor early results of cemented acetabular revision reflect the technical challenge of gaining fixation against sclerotic, deficient bone. Loosening approaches 25% in cemented acetabular revision after only 4.5 years. Re-revision with cement leads to even higher failure rates. Improved cement techniques on the acetabular side have not had the success seen with improvements on the femoral side. One study of improved cement techniques (porosity reduction and pressurization) in 113 revision cases showed improved clinical and radiographic results at 4.1 years follow-up with acetabular loosening of only 5% and a 1% revision rate. Addition of compressed morcellized allograft may contribute to longevity, as reported in 24 cases with only an 8% migration rate and none requiring revision at intermediate follow-up (4 to 8 years).

Constrained Socket The use of a constrained socket may be beneficial in the patient at high risk for dislocation. In a series of 55 patients at high risk (neuromuscular/neurologic conditions, unstable hips, and hips that underwent multiple operations), it was successful in 91% (50/55) at a short follow-up. Important criteria for longer-term success with the constrained socket include adequate soft-tissue structures and correct positioning of the component in the acetabulum. The most common problem with the constrained socket is poor socket orientation that may lead to impingement of the femoral component against the socket rim. This impingement can result in dissociation of the locking ring, which requires another operation to replace the locking mechanism.

Structural Allografts

The long-term success of bulk structural allografts, used for loadbearing in cementless socket revision, has been poor. The fact that the allograft bone will not support ingrowth, coupled with the problem of eventual graft resorption in a high percentage of patients, frequently leaves the socket unsupported, with eventual loss of fixation. Half of a series of 78 proximal femoral allografts used to support cementless revision acetabular components had significant resorption after only 3 years (range: 29 to 68 months). A series of 316 acetabular revisions had a 70% failure rate at 5 years, when more than 60% of the implant surface was in contact with structural allograft.

Due to the late onset of failure, long-term follow-up is required when evaluating the success of structural allografts. In cemented sockets with structural grafts, complications are rare before 4 years. A series of 30 structural allografts at a minimum 8-year follow-up (8 to 13.3 years, avg: 10 years) had failure of cemented socket fixation in 47%. Although a previous report of the same group at 4 years showed no failures, this increased to 32% at 6 years, and finally 47% at 10 years. Structural allografts play a continued useful role in complex THAs, but their use is tempered by long-term data showing unpredictable success.

Failure of bulk allografts in cementless sockets appears to occur earlier than in cemented sockets. The average onset of cemented allograft socket failures is about 5 years, but about half of cementless sockets placed with structural allografts are seen to migrate before 2 years. As contrasted to the catastrophic failure of bulk allografts in cemented series, the cementless devices seem to fail by progressive migration.

The long-term benefit of allograft may ultimately be the restoration of bone stock, making re-revision less complex and avoiding further allografts at re-revision. One report showed 80% salvage of the failed allograft without further graft needed for the repeat revision surgery. Another series of full loadbearing allografts had a 57% success rate (4/7) when re-revising the failures to a cementless socket onto the revascularized, viable allograft bed.

Augmentation Devices

The use of an antiprotrusio cage, which is larger than the classic protrusio shell or acetabular reinforcement ring, is a potentially useful adjunct to bridging large acetabular defects and gaining fixation to the pelvis by extensive screw fixation. This procedure may provide fixation that may not be possible by the conventional large hemispheric cementless socket. It may also eliminate the need for bulk allograft in salvage cases or may be used to protect large grafts from forces that may contribute to failure. In an intermediate follow-up of antiprotrusio cages at 5 years (2 to 11 years) in a series of 42 revisions with massive acetabular bone loss, there was success in 76%, but aseptic loosening in 12%.

A 5-year minimum (avg: 7 years, 10 months) follow-up report of 43 patients with 21 revisions using a cemented support ring showed a high incidence of nonprogressive bone-cement radiolucencies (as opposed to progressive radiolucencies usually associated with failure). In another study of 46 reinforcement rings and 20 antiprotrusio cages at a mean follow-up of 5 years the majority of failures occurred when using the ring in extensive cavitary defects, combined deficiencies, or medial defects. Thus, the ring should not be used when two or more combined deficiencies are present (in the medial wall, anterior column, or posterior acetabular column). In these combinations, an antiprotrusio cage should be considered.

Annotated Bibliography

Alternatives to Total Hip Arthroplasty

General

Duncan CP (ed): Symposium on surgical management of hip disease in young adults. *Can J Surg* 1995;38(suppl 1): S4-S68.

Contributions from multiple authors cover radiologic evaluation, clinical assessment, and surgical procedures for the management of arthritic conditions in young patients. Subjects include hip arthroscopy, core decompression, pelvic osteotomy, femoral osteotomy, hip arthrodesis, and primary cemented and cementless arthroplasty.

Osteotomy

Bombelli R (ed): *Structure and Function in Normal and Abnormal Hips: How to Rescue Mechanically Jeopardized Hips,* ed 3. Berlin, Germany, Springer-Verlag, 1993.

This book reviews theoretical mechanics of the hip and

numerous examples of osteotomy technique in dysplastic hips, including varus and valgus osteotomies and combined intertrochanteric Chiari osteotomies.

Millis MB, Murphy SB, Poss R: Osteotomies about the hip for the prevention and treatment of osteoarthrosis. *J Bone Joint Surg* 1995;77A:626–647.

This is an excellent overall review of the clinical evaluation in patient selection for pelvic and intertrochanteric osteotomies. It has an excellent bibliography.

Trousdale RT, Ekkernkamp A, Ganz R, et al: Periacetabular and intertrochanteric osteotomy for the treatment of osteoarthrosis in dysplastic hips. *J Bone Joint Surg* 1995;77A:73–85.

Minimum 5-year results of 42 patients with osteoarthritis at the time of rotational pelvic osteotomy are reported. Osteoarthritis was graded into three levels according to Tönnis. Thirty-two of 33 patients with grade I (minimal) or grade II (moderate) osteoarthritis had good or excellent results. Eight of the nine patients with grade III osteoarthritis preoperatively fared poorly. Pelvic osteotomy is contradictory in patients with significant osteoarthritis. The complication rate was 33% for heterotopic ossification, 5% for pubic nonunion, 21% for hardware bursitis. Nine of the 42 patients required a subsequent operation within 5 years, either for a THA or adjunctive intertrochanteric osteotomy.

Osteonecrosis

Katz RL, Bourne RB, Rorabeck CH, et al: Total hip arthroplasty in patients with avascular necrosis of the hip: Follow-up observations on cementless and cemented operations. *Clin Orthop* 1992;281:145–151.

This review of 42 total hips, including cemented and cementless techniques, demonstrated high success rate using modern cement technique and cementless technology in a group of patients with osteonecrosis. The overall postoperative Harris scores at minimum 2-year and average 46-month follow-up were 88 in the cemented group and 84 in the noncemented group. Thigh pain was a problem in 29% of the patients in the cementless group.

Total Hip Arthroplasty

Introduction/Historical

Huiskes R: Failed innovation in total hip replacement: Diagnosis and proposals for a cure. *Acta Orthop Scand* 1993;64:699–716.

This is a thoughtful and thought-provoking review of past implant design efforts and the factors leading to many of the failures observed. The author discusses the importance of incompatible design goals, tolerance for a trial and error approach without adequate testing, and lack of appropriate regulation of marketing approval.

Demographics/Utilization

Peterson MG, Hollenberg JP, Szatrowski TP, et al: Geographic variations in the rates of elective total hip and knee arthroplasties among Medicare beneficiaries in the United States. *J Bone Joint Surg* 1992;74A:1530–1539.

This article documents the geographic differences in hip arthroplasty rates in the United States. This study also shows that an unexpected inverse relationship exists between the percentage of the population on Medicare and regional arthroplasty rates, suggesting that financial disincentives may be limiting utilization of this procedure in Medicare recipients.

Cost Effectiveness/Outcome Assessment

Barber TC, Healy WL: The hospital cost of total hip arthroplasty: A comparison between 1981 and 1990. *J Bone Joint Surg* 1993;75A:321–325.

The authors detail the change in overall costs and in distribution of costs associated with hip arthroplasty. Expenditures were reduced because of shorter hospital stays and use of less resources, while costs of the implants increased in real terms and as a percentage of the total spent from 11% to 24% by 1990. This was largely due to actual dollar increases of 212% in the cost of the prosthesis, which corresponds to an inflation adjusted increase of 117% over 10 years.

Laupacis A, Bourne R, Rorabeck C, et al: The effect of elective total hip replacement on health-related quality of life. *J Bone Joint Surg* 1993;75A:1619–1626.

This prospective outcome study quantitates the dramatic benefit produced by hip arthroplasty on patient physical function, social interaction, and overall health, most of which is realized within 3 months after surgery. This study serves as a model for similar outcome study efforts in this area.

Fixation Issues

Rorabeck CH, Bourne RB, Laupacis A, et al: A double-blind study of 250 cases comparing cemented with cementless total hip arthroplasty: Cost-effectiveness and its impact on health-related quality of life. *Clin Orthop* 1994;298:156–164.

The authors report a prospective double blind study of cemented versus cementless THA. There was no difference in overall health-related quality of life at 2 years postsurgery.

First-Generation Cement Fixation

Joshi AB, Porter ML, Trail IA, et al: Long-term results of Charnley low-friction arthroplasty in young patients. *J Bone Joint Surg* 1993;75B:616–623.

Two hundred eighteen THA cases in patients under age 40 years at surgery were followed up a minimum of 10 years postsurgery, with a mean follow-up of 16 years. Twenty-year survivorship probability was 86% for the femoral stem and 84% for the acetabular component overall, but was affected by diagnosis. For rheumatoid patients, 20-year survivorship for both cup and stem was 96% but for osteoarthritic patients only 51%.

Kavanagh BF, Wallrichs S, Dewitz M, et al: Charnley low-friction arthroplasty of the hip: Twenty-year results with cement. *J Arthroplasty* 1994;9:229–234.

This is a report of 20-year follow-up of the first 333 Charnley THA cases performed at the Mayo Clinic. For the surviving 112 patients, clinical results remained excellent overall. Probability of component survival 20 years without revision was 84%, with linear rates of loosening, revision, and failure noted. Probability of revision was effected by age with revision in 27% of those 59 years or less, 13% for those 59 to 65 years, and 7.5% for those 65 to 70 years of age at surgery.

Schulte KR, Callaghan JJ, Kelley SS, et al: The outcome of Charnley total hip arthroplasty with cement after a minimum twenty-year follow-up: The results of one surgeon. *J Bone Joint Surg* 1993;75A:961–975.

Twenty-year follow-up of 330 cases performed by one surgeon is reported. At the minimum 20-year follow-up, 10% had been revised, with 2% for infection, 7% for loosening, and 1% for dislocation. Revision of a loose cup was required in 6% of the original patients (10% of the 98 patients still alive at follow-up) and revision for a loose stem in 2% overall (3% of the survivors alive at follow-up).

Sullivan PM, MacKenzie JR, Callaghan JJ, et al: Total hip arthroplasty with cement in patients who are less than fifty years old: A sixteen to twenty-two-year follow-up study. *J Bone Joint Surg* 1994;76A:863–869.

This is a report on 89 THAs performed by a single surgeon on 67 patients, all under 50 years of age at arthroplasty. Follow-up averaged 18 years (range 16 to 22 years). Thirteen percent were revised for a loose cup and 2% for a loose stem. If revision and radiographic loosening rates are combined, the mechanical failure rate of the cups was 50%, and of the femoral stem, only 8%.

Second-Generation Cement Fixation

Ballard WT, Callaghan JJ, Sullivan PM, et al: The results of improved cementing techniques for total hip arthroplasty in patients less than fifty years old: A ten-year follow-up study. *J Bone Joint Surg* 1994;76A:959–964.

Ten-year results of a single surgeon series of 42 hips reveals a revision rate for aseptic loosening of 5% for femoral components and 24% for acetabular components. An additional 12% of cups and 12% of stems were definitely radiographically loose. Thus, excellent stem fixation and disappointing cup fixation were observed with second-generation methods in this series.

Third-Generation Cement Fixation

Star MJ, Colwell CW Jr, Kelman GJ, et al: Suboptimal (thin) distal cement mantle thickness as a contributory factor in total hip arthroplasty femoral component failure: A retrospective radiographic analysis favoring distal stem centralization. *J Arthroplasty* 1994;9:143–149.

The authors document the adverse effect of thin cement mantles at the medial diaphysis (Gruen zones 5 and 6) on femoral loosening rates and failure.

Cemented Acetabular Cups

Cates HE, Faris PM, Keating EM, et al: Polyethylene wear in cemented metal-backed acetabular cups. *J Bone Joint Surg* 1993;75B:249–253.

Results with metal-backed versus all polyethylene cups and a 28-mm titanium one-piece stem were compared in 233 hips. A 37% increase in wear rate was seen in the metal-backed cups, with a linear wear rate of 0.11mm/yr versus 0.08 mm/yr for the all polyethylene cups, and a volumetric wear rate of 66.2 mm^3/yr versus 48.2 mm^3/yr.

Uncemented Total Hip Arthroplasty

Heekin RD, Callaghan JJ, Hopkinson WJ, et al: The porous-coated anatomic total hip prosthesis, inserted without cement: Results after five to seven years in a prospective study. *J Bone Joint Surg* 1993;75A:77–91.

Five- to seven-year follow-up study of 100 PCA THA cases shows a femoral subsidence rate of 5%, a cup migration rate of 6%, and thigh pain rates of 18% at 1 year, 19% at 2 years, 23% at 3, 26 at 4, and 15% at 5 years postsurgery.

Owen TD, Moran CG, Smith SR, et al: Results of uncemented porous-coated anatomic total hip arthroplasty. *J Bone Joint Surg* 1994;76B:258–262.

Five-year follow-up (range: 2 to 9 years) of 241 PCA THA cases indicated a 13% failure rate, 11% on the cup side and 2% on the stem side. Survivorship analysis revealed a 91% survivorship at 6 years, but only 73% at 7 years, and 57% at 8 years, mainly due to a high incidence of significant polyethylene wear and osteolysis on the cup side. Close radiographic follow-up.

Porous Coated Cups

Maloney WJ, Peters P, Engh CA, et al: Severe osteolysis of the pelvis in association with acetabular replacement without cement. *J Bone Joint Surg* 1993;75A:1627–1635.

Fifteen hips in 14 patients were reported with osteolysis on the cup side. Eight of the cups were titanium alloy and seven were cobalt-chrome. All polyethylene liners were less than 10 mm thick and 12 of the 15 were 8 mm or less in thickness. All patients were functioning well and the diagnosis was made radiographically in the absence of significant symptoms. The osteolysis first appeared on radiographs at 53 to 84 months postoperation. The importance of regular radiographic follow-up of all such patients after THA is stressed.

Sumner DR, Jasty M, Jacobs JJ, et al: Histology of porous-coated acetabular components: 25 cementless cups retrieved after arthroplasty. *Acta Orthop Scand* 1993;64: 619–626.

The authors report a retrieval study of 25 H-G cups originally fixed with screws, at 1 to 140 weeks postimplantation (mean 30 weeks). None were removed for infection or failure of fixation. Eighteen of the 25 showed histologic evidence of bone ingrowth, with up to 80% of the area of the bone-implant interface involved with bone ingrowth and up to one third of the available void space filled with bone. Metal debris was observed within histiocytes adjacent to screw holes in longer-term cases.

Threaded Cups

Capello WN, Colyer RA, Kernek CB, et al: Failure of the Mecron screw-in ring. *J Bone Joint Surg* 1993;75B:835–836.

A high failure rate of 17% (9 of 54) after primary THA and 50% (16 of 32) of revisions at a mean follow-up of 42 months (range 26 to 51) were reported. Survivorship at 4 years was only 71% overall, and 85% for primaries. The authors have abandoned this type of design.

Fox GM, McBeath AA, Heiner JP: Hip replacement with a threaded acetabular cup: A follow-up study. *J Bone Joint Surg* 1994;76A:195–201.

Sixty-eight threaded titanium cups were placed in 52 primary and 16 revision THA cases. At 5 to 9 years of follow-up, 17 cups had been revised and more were loose with revision pending; thus, 26 (38%) had experienced mechanical failure overall. In the revision group, 10 of 16 (63%) failed versus 16 of 52 (31%) for the primaries. The authors believe that use of this cup is not warranted.

Hydroxyapatite-Coated Cups

Capello WN, D'Antonio JA, Manley MT, et al: Abstract: Hydroxyapatite versus porous coated cups in conjunction with hydroxyapatite coated stems: Five-year minimum follow-up. Proceedings of the American Academy of Orthopaedic Surgeons 62nd Annual Meeting, Orlando,

FL. Rosemont, IL, American Academy of Orthopaedic Surgeons, 1995, p 247.

Authors compare multicenter data on 129 HA-coated and 121 porous-coated cups of similar design at minimum 5-year follow-up. Mechanical failure rates were higher in the HA-coated group at 10.1% (12 revisions, one migrated), compared to a mechanical failure rate of 3.3% for the porous-coated cups (four revisions, none loose or migrated).

Proximally Porous-Coated Stems

Kim YH, Kim VE: Uncemented porous-coated anatomic total hip replacement: Results at six years in a consecutive series. *J Bone Joint Surg* 1993;75B:6–13.

One hundred eight hips were followed up for at least 6 years, with a 33% incidence of osteolysis at final follow-up. Excessive wear of 5 mm or greater was present in 20 out of 108 cups by 6 years. Thigh pain correlated with an undersized femoral stem; no patient with a well-fitting stem had disabling thigh pain.

Martell JM, Pierson RH III, Jacobs JJ, et al: Primary total hip reconstruction with a titanium fiber-coated prosthesis inserted without cement. *J Bone Joint Surg* 1993;75A: 554–571.

The authors report a prospective study of 121 uncemented Harris-Galante THAs followed up for a mean of 67 months (range 55 to 79). Survivorship at 5 years was 97% for the femoral stem, with four revised for loosening in this series; however, another seven were radiographically loose, for a total of 11 out of 121 loose or revised (9%). Only one cup was revised, and that was for dislocation.

Extensively Porous-Coated Stems

Engh CA, Hooten JP Jr, Zettl-Schaffer KF, et al: Porous-coated total hip replacement. *Clin Orthop* 1994;298:89–96.

This report on the first 15 years experience with the AML prosthesis gives details regarding the first 393 cases implanted prior to 1985. Six of these 393 stems (1.5%) have required revision: three for loosening, two for stem breakage, and one for infection. Retrievals from autopsy specimens with hips in place were also reported. Specimens showed very little micromotion (40 μm or less), and bone remodeling as measured via dual x-ray absorptiometry showed 5% to 52% loss of bone mineral content. The greatest bone loss occurred in those already osteoporotic.

Hydroxyapatite-Coated Stems

D'Antonio JA, Capello WN, Jaffe WL: Hydroxylapatite-coated hip implants: Multicenter three-year clinical and roentgenographic results. *Clin Orthop* 1992;285:102–115.

Three hundred twenty cases with 2-year follow-up and 142 with 3-year follow-up show continued excellent short-term results and a hip score of 96 at 3 years. Activity-related thigh pain was noted in only 1.4% of patients at 3 years. Two stems were revised and none were radiographically loose, for a mechanical failure rate of 0.46%.

Hybrid Fixation

Schmalzried TP, Harris WH: Hybrid total hip replacement: A 6.5-year follow-up study. *J Bone Joint Surg* 1993;75B:608–615.

This is a review of 97 consecutive cases performed with a porous-ingrowth cup and a cemented stem inserted with third-generation cement technique, at 5 years minimum (mean 6.5 years) postsurgery. Average Harris hip score was 93. No cups and one stem were revised for loosening. This study suggests extremely durable results can be expected over the first decade, at least, with this approach.

Evaluation of the Failed Total Hip Arthroplasty

Barrack RB, Harris WH: The value of aspiration of the hip joint before revision total hip arthroplasty. *J Bone Joint Surg* 1993;75A:66–76.

In a series of 270 revision hips, a low incidence of true infection (2%) was ultimately determined. Unfortunately, the preoperative aspirations were misleading, with 13% false positive and only 6% true positive. No hip had a true positive preoperative aspiration that did not already have clinical and radiographic evidence of infection (focal lysis, aggressive nonfocal lysis, or periostitis).

Complications of Total Hip Arthroplasty

Osteolysis

Albores-Saavedra J, Vuitch F, Delgado R, et al: Sinus histiocytosis of pelvic lymph nodes after hip replacement: A histiocytic proliferation induced by cobalt-chromium and titanium. *Am J Surg Pathol* 1994;18:83–90.

This pathologic analysis of ipsilateral pelvic lymph nodes in patients with prostheses of the hip has demonstated a histiocytic response within the nodes with evidence of both cobalt-chrome and titanium metals, as well as polyethylene particles. This response demonstrates the metastatic nature of particle disease in the hip.

Boehler M, Knahr K, Plenk H Jr, et al: Long-term results of uncemented alumina acetabular implants. *J Bone Joint Surg* 1994;76A:53–59.

In this long-term (12-year mean) follow-up of ceramic on ceramic cementless THA in 67 hips, there was a 12.4% revision rate. Stable implants had extremely low wear rates (0.9 μm on the socket), but there was extreme wear in loose prostheses (27 μm). The nature of the membranes indicates ceramic on ceramic is not immune from the particle disease seen with polyethylene articulations.

Buly RL, Huo MH, Salvati E, et al: Titanium wear debris in failed cemented total hip arthroplasty: An analysis of 71 cases. *J Arthroplasty* 1992;7:315–323.

Cemented titanium alloy stems that were removed underwent analysis. Metal levels were measured. The presence of titanium metallic particles was noted to accelerate bone loss and loosening.

Cates HE, Faris PM, Deating EM, et al: Polyethylene wear in cemented metal-backed acetabular cups. *J Bone Joint Surg* 1993;75B:249–253.

A series of 233 cemented hips analyzed for polythylene wear showed a 37% higher rate of wear in metal-backed cups than in all-polythylene cups. This rate raises concern over the fate of uncemented metal-backed sockets.

Haynes DR, Rogers SD, Hay S, et al: The differences in toxicity and release of bone-resorbing mediators induced by titanium and cobalt-chromium-alloy wear particles. *J Bone Joint Surg* 1993;75A:825–834.

This in-vitro animal study shows a differential response between metal particles generated by titanium-aluminum-vanadium (TiAlVa) alloy and cobalt-chrome alloy. The TiAlVa particles induced more prostaglandin E_2, interleukin-1, tumor necrosis factor, and interleukin-6, indicating a more potent inflammatory stimulation and lysis response in bone than the response to cobalt-chrome.

Horowitz SM, Doty SB, Lane JM, et al: Studies of the mechanism by which the mechanical failure of polymethylmethacrylate leads to bone resorption. *J Bone Joint Surg* 1993;75A:802–813.

This retrieval study of 18 aseptically loose femoral components demonstated an important effect of particle size on the membrane activity and subsequent bone resorption. Particle size small enough to be phagocytized by macrophages (1 to 12 μm) was the critical factor in this reactive mechanism.

Jiranek WA, Machado M, Jasty M, et al: Production of cytokines around loosened cemented acetabular components. *J Bone Joint Surg* 1993;75A:863–879.

This retrieval study of 10 hip membranes surrounding loose cemented acetabular components demonstrated production of two potent cytokines, interleukin-1-B and platelet derived growth factor. These cytokines appear to be involved in the loosening process.

Maloney WJ, Peters P, Engh CA, et al: Severe osteolysis of the pelvis in association with acetabular replacement without cement. *J Bone Joint Surg* 1993;75A:1627–1635.

Analysis of a series of 14 patients with large osteolytic defects surrounding the acetabular component emphasizes the silent nature of the process and the need for regular follow-up radiographs.

Schmalzried TP, Guttmann D, Grecula M, et al: The relationship between the design, position, and articular wear of acetabular components inserted without cement and the development of pelvic osteolysis. *J Bone Joint Surg* 1994;76A:677–688.

This study in the behavior of lysis surrounding acetabular components demonstrated a biologically erosive process that can extend through the peripheral margin of a cementless socket and gain access to the pelvic bone. This study challenges the concept that peripheral rim fit will somehow seal the acetabular bone from particle disease.

Infections

Nelson CL, Evans RP, Blaha JD, et al: A comparison of gentamicin-impregnated polymethylmethacrylate bead implantation to conventional parenteral antibiotic therapy in infected total hip and knee arthroplasty. *Clin Orthop* 1993;295:96–101.

A prospective randomized protocol of two (two stage) treatment protocols comparing debridement and PMMA beads with debridement and conventional antibiotics showed no differences in outcomes. Common conditions associated with recurrence were (1) multiple previous surgeries, (2) host compromise and malnutrition, (3) extensive infection, and (4) inadequate debridement.

Stress Shielding

Kilgus DJ, Shimaoka EE, Tipton JS, et al: Dual-energy x-ray absorptiometry measurement of bone mineral density around porous-coated cementless femoral implants. *J Bone Joint Surg* 1993;75B:279–287.

Dual energy x-ray absorptiometry measurement of bone mineral density of 72 cementless femoral implants with varying stiffness and extent of porous coatings showed that the greatest decrease (34.8%) occurred in the relatively stiff, extensively porous-coated implants. Progressive decreases in density continued for 5 to 7 years after implantation.

Neurovascular

Rasmussen RJ, Black DL, Bruce RP, et al: Efficacy of corticosomatosensory evoked potential monitoring in predicting and/or preventing sciatic nerve palsy during total hip arthroplasty. *J Arthroplasty* 1994;9:53–61.

This study was performed on 290 consecutive patients to try and prevent sciatic nerve palsy (SNP) during hip replacement surgery. Corticosomatosensory evoked potential monitoring was neither predictive nor helpful in preventing SNP.

Femoral Component Revision

Cameron HU: The two- to six-year results with a proximally modular noncemented total hip replacement used in hip revisions. *Clin Orthop* 1994:298:47–53.

Two- to 6-year results are reported of femoral revision using a proximally modular uncemented total hip stem in 91 cases. Ten cases required repeat revision, four because of distal femoral perforation by the stem tip, three for deep infection, one because of trochanteric nonunion, and two because of acetabular problems. No stem or sleeve fractures, implant dissociations, or progressive osteolysis problems were noted, and in failed cases, no metallosis was noted at the modular junction.

Chandler H, Clark J, Murphy S, et al: Reconstruction of major segmental loss of the proximal femur in revision total hip arthroplasty. *Clin Orthop* 1994;298:67–74.

Use of a modular long-stem implant cemented to the allograft proximally and press fit to the host bone distally for reconstruction of major proximal femoral bone deficiencies is described. Follow-up for this series of 30 hips was an average of 22 months over the short term. Twenty-eight of 30 hips appeared to show healing of the allograft to the host. One deep infection was observed.

Elting JJ, Zicat BA, Mikhail WEM, et al: Impaction grafting: Preliminary report of a new method for exchange femoral arthroplasty. *Orthopedics* 1995;18:107–112.

This is a report of 100 femoral revisions using impaction cancellous bone grafting. Two-year follow-up was reported on 31 of these cases with the short-term preliminary results believed to be quite promising but with slight subsidence of a few millimeters noted in over 50% of the stems within the cement column and subsidence of a minimal degree involving the cement within the allograft noted in approximately 11% in the series. Graft incorporation was felt to have occurred radiographically in 77%.

Estok DM II, Harris WH: Long-term results of cemented femoral revision surgery using second-generation techniques: An average 11.7-year follow-up evaluation. *Clin Orthop* 1994;299:190–202.

Thirty-eight hips in 36 patients were reviewed at a mean of 11.7 years after revision THA using second-generation methods. Results were relatively durable on the femoral side with a repeat revision required in 10.5%, and an additional 10.5% showing definite radiographic loosening despite the revision setting at the time of the original operation.

Gie GA, Linder L, Ling RS, et al: Impacted cancellous

allografts and cement for revision total hip arthroplasty. *J Bone Joint Surg* 1993;75B:14–21.

The authors report results following impaction cancellous grafting and cemented stem fixation within the column of graft. Fifty-six hips were reviewed 18 to 49 months following surgery with subsidence of several millimeters noted in approximately 50% of the series but with satisfactory clinical results in the majority of patients and radiographic evidence of graft incorporation.

Head WC, Wagner RA, Emerson RH Jr, et al: Revision total hip arthroplasty in the deficient femur with a proximal load-bearing prosthesis. *Clin Orthop* 1994; 298:119–126.

One hundred seventy-four revision total hip arthroplasties were treated with onlay cortical strut allografts and a proximally porous-coated calcar replacement femoral stem. Graft union was noted in 98%. Six revisions for failure on the femoral side have been required.

Katz RP, Callaghan JJ, Sullivan PM, et al: Abstract: Cemented revision total hip arthroplasty using contemporary techniques: A minimum ten year follow-up study. *J Arthroplasty* 1994;9:103.

This is a review of 82 hips followed up a minimum of 10 years with original implantation employing second-generation cemented methods. Re-revision rate was 6% and there was a 10% incidence of radiographic femoral loosening.

Klein AH, Rubash HE: Femoral windows in revision total hip arthroplasty. *Clin Orthop* 1993;291:164–170.

The authors report 21 revision procedures performed with femoral windows to facilitate cement removal. Cortical windows were replaced, grafted with autogenous cancellous bone and fixed with cerclage wires. A noncemented revision stem was used that extended at least two cortical diameters past the defect. No intraoperative fractures or inadvertent perforations were noted, no thigh pain or loosening occurred at a mean follow-up of 22 months, and all windows healed at a mean of 17 weeks.

Lawrence JM, Engh CA, Macalino GE, et al: Outcome of revision hip arthroplasty done without cement. *J Bone Joint Surg* 1994;76A:965–973.

Ninety-three femoral revision arthroplasties performed because of symptomatic loosening of a prior femoral component were followed up for 5 to 13 years (mean 9 years). The re-revision rate for the extensively coated femoral stem used at the time of revision was 10% and the rate of mechanical loosening was 11%.

Malkani AL, Settecerri JJ, Sim FH, et al: Long-term results of proximal femoral replacement for non-neoplastic disorders. *J Bone Joint Surg* 1995;77B:351–356.

The authors report long-term results of proximal femoral replacement stem use for nontumor, revision arthroplasty cases in which major bone loss problems had occurred. Overall survivorship was 64% at 12 years postrevision, and complications included dislocation in 11 of the original 50 patients.

Pierson JL, Harris WH: Cemented revision for femoral osteolysis in cemented arthroplasties: Results in 29 hips after a mean 8.5-year follow-up. *J Bone Joint Surg* 1994; 76B:40–44.

This is a report of second generation cemented revisions in 29 patients in whom the indication for revision involved significant femoral osteolysis following a previously cemented implant. At 8.5 years average follow-up, osteolysis had recurred in only two patients (6.9%) and 86% of stems remained solidly fixed.

Acetabular Revision

Berry DJ, Müller ME: Revision arthroplasty using an anti-protrusio cage for massive acetabular bone deficiency. *J Bone Joint Surg* 1992;74B:711–715.

This report on the 2- to 11-year results (mean: 5 years) of 42 cemented revision sockets secured by the Burch-Schneider antiprotrusio cage shows 12% aseptic failure, 12% septic failure, and 76% success.

Haentjens P, de Boeck H, Handelberg F, et al: Cemented acetabular reconstruction with the Müller support ring: A minimum five-year clinical and roentgenographic follow-up study. *Clin Orthop* 1993;290:225–235.

The use of a Müller reinforcement ring in cemented acetabular reconstruction is advocated in cases of bone deficiency or poor quality. In this series of 21 revisions and 22 primary cases in the longest follow-up series to date, three cases overall required revision (7%), and two cases (11%) in the revision group had migrated.

Hooten JP Jr, Engh CA Jr, Engh CA: Failure of structural acetabular allografts in cementless revision hip arthroplasty. *J Bone Joint Surg* 1994;76B:419–422.

This series of 31 patients with structural allografts used to support cementless sockets showed a 44% failure rate after only 29 months average follow-up. These poor results parallel the poor results that are seen with structural allografts and cemented sockets, and thus continue to argue against structural allograft in all but salvage situations.

Kwong LM, Jasty M, Harris WH: High failure rate of bulk femoral head allografts in total hip acetabular reconstructions at 10 years. *J Arthroplasty* 1993;8:341–346.

This is the longest follow-up of structural allografts. This study of 30 patients, mostly revisions, at 10-year follow-up (range: 8 to 13 years) with cemented sockets showed 47% failure. But eight of 14 cases (57%) that failed were revised without further allograft.

Padgett DE, Kull L, Rosenberg A, et al: Revision of the acetabular component without cement after total hip arthroplasty: Three to six-year follow-up. *J Bone Joint Surg* 1993;75A:663–673.

A 3- to 6-year follow-up of 129 cementless revision sockets showed no revisions for aseptic loosening. Four hips were revised for sepsis and three for instability. None migrated in the absence of infection. This shows tremendous improvement in results with a fixed porous device at intermediate follow-up.

Paprosky WG, Magnus RE: Principles of bone grafting in revision total hip arthroplasty: Acetabular technique. *Clin Orthop* 1994;298:147–155.

This intermediate-term follow-up of 2 to 10 years (avg: 5.1 years) describes major structural reconstruction using a notched distal femur allograft in the shape of a "7." A high failure rate (70%) was noted in those cases where Kohler's line was broken, indicating anterior column deficiency.

Tanzer M, Drucker D, Jasty M, et al: Revision of the acetabular component with an uncemented Harris-Galante porous-coated prosthesis. *J Bone Joint Surg* 1992;74A:987–994.

This 140 hip revision socket series with a 2- to 6-year follow-up shows dramatic results for acetabular loosening. Detectable loosening was found in only 1%, and only one revision was performed for socket loosening.

Classic Bibliography

Alternatives to Total Hip Arthroplasty

Aronson J: Osteoarthritis of the young adult hip: Etiology and treatment, in Anderson LD (ed): American Academy of Orthopaedic Surgeons *Instructional Course Lectures XXXV.* St. Louis, MO, CV Mosby, 1986, pp 119–128.

Callaghan JJ, Brand RA, Pedersen DR: Hip arthrodesis: A long-term follow-up. *J Bone Joint Surg* 1985:67A: 1328–1335.

Ganz R, Klaue K, Vinh TS, et al: A new periacetabular osteotomy for the treatment of hip dysplasias, technique and preliminary results. *Clin Orthop* 1988;232:26–36.

Glimcher MJ, Kenzora JE: The biology of osteonecrosis of the human femoral head and its clinical implications: I. Tissue biology. *Clin Orthop* 1979;138:284–309.

Harris WH: Etiology of osteoarthritis of the hip. *Clin Orthop* 1986;213:20–33.

Liechti R (ed): *Hip Arthrodesis and Associated Problems.* Berlin, Germany, Springer-Verlag, 1978.

Marti RK, Schuller HM, Raaymakers EL: Intertrochanteric osteotomy for non-union of the femoral neck. *J Bone Joint Surg* 1989;71B:782–787.

Morscher E, Feinstein R: Results of intertrochanteric osteotomy in the treatment of osteoarthritis of the hip, in Aronson J, Schatzker J (eds): *The Intertrochanteric Osteotomy.* Berlin, Germany, Springer-Verlag, 1984, pp 169–177.

Sponseller PD, McBeath AA, Perpich M: Hip arthrodesis in young patients: A long-term follow-up study. *J Bone Joint Surg* 1984;66A:853–859.

Steel HH: Triple osteotomy of the innominate bone. *J Bone Joint Surg* 1973;55A:343–350.

Steinberg ME, Hayken GD, Steinberg DR: A new method for evaluation and staging of avascular necrosis of the femoral head, in Arlet J, Ficat RP, Hungerford DS (eds): *Bone Circulation.* Baltimore, MD, Williams & Wilkins, 1984, pp 390–403.

Stulberg BN, Bauer TW, Belhobek GH: Making core decompression work. *Clin Orthop* 1990;261:186–195.

Total Hip Arthroplasty

Barrack RL, Jasty M, Bragdon C, et al: Thigh pain despite bone ingrowth into uncemented femoral stems. *J Bone Joint Surg* 1992;74B:507–510.

Barrack RL, Mulroy RD Jr, Harris WH: Improved cementing techniques and femoral component loosening in young patients with hip arthroplasty: A 12-year radiographic review. *J Bone Joint Surg* 1992;74B:385–389.

Bauer TW, Geesink RC, Zimmerman R, et al: Hydroxyapatite-coated femoral stems: Histological analysis of components retrieved at autopsy. *J Bone Joint Surg* 1991;73A:1439–1452.

Bauer TW, Stulberg BN, Ming J, et al: Uncemented acetabular components: Histologic analysis of retrieved hydroxyapatite-coated and porous implants. *J Arthroplasty* 1993;8:167–177.

Callaghan JJ, Heekin RD, Savory CG, et al: Evaluation of the learning curve associated with uncemented primary porous-coated anatomic total hip arthroplasty. *Clin Orthop* 1992;282:132–144.

Coventry MB: Lessons learned in 30 years of total hip arthroplasty. *Clin Orthop* 1992;274:22–29.

Davies JP, Harris WH: In vitro and in vivo studies of pressurization of femoral cement in total hip arthroplasty. *J Arthroplasty* 1993;8:585–591.

Ebramzadeh E, Sarmiento A, McKellop HA, et al: The cement mantle in total hip arthroplasty: Analysis of long-term radiographic results. *J Bone Joint Surg* 1994;76A: 77–87.

Engh CA, Glassman AH, Suthers KE: The case for porous-coated hip implants: The femoral side. *Clin Orthop* 1990;261:63–81.

Engh CA, McGovern TF, Bobyn JD, et al: A quantitative evaluation of periprosthetic bone-remodeling after cementless total hip arthroplasty. *J Bone Joint Surg* 1992;74A:1009–1020.

Engh CA, Zettl-Schaffer KF, Kukita Y, et al: Histological and radiographic assessment of well functioning porous-coated acetabular components: A human postmortem retrieval study. *J Bone Joint Surg* 1993;75A:814–824.

Goldring SR, Clark CR, Wright TM: Editorial: The problem in total joint arthroplasty: Aseptic loosening. *J Bone Joint Surg* 1993;75A:799–801.

Harris WH: Is it advantageous to strengthen the cement-metal interface and use a collar for cemented femoral components of total hip replacements? *Clin Orthop* 1992;285:67–72.

Hernandez JR, Keating EM, Faris PM, et al: Polyethylene wear in uncemented acetabular components. *J Bone Joint Surg* 1994;76B:263–266.

Huiskes R: Failed innovation in total hip replacement: Diagnosis and proposals for a cure. *Acta Orthop Scand* 1993;64:699–716.

Jasty M, Bragdon CR, Maloney WJ, et al: Ingrowth of bone in failed fixation of porous-coated femoral components. *J Bone Joint Surg* 1991;73A:1331–1337.

Jasty M, Maloney WJ, Bragdon CR, et al: Histomorphological studies of the long-term skeletal responses to well fixed cemented femoral components. *J Bone Joint Surg* 1990;72A:1220–1229.

Johanson NA, Charlson ME, Szatrowski TP, et al: A self-administered hip-rating questionnaire for the assessment of outcome after total hip replacement. *J Bone Joint Surg* 1992;74A:587–597.

Kelley SS, Fitzgerald RH Jr, Rand JA, et al: A prospective randomized study of a collar versus a collarless femoral prosthesis. *Clin Orthop* 1993;294:114–122.

Levitsky KA, Hozack WJ, Balderston RA, et al: Evaluation of the painful prosthetic joint: Relative value of bone scan, sedimentation rate, and joint aspiration. *J Arthroplasty* 1991;6:237–244.

Liang MH, Katz JN, Phillips C, et al: The total knee arthroplasty outcome evaluation form of the American Academy of Orthopaedic Surgeons: Results of a nominal group process. The American Academy of Orthopaedic Surgeons Task Force on Outcome Studies. *J Bone Joint Surg* 1991;73A:639–646.

Ling RS: The use of a collar and precoating on cemented femoral stems is unnecessary and detrimental. *Clin Orthop* 1992;285:73–83.

Maloney WJ, Harris WH: Comparison of a hybrid with an uncemented total hip replacement: A retrospective matched-pair study. *J Bone Joint Surg* 1990;72A:1349–1352.

Neumann L, Freund KG, Sorenson KH: Long-term results of Charnley total hip replacement: Review of 92 patients at 15 to 20 years. *J Bone Joint Surg* 1994;76B: 245–251.

Ritter MA, Keating EM, Faris PM, et al: Metal-backed acetabular cups in total hip arthroplasty. *J Bone Joint Surg* 1990;72A:672–677.

Rorabeck CH, Bourne RB, Laupacis A, et al: A double-blind study of 250 cases comparing cemented with cementless total hip arthroplasty: Cost-effectiveness and its impact on health-related quality of life. *Clin Orthop* 1994;298:156–164.

Schmalzried TP, Harris WH: The Harris-Galante porous-coated acetabular component with screw fixation: Radiographic analysis of eighty-three primary hip replacements at a minimum of five years. *J Bone Joint Surg* 1992;74A:1130–1139.

Schmalzried TP, Kwong LM, Jasty M, et al: The mechanism of loosening of cemented acetabular components in total hip arthroplasty: Analysis of specimens retrieved at autopsy. *Clin Orthop* 1992;274: 60–78.

Schmalzried TP, Maloney WJ, Jasty M, et al: Autopsy studies of the bone-cement interface in well-fixed cemented total hip arthroplasties. *J Arthroplasty* 1993; 8:179–188.

Schmalzried TP, Wessinger SJ, Hill GE, et al: The Harris-Galante porous acetabular component press-fit without screw fixation: Five-year radiographic analysis of primary cases. *J Arthroplasty* 1994;9:235–242.

Schwartz JT Jr, Engh CA, Forte MR, et al: Evaluation of initial surface apposition in porous-coated acetabular components. *Clin Orthop* 1993;293:174–187.

Wiklund I, Romanus B: A comparison of quality of life before and after arthroplasty in patients who had arthrosis of the hip joint. *J Bone Joint Surg* 1991;73A:765–769.

Wixson RL: Do we need to vacuum mix or centrifuge cement? *Clin Orthop* 1992;285:84–90.

Wixson RL, Stulberg SD, Mehlhoff M: Total hip replacement with cemented, uncemented, and hybrid prostheses: A comparison of clinical and radiographic results at two to four years. *J Bone Joint Surg* 1991;73A: 257–270.

Complications of Total Hip Arthroplasty

Abraham WD, Dimon JH: Leg length discrepancy in total hip arthroplasty. *OCNA* 1992;23:201–209.

Barrack RL, Burke DW, Cook SD, et al: Complications related to modularity of total hip components. *J Bone Joint Surg* 1993;75B:688–692.

Garcia-Cimbrelo E, Munuera L: Early and late loosening of the acetabular cup after low-friction arthroplasty. *J Bone Joint Surg* 1992;74A:1119–1129.

Hodgkinson JP, Maskell AP, Paul A, et al: Flanged acetabular components in cemented Charnley hip arthroplasty: Ten-year follow-up of 350 patients. *J Bone Joint Surg* 1993;75B:464–467.

Krushell RJ, Burke DW, Harris WH: Elevated-rim acetabular components: Effect on range of motion and stability in total hip arthroplasty. *J Arthroplasty* 1991; 6(suppl):S53-S58.

Morrey BF: Instability after total hip arthroplasty. *OCNA* 1992;23:237–248.

Pagnani MJ, Pellicci PM, Salvati EA: Effect of aspirin on heterotopic ossification after total hip arthroplasty in men who have osteoarthritis. *J Bone Joint Surg* 1991;73A;924–929.

Santavirta S, Konttainen YT, Hoikka V, et al: Immunopathological response to loose cementless acetabular components. *J Bone Joint Surg* 1991;73B: 38–42.

Schmalzried TP, Harris WH: The Harris-Galante porous-coated acetabular component with screw fixation: Radiographic analysis of eighty-three primary hip replacements at a minimum of five years. *J Bone Joint Surg* 1992;74A:1130–1139.

Schmalzried TP, Jasty M, Harris WH: Periprosthetic bone loss in total hip arthroplasty. *J Bone Joint Surg* 1992; 74A:849–863.

Schulte KR, Callaghan JJ, Kelley SS, et al: The outcome of Charnley total hip arthroplasty with cement after a minimum twenty year follow-up. *J Bone Joint Surg* 1993; 75A:961–975.

Tanzer M, Maloney WJ, Jasty M, et al: The progression of femoral cortical osteolysis in association with total hip arthroplasty without cement. *J Bone Joint Surg* 1992; 74A:404–410.

Femoral Component Revision

Allan DG, Levoi GJ, McDonald S, et al: Proximal femoral allografts in revision hip arthroplasty. *J Bone Joint Surg* 1991;73B:235–240.

Bargar WL, Murzic WJ, Taylor JK, et al: Management of bone loss in revision total hip arthroplasty using custom cementless femoral components. *J Arthroplasty* 1993;8: 245–252.

D'Antonio J, McCarthy JC, Bargar WL, et al: Classification of femoral abnormalities in total hip arthroplasty. *Clin Orthop* 1993;296:133–139.

Emerson RH Jr, Malinin TI, Cuellar AD, et al: Cortical strut allografts in the reconstruction of the femur in revision total hip arthroplasty: A basic science and clinical study. *Clin Orthop* 1992;285:35–44.

Glassman AH, Engh CA: The removal of porous coated femoral hip stems. *Clin Orthop* 1992;285:164–180.

Gustilo RB, Pasterrak HS: Revision total hip arthroplasty with titanium ingrowth prothesis and bone grafting for failed cemented femoral componenet loosening. *Clin Orthop* 1988;235:111–119.

Kavanagh BF, Wallrichs S, Ilstrup D, et al: Abstract: Ten year follow-up of cemented revision total hip replacement. *Orthop Trans* 1993;17:943.

Malkoni AL, Lewallen DG, Cabanela ME: Two to 5 year follow-up of femoral component revisions using an uncemented, proximally-coated chrome cobalt, long-stem curved prothesis. *Orthop Trans* 1993;17:940–941.

Mulroy WF, Estok DM II, Harris WH: Fifteen year results of cemented femoral revisions using second-generation cementing technique. Proceedings of the American Academy of Orthopaedic Surgeons 61st Annual Meeting, New Orleans, LA. Rosemont, IL, American Academy of Orthopaedic Surgeons, 1994, p 251.

Pak JH, Paprosky WG, Jablonsky WS, et al: Femoral strut allografts in cementless revision total hip arthroplasty. *Clin Orthop* 1993;295:172–178.

Pellicci PM, Wilson PD Jr, Sledge CB, et al: Long-term results of revision total hip replacement: A follow-up report. *J Bone Joint Surg* 1985;67A:513–516.

Rubash HE, Harris WH: Revision of non-septic loose cemented femoral components using modern cementing techniques. *J Arthroplasty* 1988;3:241–248.

Trousdale RT, Morrey BF: Uncemented femoral revision of total hip arthroplasty. *Orthop Trans* 1993;17:964–965.

Acetabular Revision

Pollack FH, Whiteside LA: The fate of massive allografts in total hip acetabular revision surgery. *J Arthroplasty* 1992;7:271–276.

Rosson J, Schatzker J: The use of reinforcement rings to reconstruct deficient acetabula. *J Bone Joint Surg* 1992; 74B:716–720.

Russotti GM, Harris WH: Proximal placement of the acetabular component in total hip arthroplasty: A long-term follow-up study. *J Bone Joint Surg* 1991;73A:587–592.

37

Femur: Trauma

Femoral Shaft Fractures

Introduction

Fractures of the femoral shaft are severe injuries that require emergent orthopaedic treatment. These fractures usually result from a directly applied high-energy force, often pose an immediate threat to life and limb, and have a significant impact on the patient's ultimate functional outcome. Important initial concerns, such as limb deformity and injury to the surrounding soft tissues, can be overshadowed by other associated injuries and systemic complications.

Classification

Femoral shaft fractures are classified by their bony configuration as well as by the degree of injury to the surrounding soft tissues. Fracture location, fracture pattern, and the amount of comminution are the important parameters in the commonly used classification developed by Winquist, Hansen, and Clawson (Fig. 1). In this classification scheme, fractures are described as proximal, distal (infraisthmal), or middle third in location with a transverse, oblique, spiral, segmental, or comminuted fracture pattern. Fracture comminution is further defined by degree. Type I comminution denotes a small butterfly fragment involving 25% or less of the bony circumference. In type II comminution, the fragment involves up to 50% of the width of the bone. In type III, there is a large butterfly segment (more than 50%) that leaves only a small area of contact between the main proximal and distal fracture fragments. Type IV comminution involves the entire bony circumference. In type V, which has been added, there is segmental bone loss. This classification system was developed to assess the degree of bony stability and its relationship to standard and interlocking intramedullary nailing techniques. Types I and II comminuted fractures located in the middle third of the femoral diaphysis are axially and rotationally stable after standard reamed intramedullary nailing. Fractures with a proximal or distal location are rotationally and, in some cases, axially unstable, requiring interlocking intramedullary nailing. Spiral fractures and those with types III, IV, and V comminution are axially and rotationally unstable (Fig. 1).

The AO/ASIF group, as part of their Comprehensive Classification of Fractures of Long Bones, have also presented a classification scheme for femoral shaft fractures that, at first glance, with 27 different categories, appears to be extremely complex and cumbersome. In actuality, it is a modification, albeit a complicated one, of that developed by Winquist and associates. The categories are similarly based on fracture location, pattern, and comminution. A major difference lies in its increased emphasis on various spiral and comminuted fracture configurations. Although the added information may be helpful for documentation purposes, at the present time it does not appear to offer any additional therapeutic or prognostic advantage.

Classification systems also exist for the grading of the soft-tissue injury in both open and closed fractures. For open fractures, the method of Gustilo and Anderson, later modified by Gustilo and associates, is commonly used. Fractures are categorized as type I, II, or III, and type III is further divided into three groups, A, B, and C, which depend mainly on the magnitude of the observed soft-tissue wound (Table 1). The accepted supposition that these subdivisions correlate with the level of wound contamination and/or impaired vascularity allows them to serve as a basis for decision-making and prognosis. Because this method is subjective, it now appears that determination of the "type" for each individual injury is subject to a high degree of interobserver variability and is not consistently reproducible. Grading of the soft-tissue injury in closed fractures has had limited applicability for fractures of the femoral shaft. The AO/ASIF group has proposed an extensive soft-tissue grading system that incorporates specific skin, muscle–tendon, and neurovascular injury groups (Table 2). Used in conjunction with their fracture classification, this system may prove useful in eliminating the deficiencies of other methods.

Patient Evaluation

Overview In most cases, patients with a femoral shaft fracture have sustained high-energy trauma. Therefore, examination of the injured extremity, even in those with an apparent isolated injury, should be just one part of a well-organized comprehensive approach. Associated injuries can be life- or limb-threatening. The recommended Advanced Trauma Life Support evaluation sequence (Outline 1) should be followed.

Examination of the injured extremity is carried out during the secondary survey except in cases of obvious exsanguinating hemorrhage. A closed fracture of the femoral shaft, occurring alone or in combination with other extremity fractures, should not be considered the cause of hypotensive shock. An alternative source of hemorrhage should always be sought.

Multiple System Injury Patients with multiple injuries in association with a femoral shaft fracture are best treated

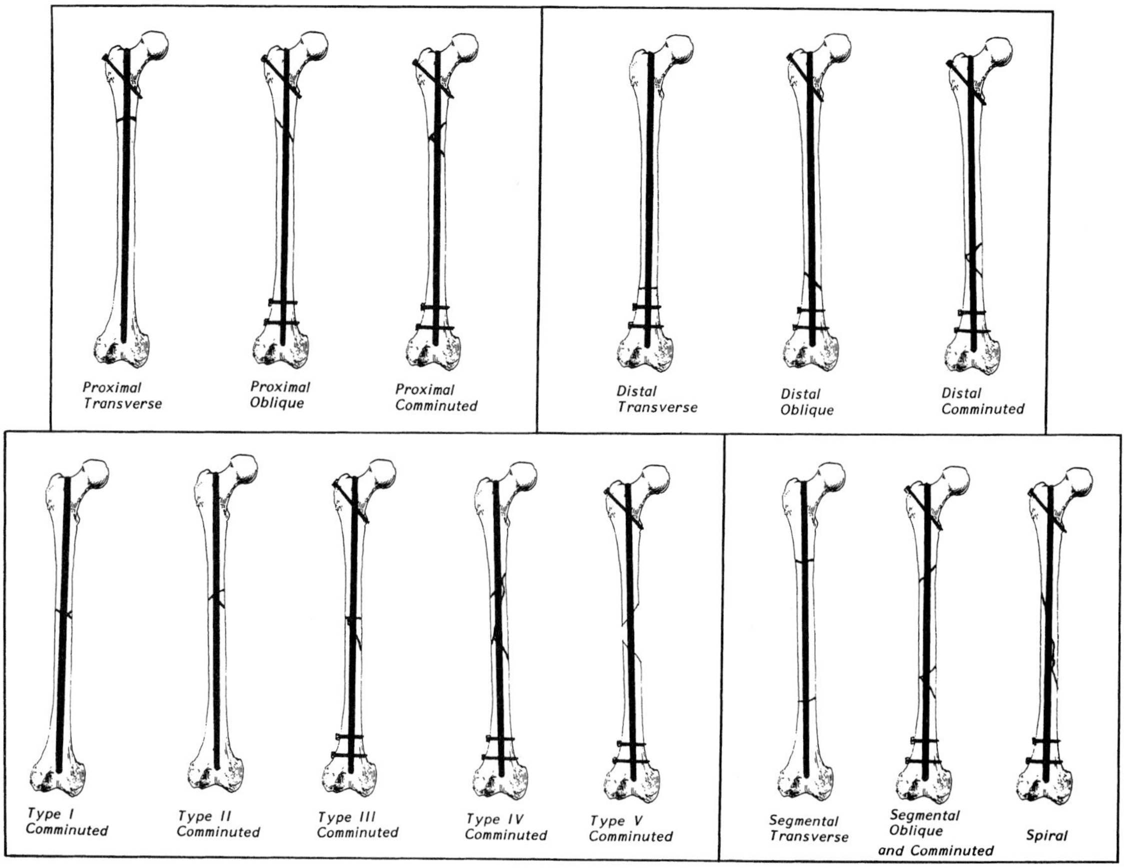

Fig. 1 Winquist classification of femoral shaft fractures and recommended method of nail fixation.

Table I. Gustilo classification of open fractures

Type	Description
I	A wound less than 1 cm long with little soft tissue damage; fracture pattern is simple with little comminution
II	A wound more than 1 cm long without extensive soft tissue damage, flaps, or avulsion; contamination and fracture comminution are moderate
III	Extensive soft tissue damage, contamination and fracture comminution
	A. Soft tissue coverage is adequate; comminuted and segmental high-energy fractures are included regardless of wound size.
	B. Extensive soft tissue injury with massive contamination and severe fracture comminution requiring a local or free flap for coverage
	C. Arterial injury requiring repair

by fracture stabilization within 24 hours of injury. Surgical intervention should proceed as soon as possible after completion of the initial resuscitation and treatment of any head, chest, or abdominal injuries. This approach allows early mobilization of the multiply-injured patient and is instrumental in preventing pulmonary complications.

Open Fractures Irrigation and debridement of an open fracture with the institution of appropriate intravenous antibiotics should be performed on an emergent basis. Initially, the traumatic wounds should remain open. Subsequent treatment depends on the time delay from injury to surgical intervention, the magnitude of the soft-tissue injury, and the presence of any additional injuries.

As noted above, patients with multiple injuries require early fracture stabilization. If the treatment delay is less than 8 hours, intramedullary nailing is preferred for fixation of types I, II, and IIIA open fractures (Table 1). Otherwise, alternative methods that allow early patient mobilization should be considered. For types IIIB and IIIC injuries, treatment must be individualized. External fixation, plating, and intramedullary nailing all have a place in the treatment armamentarium.

In patients with an isolated open femur fracture, an accepted treatment method is the traditional sequence of tibial pin traction for temporary fracture stabilization, delayed primary wound closure 5 to 7 days after the initial debridement, and closed intramedullary nail fixation 5 to 7 days later. However, it is preferable to treat types I, II,

Table 2. AO/ASIF classification of soft tissue injury

Skin Injury			
Integument Closed (IC)	**Integument Open (IO)**	**Tendo-Muscle Injury (M-T)**	**Neurovascular Injury (NV)**
IC1 No injury	IO1 Inside out puncture	MT1 No injury	NV1 No injury
IC2 Contusion	IO2 Outside in < 5 cm	MT2 Localized injury, one compartment	NV2 Isolated nerve injury
IC3 Local degloving	IO3 > 5 cm with contused devitalized edges, local degloving	MT3 Two compartment involvement	NV3 Localized vascular injury
IC4 Extensive degloving	IO4 Full-thickness contusion, abrasion, or skin loss	MT4 Extensive muscle defect, tendon laceration	NV4 Combined neurovascular injury
IC5 Skin necrosis from contusion	IO5 Extensive degloving	MT5 Crush or compartment syndrome	NV5 Subtotal or complete amputation

(Adapted with permission from Müller ME, Allgöwer M, Schneider R, et al (eds): *Manual of Internal Fixation.* Berlin, Germany, Springer-Verlag, 1991, pp. 151–158.)

Outline 1. Recommended advanced trauma life support evaluation sequence

1. Primary survey and resuscitation
   a. Airway with control of the cervical spine
   b. Breathing
   c. Circulation with control of hemorrhage
   d. Disability: brief neurologic exam
   e. Exposure: undress the patient
2. Secondary survey
   a. Perfusion
   b. Alignment
   c. Function
3. Definitive care

and IIIA open fractures by emergent debridement and intramedullary nailing. Types IIIB and C open fractures require careful individual assessment, but emergent fracture fixation is preferable.

Open fractures caused by gunshots present a special situation. Low-velocity gunshot fractures do not require formal debridement, but should otherwise be handled as type I injuries. High-energy injuries, such as close-range shotgun blasts and high-velocity gunshots, should be managed as type IIIB injuries.

Vascular Injury Although concomitant vascular (arterial or venous) injury is uncommon (less than 2%), it can occur with any of the fracture types. It is most commonly associated with fractures caused by penetrating trauma. In general, evidence of vascular injury can be divided into hard and soft signs. The specific hard signs include distal ischemia or a pulse deficit, presence of a bruit, an expanding or pulsatile hematoma, and obvious arterial bleeding. The less specific soft signs include a small stable hematoma, adjacent nerve injury, unexplained hypotension, and proximity of a penetrating wound or displaced fracture, such as fracture at the level of the adductor hiatus. Although the finding of any of the hard signs reliably indicates the presence of arterial injury, their absence does not exclude injury. Arteriography is indicated in patients with overt signs of arterial injury only when needed to further define or localize the lesion prior to surgical intervention, such as in patients with preexisting peripheral arterial disease. Arteriography is also indicated to exclude injury in patients with equivocal findings or soft signs. Although noninvasive studies, such as the Doppler-derived arterial pressure index and duplex ultrasonography, have been found to be helpful as screening tests for occult arterial trauma, their use in place of arteriography remains controversial.

The treatment of an arterial injury depends on a number of factors including amount of blood loss, quality of limb perfusion, and duration of ischemia. Ideally, distal limb ischemia should be limited to less than 6 hours. This limitation requires a team approach. Installation of temporary vascular shunts can be helpful in limiting ischemia time and will allow the femoral shaft fracture to be stabilized without the risk of disrupting vessel repair. External fixation, plate fixation, and, to a lesser extent, intramedullary nailing are fracture treatment options. Fracture fixation is followed by the definitive vascular repair. Fasciotomy is indicated if there has been any period of limb ischemia exceeding 8 hours or subsequent elevation of compartment pressures.

Nerve Injury Peripheral nerve injury is not commonly associated with femoral shaft fractures caused by blunt trauma. The incidence is higher with penetrating injury, which can result in an incomplete nerve lesion with a patchy neurologic deficit. A detailed examination is needed to define these injuries. Functional recovery is variable, depending on the type and severity of the nerve lesion. Iatrogenic nerve palsy can result from both direct pressure and stretch injury, depending on the treatment modality. The prognosis for recovery is good in these cases.

Compartment Syndrome Although uncommon, compartment syndrome of the thigh must always be considered during evaluation of a patient with a femoral shaft fracture. Predisposing factors include multiple injuries, systemic hypotension, vascular injury, coagulopathy, a history of external limb compression, and the use of military antishock trousers. Open fractures are also at risk. An associated high incidence of infection and neurologic deficit make early diagnosis mandatory in order to provide the best chance for recovery. A high index of suspicion and judicious use of compartment pressure monitoring are essential.

Ipsilateral Knee Ligament and Meniscal Injury Ipsilateral knee ligament injury should be suspected in any patient with a femoral shaft fracture. The incidence is quite high, up to almost 50% in some reported series. Often, the diagnosis is delayed for weeks or months, and this has a detrimental effect on limb rehabilitation. The presence of a femoral shaft fracture makes evaluation of the ipsilateral knee very difficult. Before any traction is applied, the knee should be clinically examined and appropriate radiographs obtained. Knee ligament injury precludes use of a tibial traction pin. After fracture fixation, the knee should be re-examined and any ligamentous injury identified should be treated.

Meniscal injury is also not uncommon. In a series of 47 closed diaphyseal fractures, ipsilateral meniscal tears requiring surgical treatment were present in 11 knees (23%). Knee effusion should be evaluated in all patients with a femoral fracture. However, there may be no acute clinical evidence of the meniscal injury, which will result in a delayed diagnosis.

Associated Extremity Fractures Patients with multiple fractures warrant the same aggressive approach as that required for the treatment of patients with multiple system injury. Bilateral fractures of the femoral shaft are usually associated with additional musculoskeletal or systemic injury. Closed intramedullary nailing is the treatment of choice. The floating knee syndrome, ipsilateral fracture of the femoral and tibial shafts, is a serious high-energy injury. Open fractures of one or both bones are common. Associated injuries involving other systems are also common with a reported mortality rate ranging from 5% to 15%. The best results are achieved when both fractures are stabilized, allowing early restoration of knee motion.

Ipsilateral fractures of the femoral neck and shaft are uncommon injuries, which are often not identified at the time of initial patient evaluation. Radiographs of the hip should be obtained in all patients with a fracture of the femoral shaft on initial presentation, after fracture fixation, and in the early (2 to 4 week) postinjury period. Furthermore, any patient complaining of groin or hip pain should have additional studies. The potential for a poor outcome is related to the complications of the femoral neck fracture. Therefore, although simultaneous fixation of both the hip and shaft fractures is desirable, optimal management of the femoral neck fracture cannot be compromised. Reduction and stabilization of the neck fracture is the first priority, followed by fixation of the femoral shaft fracture. Antegrade femoral nailing following initial screw fixation of the femoral neck fracture has not been uniformly successful. Ipsilateral intertrochanteric and diaphyseal fractures of the femur are to be differentiated from femoral neck/shaft fractures. Although technically demanding, this fracture combination does not present the same potential for complications as the ipsilateral femoral neck and shaft combination. Second-generation locked intramedullary nails allow stabilization of this ipsilateral hip/shaft fracture pattern. Care must be taken to avoid varus malposition or medial displacement of the intertrochanteric fracture component. A less demanding method is the compression hip screw and plate combination.

Treatment Methods

Nonsurgical Care Traction is mainly used for the temporary stabilization of a femoral shaft fracture if definitive surgical fixation must be delayed. Traction can be applied by means of a pin placed through either the proximal tibia or distal femur. A distal femoral pin is required in the presence of ipsilateral knee ligament injury, but should be avoided if intramedullary nailing is planned. There are very few indications for traction as the definitive treatment plan. These include the lack of equipment or expertise to perform surgical fixation, systemic contraindications to anesthesia, or a local contraindication, such as infection at the surgery site. In these cases, a variable period of traction, usually 6 weeks, is followed by hip spica cast or cast-brace application. Although this treatment method has a high fracture union rate, problems, such as prolonged recumbency and hospital stay, knee stiffness, and fracture malunion, preclude its general use.

External Fixation External fixation is not indicated for the routine treatment of fractures of the femoral shaft. It is indicated mainly for the management of open fractures with severe soft-tissue injury (types IIIB and C). An external fixator should also be considered in treatment of patients with severe burns, closed fractures with associated vascular injury, and infected fractures previously treated by internal fixation. The surgical procedure can be performed quickly. Therefore, external fixation can also be of use for the patient, multiply-injured or otherwise, who cannot tolerate prolonged anesthesia. External fixators can be applied for temporary fracture stabilization, allowing healing of the soft tissues prior to delayed internal fixation, or as the definitive method of fracture management. Although early mobilization of the patient is facilitated with this technique, significant late complications are common, including knee stiffness, malunion, nonunion, pin-site infection, and osteomyelitis. Delayed conversion to internal fixation carries with it an increased risk of subsequent infection.

Plating Accurate reduction and stable fixation allowing early mobilization of the patient and the limb can be achieved using plating techniques. The disadvantages are substantial (infection, hardware failure, and delayed union) and preclude the general use of plating. Recent concern regarding an increased potential for pulmonary injury associated with reamed intramedullary nailing in the multiply-injured patient has created renewed interest in plate fixation for the polytrauma patient. However, further study is required. Current indications continue to be diaphyseal fractures associated with an ipsilateral femoral neck fracture or a vascular injury requiring repair. The surgical procedure involves the application of a single broad plate to the lateral aspect of the femur, with cancellous bone graft placed medially along the shaft. An "indirect reduction," as advocated by the AO/ASIF group, either by using an intraoperative distraction device or precontouring of the plate, is instrumental in limiting periosteal stripping and medial dissection. Comminuted fragments are not directly dissected free and anatomically reduced, but are bridged by the plating, theoretically eliminating the need for bone graft and decreasing the rate of complications.

Intramedullary Nailing

Overview Intramedullary nailing is the treatment of choice for the majority of femoral shaft fractures. Closed antegrade nailing with reaming is the preferred method. Open nailing, using a small incision at the fracture site only to allow fracture reduction and passage of the guide wire, may provide similar results to closed nailing. A formal open procedure, which exposes the bone ends for nailing or supplemental wire fixation, is to be avoided due to higher rates of infection and impaired fracture healing. The usual surgical technique requires a fracture table with the patient in a supine or lateral position. An alternative method, using the AO/ASIF distractor with the patient placed on a radiolucent operating room table, has been shown to be effective, especially in patients with multiple injuries. Although the standard cloverleaf Küntscher nail has now been essentially replaced by more rigid closed-section nails with an interlocking capability, the basic surgical technique remains unchanged.

Antegrade Locked Nailing With Reaming This method remains the treatment of choice for closed and types I, II, and IIIA open fractures. With the advent of interlocking, direct manipulation of the fracture site for cerclage wiring or any other supplemental fixation is no longer necessary. Static interlocking (insertion of cross-locking screws in both the proximal and distal fracture fragments), as dictated by the fracture configuration (Fig. 1), was at one time thought to require dynamization (removal of either the proximal or distal screws) in order to optimize fracture healing. Many reports now indicate that static interlocking does not clinically affect fracture union. Furthermore, it appears that, in most cases, only one distal locking screw is required in the interlocking nail construct; the exceptions are distal (infraisthmal) fractures. Errors in the initial radiographic assessment and subsequent locking screw decision-making can result in the unanticipated loss of fracture reduction. Therefore, initial static interlocking should be used in all cases. Dynamization is reserved for those fractures that radiographically demonstrate minimal callus formation 16 to 20 weeks after nailing.

Results The results of reamed intramedullary nailing are far superior to those of other treatment methods for closed and open types I, II, and IIIA fractures. Almost complete return of hip and knee motion and a union rate of over 95% can be expected. Infection rates are also extremely low. The reported numbers are small and the situation is not so clear-cut for types IIIB and IIIC open fractures, however. In type IIIB injuries, intramedullary nailing provides improved fracture alignment and joint motion in exchange for an increased risk of infection. Intramedullary nailing for type IIIC fractures places the vascular repair or shunt at risk. This risk, however, could be decreased by using the AO/ASIF distractor, rather than the fracture table, to restore length prior to vessel repair.

Although results of intramedullary nailing are felt to be excellent in terms of fracture union, return of joint motion, and a low overall complication rate, there are few data regarding the functional outcome from the patients' perspectives. One study indicates that this outcome is not as good as expected. Thirty-nine percent had limited walking, standing, and stair-climbing ability, and 37% had residual discomfort. Further outcome studies are needed to define the actual end results following these injuries.

Retrograde Reamed Nailing Retrograde intramedullary nailing of fractures of the femoral shaft using a distal extra-articular entry portal via the medial femoral condyle has been advocated for the treatment of patients with ipsilateral fracture of the femoral neck and shaft and those with multiple injuries. Technical difficulties and an increased potential for femoral malunion limit its use.

Complications Significant complications of reamed antegrade locked intramedullary nailing are infrequent. Infection (~ 1%, closed fractures) requires thorough debridement at the fracture site. If the nail is providing fracture stability, it may be left in place. However, if fixation is compromised, the nail should be removed, the medullary canal reamed, and a larger nail inserted. This approach is usually successful, if there is an early diagnosis, an intact soft-tissue envelope, and the absence of extensive necrotic bone and purulence. Staged, sequential reconstructive methods incorporating the use of external fixation may otherwise be required.

Although low in incidence, malunion continues to occur even with static interlocking. In a report of one series, angular deformity occurred in 2.5% of the patients and malrotation in 7%. Significant leg-length discrepancy was present in < 2%. Fracture malalignment, especially malrotation, should be evaluated in the immediate postoperative period, at which time it can usually be corrected by revision of the position of the locking screws. Aseptic nonunion can be addressed by exchange to a larger-diameter reamed nail.

Heterotopic ossification about the hip is common after reamed antegrade nailing, but only infrequently (< 5%) affects hip motion. If necessary, delayed excision is usually successful in regaining functional joint motion. Iatrogenic nerve palsy can involve one or both divisions of the sciatic nerve or, more commonly, the pudendal nerve. These problems have been related to fracture table-related problems of poor patient positioning, excessive traction, and prolonged surgery times. Prognosis for spontaneous recovery is good.

Of more serious concern are recent reports, in contradistinction to reports of earlier studies, attributing an increased risk of developing adult respiratory distress syndrome when reamed intramedullary nailing is performed in patients with concomitant severe pulmonary injury. These data are presented not to suggest that early fracture stabilization should be avoided in these patients, but that alternative fixation methods that do not require reaming may be preferable. As a treatment option, locked intramedullary nailing without reaming has shown promise, but its advantages and shortcomings have not yet been clearly defined (Fig. 2). It is still premature to conclude that any alternative treatment method is superior to reamed intramedullary nailing. Pending the publication of controlled, randomized, prospective studies indicating otherwise, early closed antegrade intramedullary nailing with reaming remains the treatment of choice, providing early patient mobilization and a decreased incidence of complications. The importance of this point cannot be overemphasized.

Supracondylar Fractures of the Femur

Introduction

Supracondylar fractures of the femur occur in a bimodal age distribution. In the younger, predominantly male patient group, the fractures result from high-energy trauma with a greater incidence of intra-articular damage and associated systemic or skeletal injuries. Fractures in the elderly, predominantly female group are low-energy injuries that often occur in association with radiographic evidence of generalized osteopenia or other "age-related fractures" of the hip, spine, or pelvis. Knee stiffness and osteoarthrosis are common sequelae of this injury. Fracture management depends on many factors, including the frac-

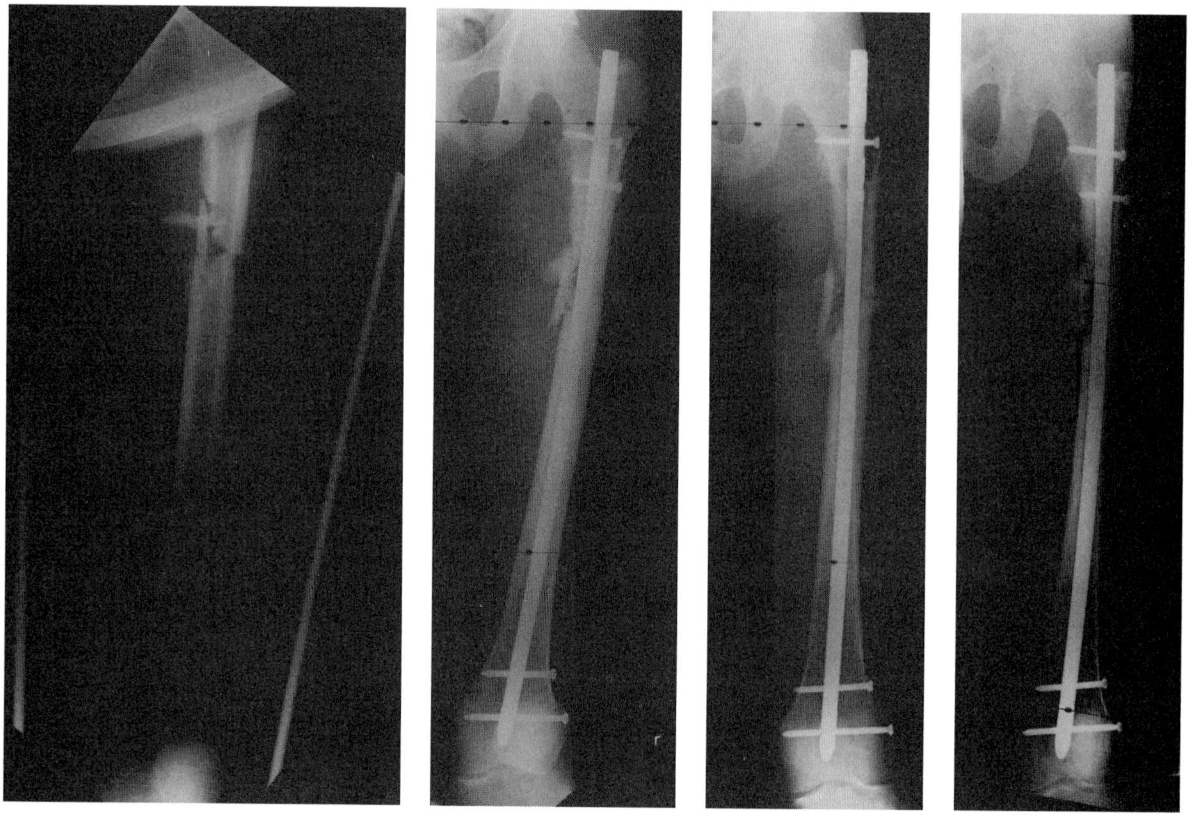

Fig. 2 Left, Comminuted closed femoral shaft fracture in a patient with multiple injuries. **Left center,** Two weeks following closed static locked nailing without reaming. **Right center,** Four months later with minimal callus evident. The nail was subsequently dynamized. **Right,** Eight months after injury the patient continued to complain of pain with ambulation. Radiographs demonstrated delayed healing. Note the retained screw in the dynamic proximal slot of the nail. Exchange to a reamed nail was required to obtain fracture union.

ture type, bone quantity, and the patient's overall medical condition. Although treatments vary, both patient groups will benefit from restoration of joint congruity and the institution of early knee motion.

Classification

Ideal prerequisites for a classification system require that it be simple enough to remember and understand, allow description of all the fracture variations, assist in formulating a treatment plan, and provide prognostic information. The AO/ASIF classification of supracondylar fractures (Fig. 3), which divides fractures into extra-articular (A), unicondylar (B), or bicondylar intra-articular (C) fracture types, appears to satisfy most of these criteria.

Treatment Methods

Nonsurgical Care Skeletal traction is not appropriate for the majority of supracondylar fractures of the femur because better results can be obtained with internal fixation. Patients with displaced fractures who present with contraindications to surgical intervention are the main candidates for this treatment method. It must be understood that these fractures are difficult to manage in traction and require constant vigilance to minimize the significant risks of malunion and knee stiffness as well as the potential complications of recumbancy. A variable period of traction is usually followed by mobilization using a cast-brace.

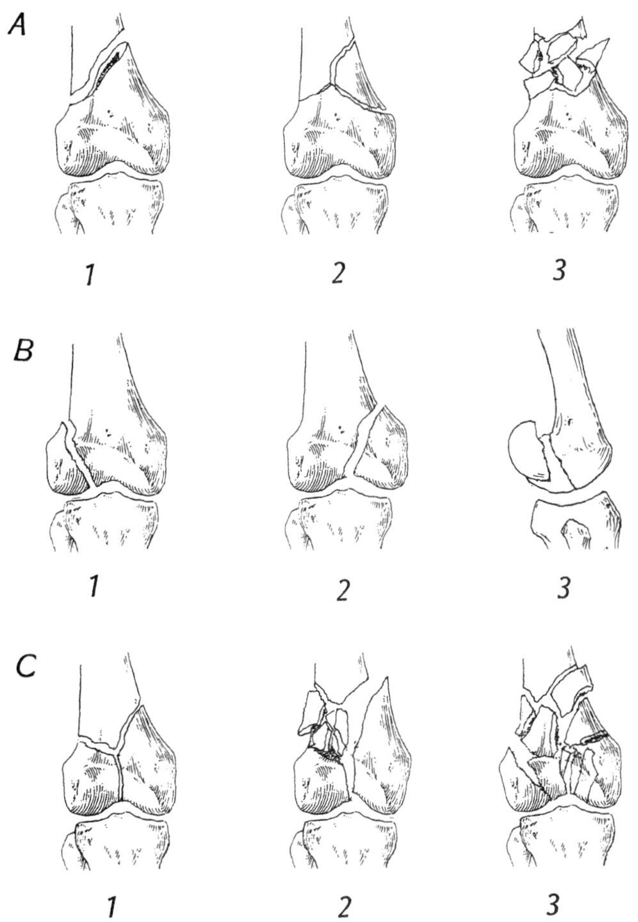

Fig. 3 Current AO/ASIF classification of supracondylar fractures. (Adapted with permission from Müller ME, Allgöwer M, Schneider R, et al (eds): *Manual of Internal Fixation.* Berlin, Germany, Springer-Verlag, 1991, pp 140–141.)

Antegrade Locked Intramedullary Nailing With Reaming This method has been successfully used to stabilize type A and selected types C1 and C2 fractures occurring both alone and in combination with ipsilateral femoral shaft fractures. Careful preoperative evaluation is required to ensure that type C3 injuries with coronal plane fracture lines are not inadvertently treated using this technique. Many modifications to the standard nailing procedure are required, including supplemental lag screw fixation of the intra-articular component in the C-type fractures and removal of the distal 15 mm of the nail to allow satisfactory purchase of the distal locking screws. The procedure is performed with the patient supine to avoid a valgus reduction. Displaced intercondylar fracture lines that cannot be anatomically reduced by closed means require either an arthrotomy for visualization and manipulation of the intra-articular component or selection of an alternative method of fixation. Overall, results are best for the type A fractures. Caution must be advised, as there is an increased risk of nail fatigue failure when the fracture line is within 5 cm of the most proximal of the distal locking screw holes. This risk is minimized by using large-diameter nails and avoiding early weightbearing.

Retrograde Interlocking Intramedullary Nailing With Reaming A relatively new device, a supracondylar intramedullary nail, allows closed locked retrograde fixation of all types A and C fractures. Published reports, which are preliminary, indicate that this implant is still under development and cannot be advocated for general use. This device may find its best application in the stabilization of type A fractures above a total knee arthroplasty.

Plate Fixation Plating techniques provide stable anatomic fracture fixation, which allows early limb mobilization. Plating is currently the standard to which all other treatment methods must be compared. The standard surgical approach uses a midlateral incision directed toward the midpoint of the lateral femoral condyle, extending, as needed, toward a point just distal to the tibial tubercle to address intra-articular fracture lines. Type C3 fractures may require additional medial exposure, which can be obtained by osteotomizing the tibial tubercle or using a second, medial incision.

A blade plate or condylar compression screw can be used for types A, C1, most C2, and selected C3 fractures. With these devices, good to excellent results are reported in over 70% of treated patients. The surgical technique is demanding, however. Careful preoperative planning and strict adherence to the described surgical details are necessary to approximate these reported results. Complications are often the result of avoidable technical errors.

The condylar buttress plate should be used when the fracture pattern does not allow insertion of the blade plate or condylar screw (type C3 and severely comminuted C2 fractures). This plate is not very strong and does not control varus–valgus alignment very well. A deficient medial cortical buttress, evident after buttress plate application, is an indication for supplemental medial plate fixation.

Special Considerations

Bone Grafting Autogenous cancellous iliac crest bone should be applied wherever there is metaphyseal comminution and medial stability cannot be obtained. This recommendation currently applies to all type A3, C2, and C3 fractures. In the future, "indirect reduction" techniques, as previously mentioned, may prove to alter the indications for bone grafting.

Type B Fractures Adequate fixation of displaced unicondylar fractures can be obtained using cancellous lag screws. Occasionally, type B1 and B2 fractures require supplemental buttress plating, especially in osteoporotic bone. Excellent long-term results have been reported in over 80% of patients.

Fractures in the Elderly

Stable internal fixation with plates and screws is difficult to achieve in osteoporotic bone. In this situation, screw purchase can be greatly improved by the use of methylmethacrylate. This technique may be applicable for selected type A and type C fractures. Alternatively, type A fractures with minimal comminution can be adequately stabilized using flexible intramedullary devices, such as the Zickel supracondylar nail, or standard locked nailing as described above. Type B1 and B2 fractures usually require a supplemental buttress plate. Other options—nonsurgical treatment and primary total knee arthroplasty—should always be carefully considered in all of these patients.

Annotated Bibliography

General References

Benirschke SK, Melder I, Henley MB, et al: Closed interlocking nailing of femoral shaft fractures: Assessment of technical complications and functional outcomes by comparison of a prospective database with retrospective review. *J Orthop Trauma* 1993;7:118–122.

As part of this study, an abbreviated functional assessment was performed in 56 patients at a minimum of 12 months postinjury. Thirty-seven percent of the patients had pain, and 39% had some limitation in ability to ambulate or stand. Nine percent had to obtain new employment or seek job modifications. The authors concluded that a significant portion of patients with femoral shaft fractures treated with interlocking nails will have permanent functional loss.

Vangsness CT Jr, DeCampos J, Merritt PO, et al: Meniscal injury associated with femoral shaft fractures: An arthroscopic evaluation of incidence. *J Bone Joint Surg* 1993;75B:207–209.

In 47 patients with closed, displaced, diaphyseal fractures of the femur caused by blunt trauma, there were 12 medial meniscal injuries (five tears) and 13 injuries of the lateral meniscus (eight tears). Examination under anesthesia revealed ligamentous laxity in 23 patients (49%), but the incidence of meniscal injuries was similar in knees with and without ligament injury.

Patients With Multiple Injuries

Bone LB, Johnson KD, Weigelt J, et al: Early versus delayed stabilization of femoral fractures: A prospective randomized study. *J Bone Joint Surg* 1989;71A:336–340.

One hundred seventy-eight acute femoral fractures in adults with both isolated and multiple injuries were randomly assigned to early or delayed fracture stabilization. When patients with multiple injuries had delayed fracture stabilization, the evidence of pulmonary complications (adult respiratory distress syndrome, fat embolism, and pneumonia) was higher, the hospital stay was longer, and the number of days in the intensive care unit was increased.

Pape H-C, Auf'm'Kolk M, Paffrath T, et al: Primary intramedullary femur fixation in multiple trauma patients with associated lung contusion: A cause of posttraumatic ARDS? *J Trauma* 1993;34:540–548.

One hundred six patients with a femoral shaft fracture and multiple injuries were retrospectively evaluated and divided into two groups depending on the timing of reamed intramedullary nailing (< 24 hours after injury versus > 24 hours). In patients with severe chest trauma there was a higher incidence of adult respiratory distress syndrome (33% versus 8%) and mortality (21% versus 4%). The authors concluded that in the presence of severe trauma and associated pulmonary injury alternative fracture fixation methods may be preferable.

Open Fractures

Brumback RJ, Ellison PS Jr, Poka A, et al: Intramedullary nailing of open fractures of the femoral shaft. *J Bone Joint Surg* 1989;71A:1324–1331.

Eighty-nine open femoral shaft fractures were treated. Nailing was within 24 hours in 33 fractures. A prerequisite for immediate nailing was that irrigation and debridement be done within 8 hours of injury. All fractures healed. No infections occurred in the 62 type I, type II, or type IIIA open fractures. In 27 type IIIB open fractures, there were three infections.

Brumback RJ, Jones AL: Interobserver agreement in the classification of open fractures of the tibia: The results of a survey of two hundred and forty-five orthopaedic surgeons. *J Bone Joint Surg* 1994;76A:1162–1166.

The reliability of the Gustilo and Anderson classification of open fractures was tested on the basis of responses to a survey by 245 orthopaedic surgeons. The average agreement was 60% (range: 42% to 94%). In the participant subgroup of those with the most experience (trauma trained academicians), average agreement was only 66%. It was concluded that interobserver agreement is poor and that this classification system may not be adequate.

Grosse A, Christie J, Taglang G, et al: Open adult femoral shaft fracture treated by early intramedullary nailing. *J Bone Joint Surg* 1993;75B:562–565.

One hundred fifteen consecutive open femur fractures (36 type I, 42 type II, 20 type IIIA, 12 type IIIB, 5 type IIIC) were treated by debridement of the wound and early nailing. The procedure was performed on the day of injury in 106. Union was delayed in four, and bone grafting was required in three of these. Infection occurred in three. The authors concluded that early intramedullary nailing is a safe and efficient treatment method.

Intramedullary Nailing

Brumback RJ, Reilly JP, Poka A, et al: Intramedullary nailing of femoral shaft fractures: Part I. Decision-making errors with interlocking fixation. *J Bone Joint Surg* 1988; 70A:1441–1452.

Brumback RJ, Uwagie-Ero S, Lakatos RP, et al: Intramedullary nailing of femoral shaft fractures: Part II. Fracture-healing with static interlocking fixation. *J Bone Joint Surg* 1988;70A:1453–1462.

Brumback RJ, Ellison TS, Poka A, et al: Intramedullary nailing of femoral shaft fractures: Part III. Long-term effects of static interlocking fixation. *J Bone Joint Surg* 1992;74A:106–112.

This three-part series sequentially examines the decision-making criteria, fracture healing, and long-term effects associated with locked, reamed intramedullary nailing of femoral shaft fractures. Basic conclusions are that the threshold for static interlocking nails even in apparently stable fracture patterns should be extremely low and that routine dynamization is not desirable or required.

Hajek PD, Bicknell HR Jr, Bronson WE, et al: The use of one compared with two distal screws in the treatment of femoral shaft fractures with interlocking intramedullary nailing: A clinical and biomechanical analysis. *J Bone Joint Surg* 1993;75A:519–525.

From a biomechanical study and a clinical evaluation of 27 patients using the Grosse-Kempf nailing system, it was concluded that one distal screw provides adequate distal fixation of fractures of the femoral shaft treated with locked intramedullary nailing. The authors caution that this conclusion does not apply to distal infra-isthmal or supracondylar fractures and may not apply to other, dissimilar nailing systems.

McFerran MA, Johnson KD: Intramedullary nailing of acute femoral shaft fractures without a fracture table: Technique of using a femoral distractor. *J Orthop Trauma* 1992;6:271–278.

The technique and advantages of using a femoral distractor was evaluated. The authors concluded that the method was of benefit, especially in patients with ipsilateral axial skeletal injury, bilateral extremity fracture, multiple ipsilateral lower extremity injury, and obesity.

Wiss DA, Sima W, Brien WW: Ipsilateral fractures of the femoral neck and shaft. *J Orthop Trauma* 1992;6:159–166.

Thirty-three patients with ipsilateral femoral neck and shaft fractures were treated with a "reversed" nail construct (13), a conventional interlocked nail (six), and a reconstruction nail (14). Twenty-seven (82%) of the femoral neck fractures healed. The authors concluded that closed reamed antegrade intramedullar nailing with supplemental screw fixation of ipsilateral femoral neck and shaft fractures did not produce uniformly successful results because of high rates of varus nonunion of the femoral neck.

Supracondylar Fractures

Butler MS, Brumback RJ, Ellison TS, et al: Interlocking intramedullary nailing for ipsilateral fractures of the femoral shaft and distal part of the femur. *J Bone Joint Surg* 1991;73A:1492–1502.

Twenty-three patients with a femoral shaft fracture and an ipsilateral supracondylar femur fracture were treated using locked intramedullary nailing with the addition of an arthrotomy to visualize the reduction of displaced intra-articular components prior to supplemental lag screw fixation. Nail length was critical. Complications included angular deformity in two patients, residual intra-articular displacement in one, and repeated surgery for a missed intra-articular coronal fracture line in two. The presence of a fracture in the coronal plane is a relative contraindication to the use of this method.

Iannacone WM, Bennett FS, DeLong WG Jr, et al: Initial experience with the treatment of supracondylar femoral fractures using the supracondylar intramedullary nail: A preliminary report. *J Orthop Trauma* 1994;8:322–327.

A retrograde supracondylar intramedullary nail was used to treat 38 patients with 41 supracondylar femur fractures (three type A2, 16 type A3, six type C1, six type C2, and ten type C3). Nineteen fractures were closed and 23 were open. Complications included four nonunions and five delayed unions, seven of which required revision surgery. Four patients developed fatigue failure of the nail, which was subsequently redesigned. The authors concluded that further clinical trials and additional biomechanical testing should be performed prior to general use of this implant.

Ostermann PA, Neumann K, Ekkernkamp A, et al: Long term results of unicondylar fractures of the femur. *J Orthop Trauma* 1994;8:142–146.

Twenty-four high-energy unicondylar fractures (16 B, five B2, and three B3) were treated with open reduction and lag screw fixation and followed for an average of 62 months. Fractures were closed in 23 patients and open (type IIIB) in one. Results were excellent in 20, satisfactory in three, and unsatisfactory in the one open fracture. Less than excellent results could be attributed to associated musculoskeletal injury in all four cases.

Sanders R, Swiontkowski M, Rosen H, et al: Double-plating of comminuted, unstable fractures of the distal part of the femur. *J Bone Joint Surg* 1991;73A:341–346.

Nine patients with a complex (comminuted type C2 or C3) supracondylar fracture and a deficient medial cortical buttress were reviewed. Four fractures were closed and five open. A lateral condylar buttress plate was applied, and stability of this fixation was then assessed intraoperatively. Motion at the bone-screw or the screw-plate interface indicated the need for supplemental medial plate fixation and bone graft. Of the five open fractures, medial plating was delayed until the open wound was "clean" in three, and bone grafting was delayed until wound closure in five. All fractures healed. Results were good in five patients and fair in four. Knee range of motion was limited (< 100° of flexion) in all nine.

Tornetta P III, Tiburzi D: Anterograde interlocked nailing of distal femoral fractures after gunshot wounds. *J Orthop Trauma* 1994;8:220–227.

Thirty-eight Type A fractures caused by a low-velocity gunshot wound (GSW) in 36 (type I, open) and a high-velocity GSW in two were treated by reamed anterograde nailing. Nailing was performed an average of 1.7 days following injury. All fractures healed, with 36 patients having excellent or good results and two fair. There were no infections. Of the six fractures operated on in the lateral position, three were nailed in valgus. A subsequent switch to the supine position using a described "joy stick" reduction technique eliminated residual angular deformity.

Classic Bibliography

Femur Fractures

Bucholz RW, Ross SE, Lawrence KL: Fatigue fracture of the interlocking nail in the treatment of fractures of the distal part of the femoral shaft. *J Bone Joint Surg* 1987; 69A:1391–1399.

Carr CR, Wingo CH: Fractures of the femoral diaphysis: A retrospective study of the results and costs of treatment by intramedullary nailing and by traction and a spica cast. *J Bone Joint Surg* 1973;55A:690–700.

Connolly JF, Whittaker D, Williams E: Femoral and tibial fractures combined with injuries to the femoral or popliteal artery: A review of the literature and analysis of fourteen cases. *J Bone Joint Surg* 1971;53A:56–68.

Feliciano DV, Herskowitz K, O'Gorman RB, et al: Management of vascular injuries in the lower extremities. *J Trauma* 1988;28:319–328.

Johnson KD, Cadambi A, Seibert GB: Incidence of adult respiratory distress syndrome in patients with multiple musculoskeletal injuries: Effect of early operative stabilization of fractures. *J Trauma* 1985;25:375–384.

Kempf I, Grosse A, Beck G: Closed locked intramedullary nailing: Its application to comminuted fractures of the femur. *J Bone Joint Surg* 1985;67A:709–720.

Winquist RA, Hansen ST Jr, Clawson DK: Closed intramedullary nailing of femoral fractures: A report of five hundred and twenty cases. *J Bone Joint Surg* 1984; 66A:529–539.

Wiss DA, Fleming CH, Matta JM, et al: Comminuted and rotationally unstable fractures of the femur treated with an interlocking nail. *Clin Orthop* 1986;212:35–47.

Supracondylar Fractures

Giles JB, DeLee JC, Heckman JD, et al: Supracondylar-intercondylar fractures of the femur treated with a supracondylar plate and lag screw. *J Bone Joint Surg* 1982;64A:864–870.

Mize RD, Bucholz RW, Grogan DP: Surgical treatment of displaced, comminuted fractures of the distal end of the femur. *J Bone Joint Surg* 1982;64A:871–879.

Neer CS II, Grantham SA, Shelton ML: Supracondylar fracture of the adult femur: A study of one hundred and ten cases. *J Bone Joint Surg* 1967;49A:591–613.

Olerud S: Operative treatment of supracondylar-condylar fractures of the femur: Technique and results in fifteen cases. *J Bone Joint Surg* 1972;54A:1015–1032.

Schatzker J, Home G, Waddell J: The Toronto experience with the supracondylar fracture of the femur, 1966–72. *Injury* 1974;6:113–128.

Stewart MJ, Sisk TD, Wallace SL Jr: Fractures of the distal third of the femur. *J Bone Joint Surg* 1966;48A:784–807.

38

Knee and Leg: Pediatric Aspects

Abnormalities of the Knee

Congenital Dislocation

Congenital dislocation or subluxation of the knee is rare in children. The incidence is approximately 1% of the incidence of congenital dislocation of the hip.

Etiologic factors proposed include positioning in utero, contracture of the quadriceps mechanism, and absence of the cruciate ligaments. Absence of the cruciate ligaments and fibrosis of the quadriceps mechanism are generally believed to be secondary to the dislocation rather than its cause. The most frequent associated deformity is congenital dislocation of the hip, which occurs in approximately 50% of children with congenital dislocation or subluxation of the knee.

Clinically, the lower extremity is positioned with the knee held in hyperextension. The severity of the deformity is variable. In type I, subluxation and hyperextension are minimal, and the knee can be passively flexed to 90°. In type II, or moderate, in which there is subluxation of the tibia anteriorly on the femoral condyles, the knee can be flexed up to 45°. In type III, there is complete anterior dislocation of the proximal tibia on the femoral condyles with no contact between the tibia and the femur.

The treatment varies according to the severity. Gentle manipulation and serial casting or placement in a Pavlik harness will correct a type I deformity quickly. Type II deformity with moderate subluxation is treated by gentle manipulation and serial casting. If the knee can be flexed to 90°, then splinting may be used up to 6 months of age.

For irreducible type II and type III dislocations of the knee, the treatment is surgical, and the surgery generally is performed when the child is between 6 and 12 months of age. Surgical techniques include an anterior skin incision, medial and lateral parapatellar incisions, lengthening of the quadriceps-patellar tendon complex, and comprehensive anterior capsulotomy extended both medially and laterally. Postoperative management includes initial positioning of the knee in slight flexion to remove tension on the skin incision and then subsequent positioning of the knee into progressive flexion to obtain at least 90° of knee flexion.

Discoid Meniscus

Discoid meniscus is an infrequent congenital anomaly of the knee in which the lateral meniscus is discoid in shape rather than having the normal semilunar configuration. Discoid menisci have been classified into two types. In the Wrisberg-ligament type, the lateral meniscus has no posterior ligamentous attachment to the tibial epiphysis. In the complete type, the peripheral capsular attachment to the lateral meniscus is intact, and the discoid meniscus may be complete or incomplete.

Clinical symptoms include a history of snapping, clicking, catching, or giving way at the knee; symptoms typically occur in children younger than 6 to 8 years of age, but occasionally may occur in adolescents. Magnetic resonance imaging (MRI), the diagnostic tool of choice, generally yields information about the size and shape of the discoid lateral meniscus (Fig. 1).

Partial meniscectomy, or sculpting of the meniscus, is the preferred treatment of a complete or incomplete discoid meniscus when there are symptoms of internal derangement of the knee and the peripheral capsular attachments are intact. In the Wrisberg type discoid meniscus, in which the posterior ligamentous attachments are not intact, treatment options include peripheral repair of the discoid meniscus and partial meniscectomy to a more normally-shaped meniscus or total meniscectomy. Preferred treatment is total meniscectomy if the peripheral

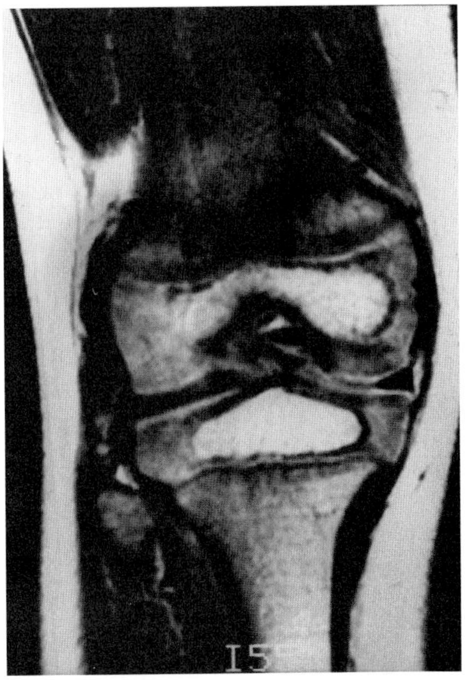

Fig. 1 Magnetic resonance imaging scan of discoid meniscus in a 4-year-old child.

attachments cannot be adequately repaired and the discoid meniscus cannot be converted to a functioning lateral meniscus that has a more normal size and shape.

Osteochondritis Dissecans

Osteochondritis dissecans (OCD) is a condition in which a portion of the articular cartilage of the knee and its underlying subchondral bone becomes separated from the remaining articular cartilage. The etiology is multifactorial but may include both ischemia and trauma to the articular surface of the femoral condyles in a skeletally immature patient.

Clinical symptoms include pain, knee effusion, and, occasionally symptoms of locking or catching of the knee when an OCD fragment has become a free loose body. Diagnostic studies include radiographs and MRI. When the medial femoral condyle is involved, the OCD lesion generally is on its most lateral and posterior aspect. When the lateral femoral condyle is involved, the lesion is "saucer-shaped" and involves the articular surface.

Treatment is directed toward healing the lesion in skeletally immature patients. In children and adolescents in whom the OCD lesion is not yet separated from the remaining subchondral bone, cast immobilization for a period of 6 to 12 weeks is warranted, with healing in most patients. When the fragment has separated from the surrounding subchondral bone or is not healed after a period of 6 to 12 weeks of cast immobilization, surgical intervention is warranted. Arthroscopic or open drilling and Kirschner-wire or screw fixation is warranted to correct large osteochondral defects in teenagers or young adults. In young adults, treatment remains controversial. If articular cartilage over the lesion is intact on MRI or arthroscopy, drilling often is used to accelerate healing. Loose fragments may be pinned in place with wires, Herbert screws, or resorbable pins in hopes of reestablishing an intact articular surface. Excision of irregular lesions with curretage of the underlying bone may be of value in some cases. Repair of articular cartilage, although experimental, may play a role in management of large displaced lesions involving the weightbearing surface (see Chapter 1, "Soft-Tissue Physiology and Repair").

Quadriceps Contracture

Contracture of the quadriceps may cause limited motion or patellar dislocation and occurs most often after fibrosis as a result of multiple injections into the muscle, although the cause may be blunt trauma, a mild form of arthrogryposis, spinal dysraphism, or idiopathic. The fibrosis usually is greatest in the vastus intermedius, occasionally in the vastus lateralis, and rarely in the vastus medialis. The iliotibial band may be scarred to the muscles as well. The fibrosis is usually greatest distally. Secondary changes may occur, such as flattening of the femoral condyles, contracture of the knee joint capsule, and patella alta.

On physical examination, there usually is atrophy and sometimes dimpling of the skin in the area of the fibrosis. The patella is more likely to sublux if the fibrosis involves the vastus lateralis. When the patella is held in place, flexion is limited. When it is allowed to sublux laterally, the knee can flex more. Knee range of motion should be checked with the hip in both flexion and extension to assess for contracture of the rectus. Patients present with one of the following patterns: (1) a stiff, extended knee at birth, in some cases with recurvatum, (2) progressive decrease in range of knee motion during the first few years of childhood, (3) habitual dislocation of the patella, or (4) degenerative joint disease later in adulthood due to the habitual dislocation.

Conservative treatment usually succeeds only in mild contractures in patients with a range of flexion of more than 60°. Surgery should be done before the age of 10 years to prevent flattening of the femoral condyles. Surgery includes the following steps to obtain a minimum of 90° knee flexion: (1) quadricepsplasty, or elevation of the functioning quadriceps components; (2) dissection and excision of the scarred muscle; and (3) z-plasty of the rectus. The iliotibial band should be divided when tight. Medial plication and transfer of lateral half of patella tendon are sometimes needed. The knee is immobilized in 90° flexion for several weeks.

Abnormalities of the Lower Extremity

Fibular Hemimelia

Fibular hemimelia (hypoplasia or aplasia of the fibula) is the most common longitudinal deficiency of the lower extremity. The spectrum varies from complete absence of the fibula, with missing lateral rays, to a fibula that is slightly short, with a ball and socket type ankle joint (Fig. 2). The magnitude of the projected shortening usually is related to the severity of fibular and lateral ray absence. An associated abnormality commonly found with fibular hypoplasia or aplasia is anteromedial bowing of the tibia, with a skin dimple overlying the deformity. Abnormalities of the ankle joint, such as a ball and socket ankle and valgus position of the hindfoot, are common. Tarsal coalition may exist, with a mass representing the talus and calcaneus. These patients almost always have some mild shortening of the femur, valgus of the distal femur, and anteroposterior knee instability (Fig. 3).

In severe deformities in which the foot cannot be rendered a stable weightbearing surface and/or there is excessive predicted leg-length discrepancy, Syme or Boyd amputation is recommended. Some authors recommend resection of the fibular anlage and posterolateral release in infancy, followed by bracing in an articulated ankle-foot orthosis (AFO) to try to maintain a reasonable position of the foot. It is not, however, possible to replace the hindfoot directly under the tibia because it will not remain in this position without an ankle arthrodesis. This procedure may be required in late adolescence or adult life to centralize the foot under the tibia in patients with severe deformities. Staged limb lengthenings have been demonstrated in some

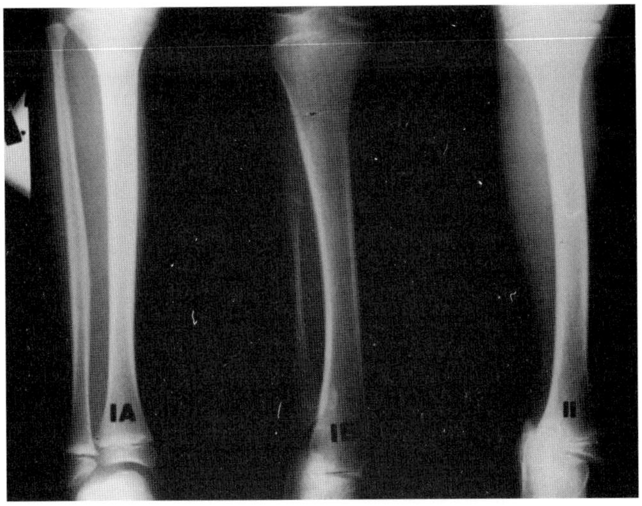

Fig. 2 Classification of fibular hypoplasia according to Kalamachi from minimal shortening of the fibula with a ball and socket ankle (A) to complete absence of the fibula (B).

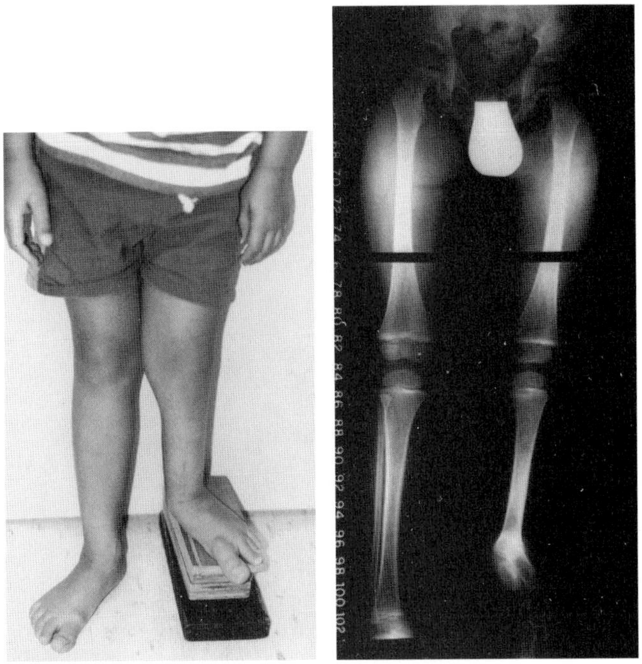

Fig. 3 Clinical appearance (**left**) and radiograph (**right**) of patient with complete fibular hemimelia, valgus ankle with tarsal coalition and femoral hypoplasia.

cases to be successful in achieving limb length equality in children with less than 35% projected shortening of the tibia and fibula, when undertaken carefully with protection of the ankle and foot to avoid exacerbation of the valgus position of the hindfoot (Fig. 4).

Tibial Hemimelia

Tibial hemimelia is a rare condition, which is reported to occur only once in a million live births. It is the only limb deficiency that may be genetic. When the condition occurs bilaterally with an associated lobster-claw hand or upper extremity abnormality, genetic evaluation is recommended.

As with other congenital deficiencies of the lower extremities, the spectrum varies from incomplete formation of the tibia to its complete absence. An associated anomaly is severe varus of the foot that superficially gives the appearance of a clubfoot (Fig. 5). In severe deformities in which the knee does not have an intact quadriceps-patellar tendon complex, a significant fixed flexion deformity of the knee causes the fibula to be positioned proximal to the knee joint adjacent and lateral to the distal femur. Occasionally, a partial reduplication of the foot or mirror foot is seen.

Treatment is related to the severity of the condition and the presence of a competent knee extensor mechanism. The standard treatment in patients who have poor active or absent knee extensor mechanisms is a knee disarticulation and prosthetic fitting. This has the advantage of avoiding a through-bone amputation in a young child, as well as allowing the distal femoral physis to remain intact. When the proximal tibial anlage is present and the distal tibia is absent (type II), a tibia-fibular synostosis may be performed. Fibular centralization, or the Brown procedure, associated with a foot release and lengthening may be fraught with complications and is not recommended. The Brown procedure accompanied by Symes amputation may rarely have a role in the management of type III tibial deficiency. Success of the Brown procedure totally depends on a competent knee extensor mechanism.

In mild deformities, in which the knee extensor mechanism is competent, knee instability is minimal, and shortening is not severe, staged tibial lengthenings can be performed to restore the normal relationship between the tibia and fibula and to lengthen the extremity. These must be undertaken with extreme caution, and long-term results are not yet proven.

Angular Deformities

Congenital Posteromedial Bowing of the Tibia

Congenital posteromedial bowing of the tibia has an unclear etiology. In its mildest form it may simply represent a deformity caused by intrauterine positioning. In patients who have growth inhibition, however, it may represent a congenital disturbance of physeal growth.

The findings at birth are that of a lower extremity apparently shortened below the knee with a calcaneovalgus foot; the foot often is positioned with its dorsum lying against the anterior leg. Radiographically, there is posteromedial angulation of the tibia (Fig. 6), which may be up to 60°.

The natural history of this disorder is gradual resolution of the foot deformity and the tibial bowing with growth.

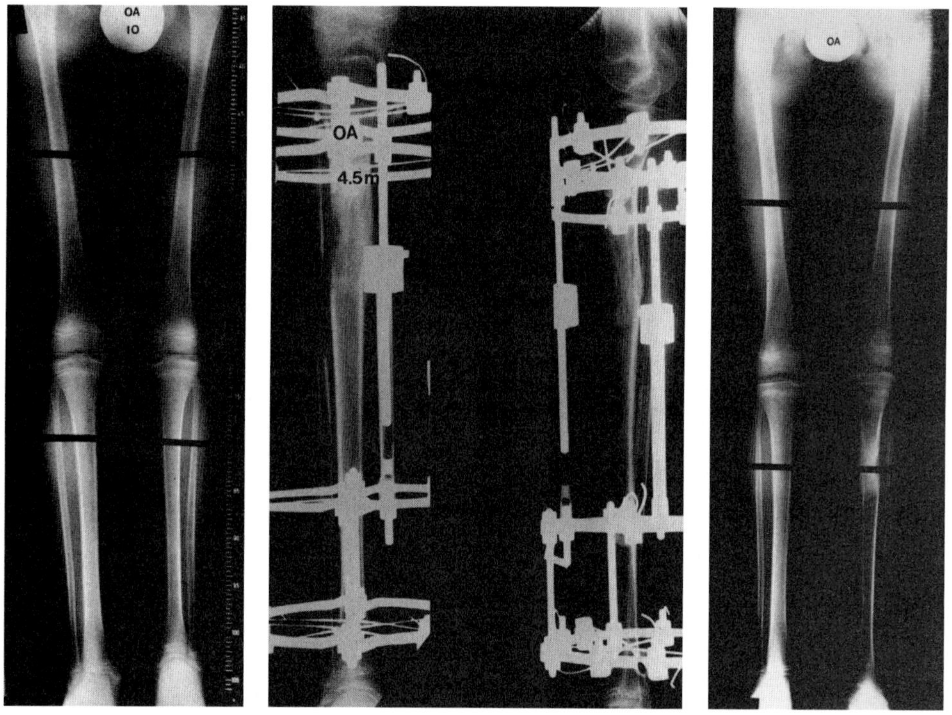

Fig. 4 Radiographs preoperative (**left**), during Ilizarov lengthening (**center**), and postoperatively (**right**) of patient with fibular hypoplasia and projected 7 cm shortening.

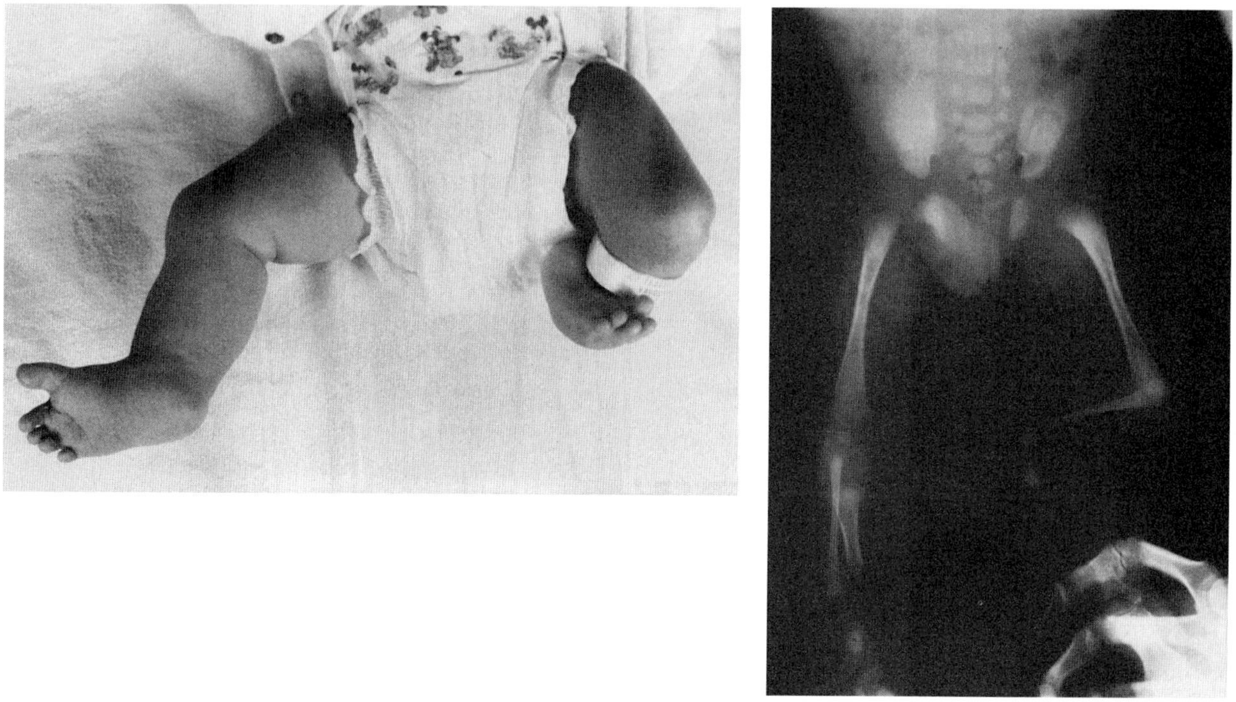

Fig. 5 Clinical appearance (**left**) and radiograph (**right**) of infant with bilateral tibial hemimelia. The patient's right lower limb has incomplete absence of the tibia whereas on the left, the tibia is completely absent.

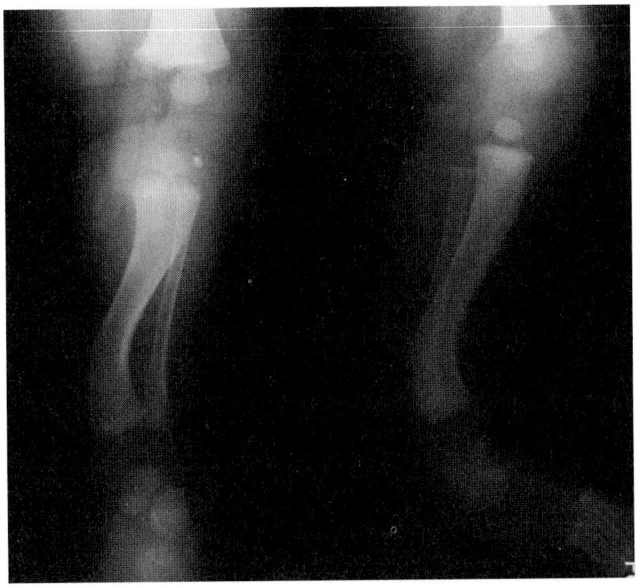

Fig. 6 Radiographs of infant with congenital posteromedial bow of the tibia.

There may be residual tibial deformity in the range of 6° to 8°, with a potential limb length inequality of up to 5 cm at maturity. These patients should have sequential follow-up in childhood for assessment of their limb length inequality, and epiphysiodesis or limb lengthening should be performed if the discrepancy is projected to exceed 2 cm at maturity.

Congenital Anterolateral Bowing of the Tibia

Congenital anterolateral bowing of the tibia, as opposed to congenital posteromedial bowing, is not a benign condition; it is the heralding physical sign of actual or impending fracture with subsequent pseudarthrosis of the tibia. Patients with this problem must be examined carefully for evidence of neurofibromatosis. Fifty percent or more of patients with congenital pseudarthrosis of the tibia have stigmata of neurofibromatosis; however, few neurofibromatosis patients have congenital pseudarthrosis of the tibia. The tibia may or may not be intact at the time of presentation and may have associated shortening and a calcaneus ankle position. The natural history of this condition, if the bone is intact at diagnosis, is for fracture with subsequent nonunion (Fig. 7). In patients with neurofibromatosis and pseudarthrosis of the tibia, bony union rarely is obtained by nonsurgical means. Even if union is obtained, refracture is common in childhood.

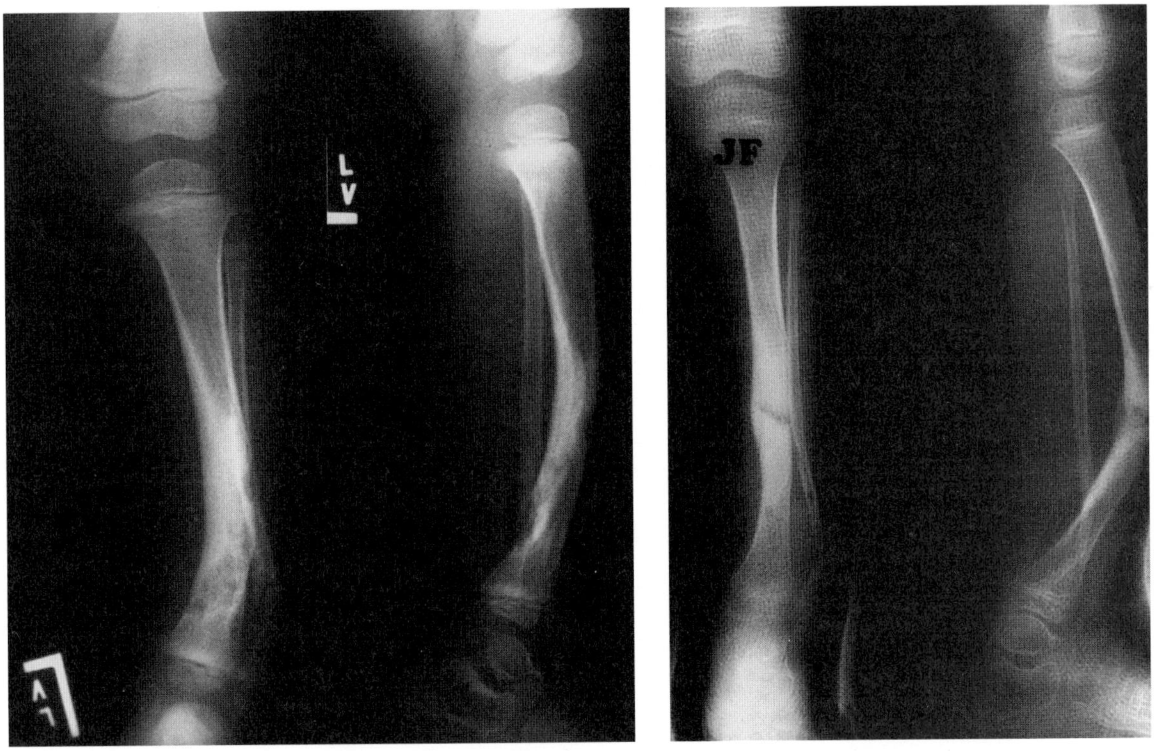

Fig. 7 Two radiographs of the same patient with congenital tibia pseudoarthrosis demonstrating pre-pseudarthrosis (**left**) and subsequent fracture (**right**).

The treatment of type II anterolateral bowing of the tibia in infants and children (narrow or sclerotic canal, high risk tibia) usually involves use of a total contact AFO to try to prevent fracture for as long as possible. Elective osteotomy or correction of the angular deformity is contraindicated because it will precipitate nonunion. The initial surgical option for this condition following fracture is intramedullary rodding with cancellous bone graft, which has a success rate approaching 80%. Multiple surgical failures may be treated by vascularized fibular graft or the Ilizarov technique. Amputation is indicated when surgery has failed, shortening is greater than 7.5 cm, and the patient has a stiff, painful foot. Treatment and follow-up through adolescence are appropriate because a high rate of refracture (throughout adolescence) often results in the need for retreatment, and delayed fracture of the tibia in late adolescence is frequent.

Developmental Angular Variations of the Lower Extremity

Genu Varum Genu varum is physiologic in infants and young children. Its appearance is maximal at approximately 12 to 18 months of age (Fig. 8, *left*) and usually resolves by the age of 3 years, with a change to physiologic genu valgum. The appearance of genu varum frequently is exacerbated or accentuated by concurrent internal tibial torsion or femoral torsion. Genu varum should not routinely be evaluated radiographically; however, if there is concern that this falls outside the range of normal in a child 18 to 36 months old, radiographs should be obtained to rule out infantile Blount disease or metabolic bone disease (Fig. 8, *right*).

Blount Disease Blount disease is excessive and abnormal tibial varus of debatable etiology. It exists in infantile (newborn to 3 years old), juvenile (4 to 8 years), and adolescent (9 to 16 years) forms. Infants afflicted by this condition usually are of black or Mediterranean origin, often have a history of early walking, and are in the upper percentile of weight for height.

Infantile Blount disease may be difficult to diagnosis in its early form because it often occurs during the age of physiologic bowing. The diagnosis is made radiographically, according to the metaphyseal–diaphyseal angle and the appearance of the medial proximal tibial physis. If the metaphyseal–diaphyseal angle is less than 11°, true Blount disease is unusual; whereas, with angles of more than 15°, the diagnosis is almost certain (Fig. 9). Currently the value of bracing is controversial. If bracing is used, it must be implemented during weightbearing hours, but its value is questionable in true Blount disease. Early valgus osteotomy (before the age of 4 years) is strongly recommended to try to minimize deformity of the proximal medial physis.

In patients with recurrent deformity, completion of the proximal tibial epiphysiodesis may be indicated to prevent recurrence of the deformity, or multiplanar osteotomy may be indicated to correct the deformity. Preliminary re-

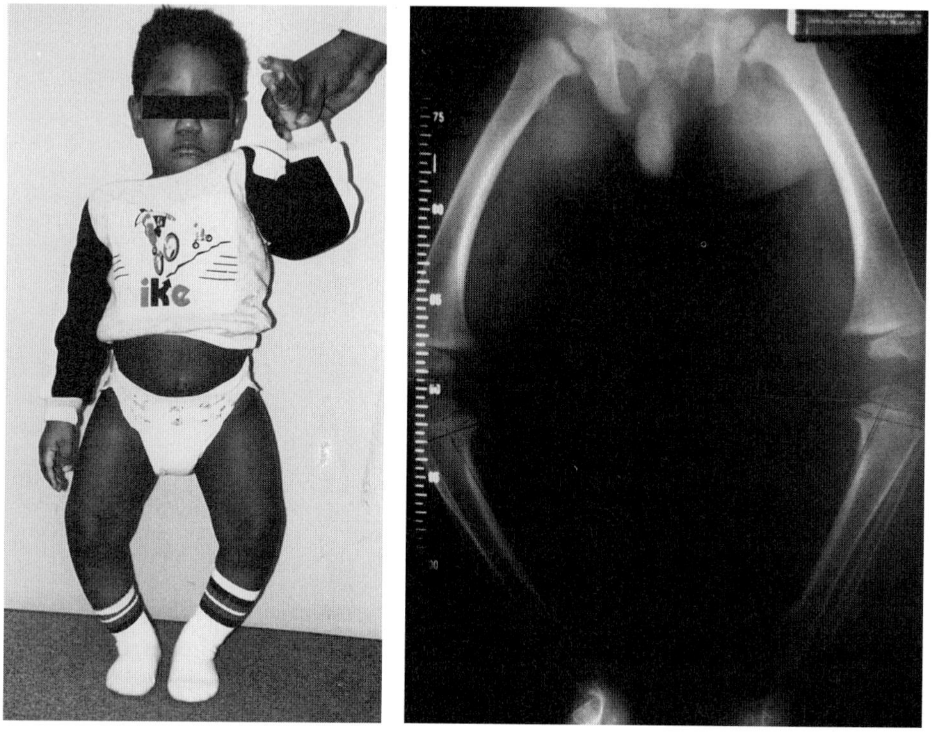

Fig. 8 Photograph (**left**) and radiograph (**right**) of physiologic bow in a 20-month-old infant.

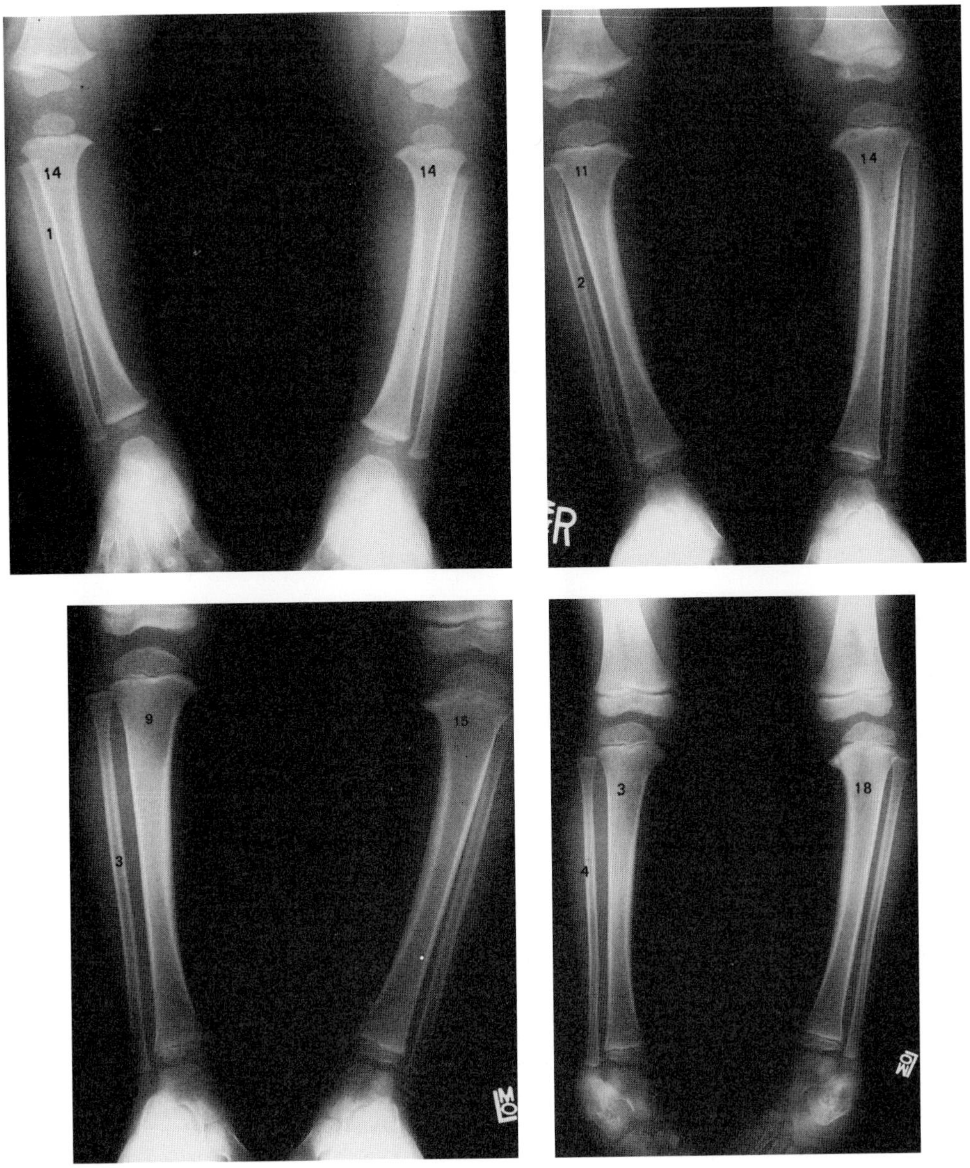

Fig. 9 Sequential radiographs of patient who eventually developed infantile Blount's disease at ages 1 through 4. Initial radiographs showed bilateral metaphyseal-diaphyseal angles of 14°. Radiographs at ages 2, 3, and 4 years demonstrated gradual improvement on the right and evident Blount's disease on the left.

ports recommend lateral tibial hemiepiphysiodesis for adolescent Blount disease. Complex Blount disease may be accompanied by limb-length inequality and severe angular deformity of the knee caused by inhibition of the growth of the proximal tibia.

Genu Valgum What appears to be excessive genu valgum may be seen after the resolution of physiologic bowing and often is maximal around the age of 3.5 to 4 years. It is more common and more pronounced in girls and in obese children. This condition must be differentiated from other causes of angular deformities in the lower extremities, such as metabolic bone disease, skeletal dysplasias, or any posttraumatic etiology. In rare cases of uncorrected physiologic genu valgum greater than 15° to 20° in an adolescent, hemiepiphysiodesis or osteotomy may be indicated.

Other Causes of Angular Deformity Metabolic bone disease is an infrequent cause of angular deformity. Dietary rickets, although less common than in the past, may occur in infants and young children who are exclusively breastfed. Other forms of rickets may coexist with renal disease, and Vitamin D-resistant rickets or hypophosphatemic rickets may escape diagnosis for several years. When it is suspected, serum calcium, phosphate, and alkaline phosphatase values should be obtained.

Skeletal dysplasias, such as metaphyseal dysplasias, achondroplasia, and hydrochondroplasia often are associated with angular deformities of the lower extremities. Many of these disorders are not apparent at birth and only become obvious within the first few years of life. A skeletal survey usually will exclude these as causes of deformities of the lower extremities.

Limb Length Inequality

A host of conditions, both congenital and acquired, are responsible for limb length inequality. The most common congenital causes are limb deficiencies, such as the spectrum of proximal focal femoral deficiency, congenital short or hypoplastic femur, tibial hypoplasia or aplasia, and fibular hypoplasia or aplasia. Idiopathic hemihypertrophy also is common and may or may not be associated with hemangiomata or other soft-tissue malformations, such as those seen in Klippel-Trénaunay-Webber syndrome, neurofibromatosis, or Proteus syndrome. A variety of skeletal dysplasias also may be responsible for limb length inequality. These most commonly include Ollier disease, fibrous dysplasia, osteochondromatosis (multiple hereditary exostoses), and Conradi-Hünermann syndrome.

The most common causes of acquired limb length inequality are infection, inflammation, and trauma. Septic growth arrest is still common today as a sequel of neonatal or childhood sepsis of the hip, knee, and ankle. Juvenile rheumatoid arthritis and hemophilia often cause mild growth stimulation in the affected limb due to joint inflammation adjacent to the physis. Trauma to the physis, from fracture, radiation, or burn, may result in limb length inequality, with or without associated angular deformity, and acute bone loss due to open fracture may cause limb length inequality.

Assessment of limb length inequality involves careful clinical and radiographic evaluation. The standing pelvic height should be examined with blocks under the short limb. In a child with congenital limb length deformity, special care should be taken to evaluate the height of the foot, as well as the presence or absence of any knee or hip contracture. Using a tape measure to determine the distance from the anteroinferior iliac spine to the medial malleolus is at best a conservative estimate. Radiographic evaluation should include scanogram, orthogram, or computed tomography (CT) scanogram. A scanogram does not assess the entire limb in terms of axial alignment and may be subject to error if the patient moves between films (Fig. 10). A standing teleoroentgenogram with a ruler allows assessment of length and axial alignment and must be done with the patellae pointing forward (Fig. 11). A CT scanogram is the most accurate; however, access and cost are important considerations (Fig. 12). A bone age should be obtained with each limb length measurement film, although bone age calculations may err by 12 to 18 months. At least three or four sequential limb measurements (using the same technique) should be obtained before any decisions are reached as to projected discrepancy and appropriate treatment. The Mosely graph or Green-Anderson tables are used to track limb length growth and predicted discrepancy.

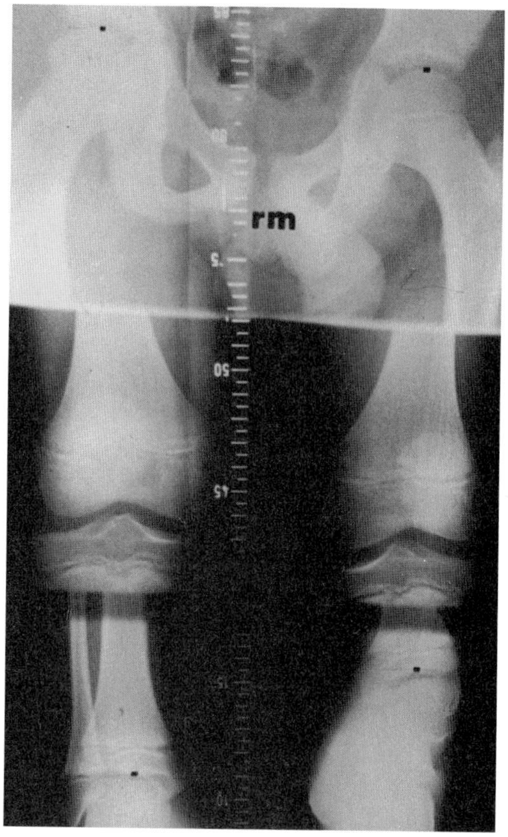

Fig. 10 Standard scanogram.

The treatment of limb length inequality may involve the use of orthotics or lifts, epiphysiodesis, limb lengthening, or femoral shortening. Lifts may be indicated in a child to avoid fixed equinus contracture, but otherwise usually are unnecessary. Epiphysiodesis requires good longitudinal growth data over 3 to 4 years to make a reasonably accurate prediction and may be subject to bone age determination errors. It is indicated for projected discrepancies of less than 5 cm in patients of normal stature who do not have significant angular limb deformity. If possible, the physis to be obliterated should be chosen so as not to result in significant knee height difference. Techniques include percutaneous epiphysiodesis, using small medial and lateral incisions and drilling through a tissue protector, and open excision of the physis. Postoperative dressings are used without casting.

Femoral shortening may be indicated in a patient who is near or at skeletal maturity, has less than a 5 to 6 cm discrepancy, and has normal alignment of the lower extremities. It also may be indicated in a patient who presents in adolescence with insufficient time to perform an

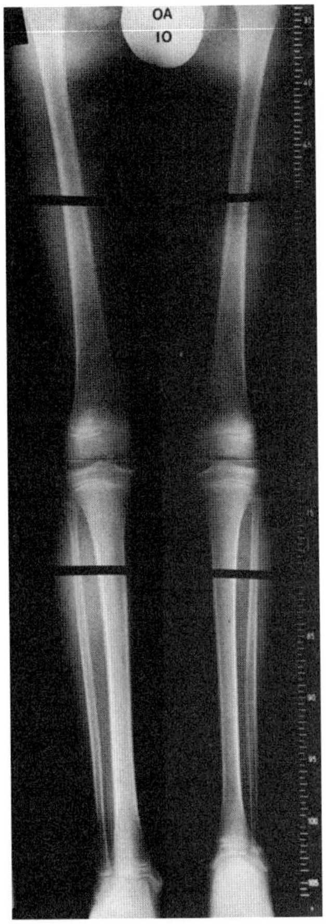

Fig. 11 Standing teleoroentgenogram with ruler demonstrating limb lengths and axial alignment.

epiphysiodesis to achieve limb length equality. Femoral shortening may be performed by an open subtrochanteric osteotomy with blade plate fixation or closed shortening with an intramedullary saw and a proximally and distally locked intramedullary nail.

Limb lengthening is indicated in patients with predicted discrepancies of greater than 5 cm at maturity, with or without angular deformity and/or short stature. Current techniques all use gradual incremental distraction after an open or percutaneous osteotomy. The bone may be predrilled with a small bit to avoid crack propagation into pins, and metaphyseal lengthening generally is preferred to provide a broader surface and more rapid bone formation.

The two most common fixation techniques are monolateral external fixation using half pins and circular external fixation with small wires, such as the Ilizarov technique. The former requires the use of three half pins proximally and two or three half pins distally to avoid cantilever bending and deformation of the bone during lengthening (Fig. 13). The advantages over circular fixation are less bulk to the apparatus, more limited muscle transfixation, and fewer pin sites. The difficulties involve inability to correct large angular or rotational deformities, which must be corrected at the time of surgery. Additionally, an angular deformity or joint subluxation that appears during lengthening may require changing or adjusting the fixator. There also are some size limitations, especially in small children.

Circular fixation using the Ilizarov technique generally is done through small tensioned wire fixation in conjunction with rings (Fig. 14). Its advantage is that simultaneous correction of angular, rotational, or translational deformities is possible during lengthening. Additionally, any deformities that develop during lengthening can be corrected without additional surgery. Adjacent joints can be controlled to avoid contracture or prevent subluxation, and there are no size limitations. Difficulties involve the bulk of the fixator, a steeper learning curve for the physician, more soft-tissue transfixation, and more pin sites.

Traumatic Disorders of the Knee and Leg

Distal Femoral Epiphyseal Fractures

Distal femoral epiphyseal fractures, especially Salter-Harris type II, have unexpectedly higher incidences of physeal arrest than epiphyseal fractures in other locations. Closed reduction and pin fixation are appropriate for most displaced types I and II distal femoral epiphyseal fractures, but repeated manipulations should be avoided for fear of physeal damage. Closed reduction often can be obtained, but because of inherent instability, percutaneous internal fixation with the aid of an image intensifier may be necessary to maintain the reduction of Salter-Harris types I and II fractures. Because of the increased incidence of bony bar formation, Salter-Harris types III and IV fractures require anatomic reduction and internal fixation.

Knee Ligament Injuries

Ligamentous injuries of the knee in children and adolescents are being recognized more frequently, and tears of both cruciate and collateral ligaments have been reported. Hemarthrosis without fracture in an adolescent or child implies significant soft-tissue injury. A recent report of arthroscopic evaluation of hemarthrosis in children reported that 47% had anterior cruciate ligament (ACL) tears, 47% had meniscal tears, and 6% had both ACL and meniscal tears. If an accurate diagnosis cannot be made by serial physical examinations and radiography, arthroscopy should be considered in a child with a traumatic hemarthrosis. There is a variable risk of concomitant meniscal injury in young ACL-injured patients, with the various series of acute ACL injuries in children and adolescents reporting rates of meniscal tears from 6% to 100%. The nonsurgical treatment of ACL tears in this young population has been unsuccessful; data from a number of studies show virtually 100% failure of rehabilitation and bracing if the

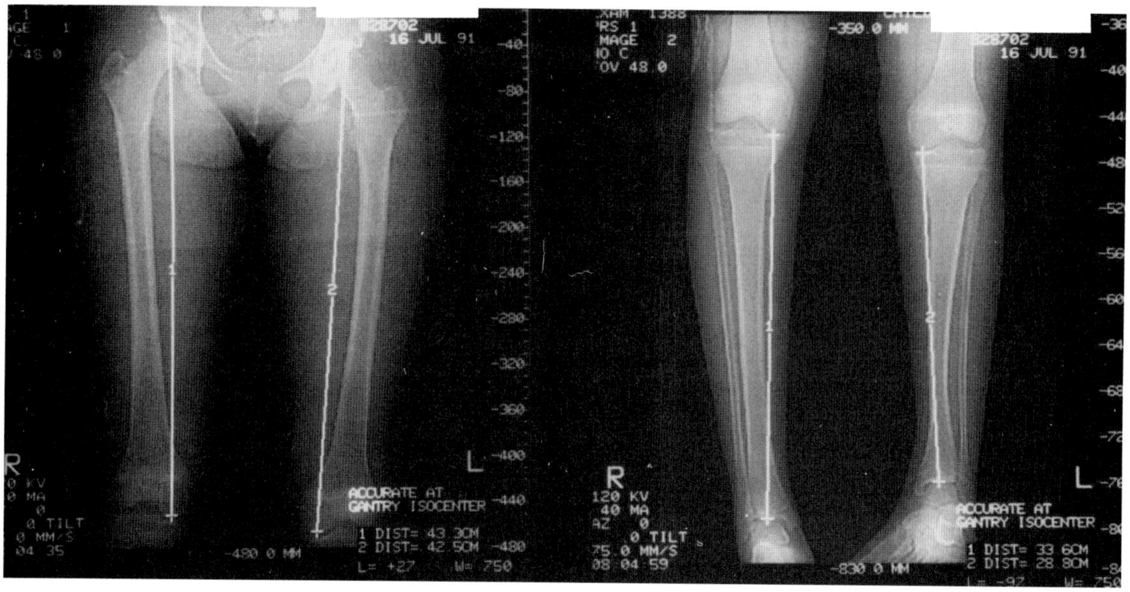

Fig. 12 CT scanogram.

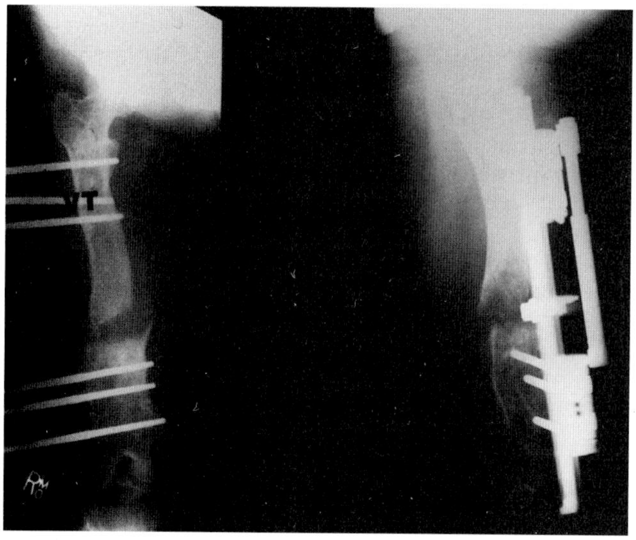

Fig. 13 Orthofix lengthening in progress with half pin fixation.

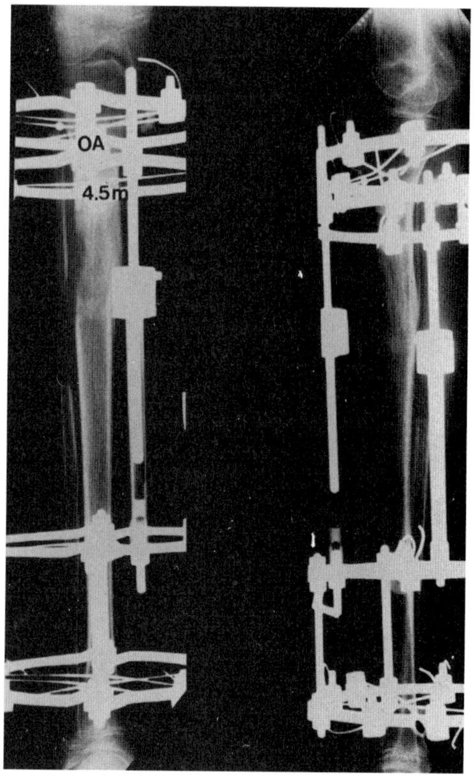

Fig. 14 Ilizarov tibial lengthening using transosseous wire fixation to rings.

patient returns to pivoting sports. These youngsters have an alarmingly high incidence of new meniscal tears after episodes of instability, which ranges from 60% to 90% before reconstruction.

Extra-articular reconstruction with iliotibial band tenodesis has not had great success in this population; 50% to 100% of patients have recurrent instability, and primary repair of ACL tears has not been satisfactory. Intra-articular ACL reconstruction has often been avoided in this population because of the theoretic potential for growth disturbances. This avoidance is in spite of the fact that only one significant growth disturbance, which was caused by hardware bridging the physis, has been reported. In a large series of adolescents (after the adolescent growth spurt and with closing physes and Tanner stage 4 or 5) treated with bone-patellar tendon-bone intra-articular reconstruction, bridging both femoral and tibial physes, there were no growth disturbances and 95% of the knees were stable. Limited numbers of younger patients have had ACL reconstructions with hamstring tendons through a tibial drill hole and over-the-top of the femur without growth disturbance. This procedure should be considered for the young ACL-injured patient who is unwilling to modify activities until nearer the end of growth.

Skeletally immature patients with combined ligamentous (ACL and medial or lateral collateral ligaments) injuries can be successfully managed with cast or brace treatment to allow healing of the collateral ligament, followed by possible intra-articular reconstruction of the ACL.

Meniscal Lesions

Diagnosis of a meniscal lesion in a young athlete is difficult because, generally, children are poor historians. Medial lesions appear to be more common, and in younger children they appear to be more peripheral than in adolescents, who usually have bucket-handle tears. Arthroscopy may be beneficial in diagnosing meniscal lesions in children. Total meniscectomy should be avoided if at all possible; partial meniscectomy can be performed in areas where meniscal repair is not possible. Meniscal repair should be considered in a child with a vertical tear in the peripheral 10% to 25%. Repair can be done with arthroscopic or open technique or a combined technique. Patient compliance is extremely important to improve healing after meniscal repair, and children should be in a supervised rehabilitation program.

Patellar Fractures

Patellar fractures usually occur in older children. Some fractures, especially osteochondral fractures, small peripheral fractures, and sleeve type fractures can be associated with acute dislocation of the patella. In adolescents, jumper's knee and Sinding-Larsen-Johansson syndrome are frequent. These avulsion injuries of the proximal and distal poles of the patella should be considered chronic repetitive ligamentous injuries. A bipartite patella occasionally causes pain in an adolescent athlete and should not be confused with a patellar fracture. Asymptomatic dorsal defects of the patella should not be confused with osteochondritis dissecans or bipartite patella. A sleeve type fracture of the distal pole of the patella often appears benign on a radiograph because only a fleck of bone is seen. However, a rather large cartilaginous sleeve is attached to the patellar tendon, and if it is not recognized and repaired, the patellar tendon extensor mechanism will become abnormally elongated.

Patellar fractures are classified according to location, type, and amount of displacement. Although treatment of patellar fractures in children follows the same guidelines as for patellar fractures in adults, associated ipsilateral lower extremity fractures often dictate treatment. For example, fractures of the femur and patella may require fixation of the femoral fractures and open reduction and internal fixation of the patellar fracture to allow early motion instead of prolonged traction and spica immobilization, which may result in a stiff patellofemoral joint.

Osteochondral Fractures

Osteochondral fractures of the knee occur primarily on the cartilaginous surface of the medial or lateral femoral condyles or the patella. Approximately a third occur after acute patellar dislocations. Half of these are capsular avulsions of the medial patellar margin, and half are loose intra-articular fragments from the lateral femoral condyle and the patella. If a significant sanguinous aspirate (hemarthrosis) is present after a traumatic episode, but ligamentous instability is not, an osteochondral fracture should be suspected, although the fragment may be more cartilage than bone and cannot be seen on radiographs. Arthroscopy generally is indicated to locate, identify, and remove the loose body. All fragments other than exceptionally large fragments from weightbearing surfaces should be excised. If recently displaced from an osseous crater, these large fragments can be replaced and internally fixed.

Tibial Intercondylar Eminence Fractures

Tibial intercondylar eminence fractures are classified according to the amount of displacement. The classic Meyers and McKeevir classification is type I, nondisplaced; type II, anterior displacement and posterior hinge intact; and type III, complete displacement. A number of reports have associated ligamentous injuries in children with fractures of the tibial eminence, and most children have objective evidence of ACL laxity at long-term follow-up regardless of treatment methods. In a study of 45 tibial intercondylar eminence fractures, 51% of patients had positive anterior drawer signs at follow-up, and all patients had some measurable loss of extension, ranging from 4° to 15°. Sixty-four percent were aware of the difference in their knees. Open reduction did not eliminate the cruciate ligamentous laxity or persistent loss of extension. Presently, closed reduction and immobilization in mild flexion is the treatment of choice for types I and II fractures. Open reduction and internal fixation should be reserved for displaced type III fractures. Arthroscopy may be used to ensure adequate reduction of the fragment. The long-term prognosis of these fractures remains guarded because of persistent anterior ligamentous laxity.

Proximal Tibial Epiphyseal Fractures

Fractures of the tibial tuberosity are most common just before cessation of growth. Watson-Jones classified this injury into three types: type I is a small fragment displaced superiorly; type II is a larger fragment involving the secondary center of ossification and proximal tibial epiphysis, which is hinged upward; and type III is a fracture passing proximally and posteriorly across the physis and proximal articular surface of the tibia (Salter-Harris type III).

In adolescents, displaced types II and III fractures generally require open reduction and screw fixation. Growth disturbance is uncommon because of the older age of these patients. In younger children, smooth pins are used to prevent premature anterior closure of the apophysis and the physis and secondary genu recurvatum deformity.

Fractures of the proximal tibial epiphysis can be classified according to the Salter-Harris system. In Salter-Harris types I and II fractures, the metaphysis can be displaced posteriorly, and peripheral ischemia occurs in 10% to 15% of patients. Most Salter-Harris types I and II fractures can be treated by closed methods. Salter-Harris type III fractures are not considered avulsions of the tibial tuberosity, but rather fractures of the physis that extend into the knee joint and require open reduction and fixation. These fractures are tongue-type fractures that extend medially and laterally, and extensive exposure is required for anatomic reduction. Salter-Harris type IV fractures generally are considered tibial plateau fractures, and the treatment recommendations for older children are the same as for adults. In younger children, anatomic reduction is mandatory to try to prevent malreduction and bony bridge formation.

Proximal Tibial Metaphyseal Fractures

Fractures of the proximal tibial metaphysis, even those that are nondisplaced, with or without associated fibular fracture, may result in a valgus angular deformity, the mechanism of which is unknown. These fractures usually occur in children between the ages of 3 and 8 years when the normal physiologic valgus of the lower extremity is at a maximum. Radiographs may reveal only a benign greenstick or nondisplaced fracture pattern. The greenstick fracture should be anatomically reduced by closed manipulation and placed in a straight leg, long leg cast. If closed manipulation is unsuccessful, soft tissue may be interposed in the fracture site, and open reduction may be required. Asymmetric growth often occurs with progressive valgus deformity following healing of this fracture. In most children the valgus deformity improves spontaneously after several years during the period of correction for physiologic genu valgum. Osteotomy of the proximal tibia should be performed only for significant deformity that does not correct. If, after many years of observation, more than 15° of increased valgus angulation is present with little potential for spontaneous correction, an osteotomy should be considered as the child approaches skeletal maturity. After early osteotomy in a younger child, the valgus deformity may recur.

Middle and Distal Tibial Shaft Fractures

Isolated tibial shaft fractures usually can be treated by closed methods. Isolated transverse fractures usually do not displace early or late while in plaster, but spiral and oblique fractures are prone to varus displacement for as long as 2 weeks after injury and require careful follow-up. Although varus deformities appear to spontaneously correct somewhat in younger children, varus angulation of more than 5° to 10° is unacceptable, especially in an older adolescent. If this occurs in the first 2 weeks after injury, manipulation is indicated. In children, fractures manipulated at 2 weeks are still mildly malleable, but at 3 to 4 weeks, the fracture callus is abundant.

Surgical treatment is indicated for tibial and fibular shaft fractures that cannot be managed by closed methods, such as in children with polytrauma, grossly unstable closed fractures, open fractures with significant soft-tissue injury, and floating-knee injuries. Open diaphyseal fractures of the tibia usually heal uneventfully; however, it has been recently noted that Gustilo-Anderson types II and III fractures appear to have an increased incidence of delayed union and nonunion. The same factors that predispose to complications in adults, such as amount of displacement, comminution, soft-tissue damage, and periosteal stripping, also contribute to nonunion and delayed union in children. Reports also indicate that the incidence of compartment syndrome, vascular injury, infection, and delayed union in children is similar to that in adults.

Open tibial fractures with extensive wounds (types II, IIIA, and IIIB) can be treated with external fixation and delayed wound closure. Intramedullary nailing occasionally is indicated for adolescents in whom reduction cannot be maintained or for children with multiple pathologic fractures, as in osteogenesis imperfecta and congenital pseudarthrosis. The proximal and distal physes should be avoided if possible.

Annotated Bibliography

Quadriceps Contracture

Gao G-X, Lee EH, Bose K: Surgical management of congenital and habitual dislocation of the patella. *J Pediatr Orthop* 1990;10:255–260.

The surgical techniques are described; there were 88% good results.

Sasaki T, Fukuhara H, Iisaka H, et al: Postoperative evaluation of quadriceps contracture in children: Comparison of three different procedures. *J Pediatr Orthop* 1985;5:702–707.

Seventy-five patients were reviewed; release of fibrosis is key element in correction.

Fibular and Tibial Hemimelia

Achterman C, Kalamachi A: Congenital deficiency of the fibula. *J Bone Joint Surg* 1979;61B:133–137.

A good review of the spectrum of fibular hypoplasia to aplasia and the associated anomalies with presentation of a simple, easily applicable classification system.

Loder RT, Herring JA: Fibular transfer for congenital absence of the tibia: A reassessment. *J Pediatr Orthop* 1987;7:8–13.

Results of the Brown procedure in six children are presented. Despite adequate knee extensor mechanisms in 3 children, long-term follow-up revealed significant instability and poor active range of motion. Knee disarticulation is recommended as the initial procedure of choice.

Miller LS, Bell DF: Management of congenital fibular deficiency by Ilizarov technique. *J Pediatr Orthop* 1992; 12:651–657.

This paper reviews results obtained by current methods of gradual distraction limb lengthening for patients with fibular hemimelia. The results suggest that many patients who previously would have required amputation and prosthetic fitting may be suitable candidates for limb salvage surgery.

Westin GW, Sakai DN, Wood WL: Congenital longitudinal deficiency of the fibula: Follow-up of treatment by Syme amputation. *J Bone Joint Surg* 1976; 58A:492–496.

A classic study of 42 patients describing excellent functional results obtained by early Syme amputation. This is a useful paper to review for those patients requiring or electing Syme amputation.

Angular Deformities

Boyd HB: Pathology and natural history of congenital pseudarthrosis of the tibia. *Clin Orthop* 1982;166:5–13.

A complete description of Boyd's classification system. Type II, characterized by an hourglass constriction of the tibia at birth, was the most common encountered.

Hoffman A, Wenger DR: Posteromedial bowing of the tibia: Progression of discrepancy in leg lengths. *J Bone Joint Surg* 1981;63A:384–388.

In 13 children with a mean limb length inequality of 3.1 cm, the degree of initial bowing correlated directly with the severity of ultimate leg length difference.

Paley D, Catagni M, Argnani F, et al: Treatment of congenital pseudoarthrosis of the tibia using the Ilizarov technique. *Clin Orthop* 1992;280:81–93.

This paper describes early results using the Ilizarov technique. The ability to obtain union appears equal or superior to that of free fibular transfer. The long-term prognosis is unclear.

Salenius P, Vankka E: The development of the tibiofemoral angle in children. *J Bone Joint Surg* 1975; 57A:259–261.

This study demonstrates that children are born with genu varum and progress to excessive genu valgum in the first few years of life. Changes in radiographic measurements lagged behind those in clinical appearance.

Yadav SS, Thomas S: Congenital posteromedial bowing of the tibia. *Acta Orthop Scand* 1980;51:311–313.

The calcaneovalgus foot position can be readily corrected in most patients by serial casting. Conservative treatment is recommended.

Limb Length Inequality

Epps CH Jr: Proximal femoral focal deficiency. *J Bone Joint Surg* 1983;65A:867–870.

Good topic review with reference to Aitken's classification and standard treatment recommendations.

Winquist RA: Closed intramedullary osteotomies of the femur. *Clin Orthop* 1986;212:155–164.

This article reviews the results of femoral shortening in 154 patients with discrepancies of 2 to 12 cm. The technique and complications are discussed.

Traumatic Disorders of the Knee and Leg

Briggs TW, Orr MM, Lightowler CD: Isolated tibial fractures in children. *Injury* 1992;23:308–310.

Of 65 tibial fractures in children, transverse isolated fractures did not displace early or late while in plaster, but spiral and oblique fractures were prone to displacement into varus for as long as 2 weeks after injury. Contrary to others, the authors believe that 5° of varus is unacceptable and recommend manipulation of the varus displacement during the first 2 weeks after injury.

Buckley SL, Smith G, Sponseller PD, et al: Open fractures of the tibia in children. *J Bone Joint Surg* 1990;72A:1462–1469.

The incidence of compartment syndrome, vascular injury, infections, and delayed union was similar to that in adults; however, two complications occurred that made this injury different in children. Four developed angular deformities of more than 10°, three of which corrected spontaneously, and four patients with severe fractures treated with external fixation had more than 1 cm of tibial overgrowth.

Cramer KE, Limbird TJ, Green NE: Open fractures of the diaphysis of the lower extremity in children: Treatment, results, and complications. *J Bone Joint Surg* 1992;74A: 218–232.

The authors reported on 40 open diaphyseal fractures that refute the general assumption that types II and III open diaphyseal fractures in children heal readily. Fifty-five percent (22 fractures) healed primarily, 30% had delayed union, and 7.5% were classified as a nonunion. They postulated that the same factors that predispose to complications in adults, such as degree of displacement, comminution, soft-tissue damage, and periosteal stripping, also contributed to delayed and nonunions in children.

Graf BK, Lange RH, Fugisaki CK, et al: Anterior cruciate ligament tears in skeletally immature patients: Meniscal pathology at presentation and after attempted conservative treatment. *Arthroscopy* 1992;8:229–233.

One hundred percent of nonoperatively (rehabilitation and brace) treated patients developed instability with seven of eight sustaining new meniscal tears. Three patients treated with extra-articular reconstructions had further instability and sustained new meniscal tears.

Hope PG, Cole WG: Open fractures of the tibia in children. *J Bone Joint Surg* 1992;74B:546–553.

Results from open tibial fractures in children treated with external fixation for extensive wounds with delayed wound closure were described. Less severe wounds, types I and II, were treated with primary wound closure and casting. Early complications included compartment syndrome, superficial and deep infection, delayed union, and malunion. They concluded that open tibial fractures are associated with a high incidence of early and late complications, especially in Gustilo-Anderson type III injuries.

Maguire JK, Canale ST: Fractures of the patella in children and adolescents. *J Pediatr Orthop* 1993;13: 567–571.

Sixty-seven patellar fractures were reviewed with the results of 24 patients analyzed at 2-year follow-up. Open reduction and internal fixation produced good results and no growth disturbance after the use of cerclage wires. However, a large number of these patients were near skeletal maturity. The wires were removed after the fracture healed. Total patellectomy for displaced comminuted fractures without ipsilateral tibial fractures was not associated with a poor result.

McCarroll JR, Shelbourne KD, Porter DA, et al: Patellar tendon graft recontruction for midsubstance anterior cruciate ligament rupture in junior high school athletes: An algorithm for management. *Am J Sports Med* 1994; 22:478–484.

Recommend patellar tendon ACL reconstruction for adolescents with closing physes. For patients with open physes, the authors recommend activity modification to nonpivoting sports until physes close.

Safran MR, McDonough P, Seeger L, et al: Dorsal defect of the patella. *J Pediatr Orthop* 1994;14:603–607.

A benign subchondral lesion of unknown etiology located in the superolateral region of the patella may be an incidental finding on knee radiographs, although occasionally it may be symptomatic. This lesion most frequently is found in adolescents. Eight dorsal lesions of the patella in five patients are described.

Stanitski CL, Harvell JC, Fu F: Observations on acute knee hemarthrosis in children and adolescents. *J Pediatr Orthop* 1993;13:506–510.

Arthroscopy on 15 children (ages 7 to 12 years) with hemarthrosis revealed 47% ACL tears, 47% meniscal tears, and 6% with both. In 55 adolescents, (ages 13 to 15), 55% had ACL tears, 27% had meniscal tears, and 18% had both.

Wester W, Canale ST, Dutkowsky JP, et al: Prediction of angular deformity and leg-length discrepancy after anterior cruciate ligament reconstruction in skeletally immature patients. *J Pediatr Orthop* 1994;14:516–521.

Using a Moseley graph, scanograms, and bone age, as well as radiographs of the distal femur and proximal tibia, the amount of shortening, valgus deformity of the distal femur, and recurvatum deformity of the proximal tibia can be predicted based on trigonometric principles and placed in graph form. The calculations assume that large 10-mm holes are drilled laterally through the distal femur and anteriorly through the proximal tibia for anterior cruciate ligament reconstruction in a skeletally immature patient.

Willis RB, Blokker C, Stoll TM, et al: Long-term follow-up of anterior tibial eminence fractures. *J Pediatr Orthop* 1993;13:361–364.

These authors found that regardless of the type of treatment, anterior cruciate ligamentous laxity after fracture was noted at long-term follow-up, although few patients had subjective complaints. Treatment recommendations include open reduction and internal fixation.

Wozasek GE, Moser KD, Haller H, et al: Trauma involving the proximal tibial epiphysis. *Arch Orthop Trauma Surg* 1991;110:301–306.

Four of 30 patients (13%) with injuries of the proximal tibial epiphysis, half of which were displaced, presented with peripheral ischemia. This benign looking fracture can cause catastrophic vascular insult.

Classic Bibliography

Choi IH, Kumar SJ, Bowen JR: Amputation or limb-lengthening for partial or total absence of the fibula. *J Bone Joint Surg* 1990;72A:1391–1399.

Kling TF Jr, Hensinger RN: Angular and torsional deformities of the lower limbs in children. *Clin Orthop* 1983;176:136–147.

Mosely CF: Assessment and prediction in leg-length discrepancy, in Barr JS (ed): *Instructional Course Lectures XXXVIII.* Park Ridge, IL, American Academy of Orthopaedic Surgeons, 1989, pp 325–330.

Paley D: Current techniques of limb lengthening. *J Pediatr Orthop* 1988;8:73–92.

Pirani S, Beauchamp RD, Li D, et al: Soft tissue anatomy of proximal femoral focal deficiency. *J Pediatr Orthop* 1991;11:563–570.

Schoenecker PL, Capelli AM, Millar EA, et al: Congenital longitudinal deficiency of the tibia. *J Bone Joint Surg* 1989;71A:278–287.

Shapiro F: Developmental patterns in lower-extremity length discrepancies. *J Bone Joint Surg* 1982;64A:639–651.

Steel HH, Lin PS, Betz RR, et al: Iliofemoral fusion for proximal femoral focal deficiency. *J Bone Joint Surg* 1987;69A:837–843.

Thompson GH, Carter JR: Late onset tibia vara (Blount's disease): Current concepts. *Clin Orthop* 1990;255:24–35.

Timperlake RW, Bowen JR, Guille JT, et al: Prospective evaluation of fifty-three consecutive percutaneous epiphysiodeses of the distal femur and proximal tibia and fibula. *J Pediatr Orthop* 1991;11:350–357.

Weiland AJ, Weiss AP, Moore JR, et al: Vascularized fibular grafts in the treatment of congenital pseudarthrosis of the tibia. *J Bone Joint Surg* 1990;72A:654–662.

Traumatic Disorders of the Knee and Leg

Houghton GR, Ackroyd CE: Sleeve fractures of the patella in children: A report of three cases. *J Bone Joint Surg* 1979;61B:165–168.

Lipscomb AB, Anderson AF: Tears of the anterior cruciate ligament in adolescents. *J Bone Joint Surg* 1986; 68A:19–28.

Meyers MH, McKeever FM: Fracture of the intercondylar eminence of the tibia. *J Bone Joint Surg* 1959;41A: 209–222.

Salter RB, Best TN: Pathogenesis of progressive valgus deformity following fractures of the proximal metaphyseal region of the tibia in young children, in Eilert RED (ed): *Instructional Course Lecture XLI.* Park Ridge, IL, American Academy of Orthopaedic Surgeons, 1992, pp 409–411.

Wiley JJ, Baxter MP: Tibial spine fractures in children. *Clin Orthop* 1990;255:54–60.

39

Knee and Leg: Bone Trauma

This chapter covers injuries of the extensor mechanism (ie, quadriceps tendon rupture, patellar fracture, and patellar tendon rupture), tibial plateau fractures, tibial shaft fractures, and compartment syndromes. Areas in which there is significant new information are the management of tibial plateau fractures, the classification of open and closed tibial diaphyseal fractures, trends in the management of grades II and III open tibial diaphyseal fractures, and the management of nonunions of the tibial diaphysis.

Patellar Fractures

Diagnosis

The diagnosis of extensor mechanism injuries is based on a history of injury, pain localized to the area of injury, pain with attempted active extension of the knee, and often, a large hemarthrosis. Complete disruption of the extensor mechanism is characterized by inability to actively extend the knee and a palpable gap at the site of injury. Radiographic signs of extensor mechanism injury are fracture of the patella, patella alta, patella baja, avulsion fracture of the tibial tubercle, or an avulsion fracture of the distal pole of the patella. Magnetic resonance imaging (MRI) is of value in determining whether a quadriceps tendon or patellar tendon rupture is complete or partial.

Patellar Fractures

Patellar fractures result from a blow to the anterior aspect of the knee or eccentric contraction of the quadriceps muscle. When the cause of the fracture is a blow to the anterior aspect of the knee, associated injuries of the hip and femoral shaft must be ruled out (dashboard injury complex). Patellar fractures are classified as minimally displaced or displaced. When a step off is present, the articular surfaces of the proximal and distal segments are not in the same plane. When distraction is present, the fragments are separated but the articular surfaces are in the same plane. The distinction between step off and distraction of the articular surface is key. Minimally displaced fractures have 1 mm or less of a step off involving the articular surface and less than 3 mm of distraction. Displaced fractures are further classified as simple (eg, transverse), as comminuted, or as involving the distal pole. When displacement exceeds 1 cm, there is an associated tear of the extensor retinaculum.

Minimally Displaced Fractures Management of minimally displaced fractures consists of casting or splinting with the knee in full extension. Despite splinting of the knee, the quadriceps exerts a distracting force across the fracture with hip flexion; therefore, the patient is followed closely for the first 3 weeks for increasing displacement. A lateral radiograph of the gently flexed knee prior to cast application indicates the tendency of a minimally displaced fracture to displace further. At 6 to 8 weeks, if the position of the fracture fragments has remained unchanged, immobilization of the knee is discontinued and active range of motion exercises are initiated.

Displaced Fractures These fractures are managed surgically. The goals of surgical management are anatomic reduction of the articular surface and restoration of the extensor mechanism. Exposure is via a vertical midline incision to facilitate future reconstructive procedures, if they are necessary. After reduction of the articular surface, ignore the anterior surface of the patella and confirm the reduction by feel through the tear in the retinaculum, or if the retinaculum is not torn, incise it vertically at the level of the fracture on the medial and lateral sides of the patella. Then stabilize the fracture; in the rare case in which reduction cannot be achieved, all or part of the patella is excised. The stability of fixation is reinforced by repairing the retinaculum or by inserting a "neutralization cable" from the tibial tubercle to the superior pole of the patella (Fig. 1).

The method of fixation is chosen by the surgeon. Good results have been reported with cerclage wires and with tension band wires. Usually, multiple screw fixation or a tension band is used with transverse fractures, cerclage wires with comminuted fractures, and a single screw with a fracture of the distal pole. A technique has recently been described in which a transverse fracture is stabilized with interfragmentary cannulated lag screws; wires are threaded through the screws and crossed in front of the patella as a tension band. Addition of an adjunctive neutralization cable increases the stability of fixation, making postoperative immobilization unnecessary. When a neutralization cable is used, gentle active range of motion is begun 1 to 2 weeks after surgery. When a cable is not used, unless fixation is extremely stable, the knee is immobilized in extension for 4 to 6 weeks.

Tibial Plateau Fractures

Tibial plateau fractures involve the proximal articular surface of the tibia. Clinically the diagnosis of tibial plateau fracture is based on a history of injury, pain localized to

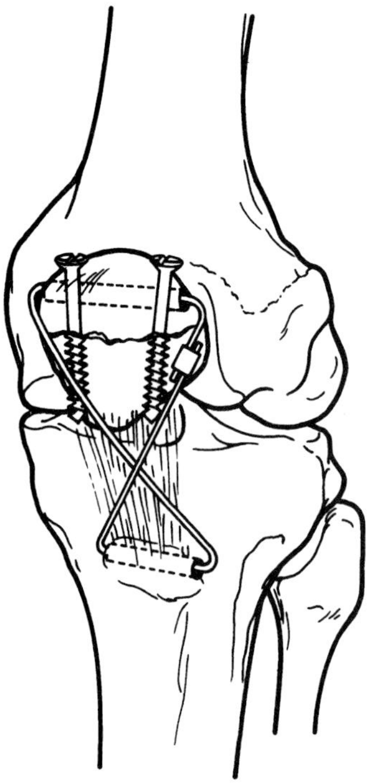

Fig. 1 A line drawing of a transverse patellar fracture treated with interfragmentary screws and a neutralization cable.

the proximal tibia, and a lipohemarthrosis. Routine radiographic evaluation consists of anteroposterior (AP), lateral, and oblique radiographs. Computed tomography (CT) scans aid in the evaluation of more complex fracture patterns (eg, bicondylar fractures). Tibial plateau fractures are classified according to a system described by Schatzker into six groups: split, depressed, split depressed, medial plateau, bicondylar, and any of the above associated with a metaphyseal fracture. It is useful to further divide medial plateau fractures into low- and high-energy fractures (Fig. 2). There is an increasing awareness of the importance of fractures in the coronal plane that involve the posterior portion of the plateau. These fractures are associated with split depressed, high-energy medial condyle, and bicondylar fractures. They are best seen on the lateral radiograph or CT scan and have been referred to as "triplane fractures." Their significance is that they are difficult to reduce and stabilize via an anterior approach.

Split fractures always involve the lateral plateau. These fractures occur in young adults with dense bone. The fracture is best seen on the AP projection and is distinctive in that it is vertical and seldom displaced more than 3 mm. The lateral meniscus may be torn at its periphery and dislocated into the fracture site.

Depressed fractures occur in osteopenic bone. The lateral femoral condyle impacts the lateral surface of the tibia, driving the entire articular surface distally. On the AP radiograph, the articular surface appears to be tilted. In cases in which the lateral metaphyseal cortex is fractured, displacement is minimal.

Split depressed fractures make up over 50% of all tibial plateau fractures. The fracture is caused by valgus stress

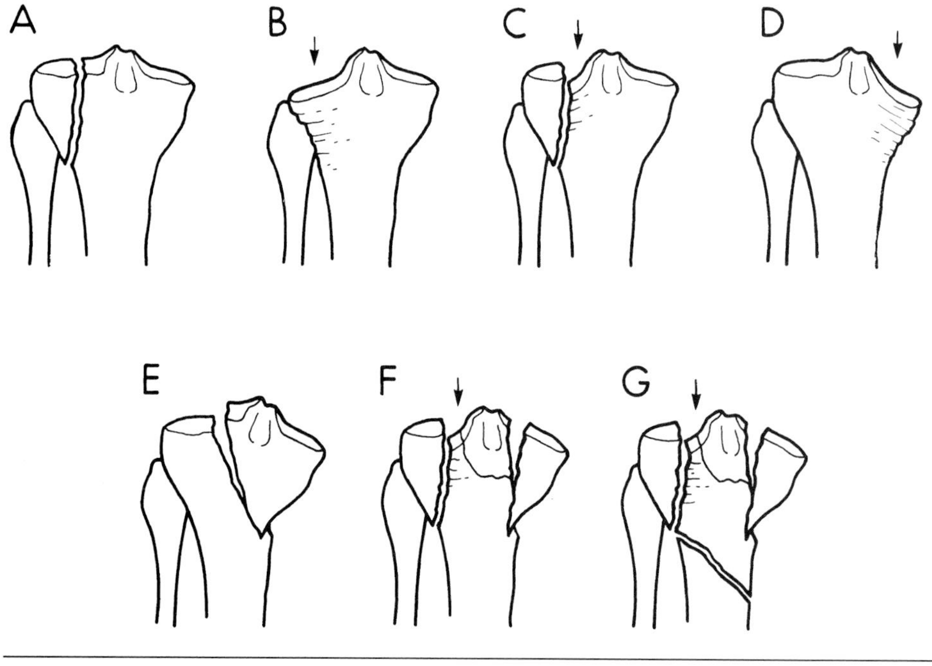

Fig. 2 Classification of tibial plateau fractures: **A:** split; **B:** lateral plateau depressed; **C:** split depressed; **D:** medial plateau low energy; **E:** medial plateau high energy; **F:** bicondylar; and, **G:** plateau fracture associated with a metaphyseal fracture. (Adapted with permission from Schenck RC Jr, Perry CR: Injuries about the knee, in Perry CR, Elstrom JA, Pankovich AM (eds): *Handbook of Fractures.* New York, NY, McGraw-Hill, 1995, pp 262–263.)

to the knee. The lateral femoral condyle impacts the lateral tibial plateau, splitting it. As the femoral condyle continues to impact the lateral plateau, it drives a segment of the articular surface into the metaphysis. This depressed segment is always on the medial fragment, not the split fragment. Fractures of the anterior plateau occur with the knee extended; fractures of the posterior plateau occur with the knee flexed.

Low-energy medial plateau fractures, like depressed fractures of the lateral plateau, occur in osteopenic bone. On the AP radiograph, the articular surface is seen to be tilted medially.

High-energy fractures of the medial plateau are the result of axial and valgus loads applied to the knee (Fig. 3, *left*). The lateral femoral condyle impacts the tibial spines resulting in a fracture line that, when viewed in the AP projection, runs obliquely from the base of the tibial spines in a medial and distal direction. The lateral collateral ligament is ruptured; the cruciates and medial collateral ligament are intact.

Bicondylar fractures are the result of complex high-energy loads applied across the knee. They are associated with neurovascular and ligamentous injuries. Plateau fractures with metaphyseal dissociation are similar to bicondylar injuries in that they are high-energy injuries and frequently are associated with neurovascular and ligamentous injuries.

Ligamentous and neurovascular injuries can be associated with any type of tibial plateau fracture, but are more commonly associated with high-energy injuries. Fracture of the medial or lateral plateau may be associated with injury of the contralateral collateral ligament. Apparent ligamentous instability with varus or valgus stressing may be due to displacement of the plateau. To definitively determine whether there is an associated ligamentous rupture, the knee is stressed under fluoroscopy. Injuries of the peroneal and tibial nerves are usually traction injuries. In cases in which sensation and motor function do not return, an electromyogram (EMG) obtained 3 to 6 weeks following injury will define the prognosis of recovery. Vascular injury is indicated by decreased or absent distal pulses. The diagnosis is confirmed with an arteriogram.

Nonsurgical Management

Nonsurgical management of tibial plateau fractures is indicated when the fracture is undisplaced, when there is preexisting osteoarthritis (considering the anticipated future total knee replacement), or when the skin and soft tissue overlying the fracture are so badly damaged that the risk of necrosis followed by infection precludes surgery. The methods of nonsurgical management are casting and traction. Casting is reserved for undisplaced fractures and fractures with preexisting osteoarthritis, and consists of application of a long leg cast followed by a cast brace at approximately 4 weeks. Traction is reserved for displaced fractures with severely damaged overlying soft tissue, and consists of inserting a distal tibial pin and placing the leg

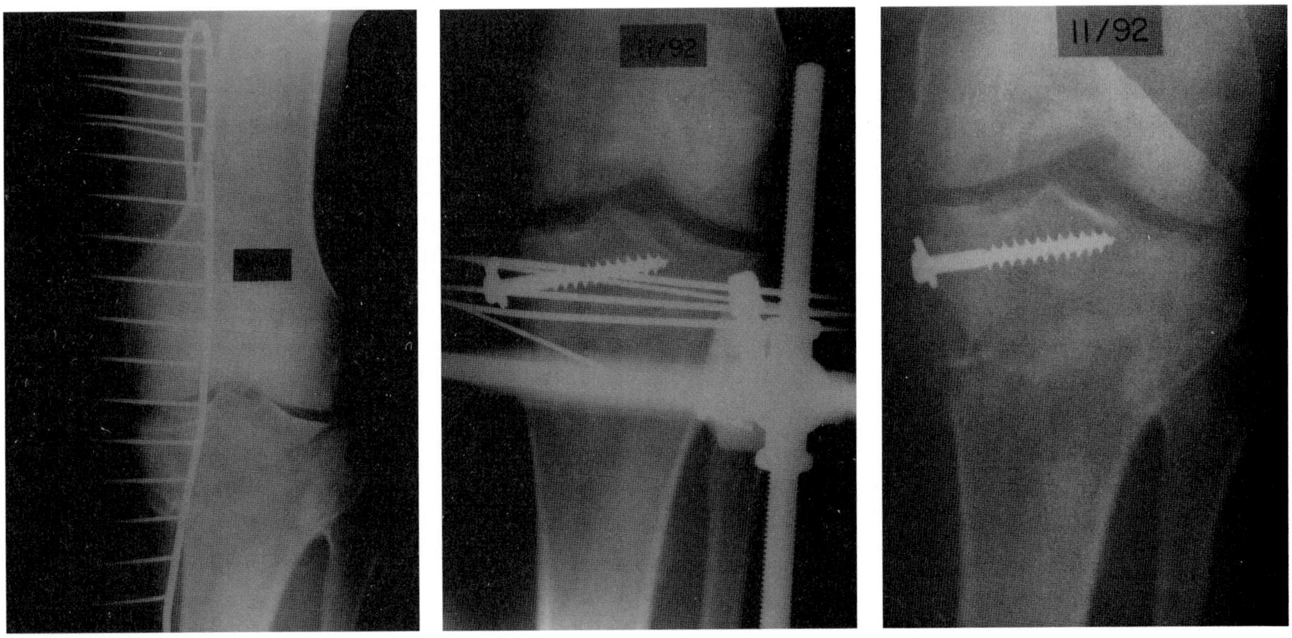

Fig. 3 **Left,** High-energy medial plateau fracture. **Center,** Fracture following limited internal fixation and application of a small wire circular frame external fixator. **Right,** Fracture following removal of the external fixator.

in balanced suspension. When traction is used, passive range of motion is initiated when initial pain becomes tolerable (2 to 3 weeks). At 4 to 6 weeks, a cast brace is applied.

Surgical Management

Indications for surgical management of closed tibial plateau fractures are an intra-articular step off that can be improved (although step-off criteria were 10 or 5 mm, more recent indications have focused on any "correctable" step off), increased valgus or varus angulation when the knee is extended, associated ligamentous injury, and floating knee. Methods of surgical management are closed or limited open reduction with percutaneous fixation and open reduction with internal fixation (ORIF).

Closed or Limited Open Reduction This reduction is achieved with indirect reduction techniques or by means of relatively small incisions. Reduction is assessed arthroscopically or fluoroscopically. A potential pitfall of arthroscopy is that the fluid used to distend the joint can extravasate, causing a compartment syndrome. Therefore, a pump is not used. In a study of the success of indirect reduction techniques (ie, ligamentotaxis, percutaneous reduction with a tenaculum clamp, and percutaneous elevation of a depressed articular segment through a metaphyseal window), the investigators found that only 13 of 20 fractures were anatomically reduced. Indirect reduction was consistently successful only in reducing split fractures. Elevation of an articular segment through a metaphyseal window with a bone tamp was uniformly unsuccessful. Small wire circular frames have been used to stabilize tibial plateau fractures following closed or limited open reduction. (Fig. 3, *center* and *right*) These fixators stabilize the reduced fracture but require less dissection than plates, therefore, the incidence of postoperative wound complications is minimized. When stability is limited, a temporary bridging frame is applied across the knee. This frame, which is an extension of the external fixator, distracts and immobilizes the femoral tibial articulation and is removed after around 6 weeks. Long-term follow-up of tibial plateau fractures treated with a small wire circular frame fixator is not yet available; however, short-term follow-up indicates that this is a promising method of management if the fracture is reduced anatomically.

Open Reduction With Internal Fixation ORIF is the standard management of displaced tibial plateau fractures. Exposure is via a vertical midline skin incision. A parapatellar incision provides access to the articular surface. Exposure can be improved by excision of the fat pad and incision of the anterior horns of the lateral and medial menisci. Recently, five cases were reported in which, in addition to the anterior approach, a medial posterior approach, identical to that used to approach the posterior cruciate ligament, was used to expose a posterior medial fragment. Following surgical exposure, depressed articular segments are elevated and bone grafted, and split fragments are reduced. In addition to a medial or lateral plate, an antiglide plate applied to the posterior medial corner of the metaphysis increases stability of fixation of bicondylar and medial plateau fractures without further devascularization of the metaphysis.

Stability of fixation is key; however, to limit devascularization there has been a trend to minimize the use of plates. If stable fixation can be obtained, screws alone are used. Ideally, they are applied to only one side of the metaphysis. Bicondylar fractures and plateau fractures with metaphyseal dissociation are stabilized with a plate on one side and screws on the other side of the metaphysis. Plates are applied to both sides of the metaphysis only as a last resort.

Tibial Shaft Fractures

Fractures of the tibial shaft are classified according to three parameters: their location, their configuration, and severity of the associated soft-tissue injury. Location is described as being proximal, mid, or distal third, and it has implications regarding prognosis (distal third fractures are thought to have a higher incidence of nonunion) and treatment (proximal third fractures are more difficult to treat with an intramedullary nail). The concept of bifocal tibial fractures has been described recently. These are two-level fractures, ie, fracture of the ankle and plateau, shaft and plateau, or shaft and ankle. Bifocal fractures of the shaft and plateau have a poor prognosis. In one report, two of 13 patients with this fracture pattern required primary amputation. Fracture configuration is described as simple or comminuted. Simple fractures are further classified as transverse, short oblique, and spiral or long oblique. Long oblique fractures are axially unstable when managed with dynamic intramedullary nails. Comminuted fractures are classified into three groups based on the extent of comminution: group 1, less than 50% of the circumference of the cortex comminuted; group 2, more than 50% but less than 100% of the circumference of the cortex comminuted; and group 3, segmental comminution. Group 1 fractures are stable when reduced. Group 2 fractures are axially stable but may be rotationally unstable, and group 3 fractures are axially and rotationally unstable.

The severity of soft-tissue injury is directly related to the incidence of nonunion; infection; and residual stiffness of the knee, ankle, and foot. Indicators of the severity of the soft-tissue injury are the amount of initial displacement and the fracture configuration. Displacement greater than the diameter of the tibia, the presence of comminution, or a transverse fracture pattern are indicators of a high-energy fracture and extensive soft-tissue injury. Whether the fracture is open or closed is an important guide to initial management, but not necessarily an indicator of the severity of the soft-tissue injury. The severity of soft-tissue injury is graded according to a system described by Oestern and Tscherne as: grade 0, indirect injury with minimal soft-tissue damage; grade I, low/moderate-energy injury with skin abrasions and contusions; grade II, high-energy injury with muscle contusion and contaminated skin abrasions; and grade III, high-energy with degloving, compartment syndrome, and possible arterial injury. The severity of soft-tissue injury of open fractures is graded according to the modified Gustillo Anderson system. This system divides open fractures into five groups: grade I, laceration less than 1 cm in length; grade II, laceration greater than 1 cm and less than 10 cm, but no flaps or contamination; grade IIIA, laceration greater than 10 cm with adequate soft-tissue coverage and no periosteal stripping; grade IIIB, soft-tissue loss usually requiring local or free tissue transfer to obtain coverage and usually grossly contaminated; and grade IIIC, any open fracture with an associated vascular injury requiring repair.

Treatment

Treatment of tibial shaft fractures is designed to restore function as quickly as possible while minimizing the incidence of nonunion, malunion, and infection. Tibial shaft fractures are managed by cast immobilization or by fixation with a plate, nail, or external fixator. Closed reduction and cast immobilization is commonly used for management. As described in a series of 780 tibial shaft fractures, the technique consists of reduction and application of a long leg cast. When initial pain and swelling subsided (at a mean of 3.8 weeks), the cast was removed and a functional brace applied. Weightbearing as tolerated and active range of motion of the knee and ankle were encouraged. In this series, there was a 2.5% incidence of nonunion, 37% of tibiae healed with 5° or more of varus or valgus angulation, 10% with 10° or more of apex anterior or posterior angulation, and 10% with at least 1 cm of shortening. Best results were achieved for low-energy fractures. Data from two prospective, randomized studies comparing closed management with nailing indicate that time to healing, residual deformity, and loss of motion of surrounding joints are minimized by intramedullary nailing. In one of these studies, 52 patients were randomized prospectively to cast or nail management. In the nail group, there were no varus or valgus malunions and two cases in which the fracture shortened. In the casted group, there were nine varus or valgus nonunions and 15 cases in which the fracture shortened. The authors considered these data so significant that they discontinued enrollment prior to completion of the study.

Plate Osteosynthesis This treatment of tibial shaft fractures is seldom indicated because casting, nailing, and external fixation have a lower risk of infection and nonunion. Relative indications for plating of a tibial shaft fracture are an associated plateau or plafond fracture (bifocal fracture), certain grade IIIC fractures in which the bone is already exposed and rapid stabilization is required to expedite an arterial repair, and multiple trauma when the patient cannot be positioned on the fracture table. These are relative indications; in most cases, nailing or external fixation are better methods of management than plating.

Closed Intramedullary Nailing In the management of closed tibial shaft fractures, this treatment has been shown to result in a high incidence of healing with a low incidence of malunion and infection. Locking obviates the need for a postoperative cast, and it extends the indications for nailing to fractures that are axially or rotationally unstable and within 6 cm of the plafond, providing good fixation is achieved with at least one distal locking screw (Fig. 4). Nailing of fractures of the proximal metaphysis is a difficult technique and frequently results in unacceptable apex anterior angulation. Closed intramedullary nailing is usually performed with the patient on a fracture table with the knee flexed. The fracture is reduced under fluoroscopic control. The patellar tendon is split or retracted laterally. The tibia is sequentially reamed through the proximal insertion portal with the tourniquet deflated to minimize heat necrosis of the cortical bone. In one study of 20 tibial shaft fractures, a femoral distractor was used to reduce the fracture instead of a fracture table. There were no complications and the authors conclude that use of a femoral distractor minimizes the incidence of traction complications and facilitates the procedure because rotation of the C-arm is unnecessary for distal locking. Compartment syndrome has been described as a sequela of reducing, reaming, and nailing of tibial fractures. That this complication is uncommon is illustrated by a study in which the

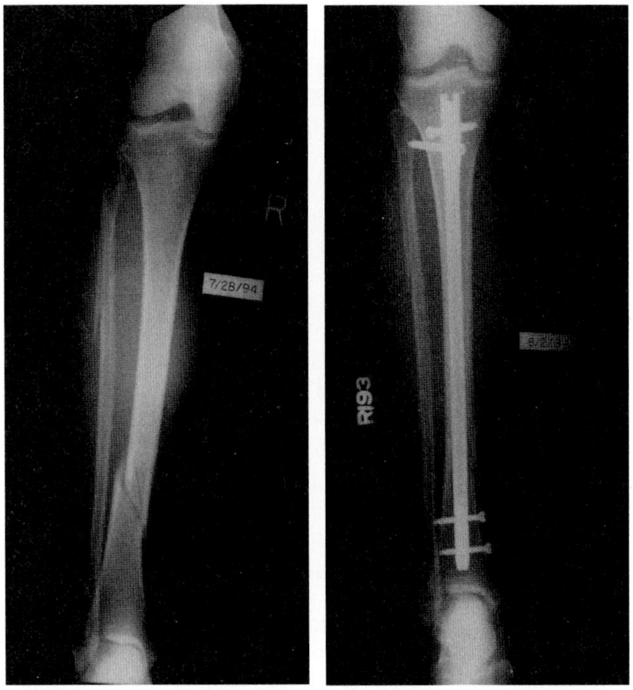

Fig. 4 **Left,** Spiral fracture of the distal third of a tibial diaphyseal fracture. **Right,** Fracture following statically locked intramedullary nailing.

compartment pressure was monitored during reduction, reaming, and nailing of 67 tibial fractures. An increase in pressure was seen when traction was applied to the leg and during reaming; however, these increases were transient and did not result in compartment syndrome. Several case reports of heterotopic bone forming posterior to the patellar tendon possibly mitigate against the use of the patellar tendon splitting approach to the proximal tibia.

External Fixation In the management of tibial shaft fractures, external fixation has the unique attributes of not requiring an extensive surgical exposure and of stabilizing the bone without leaving a foreign body in the proximity of the fracture site. These attributes are of potential benefit in two situations: periarticular fractures with compromised soft tissue, in which an extensive surgical approach is accompanied by a high incidence of skin necrosis and infection, and open fractures, in which a retained foreign body in the contaminated fracture site may increase the incidence of infection.

Open Fractures Open fractures of the tibia are managed by immediate debridement, stabilization of the bone, systemic antibiotic administration for at least 36 hours postinjury, and early soft-tissue coverage of exposed bone. In the last several years, intramedullary nailing has been used to stabilize open tibia fractures. On the surface this procedure is a simple extension of a technique used to manage closed tibia fractures. However, complex issues arise when nailing open tibial shaft fractures. A major issue is that reaming disrupts the already damaged blood supply to the bone in the proximity of the fracture, thus slowing healing and increasing the incidence of infection. Animal studies have shown that reamed nailing reduces the diaphyseal cortical circulation by about 70%, whereas unreamed nailing reduces the circulation by only about 30%. Because of this concern, most studies of intramedullary nailing of open tibia fractures have used unreamed nails, raising a second issue. Open fractures heal more slowly than closed fractures, yet compared with reamed nails, unreamed nails have a smaller diameter and are, therefore, weaker and more likely to fail. In an effort to increase the strength of unreamed nails, they are manufactured with a solid cross section. Because unreamed nails are solid, a slightly different technique is used for insertion (ie, no guide wire), and in the event of nail failure, extraction through the medullary canal may not be possible.

A third issue relates to the severity of postoperative complications. It is not accurate to equate localized osteomyelitis that occurs following external fixation with intramedullary osteomyelitis that occurs following intramedullary nailing. Despite these concerns, two studies indicate that nails are an acceptable method of stabilization of open tibial fractures. In one study, 50 open fractures of the tibia were managed with unreamed locked nails. There were no malunions. Forty eight fractures united, two grade III fractures did not unite. Locking screws broke in five patients; nails broke in three. There were no infections in the grades I and II fractures. Grade IIIB fractures had a 25% rate of infection (three of 12). These data support the use of unreamed intramedullary nailing in the management of grades I and II open tibial shaft fractures. In a second study, investigators looked more closely at the management of grade IIIB fractures with unreamed nails. Twenty-nine patients with grade IIIB tibial fractures were prospectively randomized to management with an external fixator (n = 14) or an unreamed nail (n = 15). The incidence of complications was similar in the two groups. There was one deep infection in each group, and no nonunions. The salient points of the study protocol, which may explain the remarkably low incidence of complications, are early (3 to 10 days) coverage with free or local soft-tissue transfer in 24 patients, bone grafting at 6 to 9 weeks in 19 patients, and liberal use of antibiotics (ie, a mean of 13 days in patients with soft-tissue transfers). The authors conclude that nailing is as good a method of stabilization of grade IIIB tibial fractures as external fixation.

Antibiotic Therapy Initially, this therapy consists of systemic administration of a second generation cephalosporin for grades I, II, and IIIA fractures. Penicillin is added for farm injuries, and an aminoglycoside is added for grades IIIB and IIIC injuries. A bead pouch technique of local antibiotic administration to the fracture site and surrounding soft tissue has been described. Following debridement and stabilization of the fracture, the soft-tissue defect is filled with polymethylmethacrylate-antibiotic beads. The wound is sealed over a drain by closing it primarily or covering it with an impermeable plastic drape. Extremely high levels of antibiotic are achieved locally and the incidence of infection is low when this method is used.

The results of limb salvage versus amputation in the management of severe open tibial shaft fractures has been scrutinized. In one study, 45 patients with IIIB and IIIC fractures were studied. Twenty-seven underwent limb salvage with a free tissue transfer, and 18 underwent early amputation (within 3 weeks). In the limb salvage group, five patients eventually underwent an amputation, the average hospital stay was 71 days, and cost was $109,000. The amputation group had an average hospital stay of 48 days at a cost of $66,000. Significantly more of the patients in the limb-salvage group thought that they were severely disabled (seven of 13 tested) than in the amputation group (three of 16). This study highlights the tremendous expense of management of grade IIIB and IIIC tibial fractures and demonstrates that successful limb salvage does not always equal a successful outcome.

Complications

Complications of tibial shaft fractures are nonunion, malunion, and infection. The diagnosis of nonunion is made when the healing process has slowed to the point at which consolidation of the fracture will not occur without further intervention. Most reports on studies of the management of nonunions define a nonunion as the absence of clinical and radiographic signs of healing for the prior 3 months, at least 9 months after injury. In fact, the diagnosis is usually obvious well before 9 months. Nonunions are managed nonsurgically, with electrical stimulation (direct current, electromagnetic fields, or capacitive coupling), or surgically. Surgical methods include fibulectomy, dynamic external fixation, bone grafting, and stabilization with plates or nails. Fibulectomy has the advantage of leaving the nonunion site undisturbed, but is contraindicated for hypertrophic nonunions. Dynamic external fixation uses sequential compression to stimulate hypotrophic and oligotrophic nonunions to heal, and it uses distraction alternated with compression to stimulate stiff hypertrophic nonunions to heal. Autogenous cancellous bone graft induces bone formation. The graft is placed posterolaterally in the nonunion site and between the fibula and tibia on the interosseous membrane, or simply directly in the nonunion site. The advantage of the posterolateral location is a higher rate of consolidation of the nonunion. The disadvantage is that the exposure can be difficult due to scarring from the injury and previous surgery. Plating and nailing rigidly stabilize the nonunion and are necessary when there is malalignment. Reports of two remarkably similar studies indicated the effectiveness of plate osteosynthesis in the management of a total of 83 tibial nonunions. Eighty-one nonunions eventually healed. Complications included plate failure (five), superficial wound breakdown (four), and deep infection (four). Details of the technique, which account for the high success rate, are limiting the surgical exposure to one side of the tibia, indirect reduction of deformity with a femoral distractor, application of the plate to the tension side of the bone, use of the tension device, and use of a lag screw for interfragmental compression when possible.

Malunion is defined as 5° of varus, valgus, or rotational malalignment, 10° of apex anterior or posterior angulation, and more than 1 cm of shortening. These absolute values are guidelines and are not always clinically applicable (eg, angulation is better tolerated in the mid-diaphysis than it is near the ankle or knee, and external rotation is better tolerated than internal rotation). Malunion alters the biomechanical axis of the leg and may accelerate the onset of arthritis in the knee and ankle. Symptomatic malunions are osteotomized, realigned, and stabilized with a nail or plate.

The diagnosis of infection of a tibial shaft fracture is made when there is erythema, increased pain, and culture positive drainage. When fixation is providing stability, it is left in place. When the fracture heals, the implants, necrotic bone, and soft tissue are removed. Dead space resulting from the debridement is managed with antibiotic beads or a soft-tissue transfer, and systemic antibiotics are administered for 4 to 6 weeks. In the case of an infected fracture of the tibia with fixation that has failed, the implant and necrotic tissue are removed. This removal often results in a segmental defect of the tibia. Stability is achieved most commonly with an external fixator. Dead space is managed with beads, and coverage is obtained with local or free soft-tissue transfer. Reconstruction of a bony defect is undertaken after the infection has been suppressed.

Compartment Syndrome

Compartment syndrome is defined as an increase in hydrostatic pressure in a closed osteofascial space, or compartment, resulting in decreased perfusion of the intracompartmental muscles and nerves.

Decreased perfusion of the intracompartmental structures is central to the pathophysiology of compartment syndrome. Blood flow to the muscles and nerves in the compartment is directly proportional to the arteriovenous gradient and inversely proportional to the resistance to flow (ie, local flow = [arterial pressure − venous pressure]/resistance). Increasing the intracompartmental pressure increases the venous pressure, thus lowering the arteriovenous gradient. Small increases in intracompartmental pressures are compensated for by a local decrease in resistance to flow. Lowered resistance fails to maintain local blood flow as the arterial venous gradient continues to drop, thereby resulting in shunting of blood through the compartment via larger vessels and bypassing of intracompartmental muscles and nerves. The ischemia that follows damages the capillary endothelium, allowing leakage of fluid and proteins from the intravascular space into the interstitial space, further raising intracompartmental pressure, and setting in motion a self-perpetuating cycle. The threshold intracompartmental pressure which results in the ischemia that initiates this cycle is called the critical pressure.

In clinical terms, compartment syndrome is caused by an increase in the volume of fluid within the compartment and is exacerbated by a decrease in the size or elasticity of the compartment. Causes of increased fluid volume are an intracompartmental bleed due to trauma, muscle contusion leading to extravasation of fluid, inadvertent extravasation of intravenous fluids into the compartment, or hypoxemia secondary to arterial or venous occlusion. A circumferential dressing or cast may decrease the volume of a compartment and, more importantly, prevent expansion of the compartment when there has been an increase in the intracompartmental fluid volume. Thus, in the presence of a circumferential dressing or cast, small increases in intracompartmental fluid volume result in large increases in intracompartmental pressure.

The diagnosis of compartment syndrome is based on clinical signs and measurements of the intracompartmental pressure. The physical signs of compartment syndrome are significant pain at rest, exacerbation of pain with gentle passive stretch of muscles in the compartment, decreased sensation in areas supplied by nerves that traverse the compartment, and palpably firm compartments. Of all these signs, hardness of the compartment is the most subjective. An objective method of measuring hardness of a compartment has been described. A piston probe is applied to the extremity over the compartment. As fluid is injected into the probe the volume of tissue displaced is quantified. The pressure applied divided by the volume of tissue displaced is the quantitative hardness. A potential shortcoming of this method is that surface hardness may not be representative of the pressure in a deep compartment. The signs of compartment syndrome should not be confused with the signs of arterial occlusion: pain, pallor, and pulselessness. Pulses are rarely absent secondary to a compartment syndrome because the critical pressure is less than the systolic pressure. Unless there has been an arterial injury, peripheral pulses will be present until the intracompartmental pressure exceeds the systolic pressure; therefore, peripheral pulses are present even when a full-blown compartment syndrome is present.

Actual measurement is the most objective assessment of intracompartmental pressure. However, the exact value of the critical pressure is controversial. There are two basic definitions of critical pressure: (1) an absolute value ($\geq$ 30 to 45 mm Hg); or (2) a derived value (diastolic blood pressure minus compartment pressure $\leq$ 20 mm Hg). Compartment pressures are measured by inserting a needle or catheter into the compartment. The needle or catheter is connected to a manometer. A small amount of fluid is injected into the compartment, the pressure at which the fluid enters the compartment is the intracompartmental pressure. Single measurements are made with side port or simple needles. Catheters can be left in place for long-term monitoring and are useful in the diagnosis of exercise-induced compartment syndrome. When slit catheters, side port needles, and simple needles were used to measure experimentally elevated compartment pressures in dogs, the side port needle and slit catheter gave nearly identical values. Values obtained with the simple needle were less consistent and indicated pressures 15 to 20 mm Hg greater than those obtained with the slit catheter and side port needle. Needle location in relation to the fracture is important. When pressures were measured at varying distances from the fracture, the highest pressures were found adjacent to the fracture in the anterior and deep posterior compartments.

Management of compartment syndrome is surgical decompression. This is usually accomplished through medial and lateral incisions. The deep and superficial posterior compartments are decompressed through the medial incision, the lateral and anterior compartments through the lateral incision. Alternatively, all four compartments can be decompressed through a single lateral incision. (Fig. 5) The benefit of a single incision is balanced by the risk of incomplete decompression. It has been suggested that the posterior tibialis muscle was in a separate fifth compartment, which also should be decompressed. However, in a study in which 51 cadaver legs were dissected, this was found not to be the case; therefore, individual decompression of the posterior tibial muscle is not necessary. The importance of long skin incisions is illustrated by a study in which eight patients with compartment syndrome underwent surgical decompression while their intracompartmental pressures were being monitored. Initial decompression was through a skin incision 8 cm in length. The pressure remained over 30 mm Hg in nine compartments of the eight patients, and it dropped below 30 mm Hg only after the length of the skin incision was increased to 16 cm. Following surgical decompression, the leg is elevated until swelling decreases. Occasionally a delayed primary closure is possible; usually a split thickness skin graft is required.

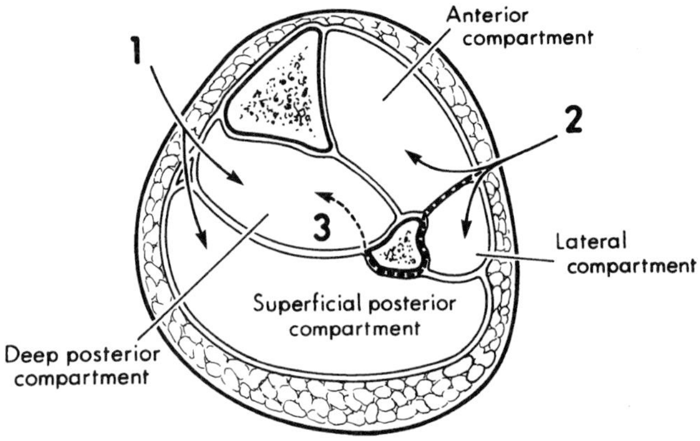

Fig. 5 Decompression of compartments of the calf is accomplished with a medial and lateral incision (1 and 2) or a single lateral incision (3).

Complications of compartment syndrome include decreased function of nerves that traverse the compartment and development of contractures. Late decompression of nerves and excision of contracted scarred muscle can be partially effective in the management of these complications.

Annotated Bibliography

Tibial Plateau Fractures

Georgiadis GM: Combined anterior and posterior approaches for complex tibial plateau fractures. *J Bone Joint Surg* 1994;76B:285–289.

Combined anterior and posterior approaches for fractures with a large posteromedial fragment are described. The posterior approach is done with the patient supine. The incision is over the medial head of the gastrocnemius, which is then retracted laterally. Reduction of the joint surface is achieved, and the fragment is held in place with a buttress plate.

Koval KJ, Sanders R, Borrelli J, et al: Indirect reduction and percutaneous screw fixation of displaced tibial plateau fractures. *J Orthop Trauma* 1992;6:340–346.

Twenty tibial plateau fractures were managed with percutaneous reduction (ie, ligamentotaxis, tenaculum clamp, and elevation of articular segment through a metaphyseal window). Only split fractures were consistently reduced. Depressed articular segments could not be reliably elevated.

Tibial Shaft Fractures

Eckman JB Jr, Henry SL, Mangino PD, et al: Wound and serum levels of tobramycin with the prophylactic use of tobramycin-impregnated polymethylmethacrylate beads in compound fractures. *Clin Orthop* 1988;237:213–215.

Bead pouch technique was used in 27 patients with open fractures. Levels of drug were determined in the serum and wound drainage. Locally, the levels were in excess of the therapeutic range of tobramycin. Systemically, the levels were well below recommended trough levels. There were no signs of infection in any of the patients managed with this technique.

Georgiadis GM, Behrens FF, Joyce MJ, et al: Open tibial fractures with severe soft-tissue loss: Limb salvage compared with below-the-knee amputation. *J Bone Joint Surg* 1993;75A:1431–1441.

The cost and effectiveness of limb salvage is compared with that of amputation in the management of IIIB and IIIC fractures. The authors found that saving the limb frequently resulted in more disability than amputation.

Helfet DL, Jupiter JB, Gasser S: Indirect reduction and tension-band plating of tibial non-union with deformity. *J Bone Joint Surg* 1992;74A:1286–1297.

Thirty three patients were managed with limited open reduction and tension band plating. Oligotrophic and hypotrophic nonunions were grafted with autogenous bone. A lag screw was inserted obliquely for interfragmentary compression. All nonunions healed. Complications included one deep infection, four cases of skin necrosis, and one plate failure.

Keating JF, Kuo RS, Court-Brown CM: Bifocal fractures of the tibia and fibula: Incidence, classification and treatment. *J Bone Joint Surg* 1994;76B:395–400.

Bifocal fractures of the tibia are fractures of the ankle and plateau (group 1) or fractures of the diaphysis with either a plateau (group 2) or ankle fracture (group 3). Bifocal fractures with a fracture of the plateau (group 2) had the worst prognosis with two primary amputations and the greatest loss of motion of the knee. The authors recommend reduction and stabilization of bifocal fractures with early bone grafting.

Tornetta P III, Bergman M, Watnik N, et al: Treatment of grade-IIIB open tibial fractures: A prospective randomised comparison of external fixation and non-reamed locked nailing. *J Bone Joint Surg* 1994;76B:13–17.

This prospective, randomized study compared the efficacy of reamed intramedullary nailing with that of external fixation in the management of grade IIIB open tibia fractures. The incidence of complications was similar in the two groups. The authors conclude that nailing is a better method of management because it is better tolerated by the patient.

Whittle P, Russell TA, Taylor JC, et al: Treatment of open fractures of the tibial shaft with the use of interlocking nailing without reaming. *J Bone Joint Surg* 1992;74A: 1162–1171.

In a consecutive series, 50 patients with open tibia fractures were managed with unreamed nails. Complications were limited almost exclusively to those patients with grade III fractures. The authors conclude that when grade I and II fractures are managed with unreamed nails, there is a low incidence of complications.

Compartment Syndrome

Cohen MS, Garfin SR, Hargens AR, et al: Acute compartment syndrome: Effect of dermotomy on fascial decompression in the leg. *J Bone Joint Surg* 1991;73B: 287–290.

This report clinically documents that the skin envelope can prevent expansion of a compartment, thereby contributing to increased intracompartmental pressure. This study supports the use of long skin incisions.

Heckman MM, Whitesides TE Jr, Grewe SR, et al: Compartment pressure in association with closed tibial fractures: The relationship between tissue presssure, compartment, and the distance from the site of the fracture. *J Bone Joint Surg* 1994;76A:1285–1292.

Twenty-five patients with closed tibia fractures had compartment pressures measured in all four compartments at 5 cm intervals from the fracture. The pressures were highest at the fracture site, decreasing about 20 mm Hg per 5 cm of distance from the fracture. Pressures were highest in the anterior and deep posterior compartment. The critical threshold was 20 mm Hg less than the diastolic pressure.

Classic Bibliography

Patellar Fractures

Weber MJ, Janecki CJ, McLeod P, et al: Efficacy of various forms of fixation of transverse fractures of the patella. *J Bone Joint Surg* 1980;62A:215–220.

Perry CR, McCarthy JA, Kain CC, et al: Patellar fixation protected with a load-sharing cable: A mechanical and clinical study. *J Orthop Trauma* 1988;2:234–240.

Tibial Plateau Fractures

Hohl M: Tibial condylar fractures. *J Bone Joint Surg* 1967;49A:1455–1467.

Perry CR, Evans LG, Rice S, et al: A new surgical approach to fractures of the lateral tibial plateau. *J Bone Joint Surg* 1984;66A:1236–1240.

Schatzker J, McBroom R, Bruce D: The tibial plateau fracture. The Toronto experience 1968–1975. *Clin Orthop* 1979;138:94–104.

Tibial Shaft Fractures

Bone LB, Johnson KD: Treatment of tibial fractures by reaming and intramedullary nailing. *J Bone Joint Surg* 1986;68A:877–887.

Caudle RJ, Stern PJ: Severe open fractures of the tibia. *J Bone Joint Surg* 1987;69A:801–807.

Gustilo RB, Gruninger RP, Davis T: Classification of type III (severe) open fractures relative to treatment and results. *Orthopedics* 1987;10:1781–1788.

Lottes, JO: Medullary nailing of the tibia with the triflange nail. *Clin Orthop* 1974;105:53–66.

Oestern HJ, Tscherne H: Pathophysiology and classification of soft tissue injuries associated with fractures, in Tscherne H, Gotzen L (eds): *Fractures With Soft Tissue Injuries.* Berlin, Germany, Springer-Verlag, 1984, pp 1–9.

Sarmiento A, Gersten LM, Sobol PA, et al: Tibial shaft fractures treated with functional braces: Experience with 780 fractures. *J Bone Joint Surg* 1989;71B:602–609.

Compartment Syndrome

Mubarak SJ, Owen CA, Hargens AR, et al: Acute compartment syndromes: Diagnosis and treatment with the aid of the wick catheter. *J Bone Joint Surg* 1978; 60A:1091–1095.

40

Knee and Leg: Soft-Tissue Trauma

The purpose of this chapter is to review knee ligamentous injuries, knee bracing, meniscal injuries, patellofemoral disorders, and extensor mechanism disruptions.

Anterior Cruciate Ligament Injuries

Nearly 100,000 new ACL injuries occur annually. A recent study of NCAA (National Collegiate Athletic Association) Division I basketball players concluded that female basketball players had a twentyfold greater likelihood of sustaining an ACL injury than their male counterparts. ACL injury may occur from a contact force, but the most common mechanism of injury is noncontact deceleration secondary to a valgus external rotation, varus internal rotation, or hyperextension mechanism. An ACL injury is usually accompanied by a rapid hemarthrosis, which generally occurs within 3 hours in approximately 80% of patients. A minor effusion does not preclude an ACL injury. Forty percent to 50% of patients will recall a tearing or "pop" sensation. Inability to continue sports participation immediately following the injury is the rule rather than exception. If the menisci are uninjured, improvement of symptoms will often occur within a 10-day period, and patients may perceive that they have fully recovered from their injury, only to subsequently experience a reinjury.

Physical Examination

The Lachman, anterior drawer, and pivot shift tests are used to establish a diagnosis of ACL deficiency. The uninjured knee should always be examined for a baseline comparison. The Lachman test is the most sensitive in an awake patient. Subtle differences in the anterior translation, particularly with the presence of a soft endpoint, are highly suggestive of an ACL injury. Grading classification is defined by increased translation compared with the opposite normal knee: grade 1 (1 to 5 mm), grade 2 (6 to 10 mm), grade 3 (11 to 15 mm), grade 4 (>15 mm). The Lachman test is performed with the patient supine and the knee flexed to approximately 20° to 30°. Sensitivity for the Lachman test approaches 95% to 98%. An alternative method of performing the Lachman test in a larger individual is with the patient in a prone position so that gravity assists in the anterior translation.

The anterior drawer test has historically been used to establish the diagnosis of ACL deficiency, but it has poor sensitivity for ACL injury. Performing this test with the foot internally or externally rotated may give information regarding posteromedial or posterolateral corner associated injuries. When performing the anterior drawer test, it is important to exclude a posterior cruciate ligament (PCL) injury. The examiner must determine whether an increased translation is occurring because the tibia comes from posterior to its neutral resting position. In general, with ACL injury, the Lachman test will have a greater anterior translation than the anterior drawer test. If the perceived anterior translation on the anterior drawer test exceeds that on the Lachman test, the examiner must consider a PCL injury.

The pivot shift phenomenon is pathognomonic of ACL deficiency. The term anterolateral rotatory instability should be abandoned. A variety of tests have been popularized, all of which elicit the subluxation-reduction phenomenon when the ACL is functionally deficient. If the ACL is torn, the tibia will sublux in extension and reduce in flexion. The magnitude of the pivot shift varies with position of the thigh and tibial rotation. Internal rotation will dampen the grade of the pivot shift as will thigh adduction. The classic description of Galway's pivot shift, performed with tibial internal rotation, may yield a false-negative result in up to 30% of patients examined under anesthesia. The pivot shift phenomenon is graded as a 1+ (glide), 2+ (jump), and 3+ (transient lock). Although the pivot shift test is pathognomonic of ACL deficiency, it may be difficult to perform in the office setting secondary to patient discomfort or apprehension, particularly in those patients who are acute or subacute. In chronic situations, the pivot shift is more easily elicited. The presence of a pivot shift phenomenon, regardless of the grade, providing it is asymmetric to the opposite knee, indicates ACL injury. A negative pivot shift test under anesthesia, despite arthroscopic evidence of an ACL injury, meets the definition of a partial ACL injury, provided there is no mechanical block (eg, displaced meniscal tear).

Imaging Studies

A radiographic series consisting of anteroposterior (AP), lateral, tunnel, and skyline views should be obtained when evaluating the patient with an ACL-injured knee. Occasionally, a concomitant osteochondritis dissecans lesion may be noted on the medial femoral condyle with a tunnel view. Additionally, intercondylar notch stenosis may be assessed with this view in chronic ACL deficiencies. A standing AP or 45° posteroanterior (PA) view will give information regarding medial or lateral compartment narrowing in the chronic ACL-deficient situation as well as detect a lateral capsular sign (Segond fracture). The normal indentation noted at the sulcus terminalis on the lateral femoral condyle may be accentuated (lateral notch sign) in a chronic ACL-deficient knee, secondary to repetitive episodes of giving way with impingement within this region. This phenomenon has been substantiated in MRI studies, which have demonstrated bone bruises in this region as well as the posterior region of the lateral tibial condyle. MRI is a very sensitive (95% to 100%) method of assessing ACL injury. However, the diagnosis of ACL injury should be confirmed by history and physical examination rather than MRI.

Instrumented arthrometry is helpful to quantify the anterior translation of ACL-deficient and reconstructed knees. Absolute anterior translation of > 10 mm at 20 lbs or maximum manual, or a maximum manual side-to-side difference of ≥ 3 mm are highly suggestive of an ACL-injured knee. Compliance index determination (20 lbs − 15 pound reading) is ≤ 2 mm in 98% of normal knees. A combination of an anterior translation > 10 mm and a maximum manual difference of ≥ 3 mm has a sensitivity of 99% for ACL injury.

Treatment Options

Nonsurgical Treatment Based on improved results of surgical treatment, there are changing perspectives on the part of patients and orthopaedic surgeons regarding treatment of ACL-deficient knees. The 1980s literature on nonsurgical treatment of the ACL-deficient knee has come under review. More recent literature suggests that patients have more disability than is suggested by Noyes' classic rule of thirds. Noyes demonstrated that one third of ACL-deficient patients who underwent rehabilitation and ACL orthosis bracing were able to fully compete in athletics, one third had to modify their sports activity, and one third continued to have problems of instability, necessitating either subsequent meniscal surgery or ACL reconstruction. Another author demonstrated a much higher incidence of disability related to ACL deficiency. The author of a prospective study concluded that activity modification must be required of all patients who are considering nonsurgical treatment. Although older patients may be more willing to modify their activities, only 8% to 10% of patients undergoing ACL reconstruction are over 35 years of age.

The patients who sustain an ACL injury must be educated on the available nonsurgical and surgical options. In general, surgical treatment should be considered for the younger, more active individual who, regardless of athletic skill level, participates in cutting, jumping, landing, and deceleration sporting activities and is unwilling to modify these activities. The patient with generalized ligamentous laxity poses a challenging problem; these individuals are frequently the ones who tolerate their ACL deficiency least well. A repairable meniscal lesion should be considered as a relative indication for ACL reconstructive surgery because most authors report a higher success rate in meniscal healing in ACL-stabilized knees.

Timing of Surgical Treatment The advantage of early surgical treatment is a reduced incidence of secondary chondral injuries and meniscal tears that may occur in the more chronic situation. Secondary restraints are less likely to be injured. This patient population has not had an opportunity to experience instability associated with ACL deficiency. Furthermore, they may have differing expectations with regards to surgical outcome compared to an individual who has chronic ACL deficiency and has experienced episodes of instability, or who has modified his/her lifestyle secondary to knee instability.

The timing of surgery is an important factor when minimizing postoperative knee-motion complications. A higher incidence of arthrofibrosis was noted in patients who underwent reconstruction via open arthrotomy less than 3 weeks after injury. In another retrospective study, it was noted that motion complications were associated with surgery performed less than 4 weeks after injury, and that they occurred in males and in those individuals who had associated medial collateral ligament (MCL) or posterior oblique ligament surgical treatment. Data from other studies have implicated locked displaced meniscal tears as a contributing factor when meniscal repair was performed concomitantly with ACL reconstruction. The current treatment principle is to defer early surgical reconstruction until the patient has nearly normal motion (0 to 120°) and the knee has a noninflamed appearance and a minimal effusion. The time from injury to early surgical reconstruction is probably less critical than the overall appearance of the knee and its range of motion.

Surgical Treatment The goals of ACL surgical treatment are to provide a stable knee, to eliminate the pivot shift phenomenon, to protect the menisci, to maintain full symmetric range of motion, to rehabilitate the knee while minimizing the likelihood of postoperative patellofemoral symptoms, and to return the patient to an appropriate level of athletics. The consensus among most knee-ligament surgeons is that intra-articular bone-tendon-bone, middle third patellar, or hamstring tendon autograft reconstructions provide the most predictable results. Nevertheless, there are proponents of allograft Achilles tendon, patellar tendon, or rolled fascia lata. Acute primary unaugmented repair or extra-articular reconstructions alone have few, if any, indications. Data from several studies have demonstrated that extra-articular augmentation is unnecessary with the use of intra-articular patellar tendon autograft. A higher complication rate with regards to lateral knee pain and hardware problems was associated with extra-articular augmentation, and there were no statistically significant differences in clinical or instrumental ligament-laxity testing. Noyes has recommended extra-articular augmentation when using an intra-articular patellar tendon allograft. The symptomatic ACL-deficient patient who has early degenerative joint disease or who has had a meniscectomy can predictably be stabilized by ACL reconstruction; however, the patient should be counseled with regard to protecting the knee and voluntarily modifying activities.

Standard surgical treatment includes the use of a high-strength graft that can be rigidly secured to allow an early range of motion and accelerated rehabilitation. Patellar tendon proponents advocate its use because of its high strength and ability to achieve rigid fixation. Data from a recent biomechanical study demonstrated that the mechanical properties of patellar tendon are greater than previously reported and that a 10-mm wide graft approximated the larger graft widths reported by Noyes and associates. Alternatively, hamstring tendon proponents claim decreased morbidity associated with donor site harvesting, apparently decreased incidence of patellar pain symptoms, less stiff material properties, and a more circular cross-sectional appearance. Hamstring advocates have also popularized the ability to double, triple, and quadruple the hamstring tendon, thus making the graft theoretically stronger than the patellar tendon autograft. The weak link with hamstring tendon usage is its fixation, although data from a recent biomechanical study indicated that a figure-of-eight fixation about two femoral screws was equivalent when compared to interference screw fixation in elderly cadaveric bone.

Regardless of graft source, intra-articular ACL reconstructive surgery must include anatomic positioning of the graft. There has been a tendency to move the tibial tunnel slightly more posterior within the middle third of the ACL insertion site to minimize impingement of the graft on the intercondylar roof in extension. The term isometry, popularized in the mid 1980s, has been replaced by anatomic placement. It is generally accepted that the 11 o'clock position on a right knee and the 1 o'clock position on a left knee are appropriate regions for femoral tunnel placement, and that an appropriate femoral tunnel leaves 1 to 2 mm of posterior cortex intact (Figs. 1 and 2). A variety of fixation devices are currently available. Some authors continue to secure patellar tendon grafts with sutures tied over buttons and report excellent stabilization results. Many authors report the use of a headless interference screw, initially popularized by Kurosaka as a form of femoral and tibial fixation. When using interference screws, care must be taken because screw divergence/convergence, graft translocation, suture laceration, or tendon laceration may occur. The graft should be secured in extension to minimize the likelihood of capturing the knee joint. Hamstring grafts are generally secured with staples or a screw and spiked washer form of fixation.

Two-incision arthroscopically assisted or miniarthrotomy techniques remain the most common for ACL reconstructive surgery. The single-incision endoscopic technique has become popularized since the late 1980s (Fig. 3). This technique is technically demanding and fraught with potential pitfalls, such as graft construct mismatch, graft laceration, and screw divergence. In a recent prospective study comparing two-incision versus single-incision procedures, no differences were noted in intermediate-term results. Although it appears that there may be no long-term differences in the single- versus double-incision techniques, patients appear more comfortable in the early postoperative course, following single-incision techniques.

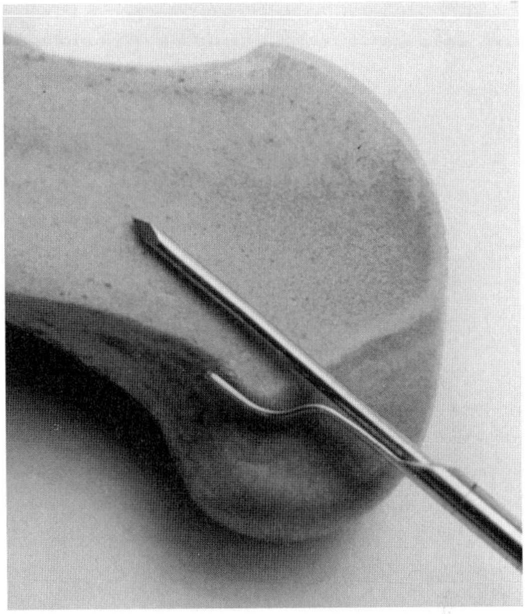

Fig. 1 Several commercially available femoral aimer guides are available. This guide keys off the "over-the-top" position. The 7-mm offset, when overreamed, will leave a 2-mm cortical rim. This aimer may be used to create provisional pilot half prior to placement of a rear entry guide if the surgeon performs two-incision techniques. (Reproduced with permission from Hardin GT, Bach BR Jr, Bush-Joseph CA, et al: Endoscopic single incision ACL reconstruction using patellar tendon autograft: Surgical technique. *Am J Knee Surg* 1992;5:144–155.)

Postoperative Management

Controversies remain considering the usage and duration of continuous-passive-motion (CPM) machines postoperatively. There is no advantage to prolonged outpatient CPM usage for routine ACL reconstructions. CPM can be helpful to initiate early flexion of the knee but is not helpful for obtaining extension, which is a more critical factor. The use of compression cryotherapy devices has received considerable attention since the late 1980s. A variety of variably priced devices are commercially available. Although they appear to be subjectively acceptable to patients and physicians and appear to be a contributing factor to reduced hospitalization, there is minimal literature to suggest their efficacy. In a recent prospective study evaluating cryotherapy devices, no effect was reported on range of motion, swelling, or pain reduction.

One of the major differences in postoperative care has been splinting the knee in complete extension and attempting to achieve complete early extension, thus reducing the incidence of knee flexion contractures. Despite the basic science literature that suggests increased strain on the ACL during the terminal 30° of extension, clinical evidence demonstrates that patients can perform straight leg raises and actively use the quadriceps in the terminal 30° of extension without causing graft attenuation. In general,

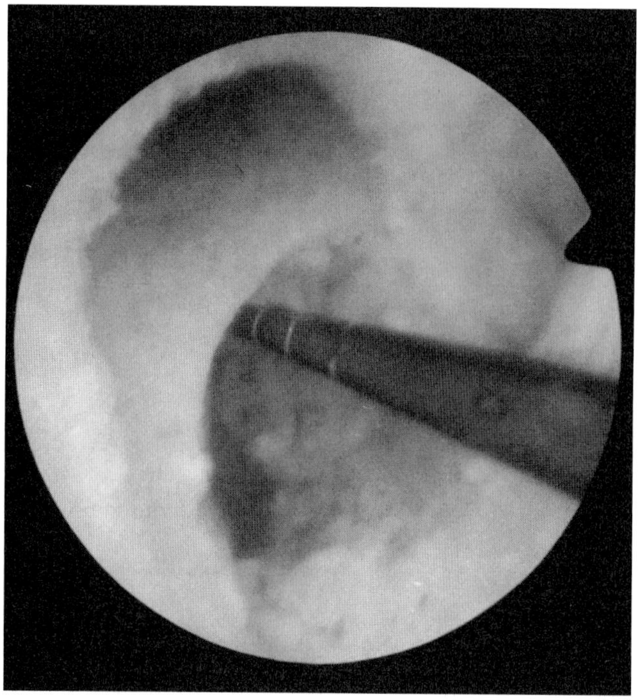

Fig. 2 Femoral tunnel placement is critical to the success of ACL reconstructive surgery. In this right knee, the femoral tunnel is located at the 11:00 to 11:15 position. The probe is palpating the posterior cortical "over the top" position. A 1- to 2-mm bridge should remain.

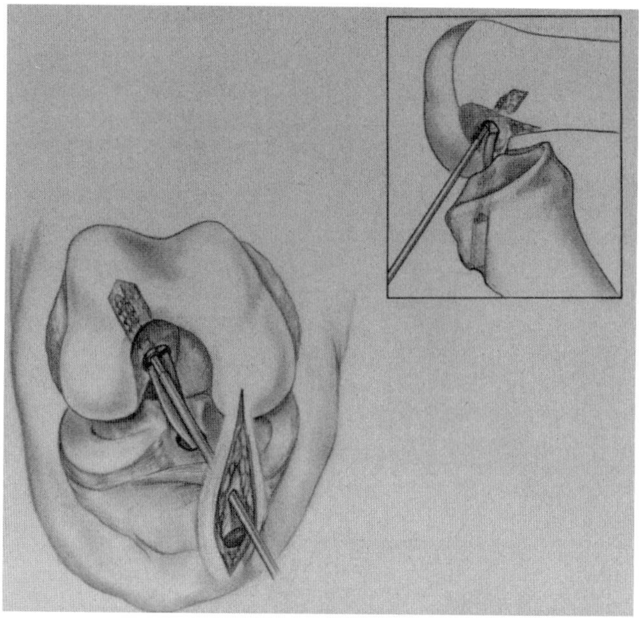

Fig. 3 The schematic illustration depicts the "push-in" technique for graft placement using a single incision endoscopic technique. Parallel femoral interference screw placement is facilitated by flexing the knee in the 100° to 110° range. (Reproduced with permission from Hardin GT, Bach BR Jr, Bush-Joseph CA, et al: Endoscopic single incision ACL reconstruction using patellar tendon autograft: Surgical technique. *Am J Knee Surg* 1992;5:144–155.)

most ligament surgeons advise weightbearing as tolerated, with many patients using crutches for less than 1 week postoperatively. Early accelerated rehabilitation is currently the standard rehabilitation protocol for patellar tendon autografts. Although some ligament surgeons are not protecting the knees in the early postoperative course, many surgeons will use a drop-lock brace or knee immobilizer to splint the knee in extension for weightbearing to protect the donor site. Splinting of the knee in extension while the patient sleeps can be helpful for maintaining extension during the first 6 weeks postoperatively. Active motion is allowed as tolerated.

Another current concept regarding rehabilitation is the use of closed kinetic chain strengthening exercises, such as bicycling, stair-stepper, slide board, leg press, and squat machine, which are performed when the affected foot is placed against a pedal, platform, or surface. Open-chain exercise, such as quadriceps extension or isokinetic strengthening, has been associated with increased patellofemoral symptoms. Therefore, occasional isokinetic testing is preferable to isokinetic strengthening. Guidelines for postoperative range of motion goals should be approximately 0 to 90° of motion by 2 weeks, 0 to 120° by 6 weeks, and full range of motion by 3 months postoperatively. However, patients with small flexion contractures can gain complete extension without requiring early surgical intervention. If a patient develops a knee flexion contracture after a graft has been properly placed and secured, the most common reason is secondary to scar formation in the intercondylar notch. A fibroproliferative scar nodule (cyclops lesion) may occur near the anterior base of the ACL insertion and impinge within the patellofemoral region as the knee is extended. Painful crepitation or an audible clunk may be associated with this syndrome. Outpatient arthroscopic resection and expansion notchplasty as needed can be helpful for regaining extension; extension splinting or casting may be necessary.

Guidelines for activities include stationary bicycling at 2 weeks, stair-stepper activities at 4 to 6 weeks, running at 3 months, and potential return to athletics between 4 and 6 months after reconstruction. Patients should use an ACL orthosis when they return to sports until 1 year postoperatively. If patients are returning to sports before 6 months, they should be counseled that there is a slight chance that they can injure the graft.

Complications

In arthroscopically assisted reconstructive techniques, the incidence of infection, patellar fractures, and patellar tendon ruptures individually are less than 1%. Intraoperatively induced patellar fractures are sagittally oriented in nature, whereas patellar fractures sustained postoperatively secondary to a fall will generally have a transverse or triradiate pattern of fracture. Patellar tendon ruptures are rare and have been reported at the tibial tubercle, distal patellar pole, and within the quadriceps tendon region. Meniscal repairs performed at the time of ACL reconstructive surgery appear to have a failure rate of approximately 10%. With the current concepts of accelerated rehabilitation, early extension, and early complete range of motion, the incidence of symptomatic knee flexion contractures has been substantially reduced. Repeated surgery for symptomatic knee flexion contractures should be less than 4%. Stabilization failures appear to be within the 8% to 10% range at intermediate (3 to 5 year) follow-up. Graft failure can occur secondary to improper placement of the femoral tunnel because the femoral side is more sensitive to position than the tibial side. However, if the tibial tunnel is placed too anteriorly, the graft may impinge in extension, resulting in either knee flexion contracture or graft attenuation. Patellar tendinitis symptoms characterized by localized tenderness at the distal patellar pole occur in less than 5% of patients during the postoperative rehabilitation period; this problem is self-limited.

Patellar pain during ascending and descending stairs or stiffness when sitting for periods of time are the most common complications of ACL surgery regardless of graft usage. In two separate studies in which hamstring tendons were used, a 12% incidence was reported. Patellar pain with patellar tendon use has been reported from 18% to 57%. A number of factors may contribute to patellar pain, including preexistent patellofemoral chondromalacia, open-chain rehabilitation, a period of immobilization or use of extension block braces, delayed quadriceps strengthening, and tourniquet time. With contemporary rehabilitation protocols, the incidence of patellar pain is far less than noted in the late 1980s.

Results of ACL Surgery

Contemporary techniques of ACL reconstruction, whether using autograft patellar tendon or hamstring tendons, when properly performed, should eliminate the pivot shift phenomenon in over 90% of patients at intermediate (3 to 5 year) follow-up. Instrumented laxity testing is helpful in the postreconstructive setting. Most authors report the maximum manual difference. Stratification of ≤ 3 mm, 3 to 5 mm, and ≥ 5 mm side-to-side differences are frequently reported, along with absolute translations. Contemporary methods of reconstruction indicate that 85% to 95% of patients should have ≤ 3 mm of maximum manual difference postoperatively. A postoperative maximum manual difference of ≥ 5 mm defines an arthrometric failure of surgical reconstruction.

In a prospective study comparing arthroscopically assisted hamstring and ACL reconstruction techniques, no statistically significant differences were found in clinical examination (Lachman and pivot shift), instrumented laxity, or functional results. No differences in surgical results were reported for a recent study in which hamstring tendon reconstructions performed via a femoral drill tunnel were compared with those placed in an "over the top" position. In another prospective study of hamstring and patellar tendon surgical procedures, the results of hamstring reconstruction were slightly more lax than patellar tendon. The authors concluded that the patellar tendon reconstruction, although there was slightly more morbidity with the procedure, was a more durable procedure with results that actually improved over time. In another recent study in which an arthroscopically assisted two-incision technique with patellar tendon autograft was used, researchers noted a 92% negative pivot shift rate, an instrumented maximum manual laxity difference of ≤ 3 mm in 92%, excellent quadriceps recovery (8% to 10% quadriceps deficit per isokinetic testing), and excellent functional recovery with single leg jump, vertical jump, and timed single leg jumps (8% to 10% deficits). Patients' subjective satisfaction appears to range in the area of 90% to 95% for ACL reconstructive procedures performed in a contemporary fashion.

Posterior Cruciate Ligament Injuries

Treatment of the isolated PCL-deficient knee continues to be controversial. This vertically oriented ligament, which is stronger than the ACL and is the primary restraint to posterior translation of the knee, is less commonly injured. The natural history of PCL injury is not well understood secondary to its relative infrequency; the ACL is injured 10 to 20 times more frequently. The mechanism of injury is varied. A direct posterior blow is one mechanism; a fall onto the ground with the foot plantarflexed results in striking the tibial tubercle, rather than the patella, with a resultant posteriorly directed force. A direct posterior blow to a flexed knee (eg, motorcycle) or severe hyperextension injury may result in an injury to the PCL. Complicating factors, other than the relative infrequency, include the pathologies—MCL, ACL, or posterolateral complex—frequently associated with a PCL-deficient knee. A low versus high velocity mechanism of injury also may affect the long-term prognosis and surgical treatment recommendations. Finally, the PCL is injured in the majority of knee dislocations.

An isolated PCL injury will generally result in a hemarthrosis, which is less than the one associated with an ACL injury. There may be an associated popliteal region ecchymosis. A pop or tear sensation is less frequently appreciated. A proximal anterior tibial abrasion should raise clinical suspicion of a potential PCL injury. Asymmetric knee hyperextension is another finding. Although patients may have complaints of instability, it is noted far less frequently than in an ACL injury. PCL injuries are more frequently associated with pain. In chronic situations, patients may have complaints of associated patellofemoral or medial compartment symptoms, because studies have shown a predilection to premature articular wear in these compartments. If the injury is associated with a posterolateral injury, the patient frequently may complain of instability when descending ramps.

Clinical diagnosis of the PCL injury is established by an asymmetric posterior drawer or posterior sag test. The external rotation recurvatum test may be an associated finding in PCL–posterolateral complex injured knees. Associated posterolateral laxity must be excluded (see Posterolateral Complex Injuries).

Standard radiographic series should be obtained when evaluating PCL-injured patients. An avulsion fracture of the PCL insertion site may be noted on the lateral radiograph, and if it is larger than 1.5 cm and displaced, this fracture may be an indication for primary surgical fixation. In the more chronic situations, medial compartment or patellofemoral compartment degeneration may be noted. A mechanical axis view is recommended in patients who have an associated posterolateral injury, particularly in more chronic situations in which high tibial osteotomy should be considered in the varus knee. Although the MRI is extremely sensitive for determining PCL injury, diagnosis should be established by history and physical examination rather than by MRI.

Treatment considerations for PCL injuries are not well defined. In the acute setting, it is extremely unusual to surgically repair/reconstruct a PCL injury unless it is a grade 3 or 4 injury. In one survey, 90% of the respondents indicated that they would conservatively treat and observe the vast majority of acute isolated PCL injuries, regardless of the grade. In chronic situations, the symptomatic grade 2 or higher lesions were considered potential surgical candidates. Triple phase bone scans have been recommended for following up conservatively treated patients to assess for any early articular surface wear that may be considered for surgical reconstruction. Many surgeons have observed that long-term results of reconstruction at best approach a 1+ posterior drawer and that it is extremely unusual to restore the posterior drawer test to normal. This problem is one of the major reasons why only higher-grade lesions have been considered for surgical treatment. The grade 1 lesions generally represent incomplete injuries.

Considerable controversy continues in regard to the choice of graft tissues, the location of tunnel placements, the position of knee flexion when securing a graft, and the methods of fixation. Other factors affecting static ligament examination may be the early range of motion and the extent of range of motion used postoperatively. Patellar tendon autograft is preferable to hamstrings for surgical reconstruction, but passage of the bone-tendon-bone construct is difficult due to the orientation of the tunnels (Fig. 4). Allograft tissues have played an important role in the surgical treatment of PCL deficiencies. Bone-patellar tendon-bone, allograft, and, more commonly, Achilles tendon allograft have been frequently used.

There are few studies on the surgical results of PCL reconstruction using contemporary techniques. Clancy's study remains the benchmark for comparison as over 90% of his patients had a trace to 1+ posterior drawer at follow-up. This should be juxtaposed to the observation of Bergfeld and Fowler, who noted that, despite static laxity, patients functioned reasonably well without reconstruction. A recent study of nonsurgically treated PCL patients noted a higher degree of disability than reported by these authors.

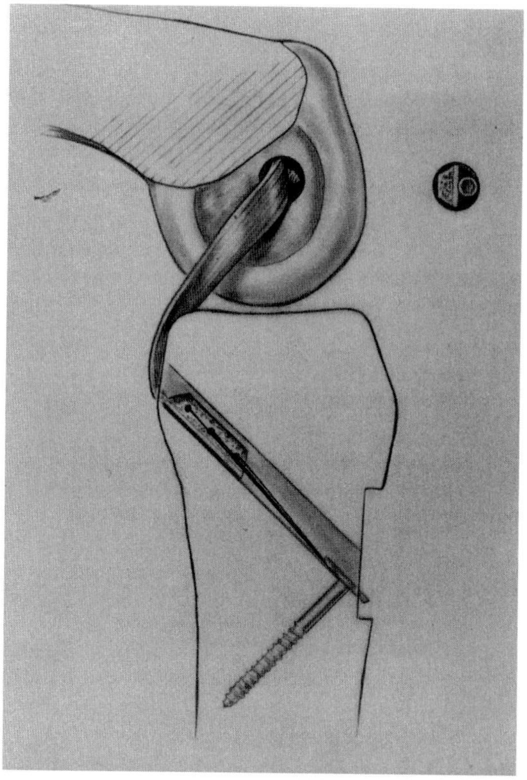

Fig. 4 This lateral schematic illustration depicts appropriate tunnel location of a PCL reconstruction. On the femoral side an interference screw is placed anterior to the bone plug to minimize graft injury if the screw protruded beyond the tendo-osseous junction. On the tibial side, the length of the construct results in the bone plug residing deep within the tibial tunnel. Fixation with a standard interference screw would make any future reconstructive procedure (eg, HTO) extremely different. Note the "zig-zag" course the graft passes prior to fixation. (Reproduced with permission from Bush-Joseph CA, Bach BR Jr: Arthroscopic assisted posterior cruciate reconstruction using patellar tendon autograft. *Sports Med Arthroscopy Rev* 1994;2: 106–119.)

Posterolateral Complex Injuries

Injuries to the posterolateral complex involve the popliteus tendon, arcuate complex, and the lateral collateral ligament (LCL). These infrequent injuries are often associated with ACL or PCL injuries or with knee dislocations, but they may occur as an isolated entity. Understanding of these injuries probably lags behind even that of the PCL. The mechanism of injury is frequently an anteromedial blow to the tibia. Patients who sustain this injury may have complaints of knee instability, particularly when descending ramps. At the time of injury, even if confined to the posterolateral complex, there may be a hemarthrosis. A popliteus tendon avulsion fracture from its origin on the lateral femoral condyle is a rare cause of a knee hemarthrosis. The specific examination for posterolateral complex injuries include varus laxity at 0 or 30° and asymmetric thigh–foot angles greater at 30° than at 90°. Posterolateral spin is greater at 30° than 90° in the isolated posterolateral complex injury. Thigh–foot angles may be measured with the patient supine or prone (Fig. 5). The reverse pivot shift is felt to be an indicator of a posterolateral complex injury.

There are no prospective studies available on the natural history of posterolateral complex injuries. However, biomechanically, loss of lateral and posterolateral soft-tissue restraints results in increased tensile forces on the lateral side of the knee and subsequent increased compressive forces on the medial aspect of the knee. Data from gait analysis studies have indicated that patients with posterolateral complex injuries in association with varus aligned knees and ACL deficiencies have increased adduction moments within the medial compartment. Injuries to the posterolateral complex may result in accelerated wear of the medial compartment or increased articular surface injury to the lateral compartment because of the excessive spin. A recent study demonstrated that cadavers with combined posterolateral–PCL injuries will have greater patellofemoral contact pressures than an isolated PCL-deficient knee.

The treatment of posterolateral complex injuries is controversial. No long-term studies have demonstrated a superior result of specific surgical techniques. In the acute situation, direct primary repair of injured posterolateral complex structures had been advocated. A procedure has become popular in which the long head biceps tendon is tenodesed to the origin of the LCL, the posterolateral complex is tightened, and the flexion and external rotation deforming forces of the long head biceps are reduced (Fig. 6). Popliteus tendon bypass procedures, split biceps tendon advancements, and the use of split Achilles tendon allograft to address the lateral collateral and popliteus pathologies have been advocated. If a patient has a varus aligned knee, soft-tissue reconstructions are likely to stretch in this situation, and valgus high tibial osteotomy (HTO) is indicated. Once an HTO has been performed, placing the patient's knee in a valgus alignment, posterolateral tissues that have been subjected to tensile forces may contract and tighten. There are few reports available on the results of posterolateral repairs/reconstructions.

Medial Collateral Ligament Injuries

Since the mid 1980s, the accepted form of treatment of an isolated MCL injury, regardless of its magnitude, has been nonsurgical. Recent literature continues to substantiate this treatment method. The classification scheme comprises three grades of valgus laxity: grade 1 (1 to 5 mm), grade 2 (6 to 10 mm), and grade 3 (11 to 15 mm). The MCL is the primary restraint both at 0 and 30° of knee flexion, but it is a more important primary restraint at 30°. Valgus laxity in extension implies injuries to secondary restraints such as the ACL, PCL, or posterior capsule. The best position for identification of an MCL sprain is with the knee flexed at between 25° and 30°. An associated

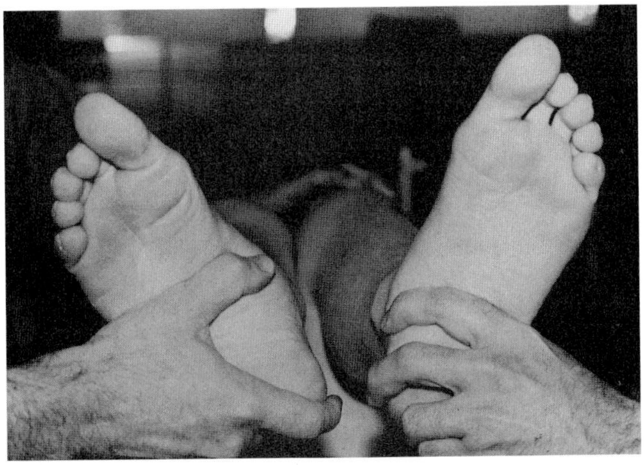

Fig. 5 This intraoperative photograph demonstrates asymmetric thigh foot angles in an affected right knee in a patient with a combined PCL-posterolateral complex injury.

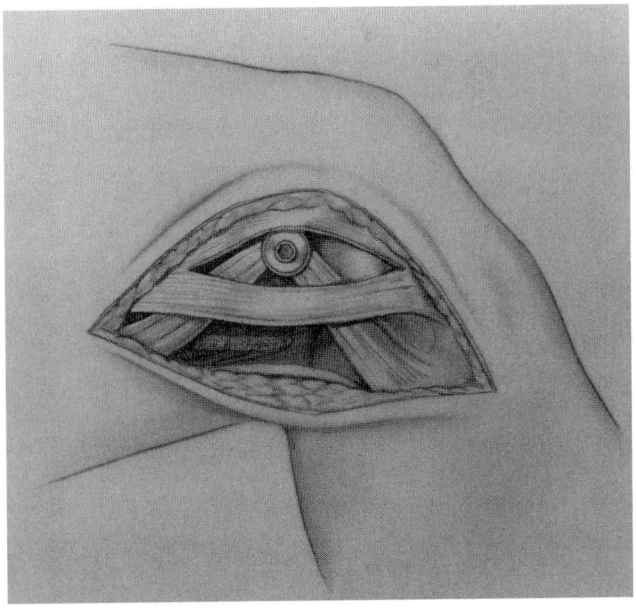

Fig. 6 This schematic illustration depicts the biceps tenodesis procedure used for valgus aligned patients with symptomatic posterolateral laxity. (Reproduced with permission from Bach BR Jr: Posterolateral reconstruction using Clancy biceps tenodesis: Surgical technique. *Am J Knee Surg* 1993;6:97–103.)

meniscal tear is unusual with an isolated MCL injury in contrast to a combined ACL/MCL sprain. O'Donoghue's triad (ACL, MCL, medial meniscal tear) has been questioned recently. A higher incidence of lateral meniscal tears than medial meniscal tears in ACL/MCL injuries were observed in one study. The meniscus was more likely to sustain a grade 2 injury in contrast to a grade 3 MCL sprain.

Long leg casts are currently infrequently used for treatment of MCL sprains. Patients with a grade 1 MCL sprain may be treated in a knee immobilizer or Neoprene knee sleeve with medial–lateral hinges. Usual recovery is in 2 to 3 weeks. A grade 2 MCL sprain is better treated in a hinged postoperative knee motion brace. Weightbearing can be progressed as tolerated, but usually patients may require 1 week of nonweightbearing. Patients with grade 3 injuries may be treated in a long leg cylinder cast or, preferably, a hinged knee brace for 3 to 4 weeks. Standard MCL treatment includes early range of motion, muscle rehabilitation, and avoidance of patellofemoral symptoms. Weightbearing should be deferred in the grade 3 injuries, particularly if the patient has an anatomic valgus alignment. Return to athletics is based on range of motion, strength recovery, and ability to perform functional agility drills. Knee bracing continues to remain controversial with regard to MCL injuries. It is common to use a functional knee brace when returning an MCL-injured athlete to sports during the season of injury.

Controversy exists in regard to the more significant grade 3 MCL injuries with associated posterior-oblique ligament complex injuries. Some advocate surgical treatment for this lesion, and others recommend, based on selective cutting cadaveric studies, that it can be treated nonsurgically. In a recent study, the importance was demonstrated of differentiating whether the MCL injury is proximal or distal; the authors noted an increased likelihood of knee stiffness and delayed motion recovery following surgery with injuries involving the MCL origin or the midsubstance.

The treatment of combined ACL/MCL injuries also remains controversial. Most knee ligament surgeons will recommend surgical treatment of the ACL and nonsurgical treatment of the MCL. In one study, untreated MCL injuries were found to be an associated factor in patients who had less than optimal results, whereas in another study, a series of patients treated nonsurgically had excellent results. A more important consideration is the timing of surgical treatment. An associated MCL injury places the knee at increased risk for stiffness. This risk is the rationale for nonsurgical treatment of the MCL when addressing the ACL injury. In this situation, it is advantageous to begin early rehabilitation of the knee, aggressive range of motion, and a delayed ACL surgical reconstruction. Combined ACL/MCL injury, however, is not an absolute indication for surgical treatment if patients are not considered good surgical or compliant rehabilitation candidates.

When conservatively treating a patient with an MCL injury and associated joint line tenderness, the surgeon must be cognizant of the possibility of a concomitant medial meniscal tear. A delay in recovery or prolongation in a patient's symptoms with specific joint line tenderness and rotational findings should make the physician suspicious of an associated medial meniscal tear.

Knee Dislocations

Uncommon, although not rare, traumatic knee dislocations are an orthopaedic emergency. Knee dislocations are classified relative to the position of the tibia, and there are five types: anterior, posterior, medial, lateral, and rotational. The rotational classification may be subcategorized into anteromedial, anterolateral, posteromedial, and posterolateral. Some knee dislocations may not be classifiable. Anterior knee dislocations occur most frequently (40%), followed by posterior knee dislocations (33%), lateral knee dislocations (18%), medial knee dislocations (< 5%), and rotatory dislocations (< 5%). Low- or high-velocity mechanisms of injury may be involved. Hyperextension injuries may result from a low-velocity injury but, generally, posterior knee dislocations are the result of high-velocity trauma.

Vascular injury is more frequently noted with anterior and posterior dislocations. An overall incidence of vascular injury is in the 20% to 35% range in most studies. Currently, the incidence of amputation secondary to vascular injury is approximately 10%. Recognition of a vascular injury is essential. Normal pulses or normal capillary refill do not preclude an arterial injury, and arteriography should be considered in all knee dislocations. If the leg is ischemic, the arteriogram should be circumvented and the patient taken directly to the operating room. In a classic study, the amputation rate was 11% if vascular repair was performed within 6 hours, and increased to 86% if repair was delayed beyond 8 hours. Muscle fibrosis, contracture, and chronic vascular insufficiency commonly occur in 66% of patients when ischemia exceeds 6 hours.

Neurologic injuries most frequently involve the common peroneal nerve because of its tethered proximity to the fibular head. Lateral and posterolateral dislocations are the most frequent causes of common peroneal nerve injury. Overall, incidence of neurologic injuries varies between 16% and 40%. Less than 50% of patients will have partial or complete recovery from a peroneal nerve palsy. The examiner must be cognizant that the multiligament knee injury may represent a reduced knee dislocation.

Currently, concurrent repair of ligaments and vascular injury is not recommended. Vascular injury must take precedence, and it is advisable to defer ligamentous reconstruction until vascular stability has been achieved. Indications for immediate surgery include: popliteal vascular injury, open dislocation, and irreducible dislocations. Irreducible dislocations most frequently are lateral and posterolateral with entrapment of the MCL or capsule. Skin dimpling may confirm this diagnosis.

There are no prospective studies in which the results of

surgical treatment of knee dislocations have been evaluated. Reports of most recent studies suggest that knee motion, stability, and overall knee ratings are superior with early surgical treatment. Reports of other retrospective studies contradict this concept, however. The common complication of knee stiffness following knee dislocations has resulted in rethinking of the surgical treatment of this problem. Some surgeons are deferring surgery until motion has been regained and then performing early arthroscopically assisted multiligament reconstructions for the ACL and PCL. Some knee dislocations may occur without injury to three or four ligaments. Posterior or posterolateral dislocation may occur without an ACL injury, and anterior dislocation may occur without PCL disruption. External fixators and transpatellar olecranonization (fixation by a pin from patella to tibia) are currently used less frequently due to the high incidence of articular surface damage associated with their use. In contrast to an isolated cruciate ligament injury, the ACL and/or PCL pathology associated with knee dislocation may frequently be avulsion rather than midsubstance tears. Primary repair with augmentation may be considered in this situation. Midsubstance ligament injuries should be reconstructed. Allograft tissues have an important role in the surgical treatment of knee dislocations when tissue availability is a concern. Most authors advocate surgical treatment of all ligamentous pathology; others are more conservative and will reconstruct/repair the ACL and/or PCL.

Synthetic Grafts

Synthetic replacements for knee ligaments are categorized as stents, prostheses, and scaffolds. An example of a stent is the polyester ligament augmentation device (LAD) designed to protect autogenous or allograft tissues as they regain their mechanical strength following reconstruction. A prosthesis is a permanent device that is secured at both ends of the articular surface to replace the ligament. Polytetrafluoroethylene and polyester are other materials used for permanent prostheses. The Leeds-Keio device is a polyster scaffold that functions to provide biologic ingrowth.

The Gore-Tex graft is not recommended for primary ACL surgery. Numerous reports have indicated a deterioration of results over time, with an anticipated success rate of approximately 50% at 5-year follow-up. Its current use is limited for revision ACL surgery. It has recently been revised into a compact diameter graft. There are no clinical results reported on use of this second-generation device.

The LAD was initially approved by the FDA to supplement the quadriceps tendon expansion. Some surgeons had expanded its use to augment the hamstring tendons and patellar tendon auto- or allograft. Recent prospective studies have demonstrated that there is no advantage to using an LAD when compared to autogenous tissues.

Results for use of a Dacron polyester prosthesis (polyethyleneterephthalate) appear to be better than those for the Gore-Tex graft. Data from recent studies have indicated that one third of the grafts were nonfunctional at 5 years.

Allograft Tissues

The most common allograft tissues used for knee reconstruction include patellar tendon, fascia lata, Achilles tendon, and hamstring tendons. The advantages of allograft use include reduced donor site morbidity, smaller surgical incisions, enhanced early postoperative rehabilitation, and tissue availability for multiligament-injured knees. The disadvantages include potential for disease transmission, a slower mechanical remodeling rate, and less successful results than those for autograft tissues. Currently, few ligament surgeons initially choose allograft tissues for ACL reconstruction. Allograft tissue should be used on an individualized basis. Relative indications include revision surgery, tissue access in multiple-ligament injuries, older patients with symptomatic instability, patients who may not be ideal candidates for rehabilitation but have symptoms of instability that warrant reconstruction, or the patient who has moderate patellofemoral symptoms. The patellar tendon is the allograft tissue of choice for ACL reconstruction, whereas the Achilles tendon allograft appears to be used most frequently for PCL reconstruction.

The patient for whom allograft reconstructive surgery is being considered must be apprised of the potential for disease transmission. Currently, the potential for human immunodeficiency virus (HIV) transmission is estimated as 1:667,000; and the use of polymerase chain reaction (PCR) testing should further reduce this potential. Testing for hepatitis A is no longer performed, whereas testing for hepatitis B and C is routinely performed. The surgeon must understand the types of ligament processing and testing performed by the tissue bank from which the tissue is procured. Biomechanical alterations in collagen are noted with less than 3 Mrad of irradiation; however, more than 3 Mrad are required to kill the HIV virus. Some surgeons will use freeze-dried or deep frozen allograft tissues that have not been irradiated because there appear to be fewer mechanical alterations in the tissue. The deep-freezing technique appears to reduce the antigenicity of the allograft by reducing major histiocytic antigens.

Knee Bracing

Knee braces are classified as prophylactic, postoperative (rehabilitative), functional, and patellofemoral. Lateral prophylactic knee braces, which were designed with the hopes of reducing the incidence and severity of MCL and/or ACL injuries, have been controversial. Variations in coaching techniques and game rules, nonstandardization of injury diagnosis, changes in shoe wear, artificial versus natural turf, position-specific factors, athlete compliance, and inaccurate data collection methods are among the multitude of factors that contribute to conflicting results. Although the AAOS position statement on prophylactic knee braces is that they are not efficacious in preventing knee injuries, data from a well-designed, prospective, randomized controlled West Point study demonstrated reduced incidence and severity of MCL injuries in defensive backs using lateral prophylactic knee braces. There remains no clear mandate to recommend lateral prophylactic knee braces.

Functional knee braces are designed to protect the ACL-deficient and ACL-reconstructed knee. Current literature seems to indicate that functional braces may diminish anterior translation in cadaveric knees, but not at the physiologic loads to which the knee is subjected in vivo. Functional brace use may adversely affect oxygen consumption, agility, and speed. There are no data available that suggest an ACL functional brace will prevent an ACL injury in an otherwise normal knee. Clinically, it is best to educate patients that an ACL functional brace will reduce, but not eliminate, episodes of instability. Because it appears that the functional ACL orthosis will not prevent anterior translation at high physiologic loads, the current explanation is that these braces provide neuromuscular, proprioceptive feedback. Most surgeons use an ACL orthosis to protect the ACL during the first year following surgery. Increasing numbers of investigators are prospectively evaluating patients who do not use a postoperative ACL functional brace, and they are encouraged by early short-term results. The use of high-strength, rigidly fixed grafts, frequent noncompliance of patients in regard to brace usage, and the expense ($800 to $1,200) of custom ACL orthoses makes this an intense area of interest.

Meniscal Tears

Rotational twisting injuries are generally the cause of meniscal tears. The cause may be as trivial as arising from a kneeling or squatting position or any type of athletic activity resulting in rotation of the knee. A pop or tearing type of sensation, joint line tenderness, mild effusion in most meniscal tears, and a mild to moderate hemarthrosis in peripheral tears may be noted. Patients frequently note that rotation of the leg resulting from rolling over in bed, crossing a leg, or catching one's foot on the carpet causes pain in the knee with a torn meniscus. Many individuals may tolerate uniplane activities quite well. The majority of meniscal tears noted in adult recreational athletes are posterior horn flap patterns with an anterior based axilla.

The clinical diagnosis of a meniscal tear should be established by history and physical examination in 90% of patients. A standard radiographic series (standing PA, lateral, tunnel, and skyline views) should be obtained initially on all patients. MRI is more sensitive for medial than lateral meniscal tears. Although it is extremely sensitive, routine MRI for meniscal tear pathology is unwarranted because it does not affect surgical decision making in the vast majority of situations. MRI is not helpful in assessing the affected meniscus after meniscal surgery because although it will demonstrate an abnormal meniscal configuration, it cannot differentiate between postsurgical changes and a retear. MRI is not indicated in assessing healing because signal changes are noted long-term.

The medial meniscus is more frequently torn than the lateral meniscus in normal and ACL-deficient knees. In acute ACL injuries, however, the lateral meniscus is more frequently torn. Peripheral longitudinal meniscal tears, which are amenable to repair, are more frequently noted medially than laterally, and approximately 80% of patients who undergo meniscal repair have an acute or chronic ACL-deficient knee. Radial split tears are more frequently noted in the lateral meniscus and, if they extend to the periphery, have the potential to heal. Therefore, they may be considered for repair. Horizontal cleavage pattern tears also are more frequently noted in the lateral meniscus and may be associated with lateral meniscal cysts. Most meniscal tear patterns involve the posterior one third of the meniscus. Partial thickness tears of 10 mm or less, which are stable to probing, may not require resection or repair.

In general, meniscal repair is indicated for lesions greater than 1 cm in length that are located within the vascular zone. Repair of the meniscus may be performed using a variety of techniques. In most cases, arthroscopic repair is feasible—either by an "outside-in" or an "inside-out" technique. Recently, "all-inside" systems have been developed that require intra-articular knot tying techniques. Long-acting absorbable or, preferably, nonabsorbable sutures should be used for meniscal repair. The use of stacked sutures with alternating placement on the superior and inferior surfaces of the meniscus is recommended (Fig. 7). Reconstruction of the ACL at the time of meniscal repair has a favorable effect on meniscal healing. In one recent series, the success rate of meniscal repair was 50% in patients with normal ACLs who had isolated repair compared to 93% in patients who underwent a concomitant reconstruction of the ACL. If meniscal repair is attempted in the ACL-deficent knee without reconstructing the ACL, failure rates of 13% to 30% have been reported.

Patellar Disorders

Patellofemoral disorders, including patellofemoral pain, instability, malalignment, quadriceps tendinitis, distal patellar tendinitis, patellofemoral arthrosis, and symptomatic plica syndrome, are the clinical entities most frequently noted about the knee joint. Standard treatment is conservative care. The history and physical examination are critical to the diagnosis of patellofemoral pain disorder. If the patient has been involved in a conditioning program, the physician must clarify whether there had been any component of open kinetic chain strengthening, such as quadriceps extension exercises, or, in a supervised physical therapy setting, isokinetic strengthening, which may have aggravated the patient's patellofemoral symptoms. Localization of pain is important and helps to diagnose

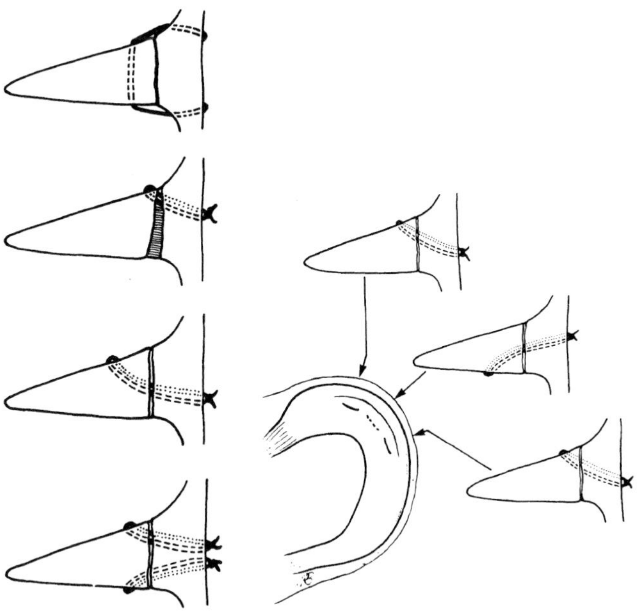

Fig. 7 **Left,** Diagram demonstrating suture placement patterns for meniscal repair. Note that the vertical and centrally placed horizontal sutures will reapproximate the tear surfaces, whereas a suture placed off-center superiorly or inferiorly may inadequately close the tear. **Right,** Diagram illustrating "stacking" of horizontal mattress sutures on the superior and inferior surfaces of the meniscus. (Reproduced with permission from Cooper DE: Arthroscopic meniscal repair: "Outside-in" technique. *Oper Tech Sports Med* 1994;2:190–200.)

quadriceps tendinitis, distal pole patellar tendinitis, or symptomatic plica syndrome. Clinical lateral tilt, ability to evert the lateral patellar edge, the dynamic Q angle, seated 90° Q angle, apprehension signs, generalized ligamentous laxity findings, and flexibility of quadriceps and hamstrings are critical components of the physical examination. The examiner must be cognizant of a superimposed reflex sympathetic dystrophy (RSD), particularly in the patient who has had previous patellofemoral surgery. Referred sources of pain from the back and hip must be excluded.

Radiographic evaluation should include a standardized patellofemoral axial view; although axial views are not particularly sensitive, a Merchant view is easily standardized, and the congruence angle may be determined. Radiographic evidence of subluxation (lateral translation) is easier to determine than patellar tilt. Computed tomography (CT) of the patellofemoral joint performed at 15°, 30°, and 45° is preferable to MRI; however, routine CT evaluation of the patellofemoral joint is not indicated. Standardized cuts through the midpatellar region should be obtained. Patella baja or alta may be radiographically diagnosed with 30° flexion lateral radiographs. Contralateral films should be considered if postoperative patella baja is considered. Data from a recent study suggest that a true lateral view with the knee extended and the quadriceps contracted can provide additional information with regard to patella alta. Radionuclide scanning may localize patellofemoral pathology and is useful in the assessment of RSD.

The treatment of patellofemoral disorders includes the use of anti-inflammatory medication and icing. Open chain quadriceps resistance exercises should be minimized or avoided in contrast to closed chain strengthening. Quadriceps and hamstrings flexibility is critical. Straight leg raises with and without ankle weights, as well as variable angle leg raises are important aspects of treatment. Isokinetic exercises should be avoided. Patellar taping, simple bracing with a patellar cutout, and general aerobic conditioning are other components of conservative treatment. Strengthening should be performed through a pain-free arc. The patient should exhaust conservative measures before surgical treatment is considered.

Arthroscopic debridement should be reserved for chondral lesions that may further fragment. Localization of articular lesions is extremely important to specific treatment. It is generally recommended that, if debridement is performed, the edges should not be bevelled. Overzealous treatment of grade 1 (blistering) and grade 2 (linear fissures) disorders should be avoided.

Arthroscopic lateral release may be considered for patients with lateral patellar tilt and recalcitrant patellar pain who have minimal articular surface damage. Lateral release is variably effective for subluxation; if subluxation is combined with lateral tilt, it may reduce the tilt and clinical symptoms related to patellar pain. Lateral release is generally ineffective in patients with more severe patellofemoral chondromalacia (grades 3 or 4) and may worsen symptoms in patients with distal medial patellar chondromalacia. In a recent study, improved results were noted with lateral release in patients with a medial congruence angle. Overzealous extension of lateral release may result in a postoperative complication of medial patellar instability; the surgeon should avoid extending it into the vastus lateralis musculature. The recommended intraoperative achievement of 45° of lateral tilt can be difficult to determine secondary to soft-tissue swelling. Lateral release should not be performed in a patient who has had previous dislocation with medial patellar facet chondromalacia. Hemarthrosis is the most common complication following a lateral release. Meticulous hemostasis should be achieved with electrocautery. The tourniquet, if used, should be released to assess control. A hemovac should be considered as well. The knee should not be splinted in extension because the released tissues may coapt. Early motion should be encouraged.

Distal realignment may be considered in patients with increased Q angles and subluxation or dislocation. The Elmslie-Trillat procedure, a medialization of the tibial tubercle without posteriorization, which unloads the distal and lateral facets of the patella, should be considered if there is minimal or absent articular injury. Lateral release should be performed concurrently. Fulkerson's anteromedial tibial tubercle transfer should be considered in patients with malalignment and more extensive lateral facet involvement. This procedure has less successful results if there is medial patellar chondromalacia. A direct tibial tubercle anteriorization procedure may be considered in patients who have extensive patellofemoral involvement without an abnormal Q angle. Most surgeons attempt to elevate the tibial tubercle 10 to 12 mm. This procedure should be considered a salvage procedure and has less predictable results. In the most severe situations, patellectomy may be considered. Patients should clearly understand that there will be a significant loss of quadriceps strength following patellectomy. Satisfactory alignment should be achieved prior to patellectomy.

Regardless of the technique selected, patient and physician expectations must be clearly understood by each party. Patients should understand that patellofemoral crepitation cannot be eliminated with surgical procedures, that surgical treatment for patellofemoral disorders is not a quick fix, that the patient's commitment to physical therapy is critical, and that the recovery period following, for example, an arthroscopic lateral release is much longer than that after arthroscopic partial meniscectomy.

Distal patellar tendinitis (jumper's knee) is characterized by tenderness at the distal patellar pole. Quadriceps and hamstring tightness are frequently observed and should be appropriately treated with flexibility exercises. Eccentric quadriceps strengthening and a patellar tendon strap are helpful. In chronic situations, MRI may reveal a tendon necrosis within the patellar tendon, proximally. However, MRI is not absolutely essential if the physician is considering surgical treatment. Ulstrasonography is an alternative imaging modality. Patients should be treated conservatively for a minimum of 6 months before surgical treatment is considered. Local corticosteroid injection of the tendon should be avoided. Localized debridement of the patellar tendon in the region of localized tenderness can be beneficial.

Plica Syndrome

There are four synovial plica folds in the knee joint. The most clinically important synovial fold is the medial plica. It arises from the medial edge of the intercondylar fat pad and swings along the medial edge of the femoral condyle. Approximately 40% to 70% of patients undergoing arthroscopy will have a medial plica shelf. Its presence does not signify pathology nor does it warrant routine surgical debridement. Overall, clinical plica syndrome is uncommon. However, certain mechanisms of injury and sport-specific activities may place a patient at risk for irritating the medial plica shelf. Direct blunt trauma to the anteromedial aspect of the knee and repetitive flexion–extension sports, such as stair-stepper, bicycling, and running, may irritate the medial plica shelf, resulting in inflammation, localized synovitis, and subsequent fibrosis. Patients may complain of snapping and rub a hand along the anteromedial aspect of the knee in a band-like distribution. Occasionally, patients may have meniscal-like symptoms, rotational findings, and joint line tenderness.

During physical examination of a symptomatic medial plica shelf, rubbing directly in the area of the medial retinacular structure will reveal tenderness and a band tender to palpation. Most patients respond to conservative care. A cortisone injection into the plica band region was helpful in approximately 50% of patients. In patients with persistent pain who have not responded to the conservative modalities of ice, activity modification, and anti-inflammatory medication, arthroscopic debridement may be warranted. The medial plica shelf may make direct contact with the peripheral edge of the medial femoral condyle. There may be synovitis noted upon the superior shelf. Resection may be best achieved with the arthroscope in the inferolateral portal and a midpatellar or superolateral working portal with the knee in extension. In patients who have a symptomatic medial plica that warrants surgical excision, recovery is usually rapid and results excellent.

Reflex Sympathetic Dystrophy

RSD involving the knee region does not always follow the classic description associated with upper extremity RSD. Severe pain out of proportion to physical findings should make the orthopaedist suspicious of this disorder. Recent studies suggest that up to 30% of RSD involving the knee occurs subsequent to arthroscopic surgical intervention. This exaggerated response to injury is generally characterized by four findings: (1) pain out of proportion, (2) delayed functional recovery, (3) vasomotor disturbances (vasodilation/vasoconstriction), and (4) trophic changes. The classic clinical signs include decreased temperature, skin hypersensitivity, swelling, hyperhydrosis, and atrophic skin changes. Vasodilatation may result in decreased sympathetic activity, whereas vasoconstriction will result from increased sympathetic activity. Loss of flexion occurs more frequently than loss of extension, and the patellofemoral joint is frequently involved. RSD involving the knee joint may vary markedly from the classic description of this entity. It is important to recognize this disorder, because if the patient's pain is attributed to an intra-articular disorder a subsequent procedure might be performed that could worsen the RSD symptoms.

Treatment of the RSD should be initiated before any surgical treatment and should be considered even if there is a mechanical disorder. If the RSD is of a short duration (less than 6 weeks), treatment should consist of anti-inflammatory medication, contrast baths, muscle stimulation, supervised physical therapy, and weightbearing. If the symptoms persist for more than 6 weeks, a sympathetic block should be performed. It will confirm the diagnosis and may terminate symptoms. A continuous indwelling epidural block should be considered if symptoms persist or recur. An indwelling catheter may be used if manipulation or surgical treatment is indicated. Most authors consider flexion of less than 90° an indication for manipulation. A bupivicaine epidural block may be followed by the use of a narcotic epidural agent (meperidine, morphine, fentanyl), which may provide pain relief without producing a complete motor block. Using this protocol, an 80% success rate was achieved. An epidural protocol should be performed at least twice before surgical sympathectomy is considered. Chemical sympathectomy has a greater risk of complication and is more controversial. The key principle to treatment of RSD is early recognition, aggressive treatment, and avoiding unnecessary surgical procedures. The patient with multiple operations and severe pain may have an underlying RSD, and salvage procedures, such as Maquet patellofemoral decompression, total knee arthroplasty, and even knee arthrodesis, may not produce a pain-free extremity.

Extensor Mechanism Disruption

Soft-tissue extensor mechanism disruptions include quadriceps and patellar tendon ruptures. Quadriceps tendon ruptures occur generally in patients older than 40 years, whereas 80% of patients who sustain a patellar tendon rupture are younger than 40 years. Systemic medical diseases, such as diabetes, systemic lupus erythematosus, renal dysfunction, and gout, have been associated with both entities. Obesity is frequently associated with quadriceps tendon ruptures. The mechanism of injury is generally an eccentric contraction of the quadriceps on a partially flexed knee. Physical examination establishes the diagnosis for both entities. In each situation, the patient will be unable to actively extend the knee into terminal extension. If the extensor retinaculum is maintained, then patients may be able to actively extend the knee but will be unable to achieve full terminal extension. A palpable defect is diagnostic, and radiographs demonstrate either patella baja for quadriceps tendon ruptures or patella alta for patellar tendon ruptures. MRI is not necessary to establish a diagnosis, but generally gives visualization of the disruption.

In each entity, early surgical treatment is warranted. The results of early treatment are superior to those of delayed secondary reconstructive procedures. In the quadriceps tendon subgroup, age is an important factor affecting surgical results because these injuries may occur in the elderly patient population as well. Patellar tendon rupture patients may have some preexisting Osgood Schlatter or chronic patellar tendonitis symptoms. Steroid injections into the quadriceps or patellar tendons should be avoided because they have been implicated in tendon disruption. For quadriceps tendon ruptures, direct primary repair with nonabsorbable sutures through drill holes is performed most commonly. In chronic situations, a Scuderi quadriceps turndown, or Codivilla or Mason-Allen repair may be performed. With patellar tendon disruption, primary repair through longitudinal drill holes is most commonly performed. Reinforcement of the repair with semitendinosus tendon (Kelikian) has been reported. Although the standard postoperative treatment has been cast immobilization for quadriceps and patellar tendon repairs, early range of motion protocols may be used safely and effectively. Zero to 30°, 0 to 60°, and 0 to 90° increments of range of motion can safely be performed over 2-week intervals and will dramatically reduce knee motion complications. Most authors use cerclage wiring to protect the tendon repair with early range of motion protocols. In a delayed recognition of a patellar tendon rupture, preoperative traction via a Steinmann pin through the patella may be indicated. When performing repairs to the disrupted patellar tendon, the surgeon should avoid creating an iatrogenic patella baja. Preoperative radiographs of the opposite knee can be helpful for estimating the appropriate Insall-Salvati ratio.

Arthroscopy of the Knee

The evolution of arthroscopy of the knee has allowed the development of multiple techniques that were previously done with an open procedure. Procedures such as ligament reconstruction and meniscal repair are routinely done arthroscopically, thus making rehabilitation less painful and quicker. Many of these procedures are routinely performed on an outpatient basis. Arthroscope size has decreased, and the optics have continued to improve dramatically.

Although history and physical examination are the foundation of diagnosis of knee injuries, arthroscopy has improved accuracy and identified associated injuries. Treatment of meniscal and cruciate ligament injuries is vastly improved using arthroscopic techniques. Minimal resection of meniscal tears and repair of unstable tears near the peripheral vascular supply are the current standards and are technically feasible because of arthroscopy. The principles of anatomic placement of high strength anterior cruciate ligament (ACL) grafts with rigid fixation techniques are facilitated by use of the arthroscope.

A standard operating table that has an assortment of leg holders is generally used. Leg holders or a post allow medial and lateral stress to be applied to the knee in order to open the medial or lateral compartments for better visualization. An extremity tourniquet may be used, but it can be avoided by use of higher hydrostatic pressure or an arthroscopy pump. Both of these techniques produce a bloodless video field. Standard video cameras and equipment are used. Any procedure can be performed either with the leg suspended in the leg holder with the foot of the table down or with the table up and the foot in a holder. Diagnostic arthroscopy is then performed.

Arthroscopic Pumps

Arthroscopic pumps have been used to maintain a constant pressure in a joint and thus keep it inflated for better visualization. The inflow and outflow setup and the pump itself are much more complicated than a gravity feed system and require more training for hospital personnel. These devices should be monitored very carefully for complications that can occur, such as compartment syndromes. Immediate compartment fasciotomy and decompression are indicated if this complication occurs. In the knee with multiple ligament injury (medial collateral ligament, lateral collateral ligament complex) and in the shoulder, this possibility should be carefully checked. Whether a surgeon uses a pump or gravity feed for inflation of a joint depends on training and preference, but patient safety should always come first.

Office Arthroscopy and Outpatient Surgery

With improved optics and the size of arthroscopes decreasing, more patients are undergoing arthroscopy in the orthopaedist's office. Local anesthetics, anti-inflammatory medications, preoperative and postoperative patient education, smaller arthroscopes, and improved instruments make office arthroscopy feasible. Diagnostic examination, removal of loose bodies, local synovectomy (plica), and even partial meniscectomy can be performed as an office procedure.

Procedures such as ACL reconstruction and meniscus repair are routinely done on an outpatient or short-stay (< 24 hour) basis. Smaller incisions for graft harvest and newer arthroscopic techniques allow this to be done in a manner that involves minimal pain.

Lasers in Arthroscopic Surgery

Orthopaedic surgeons must become more aware of laser principles, selection, indications for use, limitations, and safety factors in arthroscopic surgery. A laser beam is an intense beam of light of any wavelength in the electromagnetic spectrum and includes visible, ultraviolet, and infrared light. Those used most commonly in arthroscopy include the CO_2 laser, the neodymium YAG (Nd YAG) laser, and the holmium laser. The holmium laser has gained more acceptance in arthroscopic surgery. Lasers can reach the inaccessible areas of the joint that cannot be reached by standard instruments. They can remove or coagulate tissue and thermally smooth tissue. Frayed or degenerative meniscus tears are approached by ablating the tissue. Flap tears or large fragments can be cut and removed. Laser use for chondromalacia (grades I-II) may be superior to mechanical methods of debridement. The smoothing effect produced by laser debridement can relieve symptoms of locking, catching, and crepitus produced by these lesions. Laser synovectomy can decrease bleeding and pain associated with this procedure.

However, lasers have considerable limitations. They lack the ability to remove or vaporize large volumes of tissue that can easily be removed with mechanical instruments. At present, laser ablation of tissue is not time efficient. Also, the cost of laser systems is prohibitive at the present time. The problems with safety and the cost of training hospital personnel cannot be overlooked. Eye protection must be worn at all times by all operating room personnel in order to avoid retinal or corneal damage. Because of these potential problems, the surgeon should become familiar with the use of lasers before attempting a surgical procedure.

Annotated Bibliography

ACL Injuries

Bach BR Jr, Jones GT, Sweet FA, et al: Arthroscopy-assisted anterior cruciate ligament reconstruction using patellar tendon substitution: Two- to four-year follow-up results. *Am J Sports Med* 1994;22:758–767.

Sixty-two patients were retrospectively evaluated at a minimum 2-year follow-up after two-incision arthroscopically assisted patellar tendon autograft reconstruction for ACL deficiency.

Daniel DM, Stone ML, Dobson BE, et al: Fate of the ACL-injured patient: A prospective outcome study. *Am J Sports Med* 1994;22:632–644.

A prospective outcome study of 292 patients at a median 64 months following acute arthrosis was reported. Patients were divided into four groups: early stable, no reconstruction; early unstable, no reconstruction; early reconstruction; and late reconstruction. The authors noted that sports participation hours per year and sports participation levels diminished in all four groups.

Howell SM, Taylor MA: Failure of reconstruction of the anterior cruciate ligament due to impingement by the intercondylar roof. *J Bone Joint Surg* 1993;75A:1044–1055.

Intercondylar roof impingement secondary to anterior tibial tunnel placement for ACL reconstructive surgery was evaluated. This diagnosis may be established with a lateral radiograph of a fully extended knee. In knees without impingement, extension without loss of stability was consistently obtained.

Karlson JA, Steiner ME, Brown CH, et al: Anterior cruciate ligament reconstruction using gracilis and semitendinosus tendons: Comparison of through-the-condyle and over-the-top graft placements. *Am J Sports Med* 1994;22:659–666.

Arthroscopy-assisted gracilis-semitendinosus reconstructions in 64 patients were retrospectively reviewed. The graft was placed through a femoral drill hole or in an over-the-top position. The authors noted no statistical differences between these groups in overall knee rating, range of motion, and KT-1000 arthrometer measurements.

Sgaglione NA, Del Pizzo W, Fox JM, et al: Arthroscopically assisted anterior cruciate ligament reconstruction with the pes anserine tendons: Comparison of results in acute and chronic ligament deficiency. *Am J Sports Med* 1993;21:249–256.

A retrospective study of 50 ACL reconstructions with hamstring tendons performed with an arthroscopically assisted technique was reported at a mean follow-up of 37 months. Objective outcome was superior in the acutely treated group.

Steiner ME, Hecker AT, Brown CH Jr, et al: Anterior cruciate ligament graft fixation: Comparison of hamstring and patellar tendon grafts. *Am J Sports Med* 1994;22:240–247.

Mechanical testing on older cadaveric knees was performed to assess a variety of fixation techniques for hamstring tendons and compare them to standard patellar tendon fixation techniques. Failure characteristics of a gracilis semitendinosus doubled tendon construct secured with soft tissue washers approximated those of interference screw fixation.

Magnetic Resonance Imaging

Speer KP, Spritzer CE, Bassett FH III, et al: Osseous injury associated with acute tears of the anterior cruciate ligament. *Am J Sports Med* 1992;20:382–389.

In a retrospective study, 54 patients with acute ACL injuries were studied by MRI within 45 days following the injury. Eighty-three percent of the patients were noted to have an osseous contusion over the lateral femoral condyle terminal sulcus.

Spindler KP, Schils JP, Bergfeld JA, et al: Prospective study of osseous, articular, and meniscal lesions in recent anterior cruciate ligament tears by magnetic resonance imaging and arthroscopy. *Am J Sports Med* 1993;21:551–557.

Within 3 months of initial injury, 54 patients with ACL injuries were prospectively reviewed. Eighty percent of the patients were noted to have a "bone bruise." Sixty-eight percent were noted on the lateral femoral condyle. The lateral meniscus was normal in 56%, the medial meniscus in 37%.

Complications of Knee Ligament Surgery

Fisher SE, Shelbourne KD: Arthroscopic treatment of symptomatic extension block complicating anterior cruciate ligament reconstruction. *Am J Sports Med* 1993;21:558–564.

In a series of 959 consecutive open ACL reconstructions, 42 patients in whom subsequent surgery was required for loss of extension were retrospectively identified and reviewed. Function and symptoms, specifically activity-related anterior knee pain, femoral extension crepitus, and knee stiffness, were markedly improved following surgical excision of extension block.

Harner CD, Irrgang JJ, Paul J, et al: Loss of motion after anterior cruciate ligament reconstruction. *Am J Sports Med* 1992;20:499–506.

To evaluate risk factors in patients who develop restricted motion following ACL surgery, 244 patients were retrospectively reviewed at a minimum of 1 year after surgery. Risk factors included acute reconstruction at less than 4 weeks from injury, male gender, concomitant MCL repair, and/or posterior oblique repair.

PCL Injuries

Covey CD, Sapega AA: Injuries of the posterior cruciate ligament. *J Bone Joint Surg* 1993;75A:1376–1386.

This review describes the morphology, blood supply, and innervation of the PCL anatomy; functional biomechanics of the PCL and posterolateral complex; mechanisms of clinical injuries; natural history of PCL injuries; and diagnosis via physical examination, imaging, and arthroscopic evaluation. Both nonsurgical and surgical treatment for osseous avulsion injuries, isolated injuries, and combined injuries are discussed.

Posterolateral Complex Injuries

Noyes FR, Schipplein OD, Andriacchi TP, et al: The anterior cruciate ligament-deficient knee with varus alignment: An analysis of gait adaptations and dynamic joint loadings. *Am J Sports Med* 1992;20:707–716.

Thirty-two ACL-deficient patients with varus alignments were evaluated with gait analysis. Twenty demonstrated abnormal high adduction moments on the affected knee. Fifteen of 32 knees had abnormally high lateral soft-tissue forces suggestive of lateral compartment tensile forces and medial compartment compressive forces.

Skyhar MJ, Warren RF, Ortiz GJ, et al: The effects of sectioning of the posterior cruciate ligament and the posterolateral complex on the articular contact pressures within the knee. *J Bone Joint Surg* 1993;75A:694–699.

Patellofemoral knee compartment contact pressures were measured with prescale, low pressure Fuji film in 10 fresh-frozen cadaver knees. Effects of sectioning of the PCL and posterolateral complex were studied. Combined sectioning of the PCL and posterolateral complex resulted in the most significant elevation of patellofemoral contact pressures. Medial compartment pressures were most significantly elevated after PCL sectioning.

Veltri DM, Warren RF: Posterolateral instability of the knee, in Jackson DW (ed): *Instructional Course Lectures 44*. Rosemont, IL, American Academy of Orthopaedic Surgeons, 1995, pp 441–453.

Posterolateral corner anatomy, biomechanics, and clinical application are described along with mechanisms of posterolateral injuries, clinical presentation, and physical examination findings. Surgical reconstruction in the acute and chronic settings are described.

MCL Injuries

Robins AJ, Newman AP, Burks RT: Postoperative return of motion in anterior cruciate ligament and medial collateral ligament injuries: The effect of medial collateral ligament rupture location. *Am J Sports Med* 1993;21:20–25.

A retrospective review of 20 patients with complete ACL/MCL injuries was performed. Motion problems occurred more frequently in proximal MCL injuries. At follow-up, patients with distal MCL injuries obtained significantly more flexion.

Shelbourne KD, Porter DA: Anterior cruciate ligament: Medial collateral ligament injury. Non-operative management of medial collateral ligament tears with anterior cruciate ligament reconstruction: A preliminary report. *Am J Sports Med* 1992;20:283–286.

Between 1983 and 1989, 84 patients were retrospectively reviewed following surgical reconstruction of the ACL and nonsurgical management of the MCL injury. Although the MCL injuries were not stratified, nonoperative management of the MCL in association with acute ACL reconstructive surgery had predictably good and excellent results.

Synthetic Grafts

Gillquist J, Odensten M: Reconstruction of old anterior cruciate ligament tears with a Dacron prosthesis: A prospective study. *Am J Sports Med* 1993;21:358–366.

A review of 70 patients in a prospective study at 5-year follow-up revealed a success rate of approximately 50%. The authors concluded that this was not a satisfactory result. A 23% incidence of graft rupture was noted within the 5-year follow-up period.

Paulos LE, Rosenberg TD, Grewe SR, et al: The GORE-TEX anterior cruciate ligament prosthesis: A long-term follow-up. *Am J Sports Med* 1992;20:246–252.

The authors retrospectively reviewed 188 of 268 patients in whom a Gore-Tex ACL prosthesis was implanted. Minimum 2-year, average 4-year follow-up noted that acceptable results were noted in only 44% of the patients; 34% experienced effusions.

Santi MD, Richardson AB: The ligament augmentation device in hamstring grafts for reconstruction of the anterior cruciate ligament. *Am J Sports Med* 1994;22: 524–530.

Twenty-eight patients in whom ACL reconstruction with an LAD was used in conjunction with semitendinosus and gracilis reconstruction were compared to 32 patients reconstructed with STG grafts without the LAD at an average of 31 months postoperatively, with no differences noted.

Allografts

Indelicato PA, Linton RC, Huegel M: The results of fresh-frozen patellar tendon allografts for chronic anterior cruciate ligament deficiency of the knee. *Am J Sports Med* 1992;20:118–121.

A prospective review of 73 patients undergoing fresh-frozen and patellar tendon allograft ACL reconstruction was performed. At follow-up, 78% of the patients had a negative pivot shift, and 92% have ≤ 5 mm KT-1000 side-to-side difference at 20 lbs.

Noyes FR, Barber-Westin SD, Roberts CS: Use of allografts after failed treatment of rupture of the anterior cruciate ligament. *J Bone Joint Surg* 1994;76A:1019–1031.

A prospective study of 66 patients using irradiated bone-tendon-bone allograft with a 23 to 78-month follow-up was reported. In this group, 32 patients had concurrent LAD. No difference was noted in anteroposterior translations in those who underwent allograft reconstruction and those who underwent allograft supplemented with a LAD.

Knee Bracing

France EP, Paulos LE: Knee bracing. *J Am Acad Orthop Surg* 1994;2:281–287.

The biomechanics of knee bracing with discussions regarding knee mechanics and stability are presented. Rationale for brace function; design, including mechanical properties; and brace hinge design is discussed. Functional characteristics, efficacy, and recommendations of brace types are summarized.

Meniscal Tears/Repairs

Cannon WD, Morgan CD: Meniscal repair: Arthroscopic repair techniques, in Schafer M (ed): *Instructional Course Lectures 43.* Rosemont, IL, American Academy of Orthopaedic Surgeons, 1994, pp 77–96.

Henning inside-outside technique and description of fibrin clot are discussed. Preoperative planning and details regarding surgical techniques of medial and lateral meniscal repair are described. An increased incidence of meniscal healing was noted with synchronous ACL reconstruction, shorter tears, lateral repairs, and more normal rims.

DeHaven KE, Arnoczky SP: Meniscus repair: Basic science, indications for repair, and open repair, in Schafer M (ed): *Instructional Course Lectures 43.* Rosemont, IL, American Academy of Orthopaedic Surgeons, 1994, pp 65–76.

The basic science, gross anatomy, ultrastructure, biochemistry, function, vascular anatomy, and healing of the menisci and indications for arthroscopic and open meniscal repair are reviewed. Survival rates of 89% at 5 years and 79% at 10 years were reported. A higher failure rate was noted in unstable knees: 38% at 5 years, and 54% at 10 years.

Keane GC, Bickerstaff D, Rae PJ, et al: The natural history of meniscal tears in anterior cruciate ligament insufficiency. *Am J Sports Med* 1993;21:672–679.

This retrospective study reviewed 176 consecutive patients undergoing ACL reconstruction acutely, subacutely, and chronically. The incidence of medial meniscal tears increased with chronicity. A 92% meniscal repair survivorship was noted at an average follow-up of 40 months with an 8% repeated surgery rate.

Neyret P, Donell ST, DeJour D, et al: Partial meniscectomy and anterior cruciate ligament rupture in soccer players: A study with a minimum 20-year follow-up. *Am J Sports Med* 1993;21:455–460.

The authors retrospectively reviewed 77 soccer athletes in whom 91 knees underwent rim preserving meniscectomy, with an average 27-year follow-up. The patients were divided into ACL intact and ACL deficient subgroups. Radiographic osteoarthritis was noted in 24% of the ACL intact versus 77% of the ACL deficient patients. Sports participation and patient's subjective satisfaction were statistically different among these two subgroups.

Patellar Pain

Fulkerson JP: Patellofemoral pain disorders: Evaluation and management. *J Am Acad Orthop Surg* 1994;2:124–132.

The author reviews the history and physical examination of patellofemoral pain disorders, and discusses imaging techniques. Nonsurgical and surgical approaches are reviewed.

Reflex Sympathetic Dystrophy

Cooper DE, DeLee JC: Reflex sympathetic dystrophy of the knee. *J Am Acad Orthop Surg* 1994;2:79–86.

This review summarizes the literature and discusses epidemiology, pathophysiology RSD stages, clinical signs and symptoms, diagnostic evaluation and work-up, and treatment. A treatment algorithm for RSD of the knee is presented.

Knee Biomechanics

Anderson AF, Snyder RB, Federspiel CF, et al: Instrumented evaluation of knee laxity: A comparison of five arthrometers. *Am J Sports Med* 1992;20:135–140.

The authors prospectively reviewed 50 normal control knees in 50 patients with chronic unilateral ACL deficiency. The study demonstrated differences among testing devices and the authors concluded that anterior knee laxity could not be generalized from one device to another. Maximum manual tests improved the accuracy of each device.

Cooper DE, Deng XH, Burstein AL, et al: The strength of the central third patellar tendon graft: A biomechanical study. *Am J Sports Med* 1993;21:818–824.

Mechanical testing was performed in human cadaveric knee preparations whose average donor age was 28 years. Effects of twisting the graft 90° and 180° were reported. Rotating the graft 90° increased strength, but rotation of 180° had no significant effect. Increased mean ultimate loads of 2,977 for 10-mm grafts support the practice of using smaller grafts in clinical situations.

Advances in Arthroscopy

Austin KS, Sherman OH: Complications of arthroscopic meniscal repair. *Am J Sports Med* 1993;21:864–869.

Damage to the medial side of the knee (saphenous) is at greatest risk. However, most of these complications resolve and will have satisfactory result after appropriate treatment.

Buss DD, Warren RF, Wickiewicz TL, et al: Arthroscopically assisted reconstruction of the anterior cruciate ligament with use of autogenous patellar-ligament grafts: Results after twenty-four to forty-two months. *J Bone Joint Surg* 1993;75A:1346–1355.

Combined with early aggressive rehabilitation, arthroscopic anterior cruciate ligament reconstruction was as effective as open surgery, and the likelihood of patellofemoral pain and stiffness decreased.

O'Brien SJ, Miller DV, Fealy SV, et al: Lasers and the meniscus, in Mow VC, Arnoczky SP, Jackson DW (eds): *Knee Meniscus, Basic and Clinical Foundations.* New York, NY, Raven Press, 1992, pp 153–164.

This chapter summarizes laser principles and their application in arthroscopy. Different lasers that are available (CO_2, Excimer, KTP, Ho YAG) are discussed with their advantages and disadvantages.

Classic Bibliography

Albright JP, Powell JW, Smith W, et al: Medial collateral ligament knee sprains in college football: Brace wear preferences and injury risk. *Am J Sports Med* 1994;22: 2–11.

Albright JP, Powell JW, Smith W, et al: Medial collateral ligament knee sprains in college football: Effectiveness of preventive braces. *Am J Sports Med* 1994;22:12–19.

Bach BR Jr, Warren RF, Flynn WM, et al: Arthrometric evaluation of knees that have a torn anterior cruciate ligament. *J Bone Joint Surg* 1990;72A:1299–1306.

Belzer JP, Cannon WD Jr: Meniscus tears: Treatment of the stable and unstable knee. *J Am Acad Orthop Surg* 1993;1:41–47.

Beynnon BD, Pope MH, Wertheimer CM, et al: The effect of functional knee-braces on strain on the anterior cruciate ligament in vivo. *J Bone Joint Surg* 1992;74A: 1298–1312.

Bolano LE, Grana WA: Isolated arthroscopic partial meniscectomy: Functional radiographic evaluation at five years. *Am J Sports Med 1993;*21:432–437.

Cannon WD Jr, Vittori JM: The incidence of healing in arthroscopic meniscal tears in anterior cruciate ligament-reconstructed knees versus stable knees. *Am J Sports Med* 1992;20:176–181.

Clancy WG Jr, Pandya RD: Posterior cruciate ligament reconstruction with patellar tendon autograft. *Clin Sports Med* 1994;13:561–570.

Clancy WG Jr, Shelbourne KD, Zoellner GB, et al: Treatment of knee joint instability secondary to rupture of the posterior cruciate ligament. *J Bone Joint Surg* 1983; 65A:310–322.

Cosgarea AJ, DeHaven KE, Lovelock JE: The surgical treatment of arthrofibrosis of the knee. *Am J Sports Med* 1994; 22:184–191.

Daniel BM, Stone ML, Sachs R, et al: Instrumented measurement of anterior knee laxity in patients with acute anterior cruciate ligament destruction. *Am J Sports Med* 1985; 13:401–407

Johnson RJ, Beynnon BD, Nichols CE, et al: Current concepts review: The treatment of injuries of the anterior cruciate ligament. *J Bone Joint Surg* 1992;74A:140–151.

Keller PM, Shelbourne KD, McCarroll JR, et al: Nonoperatively treated isolated posterior cruciate ligament injuries. *Am J Sports Med* 1993;21:132–136.

Larson RL, Taillon M: Anterior cruciate ligament insufficiency: Principles of treatment. *J Am Acad Orthop Surg* 1994; 2:36–43.

Noyes FR, Barber SD, Simon R: High tibial osteotomy and ligament reconstruction in varus angulated, anterior cruciate ligament-deficient knees: A two- to seven-year follow-up study. *Am J Sports Med* 1993;21:2–12.

O'Brien SJ, Warren RF, Pavlov H, et al: Reconstruction of the chronically insufficient anterior cruciate ligament with the central third of the patellar ligament. *J Bone Joint Surg* 1991;73A:278–286.

Parolie JM, Bergfeld JA: Long-term results of nonoperative treatment of isolated posterior cruciate ligament injuries in the athlete. *Am J Sports Med* 1986:14:35–38.

Paulos LE, Rosenberg TD, Grewe SR, et al: The GORE-TEX anterior cruciate ligament prosthesis: A long-term followup. *Am J Sports Med* 1992;20:246–252.

Paulos LE, Wnorowski DC, Greenwald AE: Infrapatellar contracture syndrome: Diagnosis, treatment, and long-term follow-up. *Am J Sports Med* 1994;22:440–449.

Shelbourne KD, Wilckens JH, Mollabaschy YA, et al: Arthrofibrosis in acute anterior cruciate ligament reconstruction: The effective timing of reconstruction and rehabilitation. *Am J Sports Med* 1991;19:332–336.

Steiner ME, Brown C, Zarins B, et al: Measurement of anterior-posterior displacement of the knee: A comparison of the results with instrumented devices and with clinical examination. *J Bone Joint Surg* 1990;72A: 1307–1315.

Wascher DC, Grauer JD, Markoff KL: Biceps tendon tenodesis for posterolateral instability of the knee: An in vitro study. *Am J Sports Med* 1993;21:400–406.

Wasilewski SA, Covall DJ, Cohen S: Effect of surgical timing on recovery and associated injuries after anterior cruciate ligament reconstruction. *Am J Sports Med* 1993; 21:338–342

41

Knee: Reconstruction

Introduction

The adult who has severe knee arthritis suffers from pain and the inability to function physically. Fortunately, orthopaedic treatment approaches have much to offer such a patient. This chapter summarizes the patient presentation, diagnostic evaluations, and options in management. The benefits, risks, outcomes, and surgical aspects of management will be discussed. A prosthetic categorization system is presented (Fig. 1).

Evaluation of the Knee

Pain and Tenderness

The patient suffering from osteoarthritis of the knee has pain about the articulating surfaces of the knee joint. This pain is typically aggravated by weightbearing. In comparison, patients with inflammatory arthritis tend to experience persistent and more diffuse pain. The patients with inflammatory arthritis, in active phases of their disease, will have a greater synovial reaction and diffuse tenderness about the joint.

Less common pathologies that affect the knee joint, such as osteonecrosis, posttraumatic arthritis, gout, calcium pyrophosphate dihydrate (CPPD) disease, and hemophilia are important to recognize because they have different clinical presentations, natural histories, and therapeutic considerations. The patient with osteonecrosis will tend to have night pain and will usually have maximal tenderness overlying osseous surfaces remote from the articulating surfaces. Patients with posttraumatic arthritis may have been treated surgically and have tender cutaneous neuromas from scarring in previous incisions. Patients with acute gout or CPPD disease will have severe pain, which is disproportionate to the severity of their radiologic findings, during a disease flare. Aspiration and pharmacologic treatment of the underlying inflammatory condition will usually result in symptomatic relief.

Local soft-tissue disease, including pes anserine bursitis, iliotibial band syndrome, patellar tendonitis, and hamstring tenosynovitis, should be differentiated from joint surface pathology. Patients with bursitis will usually have significant intrabursal swelling of the involved region. Patients with tendonitis will have localized tenderness and, usually, pain with loading maneuvers of the involved structure. Radiating pain from remote pathology at the hip and occasionally the back may be difficult to differentiate from primary knee pathology.

The accurate measurement of pain has become increasingly important in patient management. Regulatory organizations have suggested that the patient should actively participate in the systematic recording of his or her pain state. Several tools, including visual analog and Likert scales have been created to facilitate this process. Patient-based outcome assessment instruments, such as the Medical Outcomes Study Short Form—36 questions (SF-36), have global scales to assess this health dimension. The Western Ontario MacMasters (WOMAC), a hip and knee arthritis-specific outcome tool, has the advantage of adding sensitivity in the systematic assessment of this patient group.

Mechanical Symptoms

The patient who presents with the mechanical symptom of true knee joint locking or catching should be carefully assessed for intra-articular pathology. These patients may have a mechanical lesion that effectively results in an unstable loose body. It then becomes lodged between the femorotibial or the patellofemoral articulations. This mechanical interference with normal knee kinematics will cause intermittent episodes of catching or even true joint locking.

Intra-articular lesions that can result in mechanical symptoms include torn menisci, articular cartilage flap tears, and intra-articular loose bodies. Meniscal tears are usually caused by an acute traumatic event. Young patients will usually present with a history of intra-articular swelling from the bleeding of a peripheral tear. However, older patients with preexisting meniscal degeneration and devascularization will require less energy to cause a tear and may not have significant bleeding or swelling.

Articular cartilage flap tears and loose bodies may be associated with patellar dislocation or osteonecrosis. Articular cartilage flap tears are more likely associated with progression of osteoarthrosis in the older patient. The identification of radiolucent intra-articular loose bodies may require the use of arthroscopic techniques due to the lack of diagnostic accuracy of noninvasive imaging. Rarely, synovial chondromatosis can be the source of intra-articular loose bodies.

Symptoms of giving way of the knee are nonspecific. This symptom complex may be associated with patellofemoral symptoms or the aforementioned intra-articular pathologies of meniscal tears or loose bodies. In highly active patients, ligamentous insufficiency should be identified through clinical evaluation and, occasionally, through the use of magnetic resonance imaging (MRI) or arthroscopic techniques. More commonly, especially in the

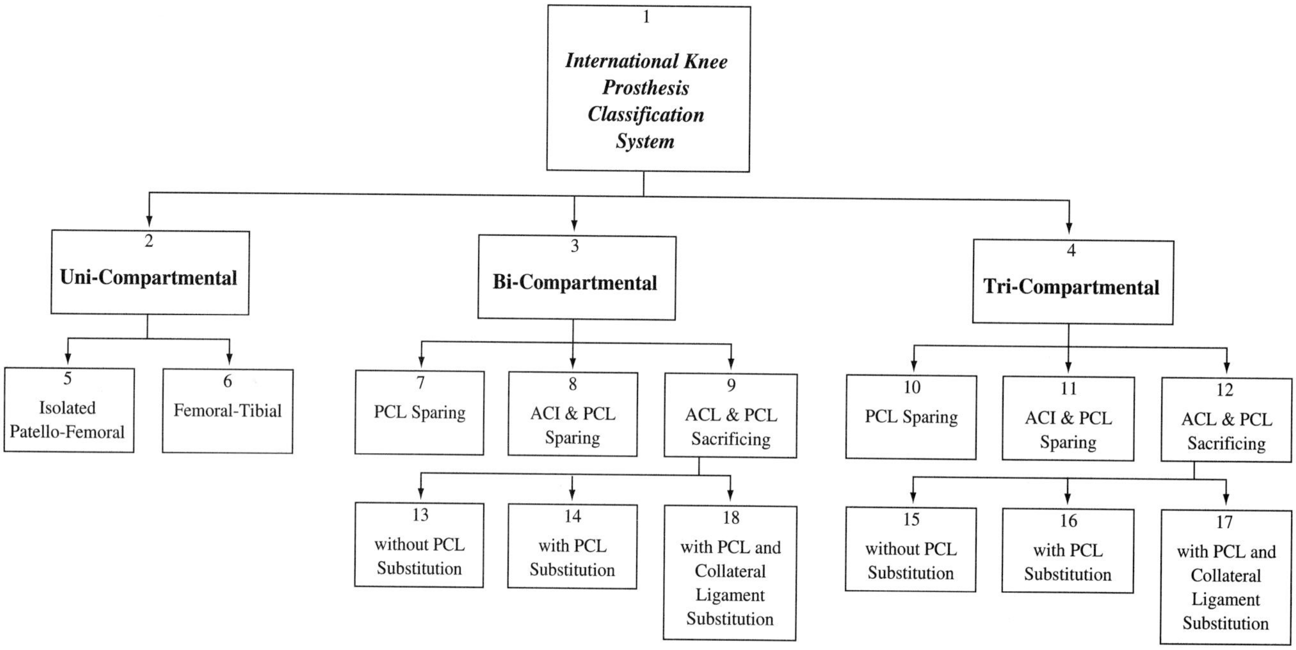

Fig. 1 International Knee Prosthesis Classification System. (Reproduced with permission from the International Knee Society.)

adult, giving way is associated with rehabilitative deficiencies of the quadriceps and hamstring muscle groups.

Gait abnormalities in the patient with significant knee pathology are being better understood. In particular, the presence of an adductor pattern is associated with premature repeated surgery in patients after osteotomy. These patients may be better treated with placement of the limb in more valgus alignment to enhance longevity. Scientific proof of the effectiveness of this postulate is pending.

Neurovascular Status

The patient's neurovascular status should be delineated at baseline and at periodic intervals. Clinical assessment of extremity vascularity is a prerequisite to surgical intervention. In the patient with vascular compromise, preoperative Doppler ultrasound evaluation and calculation of ankle:brachial ratios may be helpful to allow detection of the patient at risk for postoperative arterial insufficiency. Duplex Doppler ultrasound evaluation can be helpful in the detection of proximal thigh venous thrombi.

Outcome Assessments

The use of structured patient evaluation is becoming increasingly important. The principal components of outcome assessment as applied to the adult reconstructive patient include the systematic evaluation of demography, access to care, satisfaction with care, patient-based general health status (SF-36), patient-based disease-specific measures (WOMAC), comorbidity stratification measures (Greenfield, Charlson), and the processes of care utilized. Assessment tools are discussed in the chapter on Outcomes Assessment.

Radiographic Evaluation

Plain radiographic evaluation of the patient with knee pain undergoing diagnostic evaluation should include standing anteroposterior (AP) views of both knees, lateral view, Merchant's (sunrise) view, and tunnel views. Additional views that may be helpful include obliques, the standing posteroanterior (PA) notch view, and the standing lateral radiograph. The flexed knee standing views allow evaluation of the posterior aspect of the tibiofemoral articulation. Although these investigations can add sensitivity in the identification of clinical disease, complete statistical characterization demonstrating the utility of these additional views is lacking.

In addition to the objective identification and compartmental localization of knee arthritis, the plain radiographic views are helpful in identification of the less common diseases that afflict the knee. Of particular value is the identification of diseases that are relative or absolute contraindications to particular surgical therapies. For example, calcium pyrophosphate disease, which is identified through meniscal calcification, is one of the less common diseases and is considered a relative contraindication to the performance of unicompartmental arthroplasty or osteotomy.

To obtain the maximum benefit of a major knee reconstruction, restoration of appropriate limb and joint alignment is important. Extremes of postoperative malalignments are associated with instability, premature loosening, and excessive wear. Identification of limb malalignment factors, such as bowing or previous fractures, that adversely affect the surgeon's ability to achieve an appropriate postoperative alignment is essential. Preoperative radiographic evaluation extends the basic diagnostic evaluation to the determination of femoral geometry, tibial geometry, and the resultant overall extremity alignment. Frontal plane alignment details can be obtained through the use of long leg radiographs or independent films of the femur and tibia.

In the patient with complaints following total knee replacement, fluoroscopically positioned radiographs may be valuable. Due to the geometry of the knee replacement components, if the x-ray beam is not parallel to the surface, the bone–prosthesis interface will not be demonstrated. Careful positioning, using fluoroscopy, can overcome this limitation (Fig. 2).

Nonsurgical Alternatives in the Management of the Patient with Knee Arthritis

Medical management of the patient with early stages of knee arthritis can be helpful. It has been noted that the patient with knee arthritis can have substantial symptomatic improvement through the use of nonimpact muscle strengthening. Statistically significant pain reduction has been noted in patients entered into a supervised course of rehabilitation.

The use of acetaminophen has been found to be equal to the use of non-steroidal anti-inflammatory agents (NSAIDs) in the short-term management of the patient with knee osteoarthritis. Investigations using patient reporting (visual analogue scale) have demonstrated that both classes of medication will result in a pain reduction of approximately 33%. In light of the high gastrointestinal complication rates associated with chronic use of NSAIDs, the initial use of acetaminophen as a pain reliever is justified. Nevertheless, NSAIDs will remain a valuable medical alternative in the long-term management of patients with knee arthritis.

Both the usage and the usefulness of intra-articular injections of corticosteroids have been evaluated. In one long-term follow-up study of patients with primary knee osteoarthritis, it has been noted that those patients treated with corticosteroid injections had a greater likelihood of developing a varus deformity and more advanced radiographic degeneration. Also, the use of intraoperative steroids after arthroscopy has been demonstrated to be associated with an increased likelihood of postoperative infection.

Arthroscopy

Whereas the benefits of knee arthroscopy to address intra-articular pathology are clear and complications are infrequent, its role in the patient with knee arthritis remains controversial. Although knee synovectomy in the treatment of rheumatic disease may benefit the patient by reducing soft-tissue swelling and slowing articular destruction, the incremental impact of surgery is less clear at 5 years.

One study has demonstrated the prognostic value of arthroscopy and synovial biopsy in patients being treated for rheumatoid arthritis. In this investigation, arthroscopic findings were combined with clinical, histologic, hematologic, and immunohistologic analysis. Positive factors associated with disease progression included the clinical score, arthroscopic findings of synovitis, arthroscopic extent of cartilage damage, the immunohistologic demonstration of immunoglobulin A (IgA) positive cells and antifibrinogen positive deposits in the synovial lining.

The role of arthroscopy in the management of the older patient with knee osteoarthritis is less clear. Recent long-term follow-up studies have demonstrated the unpredictable nature of abrasion arthroplasty as a therapeutic procedure. In one study, 50% of those patients who had undergone arthroscopic abrasion arthroplasty had required knee replacement at 3 years. In the patient with coexisting meniscal pathology and osteoarthritis, abrasion arthroplasty of grade III and IV lesions has not been found to be helpful. Recently, one randomized controlled trial has even brought into question the incremental benefit of meniscal debridement in comparison to simple lavage for the patient with coexisting degenerative arthritis and meniscal pathology. Nevertheless, for the patient with mechanical symptoms superimposed on the clinical picture of osteoarthritis, arthroscopy appears to be of benefit.

Unicompartmental Knee Disease

Unicompartmental osteoarthritic involvement of the knee is common. Inflammatory arthritis is by definition not unicompartmental. Thus, techniques developed to address unicompartmental osteoarthritis are not usually helpful in the more generalized inflammatory conditions of rheumatoid arthritis, gout, and calcium pyrophosphate disease. Even in the case of osteoarthritis, by the time that the patient presents to the orthopaedic surgeon, knee arthritis has frequently progressed beyond unicompartmental involvement. Several large case series of patients presenting to the orthopaedist have revealed that the number of patients who could be considered candidates for unicompartmental therapies is low—usually below 10%.

Osteotomy

The use of both tibial and femoral osteotomy for management of adults with knee arthritis is declining, and the reasons are multiple. Data from several long-term follow-up investigations have demonstrated that the return of knee pain and dysfunction after osteotomy is time dependent. Although early favorable results exceed 85%, multiple groups have reported increasing failure rates in the long

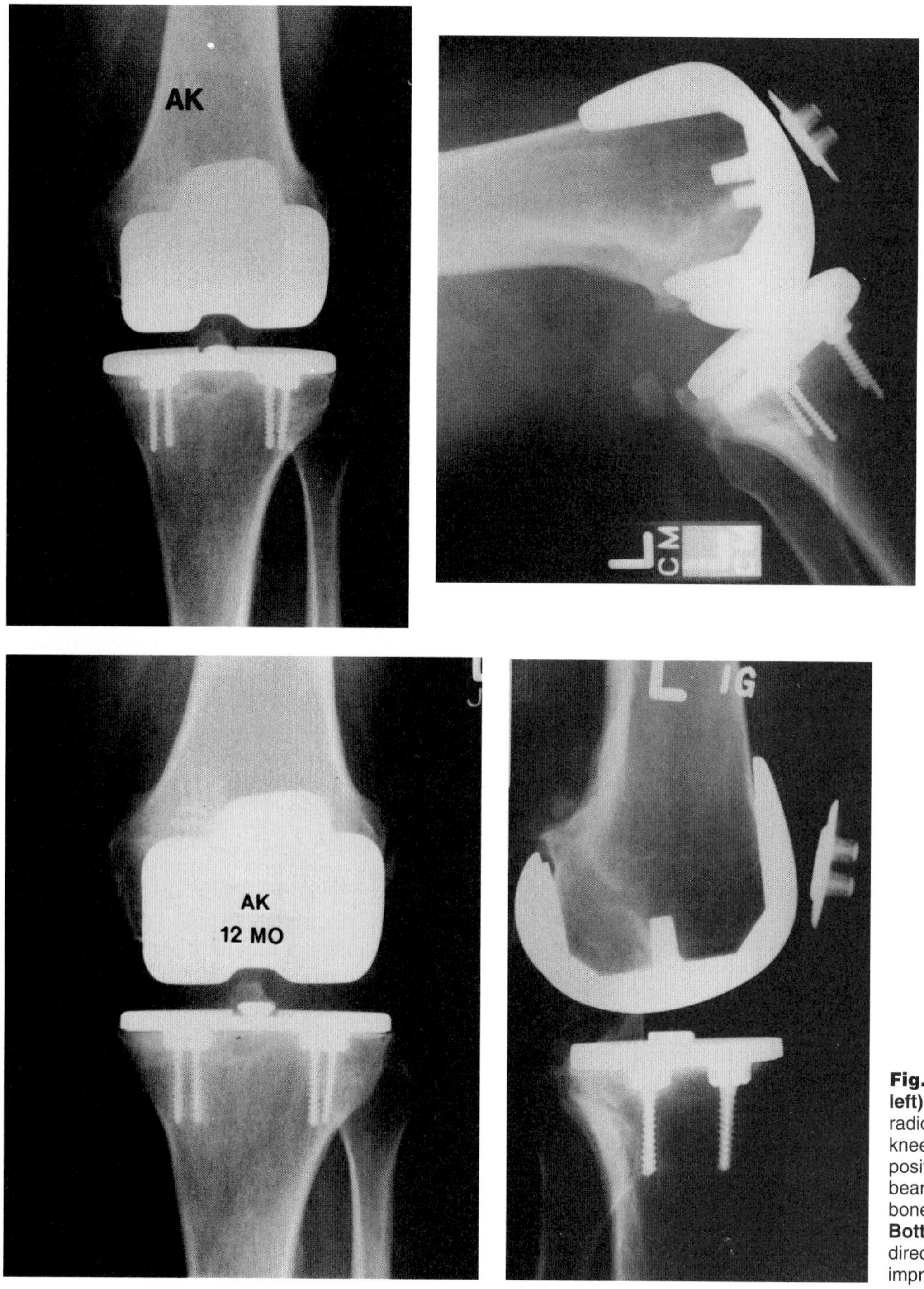

Fig. 2 Anteroposterior **(top left)** and lateral **(top right)** radiographs of a cementless total knee arthroplasty. Routine positioning of the knee and x-ray beam does not demonstrate the bone–prosthesis interface. **Bottom,** Fluoroscopically directed radiographs allow for improved interface visualization.

term. The actual late failure rate is uncertain because of the variable methods of assessment and the range of reporting styles.

One investigation with consistent endpoints and careful follow-up has reported on 40 patients treated for osteoarthritis by proximal tibial osteotomy. Risk factors for early failure included obesity, advanced age, and the extremes of frontal plane malalignment. Continued useful function of the knee was identified in only 86% at 1 year, 50% at 5 years, and 28% at 9 years.

Both early and late tibial and femoral osteotomy failure rates are substantially greater than those of either unicompartmental or tricompartmental knee replacement. As a result of this experience, the indications for osteotomy in the adult are narrowing. It remains most useful in the younger patient with osteoarthritis or posttraumatic arthritis and accompanying malalignment in whom it is expected to be a temporizing procedure.

Preoperative planning is an integral part of successful osteotomy surgery. The surgeon must first determine the principal site of deformity. In the most common presentation, a patient will have medial compartmental disease with associated tibia vara. This disease pattern is best treated with a valgus producing, proximal tibial osteotomy. In general, the osteotomy itself should be performed in the well-vascularized, metaphyseal portion of the proximal tibia. Both laterally based, closing wedge osteotomies and cylindrical osteotomies have been described. The cylindrical osteotomy is generally preferred because this technique is bone conserving, and it allows the surgeon to address a wider range of frontal plane malalignments. For lesser deformities, the closing wedge technique is an acceptable alternative.

Multiple approaches to fixation of the osteotomy have been described, including cast immobilization, staple fixation, screw and wire fixation, blade plates, and external fixation. No one technique of internal fixation has demonstrated clear superiority over the alternatives. The use of external fixation has fallen out of favor due to the recognized complication of pin tract infection. Because many of the patients treated with osteotomy will require subsequent knee replacement, this risk of infection should be avoided. The use of secure internal fixation will allow early mobilization and range of motion exercises.

Supracondylar femoral osteotomy is rarely performed. It is most frequently indicated in the patient with lateral compartment osteoarthritis and femoral valgus. Most commonly, a closing wedge technique with stapling or blade plate fixation is used. The late outcomes in patients who have received this treatment approach appear similar to those of proximal tibial osteotomy for varus deformity.

Unicompartmental Knee Replacement

Initial clinical reports involving unicompartmental knee replacement were encouraging but quickly underwent reassessment with subsequent reports of less durable outcomes. Internationally, however, the Swedish National Registry demonstrated encouraging results with unicompartmental replacement. Further clarification of the factors associated with success and failure have led to the rekindled interest in the United States. Recent meta-analyses have demonstrated that unicompartmental results rival those of tricompartmental arthroplasty. Ten-year follow-up investigations have demonstrated durability of over 91%. Good to excellent results were seen in 80% of patients. The reasons for failure are evenly distributed between aseptic loosening and disease progression in the unreplaced compartment. The use of unicompartmental replacement allows the implementation of a patient–prosthesis matching program that minimizes short-term patient morbidity, provides an improved postoperative range of motion, and has comparable 10-year durability.

Several authors have suggested that the ideal candidate for unicompartmental replacement is the elderly male patient with low activity demands who is not obese, and who has predominately medial or lateral compartmental osteoarthritis, intact cruciate ligaments, frontal plane malalignment of less than 15°, and a range of motion of at least 90°. The observation that the male patient has better outcomes is somewhat paradoxical and may be related to bone quality. A recent meta-analysis has suggested that the improved results of unicompartmental arthroplasty since 1987 may be associated with improved patient selection. Although unicompartmental arthroplasty can be performed in patients who deviate from the ideal, the greater the deviation, the higher the anticipated failure rate.

The surgical technique of unicompartmental arthroplasty is demanding. Because of the infrequency of performance, many surgeons have not had the opportunity to develop familiarity with the technique. Several factors are key to long-term success in this procedure. The prosthesis selected should be of low surface constraint and of a resurfacing design. Thin (< 8 mm) polyethylene components should be avoided.

During preparation for femoral component insertion, care should be taken to avoid patellar impingement by making certain that the anterior flange is recessed. To minimize femoral component loosening and fracture, the entire component should be well supported by bone. Care should be taken to be certain that there are no gaps between the posterior flange and the condyle. The frontal plane position should be perpendicular to the femoral mechanical axis. The transverse plane position should parallel the condylar axis. The femoral component should not impinge on the tibial spine in extension.

The tibial component frontal plane alignment should be perpendicular to the tibial mechanical axis. The sagittal plane position should parallel the normal posterior inclination of the tibial plateau. With flexion and extension of the knee, the tibial component should remain stable and not elevate anteriorly with knee flexion. The tibial component should be placed on a firm cancellous bed with anchoring holes for methacrylate interdigitation. All osteophytes should be removed. Methylmethacrylate fixation of the components is preferred because it has resulted in more predictable success than porous biologic fixation. Overall frontal plane limb alignment should be in neutral. Both over- and undercorrection have been associated with premature failure.

By paying close attention to both patient selection and technical execution, prosthetic longevity rates can easily exceed 90% at 10 years. Even should a failure occur, the difficulties of salvage have been reduced with the development of improved revision knee replacement systems.

Total Knee Arthroplasty

The number of total knee arthroplasties (TKAs) performed in North America continues to increase; it is now estimated to be over 150,000 annually. Total knee prosthesis designs have continued to converge on a tricompartmental replacement similar to the early total condylar prosthesis. Improvements in instrumentation have emphasized the correct placement of the prosthetic components in all three planes (coronal, sagittal, and transverse), while changes in the articulation itself have attempted to decrease contact stress. In spite of design changes, however, failure associated with polyethylene failure and the effects of wear debris has dominated discussion of the long-term outcome of this operation.

Patient Selection

Patient selection is based on a series of factors including age, weight, gender, patient expectations, and clinical diagnosis. Pain and functional impairment coupled with imaging studies (most often plain radiograph), which confirm the loss of articular surfaces (usually due to osteoarthrosis or rheumatoid arthritis), are the most common indications. Other causes of articular surface degeneration (such as posttraumatic arthrosis and osteonecrosis) have been successfully treated with TKA; however, the extension of this operation to these younger and more active patients must be tempered by understanding that the production of wear debris may limit the functional lifetime of a prosthesis.

The thin, elderly patient with low functional demands is the ideal candidate for TKA. Many older patients wish to maintain an active lifestyle, and functional demands of today's 65-year-old and older patient are greater than those in the past. The orthopaedist is frequently confronted with younger and heavier patients who desire a greater degree of function in whom arthrosis has severely limited the patient's lifestyle. Careful attention to the alternatives to replacement arthroplasty can result in effective treatment of some, but the rest of these patients represent the "edge of the envelope" of knee replacement arthroplasty. It is the orthopaedist's duty to spend the time necessary to inform the patient of the pros and cons of arthroplasty. The patient's knowledge of the limitations of technology coupled with reasonable expectations allow him or her to decide about treatment and lifestyle following replacement.

Strong contraindications for TKA include active sepsis and lack of extensor function. Relative contraindications, such as neuropathic arthropathy (leading to an increased risk of loosening), a functioning arthrodesis (after which TKA may lead to less satisfactory function because of lack of motion and quadriceps weakness), history of bone infection around the knee (leading to an increased incidence of periprosthetic infection), peripheral vascular disease (which may lead to poor wound healing or poor postoperative function due to claudication), and general medical condition must be taken into account in the decision to offer surgery. TKA is an elective procedure and, ultimately, it is the patient who must carefully weigh the potential benefits of the procedure against the risks, including the functional limitations imposed by an arthroplasty.

Surgical Approaches

The joint must be exposed widely enough to allow accurate bone cuts, proper ligament tensioning, and alignment of the extensor mechanism. Previous incisions should be incorporated whenever possible. Occasionally, consultation may be required to provide for durable, appropriate soft-tissue coverage. The joint itself is most often entered through a medial parapatellar incision in the capsule; however, other approaches have been advocated. The subvastus approach, which does not remove the vastus medialis from its attachment to the rectus tendon, is claimed to improve patellar tracking and to reduce postoperative pain. Exposure with this technique is more difficult in obese or heavily muscled patients. The lateral approach is used infrequently, usually in association with a severe valgus deformity. Advocates of the lateral approach point to improved patellar tracking and improved patellar vascularity. Detractors note that patellar tendon problems and difficulty of exposure leading to component malposition may be problematic with the lateral approach. For scarred knees, such as after proximal tibial fracture, proximal tibial osteotomy, anterior cruciate ligament (ACL) reconstruction, or soft-tissue trauma, a "rectus snip" or formal V-Y quadricepsplasty provides exposure while preserving the attachment of the patellar tendon into the tibial tubercle. A long tibial tubercle osteotomy done with careful preservation of the blood supply of the osteotomized fragment has been reported to have low complication rates. Potential complications include nonunion of the osteotomized fragment and tibial fracture at the osteotomy site.

Bone Resection and Limb Alignment

Bone resection should be minimized, while making certain that sufficient space exists to fit a polyethylene component at least 8 mm thick. Previous recommendations to resect the least amount of tibia to maintain the strongest bone, which is in the more proximal part of the tibia, have been supplanted by the suggestion that polyethylene thickness should be at least 8 mm, even at the sacrifice of more tibial bone, to limit wear debris or gross polyethylene failure. In most total knee systems today, a known amount of bone is resected from the distal and posterior aspects of the femur, and the bone removed is replaced with femoral component. (This technique is often called measured resection.) After ligamentous release, the tibia is resected to allow enough room for adequate polyethylene thickness. An alternative to measured resection involves tensing the collateral ligaments, and to a lesser degree the posterior cruciate ligament (PCL) when it is retained, to equal tension in flexion and extension before making the bone cuts. This technique (frequently called the balanced flexion–extension gap technique) requires careful ligamentous release to give appropriate ligamentous balance. Regardless of the technique used, the flexion and extension spaces must be nearly identical to provide for proper ligamentous tension and joint stability.

The overall alignment of the limb in the coronal plane is considered important for proper load transmission and long-term success of TKA. Based on preoperative radiographs, the surgeon places the femur and tibia at an anatomic valgus angle (usually 5° to 7°) to replace the mechanical axis through the midline of the proximal tibia.

Intramedullary alignment guides are used most often on the femur. These guides are prone to some varus–valgus and flexion–extension error, which is based on the placement of the starting hole on the distal femur and the possibility of placing the guide against the cortex in the medullary canal. Rotational position of the femoral component is critical for proper functioning of the extensor mechanism, and proper position is attained by placing jig-locating holes in at least 3° of external rotation compared to the posterior condyles of the distal femur. In some patients, 3° may be inadequate and the attempt to align the component to duplicate the transepicondylar axis or to be perpendicular to the trochlear groove may require more external rotation.

Extramedullary femoral alignment guides are available and are necessary in those cases in which the medullary canal is not accessible because of long stemmed total hip arthroplasty, deformity of the femur, or in cases of previous femoral fracture. Extramedullary guides require identification of the femoral head. The femoral component must be sized appropriately in its AP dimension to prevent over stuffing of the knee, which can create stiffness.

Extramedullary alignment guides are most commonly used on the tibia. Various systems direct the surgeon to cut either perpendicular to the shaft in both planes or with slight varus, which must be coupled with slight valgus of the femoral component, and/or posterior slope. A given total knee system is based on a specific philosophy of pairing femoral and tibial components, and the surgeon must understand the kinematics of the system in use to assure that the instruments are directing the proper cuts. Achieving proper rotational position of the tibial component will often lead the surgeon to compromise between maximum area for load transfer (with slight internal rotation of the component) on the tibia and proper tracking of the extensor mechanism (with more external rotation of the component). Care must be taken not to excessively *internally* rotate the component relative to the tibia because such rotation will lead to lateral position of the tibial tubercle and potential patellar problems.

The patella can be replaced by resecting the posterior surface of the bone or insetting the component by reaming into the bone. Patellar tracking can be improved by placing the component toward the medial side of the bone. There is general agreement that the thickness of the remaining patella and patella component should not exceed the normal thickness, which is between 20 and 25 mm, but overresection may lead to fracture. Tracking of the patella depends very much on proper rotational position of the femoral and tibial components.

Soft-Tissue Balancing

After replacement, the collateral ligaments should have equal tension throughout the range of motion of the knee. Proper ligamentous tension does not mean rigid mediolateral stability throughout the range of motion, but rather implies a knee joint that has a degree of laxity not unlike that of the normal knee. A few degrees of opening on varus–valgus stress at 20° of flexion is expected. For AP stability, a total travel of less than 1 cm is appropriate, with an endpoint either from a retained PCL or the constraint of the component design itself.

Although there is agreement that ligamentous release for the concave side of the deformity is necessary, there is no consensus regarding technique or even the sequence of releases. In the release of any ligament, underlying osteophytes must be removed and adhesion of the ligament to the underlying bone released. In varus deformity, some surgeons prefer release of the medial collateral ligament before bone resection, with additional release after trial component implantation, if necessary. Others favor release only with trial components or spacer blocks in place as guides. For valgus knees, the sequence and timing of releases varies with individual surgeons, but it generally proceeds in three stages: (1) release of the lateral collateral ligament subperiosteally at the femoral epicondyle and release of the popliteus tendon from the femur; (2) release of the iliotibial band either at the level of the joint or more proximolaterally; and (3) release of the lateral head of the gastrocnemius by elevation from the lateral aspect of the femur.

Removal of posterior osteophytes and release of adhesion of the posterior capsule should be considered to improve extension and flexion, and if performed with the knee in full flexion, there should be little chance of damage to the posterior structures.

Component Selection

The knee joint undergoes motion in all six degrees of freedom. The usual position of the axis around which the knee rotates is approximated by the transepicondylar axis—the line between the medial and lateral epicondyles (Fig. 3). This axis is rotated externally compared to the posterior aspect of the femoral condyles, but is approximately at right angles to the intercondylar notch and the trochlear groove. In one study, there was a 5° difference between the condyles and the transepicondylar line with little right to left difference in paired specimens. In a second study using 75 cadavers, there was a 3.5° difference for men and less than 1° for women. A mechanical study of five cadaver specimens showed the most normal extensor stability, with a 5° externally rotated position of the femoral component. The surgeon must take into account these variations in anatomy and place the components in the kinematically correct position.

Decision Based on the Problem of Wear Debris Component design is increasingly driven by the problem of wear debris. The generation of debris from the articular surface (mostly polyethylene), from modular adjoining surfaces (metal debris), and from fixation holes from screws (metal debris), is a major concern (Fig. 4). There is considerable variability in the opinions expressed regarding issues of design, including articular geometry (conformity and constraint versus freedom of movement and lack of constraint), cruciate ligament retention or sacrifice, metal support for polyethylene components, and method of fixation (cemented or cementless).

The first component selection dilemma involves the tibial polyethylene component. Polyethylene defects, certain manufacturing processes, and gamma sterilization in an oxygen environment are associated with premature failure. To minimize wear, maximum area of contact is necessary. However, large contact areas imply constraint, not allowing all the degrees of freedom of knee kinematics, and, at least in theory, expose the fixation interfaces to increased shear stresses. Meniscal bearing components have been suggested as a compromise to solve the dilemma of constraint and motion. If the PCL is removed, some means of limitation of AP translation is necessary, either from a central projection from the tibial component into a box on the femoral component or by "dishing" the tibial bearing surface to provide stability. If the PCL is retained, the tibial component must allow the posterior translations thought to be caused by the PCL (ie, rollback). Reports of significant wear, loosening, and osteolysis, especially with the flatter, less constrained but higher contact stress designs, have appeared in the literature. However, some of this wear could have been from problems with the polyethylene material itself. One study of 487 total knee replacements having minimal conformity between the femoral and tibial components showed a significant problem of polyethylene wear in heavier and younger patients and those in whom a thinner polyethylene insert was used.

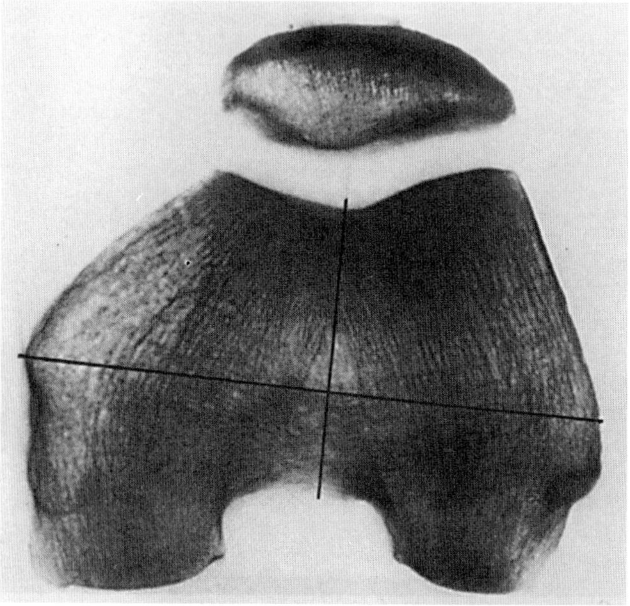

Fig. 3 Radiograph of the distal femur taken in the transverse plane. The transverse line joins the regions of the epicondyles. Note that the axis of the trochlear groove is perpendicular to the transepicondylar axis. (Reproduced with permission from Maquet PGJ (ed): *Biomechanics of the Knee*, ed 2. Berlin, Germany, Springer-Verlag, 1984.)

The patellar component is exposed to contact stresses as high as those on the tibial component. Conformity in the patellar groove of the femoral component and the tendency to tilt because of the pull of the quadriceps combined with tightness in the retinaculum (usually laterally) lead to high shear stresses. Placement of the femoral component, particularly the rotational position in the transverse plane, markedly affects these stresses. Most available patellar components are dome-shaped buttons. Although it is known that the dome design has high contact stresses, the actual amount of stress encountered depends on the design of the femoral component used.

The problems associated with patellar replacement have led to studies of the results of leaving the native patella unresurfaced against the femoral component. In a study of 891 knees for which the surgeon made a subjective decision about patella resurfacing at the time of implantation, at 2 to 15 years follow-up there was an overall complication rate of 4% in the group that had resurfacing and 12% in the group that did not. If the patella was not resurfaced, there was an increased rate of pain in patients with inflammatory disease, which led to the recommendation for patellar resurfacing in inflammatory arthritis and osteoarthrosis. Another study of 66 patients led to the conclusion that for younger, more active patients with satisfactory cartilage, no eburnated bone, satisfactory tracking, and no crystalline disease or inflammatory synovium, not resurfacing the patella can lead to a low complication and revision rate.

Metal backing of polyethylene components has been critically reevaluated because this practice decreases the thickness of the polyethylene for a given line of resection and exposes the polyethylene to higher stresses as it is sandwiched between two metal surfaces. In a study of 78 knees in 63 patients with average follow-up of 10 years, no difference was found between metal-backed and all polyethylene tibial components. However, in other studies there has been a higher failure in nonmetal-backed tibial components. The difficulty of providing adequate polyethylene thickness over the metal-backed patellar components led to high rates of early failures, with patellar wear through, metal-on-metal contact, and the generation of very large quantities of metal wear debris. For patellar replacement, most systems no longer have metal backing.

Femoral component design has shown remarkably little change as the trend of the 1980s to condylar type design has continued. A more pronounced trochlear groove is a design feature that places the patellofemoral articulation

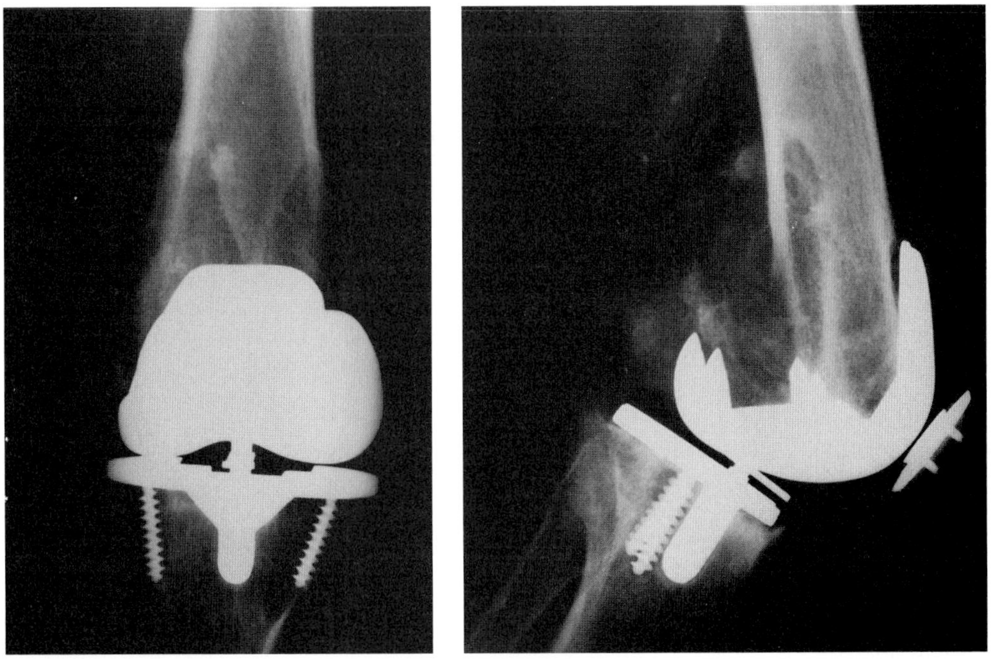

Fig. 4. These radiographs were obtained 8 years after initial prosthetic implantation. Although the patient had good knee function and no symptoms, the medial tibial metaphysis and almost the entire posterior half of the distal 8 cm of the femur have been resorbed by wear granuloma.

deeper into the anterior femur and decreases tightness of the retinaculum. Because of varus–valgus motion in gait, flat-on-flat articulation in the coronal plane, which has shown a high wear and failure rate, has been replaced with a more conforming curved-on-curved articulation. Some femoral components have a build up on the lateral side of the patellar groove to inhibit lateral subluxation of the patella, but some authors have stressed that proper rotational position of the femoral component in the transverse plane makes this component design unnecessary.

The Choices Available For knees with competent ligamentous structures, the choice is limited to a PCL-retention or substituting design, metal-backed or all polyethylene tibia, and, in some designs, a meniscal-bearing tibial component. The debate over the PCL-retaining and substituting designs continues with no convincing data yet generated to suggest superiority of one over the other. Both designs have had satisfactory and essentially equivalent long-term results. In analyzing a series of 1,430 cemented replacements, a PCL-resurfacing design showed a 15-year success rate of 91% and a PCL-substituting design, a 10-year success rate of 97.3%. A report of 28 patients with bilateral arthroplasties, one retaining the PCL and one excising it, showed no difference in knee score, but some patients who climbed stairs one at a time preferred the knee with the retained PCL. Laboratory findings that gait is more normal with the PCL-preserving designs have not proven significant in influencing patient satisfaction or function in everyday living. Most systems now offer a posterior-stabilized design that relies on a central prominence on the tibial component, which engages a box in the femoral component to provide AP stability starting at about 60° of flexion. The option of a more congruent tibiofemoral articulation with the polyethylene raised anteriorly is available. When collateral ligaments are incompetent, varus–valgus constraint must be built into the components. Extension of the tibial eminence into the femoral component without linking the two is one option for enhancing varus–valgus and rotational stability. This type of component system has limited application in the primary TKA. Reports of such constrained devices are usually combined with revision arthroplasty. However, in one report, six of 61 cases were primary replacement with satisfactory results, although radiolucent lines were found in at least one of the interfaces in 71% of cases. For completely absent collateral ligaments, reconstruction of the ligaments or placement of a linked (ie, hinged) prosthesis are other available but rarely reported choices.

Fixation Methods Fixation without cement is increasingly being replaced with a return to cemented fixation. The excellent results reported for use of the condylar system from the early 1970s with cement around all parts of all components encourage a return to this type of fixation. Femoral components placed without cement have done very well, however, and some surgeons suggest hybrid (ie, cemented tibia, cementless femur) fixation as an option. Cementless implantation in almost all instances implies a porous-coated device. Additional fixation of tibial components with screws to prevent lifting off of the component has been successful from the point of view of fixation; however, fretting of the screw against the tray has led to wear debris, which have been reported around fixation screws. Migration of implants by posterior subsidence was seen in six of seven cases studied with very sensitive radiographic technique. Although migration was minimal, it was potentially large enough to cause concern about the generation of debris from fretting. Although cementless fixation is still an option and many successful results have been reported, the promise of elimination of problems thought to be related to cement has not materialized, and the trend would appear to be increasingly to cemented fixation. Hybrid fixation has demonstrated up to 93% good results with follow-up of 8 years. In a study comparing cementless fixation (182 knees) with hybrid fixation (209) no difference was found between the groups with average follow-up of 3 years, although extensor mechanism problems were high in this series.

Patellar component fixation is almost entirely with cement, although some surgeons continue (on the basis of excellent results in their personal series) to recommend cementless fixation with metal backing.

Complications of Total Knee Arthroplasty

Infection

Deep infection rates have changed little from the already low rate of 2% reported in the literature with variation (0 to 14.8% superficial and 0 to 11.4% deep, from meta-analysis) based on specific population risk factors including malnutrition, immunocompromise, diabetes, psoriatic arthropathy, and previous periarticular sepsis. The cost of treating an infection and the severe compromise in function that results suggest that aggressive prophylaxis is indicated. Medical diseases, such as rheumatoid arthritis, should be well controlled and immune-system compromising medications, such as steroids and antineoplastic drugs, should be minimized. Distant sources of infection, including skin ulcers and urinary tract infection, should be well controlled by aggressive treatment. Data from one study demonstrated that the use of foley catheters has decreased the rate of urinary tract infections. Preoperative antibiotics administered at least 5 minutes before tourniquet inflation and measures to improve operating room air quality, such as laminar flow, ultraviolet light, and body exhaust suits, have been shown to be effective in reducing infection.

Postoperative care should include a high index of suspicion for wound infection. If the common early postoperative course of decreasing pain and increasing range of motion is interrupted with persistent erythema, poor wound healing, fever, or more than expected pain during rehabilitation, infection should be suspected. Elevated white blood cell count, sedimentation rate, or C-reactive protein are suggestive of infection. Aspiration and evaluation of the Gram's stain and culture, in spite of a 25% false negative rate, remain the most accurate means of diagnosis. Treatment of an early infection (ie, 2 to 4 weeks following surgery) demands thorough debridement of the wound and appropriate parenteral antibiotics. If the total knee components are well fixed, they may be left in place. Multiple debridements may be necessary, but the chance of success decreases with successive operations. If cultures are still positive with successive debridements, the components should be removed. Systemic treatment with the appropriate antimicrobial agent should continue for a minimum of 4 weeks following debridement for an early infection. Successful treatment of an acute infection is associated with early diagnosis, debridement, and a susceptible gram-positive organism.

An infection diagnosed later than 4 weeks following surgery is less likely to have a successful result without removal of components and is discussed in more detail in the following section on revision TKA.

Thromboembolism

Without prophylaxis, the rate of venous thrombosis following TKA is as high as 84%. Because the diagnosis of embolism is often missed, either because the embolus is silent or the appropriate studies are not done, the true rate of pulmonary embolism is not known. Reports suggest asymptomatic pulmonary embolism in 8.2% to 17%, symptomatic pulmonary embolism in 0.5% to 3%, and death in 0.3%. A recent report of patients using only elastic stockings indicated overall pulmonary embolism in 1.3% and death from pulmonary embolism in 0.19%. In a study of 2,348 patients treated prophylactically with warfarin, ventilation/perfusion scan and pulmonary angiography proven pulmonary embolism was found in 3.45% of patients, with 89% of those being asymptomatic. In this study, there was a positive correlation with advanced age and urinary tract infection, a negative correlation with heart disease, and no correlation with vasculitis, history of phlebitis in the opposite extremity, or peripheral vascular disease. The risk of death coupled with the morbidity of thrombophlebitis and postphlebitic syndrome makes prophylaxis for thrombosis necessary.

The most commonly used prophylaxis is warfarin. Reports of the effectiveness of mechanical measures, such as simple compression stockings, sequential compression devices, pedal plexus compression devices, and continuous passive motion, can be found. In a study of major knee surgery (total knee or osteotomy) in which low molecular weight heparin (LMWH) prophylaxis was used, venographically proven thrombosis was reduced from 35% to 25% ($p = 0.02$). When compared to warfarin, LMWH reduced thrombosis from 45% to 25%, with a reduction in proximal clots of from 11.4% to 1.7%. However, there was an overall increase in the rate of hemorrhagic events in the LMWH group. When a different LMWH was used, there was a significantly lower incidence of thromboembolism from the LMWH group when compared to two different regimens of warfarin.

Neurovascular Damage

Arterial injury during TKA can occur, but is a rare event (0.05%). Careful dissection in the posterior region of the joint will minimize the occurrence, and monitoring of postoperative blood loss and/or hemarthrosis will alert the surgeon to this complication. Repeated surgery to stop bleeding is rarely necessary. Patients with poor pulses or obviously calcific vessels on preoperative radiographs should be monitored carefully for pedal pulses when concern about limb vascularity is present. Consultation with a vascular surgeon may be appropriate, and prereplacement vascular reconstruction is sometimes indicated.

Direct trauma during the procedure, traction on the nerve, or external compression can lead to peroneal dysfunction. A nerve palsy found postoperatively should be treated by flexing the knee, to relieve stretch and compression on the nerve, and by releasing any compressive dressings. If the condition is diagnosed promptly and there is only a partial palsy, most patients respond quickly to treatment, and the majority recover complete function. In a report of 26 patients with peroneal nerve palsy, a partial palsy was associated with 84% complete recovery; complete palsy led to complete recovery in only 35%.

Blood Loss

The routine use of postoperative drains has been questioned, with some authorities suggesting that blood loss can be decreased by not draining the joint after routine TKA. Others suggest that the hematoma in the joint and surrounding soft tissues, which results from not using a drain, impedes rehabilitation. None of the investigations have sufficient statistical power to address the critical issue of perioperative infection. Use of an intramedullary plug in the femur to fill the hole created by the alignment rod has led to a decrease in blood loss. Tourniquet release has not been shown to decrease the amount of blood loss or the transfusion requirement for primary TKA. No decrease in bleeding has been demonstrated from the use of cryotherapy.

Periprosthetic Fractures

Fractures within 15 cm of the joint occur in 0.6% to 1.6% of patients and are often associated with minimal trauma and osteoporosis. Because most of these injuries are low energy, they heal rapidly with immobilization if reduction can be maintained. However, the effects of immobilization may be detrimental. Internal fixation with either intramedullary locked nails or extramedullary plate and screws has been advocated. If the total knee components are loose, revision to long-stem devices that bypass the fracture can rapidly return a patient to function. In a study of 20 fractures, 18 of 20 were followed up to union without further surgery, but the authors suggest surgery for any displaced, unstable, or poorly reduced fracture that will make functional treatment impossible.

Fat Embolism

The advent of fluted intramedullary instrumentation and the use of an enlarged insertion hole in the femur have seemed to decrease the rate of occurrence of this complication, but it can still occur with the use of components that have long stems. Fat embolism may occur more often than the 3% incidence frequently reported, because the effect of embolism may be attributed to other causes, and most resolve spontaneously.

Delayed Wound Healing

Placement of the skin incision can lead to avascular or hypovascular flaps that prolong wound healing time. Medical conditions that impair healing, such as diabetes, rheumatoid arthritis, and malnutrition, correlate with increased healing times. Patients at risk should be monitored closely and rehabilitation delayed, if necessary, to allow skin healing. Hematoma formation can lead to poor healing and spontaneous drainage. For persistent drainage, surgical debridement and resuture of the wound should be strongly considered. Drainage is frequently a harbinger of infection, and aspiration and culture may be indicated. Debridement should be as extensive as necessary to control potential infection.

Extensor Mechanism Problems

Fracture of the patella around a patellar component is not rare and is seen more frequently with components that have a single central stud for fixation. Nondisplaced fractures with an intact extensor mechanism can be treated with immobilization for approximately 6 weeks. Displaced fractures without loosening of the component require fixation or excision of the fragments with reconstruction of the extensor mechanism. As the degree of comminution increases, combined with patellar component loosening, fixation and replacement of the patellar component become more difficult. If simple internal fixation methods are not adequate, excision of the fragments with repair of the extensor mechanism is a better option than complicated fixation methods.

Patellar tendon avulsion is a serious complication for which treatment is frequently not successful. Patients who have had previous knee surgery, such as high tibial osteotomy or ACL reconstruction, are at risk of avulsion of the insertion when the knee is flexed during surgery. Prevention of the complication is preferable to repair and can be accomplished with proximal V-Y plasty, rectus snip, or tibial tubercle osteotomy. If the tendon is avulsed, primary repair is the best option but it is often unsuccessful. Furthermore, with no extensor power, arthrodesis or locked-knee brace treatment are the only options. Reports of successful allograft rectus tendon-patella-patellar tendon reconstructions have demonstrated that this technique may be helpful in salvaging an otherwise severely compromised knee.

Factors predisposing to patellar component dislocation are: (1) excessive medial tibial component rotation; (2) internal femoral component rotation; (3) medial placement of the femoral component; (4) underresected patella during patellar resurfacing, which results in an overly thick construct; or (5) excessive lateral placement of the patellar component. Residual postoperative valgus limb alignment can also result in an unstable extensor mechanism. Internal rotation and medial translation of the femoral component increase medial displacement, tilting, and subluxation of the patella. The combined thickness of the patellar bone and the component should not exceed the preoperative patellar thickness. However, to avoid complications of increased patellar strain and subsequent fracture, the patella should not be cut to a thickness of less than 12 to 15 mm. It may be best to perform a complete revision if one or more of these causes are suspected. If significant patellar bone loss is observed during revision, resurfacing the patella with a new implant may not be possible. It is reasonable to avoid placing a new patellar prosthesis in this setting because premature loosening or patellar fracture usually occurs. Most unresurfaced patellar remnants function quite well with minimal symptoms in the revision setting if the remnant is balanced so that it tracks centrally. A patellectomy is rarely necessary, but may be indicated in situations where closure of the arthrotomy is difficult or impossible or there is significant patellar bone loss.

Arthrofibrosis

Occasionally patients present in the postoperative period with a painful joint with poor range of motion. These patients may never gain functional range of motion following surgery or may lose motion after initially doing well. After ruling out sepsis, such knees can be successfully treated with manipulation. However, results of long-term studies have not demonstrated a gain in motion over knees that did not require manipulation. Nonsteroidal anti-inflammatory agents and decrease in aggressive physical therapy are often as effective as manipulation. In some cases, treatment as though the patient had reflex sympathetic dystrophy (amitriptyline, sympathetic nerve blocks, etc.) has been effective. In resistant cases, arthroscopic intervention to release adhesion has been variably successful. Open arthrotomy with removal of intra-articular scar can occasionally be successful. When all else fails, revision arthroplasty with implantation of smaller components may be successful.

Arthroscopy of Total Knees

Abnormal accumulations of adhesions can cause crepitus and/or pain during range of motion or can inhibit motion so that function is difficult. Removal of the adhesions combined with manipulation has been reported to increase range of motion. Lateral retinacular release can be performed from within the joint through the arthroscope with reportedly less morbidity than in an open procedure. Inspection of the component surfaces for wear, evaluation of recurrent effusions, or the patellar clunk syndrome are other potential indications.

Wear of Arthroplasty Components

Patients with debris-induced total knee problems may present with painful swelling and synovitis, but more frequently these problems are asymptomatic and are found only on routine radiographic examination, which demonstrates polyethylene component thinning and osteolysis of the femur, tibia, and/or the patella. Aspiration shows clear to cloudy synovial fluid that can be dark in color if metal debris is present. When wear or osteolysis is found, revision should be done sooner rather than later to halt the progression of the osteolytic activity and replace worn components or the entire total knee (Figs. 4 and 5).

Evaluation of the Failed Total Knee Arthroplasty

Evaluation of the failed total knee arthroplasty (TKA) involves obtaining a careful history, clinical examination, and radiologic evaluation of the joint along with appropriate laboratory analysis. The clinician should have a thorough knowledge and understanding of the potential causes of failure so that proper methods of evaluation can be implemented.

History

Because there are many different total knee replacement systems on the market, it is important to become familiar with the implant being evaluated. It is to the surgeon's advantage to be aware of which TKA components have been reported to have specific, idiosyncratic modes of failure.

Time to failure may be an important factor. A TKA that has never functioned successfully following the original implantation implies different failure etiologies than a knee that became symptomatic after many years of successful function. Development of wide radiolucent lines within 1 year of implantation is highly suspicious for infection, whereas development of radiolucency during the tenth postoperative year indicates aseptic loosening, wear, or osteolysis. A stiff, painful knee from the time of the original surgery may indicate an excessively tight PCL or insertion of an overly large prosthesis (over-stuffing).

The original surgical report should be obtained whenever possible, because it can provide the evaluating surgeon with information that may be beneficial in the planning and performance of any subsequent surgical procedure. This information includes the design type, implant sizes, and the use of other technical maneuvers, such as lateral retinacular release, collateral ligament releases, and acrylic cement usage performed by the original surgeon during the operation.

Clinical Presentation

Symptoms of a failed TKA may include any combination of the following: pain, instability, muscular weakness, stiffness, swelling (effusion versus synovitis), and erythema. Likely causes of pain include infection, aseptic loosening, mechanical failure of the polyethylene, wear with osteolysis, excessively tight PCL, over-sized implants, patellar fracture, or component fracture. In addition, neurologic disorders, either peripheral or central, as well as reflex sympathetic dystrophy (RSD), must be considered.

Frequent causes of instability are: collateral ligament insufficiency, nonfunctioning PCL, flexion/extension space mismatch, patellar malalignment, and component subsidence. Muscular weakness and stiffness may result from the combination of pain and instability. Swelling is frequently present but is nonspecific. Erythema is usually evident with infection, but can occur with aseptic loosening and failures due to excessive wear or other causes of synovitis.

Physical Examination

A thorough physical examination is essential in assessing a failed TKA. Gross instability of the collateral ligaments may be determined by medial or lateral thrusts during walking or instability during manual varus or valgus stress of the knee. Anterior-posterior instability can be detected by visible recurvatum or gross laxity noted on anterior or posterior drawer tests. Palpable crepitus can indicate peripatellar fibrosis and/or metal-backed patellar component dissociation. Audible or visual clunks or jumps indicate patellar clunk syndrome, patellofemoral instability, or femoral-tibial component instability. Loud grating noises can indicate wear through of the polyethylene articulating surfaces, with metal-on-metal grinding. Effusion may occur in infection, wear, and aseptic loosening, and may also occur as a result of persistent synovitis in rheumatoid arthritis patients. Recurrent bloody effusions may possibly result from retained periarticular soft tissue. Erythema is frequently present during infection, but it may also occur in a grossly inflamed, unstable joint. Quadriceps muscle strength should be assessed to provide an indication of the rehabilitation potential of the patient. Flexion contracture must be differentiated from extension lag in evaluating the knee for stiffness as well as in evaluating competence of the extensor mechanism. Deep pain on forced flexion may represent an excessively tight PCL. Mechanical varus or valgus malalignment can be assessed easily in a thin leg but may be more difficult in an obese one. Point tenderness may signify individual component loosening, patellar sensitivity, neuroma formation, periarticular bursitis, or tendinitis.

Because pain can be referred from the hip and/or spine

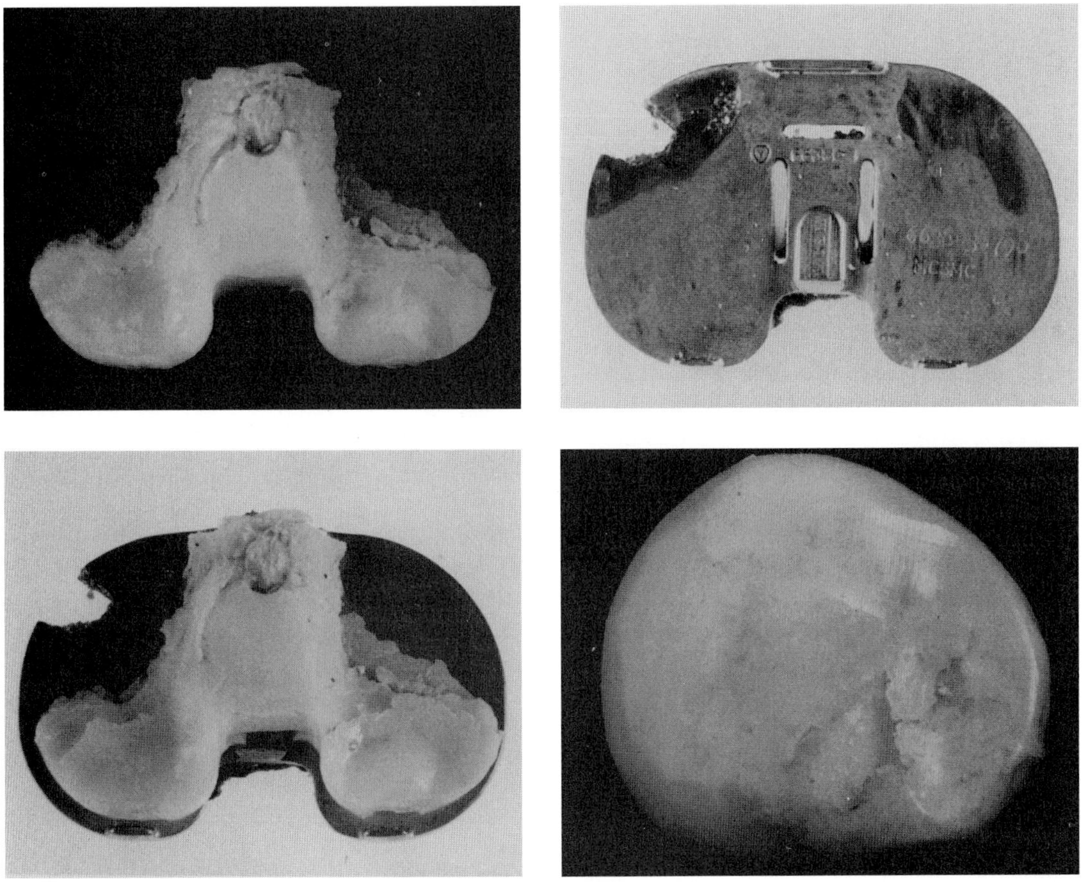

Fig. 5 Total knee components removed at revision. **Top left,** polyethylene insert; **top right,** metal back; **bottom left,** assembled tibial insert and metal back; **bottom right,** articular surface of the patellar component.

to the knee, both the hip and lumbar spine should be examined as a potential source for pain if there are any unusual aspects of the history or if the knee examination appears normal. The neurovascular status of the limb should be carefully analyzed preoperatively, both as a potential source of the underlying complaint and to ensure adequate blood supply to the leg when considering surgical intervention.

Laboratory Analysis

A painful, failed TKA should be considered infected until proved otherwise. A blood specimen should be drawn for determination of complete blood cell and differential leukocyte counts, erythrocyte sedimentation rate (ESR), and C-reactive protein to evaluate the possibility of infection. The white blood cell (WBC) count can be elevated in 50% of infections and the ESR has been reported as > 60 in 75%. An aspiration of the joint fluid should be done in all cases, with the specimen sent for culture and determination of antibiotic sensitivities of aerobic, anaerobic, and acid-fast bacteria, and fungi. An immediate gram stain should be ordered to expedite processing of the sample for plating, and cell counts of the synovial fluid may be valuable in determining the presence or absence of sepsis.

If infection is highly suspected and the patient is already taking antibiotics, these should be discontinued and the knee should be aspirated, ensuring that an adequate culture is obtained. To rule out wear debris synovitis, a sample of the aspirate should be sent to the pathology laboratory for evaluation by polarized light microscopy for the presence of polyethylene crystals.

Radiologic Evaluation

Plain AP, lateral, and patellar radiographs are all that are needed to accurately determine the failure cause in many cases. Occasionally, films of the entire limb are useful. The implant and limb alignment, patellar tracking, and adequacy of fixation as represented by periprosthetic radiolucency, as well as the underlying condition of bone stock can be assessed. Radiolucent lines have questionable significance. Incomplete radiolucent lines of 1 mm or less do not correlate with poor clinical results, whereas 2-mm radiolucent lines do. Serial films demonstrating progressive radiolucent line development are diagnostic of loosening. To accurately evaluate radiolucency, particularly with cementless components, fluoroscopically controlled radiographs (obtained parallel to the implant-bone interface) should be obtained. This procedure may be difficult in an office setting. Thus, a 1-mm radiolucent line adjacent to a polyethylene component will not appear if the prosthesis is flexed or rotated more than 5°, the roentgen beam is angulated more than 6°, or the beam is offset more than 2.5 cm (Fig. 3). These radiolucencies may represent benign fibrous tissue or a very aggressive membrane filled with macrophages and histiocytes. Careful analysis of the bony landmarks and component position with serial radiographs over time can show progressive loosening or associated bone loss and is practical from a clinical standpoint.

Radionuclide Evaluation

Technetium diphosphonate bone scans have moderate usefulness in diagnosing failure modes. Because the scan may remain active up to 2 years after implantation, scans done before this time may yield spurious results. Increased radionuclide activity may be seen in 89% of asymptomatic tibial and 63% of femoral components after 1 year. Bone remodeling adjacent to the implants accounts for the increased uptake seen within 1 year of implantation. Infection and prosthetic loosening can sometimes be differentiated by a well-done bone scan but, again, accuracy is limited when obtained within 2 years of implantation. Infection will show increased radionuclide uptake in the blood flow and pooling stages of the scan. Aseptic loosening can be determined at the acrylic-bone and porous-coated-bone interface by a complete radionuclide uptake around the limits of the prosthesis. Incomplete radionuclide uptake may or may not support the possibility of loosening.

Gallium and indium-labeled WBC scans may be helpful in evaluating infection. However, they are technician- and laboratory-dependent with regard to accuracy and often have a limited ability to determine the early presence of infection.

Revision of the Failed TKA

The revision of a failed TKA presents unique difficulties that differ from those encountered during primary TKA. Profound bone loss, flexion-extension space mismatch, and exposure difficulties are frequently encountered and require specific techniques for correction.

Causes

Although there may be one or more reasons for failure in any particular case, successful revision requires adherence to the same principles that govern successful primary TKA: establishment of correct mechanical alignment, preservation of the joint line, maintaining joint stability, maintaining extensor mechanism function, and obtaining rigid fixation of the components.

Infection

Infection represents one of the serious forms of failure due to the severe fibrosis and bone loss that may result. It is most usefully subdivided into acute and chronic types. Historically, acute infections were defined as those diagnosed within 3 months of implantation. However, current data support the concept of an acute infection as one that occurs within 2 to 3 weeks of TKA or of onset of symptoms in the case of late, apparently hematogenous infection. This time period represents the upper bounds of obtaining a potential cure of the infection by a combination of antibiotic debridement and prosthetic retention.

Chronic infections are considered to fall outside of this 2- to 3-week time period. Appropriate treatment modalities include antibiotic suppression alone, debridement and antibiotic suppression, two-stage revision TKA, single-stage revision TKA, arthrodesis, resection arthroplasty, and amputation. Data regarding the success of open debridement and antibiotic suppression are mixed, with 23% to 85% success, provided the debridement occurred within the first 3 weeks of implantation. Overall, however, the most successful results have been achieved by a two-stage revision TKA. The first stage involves removal of the implants along with all necrotic and devitalized tissue and acrylic cement and the optional use of an antibiotic-impregnated cement spacer, followed by a 4- to 6-week course of intravenous antibiotic therapy in which a serum bactericidal titer of 1:8 is maintained. The second stage is performed with a second thorough debridement and implantation of a new total knee replacement. The use of antibiotic-impregnated cement during the revision has been shown to reduce reinfection.

Preoperative Planning

The previous surgical report can alert the surgeon to specific requirements of the revision. The surgeon may anticipate areas of potential bone loss and prosthetic sizing requirements by knowing the particular design and dimensions of the respective implants. Templates can assist the surgeon in evaluating the need for metallic augments and allograft bone, as well as for the length and width requirements of intramedullary stems. Prostheses used in revision surgery may be subclassified into the following groups based on their ability to compensate for soft-tissue deficits: (1) standard PCL-retaining or substituting designs, (2) constrained condylar-type unlinked designs with intramedullary stems, and (3) linked, rotating hinges with stems. Preoperative radiographs should be obtained near the anticipated time of revision in order to properly assess the bone stock and the potential need for morcelized or bulk allograft or metallic augments.

The skin should be assessed to determine whether a muscle flap is needed to provide viable tissue coverage for the revision TKA. In particular, this requirement should not be overlooked in the treatment of the infected total knee replacement, because infection is frequently accompanied by fibrosis or necrosis of the overlying skin.

Intraoperative Decision-Making

Incision The previous incision should be used whenever possible. The incision can be lengthened proximally and distally to permit the surgeon's entrance into normal tissue planes away from scar. Creation of thin skin flaps must be avoided to preserve the skin's vascular supply, which comes from vessels perforating through the deep fascia. If the skin appears fibrotic or adherent to the underlying extensor mechanism or bone, a muscle flap transfer may be needed to assure proper skin viability. This latter procedure is best performed as a separate operation prior to the anticipated time of revision TKA. In addition, a preoperative sham incision or the use of skin expanders may be important options when potentially compromised skin is an impediment to reconstruction.

Extensor Mechanism A medial parapatellar arthrotomy is routinely performed to gain exposure of the knee. The lateral and subvastus approaches to the knee are not recommended because of the added difficulty encountered when using them in a potentially scarred environment. Ordinarily, the knee may be exposed the same way as a primary TKA. Proximal-medial, subperiosteal tibial dissection with release of the semimembranosus tendon gives sufficient freedom to flex and externally rotate the tibia and flex the knee. It is helpful but not mandatory to evert the patella. If patellar eversion is difficult, early lateral retinacular release may help. Inadvertent patellar tendon avulsion from the tibial tubercle must be avoided. If exposure is particularly difficult, secondary procedures may be done to minimize the risk of extensor mechanism disruption. These include a quadriceps snip, a V-Y quadricepsplasty, and a tibial tubercle osteotomy. The V-Y quadricepsplasty is performed by proximally transecting the quadriceps tendon that bridges the proximal limits of the medial parapatellar arthrotomy along the lines of a standard lateral retinacular release. The quadriceps snip is performed by extending the proximal portion of the medial arthrotomy in a lateral and cephalad direction across the quadriceps tendon. The tibial tubercle osteotomy is created by making a long bony flap (6 to 8 cm of the tubercle and proximal tibial crest) that is re-wired back to the tibia at the conclusion of the surgery. The purpose of these three exposures is to preserve the integrity of the extensor mechanism while obtaining exposure to the knee, because repair of a disrupted mechanism is quite difficult.

Revision Instrumentation Systems The bony architecture and landmarks present during primary TKA are often absent during revision, making the attachment of alignment guides and resection jigs difficult or impossible. Consequently, instruments used during revision TKA serve, at best, as relative guides. Trial revision components should be available to assist with proper positioning of the final implant and can also serve as guides for proper bone resection and component augmentation to allow for proper implant seating.

The actual implant may be used as a guide to aid the surgeon in obtaining the best prosthetic fit. In situations in which press fit stems are used, these stems will determine the orientation and position of the components. Consequentially, the positioning cuts on the femur and tibia should be made based on intramedullary guides that occupy the same position as the stems to be used on the prosthetic components.

A metal spacer block with alignment rod can be placed on top of the tibial implant after trial insertion to check its position and assess the need for wedge augments. Intramedullary stems can be attached to the femoral component at different valgus angles depending on the system being used. Some systems enable the stems to be placed at 3°, 5°, or 7° valgus, whereas others make use of a single valgus offset of 5°. The implant can be initially fit to properly assess joint line position and the need for bone augmentation. Overall limb alignment may be checked by placing a long alignment rod or cord across the middle of the knee and extending it from the region in the center of the malleoli to a position two finger breadths medial to the anterior superior iliac spine.

Bone Loss Management Reconstruction of deficient bone stock poses the most challenging problem during revision TKA. Choices for reconstruction include autogenous bone graft, morcelized or bulk allograft, modular metal augments, and custom-designed implants.

The only site available for autogenous bone graft in revision TKA is the iliac crest. Unfortunately, the availability of bone varies from patient to patient due to underlying osteoporosis and pelvic size, and a separate incision over the iliac crest adds to perioperative morbidity.

Allograft is the most commonly available biologic material that can be used to reconstitute bone deficiency. Contained defects are most frequently encountered on the tibia; these defects can be treated by densely packing morcelized allograft around the implant. The core implant may be cemented with press-fit intramedullary stems attached to it. Cementless systems have been implanted successfully around densely packed morcellized allograft, but this technique appears to rely primarily on the mechanical fixation of components with screws and long canal-filling stems. Uncontained bone deficits may be handled by using bulk allografts. However, this technique requires stable implant fixation that avoids direct loading of the allograft while it heals. Femoral head allografts have been used successfully to fill contained trumpet-like deficits left by excessive tibial or femoral bone loss. The allograft penetrates the deficit with an intramedullary stem attached to the femoral or tibial implant, effectively allowing the implant to sit on the "skewered" femoral head graft. Large, replacement allografts have been used in cases of profound bone loss (similar to that seen after tumor resection and clearly reflecting a salvage situation), but have shown up to a 45% failure rate (fracture, dissolution of the allograft) at intermediate-term follow-up. Supplemental metal fixation with screws and/or wires is frequently necessary to stabilize the allograft before final implantation of the revision prosthesis.

Most current revision knee replacement systems are completely modular, thereby permitting the attachment of intramedullary stems and block or wedge augments of different widths and lengths (Fig. 6). Although there is good clinical support for their use in revision situations, finite element analysis or biomechanical testing of revision arthroplasty constructs is scant. In addition, long-term evaluation of these augmentation techniques in the revision setting is not available. Most metal augments can be affixed to the prosthesis by screws or a separate batch of acrylic cement; few data are available to support one technique over the other. The proximal tibia may be augmented by metal blocks or platforms as well as half or full wedges, at various angles up to 25°. Retrieval analysis of these metal-on-metal constructs is sparse. However, mechanical testing of a retrieved prosthesis-acrylic-augment composite 6.5 years after implantation in a primary setting showed a shear strength at the interface of 77% that of a control construct.

Femoral bone loss is most easily corrected by attaching metal augments to each respective condyle of the implant. Distal as well as combined distal and posterior augments are routinely available. In addition, some systems have an anterior metal augment that can be affixed to the femoral flange of the prosthesis.

Although small augments or wedges under a stemmed tibial implant may not require the supplemental stability of a stem extension, press-fit intramedullary stem extensions are recommended whenever large wedges, metal augments, or major allografts are used. Although there are reports of stem migration following the use of constrained, unlinked revision knee designs, cementing of the stems is still broadly discouraged because of the extreme difficulty that may be encountered in revising these implants later.

Infrequently, there are cases in which modular revision systems are not applicable. Particular anatomic variations and malalignment may require special stem offsets or metal augmentation that is not available with standard systems. Computed tomographic scans can be utilized to accurately assess sizing considerations for custom-manufactured revision implants. Large bone defects may be filled with large metal distal femoral or proximal tibial replacements. However, these implants are expensive and may take a long time to manufacture. In addition, they may require additional bone resection to achieve appropriate fit at the time of implantation.

Collateral Ligament Balancing Although the principles regarding collateral ligament stability and balance are the same in primary and revision TKA, there is rarely need for collateral ligament release during revision TKA. More commonly, instability due to disrupted or attenuated collateral ligaments is encountered. Collateral ligament stability may be achieved by constrained unlinked implants, linked hinge implants, or collateral ligament repair.

Initially, the surgeon should assess the flexion (90°) and extension (0°) spaces of the knee. If they are equal, a standard implant system can be used because the collateral ligaments are most likely intact. However, if there is a significant mismatch, one or more of the above options are needed to achieve collateral ligament stability. The revision prosthesis may be needed to assess the mismatch. Tibial articular inserts of various thicknesses are put in place to check collateral ligament stability. Currently, a constrained

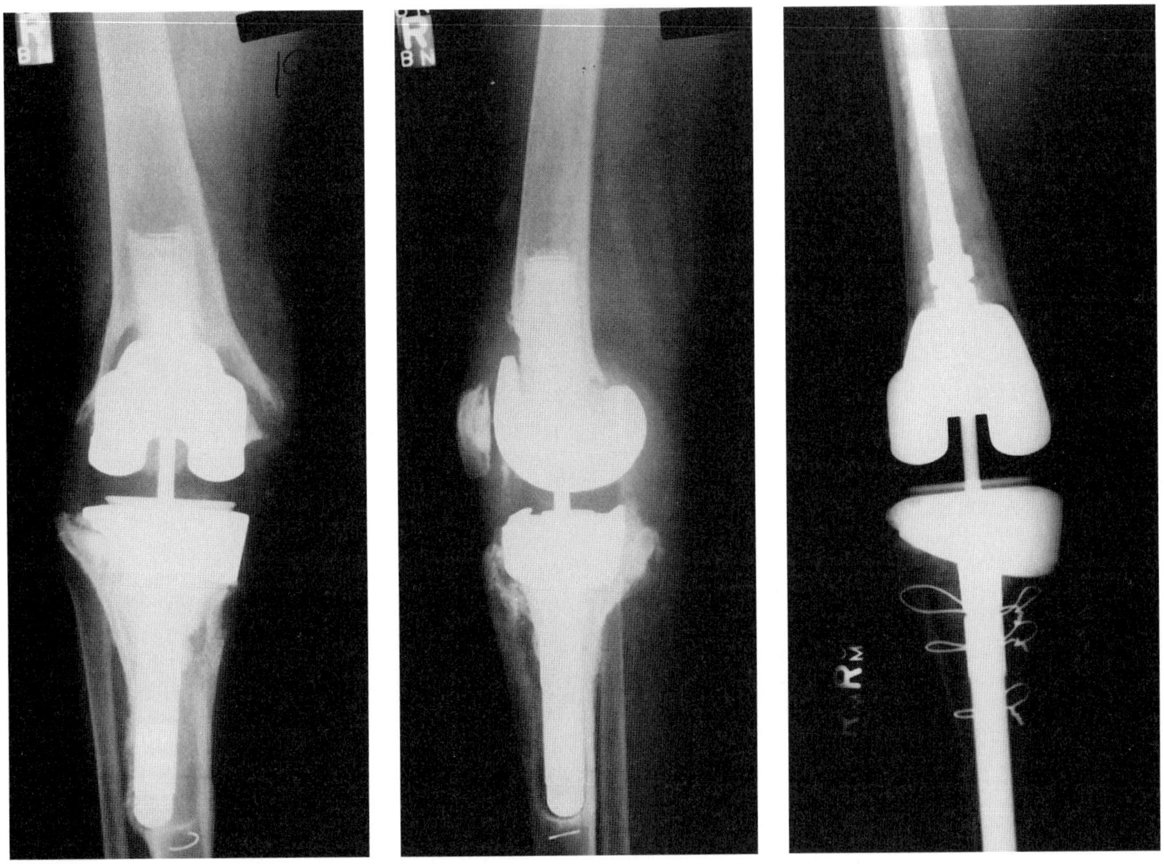

Fig. 6 **Left** and **center,** A loose infected revision total knee arthroplasty. **Right,** At a second-stage re-implantation, proximal tibial diaphyseal bone loss was augmented with cancellous allograft and metaphyseal bone loss was augmented with a wedge. Overall construct stability was augmented with an isthmus filling press-fit stem. The femoral component stem was cemented due to a patulous distal femur.

condylar unlinked implant system is most widely used to restore collateral stability to the knee. The tibial insert thickness should be chosen to avoid recurvatum. The rare indications for the use of linked hinges are recurvatum deformity with extensor mechanism weakness and revision of a failed linked hinge in a profoundly unstable knee. Although collateral ligament reconstruction using primary repair and allograft substitutes has been tried, a constrained condylar knee should also be used to provide internal stability and protect the ligament repair. It is sometimes possible to preserve the PCL during revision TKA. However, proper ligament balancing is more difficult, and its function is reliable only in cases of minimal bone and soft-tissue destruction.

Joint-Line Assessment Joint-line position affects both ligament function and patellofemoral kinematics; therefore, it is important to preserve the joint line position whenever possible during revision TKA. However, there are few anatomic landmarks to properly estimate the joint line. Knowledge of the primary implant dimensions may be helpful. It has been shown that the anatomic proximal tibia is positioned approximately 1 cm above the level of the tibial tubercle and fibular head. The femoral collateral ligament attachments are helpful in establishing the need for distal augmentation to reestablish the joint line. Although it has been shown that the knee functions best after joint line restoration, cases of profound bone loss and instability can sometimes be reconstructed only by elevating the joint line to stabilize the knee.

Clinical Outcomes of Revision TKA

The clinical results of revision TKA have been shown to be less successful and predictable than those seen after primary TKA. Whereas primary TKA can yield > 90% success rates, only 80% satisfactory results can be expected after a successful first revision. Results deteriorate with each successive revision. As a result of severe bone loss, collateral ligament instability, and scarring from multiple previous operations, second and third revisions may yield 50% satisfactory results (good and excellent Knee Society and/or Hospital for Special Surgery Scores). However, patients frequently display profound preoperative functional disability, which makes revision the only recourse. Best results can be expected when a clear cause of failure is defined preoperatively and appropriate preoperative planning is coupled with good surgical technique. Revision TKA for unexplained pain frequently results in little or no symptomatic improvement and occasionally in a clinical outcome worse than the preoperative state.

Annotated Bibliography

Outcomes Research and Assessment

American Academy of Orthopaedic Surgeons: Clinical Policies: Osteoarthritis (arthrosis) of the knee (Degenerative Joint Disease). *AAOS Bulletin* 1992;40: 49–52.

This document is the official position of the American Academy of Orthopaedic Surgeons. It is mandatory reading for all orthopaedists who treat patients with gonarthrosis.

Radiographic Assessment

Brandt KD, Fife RS, Braunstein EM, et al: Radiographic grading of the severity of knee osteoarthritis: Relation of the Kellgren and Lawrence grade to a grade based on joint space narrowing, and correlation with arthroscopic evidence of articular cartilage degeneration. *Arth Rheum* 1991;34:1381–1386.

In a careful evaluation, radiographs were found to be relatively insensitive in comparison to arthroscopy in the documentation of early cartilage change.

Nonsurgical Alternatives in the Management of the Patient with Knee Arthritis

Bradley JD, Brandt KD, Katz BP, et al: Comparison of an antiinflammatory dose of ibuprofen, an analgesic dose of ibuprofen, and acetaminophen in the treatment of patients with osteoarthritis of the knee. *N Engl J Med* 1991;325: 87–91.

In this randomized, double blind trial, patients had similar pain reductions in all groups. In light of the high rate of gastrointestinal complications associated with the use of NSAIDs, the investigators have recommended the use of acetaminophen for short-term, symptomatic relief of knee osteoarthritis.

Feinberg J, Marzouk D, Sokolek C. et al: Abstract: Effects of isometric (ISO) versus range of motion (ROM) exercise on joint pain and function in patients with knee osteoarthritis (OA). *Arthritis Rheum* 1992;35:R28.

Recent data regarding the impact of physical therapy in the management of patients with knee arthritis is limited. These authors have demonstrated the beneficial effects of rehabilitation in the management of patients with knee arthritis.

Wada J, Koshino T, Morii T, et al: Natural course of osteoarthritis of the knee treated with or without intra-articular corticosteroid injections. *Bull Hosp Jt Dis* 1993;53:45–48.

A 10-year follow-up study of 61 patients who had primary knee osteoarthritis (OA) indicated that those patients with an injection history had a 4° increase in varus and more advanced radiographic evidence of OA. Unfortunately, patients were not randomized into treatment and nontreatment groups and may have been subject to a more malignant form of OA.

Synovectomy and Arthroscopy

Bert JM, Maschka K: The arthroscopic treatment of unicompartmental gonarthrosis: A five-year follow-up study of abrasion arthroplasty plus arthroscopic debridement and arthroscopic debridement alone. *Arthroscopy* 1989;5:25–32.

At a minimum of 60-months follow-up of 126 patients who underwent abrasion arthroplasty plus arthroscopic debridement or arthroscopic debridement alone, the patients who were treated with abrasion arthroplasty had poorer results.

Chang RW, Falconer J, Stulberg SD, et al: A randomized, controlled trial of arthroscopic surgery versus closed-needle joint lavage for patients with osteoarthritis of the knee. *Arthritis Rheum* 1993;36:289–96.

With patients randomized to either knee lavage or arthroscopic knee surgery, usually partial meniscectomy, the clinical results were comparable between the two groups. The methodology used to assess more specific clinical symptoms associated with mechanically unstable meniscal tears, such as locking or catching, was lacking.

McEwen C: Multicenter evaluation of synovectomy in the treatment of rheumatoid arthritis: Report of results at the end of five years. *J Rheumatol* 1988;15:765–769.

Of 70 patients, 56 were available for evaluation at 5 years. At 5 years, limited benefits of synovectomy were demonstrated. The one exception was in the case of individual knees in which a reduction in the number of recurrences was demonstrated.

Rand JA: Role of arthroscopy in osteoarthritis of the knee. *Arthroscopy* 1991;7:358–363.

Fifty percent of those patients who had undergone arthroscopic abrasion arthroplasty had required knee replacement at 3 years. The abrasion arthroplasty was found to be unpredictable and of little benefit compared to less extensive arthroscopic surgical procedures.

Osteotomy

Matthews LS, Goldstein SA, Malvitz TA, et al: Proximal tibial osteotomy: Factors that influence the duration of satisfactory function. *Clin Orthop* 1988;229:193–200.

The authors reviewed their clinical series of 40 patients treated for osteoarthritis by proximal tibial osteotomy. Risk factors for failure included obesity, advanced age, and the extremes of frontal plane malalignment. Continued useful function of the knee was identified in 86% at 1 year, 50% at 5 years, and only 28% at 9 years.

Unicompartmental Knee Replacement

Callahan CM, Drake BG, Heck DA, et al: Patient outcomes following unicompartmental or bicompartmental knee arthroplasty: A meta analysis. *J Arthroplasty* 1995;10:141–150.

This meta-analysis provides the reader with a systematic review of the medical literature from 1966 until 1992.

Grelsamer RP: Unicompartmental osteoarthrosis of the knee. *J Bone Joint Surg* 1995;77A:278–292.

This expert review provides a summary of the medical literature regarding unicompartmental gonarthrosis. Basic science and clinical management alternatives are discussed.

Heck DA, Marmor L, Gibson A, et al: Unicompartmental knee arthroplasty: A multicenter investigation with long-term follow-up evaluation. *Clin Orthop* 1993;286:154–159.

This investigation demonstrated a 10-year prosthetic survivorship of 91.4% (± 2.8%) in 295 unicompartmental replacements.

Knutson K, Lewold S, Robertsson O, et al: The Swedish knee arthroplasty register: A nation-wide study of 30,003 knees 1976–1992. *Acta Orthop Scand* 1994;65:375–86.

This article provides an update on the Swedish national experience with knee replacement. Unicompartmental knee replacement continues to play a major role in the treatment of primary noninflammatory gonarthrosis.

Total Knee Arthroplasty

Anouchi YS, Whiteside LA, Kaiser AD, et al: The effects of axial rotational alignment of the femoral component on knee stability and patellar tracking in total knee arthroplasty demonstrated on autopsy specimens. *Clin Orthop* 1993;287:170–177.

Varus–valgus stability and tracking of the patella were tested in five cadaver specimens with a total knee femoral component implanted in neutral, 5° internal and 5° external rotation. Varus–valgus stability and patellar tracking were closest to those of the unreplaced joint when the femoral component was externally rotated.

Berger RA, Rubash HE, Seel MJ, et al: Determining the rotational alignment of the femoral component in total knee arthroplasty using the epicondylar axis. *Clin Orthop* 1993;286:40–47.

The difference between the "surgical epicondylar axis" and the line connecting the posterior condylar surfaces was found using 75 embalmed anatomic specimens. The surgical epicondylar axis was defined as a line connecting the lateral epicondylar prominence and the medial sulcus of the medial epicondyle. A mean difference of 3.5° for men and 0.3° for women was found.

Boyd AD Jr, Ewald FC, Thomas WH, et al: Long-term complications after total knee arthroplasty with or without resurfacing of the patella. *J Bone Joint Surg* 1993;75A:674–681.

This review of 891 knees with and without resurfacing of the patella using the duopatellar prosthesis has follow-up ranging 2 to 15 years with an average of 6.1 years. The authors recommended resurfacing when an unconstrained prosthesis is used in patients who have inflammatory arthritis and osteoarthrosis.

Faure BT, Benjamin JB, Lindsey B, et al: Comparison of the subvastus and paramedian surgical approaches in bilateral knee arthroplasty. *J Arthroplasty* 1993;8:511–516.

In a prospective randomized study, 20 patients having bilateral arthroplasties had one approach on one side and the other approach on the opposite knee. The knees with subvastus approach had significantly greater strength at 1 week and 1 month but not at 3 months. Patients who expressed a preference chose the subvastus approached knee 4:1. The authors concluded that the subvastus approach is a reasonable alternative to the paramedian approach.

Healy WL, Finn D: The hospital cost and the cost of the implant for total knee arthroplasty: A comparison between 1983 and 1991 for one hospital. *J Bone Joint Surg* 1994;76A:801–806.

The average cost for TKA increased 17% from 1983 to 1991 but, after adjustment for inflation, the hospital costs decreased 15% during this period. The cost of the total knee implant increased 13%. The authors conclude that hospitals and surgeons must work together to control the cost of implants if cost containment is to be achieved.

Jiganti JJ, Goldstein WM, Williams CS: A comparison of the perioperative morbidity in total joint arthroplasty in the obese and nonobese patient. *Clin Orthop* 1993;289: 175–179.

This paper reports a retrospective review of 130 patients treated with either primary total hip arthroplasty (THA) or TKA. Based on obesity, defined by weight 20% above ideal, there was no difference in the risk of perioperative complications associated with the arthroplasty surgery.

Levitsky KA, Harris WJ, McManus J, et al: Total knee arthroplasty without patellar resurfacing: Clinical outcomes and long-term follow-up evaluation. *Clin Orthop* 1993;286:116–121.

For this paper, 66 of a study group of 125 patients who had a TKA without patellar resurfacing with more than 2 years of follow-up were evaluated. The authors conclude that not resurfacing the patella can lead to low complication and revision rates for younger, more active patients who fulfill the selection criteria presented.

Mantas JP, Bloebaum RD, Skedros JG, et al: Implications of reference axes used for rotational alignment of the femoral component in primary and revision knee arthroplasty. *J Arthroplasty* 1992;7:531–535.

In a cadaver study, there was an average difference between the transepicondylar axis and the posterior condylar line of 5° with the transepicondylar line externally rotated. There was little difference between right and left knees in paired specimens.

Rand JA: Comparison of metal-backed and all-polyethylene tibial components in cruciate condylar total knee arthroplasty. *J Arthroplasty* 1993;8:307–313.

Seventy-eight knees in 63 patients were followed up for an average of 10 years following arthroplasty. Using this prosthesis, there was no significant difference between the metal-backed and the all-polyethylene tibial components. This report is one of many that present similar findings.

Rorabeck CH, Bourne RB, Lewis PL, et al: The Miller-Galante knee prosthesis for the treatment of osteoarthrosis: A comparison of the results of partial fixation with cement and fixation without any cement. *J Bone and Joint Surg* 1993;75A:402–408.

Three-hundred ninety-two total knee arthroplasties were followed prospectively; 183 had fixation without cement, and 209 were hybrid (cement for tibial and patellar components). Type of fixation was chosen based on the patient's age and the surgeon's assessment of the quality of the tibial bone. Follow-up averaged 3 years with a range of 2 to 5 years. Complications related to the extensor mechanism were high, but there was no difference in the outcome based on the type of fixation.

Ryd L, Carlsson L, Herberts P: Micromotion of noncemented tibial component with screw fixation: An in vivo roentgen stereophotogrammetric study of the Miller-Galante prosthesis. *Clin Orthop* 1993;295:218–225.

In six of seven cases, migration occurred (mean: 0.6 mm). All tilted backwards but actual subsidence along the axis of the tibia was small. Displacement under load was small (approx 0.3 mm, but one case was 1.7 mm). According to the authors, this amount of motion could be "compatible with mechanical coupling of the prosthesis to bone by bone ingrowth."

Shoji H, Wolf A, Packard S, et al: Cruciate retained and excised total knee arthroplasty: A comparative study in patients with bilateral total knee arthroplasty. *Clin Orthop* 1994;305:218–222.

Twenty-eight patients having bilateral TKA had excision of one PCL and retention of the other. Patients who ascended or descended stairs one leg at a time preferred the extremity with the retained PCL, but there was no difference in the Hospital for Special Surgery knee assessment score based on PCL retention.

Complications of Total Knee Arthroplasty

Burkart BC, Bourne RB, Rorabeck CH, et al: The efficacy of tourniquet release in blood conservation after total knee arthroplasty. *Clin Orthop* 1994;299:147–152.

This study concluded that tourniquet release for hemostasis was not effective based on the amount of postoperative blood loss or transfusion requirement when used for primary TKA.

Callahan CM, Drake BG, Heck DA, et al: Patient outcomes following tricompartmental total knee replacement: A meta-analysis. *JAMA* 1994;271:1349–1357.

This article reviews all literature contained in the MEDLARS database for the years 1966 to 1992 as well as the references cited in each article. Appropriate articles were selected for data abstraction and analysis. This represents one of the few meta-analyses available in the orthopaedic literature.

Haas SB, Tribus CB, Insall JN, et al: The significance of calf thrombi after total knee arthroplasty. *J Bone Joint Surg* 1992;74B:799–802.

This retrospective study reviewed 1,257 patients having 1,625 TKAs. Pre-and postoperative perfusion lung scans and postoperative venograms were used to determine the presence of calf or proximal thrombi. Patients with calf thrombi were found to have a significantly greater risk for both asymptomatic and symptomatic PE. The authors conclude that deep venous thrombosis places patients at greater risk for PE.

Healy WL, Siliski JM, Incavo SJ: Operative treatment of distal femoral fractures proximal to total knee replacements. *J Bone Joint Surg* 1993;75A:27–34.

The authors conclude that these fractures usually occur in osteopenic bone and recommend surgical treatment for any displaced, unstable, or poorly reduced fracture and any fracture for which functional treatment is not possible.

Khaw FM, Moran CG, Pinder IM, et al: The incidence of fatal pulmonary embolism after knee replacement with no prophylactic anticoagulation. *J Bone Joint Surg* 1993;75B: 940–941.

This is a report of 527 knee replacements done without prophylactic anticoagulation but with elastic stockings and mobilization 48 hours after surgery. The incidence of clinically significant and isotope ventilation-perfusion proven pulmonary embolism (PE) was 1.3%; death from PE was 0.19%. This study helps to define the natural history of post knee replacement pulmonary embolism without pharmacologic prophylaxis.

Lotke PA, Steinberg ME, Ecker ML: Significance of deep venous thrombosis in the lower extremity after total joint arthroplasty. *Clin Orthop* 1994;299:25–30.

The authors reported the sequellae in 920 patients. The authors concluded that asymptomatic PE occurs in 15% to 17% of patients after THA and TKA, and its incidence increases proportionally to the size of the thrombi.

Oishi CS, Grady-Benson JC, Otis SM, et al: The clinical course of distal deep venous thrombosis after total hip and total knee arthroplasty, as determined with duplex ultrasonography. *J Bone Joint Surg* 1994;76A:1658–1663.

There was a significantly higher prevalence of deep venous thrombosis after TKA than after THA. Men who had deep venous thrombosis had a higher prevalence of proximal propagation than did women. Seventeen percent of the patients who had deep venous thrombosis had the appearance of proximal thrombosis during the study period.

Raut VV, Stone MH, Wroblewski BM: Reduction of postoperative blood loss after press-fit condylar knee arthroplasty with use of a femoral intramedullary plug. *J Bone Joint Surg* 1993;75A:1356–1357.

This short report shows significant reduction in blood loss if the hole left by the intramedullary alignment rod is plugged with bone.

The RD Heparin Arthroplasty Group: RD heparin compared with warfarin for prevention of venous thromboembolic disease following total hip or knee arthroplasty. *J Bone Joint Surg* 1994;76A:1174–1185.

LMWH was compared in two doses to warfarin in THA and TKA patients. For total knees, there was a significantly lower incidence of venous thromboembolic disease for the LMWH group than the warfarin group. The rate of clinically important bleeding events was not different between the two groups.

Tsao A, Mintz L, McRae CR, et al: Failure of the porous-coated anatomic prosthesis in total knee arthroplasty due to severe polyethylene wear. *J Bone Joint Surg* 1993;75A: 19–26.

This report of 487 TKAs using the porous-coated anatomic prosthesis, which were done by a single surgeon, demonstrates the significant problem of polyethylene wear.

Vresilovic EJ Jr, Hozack WJ, Booth RE, et al: Incidence of pulmonary embolism after total knee arthroplasty with low-dose coumadin prophylaxis. *Clin Orthop* 1993;286: 27–31.

In this prospective study, PE was diagnosed by V/Q scans and pulmonary arteriograms. PE was diagnosed in 5.6% of patients. Only 0.7% were symptomatic, and none were fatal.

Evaluation of the Failed Total Knee Arthroplasty

Engh GA, Parks NL, Ammeen DJ: Tibial osteolysis in cementless total knee arthroplasty: A review of 25 cases treated with and without tibial component revision. *Clin Orthop* 1994; 309:33–43.

Revision total knee arthroplasty was performed in 25 cementless total knee replacements, which had failed by progression of tibial osteolysis that was identified radiographically and confirmed histologically. Clinical radiographic results remained excellent at a mean of 41 months postrevision. Stemmed components were utilized along with structural allograft.

Hohl WM, Crawfurd E, Zelicof SB, et al: The total condylar III prosthesis in complex knee reconstruction. *Clin Orthop* 1991;273:91–97.

Twenty-nine revision total knee arthroplasties were done using the Total Condylar III prosthesis. Radiolucent lines were observed in at least one component in 71% of patients, but few were considered significant. Follow-up averaged 6.1 years. The deep infection rate in this study was 5.7% higher than that reported in modern series of primary arthroplasties.

Mow CS, Wiedel JD: Noncemented revision total knee arthroplasty. *Clin Orthop* 1994;309:110–115.

Between 1985 and 1991, 17 revision total knee arthroplasties were done using porous-coated tibial or femoral components. Eight knees had both components inserted without cement, four the femoral component only, and five the tibial component only. The reasons for revision were aseptic loosening (15), instability (1), and infection (1). Follow-up averaged 5.6 years. The average Hospital for Special Surgery Scores were improved from a preoperative 52 to a postoperative 87. Results were comparable to cemented revision total knee arthroplasty results.

Murray PB, Rand JA, Hanssen AD: Cemented long-stem revision total knee arthroplasty. *Clin Orthop* 1994;309: 116–123.

Forty cemented long-stemmed kinematic stabilizer revision total knee arthroplasties were evaluated at an average follow-up of 58.2 months. The Knee Society pain score improved from 38 points preoperatively to 83 points postoperatively. The Knee Society function score improved from 46 preoperatively to 64 postoperatively. Initial postoperative radiographs showed tibial bone-cement radiolucencies in five knees, but at final follow-up none of these radiolucencies had progressed. Radiolucencies developed in five additional tibial components by the time of final follow-up, but they were all incomplete.

Peters PC Jr, Engh GA, Dwyer KA, et al: Osteolysis after total knee arthroplasty without cement. *J Bone Joint Surg* 1992;74A:864–876.

The prevalence and characteristics of osteolysis were studied after 174 consecutive uncemented total knee arthroplasties; 16% (27) of the implants demonstrated osteolysis. The diagnosis was made an average of 35 months after surgery. Of the 27 prostheses, 15 (56%) were revised after an average of 45 months in situ. The remaining 12 implants were still in situ 5 years or more postoperatively. In the revision group, six implants were judged stable and nine were loose. The medial aspect of the tibial metaphysis was the most common site for bone resorption (24 knees). Potential etiologies for generating particulate debris implicated in osteolysis formation are failure of thin, polyethylene inserts; abrasion of prominent polyethylene tibial eminence; metal-backed patellar component failure with polyethylene and metal debris; and corrosion between titanium screws and the cobalt-chromium base plate.

Rand JA: Revision total knee arthroplasty using the Total Condylar III prosthesis. *J Arthroplasty* 1991;6:279–284.

Twenty-one revision TKAs were done between 1980 and 1987, using the Total Condylar III prosthesis. The reasons for revision were: bone loss (10), instability (9), supracondylar femur fracture (1) and implant malposition (1). After a 4-year follow-up, the knee scores were excellent in 25%, good in 25%, fair in 25%, and poor in 25%. There was a 33% complication rate. The results were similar to those for other constrained implants used for revision in patients with severe bone loss and ligamentous instability.

Rand JA: Augmentation of a total knee arthroplasty with a modular metal wedge: A case report. *J Bone Joint Surg* 1995;77A:266–268.

Retrieval analysis of an implant augmented with a metal wedge cemented to the undersurface of the metal tibial base plate was compared to a similar construct that had never been implanted. The in vitro wedge failed at a load of 3,470 N. The wedge retrieved after 6 years of in vivo use failed at a load of 2,688 N (77% of the shear strength of the control wedge).

Rosenberg AG, Verner JJ, Galante JO: Clinical results of total knee revision using the total condylar III prosthesis. *Clin Orthop* 1991;273:83–90.

A cemented Total Condylar III prosthesis was used in 36 revision total knee arthroplasties. The reasons for revision were infection (15) and loosening or instability (21). Hospital for Special Surgery Scores improved from a mean of 36 preoperatively to a mean of 77 postoperatively. Lucent lines occurred in 60%, with 16% of the patients showing progressive tibial lucencies. This prosthesis was effective for salvaging unstable knees, but less-constrained devices should be used whenever possible.

Stuart MJ, Larson JE, Morrey BF: Reoperation after condylar revision total knee arthroplasty. *Clin Orthop* 1993;286:168–173.

Six hundred fifty-five condylar revision total knee arthroplasties performed during a 10-year period were retrospectively reviewed. Average follow-up was 7.5 years. Forty-six knees without a history of arthroplasty infection required 60 reoperations after the revision. Reoperation was performed for extensor mechanism problems in 19 knees (41%), component loosening in 10 knees (22%), deep infection in 9 knees (20%), wound problems in 9 knees (20%), tibiofemoral instability in 8 knees (17%), limited motion in 4 knees (8%), and particulate debris synovitis in 1 knee (2%). Twenty-four knees (52%) were considered clinical failures because of pain, limited motion, instability, and sepsis.

Whiteside LA: Cementless revision total knee arthroplasty. *Clin Orthop* 1993;286:160–167.

Fifty-six cementless revision total knee arthroplasties were performed using cementless technique emphasizing long-stemmed components and morcellized allograft. All knees had increasing radiodensity in the grafted areas 1 and 2 years postoperatively as compared with the 1-month radiograph. All implants except two achieved stable fixation to bone. Alignment, stability, and patient comfort were all improved with cementless revision technique.

42

Ankle and Foot: Pediatric Aspects

Congenital and Acquired Deformities

Metatarsus Adductus (Metatarsus Varus)

Metatarsus adductus is a common foot disorder that occurs in one of every 1,000 live births. One half of affected children have bilateral involvement. This deformity results from the intrauterine position of the child's foot and tibia. The forefoot is deviated medially in the transverse plane, with some degree of varus position in the frontal plane. The sole of the foot is kidney shaped with a medial plantar crease. The heel is never in equinus.

A line bisecting the heel normally passes between the second and third toes. On clinical examination, the heel bisector line passes through the third toe in a mild deformity, between the third and fourth toes in a moderate deformity, and between the fourth and fifth toes in a severe deformity. Foot flexibility is determined by abducting the forefoot against a fulcrum located at the base of the fifth metatarsal. A deep medial crease is suggestive of moderate deformity. Associated conditions include developmental dislocation of the hip.

Passively correctable metatarsus adductus resolves spontaneously. In most children with a moderate or rigid deformity, the deformity can be corrected with serial manipulation and casting. Children that require serial casts may be placed in straight or reverse last shoes for several months after casting.

Long-term results of patients who have mild to moderate residual deformity after treatment are good. Surgical treatment is indicated in children 5 years and older with severe, symptomatic residual metatarsus adductus. The deformity can be treated with a lateral shortening osteotomy (cuboid) and/or a medial cuneiform opening wedge osteotomy, or multiple metatarsal osteotomies.

Clubfoot (Talipes Equinovarus)

Clubfoot (talipes equinovarus) occurs with a prevalence of 1.5 per 1,000 live births, and the deformities are bilateral in approximately half of affected children. Most affected children are male. Idiopathic clubfoot follows a multifactorial pattern of inheritance. When one child has a clubfoot, a 2% to 6% chance exists that the next sibling will be affected. If the parent also has a clubfoot, a 25% chance exists that the subsequent offspring will have the same disorder. Clubfoot also is associated with other conditions, including myelodysplasia, arthrogryposis, amniotic band syndrome, and diastrophic dwarfism.

The pathoanatomy of clubfoot is complex. The talus of a child with a clubfoot is smaller than normal, the talar neck has a medial angulation, and the dome of the talus has a normal shape. The calcaneus is also smaller than normal, and it is positioned in equinus, varus, and medial rotation. The malposition of the anterior and medial facets form a V on which the talar head rests. The medial facet of the calcaneus lies vertically oriented because of the medial rotation of the calcaneus on the talus. The cuboid may be adducted on the calcaneus. The sheaths of the flexor digitorum longus and flexor hallux longus are adherent at Henry's knot.

The clinical appearance of the foot is a reflection of the pathoanatomy. The calf and foot are smaller than those of the contralateral extremity. The forefoot is adducted and supinated. The normal space between the navicular and the medial malleolus is not palpable, and a deep medial foot crease exists. The hindfoot is in equinus and varus.

The standard radiographic views are the stress abduction anteroposterior (AP) view and the stress dorsiflexion lateral view (Fig. 1). The latter shows little or no convergence of the talocalcaneal axis, which is normal at approximately 30° to 40°. The tibiocalcaneal alignment on a lateral radiograph reveals equinus.

The initial treatment of an infant with a clubfoot is manipulation and serial casting. The forefoot adduction is corrected first while the heel is casted out of varus. The foot is dorsiflexed progressively once the forefoot adduction has been corrected. Care must be taken not to apply the dorsiflexion force to the distal aspect of the foot because this force can produce a deformity of the midfoot (a rocker-bottom foot). The success rate of nonsurgical care depends on the initial severity of the clubfoot, the patient's gender, and whether the disorder is unilateral or bilateral. A mild unilateral clubfoot in a boy is the easiest to correct with manipulation and serial casts. Clubfoot in girls and in boys with bilateral involvement is more resistant to nonsurgical treatment and often requires a surgical correction. Surgery is indicated if satisfactory correction cannot be achieved. Timing of the surgery is variable, with recommendations ranging from 2 to 12 months of age, an 8-cm foot, or a 12-lb child.

Generally, the surgical correction is done between 4 and 8 months of age. There are two commonly used surgical approaches to the equinovarus deformity. Many surgeons perform a transverse "Cincinnati" circumferential incision with the child lying prone. Others use a small, medial approach to the foot with a second posterolateral incision. Both provide good exposure of the pathoanatomy and allow protection of the neurovascular structures. Because

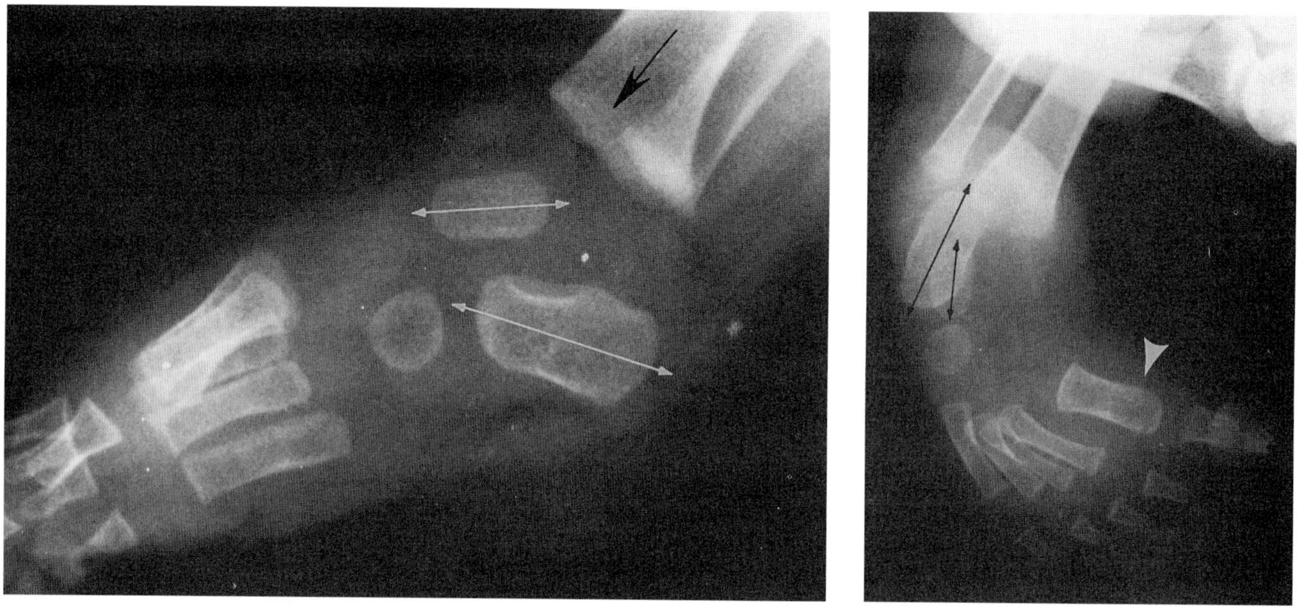

Fig. 1 **Left,** Stress dorsiflexion lateral radiograph of the foot in a child with resistant talipes equinovarus. The talus and calcaneus are in equinus relative to the tibia (arrows). The cuboid lies plantar to the calcaneus as does the first metatarsal to the talus. **Right,** Anteroposterior radiograph of the foot in a 4-month-old child with resistant talipes equinovarus. Note the decreased angle formed by the axis of the calcaneus and talus (arrows). The cuboid appears to align with the talus instead of the calcaneus. The first ray (dart) is deviated in a medial direction.

many children with equinovarus deformities have hypotrophic dorsalis pedis arteries, preservation of the posterior tibial vessels is important.

Extensive clubfoot release should include release of the flexor tendons, the Achilles tendon, and the capsules of the midfoot and hindfoot, as well as repositioning of the bony anatomy of the foot.

The foot is placed into a reduced position. Many surgeons use one or more pins to maintain the proper reduction. The initial postoperative cast normally is changed at 2 weeks to apply a better fitting cast and to manipulate the foot after the swelling has subsided. Postoperative casting is continued for 6 to 12 weeks. The pins normally are removed at 6 weeks. The foot may be placed in a night splint or orthosis until ambulation begins.

Residual forefoot adduction and cavovarus are the most common deformities that persist after clubfoot surgery. This persistence results from an incomplete release of the calcaneocuboid joint and the plantar fascia and from failure to recognize residual forefoot adduction on the intraoperative radiograph at the time of the primary surgery. Children with medial displacement of the cuboid relative to the calcaneus should have a complete calcaneocuboid release at the time of soft-tissue release.

If the deformity can be passively corrected to a neutral position, surgical correction is not required for residual heel varus, forefoot adduction, or intoeing in a young child. Excessive residual forefoot adduction in older children can be treated with lateral column shortening and/or medial column lengthening, or multiple metatarsal osteotomies. Persistent heel varus is corrected by a calcaneal osteotomy, and multiple deformities are treated with triple arthrodesis.

Cavus Foot

Patients with cavus foot deformities often present with complaints of clawtoes, metatarsal pain, a high arch, anterior ankle pain, and recurrent ankle sprains. The deformity is characterized by a pathologic elevation of the longitudinal arch that results from forefoot plantarflexion and/or an increase in dorsiflexion or varus of the calcaneus. A secondary contracture of the plantar fascia then develops. Often the first deformity seen in a patient with cavus foot is clawtoe, with other deformities, such as depression of the first metatarsal, heel varus, and heel equinus. In over two thirds of patients, the etiology of cavus foot is a neuromuscular disorder, such as hereditary sensory motor neuropathy (Charcot-Marie-Tooth), spinal cerebellar degeneration, spina bifida, poliomyelitis, polyneuritis, spinal cord tumor, and syringomyelia. Other etiologies are congenital (talipes equinovarus, arthrogryposis), traumatic (nerve injuries, fractures of foot, anterior compartment syndrome), and idiopathic. A thorough neurologic examination is essential, particularly if the deformity is unilateral. Evaluation may also include spinal radiographs, magnetic resonance imaging (MRI) of the spinal cord, and nerve conduction studies. The radiographic assessment consists of measuring the angle created by a line drawn through the axis of the talus and the first metatarsal on a standing lateral radiograph. A cavus foot is present if the first metatarsal is plantarflexed relative to the axis of the talus.

The treatment of a patient with cavus foot is based on the severity of deformity and the etiology. Patients with symptomatic, passively correctable deformities can be placed into a well-molded orthosis. Patients with moderate contractures without significant bony abnormalities may be treated by radical plantar-medial soft-tissue release and appropriate tendon transfers. Bony procedures as well as soft-tissue procedures are performed for fixed deformities. The osteotomy performed most commonly for cavus foot is a dorsal closing wedge osteotomy at the base of the first metatarsal combined with a radical plantar release. Rigid heel varus is corrected by a wedge or sliding calcaneal osteotomy. A triple arthrodesis may be required for an older adolescent with a fixed deformity. This should be viewed as a salvage procedure.

Calcaneovalgus Foot

Calcaneovalgus feet occur in one per 1,000 live births. It is believed to be secondary to intrauterine positioning and is associated with mild lateral tibial torsion. The foot can be corrected passively. This positional deformity normally resolves spontaneously. If the foot appears less flexible, plantarflexion lateral stress radiographs may help delineate this from congenital vertical talus.

Idiopathic (Flexible) Flatfoot (Pes Planus)

Idiopathic (flexible) flatfoot is a frequent, benign condition that rarely requires treatment. It has a prevalence ranging from 7% to 22%. On weightbearing, the foot is in a pronated position (abduction, eversion, dorsiflexion) with characteristic heel valgus and flattening of the medial longitudinal arch. The head of the talus is prominent medially. Extension of the great toe produces heel inversion and restoration of a visible longitudinal arch. Standing AP and lateral radiographs of the feet reveal an increase in talar plantarflexion (talar to first metatarsal angle $> 0°$), a decrease in the dorsiflexion angle of the calcaneus, and an increase in the talocalcaneal angle when compared to a normal foot (Fig. 2, *top*).

Children with asymptomatic idiopathic flatfoot generally do not require therapy. Whether a well-molded corrective orthosis in slight forefoot adduction and heel varus will affect the development of the longitudinal arch is currently controversial. Symptomatic (pain, excessive shoe wear, or progressive deformity) children with a flexible flatfoot are placed into an accommodative orthosis. Painful feet that are unrelieved by orthotics are treated with an opening wedge osteotomy of the distal lateral calcaneus or a medial calcaneal sliding osteotomy (Fig. 2, *bottom*). A heel cord lengthening often is required with bony procedures.

Accessory Navicular

The prevalence of an accessory navicular is between 4% and 21%. It often is discovered incidentally on an AP radiograph of the foot. Three types of accessory naviculars exist. Type I (os tibiale externum) is a sesamoid bone in the tendon of the posterior tibial muscle and normally is separated from the navicular by at least 3 mm (Fig. 3, *left*). The majority, 50% to 70%, of accessory naviculars are type II (Fig. 3, *right*). These measure up to 12 mm in diameter and are triangular or heart-shaped. A cartilaginous or fibrocartilaginous synchondrosis exists between the accessory navicular and the main body of the navicular. The posterior tibial tendon inserts into this prominence. The type III accessory navicular is an end-stage type II with fusion of the os tibiale externum to the main body of the navicular. This fusion forms a prominent process known as the cornuate navicular. Type I and most type III accessory naviculars are asymptomatic, although patients with type II accessory naviculars may have chronic pain. The typical patient is a physically active female in the second decade of life who has pain in the medial aspect of the foot, centered over the navicular. The patient may have an associated flatfoot.

Conservative treatment consists of 3 weeks of immobilization in a short leg cast followed by the application of padding or shoe modification. The most successful surgical treatment is a simple resection of the accessory navicular that reduces the size of the medial navicular prominence.

Congenital Vertical Talus

A vertical talus produces a rigid flatfoot deformity with a fixed dorsal dislocation of the navicular on the talar neck. It has an associated equinus ankle contracture and abduction of the midfoot and forefoot (Fig. 4). The peroneal, anterior tibial, and long toe extensor tendons are contracted. A lateral radiograph of the foot in maximum plantarflexion demonstrates an irreducible talo-navicular joint. A lateral radiograph in maximum dorsiflexion demonstrates fixed equinus. A line drawn through the axis of the talus passes plantar to the first metatarsal axis. Most vertical tali are teratologic and associated with a chromosomal disorder, arthrogryposis, or myelomeningocele. Others are neurogenic, developing secondary to a muscle imbalance in the foot. Rarely is rigid vertical talus an isolated problem.

Children with a rigid vertical talus may be casted briefly to stretch the lateral and anterior soft tissues in preparation for surgery. Surgical correction is performed between 6 and 15 months of age. In a single-stage procedure, the Achilles, peroneal, anterior tibialis, and toe extensor tendons are lengthened, and the posterior ankle–subtalar, the calcaneocuboid, and talonavicular joints are released. The posterior tibial tendon and talonavicular capsule often require plication. The talonavicular joint is pinned in the reduced position. The pin is removed at 6 weeks, and the postoperative cast is removed at 12 weeks.

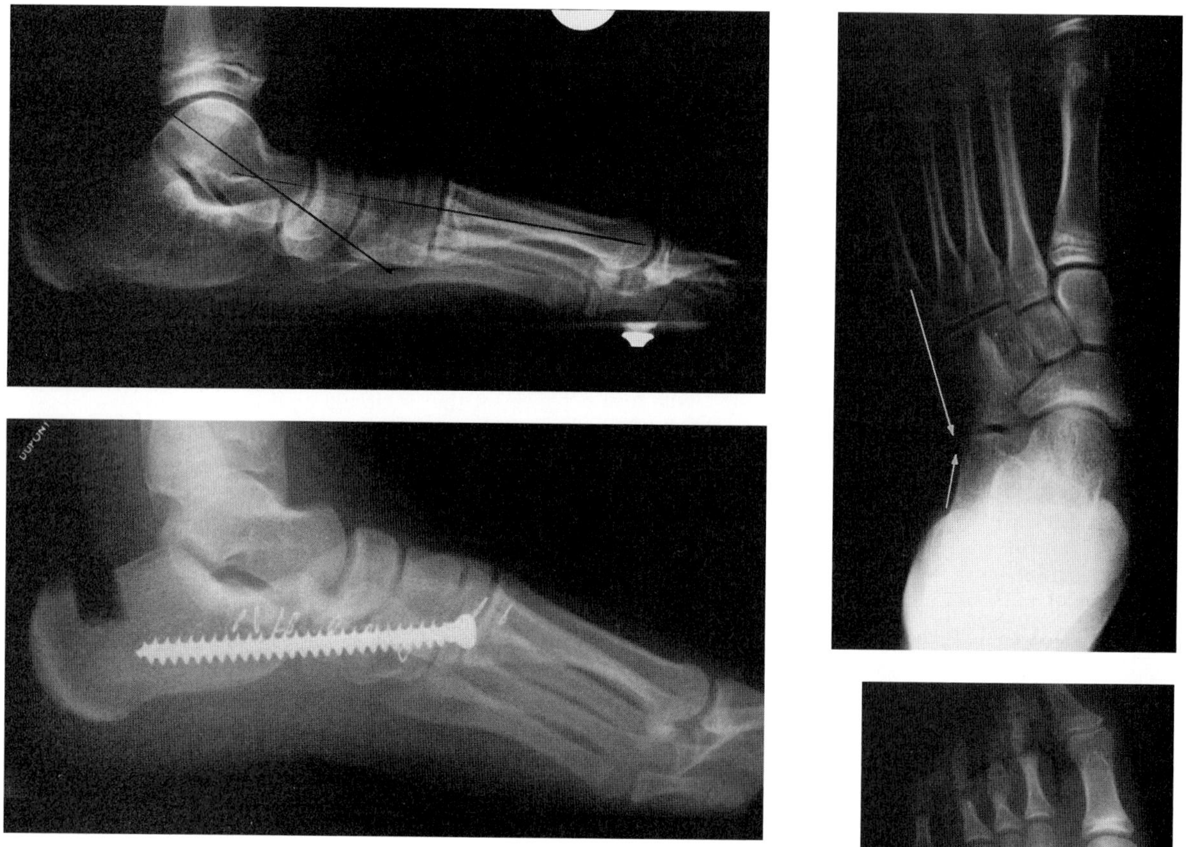

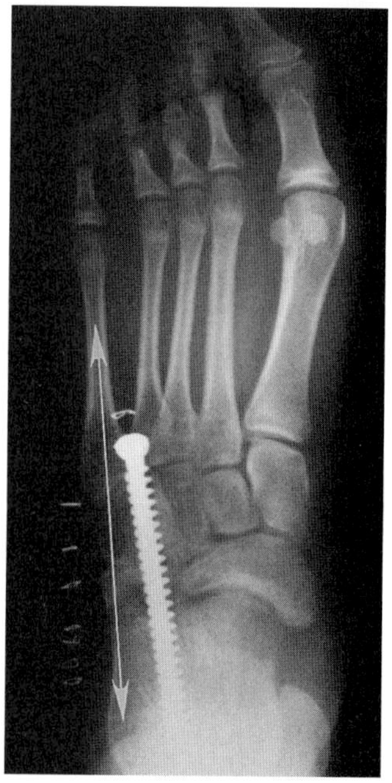

Fig. 2 **Top left,** Standing lateral radiograph of a 13-year-old with moderate pes planus. Note the talus plantarflexion in relationship to the longitudinal axis of the first metatarsal. **Top right,** Standing anteroposterior radiograph demonstrates the abduction of the midfoot (arrows). **Bottom left,** Normal alignment between the talus and the first metatarsal has been established following a lateral column lengthening arthrodesis between the calcaneus and cuboid. **Bottom right,** Anteroposterior radiograph demonstrates a normal alignment between the calcaneus, cuboid and fifth metatarsal.

Recurrent deformity in children between the ages of 2 and 6 years is corrected through a combined medial and lateral approach in which the hindfoot and midfoot capsulotomies are revised. An isolated extra-articular subtalar arthrodesis also may be necessary in an older child with residual deformity. Triple arthrodesis is a salvage procedure reserved for symptomatic adolescents.

Tarsal Coalition

Tarsal coalition, a fusion of two or more tarsal bones, may be fibrous, cartilaginous, or bony. Most tarsal coalitions are congenital, transmitted as an autosomal dominant trait with variable penetrance. Tarsal coalition also may be secondary to an intra-articular fracture, degenerative joint disease, rheumatoid arthritis, or infection. Fifty percent of

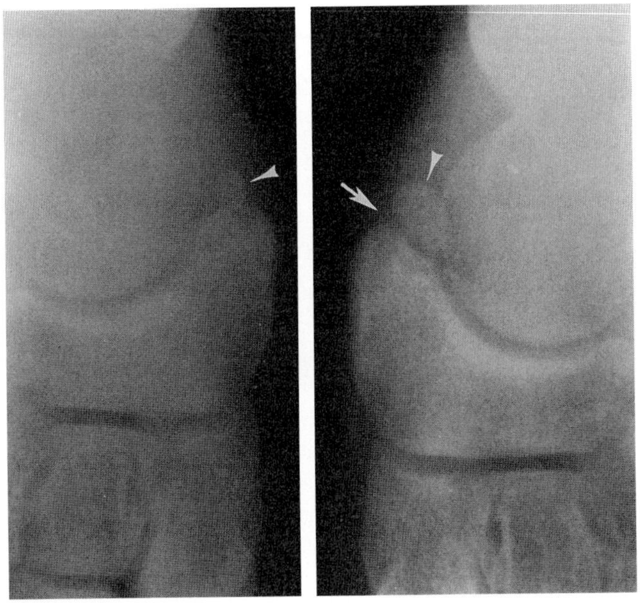

Fig. 3 Accessory navicular. **Left,** Type I (arrow). **Right,** Type II (arrows).

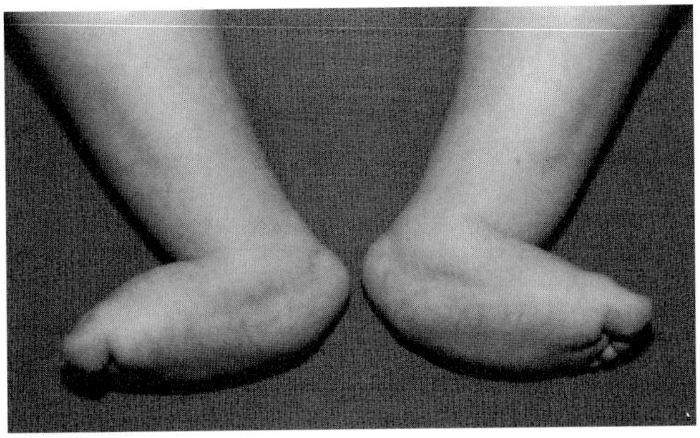

Fig. 4 Bilateral congenital vertical talus in a 9-month-old infant.

coalitions are bilateral. Talocalcaneal and calcaneonavicular coalitions occur with equal frequency and represent 90% of all tarsal fusions. Some patients may have multiple coalitions in the same foot.

The tarsal bones and the coalitions progressively ossify with increasing age; children become symptomatic when they lose motion in the foot from the bony transformation of the coalition. Patients with talocalcaneal coalitions usually present with complaints of pain between the ages of 12 and 16 years. Children with calcaneonavicular coalitions become symptomatic between the ages of 8 and 12 years. The vague aching pain in the hindfoot is aggravated by activity, and some patients complain of frequent ankle sprains. The foot examination in a patient with a coalition demonstrates decreased subtalar complex motion. The most impressive presentation is the peroneal spastic flatfoot: the hindfoot is held in rigid valgus and the forefoot is abducted. Peroneal spasm often is present as a pain reflex.

The radiographic evaluation of a patient suspected of having a tarsal coalition includes standing AP, lateral (Fig. 5, *left*), and oblique views. The radiographic signs of a coalition include blunting of the subtalar process, elongation of the anterior calcaneal process, narrowing of the posterior subtalar joint, and talar beaking. Calcaneonavicular coalitions are frequently seen on the oblique view. Computed tomography (CT) is the investigation of choice in suspected middle facet tarsal coalitions (Fig. 5, *center* and *right*). Angulation of the middle facet by more than 20° from horizontal is consistent with a coalition even if the joint appears open. Magnetic resonance imaging recently has been reported to be more sensitive for identification of a fibrous or cartilaginous coalition than CT.

Most tarsal coalitions are asymptomatic, and they often remain so into adulthood. Patients with symptomatic lesions are placed in a short leg walking cast for several weeks until symptoms resolve. Orthotic management may then be appropriate. If conservative therapy fails, surgery is indicated. Calcaneonavicular coalitions are treated with a generous excision of the coalition and interposition of the extensor digitorum brevis muscle between the calcaneus and the navicular. The surgical treatment of middle facet coalitions is more difficult and controversial. Adolescents with middle facet talocalcaneal coalitions may be treated with resection, provided that less than 50% of the facet is involved. Patients with significant posterior facet degenerative changes are treated with an isolated subtalar joint fusion, provided there are no significant midfoot degenerative changes. Patients with degenerative changes and pain in both the hindfoot and the midfoot are best treated by triple arthrodesis. Patients with persistent deformity following resection may require peroneal lengthening or hindfoot osteotomy.

Cerebral Palsy

The most common foot and ankle abnormality associated with cerebral palsy is ankle equinus. This progressive developmental condition results from the spasticity of the triceps surae muscle. Children younger than 2 years of age may have a deformity that can be corrected by serial casting. A myostatic contracture develops as the child grows older. Children with a mild equinus contracture of the ankle are treated initially with serial casting. An Achilles tendon lengthening, performed if the child fails to respond to this form of treatment, should be delayed until 4 years of age if possible. A percutaneous technique is used in young children, but open technique may be required for revision lengthenings and lengthenings in older patients. Usually, no associated capsular contractures occur with

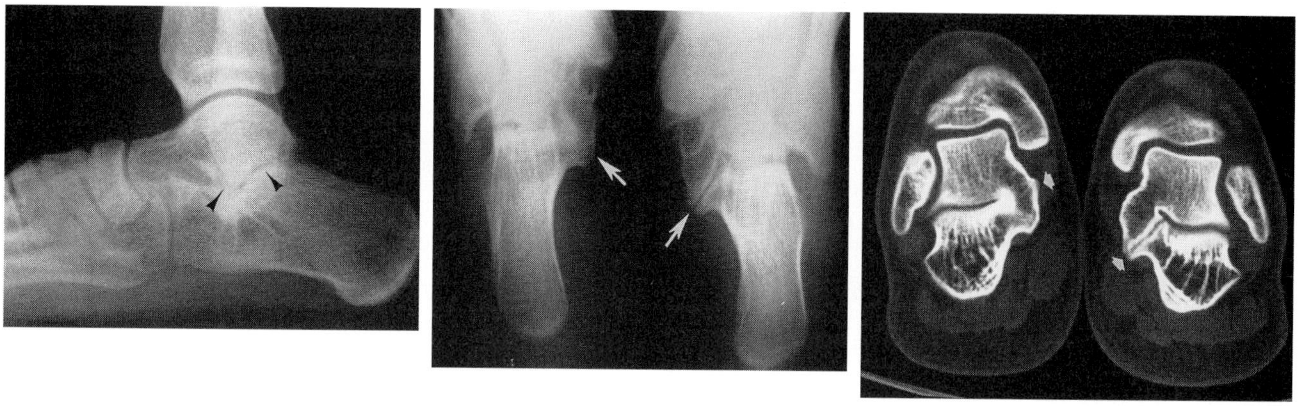

Fig. 5 **Left,** Standing lateral radiograph of a 13-year-old with a middle facet talocalcaneal coalition. Note the bony sclerosis at the site of the posterior and middle facet (darts). **Center,** Harris calcaneus view demonstrates middle facet talocalcaneal coalitions/left: bony; right: cartilaginous (arrows). **Right,** Computerized tomography demonstrates middle facet talocalcaneal coalitions.

this deformity in younger children. It is important to correct all lower extremity contractures about the hip, knee, and ankle during the same surgery. A foot or ankle deformity should not be viewed as an isolated problem. Achilles tendon lengthening alone may exacerbate crouching if knee and hip contractures are not corrected as well.

Equinovalgus is common in children with spastic diplegia and quadriplegia. A mild deformity can be corrected with a peroneal tendon lengthening (usually brevis) combined with an Achilles tendon lengthening. A medial displacement osteotomy of the calcaneus can be performed with this procedure if the heel valgus is pronounced. Marked heel valgus and subtalar pronation are treated with an opening wedge osteotomy of the anterior calcaneus. A subtalar fusion with concomitant tendon lengthening is performed if the hindfoot is in rigid valgus. The technique of Dennyson and Fulford is very reliable and involves placing a screw from the talar neck into the calcaneus. The screw holds the foot in a corrected position while a cancellous bone graft placed in the sinus tarsi consolidates.

Children with hemiplegia often have equinovarus foot deformities secondary to spasticity in the posterior tibial tendon. A split posterior tibial tendon transfer combined with an Achilles tendon lengthening provides excellent correction of this deformity if the heel varus is flexible. A split anterior tibialis transfer is performed when forefoot supination is the dominant deformity and usually is combined with a posterior tibial tendon lengthening. A complete transfer of the posterior tibial tendon to the dorsum of the foot can be performed when electromyograms show that the muscle is active only during the swing phase of gait. This procedure may be complicated by progressive calcaneovalgus deformity, particularly when associated with heel-cord lengthening. Rigid heel varus is treated with a lateral closing wedge osteotomy of the calcaneus combined with a soft-tissue balancing procedure. A triple arthrodesis is the procedure of choice for a symptomatic, rigid, deformed foot in an adolescent.

Myelomeningocele

Approximately half of the children born with a myelomeningocele have significant deformities of the feet. Secondary deformities develop with growth because of muscle imbalance and/or spasticity. The lack of sensation in these children makes it imperative that treatment modalities produce and maintain a plantigrade foot. Treatment options that leave the foot flexible are preferable. Complex tendon transfers provide inconsistent results because of the lack of selective muscle control and the tendency to create a new muscle imbalance.

Children with an equinovarus deformity require surgical correction to position the foot properly. Surgery usually is performed between 12 and 18 months of age and consists of a complete posterior medial release. The tendons normally are nonfunctioning and can be transected instead of lengthened. A talectomy rarely is indicated as the initial form of treatment for severe deformity. It may be necessary, however, for revision surgery.

A calcaneus foot deformity can have an associated cavus or valgus component, which is managed initially with bracing. In most children, a calcaneus foot deformity progresses unless the muscle imbalance in the lower extremity is corrected by early tenotomy or tendon transfer, such as transfer of the anterior tibialis tendon to the calcaneus. Older children may require a calcaneal osteotomy to decrease the plantar prominence of the calcaneal tuberosity.

Ankle and subtalar valgus deformities are common, especially in children who ambulate. These deformities often coexist with external tibial torsion. Children develop the valgus deformities because of progressive fibular shortening. In children, a mild deformity can be corrected by a partial Achilles tendon tenodesis to the fibula. Patients with more severe deformities are treated with a medial tibial epiphysiodesis or a distal tibial varus osteotomy. Children with associated calcaneus deformities secondary to unopposed anterior tibialis function are treated with a concomitant tendon release or transfer to the os calcis. The subtalar joint may be stabilized in some older children to control residual foot valgus, but this procedure can lead to a rigid foot and increase the risk of pressure sores. Stabilization normally is accomplished by performing a subtalar arthrodesis or a calcaneal osteotomy.

Lesser Toe Deformities

An overlapping fifth toe deformity usually is bilateral and asymptomatic. Contractures of the dorsal medial metatarsophalangeal joint capsule and extensor tendon cause the phalanges of the fifth ray to rotate in a lateral direction. Occasionally, callosities and abrasions occur from shoe wear. Surgical correction in symptomatic children is achieved by either a partial phalangeal resection combined with syndactylization of the fifth toe to the fourth, or by a circumferential incision allowing a capsulotomy and extensor tendon release. The latter procedure permits the toe to flex and derotate.

Congenital curly toes usually affect the fourth and fifth rays. They are familial and usually bilateral. They rarely are symptomatic, and they occasionally improve spontaneously. If necessary, correction can be obtained by releasing the long flexor tendons.

A bunionette is a lateral prominence of the fifth metatarsal head. The prominence is formed by the metatarsal head and the soft tissue at the metatarsophalangeal joint and usually is unilateral. A bunionette becomes symptomatic secondary to chronic irritation of the lateral aspect of the forefoot by shoewear. Initial treatment consists of shoewear education. If this is unsuccessful, patients are treated with a chevron osteotomy at the fifth metatarsal, which preserves the function of the fifth metatarsophalangeal joint. The thickened, inflamed soft tissue on the lateral aspect of the fifth metatarsal joint rapidly disappears after the pressure on the forefoot is relieved by the alteration in the width of the forefoot.

Hallux Valgus

A medial prominence of the first metatarsal head develops when the intermetatarsal angle between the first and second ray exceeds 10° with more than 18° of hallux valgus. Structural factors that predispose to the development of hallux valgus include metatarsus primus varus (intermetatarsal angle $\geq$ 14°), ligamentous laxity, forefoot pronation, heel cord contracture, and shoewear. Juvenile hallux valgus differs from the adult version by the less pronounced deviation of the hallux, the smaller medial eminence, and the presence of the rotational deformity of the great toe only in patients with a severe deformity. Close attention must be paid to the articular characteristics of both the tarsometatarsal and metatarsophalangeal joints (proximal hypermobility, distal metatarsal articular angle, articular congruency, interphalangeal hallux valgus).

Most pediatric and adolescent patients with hallux valgus are asymptomatic and do not require therapy. Occasionally, a child or teenager with pain or a deformity that is cosmetically unacceptable is treated with a low temperature thermoplast splint that is worn at night. The indications for surgical intervention include moderate pain, deformity, and limitation in shoewear. Patients with slightly elevated intermetatarsal angles and moderate hallux valgus can be treated with a soft-tissue procedure and a distal metatarsal chevron osteotomy. More commonly, adolescents with more severe deformities are treated with a distal soft-tissue procedure and either a proximal metatarsal osteotomy or a double osteotomy of the first metatarsal. A proximal phalangeal osteotomy can be done to correct hallux valgus interphalangeus or, in combination with other procedures, to correct all components of a hallux valgus deformity. It also can be used in patients with an asymptomatic great toe valgus deformity who have symptoms in the second toe.

Complications associated with the surgical correction of hallux valgus may be common and include overcorrection, recurrence of deformity, stiffness, and injury to the proximal first metatarsal physis. The rate of recurrence after surgical correction is inversely related to the age of the child and may approach 50% prior to skeletal maturity.

Sever's Disease

Sever's disease is a traction apophysitis at the insertion of the Achilles tendon. The patient complains of pain in the heel that is exacerbated by activities like running and activity on hard surfaces. Rest improves the symptoms. Physical examination reveals tenderness at the insertion of the heel cord, usually without swelling. Most patients have decreased ankle dorsiflexion when compared to the uninvolved side. Radiographs often are normal. Occasionally, increased radiodensity or fragmentation of the calcaneal apophysis may be present, but this may be a normal variant.

The treatment of Sever's disease begins with activity modification—rest. The child is given a one half inch heel cushion, and ice is applied to the heel cord insertion after strenuous activity. Instructions are given to stretch the heel cord after symptoms subside. This treatment is combined with administration of nonsteroidal anti-inflammatory medications. In severe cases, the patient may need cast immobilization in approximately 5° of plantarflexion. The child may return to normal activities when asymptomatic.

Köhler's Disease

Köhler's disease of the tarsal navicular is a self-limited condition characterized by flattening sclerosis and irregularities of the tarsal navicular (Fig. 6). It is more common in boys than girls. It normally appears in boys at 5 years of age and in girls at 4 years of age, and it is bilateral in approximately one third of patients. Köhler's disease probably results from repetitive compressive forces applied to the tarsal navicular. Children with Köhler's disease have an antalgic limp and bear weight on the lateral aspect of

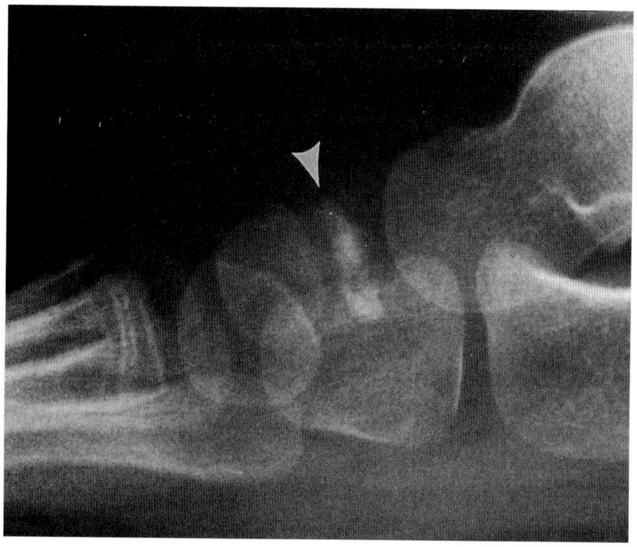

Fig. 6 Köhler's disease involving the foot navicular (dart).

the foot to relieve stress on the longitudinal arch. Pain, tenderness, and occasional swelling occur at the navicular. Hindfoot and midfoot motions are normal.

Children with mild discomfort are treated by placing the affected foot in a soft longitudinal arch support with a one eighth-inch inner heel wedge and a Thomas heel. When the child is asymptomatic, return to normal shoewear is appropriate. Patients with moderate to severe pain are treated initially with a below the knee walking cast with the foot in 10° to 15° of varus and 20° of equinus for approximately 6 weeks, followed by shoe modifications or an orthosis. The prognosis for children with Köhler's disease is excellent. The navicular normally reconstitutes itself, usually without any residual deformities.

Freiberg's Infraction

Freiberg's infraction is believed to be an aseptic necrosis of the second metatarsal head that produces an anterior metatarsalgia. This condition normally is seen in adolescents; approximately 75% of cases occur in girls. The second metatarsal head is the most common site of involvement, although other metatarsals also may be affected. The disorder occasionally is bilateral and is believed to result from vascular insufficiency secondary to chronic stress.

Patients with Freiberg's infraction complain of pain in the forefoot, normally at the second metatarsal head. The metatarsophalangeal joint has mild local swelling and limitation of motion. Radiographs demonstrate metatarsal head flattening and irregularity. Patients with Freiberg's infraction are treated by placing the affected foot in a below the knee walking cast for 4 weeks. Pressure is relieved from the metatarsal head with a metatarsal pad after the cast is removed. If conservative care does not relieve symptoms, the avascular bone is curetted and grafted with cancellous bone from the cuboid or lateral cuneiform.

Traumatic Disorders

Distal Tibial and Fibular Epiphyseal Fractures

Fractures of the ankle joint generally conform to the Salter-Harris classification. Most fibular fractures are Salter-Harris type I or II and can be treated by closed means. Salter-Harris type I or II fractures of the distal tibial physis are treated by closed reduction and application of a bent knee cast. Occasionally, a torn periosteal sleeve caught in the physeal fracture site prevents reduction, and open reduction and smooth pin fixation are required. Moderate displacement, especially in the AP plane, is acceptable and can be expected to remodel; however, varus angulation and valgus angulation of more than 10° to 15° in an older child with a type I or II fracture will not correct spontaneously. Displaced Salter-Harris types III and IV fractures, including triplane and Tillaux fractures with a 2-mm or more displacement, require open reduction and internal fixation. With the exception of triplane and Tillaux fractures, Salter-Harris types III and IV fractures usually are medial. In a young child, symptomatic ossification centers in the medial malleolus should not be mistaken for a Salter-Harris type III fracture. Premature physeal closure by formation of a bony bridge is frequent after types III and IV fractures of the medial plafond. Smooth pins or 4.0-mm cannulated screws should be inserted from medial to lateral in the epiphysis distal to the physis when possible.

Juvenile Tillaux Fractures

Juvenile Tillaux fractures occur in older adolescents, and the mechanism of injury is an external rotation force with stress placed on the anterior tibiofibular ligament, causing avulsion of the distal tibial physis anterolaterally. This avulsion generally occurs after the medial part of the physis is closed but the lateral portion is still open. Thus, the fracture courses through the physis and traverses distally across the epiphysis into the joint, creating a Salter-Harris type III or IV fracture. Open reduction and internal fixation are indicated if the fracture is displaced and cannot be reduced by closed methods (Fig. 7). More recently, percutaneous indirect reduction of the fragment and internal fixation have been recommended by some authors.

Triplane Fractures

The classic triplane fracture is a three-part fracture, although more recently the term has included two-part fractures. Three-part fractures are considered to be a combination of Salter-Harris types II and III fractures, whereas two-part fractures are considered to be Salter-Harris type

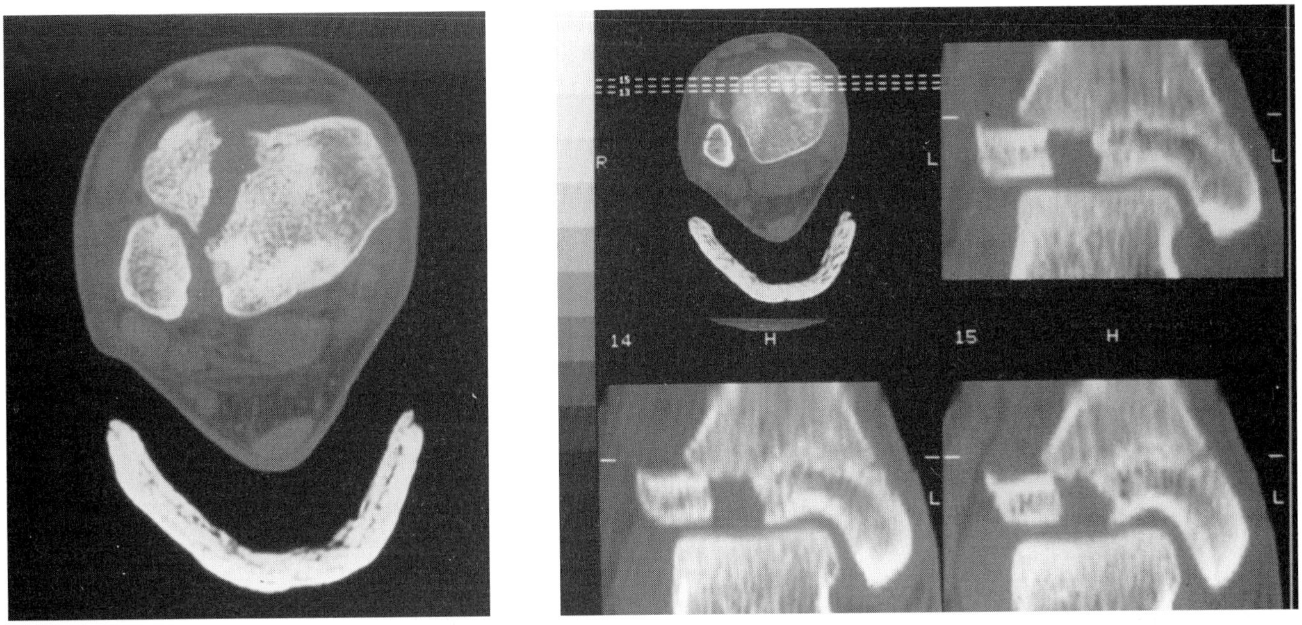

Fig. 7 Tillaux fracture. **Left,** Computed tomography (CT) scan in coronal plane shows anterior and lateral fracture. **Right,** Reformatted CT scan shows extent of displacement of fracture. (Courtesy of Dr. Alvin Crawford, Cincinnati, OH.)

IV fractures (Fig. 8). Tomograms or computed tomography (CT) scans may be helpful to determine the configuration and the amount of displacement. Closed reduction can be attempted by internal rotation of the foot, followed by immobilization in a long bent-knee leg cast. If closed reduction to 2 mm or less of displacement cannot be achieved, open reduction and internal fixation are necessary. Because of the complex fracture pattern and the large size of the fragments, the fracture is not easy to reduce, and quite often multiple incisions and extensive dissection are necessary. Attention should be focused on obtaining articular congruity.

Talar Fractures

Talar neck fractures in children should be treated in the same way as in adults. If the talar neck is severely displaced, open reduction and internal fixation are necessary. Osteonecrosis can be expected when the body of the talus is subluxed or dislocated from the subtalar or ankle joint. The prognosis of osteonecrosis in children with talar fractures differs from that in adults. It generally progresses from a sclerotic lesion in the talar dome and body to a cystic lesion on the radiograph, with resolution and little collapse of the talus 2 to 3 years after injury.

Ankles sprains occur in children as they do in adults. If swelling and disability persist 6 weeks after the original ankle injury, an osteochondral fracture or osteochondritis dissecans of the talus should be suspected. Chronic recurrent ankle sprains may suggest a tarsal coalition.

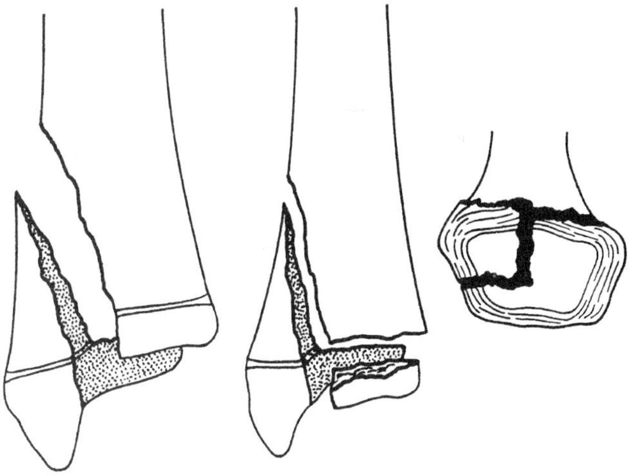

Fig. 8 **Left,** Two-fragment triplane fracture (Salter-Harris type IV). **Right,** Three-fragment triplane fracture (Salter-Harris types II and III fractures). (Reproduced with permission from Rockwood CA Jr, Wilkins KE, King RE (eds): *Fractures in Children.* Philadelphia, PA, JB Lippincott, 1984, pp 1021–1027.)

Calcaneal Fractures

Calcaneal fractures are less common in children than in adults and do not have the same fracture pattern. Also, children have some ability to remodel the fracture, especially at the subtalar joint. Sixty percent of calcaneal fractures in children are extra-articular and 40% are intra-articular, which is the opposite of the adult fracture pattern. Displacement of intra-articular fractures in most children is minimal and some remodeling can be expected. However, in an older child with involvement of the subtalar joint, a decreased "crucial" angle, and joint compression, the fracture should be treated by open reduction and internal fixation as in an adult.

Lisfranc Fracture-Dislocation

In children, fractures of the tarsal bones often are associated with severe injury to the foot, such as from a wringer, lawn mower, or severe compression injury. A subtle Lisfranc dislocation has been noted in children with a chip fracture at the base of the second metatarsal and a buckle fracture of the cuboid, and it implies significant tarsometatarsal joint injury. Closed reduction and pinning or open reduction and internal fixation are indicated as in adults.

Metatarsal Fractures

Fractures of the metatarsal phalanges are fairly common in children. Most heal uneventfully and rarely require surgical treatment. Overuse stress fractures of the metatarsal shaft or neck have been reported in children as young as 10 years of age. Jones fractures of the fifth metatarsal are rare in children and usually heal uneventfully. A small avulsion of the most proximal base of the fifth metatarsal should not be confused with the secondary ossification center or epiphysitis that occurs in Iselin's disease.

Annotated Bibliography

Metatarsus Adductus

Cook DA, Breed AL, Cook T, et al: Observer variability in the radiographic measurement and classification of metatarsus adductus. *J Pediatr Orthop* 1992;12:86–89.

The use of radiographs to classify subtypes of metatarsus adductus is error prone. Irregularity of hindfoot ossification centers makes radiographic measurements inconsistent.

Farsetti P, Weinstein SL, Ponseti IV, et al: The long-term functional and radiographic outcomes of untreated and non-operatively treated metatarsus adductus. *J Bone Joint Surg* 1994;76A:257–265.

Metatarsus adductus that is passively correctable resolved without treatment. Serial manipulation and casting produced correction of noncorrectable rigid metatarsus adductus. Patients with a mild to moderate residual deformity at follow-up were functional and had pain only after strenuous activities. Surgical treatment is not necessary.

Smith JT, Bleck EE, Gamble JG, et al: Simple method of documenting metatarsus adductus. *J Pediatr Orthop* 1991;11:679–680.

An accurate, inexpensive method of documenting metatarsus adductus with serial photocopies is described.

Clubfoot

Catterall A: A method of assessment of the clubfoot deformity. *Clin Orthop* 1991;264:48–53.

This article defines a reproducible method of analysis of clubfoot deformity after treatment.

Howard CB, Benson MK: Clubfoot: Its pathological anatomy. *J Pediatr Orthop* 1993;13:654–659.

This article describes the pathologic anatomy of clubfeet.

Ikeda K: Conservative treatment of idiopathic clubfoot. *J Pediatr Orthop* 1992;12:217–223.

Surgery is not required after cast therapy for idiopathic clubfeet if residual varus, adductus, or intoeing is passively correctable to at least a neutral position. Residual equinus without fixed varus is correctable by serial casting during childhood.

Sodre H, Bruschini S, Mestriner LA, et al: Arterial abnormalities in talipes equinovarus as assessed by angiography and the Doppler technique. *J Pediatr Orthop* 1990;10:101–104.

Preoperative angiography in 30 uncorrected clubfeet demonstrated abnormal vascular patterns in all but two limbs, with hypoplasia or premature termination of the anterior tibial and medial plantar arteries in the remainder. Because the posterior tibial artery usually provides the only arterial supply to the foot, this vessel must be preserved meticulously at surgery and during subsequent ankle dorsiflexion.

Stanitski CL, Ward WT, Grossman W: Noninvasive vascular studies in clubfoot. *J Pediatr Orthop* 1992;12:514–517.

Pulse oximetry and Doppler assessment are available, noninvasive, and reproducible means of monitoring vascular integrity in children with a talipes equinovarus after surgical correction.

Tarray YN, Carroll NC: Analysis of the components of residual deformity in clubfeet presenting for reoperation. *J Pediatr Orthop* 1992;12:207–216.

Residual forefoot adduction and supination are the most common deformities persistent in undercorrected clubfeet after surgery (95%). This results from not releasing the calcaneocuboid joint and the plantar fascia, and failure to recognize residual forefoot adduction on the interoperative radiograph at primary surgery.

Thometz JG, Simons GW: Deformity of the calcaneocuboid joint in patients who have talipes equinovarus. *J Bone Joint Surg* 1993;75A:190–195.

This report of 26 feet in children with surgically treated clubfoot and grade II calcaneocuboid deformity (central cuboid line on or medial to medial tangent of calcaneus) recommends release of the calcaneocuboid joint at the time of posterior medial release.

Pes Cavus

Price AE, Maisel R, Drennan JC: Computed tomographic analysis of pes cavus. *J Pediatr Orthop* 1993;13:646–653.

Patterns of muscle degeneration in patients with peripheral neuropathies and pes cavus are described. Abnormalities of the intrinsic muscles of the foot occur earlier and are more severe than in the extrinsic muscles

Watenabe RS: Metatarsal osteotomy for the cavus foot. *Clin Orthop* 1990;252:217–230.

This article describes the results of metatarsal osteotomies for the correction of pes cavus.

Idiopathic (Flexible) Pes Planus

Sangeorzan BJ, Mosca V, Hansen ST Jr: Effect of calcaneal lengthening on relationships among the hindfoot, midfoot, and forefoot. *Foot Ankle* 1993;14: 136–141.

A significant correction of the relationship of the navicular and talus can be achieved with a lateral column lengthening in patients with flexible pes planus.

Wenger DR, Mauldin D, Speck G, et al: Corrective shoes and inserts as treatment for flexible flatfoot in infants and children. *J Bone Joint Surg* 1989;71A:800–810.

A prospective study was performed to determine whether flexible flatfoot in children can be influenced by treatment; 129 children were stratified into four groups ($p < 0.01$) including controls. The authors concluded that wearing corrective shoes or inserts for 3 years does not influence the course of flexible flatfoot in children.

Accessory Navicular

Bennett GL, Weiner DS, Leighley B: Surgical treatment of symptomatic accessory tarsal navicular. *J Pediatr Orthop* 1990;10:445–449.

Fifty patients (75 feet) were reviewed retrospectively. Surgery consisted of excision alone with good to excellent results in 90%. A comprehensive review is presented.

Congenital Vertical Talus

Schrader LF, Gilbert RJ, Skinner SR, et al: Congenital vertical talus: Surgical correction by a one-stage medial approach. *Orthopedics* 1990;13:1233–1236.

A one-stage procedure for correction of congenital vertical talus using a medial approach is described; the operation was performed on 14 feet with good initial anatomic results in all cases.

Tarsal Coalition

Gonzalez P, Kumar SJ: Calcaneonavicular coalition treated by resection and interposition of the extensor digitorum brevis muscle. *J Bone Joint Surg* 1990;72A: 71–77.

Seventy-five feet in 48 patients with calcaneonavicular coalitions were evaluated at 2 to 23 years after resection of the coalition and interposition of the extensor digitorum brevis muscle. The best results occurred in patients with a cartilaginous coalition who were younger than 16 years of age at the time of surgery.

Kumar SJ, Guille JT, Lee MS, et al: Osseous and non-osseous coalition of the middle facet of the talocalcaneal joint. *J Bone Joint Surg* 1992;74A:529–535.

Patients with symptomatic talocalcaneal coalitions that do not resolve following conservative care should have a resection of the coalition with tendon interposition.

Pachuda NM, Lasday SD, Jay RM: Tarsal coalition: Etiology, diagnosis, and treatment. *J Foot Surg* 1990; 29:474–488.

This paper is an excellent review of tarsal coalition.

Salomao O, Napoli MM, de Carvalho AE Jr, et al: Talocalcaneal coalition: Diagnosis and surgical management. *Foot Ankle* 1992;13:251–256.

Patients with symptomatic talocalcaneal coalitions were treated with bar resection and interposition fat graft. At follow-up, 78% of the feet were painless. The remaining patients had an improvement in their pain. Approximately 69% of the feet had an improvement in the deformity, and 76% demonstrated an improved range of motion.

Cerebral Palsy

Barnes MJ, Herring JA: Combined split anterior tibial-tendon transfer and intramuscular lengthening of the posterior tibial tendon: Results in patients who have a varus deformity of the foot due to spastic cerebral palsy. *J Bone Joint Surg* 1991;73A:734–738.

A combined procedure is described for the correction of a flexible varus deformity of the foot in patients with cerebral palsy. Other procedures to correct this problem are discussed for comparison.

Gallien R, Morin F, Marquis F: Subtalar arthrodesis in children. *J Pediatr Orthop* 1989;9:59–63.

A retrospective study of 30 patients (51 feet) with valgus foot deformities who were treated by three different types of subtalar extra-articular and intra-articular arthrodesis. A combined Grice-Green-Batchelor procedure gave the best outcome (84% excellent and good results), with bony union in 96% of the feet. The results from the Grice-Green-Batchelor procedure were not as good in paralytic flatfeet of children with cerebral palsy. It is necessary to rule out ankle valgus versus subtalar valgus. Weightbearing films of the ankles in the anteroposterior plane are essential before surgery to determine the true extent of the deformity in every paralytic child.

Synder M, Kumar SJ, Stecyk MD: Split tibialis posterior tendon transfer and tendo-Achillis lengthening for spastic equinovarus feet. *J Pediatr Orthop* 1993;13:20–23.

Split tibialis posterior tendon transfer and Achilles tendon lengthening were performed on 21 patients with spastic equinovarus foot deformities. Fifteen of 18 ambulatory patients were graded as excellent or good. All nonambulatory patients had a plantigrade foot at follow-up. Indications for this procedure are a spastic varus or an equinovarus foot deformity in which the varus component is flexible and results from an overactive posterior tibialis muscle.

Myelomeningocele

Georgiadis GM, Aronson DD: Posterior transfer of the anterior tibial tendon in children who have a myelomeningocele. *J Bone Joint Surg* 1990;72A:392–398.

The technique and indications for this procedure are discussed. Surgical results are best when the child is at least 4 years of age and has a low lumbar or sacral motor level.

Sherk HH, Marchinski LJ, Clancy M, et al: Ground reaction forces on the plantar surface of the foot after talectomy in the myelomeningocele. *J Pediatr Orthop* 1989;9:269–275.

Talectomy rarely succeeds in distributing weightbearing forces uniformly over the plantar surface of the foot. This may predispose a patient to neurotrophic ulceration.

Toe Deformities

Diebold PF: Basal osteotomy of the fifth metatarsal for the bunionette. *Foot Ankle* 1991;12:74–79.

This paper describes the surgical correction of a symptomatic bunionette deformity.

Hallux Valgus

Frey C, Jahss M, Kummer FJ: The Akin procedure: An analysis of results. *Foot Ankle* 1991;12:1–6.

The Akin procedure can be used in combination with other procedures in the initial surgical treatment of hallux valgus. It can be used alone in patients with an asymptomatic great toe valgus deformities that produce symptoms in the second toe, or for residual hallux valgus after surgical correction.

Gebuhr P, Soelberg M, Larsen TK, et al: McBride's operation for hallux valgus: A 2–11-year follow-up of 46 cases. *Acta Orthop Scand* 1992;63:189–191.

The McBride bunionectomy remains an excellent treatment option for mild to moderate hallux valgus if the procedure is performed as originally described: medial capsulorrhaphy of the first metatarsophalangeal joint, exostectomy of the medial prominence, tenotomy of the adductor complex and reattachment to the first metatarsal, and excision of the lateral sesamoid.

Groiso JA: Juvenile hallux valgus: A conservative approach to treatment. *J Bone Joint Surg* 1992;74A: 1367–1374.

This article reviews the results of an office-made, low-temperature thermoplast night splint for the treatment of hallux valgus in childhood and adolescence. This was combined with both passive and active medial mobilization of the metatarsophalangeal joint. Eighty-eight percent of the patients with an initial metatarsophalangeal angle of at least 15° or an interphalangeal angle of 9° or more had an improvement.

Mann RA, Rudicel S, Graves SC: Repair of hallux valgus with a distal soft-tissue procedure and proximal metatarsal osteotomy: A long-term follow-up. *J Bone Joint Surg* 1992;74A:124–129.

This article retrospectively reviews 75 patients (109 feet) in whom a hallux valgus deformity was corrected with a distal soft-tissue release, excision of the medial eminence, plication of the medial capsule, and a crescentic osteotomy of the first metatarsal. Ninety-three percent of the patients were satisfied with the surgical result. The hallux valgus angle improved from 31° to 9° while the intermetatarsal angle improved from 14° to 6°.

Peterson HA, Newman SR: Adolescent bunion deformity treated with double osteotomy and longitudinal pin fixation of the first ray. *J Pediatr Orthop* 1993;13:80–84.

A concomitant distal and proximal first metatarsal osteotomy provides excellent correction for moderate to severe hallux valgus in the adolescent.

Freiberg's Disease

Katcherian DA: Treatment of Freiberg's disease. *Orthop Clin North Am* 1994;25:69–81.

This article is an excellent review and discussion of the treatment of Freiberg's disease.

Traumatic Disorders of the Ankle and Foot

Schlesinger I, Wedge JH: Percutaneous reduction and fixation of displaced juvenile Tillaux fractures: A new surgical technique. *J Pediatr Orthop* 1993;13:389–391.

The authors describe a technique for percutaneous reduction and fixation of Tillaux fractures when closed manipulation and reduction fails to restore the articular surface.

Classic Bibliography

Johnson GF: Pediatric Lisfranc injury: "Bunk bed" fracture. *AJR* 1981;137:1041–1044.

Stanitski CL, Micheli LJ: Observations on symptomatic medial malleolar ossification centers. *J Pediatr Orthop* 1993;13:164–168.

43

Ankle and Foot: Trauma

Ankle fractures are among the most common injuries treated by orthopaedic surgeons. An older, more active population and additional safety constraints in high-speed motor vehicle accidents have resulted in greater incidence and severity of ankle fractures. The goal of treatment is to maximize the long-term function of the ankle. The crucial decision is whether surgery is needed or desirable for precise restoration of the anatomy. There is evidence to support the notion that in ankle fractures with diastasis, the best result depends on the accuracy and stability of the reduction.

Tibial Pilon Fractures

There are two variants of pilon fractures: the first is produced by primarily rotational forces, and the second, the "explosion fracture," is produced by axial loading. Anatomically, pilon fractures can be categorized by the amount of intra-articular incongruity and comminution (Fig. 1). Type I fractures are intra-articular through the plafond without significant displacement of the articular surface. Type II fractures have incongruity of the articular surface without a great deal of comminution. Type III fractures demonstrate incongruity as well as displacement of multiple small fracture fragments involving the metaphysis of the distal tibia. Accurate classification requires computed tomography (CT).

Type I fractures do well with nonsurgical treatment and cast immobilization. Repair of explosion fractures (types II and III) usually requires open reduction and internal fixation (ORIF) because these fractures involve articular comminution and significant soft-tissue damage. Numerous difficulties have been encountered during efforts at open reduction and plate fixation of explosion fractures, with total complications ranging as high as 54% in some series. Most of these complications, such as infections and wound breakdown, relate to the soft tissues. The response to this high incidence of complications is external fixation in which the external fixator serves as a buttress to connect the joint and the shaft.

External fixation is often combined with an open reduction of the joint. The options include use of a large 1/2 pin fixator or some variance of Ilizarov frames. Although this approach has avoided disastrous soft-tissue problems, pin track infection and late shaft deformity remain difficulties peculiar to external fixation. Emphasis on a delayed approach for closed fractures and careful soft-tissue handling appear to be ingredients for success in the external fixation series. These measures are also advised for patients treated with plating, using sufficient open reduction to manipulate and reduce the joint fragments.

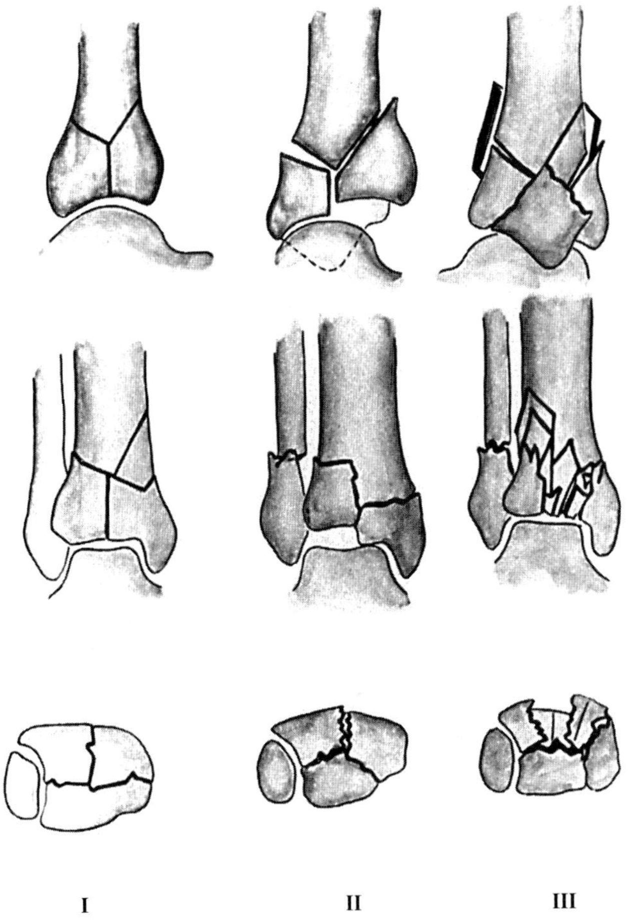

Fig. 1 Classification system for pilon fractures. Type I fractures show minimal displacement; types II and III show increasing degrees of articular displacement and comminution, respectively. (Reproduced with permission from Mast J: Pilon fractures of the distal tibia: A test of surgical judgement, in Tscherne H, Schatzker J (eds): *Major Fractures of the Pilon, the Talus, and the Calcaneus: Current Concepts of Treatment.* Berlin, Germany, Springer-Verlag, 1993, pp 7–28.)

Ankle Fractures

Although there is a tendency to radiograph the ankle of any patient who complains of pain and swelling, limiting radiography to those ankles with specific indications may reduce radiograph usage by 50% without missing any significant fractures. These indications are gross deformity, instability of the ankle, crepitus, localized bone tenderness, swelling, and inability to bear weight. A good case has also been made for obtaining only lateral and mortise views, because the anteroposterior view has not been found to add a significant amount of information.

Evaluation of ankle fracture radiographs includes classification of the fracture. The two most widely used systems are the Weber-AO system, which depends on the level of the fibula fracture, and the Lauge-Hansen system in which the first term refers to the position of the foot and the second term refers to the direction of the deforming force. In the Weber-AO system, type A fractures are below the tibial plafond and typically are transverse fractures, type B fractures begin at the level of the tibial plafond and typically extend proximally in a spiral or short oblique fashion, and type C fractures of the fibula are initiated above the tibial plafond and are associated with syndesmotic injuries. In the Lauge-Hansen system, fractures involving a supinated foot will sustain an anterolateral soft-tissue injury first, because the medial ligamentous structures are lax in the supinated foot/ankle. An example of this is seen in Figure 2, *left,* in which the common supination-external rotation fracture pattern is shown. Figure 2, *right,* shows how changing the initial foot position from supination to pronation can alter this fracture pattern. With the foot in pronation, forces start on the medial side with either rupture of the deltoid or medial malleolus followed by the lateral syndesmotic ligament group and fibula. Pilon and ankle fractures make up at least two thirds of complex foot and ankle injuries. Incidence of the supination external rotation injury is 60%, and that of the pronation external rotation injury is 12%.

It has been shown that the Weber-AO system is neither prognostic nor predictive of surgical treatment. In contrast, several studies have found that Lauge-Hansen stage II supination-external rotation injuries have equivalent outcomes whether treated surgically or nonsurgically, whereas stage IV supination-external rotation injuries have a better outcome with surgical intervention.

In an implicit recognition of the shortcomings of both the Weber-AO and earlier Lauge-Hansen classification systems, numerous investigators have published what they consider to be acceptable bony displacements that are compatible with satisfactory long-term outcome. Acceptable lateral malleolar displacement ranges between 0 and 5 mm in any direction, while a talar shift between 0 and 2 mm may be acceptable on plain radiographs. However, these plain-film measurements have been shown to overstate the amount of displacement of the lateral malleolus at its articulation with the talus. External rotation deformity of the distal fibular fragment, as seen on plain radiographs, has also been advanced as a surgical indication. Based on computed tomography (CT) studies of ankle fractures, it has been shown that this rotatonal deformity at the fracture site reflects internal rotation of the proximal

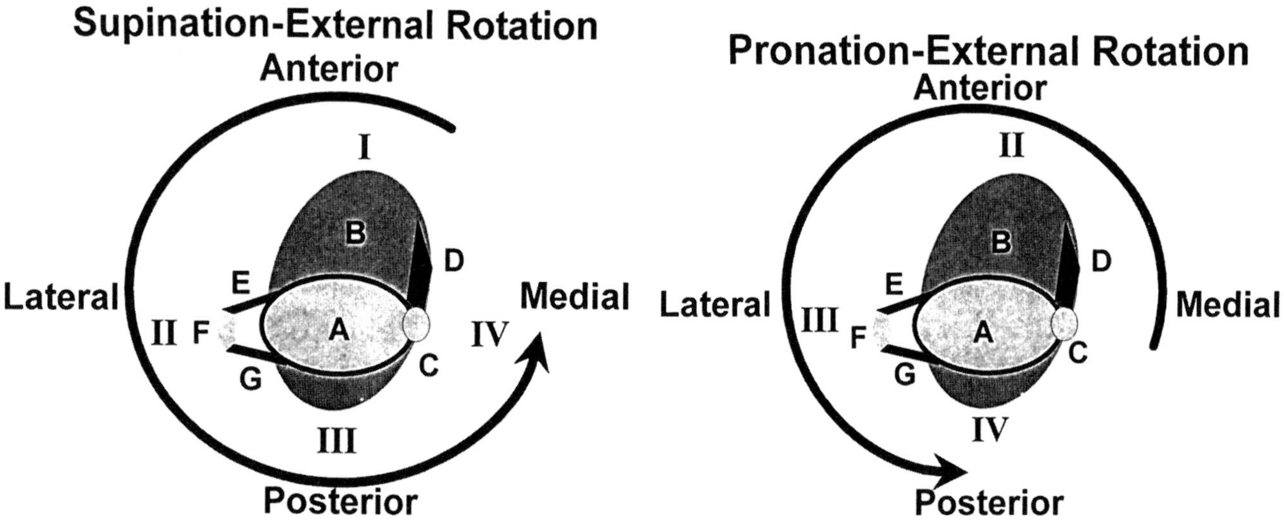

Fig. 2 The schematic diagram of the Lauge-Hansen classification system for ankle fractures. **Left,** Schematic representation of the supination-external rotation injury. The foot is held supinated and subjected to an external rotation force. The injury stages start with anterior injury to the capsule and the anterior tibiofibular ligament (E). Stage II injury involves fracture of the fibula (F). Stage III injury progresses to posterior tibiofibular ligament (G) injury. Stage IV injury involves either medial malleolus fracture (C) or deltoid ligament injury (D). This mechanism is most common, with an incidence of 60%. **Right,** Schematic diagram of the pronation-external rotation injury. The foot is held pronated while the talus (B) is rotated externally about the tibia (A). The injury begins on the medial side with either C or D. Stage II injury includes E; stage III injury progresses to F; and stage IV involves G or posterior capsular injury. (Reproduced with permission from Michelson J: Fractures of the ankle, in Lutter LD, Mizel MS, Pfeffer GB (eds): *Orthopaedic Knowledge Update: Foot and Ankle.* Rosemont, IL, American Academy of Orthopaedic Surgeons, 1994, pp 193–203.)

fibula with maintenance of normal talofibular alignment distally. Consequently, surgical intervention to correct ankle biomechanics is not warranted.

Syndesmotic space between the tibia and fibula is measured 1 cm proximal to the plafond. The criterion for a normal space is more than 1 mm of overlap between the tibia and fibula on any view, or a clear space between the medial border of the fibula and the medial border of the incisura fibularis measuring less than 6 mm on either the anteroposterior or mortise view (Fig. 3).

Treatment of Specific Fracture Types

Isolated Lateral Malleolar Fracture

There is little justification for surgery on isolated lateral malleolar fractures in the absence of medial injury. The apparent rotational and translational displacements of the lateral malleollus do not affect the tibiotalar articulation and, consequently, are not felt to alter the mechanics of the ankle joint. This has been substantiated by numerous clinical studies which have specifically examined the stage II supination-external rotation (SE-II) fractures. In follow-ups ranging from 3 to 30 years, excellent results are seen in 95% to 98% of patients treated nonsurgically. No improvement in outcome is seen for those patients who undergo surgery. Therefore, surgery generally is not indicated for SE-II fractures. Protected weightbearing, which does not cause further displacement, in a walking cast or brace can be begun as soon as the patient feels comfortable.

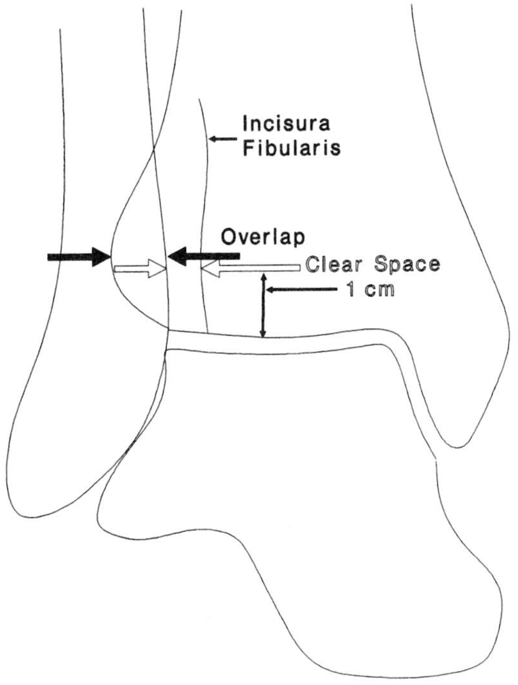

Fig. 3 Normal syndesmotic relationships. The tibiofibular clear space between the hollow arrows, 1 cm above the tibial plafond, should be less than 6 mm. The tibiofibular overlap on this simulated anteroposterior view (solid arrows) should be greater than 6 mm or 42% of the fibular width and greater than 1 mm on mortise view. (Reproduced with permission from Katcherian MD: Soft-tissue injuries of the ankle, in Lutter LD, Mizel MS, Pfeffer GB (eds): *Orthopaedic Knowledge Update: Foot and Ankle.* Rosemont, IL, American Academy of Orthopaedic Surgeons, 1994, pp 241–253.)

Bimalleolar Fractures and Equivalent Injuries

Fractures involving both medial and lateral disruption are unstable and generally require surgical intervention to restore normal joint kinematics. The goal of surgical treatment is to restore normal anatomic relationships; anatomic reduction has been shown to yield the best results. Achievement of an anatomic reduction leads to the expectation of 85% to 90% good to excellent results at 3 years or greater.

When the deltoid is ruptured in the setting of a lateral malleolar fracture, the ankle is exposed to the mechanical equivalent of a bimalleolar ankle fracture, and should be operated upon to achieve the optimal reduction of the lateral malleolus. Attempts at open repair of the deltoid are not necessary, because anatomic fixation of the lateral malleolus and treatment with a short leg cast will lead to satisfactory results in 90% of cases. The only indication for opening the medial side is if the deltoid has flipped into the ankle joint such that it prevents reduction of the talus medially. Further attempts at direct ligamentous repair are not necessary and generally lead to worse results than those treated without repair. It is not entirely clear whether all lateral malleolar fractures in the presence of any medial tenderness constitute a bimalleolar equivalent. Certainly, if any talar shift is seen on the radiographs, the ankle is considered unstable and should be operated upon.

Trimalleolar Fractures

The trimalleolar fracture occurs when the posterior injury to the ankle includes avulsion of the tibial insertion of the posterior tibiofibular ligament. If the fragment is less than 25% of the tibial articular surface, as measured on a lateral plain film, the mechanical characteristics of the ankle are unchanged and the results of nonsurgical treatment are as good as those of surgical reduction and fixation. Large displaced posterior fragments frequently reduce to near anatomic position once the lateral malleolus has been reduced and stabilized, obviating the need for internal stabilization if there is less than 2 mm residual displacement of the posterior fragment. Whether approached anteriorly or posteriorly, the fracture fragment should be attached by one or two screws to the main body of the tibia using lag technique.

Ankle Fractures With Diastasis

The syndesmotic complex is composed of the interosseus ligament, anterior and posterior tibiofibular ligaments, and the posterior transverse tibiofibular ligament. The superficial deltoid consists of the tibionavicular, posterior tibiotalar, and strong tibiocalcaneal components. The deep deltoid mainly comes off the posterior colliculus and resists the varus tilting of the talus. The tibiocalcaneal ligament is responsible for most of the stability of the ankle.

Criteria indicating the need for radiographs of an ankle injury are pain near the malleoli and inability to bear weight or tenderness on the posterior edge of the malleolar tip. Only mortise and lateral views are required. Radiographic criteria for instability include a medial clear space $\geq$ 4 mm and a tibiofibular clear space, which is measured from the posterior border of the tibia to the inner border of the fibula, $\geq$ 6 mm at the intercostal margin proximal to the plafond. The tibiofibular clear space will increase with lateral shift and internal rotation of the fibula and decrease with external rotation of the fibula.

The relative indications for stabilization of the syndesmosis after the lateral and medial structures are stabilized would be a Weber-AO type B or C injury plus a deltoid injury or poor medial fixation, a positive stress test done after ankle fixation, a Weber-AO type C injury in which the distal portion of the fibula extends more than 4.5 cm above the joint, or an avulsion fracture of the anterior tibiofibular ligament that is large enough to fix. For stabilization of the syndesmosis, a 4.5 cortical screw is placed through three cortexes with the ankle in neutral at a position 2.5 to 4 cm above the mortise and at a 30° angle anterior to the fibula. Because a syndesmotic screw does not allow for external rotation of the fibula, removal at 3 to 4 months after fixation is recommended. Surgical risk factors include hematoma, edema, fracture blisters, skin necrosis, vascular disease, or osteopenia.

Surgery should be delayed until the swelling decreases (skin starts to wrinkle) and fracture blisters are left alone. The procedure can be delayed for up to 2 weeks. The surgical technique should involve careful positioning and the use of intraoperative fluoroscopy. The fibular and medial approaches are done prior to fixation. Fixation of the fibular component usually requires a lag screw and a semitubular 3.5 buttress plate with minimal contouring. An antiglide posterior fibular neutralization plate can also be used, and screws should not enter the articular cortex of the fibula below the mortise. Severe comminution may require bone grafting. Rush rods or tension-band techniques can be used when a neutralization plate cannot be used. After stabilization of the fibula, the surgeon usuallly stabilizes the medial malleolus fracture with two metaphyseal 4.0 screws, taking care not to injure the posterior tibial tendon. Tension banding of the medial malleolus can provide stable fixation. Deltoid ligament injuries usually are not explored unless there is a large bone avulsion or reduction is blocked by the ligament. It is advisable to check the joint for articular injury and to repair a large syndesmotic avulsion.

Posterior malleolar fixation usually is required if the fragment consists of more than 25% of the bone or if the ankle is unstable as far as the anterior draw after fixation of the fibula and the medial malleolus. This fragment is usually posterolateral, and the posterolateral approach behind the fibula, using the flexor hallucis longus tendon path to the tibial dome, is recommended. Biomechanically, a screw from posterior to anterior is best. Displaced posterior colliculus fractures require special care because of the deep deltoid origin.

Postoperative care for ankle fractures involves use of walking or nonwalking short leg casts, cam walkers, or air splints. No difference in results has been reported. Elderly patients and patients with osteopenia or excessive weight require special consideration in postoperative care. No difference in long-term results has been reported for early motion versus motion delayed until 3 to 6 weeks after surgery. Outcomes for the Lauge-Hansen supination external rotation type II injury are usually 90% good to excellent with either open or closed treatment. Supination external rotation type IV injuries usually have a better prognosis with ORIF. The radiographic factors most predictive of a poor outcome were abnormal clear space and a posterior malleolar fracture > 20%. Open reductions usually have been advised for repair delayed up to 6 months. Special problems, such as the neurotrophic ankle fracture, should be treated anatomically and with long-term containment.

Open ankle injuries should be fixed early, and appropriate debridements are required at the time of injury. The ankle joint should not be left open. Antibiotic usage depends on the grade of injury. If the ankle is exposed, then early soft-tissue coverage with a free flap is necessary because no local tissue is available for transfer. CT and magnetic resonance imaging (MRI) have not been found to be helpful in the treatment of nonpilon ankle fractures. With the use of appropriate local anesthesia (ankle blocks), ankle fractures can be treated on an outpatient basis in selected cases.

Fractures of the Foot

Complex Injuries of the Talus

Motor vehicle accidents account for 43% of talar fractures. In a complex series of 1,558 ankle and foot fractures, 120 were talar fractures. Of these, 13% were open, and included associated injuries of the medial malleolus, calcaneus, and metatarsals. The anatomy of the talus is important in planning fracture repair. There are seven articular surfaces, medial deviation of the talar neck, and a strong lateral tubercle; moreover, the lateral posterior process is larger and can be disunited as in the os trigonum.

The blood supply to the head of the talus is very good, but the supply to the posterior and lateral talar body is poor. The talar body is supplied by the deltoid artery, which is a branch of the tarsal canal artery. Therefore, with any talar body manipulation, it is important to preserve the deep deltoid ligament in an attempt to preserve the deltoid artery. In most displaced talar neck fractures, the interosseus blood supply usually is disrupted, and preservation of blood supply to the talar body is critical.

The mechanism of injury of talar neck fractures is usually an axial load that causes compression of the talar neck against the tibial dome accompanied by distraction of the ankle capsule and rupture and rotation (supination) of the hindfoot with subtalar dissociation. The Hawkins classification is used for these fractures. Type I is nondisplaced, type II is a displaced talar neck with subtalar stability, type III is a displaced talar neck with subtalar instability with or without ankle dislocation, and type IV is a type III fracture with dislocation of the talonavicular. Type I talar fractures are unusual and usually are treated with cast containment until bone healing unless there is a great deal of comminution, which may require bone grafting and stabilization.

Once there is displacement of the talar neck, as in types II through IV, fixation is mandatory. The anterior medial approach can be used to provide anatomic reduction, but fixation is less stable. Anterior lateral approaches are believed to provide easy access exposure of the sinus tarsi and more biomechanical fixation, but care must be taken to preserve the neurovascular structures and the vascularity of the talar neck and body. Posterior fixation has been found to be biomechanically superior to anterior fixation, and screws have been found to be superior to Kirschner wires (K-wires). The bone density has been shown to be increased in the lateral body and decreased in the neck area.

In type III injuries, there usually is a high incidence ($> 60\%$) of osteonecrosis (ON) and open injuries. Distraction techniques are used to reduce the talar body over the posterior facet under general anesthesia. The talar neck is then stabilized with the subtalar joint. If the body of the talus is within the body cavity and not grossly contaminated, it should be reduced to restore hindfoot architecture for secondary salvage purposes. In the severely comminuted talus with no chance of osseus or vascular return, the open wound usually is treated in an external fixator for approximately 6 to 8 weeks, followed by hindfoot reconstruction. The most appropriate reconstruction is tibiocalcaneal arthrodesis using autogenous iliac block bone graft with screw fixation through a posterior approach. The Blair stabilization is technically difficult, and a talectomy is not a good option. Open injuries of the talus are susceptible to late sepsis.

Fracture healing is not a significant problem. ON occurs because of a precarious medial circulation, and its incidence increases with the severity of the fracture and dislocation. Hawkins' sign is used at approximately 2 months for evidence of revascularization. This sign has an increased sensitivity and moderate specificity with a false positive rate of 5%. Early MRI is unnecessary in the treatment of talar fractures. If, after 3 months, Hawkins' sign is negative, an MRI would be indicated. There is no standard of treatment for a partially or totally avascular talus. Alteration of activity with avoidance of severe loading and varus or valgus stress is recommended with a follow-up MRI at 1 year to see if revascularization is occurring. Use of titanium screws is recommended for talar fractures in which there may be a high incidence of ON so that diagnostic studies can be done.

Complications of talar fractures, such as ON, loss of ankle and subtalar motion, talocrural and subtalar arthritis, malunion, and nonunion, correlate with the degree of injury. Long-term follow-up studies have demonstrated that outcome decreases as the degree of injury increases. Approximately half of the normal range of motion of both the ankle and the subtalar joint is lost.

Fractures of the body of the talus can be sagittal, coronal, or transverse, and often are hidden on plain radiographs. A CT scan is needed for diagnosis and treatment. Talar body fractures occur within the articular portion of the talus, and a fibular or medial malleolar osteotomy often is necessary to approach the fracture. Fracture fragments should be reduced anatomically when possible using subarticular screw techniques. Portions of cartilage that are too small to fix or too comminuted should be removed.

Occult injuries often are missed when dealing with talar fractures. Fractures of the lateral tubercle can be missed on routine radiographs and often are treated as ankle inversion injuries. A CT scan often is needed to define the fracture. These fractures usually can be excised later or treated with reduction techniques, if necessary. Posterior process fractures are often missed, and a bone scan can help detect these occult injuries. Excision is usually the treatment of choice because the affected area is poorly vascularized. Osteochondral injuries associated with trauma usually occur on the lateral side as an avulsion or tangential injury to the lateral anterior portion of the talus. They can be reached easily by arthrotomy or arthroscopy. Medial osteochondral defects are often developmental and appear concave. They require arthroscopy or a medial malleolar osteotomy. The key to treatment is determining if there is a flap lesion, which usually needs to be excised, or if the lesion is in continuity and can be drilled arthroscopically. The outcome for these treatments, however, has not been established.

Subtalar Dislocation

Simultaneous dislocation of both the talocalcaneal and talonavicular is referred to as a subtalar dislocation. This is a rare high energy injury that occurs because the talonavicular and talocalcaneal capsules are weaker than the calcaneonavicular ligament. Ten percent of these injuries are open.

The dislocation is classified by the displacement of the distal portion, and 80% are medial. Fractures of the navicular, fibula, calcaneus, and fifth metatarsal are noted in 50%. A closed reduction usually is done under general anesthesia or intravenous sedation. Pin fixation rarely is needed. The patient usually is immobilized for 4 to 6 weeks, depending on general ligamentous laxity. This injury usually results in some loss of range of motion. Instability is a complication related to short periods of casting, and early motion is not recommended. If the subtalar dislocation is not reducible, entrapment of the anterior tibialis, posterior tibialis, or osteochondral fragments can occur.

Calcaneal Fractures

The widespread use of CT scans combined with experimental and clinical observation has improved understanding of calcaneal fracture anatomy. Shear and compression forces divide the calcaneus with two primary fracture lines. The first fracture line divides the calcaneus into medial and lateral halves, producing a superomedial fragment, fractures of the posterior facet, and fractures of the cuboid and anterior facet. The second fracture line divides the calcaneus and anterior and posterior portions at the angle of Gissane, producing the anterior lateral fragment, and crushes the lateral wall. Because of its firm ligamentous attachments, the superomedial fragment remains in anatomic relation to the talus. The tuberosity commonly is driven laterally and superiorly, and tilts into varus. The anterior lateral fragment shortens and tilts superiorly. Finally, the split lateral portion of the posterior facet is rotated and impacted into the body of the calcaneus. A double split of the facet surface may occur, producing three major pieces. The variables of foot position at impact, force factors, and degree of energy involved serve to produce the specific fracture observed.

Classifications based on CT scan have attempted to relate facet displacement with outcome. The critical threshold appears to be posterior facet displacement of 2 mm. Fractures with less displacement may be treated nonsurgically with generally good results. If the facet is displaced more than 2 mm, the nonsurgical results deteriorate, particularly if comminution is present. Pain is the most significant determinant of outcome. Despite the poor results of nonsurgical treatment, it has been difficult to prove the benefits of surgical treatment. Lack of proof may be explained by the observation that truly good to excellent results are not obtained unless anatomic (< 1 mm) reductions are obtained. Thus, if surgical treatment is chosen, the goal is as exact a reduction as possible. Caution must be exercised in the settings of diabetes, vascular disease, poor skin conditions, and noncompliance. Unresolved issues include the optimal surgical approach and the type and amount of fixation necessary.

The surgeon has the option of a medial, lateral, or combined medial–lateral approach. If a single approach is chosen, indirect reduction of the opposite column is required. The extensile lateral approach is based on the soft-tissue blood supply of the peroneal artery. Key steps include reduction of the anterolateral fragment, the tuberosity, and the superomedial fragment to facilitate accurate posterior alignment, which must be verified by Harris and Brodén views. The posterior facet is then fixated with two lag screws. A lateral column buttress plate is applied, and screws are directed to intact medial bone stock. Bone grafting is advocated by some for comminuted injuries.

The medial approach is based on the significant fracture reduction obtained by accurate medial alignment.This reduction can be held with a large threaded pin. A lateral approach through the sinus tarsi may be required to obtain an accurate posterior facet reduction. For less comminuted injury patterns, numerous authors claim success using "minimal internal fixation," which consists of screws, K-wires, and staples. Although surgical treatment series commonly lack nonsurgical controls, good to excellent results are reported in 65% to 85% of patients. The prognosis is better for displaced large piece fractures as compared to highly comminuted injuries. This observation has renewed some interest in primary fusion, although data to support this option currently are lacking.

The major complications of surgical treatment are infection and wound complications. The rates vary from 2% to 10%. The need for free flaps and, rarely, amputation have been reported. Thus, careful patient and fracture selection are required if surgical treatment is to be successful.

Tarsometatarsal Fracture Dislocations

The second and third metatarsals are the rigid keystone of this joint's stability. The dorsal ligaments are not as strong as the plantar ligaments; therefore, dorsal dislocations are more common. The Lisfranc's ligament goes from the second metatarsal to the first cuneiform bypassing the first metatarsal. Abnormal facets have been demonstrated at the proximal first metatarsal–cuneiform articulation. The plantar branch of the anterior tibial artery and the deep peroneal nerve are within the base of the first and second metatarsals.

The three most common mechanisms of injury are twisting of the forefoot, axial loading of a fixed foot in equinus, and crush. Twisting injuries occur with the forefoot held fixed and the hindfoot rotated, and crush injuries usually involve plantar dislocations. These injuries can be classified as homolateral, divergent, or isolated using the Hardcastle classification or as medial (medial cuneiform plus first metatarsal), middle (second and third cuneiform and metatarsals), and lateral (fourth and fifith metatarsal plus cuboid) using the Myerson column injuries.

An anatomic reduction will provide the best possible chance for good to excellent results. Anesthesia and traction are appropriate for closed or possible open reduction. It is important to be sure that pulses are present and that no compartment problems exist. If the fracture-dislocation is reduced percutaneously, the reduction is held with multiple 0.062 K-wires and must be fairly perfect. The second metatarsal initially should be reduced into the cuneiform complex. The lateral segment is almost always reduced with K-wires. Screws have been used for stabilization of medial and middle segments; open incisions usually are between the first and second metatarsals. The screws are left in for at least 6 months, K-wires are left in for 6 weeks, and the patient usually is in a cast for 3 months and then in a full length firm orthotic with a longitudinal and metatarsal arch.

Pitfalls to reduction can occur. Entrapment of the anterior tibial tendon in the fracture site has been described. If the reduction is not perfect to within 5 mm between the first and second metatarsals, an open reduction is in order. Metatarsal head fractures should be treated and not left displaced. Associated injuries of the navicular, first cuneiform, and cuboid should be addressed. The best results are obtained with an anatomic reduction, but any articular injury to these joints can make the outcome less than satisfactory. If the patient has pain after reduction of the tarsometatarsal fracture, a CT scan is used to find the arthritic area, and a fusion is done. Usually the fourth and fifth metatarsals are left unfused.

Occult injuries of this joint occur in athletic activities. A high index of suspicion and clinical examination lead to this diagnosis. In these injuries, the static radiographs usually are negative, but stress, traction, or standing views may demonstrate injury. A bone scan also has been used for people with persistent pain in this area. Occult injuries usually are treated by containment for long periods followed by long-term use of orthotics for support of both the metatarsal and the longitudinal arch.

Metatarsal Fractures

The blood supply to the fifth metatarsal base is supplied by an abundant metaphyseal artery network. The diaphysis is supplied by a nutrient artery that enters medially in the middle third of the bone, then sends branches distally and proximally. A proximal diaphyseal fracture (Jones fracture) may damage these proximal branches, and such damage could explain the high prevalence of nonunion in metatarsal fractures. The commonly encountered disturbances in union have led some authors to recommend outpatient screw fixation for these injuries in athletes. This approach allows a more aggressive rehabilitation program and, potentially, an earlier return to sports.

Annotated Bibliography

Ankle

Amendola A: Controversies in diagnosis and management of syndesmosis injuries of the ankle. *Foot Ankle* 1992;13:44–50.

A review of management of syndesmosis injuries is presented with highlights of biomechanical, laboratory, and clinical data.

Burns WC II, Prakash K, Adelaar R, et al: Tibiotalar joint dynamics: Indications for the syndesmotic screw. A cadaver study. *Foot Ankle* 1993;14:153–158.

Complete deltoid and syndesmosis rupture in the cadaver would cause significant increases in contact pressure, which would be decreased with the use of a syndesmotic screw.

Earle M, Adelaar RS, et al: Biomechanical study of the deltoid ligament in cadavers. *Orthop Trans,* in press.

Sectioning of the superficial tibiocalcaneal ligament caused statistical decrease in ankle contact area, increase in peak pressure, and transfer of the centroid to the lateral talus. The deep deltoid and other superficial components had no affect.

Harper MC: An anatomic and radiographic investigation of the tibiofibular clear space. *Foot Ankle* 1993;14:455–458.

This parameter represents the posterior aspect of syndesmosis and varies with lateral displacement and rotation of the distal fibula.

Michelson JD: Fractures about the ankle. *J Bone Joint Surg* 1995;77A:142–152.

A review of unstable ankle fractures with indications, techniques, and postoperative management are presented.

Michelson JD, Clarke HJ, Jinnah RH: The effect of loading on tibiotalar alignment in cadaver ankles. *Foot Ankle* 1990;10:280–284.

Application of moment forces to cadavers showed that neither displacing the fibulae laterally or sectioning the deltoid ligament influenced talar shift. The criteria for unstable ankle fracture may need a closer analysis.

Michelson JD, Magid D, Ney DR, et al: Examination of the pathologic anatomy of ankle fractures. *J Trauma* 1992;32:65–70.

Using CT, the rotational deformity of the lateral malleolar fracture was found to be internal rotation of the proximal shaft, not external rotation of the lateral malleolus. The anatomy of the ankle joint, thus, is not disrupted in these injuries.

Mont MA, Sedlin ED, Weiner LS, et al: Postoperative radiographs as predictors of clinical outcome in unstable ankle fractures. *J Orthop Trauma* 1992;6:352–357.

The radiographic factors most predictive of a poor outcome were an abnormal clear space and a large posterior fracture (> 20%). Fibular shortening, talar tilt, and a wide syndesmosis were suggestive of a poor result. A perfect radiographic result did not guarantee an excellent clinical outcome.

Stiell IG, Greenberg GH, McKnight RD, et al: Decision rules for the use of radiography in acute ankle injuries: Refinement and prospective validation. *JAMA* 1993;269:1127–1132.

Mortise and lateral radiographs are required for initial assessment. With an ankle injury, the criteria for radiography would be pain near the malleoli or an inability for weightbearing.

Tibial Pilon

Bonar SK, Marsh JL: Unilateral external fixation for severe pilon fractures. *Foot Ankle* 1993;14:57–64.

Twenty-one severe pilon fractures were treated with unilateral large screw external fixation. In 15 patients, limited internal fixation was used. Four patients required arthrodeses and one received late amputation. There were no cases of wound infection, skin slough, or osteomyelitis.

Helfet DL, Koval K, Pappas J, et al: Intraarticular "pilon" fracture of the tibia. *Clin Orthop* 1994;298:221–228.

This is a good summary of current techniques using internal fixation. These techniques include preoperative planning, atraumatic soft-tissue handling (indirect reduction), and anatomic joint reduction.

McFerran MA, Smith SW, Boulas HJ, et al: Complications encountered in the treatment of pilon fractures. *J Orthop Trauma* 1992;6:195–200.

This report documents the hazards of internal fixation for the pilon fracture. The complications were largely related to the soft tissues and fracture healing. The overall local complication rate was 54%. The majority of complications occurred during the first 6 months postinjury.

Tornetta P III, Weiner L, Bergman M, et al: Pilon fractures: Treatment with combined internal and external fixation. *J Orthop Trauma* 1993;7:489–496.

Twenty-six patients with distal tibial extra- and intra-articular fractures were treated with hybrid fixation, often combined with screw fixation of the joint. Of Reudi III fractures, 69% experienced good or excellent results. Incidence and severity of complications were less than for internal fixation series.

Talus

Daniels TR, Smith JW: Talar neck fractures. *Foot Ankle* 1993;14:225–234.

This review of talar neck fractures stresses open anatomic reduction, internal stabilization, and long-term observation for osteonecrosis. The incidence of poor results is high.

Jensen I, Wester JU, Rasmussen F, et al: Prognosis of fracture of the talus in children: 21 (7-34)-year follow-up of 14 cases. *Acta Orthop Scand* 1994;65:398–400.

A 21-year follow-up on talar neck and body fractures is presented. All fractures were treated by ORIF and immobilization. All patients with displaced fractures had exercise-induced pain and those with nondisplaced fractures were normal.

Sanders R, Pappas J, Mast J, et al: The salvage of open grade IIIB ankle and talus fractures. *J Orthop Trauma* 1992;6:201–208.

A protocol of debridement, temporary placement of antibiotic beads, soft-tissue coverage, intravenous antibiotics, and finally a fusion with an anterior plate and bone grafts was used. A majority of patients had pain, difficulty with stairs, and limited ambulation.

Swanson TV, Bray TJ, Holmes GB Jr: Fractures of the talar neck: A mechanical study of fixation. *J Bone Joint Surg* 1992;74A:544–551.

In a cadaver study all screw configurations were stronger than K-wires. Screws from posterior to anterior were biomechanically superior.

Szyszkowitz R, Seggl W, Wildburger R, et al: Late results of fractures and fracture-dislocation after ORIF, in Tscherne H, Schatzker J (eds): *Major Fractures of the Pilon, the Talus, and the Calcaneus: Current Concepts of Treatment.* Berlin, Germany, Springer-Verlag, 1993, pp 105–112.

Late results of ORIF of 108 talar fractures are reported. The severity of arthrosis, loss of range of motion, and osteonecrosis was related to the severity of injury.

Veazey BL, Heckman JD, Galindo MJ, et al: Excision of ununited fractures of the posterior process of the talus: A treatment for chronic posterior ankle pain. *Foot Ankle* 1992;13:453–457.

Excision of ununited posterior process fractures with ankle pain is discussed. Pain on forced plantarflexion and a positive bone scan helped diagnosis.

Zwipp H: Severe foot trauma in combination with talar injuries, in Tscherne H, Schatzker J (eds): *Major Fractures of the Pilon, the Talus, and the Calcaneus: Current Concepts of Treatment.* Berlin, Germany, Springer-Verlag, 1993, pp 123–135.

A 20-year period of complex foot and ankle fractures is reported from The Hanover, Germany, Medical School. This is a realistic incidence of these injuries from a modern regional trauma center.

Subtalar Dislocations

Brennan MJ: Subtalar dislocations, in Green WB (ed): *Instructional Course Lectures Volume XXXIX.* Park Ridge, IL, American Academy of Orthopaedic Surgeons, 1990, pp 157–159.

This is a review of the literature and mechanism of subtalar dislocations.

Calcaneal

Buckley RE, Meek RN: Comparison of open versus closed reduction of intraarticular calcaneal fractures: A matched cohort in workmen. *J Orthop Trauma* 1992; 6:216–222.

Using a retrospective matched cohort method, results were compared for 17 surgically and 17 nonsurgically treated calcaneal fractures. There was no statistically significant difference between the two groups. The overall clinical result was better in the surgically treated patients when an anatomic reduction of the subtalar joint was achieved.

Carr JB: Mechanism and pathoanatomy of the intraarticular calcaneal fracture. *Clin Orthop* 1993; 290:36–40.

The two primary fracture line mechanism is outlined. This produces split depressions of the posterior facet and the anterolateral and anteromedial fragments. The extra-articular pathology is also described.

Crosby LA, Fitzgibbons T: Computerized tomography scanning of acute intra-articular fractures of the calcaneus: A new classification system. *J Bone Joint Surg* 1990;72A:852–859.

Thirty calcaneal fractures were analyzed using a classification system based on posterior facet comminution and displacement. Minimally displaced (2 mm) type I fractures fared well. Only two of 17 patients with displaced and/or comminuted posterior facet fractures achieved good results with nonsurgical treatment.

Sanders R, Fortin P, DiPasquale T, et al: Operative treatment in 120 displaced intraarticular calcaneal fractures: Results using a prognostic computed tomography scan classification. *Clin Orthop* 1993; 290:87–95.

The results in 120 intra-articular calcaneal fractures treated using an extensile lateral approach with screw and plate fixation were analyzed. The results were best in type II (73%) and type III (70/%) fractures. Comminuted type IV fractures experienced only 27% good/excellent results. A distinct learning curve was evident for type II and III fractures.

Tarsometatarsal

Curtis MJ, Myerson M, Szura B: Tarsometatarsal joint injuries in the athlete. *Am J Sports Med* 1993;21:497–502.

A retrospective series of 19 patients is presented with a poor outcome for those with a delayed diagnosis and inadequate treatment. The third degree sprain would require ORIF.

Faciszewski T, Burks RT, Manaster BJ: Subtle injuries of the Lisfranc joint. *J Bone Joint Surg* 1990;72A:1519–1522.

A diastasis of 2 to 5 mm is reported between the first and second metatarsals. There is often a long delay in diagnosis, and weightbearing radiographs are helpful.

Myerson MS: Injuries to the forefoot and toes, in Jahss MH (ed): *Disorders of the Foot and Ankle: Medical and Surgical Management,* ed 2. Philadelphia, PA, WB Saunders, 1991, vol 3, pp 2233–2273.

Injury to the tarsometatarsal is classified by columns into medial, middle, and lateral. Results depend on an anatomic reduction.

Sangeorzan BJ, Veith RG, Hansen ST Jr: Salvage of Lisfranc's tarsometatarsal joint by arthrodesis. *Foot Ankle* 1990;10:193–200.

Screws were used to achieve rigid fixation and high rates of fusion. Attempts should be made to correct deformity.

Metatarsal

Mindrebo N, Shelbourne KD, Van Meter CD, et al: Outpatient percutaneous screw fixation of the acute Jones fracture. *Am J Sports Med* 1993;21:720–723.

Nine varsity athletes sustaining a Jones fracture were treated with outpatient percutaneous screw fixation. This allowed accelerated rehabilitation with an average return to running of 5.5 weeks. Full sports participation was obtained in 12 weeks. All fractures healed.

Smith JW, Arnoczky SP, Hersh A: The intraosseous blood supply of the fifth metatarsal: Implications for proximal fracture healing. *Foot Ankle* 1992;13:143–152.

Using arterial injection techniques, the blood supply to the proximal fifth metatarsal was investigated. The intraosseous blood supply to the tuberosity arose from numerous metaphyseal vessels. The proximal diaphysis was supplied primarily from a relatively poor blood supply, which contributed to the incidence of impaired osseous healing.

Classic Bibliography

Baird RA, Jackson ST: Fractures of the distal part of the fibular with associated disruption of the deltoid ligament: Treatment without repair of the deltoid ligament. *J Bone Joint Surg* 1987;69A:1346–1352.

Boden SD, Labropoulos PA, McCowin P, et al: Mechanical considerations for the syndesmosis screw: A cadaver study. *J Bone Joint Surg* 1989;71A:1548–1555.

Franklin JL, Johnson KD, Hasen SD: Immediate internal fixation of open ankle fractures. *J Bone Joint Surg* 1984; 66A:1349–1356.

Joy G, Patzakis MJ, Harvey JP Jr: Precise evaluation of the reduction of severe ankle. *J Bone Joint Surg* 1974; 56A:979–993.

Lauge-Hansen N: Fractures of the ankle: II. Combined experimental-surgical and experimental-roentgenologic investigation. *Arch Surg* 1950;60:957–985.

Leeds HC, Erlich MG: Instability of the distal tibiofibular syndesmosis after bimalleolar and trimalleolar ankle fractures. *J Bone Joint Surg* 1984;66A:490–503.

Limbard RS, Aaron RK: Laterally comminuted fracture-dislocation of the ankle. *J Bone Joint Surg* 1987;69A: 881–885.

McCullough CJ, Burge PD: Rotatory stability of the load-bearing ankle: An experimental study. *J Bone Joint Surg* 1980;62B:460–464.

Ovadia DN, Beals RK: Fractures of the tibial plafond. *J Bone Joint Surg* 1986;68A:543–551.

Phillips WA, Schwartz HS, Keller CS, et al: A prospective, randomized study of the management of severe ankle fractures. *J Bone Joint Surg* 1985;67A:67–78.

Ramsey PL, Hamilton W: Changes in the tibiotalar area of contact caused by lateral shaft talar shift. *J Bone Joint Surg* 1976;58A:356–357.

Schaffer JJ, Manoli A: The antiglide plate for distal fibular fixation: A biomechanical comparison with fixation with a lateral plate. *J Bone Joint Surg* 1987;69A:596–604.

Thomsen NO, Overgaard S, Olsen LH et al: Observer variation in the radiographic classification of the ankle fractures. *J Bone Joint Surg* 1991;73B:676–678.

Yablon IG, Heller FG, Shouse L: The key role of the lateral malleolus in displaced fractures of the ankle. *J Bone Joint Surg* 1977;59A:169–173.

Yablon IG, Leach RE: Reconstruction of malunited fractures of the lateral malleolus. *J Bone Joint Surg* 1989;71A:521–527.

Yde J, Kristensen KD: Ankle fractures: Supination-eversion fractures stage II and late results of operative and non-opeerative treatment. *Acta Orthop Scand* 1980;51:695–702.

44

Ankle and Foot: Reconstruction

Hallux Valgus

Hallux valgus is a lateral deviation of the great toe. The individual elements contributing to the deformity include varus positioning of the first metatarsal, valgus of the proximal phalanx at the metatarsophalangeal (MTP) joint, and in some cases lateral deviation of the distal phalanx at the interphalangeal (IP) joint. Physical examination includes determining the degree of flexibility of the deformity as well as noting painful motion at the MTP joint suggestive of an arthritic component. Hypermobility of the tarsometatarsal (TMT) joint and a flexible flatfoot are important in determining surgical strategy. Stabilization of the first ray will be important to establish balanced weightbearing, and correction of the flatfoot either with arch supports or surgically will be important to reestablish normal toe-off and prevent recurrence of hallux valgus.

Radiographic examination consists of bilateral weightbearing anteroposterior (AP), lateral, and oblique views of the feet. The sesamoid view can be helpful. The hallux valgus angle, the angle between the first two metatarsals, the hallux IP angle, MTP congruity, metatarsal head articular orientation (MAO), obliquity of the TMT joint, sesamoid placement, and preservation or loss of the MTP joint space are evaluated.

The initial treatment is shoewear education and modification. If an adequate trial of nonsurgical measures fails and significant pain persists, surgical intervention may be considered. Multiple surgical procedures for the correction of hallux valgus have been described. The surgical algorithm is based on the degree of deformity, intermetatarsal angle (IMA), reducibility determined during the physical examination, toe pronation, presence of a transfer lesion, joint congruity, and the presence or absence of arthritis.

The role of an isolated distal soft-tissue balancing procedure (modified McBride procedure) for correction of hallux valgus is limited, and the results have been disappointing. Distal metatarsal osteotomies (chevron, Mitchell) are used for correction of a mild to moderate deformity (hallux valgus angle $< 30°$; IMA $< 15°$). Internal fixation with a chevron osteotomy is generally used. Recent modifications of the 60° V-cut osteotomy, with the development of a longer lower limb for dorsal to plantar screw fixation, have been suggested. First web space soft-tissue release used in conjunction with distal metatarsal osteotomies risk osteonecrosis (ON) of the metatarsal head. However, a recent research study disputes this concept and suggests a plantar approach modification of the first web space release to avoid injury to the dorsolateral blood supply to the first metatarsal head. Variations in the chevron technique for special circumstances include downward angulation of the V-cuts from medial to lateral to depress the head where a transfer lesion exists and medial wedge cuts in the standard V to tilt back the head when the articular surface is laterally oriented (Fig. 1). Other Z-cut rotational osteotomies are under current study to determine their efficacy.

A distal soft-tissue procedure used in conjunction with the proximal metatarsal osteotomy (crescentic and proximal chevron) can be used to correct a hallux valgus angle greater than 35° and an IMA greater than 15°. These osteotomies at the proximal metaphyseal–diaphyseal junction involve a portion of the diaphyseal bone and require stabilization with screw or pin fixation.

Arthrodesis is indicated in patients with significant first MTP arthritis or cerebral palsy. Patient age, lifestyle, and the goals of surgery need to be clearly defined before this procedure. The recommended position of arthrodesis is 10° of dorsiflexion with reference to the first metatarsal shaft and 10° to 15° of valgus. Modification of this arthrodesis position is appropriate based on individual variation of foot alignment (pes cavus or pes planus). The incidence of nonunion with first MTP arthrodesis ranges from 5% to 25%. Asymptomatic fibrous nonunion requires no treatment. Bone grafting and revision arthrodesis are indicated in the symptomatic patient.

Resection arthroplasty (Keller procedure) is indicated in older or sedentary individuals with progressive arthritis of the MTP joint. With resection of the proximal phalangeal base, there is a loss of the flexor hallucis brevis (FHB) attachment, plantar plate, plantar aponeurosis attachments, toe shortening, the potential for a dorsal subluxation deformity, and recession and prominence of the sesamoids. With loss of the great toe windlass mechanism, a second toe transfer lesion occurs. Minimal resection of the proximal phalangeal base is recommended. The results of long-term studies using silicone arthroplasties for the MTP joint have been disappointing. Hallux valgus with hypermobility of the TMT joint may require arthrodesis of this joint (modified Lapidus).

Postoperative treatment in hallux valgus surgery is directed toward the avoidance of late surgical complications such as recurrence, hallux varus, malunion, or nonunion. Supplemental soft-tissue dressings providing maintenance of toe alignment are used for 4 to 6 weeks. A cast or stiff-soled shoe or equivalent is used for 6 to 12 weeks until the osteotomy or fusion has healed. A rocker bottom shoe may be used long term for arthrodesis patients.

Choosing the appropriate surgical procedure for the de-

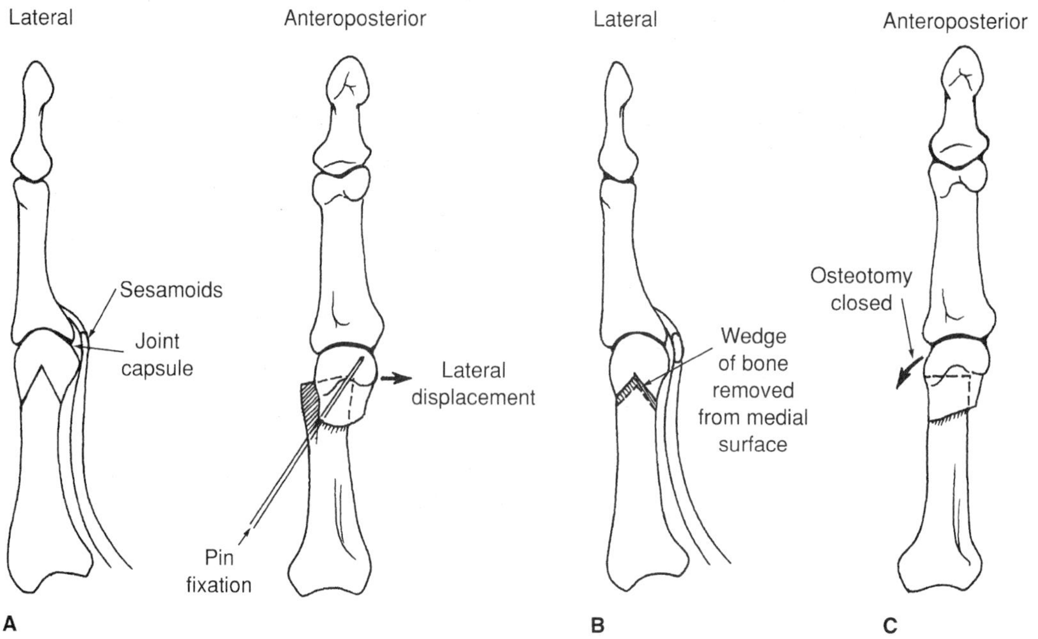

Fig. 1 Biplanar chevron osteotomy to correct a laterally sloping distal metatarsal articular surface. **A,** Placement of the normal chevron osteotomy. **B,** Removal of medial bone wedge measuring 1 to 3 mm. This permits medial deviation of the articular surface of the metatarsal head, thereby correcting the DMA angle. **C,** Distal articular surface after correction. The osteotomy site should be fixed with a pin. (Reproduced with permission from Mann RA: Disorders of the first metatarsophalangeal joint. *J Am Acad Orthop Surg* 1995;3:34–43.)

gree of deformity will decrease the risk of recurrence of hallux valgus. Biomechanical realignment is the key. Hallux varus may occur with excessive medial eminence resection or medial capsular plication, resection of the lateral sesamoid (original McBride procedure), overcorrection of the first metatarsal with osteotomy, and an excessive soft-tissue lateral release. Treatment for this complication may include first MTP joint arthrodesis when associated arthritis is present or an abductor hallucis muscle release or lengthening with an extensor hallucis longus (EHL) transfer and IP joint arthrodesis. Other soft-tissue balancing techniques have also been described.

ON of the first metatarsal head occurs to a variable degree with combined distal first metatarsal osteotomy and soft-tissue release procedures. With these combined procedures, the intramedullary blood supply is lost and the important dorsolateral vessels to the metatarsal head are at risk for injury. Avoidance of these combined procedures is warranted. Treatment of ON with partial head involvement consists of prolonged protection for 4 to 6 months to allow for revascularization. Salvage surgery includes a first MTP joint arthrodesis with the potential need for intercalary bone grafting.

Hallux Rigidus

Hallux rigidus is characterized by limited motion and arthritic changes involving the first MTP joint. Although its cause is unknown, theories include a long first metatarsal in relation to the second metatarsal (Morton's foot), dorsiflexed first metatarsal, and microtrauma involving the dorsal aspect of the first MTP joint.

Physical examination demonstrates a limited arc of dorsiflexion and plantarflexion motion, which is painful at the extremes. With dorsiflexion, impingement of dorsolateral osteophytes occurs. With plantarflexion, the dorsal capsule over the osteophytes is tethered and traction is applied to the dorsomedial cutaneous nerve to the hallux. These events can produce pain and paresthesias. Weightbearing radiographs should be obtained. AP radiographs of the foot reveal narrowing of the MTP joint space and osteophyte formation laterally. Lateral radiographs reveal dorsal osteophytes and joint space narrowing that often involves only the dorsal aspect of the joint.

Nonsurgical treatment is directed toward limitation of first MTP joint motion. Rigid soled or steel shank shoes with rocker soles may be used successfully. A high toe box is necessary to avoid contact of the dorsal osteophytes with the shoe.

Surgical intervention may include a dorsal cheilectomy. Removal of the dorsal one-third of the metatarsal head and the osteophytes involving the proximal phalanx is recommended (Fig. 2). Early physical therapy is undertaken to obtain optimal range of motion. With severe arthritic changes of the MTP joint, an arthrodesis may be necessary. Alternative procedures include a modified Keller

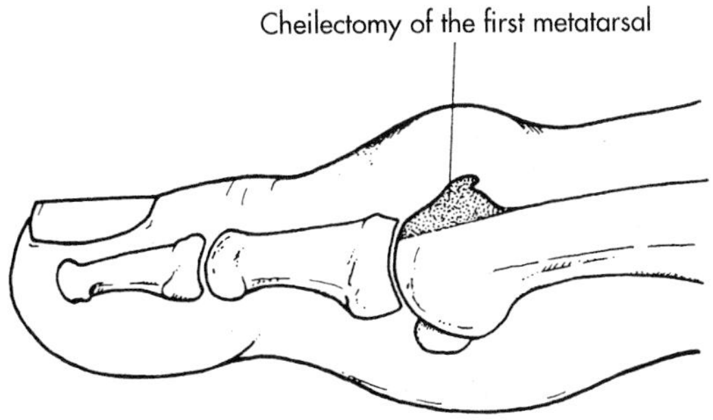

Fig. 2 Cheilectomy of the first metatarsal. The shaded area shows the amount of bone excised from the metatarsal head. (Reproduced with permission from Quirk R: Ballet injuries, in Baxter DE (ed): *Foot and Ankle in Sport.* St. Louis, MO, Mosby-Year Book, 1995, pp 287–303.)

arthroplasty with osteophyte resection from the metatarsal head with reattachment of the plantar plate to the proximal phalanx stump. A Moberg (dorsal closing wedge) osteotomy of the proximal phalanx has been used to decrease stress at the MTP joint and improve the dorsiflexion component of the arc of motion. Implant arthroplasties are currently investigational. Silicone prostheses are not recommended by most authors.

Sesamoid Problems of the Hallux

The sesamoid complex of the first MTP joint consists of medial (tibial) and lateral (fibular) sesamoids, which are located within tendinous expansions of the FHB muscle and are linked through the intersesamoidal ligament. With this ligament as its roof, the flexor hallucis longus (FHL) tendon runs between the sesamoids to attach to the base of the distal phalanx. The abductor and adductor hallucis send slips of tendon to the medial and lateral sesamoids, respectively. This complex arrangement of ligaments and tendons, with the addition of a ridge of bone and cartilage called the crista under the midplantar metatarsal head, provides the dynamic and static restraints for the sesamoid sling. The sesamoids function to alter plantar pressure, decrease friction, and improve the mechanical advantage of the tendons. Alterations in the balance of the sesamoid complex can lead to sesamoiditis, osteochondritis, arthritis, stress fractures, and skin ulceration that may lead to infection.

Pathology to the sesamoids is localized by palpating for tenderness and testing if motion at the first MTP joint causes movement and, possibly, pain from the sesamoid complex. Dorsiflexion of the IP joint may also cause pain by motion of the FHL tendon adjacent to the sesamoids. Radiographic evaluation includes medial and lateral oblique views of the foot and a sesamoid view.

Initial treatment for sesamoiditis (sesamoid–metatarsal arthrosis) is conservative. Treatment includes unweighting of the sesamoid with a metatarsal pad proximally and cutouts over the tender bone, with limitation of sesamoid motion at the first MTP joint. This can be accomplished through casting, bracing, a rigid sole shoe with a rocker sole, and/or first MTP joint taping, limiting dorsiflexion and plantarflexion.

Sesamoid excision is indicated with the fragmentation of osteochondritis, nonunion after fracture, infection, or severe arthritis. In sesamoid excision, it is important to include reconstruction of the sesamoid sling and intersesamoidal ligament to avoid hallux varus (with the removal of the fibular sesamoid) or hallux valgus (with removal of tibial sesamoid). Most authors agree a medial approach should be used to remove the tibial sesamoid; either a dorsolateral or a plantar incision in the skin creases has been suggested for fibular sesamoid excision. The latter is more direct with easier visibility. Damage to the digital hallucal nerves must be avoided. Results after sesamoid excision indicate complete pain relief in approximately 50% of patients, restricted range of motion in 33% to 58%, and plantarflexion weakness in 60%. Bone grafting for nonunion of a sesamoid has been reported to have reasonable success. An additional problem with the hallucal sesamoids is the development of a discrete plantar callus. Paring of the keratosis and unweighting is palliative, but sesamoidal shaving may be needed. A first metatarsal dorsiflexion osteotomy to elevate the sesamoids may be required after recurrent ulceration, especially with neuropathic feet.

A subhallucal sesamoid is present in 5% to 13% of the general population. It is an intra-articular bone within or juxtaposed to the FHL tendon at the IP joint of the great toe. When prominent, it can be a localized area of excessive weightbearing with subsequent painful callus formation. In the neuropathic patient, an ulcer can form. Insert modification with a proximal pad can be helpful to unweight the sesamoid area. With failure of conservative treatment, the sesamoid can be shelled out through either a medial or direct plantar zigzag approach and a longitudinal incision in the FHL. The tendon defect should be approximated prior to closure. Retracted proximal sesamoids as a complication of a Keller bunionectomy should be excised, along with arthrodesis of the first MTP joint, if conservative measures have failed.

Lesser Toe Deformities

Lesser toe MTP joint deformities are very common and can be a source of pain and disability. A hammertoe consists of a flexion deformity at the proximal IP (PIP) joint and, hyperextension at the distal IP (DIP) joint, with or without hyperextension at the MTP. A claw toe involves a flexion deformity at both the PIP and DIP joints, with hyperextension at the MTP. It is often bilateral, affects multiple toes, and is associated with neurologic conditions, including some forms of cavus deformity. A mallet toe consists of a flexion deformity of the DIP joint. The second toe is most commonly afflicted in hammer, claw, and mallet toe deformities (Fig. 3).

The deformities arise when the balance between the intrinsic and extrinsic muscles is disturbed. These muscles serve as active anatomic restraints. Passive restraints consist of the plantar aponeurosis, the plantar plate and capsule, and the collateral ligaments. The deformities can be fixed or flexible, depending on the extent and duration of involvement. In flexible deformities, an imbalance exists but the joints retain their function and, with manipulation, the deformity is passively correctable; rebalancing the toe should result in correction. Rigidity on examination implies a fixed deformity. Conservative treatment includes use of shoes with wide, deep toe boxes and lower heels, appropriate corn padding and trimming, hammertoe elastic splints, and metatarsal pads. When symptoms persist, surgical intervention is considered. Surgery should entail mobilization of the fixed segment to correct its position, then address the cause of the deformity to rebalance the toe.

Although claw toes and hammertoes differ anatomically, surgical treatment is similar. Whether MTP hyperextension needs to be corrected and to what extent is determined preoperatively. If the MTP hyperextension is minimal, percutaneous dorsal capsulotomies and extensor tenotomies are sufficient. If the deformity is more extensive, the MTP is approached dorsally in a sequential fashion. Through an oblique or Z-shaped dorsal skin incision, the extensor digitorum longus (EDL) tendon is released or lengthened, the extensor digitorum brevis (EDB) is tenotomized, the dorsal capsule is released, the collateral ligaments are released, and the plantar recess of the proximal phalanx is reestablished by easing the plantar plate from the undersurface of the plantar metatarsal condyles where adhesions can form. The Girdlestone-Taylor transfer of the flexor digitorum longus (FDL) to the extensor hood on the dorsal aspect of the proximal phalanx is performed, and if the PIP deformity is flexible, this completes the procedure. If the PIP is rigid, either a proximal phalanx distal condylectomy and tendon transfer or PIP resection arthrodesis is done. Some surgeons do not use the flexor to extensor transfer with the condylectomy or fusion, depending on Kirschner wire (K-wire) temporary stabilization or adjacent toe syndactylization to maintain alignment. A formal PIP arthrodesis is indicated in the presence of severe or recurrent deformity or when associated with neurologic disturbance in the forefoot. When K-wires are used to temporarily hold the corrected toe position and cross the MTP joint, a 0.062-in wire should be used to decrease the possibility of wire breakage. If all components of the deformity are surgically corrected, syndactylization should not be necessary. A proximal hemiphalangectomy was believed to be indicated for these deformities, but the articular contour on the proximal phalanx is thought to be critical to the stability of the MTP joint, and therefore, this procedure has limited indication. A mallet toe can be addressed by an FDL tenotomy alone or with excision of the head of the middle phalanx with or without tenotomy of the FDL. Again, a K-wire may be used as an adjunct.

The small or fifth toe may have unique deformities. Because it is the most lateral ray, skin tension plays a larger role here and must be considered in surgical correction. The cocked-up fifth toe consists of a fixed hammertoe with dorsal subluxation of the MTP. When mild to moderate, the same procedures described for the middle digits are helpful. When severe, the Ruiz-Mora procedure has been performed. This entails a partial (modified), or total proximal phalangectomy through a plantar elliptical incision with resultant dermadesis to help stabilize the MTP joint.

Disorders of the Second Metatarsophalangeal Joint

The second toe MTP joint has disease processes similar to those of the other rays, as well as several unique conditions. A long second metatarsal often is believed to contribute. Perhaps one of the most common and earliest recognizable deformities is spontaneous synovitis of the second MTP, possibly related to low-grade trauma. Some believe this is the initial stage of a continuum that involves subluxation and may end as frank dislocation of the proximal phalanx on the metatarsal head, along with the formation of a rigid claw toe deformity. Persistent synovitis allows stretching or actual rupture of the plantar plate.

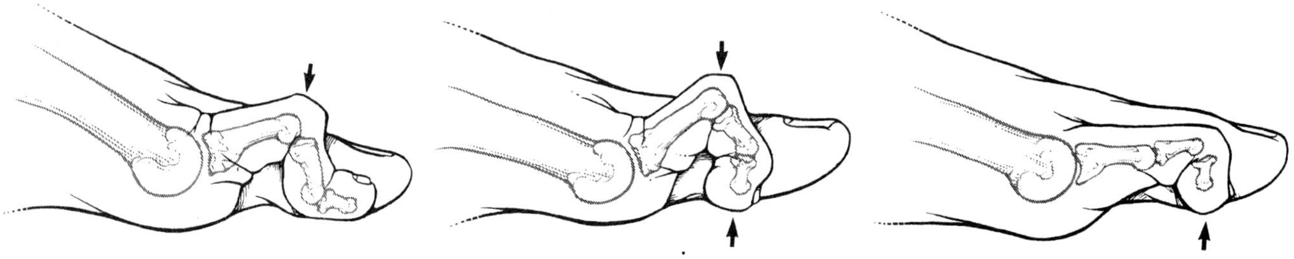

Fig. 3 Hammer toe **(left),** claw toe **(center),** and mallet toe **(right).** (Reproduced with permission from Alexander IJ: *The Foot: Examination and Diagnosis.* New York, NY, Churchill Livingstone, 1990, pp 68–71.)

The dorsal translation subluxation test described by Thompson and Hamilton is helpful in detecting subtle instability (Fig. 4).

After systemic arthritides are excluded, the stable joint is protected by metatarsal pads, extended steel shanks, soft rocker bottom soled shoes, and anti-inflammatory medications. In early instability, a hammertoe shield or taping in such a way that a plantar-directed force is applied to the proximal phalanx is recommended. If symptoms persist, surgical intervention is considered. Hallux valgus deformity should be corrected even if it is relatively asymptomatic. Synovectomy combined with a Girdlestone-Taylor flexor to extensor transfer for stability is indicated. Once fixed subluxation or dislocation occurs, the sequential steps to reduce MTP hyperextension outlined above must be followed. Again, a flexor extensor transfer can be added to restabilize the joint. In addition, bony decompression may be required to reduce the dislocation. It can be carried out at the PIP joint as a resection arthroplasty or at the MTP joint. A modified DuVries arthroplasty, which comprises removing the distal 3 to 4 mm of the metatarsal and reshaping the head to a convex surface to retain stability, is done. Creating the bone–cartilage interface may sometimes lead to painful arthritis. A K-wire traversing the MTP joint is used for 3 to 4 weeks. Partial proximal hemiphalangectomy of the second toe with subtotal syndactylization to the third also has been advocated. With this technique, MTP instability and shortening of the digit may be problematic. It is unclear which MTP joint procedure is superior, and decompression of the MTP joint by resection of the PIP is preferable to both procedures at the MTP level.

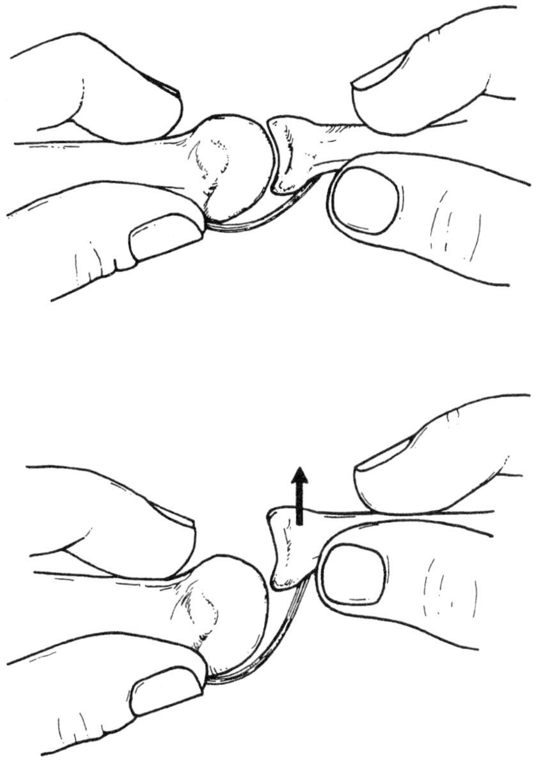

Fig. 4 Dorsal translation test for metatarsophalangeal joint instability. (Reproduced with permission from Coughlin MJ: Forefoot disorders, in Baxter DE (ed): *Foot and Ankle in Sport*. St. Louis, MO, Mosby-Year Book, 1995, pp 221–244.)

Intractable Plantar Keratosis

A callosity on the sole of the foot is termed an intractable plantar keratosis (IPK). The epidermis proliferates in response to pressure and the condition can become painful. IPKs can be localized or more diffuse. A diffuse IPK beneath several metatarsal heads, which is associated with cavus feet, plantar fat pad atrophy, and systemic arthritides such as rheumatoid arthritis, is most amenable to conservative treatment. These lesions must be differentiated from a plantar wart, which may or may not occur beneath a bony prominence, is painful with circumferential compression rather than axial, has skin lines that end abruptly at its edge, and reveals small central punctate hemorrhages after paring. Conservative measures—accommodating soft-soled shoes, appropriate metatarsal padding, and trimming of the lesion—should always be attempted initially.

If surgical intervention is considered, routine radiographs, including a sesamoid view, are needed. A prominent condyle is addressed by a modified DuVries arthroplasty (resection of the plantar condyles) of the metatarsal head. When an entire metatarsal head is responsible for the IPK, options include an oblique shortening osteotomy (for a long metatarsal) or a dorsiflexion osteotomy of the metatarsal neck or base. Multiple variations have been described; a dorsal closing wedge and a vertical chevron are currently popular. Nonunions are rare, but transfer lesions beneath adjacent metatarsals are common. Precision is critical and internal fixation is recommended. When treating IPKs, every effort should be made to save the metatarsal head.

Bunionette

The bunionette (Tailor's bunion) is characterized by prominence of the lateral condyle of the fifth metatarsal head and, often, a varus fifth toe deformity. Shoes compress the overlying skin against the prominence and lead to a lateral plantar bursa or hard corn formation. Several anatomic variants account for the metatarsal prominence. The fifth metatarsal head may have a lateral prominence, become more prominent by pronation of the metatarsal, or be enlarged. The metatarsal shaft may curve laterally resulting in prominence of the head despite a normal IMA between the fourth and fifth metatarsals or it may be straight, but diverge from the fourth metatarsal shaft resulting in an increased IMA (Fig. 5). In one study, the normal IMA

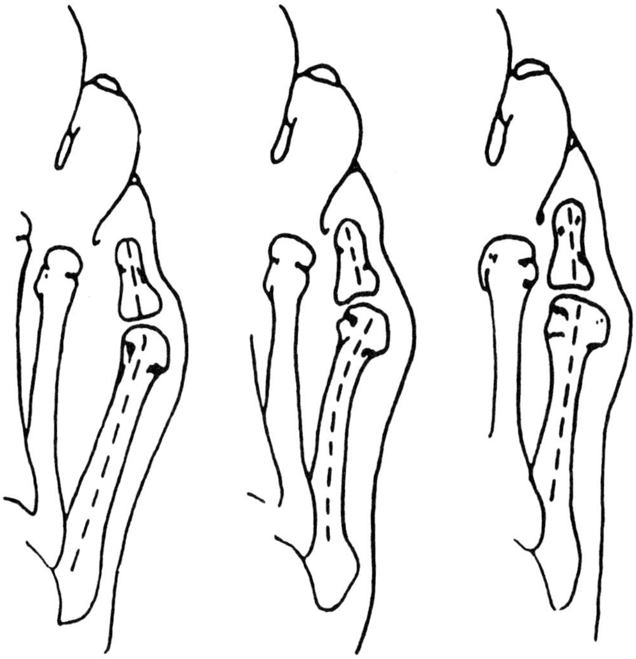

Fig. 5 The variants of bunionette. (Reproduced with permission from Coughlin MJ: Etiology and treatment of the bunionette deformity, in Greene WB (ed): *Instructional Course Lectures XXXIX*. Park Ridge, IL, American Academy of Orthopaedic Surgeons, 1990, pp 37–48).

between the fourth and fifth metatarsals measured 6.2°, whereas it measured 9.6° in patients with symptomatic bunionettes. Pes planus was noted to increase this IMA by 3° in one study, and two thirds of bunionette cases were believed to be associated with pronated feet.

Surgical intervention is indicated for a persistently symptomatic Tailor's bunion. An attempt should be made to identify the anatomic pattern. Resection of the lateral condyle is simple and effective in the presence of an isolated prominent lateral fifth metatarsal head. However, recurrence is due to inadequate resection or further MTP subluxation. Excision of the fifth metatarsal head is not recommended. In the presence of a widened IMA between the fourth and fifth metatarsals or a laterally bowed fifth metatarsal shaft, an osteotomy of the metatarsal is necessary. Several distal osteotomies, including a chevron and a medial displacement oblique technique, have been described for lateral bowing and appear to achieve satisfactory results. Complications include nonunion, malunion, or the development of transfer plantar keratotic lesions. Middiaphyseal osteotomies are used in patients with an increased IMA between the fourth and fifth metatarsals or those with large keratotic lesions on the plantar-lateral aspect of the fifth head. The best results have been reported for resection of the lateral eminence and realignment of the fifth MTP joint in conjunction with the osteotomy. Few long-term follow-up reviews exist on any of these surgical procedures for bunionettes.

Toenail and Matrix Problems

Many conditions can involve the nail plate and toenail matrix. These may be congenital, traumatic, collagen disorders, fungal infections, or even neoplasms. One of the most common causes of dystrophic nails is a dermatophytic fungal infection. This common type of infection begins distally beneath the free edge of the nail plate, with hyperkeratosis of the bed and subsequent secondary discoloration and thickening of the plate. Typically, only some of the nails are affected, unlike collagen disorders, such as psoriasis, in which all toenails may be affected. Other dystrophies include congenital varieties and those due to aging or poor arterial perfusion. Because oral griseofulvin is fungistatic rather than fungicidal, a nail must completely grow out and replace itself before treatment is stopped; this process ranges from 9 to 12 months for the great toenail. The cure rate is only 50%, and recurrences are high. Ketoconazole may be more effective, but it has a high recurrence rate and more side effects. Soaking of the nail and sanding with an emery board or dremel may be effective as palliative maneuvers. Topical agents have not been effective, nor has the use of a laser. Removal of the entire nail plate and germinal matrix (Zadik procedure) is indicated when the nail becomes so thickened that it catches in the patient's stockings or is torn accidentally from its bed.

An ingrown toenail also usually involves the hallux. Ingrowth results from a combination of direct trauma, improper nail trimming, ill-fitting shoes, and faulty biomechanics. One or both sides of the nail plate pierce the nail fold, initiate an inflammatory process, and, if allowed to persist, allow secondary bacterial infection. The condition may be resolved by a properly fitting shoe with an insert if pronation is a problem, soaks, systemic or topical antibiotics, and cotton wisp packing beneath the offending nail edge to free it from the nail fold. However, recurrence is common in patients with diabetic neuropathy, for example, and can led to deep infection or osteomyelitis. Surgical intervention often is required in chronic or recurrent cases.

Bruising of the nailbed may occur when the toe is long and the athletic shoe too short, resulting in subungual hemorrhage or the sudden appearance of a white nail after the trauma ("tennis toe," often involving the second toe). The condition will spontaneously resolve with loss of the nail. A single dystrophic nail without an obvious diagnosis, however, is of considerable concern, and the nail plate may require avulsion to properly examine the underlying matrix. Invasive or in situ squamous cell carcinoma and melanoma are the most important tumors that must be recognized. More benign conditions include a pyogenic granuloma, which can occur from a splinter under the nail, or a benign exostosis from the distal phalanx. To properly treat these benign problems, which occur under the sterile matrix, the nail plate should be avulsed gently using a freer elevator after anesthetizing the toe. The proximal sharp wings at the base of the plate should be rounded off and the plate preserved for temporary reimplantation. Using loupe magnification, the sterile matrix should be divided, typically longitudinally, over the underlying lesion or, in the case of a pyogenic granuloma, peeled off around the lesion. The granuloma is curetted away, and an exostosis is removed with a rongeur down to the plane of the original distal phalanx surface. The sterile matrix is reapproximated with fine dissolving suture (6-0) and a defect may be covered with a split matrix graft. This may be obtained from the adjacent sterile matrix using a #15 knife blade and simply layered over the defect. If the defect is large, the graft can be taken from an adjacent toenail bed. The nail plate is then repositioned in the proximal nail fold and held in place with sutures at all four corners. If the nail plate has been significantly damaged, a piece of silicone sheeting or an artificial nail can be used as a temporary cover. This is usually left in place for 3 to 4 weeks.

Surgical procedures for the removal of the nail plate or matrix may be partial or complete. Removal of a medial or lateral spike of nail might be helpful in controlling infection. A partial matrixectomy (Heifetz procedure) removes a medial or lateral segment of the nail plate and a wedge of medial or lateral side germinal and sterile nail matrix and nail fold. Curettage of the bed and closure may be sufficient. The use of phenol lowers recurrence but tends to leave a draining wound for long periods of time. The complete matrixectomy (Zadik procedure) is indicated for distressing dystrophic nail problems, such as psoriasis or chronic fungal infections. Recent studies suggest that ablation with phenol may result in a lower recurrence rate. The terminal Syme (Thompson-Terwilliger procedure) involves amputation of the tuft of the distal phalanx along with the overlying nail plate and matrix. The plantar skin flap is approximated to the dorsal aspect of the toe. It is used as a salvage for failed lesser procedures and after chronic infection. Epithelioid inclusion cyst formation and an unattractive bulbous stump of the toe are complications.

Tendinitis of the Foot and Ankle

Inflammation of tendinous units about the foot and ankle most commonly is caused by direct trauma or overuse. Inflammatory disorders, anatomic variations, infection, and degenerative tendon disease have also been implicated in tendinitis about the foot. The posterior tibial tendon and the Achilles tendon are affected most commonly; peroneal tendons, the FHL tendon (especially in dancers), and the anterior tibial tendon are less commonly involved. The inflammatory reaction may be in the midsubstance of the tendon, at the insertion, at the entrance or within a retinacular pulley area, or at the site of trauma. The initial traumatic injury or a chronic progressive inflammatory process may lead to tendon rupture.

Most tendinitis about the foot will respond to conservative management. In the acute phase, activity modification, non-steroidal anti-inflammatory medications (NSAIDs), and immobilization, if necessary, will resolve the pain. When symptoms allow, physical therapy emphasizing both eccentric and concentric contractions and proper shoe wear will help prevent further episodes. Surgery should be reserved for cases refractory to conservative management, cases involving tendinous degeneration or rupture, and osseous abnormalities. Steroid injections have been used for acute inflammation, but caution must be used because tendon rupture following steroid injection has been reported.

Achilles tendinitis, most often caused by overuse, causes tenderness in the substance of the tendon 3 to 5 cm proximal to the insertion and should be differentiated from retrocalcaneal and precalcaneal bursitis, which cause pain in the region of the insertion of the tendon. However, Achilles tendinitis, most often a result of trauma, can occur and may be associated with calcifications at the tendinous insertion. Paratendinitis that is refractory to conservative therapy may be amenable to surgical debridement of the paratenon. Nodular swelling may represent tendinosis. If tendinosis is present, the tendon should be debrided and repaired.

If left untreated, posterior tibial tendinitis may lead to fixed flatfoot deformity that requires major reconstruction. Pain and tenderness just distal to the medial malleollus signify overuse or degenerative syndromes. Pain at the insertion on the navicular usually signifies partial or complete ruptures. Tenosynovitis of the FHL tendon where it enters the sheath posteromedially, just behind the subtalar joint, results in a trigger-like phenomenon known as a "jumping toe," or hallux saltans. Release of the entrance to the sheath is curative.

Peroneal tendinitis usually results from trauma that causes stenosis of the peroneal tendon sheath. Lateral malleolar fractures, calcaneal fractures, and inversion ankle injuries have been implicated in peroneal tendinitis. Stenosis usually occurs at one of three sites: posterior to the lateral malleolus, at the peroneal tubercle, and under the cuboid. An os peroneum and a congenitally enlarged peroneal tubercle have been implicated in peroneal tendinitis.

Acquired Flatfoot

Posterior tibial tendon dysfunction is the most common cause of acquired flatfoot deformity in adults. Other causes include old Lisfranc dislocation, inflammatory arthritis of the hindfoot, neuropathic involvement of the midfoot or hindfoot, and degenerative osteoarthritis of the hindfoot. Posterior tibial tendon insufficiency may be difficult to diagnose. At first, tenosynovitis causes pain medially, and clinical findings include tenderness and swelling along the tendon and pain or inability to perform single limb heel rises. As the disease progresses, the talonavicular and subtalar joints collapse, the heel drifts into valgus, the midfoot pronates, and the forefoot becomes abducted and supinated. As the deformity progresses, symptoms usually shift from the medial to lateral side with abutment of the fibula and calcaneus. The patient exhibits the "too many toes" sign, demonstrating forefoot abduction. With longstanding deformity, a fixed flatfoot develops, limiting surgical options to arthrodesis.

Early treatment is aimed at tenosynovitis and includes NSAIDs, medial sole and heel wedges, and immobilization if symptoms are severe. Long-term nonsurgical treatment may include orthotics and bracing. Surgical options for posterior tibial insufficiency remain controversial. Options include tendosynovectomy, direct repair, direct repair with graft augmentation, flexor tendon transfer, arthrodesis, and combinations of the above. Tenosynovectomy may help to relieve pain but will not stop progression of deformity if the tendon is dysfunctional as a result of intratendinous tearing and elongation. Posterior tibial tendon reconstruction (shortening, reinforcement with graft), remains feasible by itself if the muscle still has elasticity and the static arch stabilizers retain their integrity. Among the reconstruction options are direct repair, reinforcement with tendon graft, and use of the distal half of the anterior tibial tendon, which retains its distal attachment and is woven through the distal stump of the posterior tibial tendon and into the proximal portion. When the posterior tibial muscle status is questionable, tendon transfers add strength and are quite successful. Flexor tendon transfer should be considered for dysfunctional tendons when the posterior tibial muscle is also dysfunctional and the arch static stabilizers are intact. A recent anatomic study suggests that transfer of the FDL tendon is preferable to that of the FHL because of the proximity of the transfer and minimal functional loss of toe flexion. Toe flexion is maintained by the attachments of the FHL to the distal flexor digitorum, the action of the quadratus plantae and the short flexor tendons to the toes, and by suturing the FHL to the FDL stump.

Various arthrodeses are indicated for more severe deformities secondary to stretched out static stabilizers. Isolated talonavicular, talonavicular with calcaneocuboid, or subtalar arthrodesis have all been performed based on whether there is more hindfoot valgus or midfoot abduction. More recently, combinations of posterior tibial tendon reconstruction with or without transfer, augmented by isolated arthrodeses, have been used. This approach seems necessary because flexor tendon transfers alone only occasionally are adequate for foot stabilization. Calcaneocuboid distraction arthrodesis (lengthening the lateral column), in conjunction with posterior tibial tendon reconstruction with or without flexor tendon transfer, is currently being evaluated, as is the isolated subtalar fusion with medial tendon reconstruction. Triple arthrodesis after reduction of the hind and midfoot is indicated for fixed deformity.

Plantar Fasciitis

Plantar fasciitis is a discrete clinical entity with a classic history and precise physical findings. The onset is insidious and usually is related to overuse. The pain is accentuated when the ankle and great toe are dorsiflexed, stretching the fascia, and there is point tenderness over the fascia at its origin.

Conservative treatment is successful in over 90% of patients. Triple therapy is required: oral anti-inflammatories; heel-cord stretching (at least twice a day for 20 minutes); and wearing of an orthotic that cups the heel, has a soft spot under the tender area, and supports the arch. The patient should note significant relief within 2 weeks and become essentially asymptomatic within 6 weeks. In recalcitrant cases, an ankle foot orthosis (AFO) night splint is used with the triple therapy. Plantar fascia surgical release is indicated in less than 5% of patients. Although steroid injection successfully provides temporary relief, it is not indicated because of complications—fat pad atrophy (an almost untreatable condition) and possible development of plantar fascia rupture (which is more difficult to treat).

Plantar fascia rupture occurs both spontaneously (evolves from plantar fasciitis) and after steroid injection. The complaints are similar to those of plantar fasciitis, but the pain often is more distal in the longitudinal arch and may extend up the posteromedial ankle. Night pain also is a component. The pain recedes more slowly with rest after walking. The symptoms thus become more neurogenic. Tenderness on palpation is present not only at the origin of the plantar fascia, but also more distally over the fascia and posteromedially over the neurovascular bundle. The plantar fascia medial edge is no longer distinct with dorsiflexion of the ankle and the great toe or is significantly less so than on the uninvolved normal side.

Conservative treatment is identical to that of plantar fasciitis, except that the orthotic has a soft channel added medially under the course of the nerve. The condition is more recalcitrant than plantar fasciitis, and many patients require surgical intervention, consisting of both plantar fascia release and release of the tarsal tunnel.

Nerve Entrapment Syndromes

These syndromes may be primary (developing spontaneously), related to hormonal shifts that may relax ligamentous support, or due to systemic diseases, such as an adjacent vasculitis, or neuropathy, such as that found in diabetes. A nerve may be compressed by lesions, such as a nonspecific synovitis, tenosynovitis, rheumatoid arthritis, or gouty; ganglions; and other tumors. The compression may be posttraumatic or iatrogenic. Dynamic or quasimechanical compression may occur when the patient is standing, walking, or wearing a tight shoe. The patient typically complains of pain, but also may have decreased sensibility and paresthesias. A neurapraxia may be a simple conduction block or, after time, a more extensive demyelination. Long-standing severe compression also can result in axonotmesis. The degree of resulting nerve injury varies, accounting for the variable rate of recovery following decompression.

Tarsal tunnel syndrome refers to compression of the tibial nerve and its branches behind the medial malleolus and, particularly, at more distal sites. The main nerve splits into medial and lateral plantar branches just proximal to the superior border of the abductor hallucis muscle. The calcaneal branches descend from the nerve proximal to this muscle and lie superficial to it. Deep to the abductor hallucis, the medial and lateral plantar nerves follow separate channels into the foot. A branch from the lateral plantar extends over the quadratus plantae to the lateral border of the foot. Compression of this nerve, which has sensory components and may give off a branch to the heel skin, is a recently described source of heel pain. Both the medial and lateral plantar nerves may be compressed under the superior or inferior borders of the abductor hallucis deep fascia. The lateral plantar nerve, and to some extent the medial plantar nerve, pass under the intersection of the plantar fascia and the inferior border of the abductor hallucis fascia. They also pass over the leading fascial edge of the quadratus plantae (Fig. 6). The medial plantar nerve, which lies under the fascia of the abductor hallucis as it proceeds distally, also passes under the crossing of the FHL and flexor digitorum. Synovitis in this sheath may cause compression, particularly in patients with a flexible flatfoot. Patients with posterior tibial tendon dysfunction also complain of neurogenic symptoms, which may be related to posterior tibial nerve compression.

These conditions are treated with anti-inflammatory medication, an orthotic that has an area of relief built into it medially under the nerve, and a variety of other medications, including antiepileptics and mood elevators such as amitriptyline. Magnetic resonance imaging (MRI) has been used to demonstrate space-occupying lesions within the tunnel area. A recent report has suggested good to excellent results in 44% of patients treated surgically; in another recent study on repeated surgery, there was definite evidence of an incomplete release in most cases. Electrodiagnostic tests were positive in the majority of patients treated surgically, but the test results did not correlate with the outcomes. Surgery is indicated for patients who were unresponsive to conservative treatment and in whom the symptoms have become incapacitating.

Anterior tarsal tunnel syndrome is entrapment of the deep peroneal nerve under the inferior extensor retinaculum where the nerve overlies the talus and navicular. Surgical release has generally been successful in improving the symptoms of these rare compressions. The superficial peroneal nerve may be damaged by trauma and is extremely vulnerable during surgical procedures. The sural nerve, which also is vulnerable during surgery, may be injured or entrapped in calcaneal fractures. In the severe valgus foot, there may be impingement of the nerve and peroneal tendons between the calcaneus and fibula.

Morton's neuroma represents entrapment of the intermetatarsal nerve under the distal border of the intermetatarsal ligament as the nerve splits into its digital branches. Its symptoms include pain in the webspace, with radiation and sometimes paresthesias or hypoesthesia in the adjacent toes. Palpation of a mass or the elicitation of tenderness with compression dorsally and plantarward between the metatarsal heads, especially with the awareness of a click during this palpation or during compression of the heads from medial to lateral, have been the hallmarks of diagnosis. Recently, studies have suggested use of ultrasonography and MRI for objective diagnosis. There is a wide

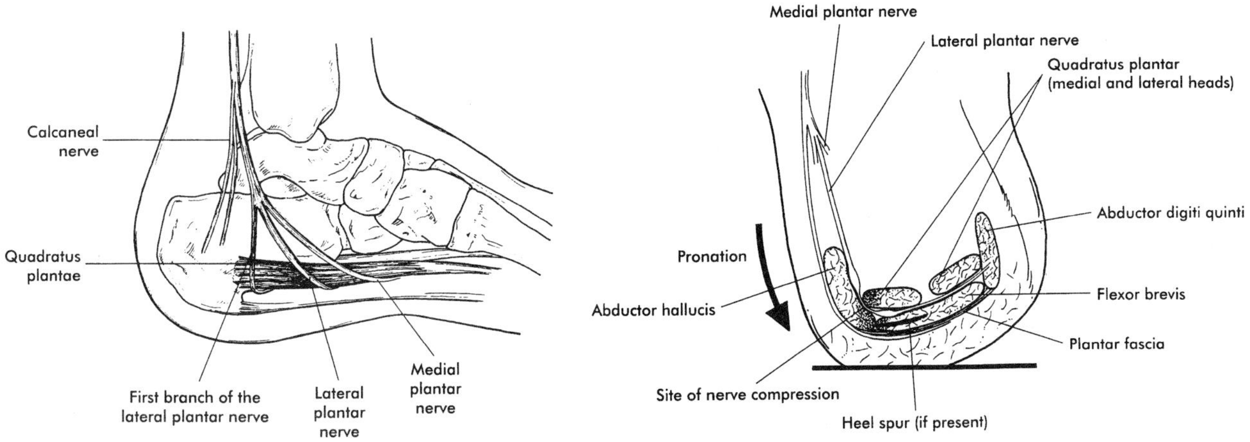

Fig. 6 Compression between the distal edge of the abductor hallucis fascia and the fascia over the quadratus plantae. (Reproduced with permission from Pfeffer GB: Plantar heel pain, in Baxter DE (ed): *Foot and Ankle in Sport.* St. Louis, MO, Mosby-Year Book, 1995, pp 195–206.)

range in the reported value of these techniques. The use of MRI with high resolution small coils and surgical confirmation seem to validate this approach in some centers. The spaces between the second, third, and fourth metatarsals appear to be the most commonly involved, as well as the third web space where branches from the medial and plantar nerves form the intermetatarsal nerve. In a recent study of histologic changes in the third web space, findings of nodular formation and fibrosis were identical in symptomatic and asymptomatic patients. The symptomatic patients, however, demonstrated demyelination. This study indicates that enlargement per se, as seen on imaging studies, may not indicate bona fide pathology.

Nonsurgical treatment consists of shoes with an adequate width and height to the toe box and the placement of a metatarsal pad proximal to the metatarsal heads of the involved web space. According to recent studies, felt pads that supinate or pronate the foot do not seem to have any long-term benefit. Injection of the intermetatarsal space with steroid preparations is reported to provide immediate good results in 30% of patients and partial relief in 50%; 80% of patients indicated complete relief at 2 years. Reports vary considerably in these estimates. For patients who do not respond to conservative treatment, surgery generally consists of division of the intermetatarsal ligament and excision of the nerve through a dorsal approach. Of patients, 60% to 80% report complete cures or significant improvement. Simple release of the intermetatarsal ligament continues to be investigated. Recurrences usually are treated surgically. Using a plantar approach, the nerve is redirected deep into the intrinsic muscles or at least proximally into the intermetatarsal space well off the plantar aspect of the foot.

Cavus Foot

Cavus foot refers to a fixed equinous deformity of the forefoot in relation to the hindfoot, which results in an abnormally high arch. The apex may be at the level of the metatarsocuneiform joints or more proximally in the mid tarsus. The first metatarsal alone or all five metatarsals may be depressed. The heel may be in neutral, varus, valgus, calcaneous, or equinus, and there often is clawing of the toes. The cause may be one of the hereditary motor and sensory neuropathies (HMSN), including Charcot-Marie-Tooth disease, Friedreich's ataxia, spinal dysraphism (eg, syringomyelia, diastomatomyelia, or spina bifida), or unknown. Cavus foot also may be secondary to poliomyelitis, cerebral palsy, club foot surgery, spinal cord injury, ankle fractures with a compartment syndrome, and other conditions. Biomechanically, the feet are rigid and unyielding, with a locked subtalar and midfoot complex. The fluid motion of these joints is absent in gait; the foot is unable to dissipate the ground reaction force. Weightbearing is not evenly distributed, and high contact areas (first and fifth metatarsal heads and the heel) develop callusing and pain.

The pathophysiology varies with the underlying condition, but muscle imbalances exist between the extrinsic muscles themselves and with the intrinsics, which are frequently nonfunctional. The heel cord may be contracted in some patients; more typically, the os calcis is in calcaneous with weakness of the triceps surae. Overpull of the posterior and anterior tibial muscles with nonfunction of the peroneus brevis leads to hind and midfoot varus. Overpull of the peroneous longus results in plantarflexion of the first metatarsal. Weakness of the anterior tibial, as in Charcot-Marie-Tooth, extenuates this plantarflexion and may add the problem of foot drop. Contracture of the abductor hallucis and the plantar fascia lead to varus and the high arch. Intrinsic weakness, plantar fascia contracture, and extrinsic muscle imbalance have all been cited as the initiating factor in the development of varus. Nonfunction of the intrinsics results in clawing of the toes as well. The heel varus on heel strike adds further strain to the lateral ankle ligaments, with stretching of these structures resulting in pain and instability. Patient symptoms vary with the underlying etiology and pathology, age, weight, and activity level. Joint surfaces and shapes have fixed shape deformities, which become incongruous with soft-tissue rebalancing, or they may already be arthritic.

Initiation of jogging or similar physical fitness efforts may be the patient's first indication of a foot problem. Typical complaints are of dorsal arch pain, metatarsalgia, and problems with shoe fitting. Leg and lateral ankle pain may also appear. After determination of the etiology of the condition, neurologic consultation may be warranted to determine if the primary condition is progressive or treatable. Joint position, flexibility, and muscle function are determined. Sensory evaluation should include Semmes-Weinstein monofilament testing, deep tendon reflex assessment, and determination of overall muscle balance. In some patients, electrodiagnostic studies may be warranted. Standing AP and lateral radiographs will demonstrate the location of the apex of the deformity, the calcaneal pitch, and the overall severity of the problem. The extent of the cavus is determined by the angle of Meary, which is found by drawing lines, which normally would be parallel, through the long axis of the first metatarsal and the talus. The angle of Hibbs (used to describe cavus) is determined from long axis of the calcaneus and the axis of the first metatarsal; it normally should not be less than 150°. The calcaneal pitch is determined by the angle formed between a line along the plantar surface of the calcaneus and the weightbearing surface of the foot. If the angle is over 30°, the calcaneus is excessively dorsiflexed.

Four approaches can be considered: conservative, soft-tissue balancing, soft-tissue balancing with osteotomies for bone realignment, and soft-tissue balancing with arthrodeses. Nonsurgical treatment includes an insert that fills the arch, places a metatarsal pad proximal to the heads, and relieves under the metatarsal heads with soft material. An extra depth shoe is warranted to accommodate a high arch; SACH material is added as a wedge in the heel to soften heel strike, and a crepe rubber rocker sole is added to absorb ground force and shift weightbearing proximal to the heads as well as to assist with toe-off. A lateral flare is added to the heel to stabilize the tendency to invert further on heel strike. In the flexible heel, a lateral wedge may be considered. In the patient with foot drop, an AFO, ranging from a simple polypropylene fixed ankle device to a dorsiflexion assist short leg brace with a T-strap to prevent varus, may be added. When surgery is necessary, soft-tissue releases are done initially to gain maximal correction. Osteotomies are subsequently carried out if necessary to obtain a plantigrade foot. If preliminary computed tomography (CT) scans demonstrate arthritic joints, or if the patient is middle aged ($\geq$ 40 years), arthrodeses often replace or are added to osteotomies. They also are used for salvage procedures.

Soft-tissue releases typically include division of the plantar fascia, short flexor origin, the abductor hallucus and its deep fascia, the deep fascia of the abductor digiti quinti, and, at times, the short and long plantar ligaments from the undersurface of the calcaneus to the level of the talonavicular and calcaneocuboid joints. The posterior tibial tendon may also be lengthened along with the peroneus longus and the EHL. The Achilles tendon occasionally is lengthened, but not in conjunction with plantar fascia release. Tendon transfers include splitting the anterior tibial, placing the lateral half into the cuboid or third cuneiform. The posterior tibial may be transferred subcutaneously or through the interosseous membrane to the midfoot for foot drop; or it has been split, routing half of the tendon posterolaterally into the cuboid or peroneus brevis. The peroneus longus may be transferred into the peroneus brevis rather than simple lengthening. All of these maneuvers are efforts to balance the hind and midfoot varus–valgus, the peroneus longus to brevis transfer is done to eliminate the former's deforming force and improve abduction. The EHL may be transferred into the neck of the first metatarsal, fusing the IP joint of the great toe (Jones procedure). This procedure is less popular because the elevation of the first metatarsal by the EHL appears to be minimal, and the lag in extension of the great toe after the procedure is undesirable.

Before transfers, but after soft-tissue releases, osteotomies to improve alignment include (1) the lateral based wedge (Dwyer) or slide osteotomy of the calcaneus to place the heel in valgus or (2) a dorsal to plantar concentric osteotomy of the calcaneus to slide the posterior tubercle superiorly to decrease accentuated pitch. A dorsal wedge or dome osteotomy is used to elevate the first metatarsal and to abduct it if necessary. The biplane wedge or dome concentric procedure may be used on the other metatarsals as well. A concentric osteotomy through the cuneiforms and cuboid as described by Weiner has been popularized to elevate and derotate the deformity in the midfoot.

Long flexor to extensor transfers (Girdlestone-Taylor) to reestablish intrinsic function have been advocated for toe clawing. Transfer can also be done for the great toe when indicated. Recession of the long extensors to the metatarsal necks is done somewhat less frequently at this time. Simple tenotomies of the extensors and long flexors may suffice in older patients with lesser goals of function, and in whom less surgery is desirable. The toes are all pinned in the corrected position after these releases, and the distal proximal phalanges may be removed to decompress the contracted toes and allow straightening after the tenotomies.

Triple arthrodesis is reserved for the patient who has arthritis in the subtalar–midtarsal complex and/or for older patients who do not seem to do well with osteotomies alone, or as an eventual salvage after prior procedures. Although results of long-term studies for triple arthrodesis in patients with polio are satisfactory, recent reports have suggested only a 24% satisfactory result in long-term follow-up of patients with HMSN. Therefore, joint preserving procedures should be considered until degenerative changes have occurred. In addition to all of the above, patients may need lateral ankle ligament reconstruction, inserts, modified shoe wear, and bracing.

Posttraumatic Arthritis

Posttraumatic arthritis of the midfoot is frequent following TMT fracture and/or dislocation and in fractures of the navicular and cuboid associated with subtalar dislocation. Arthritis will occur in virtually all cases without adequate initial reduction and may occur with reduction because of chondral damage at the time of injury. Symptoms develop within the first 6 to 9 months. NSAIDs may relieve some of the discomfort. Orthotic use and shoe modifications may be considered.

Thorough evaluation of the painful area includes CT scan to visualize the individual joints involved, bone scanning to demonstrate actively inflamed areas, and selective injections of anesthetics and radiopaque dyes under fluoroscopy to ensure adequate placement. Recommended salvage after failure of nonsurgical treatment is arthrodesis of the involved joints.

Hindfoot arthritis results most commonly from intra-articular calcaneal fractures and less commonly from talar fractures. In addition to NSAIDs, conservative treatment consists of inserts, shoe modifications, and braces designed to decrease movement at the painful articulations.

If nonsurgical treatment fails, arthrodesis of the involved joints is recommended. CT scan, bone scans, and diagnostic injections are helpful to localize symptoms. Reestablishment of alignment including varus–valgus angulation of the heel and a decrease in the talar declination angle should be part of the surgical procedure. Autogenous bone graft is typically used. In a triple arthrodesis, the subtalar, calcaneocuboid, and lateral talonavicular joints are easily exposed through a lateral incision; a medial incision is used to complete removal of articular cartilage at the talonavicular joint.

Posttraumatic arthritis of the ankle may result from ankle fracture, chronic instability, or talar injury with secondary ON or osteochondrosis. Nonsurgical treatment includes medications and bracing as described above. With the failure of nonsurgical treatment, arthrodesis is the treatment of choice. Ankle arthroplasty at this time is investigational.

An arthrodesis in situ may be carried out through the arthroscope. To obtain a solid fusion, there should be good bony apposition with rigid compression to enhance stability and healing potential. The talus should be displaced posteriorly 0.5 to 1.0 cm to reduce forces across the midtarsal joint that may lead to subsequent degenerative changes, and the foot should be externally rotated slightly for optimal ambulation. Currently popular methods for fixation include several external fixation devices, crossing cannulated cancellous screws placed from anterolateral to posteromedial, from posteromedial to midtalus, and from posterior tibia into the head and neck of the talus. A 30-mm pediatric four-hole blade plate with the flange removed has also been proposed, particularly for salvage procedures. This device also is useful for tibiocalcaneal arthrodesis. Additional tibiocalcaneal fixation devices include: 6.5 and 7.0 screws and locked and partially-locked intramedullary rod devices. Intramedullary rods are fixed to the calcaneus and may be dynamic or static proximally. The position of the fusion and hardware should be confirmed radiographically in the operating room.

Reconstruction for Complications of Calcaneal Fractures

Symptoms of pain, stiffness, and weakness are common after comminuted or intra-articular fractures of the calcaneus. Mechanical problems, soft-tissue problems, and posttraumatic arthritis can be the cause. Because most patients do not stop improving until 1 year after injury and many continue to improve for up to 4 years, nonsurgical treatment should be exhausted before surgical intervention is considered. Depending on the disabling problems, NSAIDs, corticosteroid injections, inserts, and shoe modifications, as well as weight-relieving patellar tendon bearing orthoses may be indicated. Mechanical problems result from the characteristic bony deformities of the os calcis fracture. Loss of calcaneal height and length with a shortened heel cord and shortened intrinsic muscles leads to weakened toe-off and alterations in the windlass mechanism. Translation and heel widening cause difficulty in shoe wear, and all of these factors may contribute to the appearance of a flatfoot. Anterior tibiotalar abutment may result from the altered ankle mechanics, and the transverse tarsal joint may be locked, resulting in increased stresses at Chopart's joint. Calcaneofibular abutment may result from the lateral blow-out component of the fracture, and dislocation of peroneal tendons can lead to impinging tenosynovitis under the fibula.

Any combination of mechanical problems may be present in a given patient, therefore salvage procedures must be tailored to the individual. A subtalar distraction bone block fusion, which addresses several of these problems, is done by insertion of a tricortical iliac crest graft into the arthrodesis site. This procedure will increase heel height, correct varus–valgus deformity, and eliminate tibiotalar abutment by correcting the talar declination angle. A recently described alternative method, consisting of a corrective osteotomy through the original fracture site in the os calcis, may help os calcis positioning, but subtalar arthritis still needs to be addressed. An ostectomy of the protruding bone laterally will narrow the heel, improve calcaneofibular abutment, and relieve symptoms of sural nerve entrapment and peroneal tendon encroachment. Hammertoes that have resulted due to a compartment syndrome may require management. Injuries of the sural nerve, resulting in scar entrapment or neuroma, are often best treated by nerve excision. Arthritic changes in the subtalar and calcaneocuboid joints may require arthrodesis.

Ankle and Subtalar Joint Instability

Ankle Instability

Although ligamentous injuries of the ankle are the most common athletic injury, they often are inadequately diagnosed and treated. The typical ankle sprain involves ligament(s) of the lateral ligamentous complex: the anterior talofibular ligament; in more severe cases, the calcaneofibular ligament; and rarely, the posterior talofibular ligament. Associated or isolated injuries to the subtalar joint ligaments, the distal tibiofibular ligaments (syndesmosis), or the deltoid ligament can alter treatment and prognosis. Other possible diagnoses, particularly in patients with chronic instability or pain, are peroneal tendon pathology, superficial or sural nerve injury, associated fractures, and intra-articular lesions, such as osteochondral fractures and impingement lesions.

Essentially all authors agree that grade I and II ankle sprains should be treated nonsurgically with an emphasis on early mobilization and proprioceptive exercises. Nonsurgical treatment with early functional mobilization also is indicated for grade III tears of the lateral ligament. Proper rehabilitation progresses through four stages: acute symptom management, range of motion exercises and early strengthening, aggressive strengthening and proprioception, and progressive return to functional activities. Recommendations for the first stage of treatment vary, but include casting in neutral and casting in 10° to 15° of dorsiflexion for up to 5 weeks. A more aggressive sports medicine approach aims to avoid muscle atrophy and stiffness, and most patients with acute ankle sprains can be treated with a pneumatic compression splint that allows at least partial weightbearing immediately and initiation of active range of motion exercises. While the ankle is rested in an elevated position and ice is applied, range of motion activities are encouraged as tolerated. Cast immobilization is reserved for patients with severe pain and swelling that prohibit motion. The cast is removed after 1 week and a pneumatic splint applied. Stage II of rehabilitation begins with gentle isometrics and isotonic and isokinetic progressive resistive exercises. Proprioceptive exercises are introduced as soon as strength allows. The final stage of rehabilitation includes running and activities involving agility. Heel-cord stretching is also emphasized throughout rehabilitation, and the tilt board and balance disk are helpful to restore proprioception. The pneumatic splint is used for varying periods of time and discontinued when the individual feels comfortable and confident. High-performance athletes can be treated with taping.

The kinematics of ankle instability can involve talar tilting or rotation. Talar tilting can occur, even with weighbearing, when both the anterior talofibular and calcaneofibular ligaments are torn. Rotatory instability occurs when the anterior talofibular ligament is disrupted, allowing the talus to rotate in the transverse plane "uncoupling" the ankle-subtalar complex. Acute ankle ligament injuries are diagnosed clinically by noting the amount of swelling, areas of tenderness, and degree of instability. Stress radiographs are not needed in the acute phase. With chronic instability, an anterior drawer test that shows 5 mm of anterior translation greater than that of the uninjured ankle indicates a grossly unstable ankle and is more reliable than the talar tilt test. The anterior translation is measured from the posterior lip of the tibia to the nearest part of the talus.

The anterior drawer test, performed with the patient's ankle in neutral and plantarflexion, determines the integrity of the anterior talofibular ligament and can be depicted on lateral radiographs. The inversion stress test or talar tilt evaluates the integrity of the calcaneofibular and anterior talofibular ligaments; it is performed with the ankle in neutral or slightly plantarflexed. The angle between the tibial plafond and tibial dome is measured radiographically. A talar tilt greater than 10° compared to the contralateral ankle represents significant mechanical instability.

Surgery is reserved for patients with both mechanical instability (on clinical examination) and functional instability (demonstrated by giving way) that do not respond to an aggressive rehabilitation program. Electromyographic (EMG) studies have documented prolonged peroneal reaction times in unstable ankles. Therefore, the rehabilitation must include peroneal muscle strengthening and proprioception enhancing exercises.

When nonsurgical treatment has failed, the most popular anatomic procedure is the modified Broström repair of the anterior talofibular and calcaneofibular ligaments (Fig. 7). Modifying the ligament reefing procedure by mobilizing and attaching the extensor retinaculum to the fibula reinforces the repair and helps stabilize the subtalar joint, which is often a component of the instability. Reconstruction using a portion of the peroneal brevis tendon is indicated in patients with generalized ligamentous laxity, a failed repair or reconstruction, or severe subtalar instability. Some procedures that have produced excellent results can result in too much stiffness of the ankle or subtalar joints.

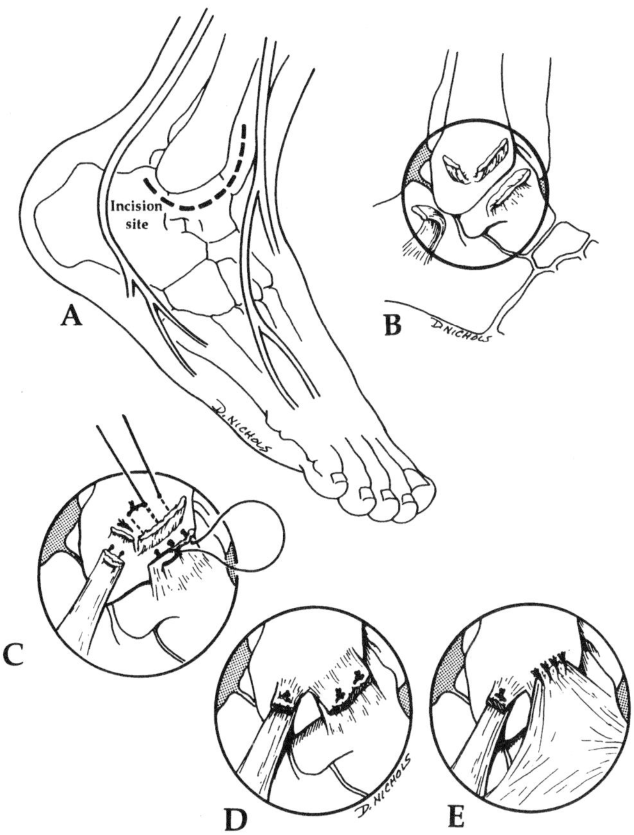

Fig. 7 Modified Broström (Broström-Gould) procedure. **A,** Anterolateral curved incision. **B,** Arthrotomy leaving a 3-mm cuff at the fibula. The proximal stump of the ligament is elevated. **C,** The distal stump of the ligament is sutured into the fibula. **D,** The proximal stump of the ligament is sutured over the distal stump in a pants-over-vest fashion. **E,** The lateral extensor retinaculum is sutured over the repair into the fibula. (Reproduced with permission from McCluskey LC, Black K: Ankle injuries in sports, in Gould JS (ed): *Operative Foot Surgery.* Philadelphia, PA, WB Saunders, 1994, pp 901–936.)

It has been reported that 10% of all ankle sprains involve rupture of the anterior inferior tibiofibular ligament. The diagnosis requires a high index of suspicion and can be confirmed by tenderness of the syndesmosis, a positive "squeeze test," and positive pain on external rotation of the ankle. Syndesmotic widening is measured on a mortise view: the clear space, measured 1 cm proximal to the ankle joint, should be less than 6 mm. If mortise view radiographs are normal, stress views with the ankle in external rotation can be used to identify a "latent" diastasis. If the stress views are normal, functional rehabilitation similar to that prescribed for more typical ankle sprains can be started. A long leg nonweightbearing cast is used to treat latent diastasis. A frank diastasis should be treated with reduction and syndesmotic screw fixation.

External rotation and abduction of the foot can produce isolated tears of the deltoid ligament, but there usually is a concomitant syndesmotic injury or fibular fracture. Because the deltoid ligament has also been shown to restrain internal rotation of the talus during axial loading, it can be injured along with the lateral ligaments. Nonsurgical treatment, consisting of protected mobilization or casting, for patients with deltoid ligament sprains is usually sufficient, but surgical treatment is necessary when extrication of the torn ligament from the joint is necessary to reduce the ankle joint to an anatomic position.

Subtalar Joint Instability

Subtalar joint instability easily can be confused with ankle or tibiotalar instability. If subtalar instability is suspected, a stress radiographic view or examination under fluoroscopy may show the instability pattern. MRI can demonstrate potential ligamentous pathology, and tenderness over the calcaneofibular ligament area may also be a clue to pathology. Giving way of the ankle or dynamic stress tests determine the need for surgery. The inversion and the anterior drawer tests can be performed under fluoroscopy. In the Broden projection, the patient is supine and the leg and foot are internally rotated 45° with the ankle at a right angle. The central ray is directed at a point 2 to 3 cm caudoventral to the lateral malleolus. Exposures are taken with the tube angle at 40°, 30°, 20°, and 10° toward the head. The anterior part of the talocalcaneal joint is seen at 40°, and the posterior aspect is shown at 10°. An inversion stress will open the unstable joint. The two sides are compared along with the stress test of the ankle.

Subtalar instability can occur independently or in conjunction with ankle instability. Most cases of subtalar joint instability accompanied by ankle instability can be treated with a Broström-Gould procedure if functional rehabilitation is not successful. In patients requiring maximum plantarflexion, such as dancers, it is the procedure of choice. However, in large athletes or individuals in whom some stiffness or lack of mobility would not be a detriment, the Broström-Gould procedure may be supplemented with reconstruction using a portion of the peroneous brevis, such as in the modified Evans or Chrisman-Snook procedures. When the subtalar instability is isolated, Broström-Gould is still recommended, although the cervical ligament of the subtalar joint could also be reconstructed. The anterior portion of the peroneous brevis is passed through a calcaneal bone tunnel and through a V-shaped tunnel around the lateral talar ridge. The procedure spares the subtalar joint. Injuries to the subtalar joint should always be considered in the evaluation of ankle sprains.

Ankle Arthroscopy

Many procedures previously performed using arthrotomy can be performed arthroscopically with less morbidity and more rapid functional return. Small diameter 2.7-mm arthroscopes available in 25° and 70° angles of view are recommended for ankle arthroscopy. Three standard operating portals are used for ankle arthroscopy. The anteromedial portal is located adjacent to the medial border of the anterior tibial tendon; the anterolateral portal is located adjacent to the lateral border of the peroneus tertius tendon; and the posterolateral portal is placed adjacent to the lateral border of the Achilles tendon slightly distal to the level of the anterior portals. The anterocentral and posteromedial portals are not recommended because of significant risk of neurovascular injury.

Accessory anteromedial or anterolateral portals may be used depending on the pathology encountered during the procedure. Attention to detail in portal creation minimizes the risk of injury to superficial nerves and vessels. It is recommended that the portal be established by skin incision and blunt dissection into the joint. A dedicated inflow system through a posterolateral cannula or an arthroscopic fluid pump can be used. A set of small joint instruments, including motorized shavers and burrs, and mechanical instruments, such as basket forceps, currettes, rongeurs, and loose body forceps, should be available.

Osteophytes are best evaluated radiographically on the lateral view of the ankle and usually demonstrate increased uptake on bone scan. Arthroscopic removal can be expected to produce good results in ankles that do not have significant degenerative changes on the weightbearing surfaces of the talus and tibia. Loose bodies in the ankle cause mechanical symptoms, such as locking and catching of the joint, along with pain and swelling. They are identified and removed individually using loose body forceps. A synovectomy also is performed for synovical chondromatosis. The most common soft-tissue impingement lesions arise in the lateral talomalleolar joint or in the distal tibiofibular joint and are noted at arthroscopy to be firm, vascular masses that can cause mechanical impingement. The lesions can be removed arthroscopically using basket forceps and currettes.

Osteochondral lesions of the talar dome are common disorders that occur in 6.8% to 22% of ankle sprains and often require surgical treatment. Poor results are reported in up to 75% of cases treated conservatively. Most authors treat stage I, II, and III lesions conservatively and operate on loose fragments (stage IV) with symptoms of crepitus, catching, or locking. If a patient is symptomatic less than 3 months and mechanical symptoms do not exist, treatment may be conservative. Symptoms longer than 3 months, mechanical symptoms, and high athletic demands are relative indications for surgery. Available arthroscopic techniques eliminate the need for open surgery.

Complications of ankle arthroscopy are relatively rare; nevertheless, they must be acknowledged and hopefully avoided. These include breaking of instruments with loose instrument fragments within the joint requiring retrieval, damage to intact articular cartilage, and ligament or tendinous injury (for example, the FHL) from failure to appreciate normal and abnormal structures. Pseudoaneurysms of popliteal vessels, nerve injury from careless techniques in opening the portals (for example, superficial peroneal nerve), and infection and persistent portal drainage are all problematic.

Compartment Syndrome of the Foot

Compartment syndrome of the foot is reported to be present in approximately 10% of calcaneus fractures and 41% of crush injuries. The nine plantar compartments were identified using injection techniques. The calcaneal compartment communicates with the deep posterior compartment of the leg through the medial retromalleolar space.

The diagnosis of foot compartment syndrome is based on a high index of suspicion, supplemented with invasive pressure monitoring. Pain and pain with passive stretch remain the cardinal signs of this syndrome. Pallor, paresthesias, pulselessness, and paralysis occur later or sometimes not at all. Because these warning signs, including pain, may not be detectable in some patients and may not correlate with the actual condition, any patient having the potential to develop this syndrome should be tested. Swelling in calcaneal fractures does not necessarily correlate with the presence or absence of foot compartment elevated pressures. Calcaneal compartment pressures routinely should be obtained for calcaneal fractures. If pressure is elevated, the medial, lateral, superficial, and interosseous compartments should be evaluated. Forefoot or crush injuries should also be monitored using multistick assessments. Compartment release is based on absolute compartment pressures higher than 30 mm Hg or, in the case of the hypotensive traumatized patient, a compartment pressure higher than the diastolic blood pressure minus 10 to 20 mm Hg.

Recommended fasciotomy incisions include two dorsal longitudinal incisions (medial aspect of the second metatarsal, lateral aspect of the fourth metatarsal) and/or one 6-cm medial incision. This incision begins at the posterior margin of the medial malleolus and continues distally, paralleling the sole of the foot. The medial, cancaneal and lateral compartments can be released through the medial incision. The remaining compartments can be released through the dorsal incisions. The fasciotomy incisions are left open initially with either delayed primary closure or split-thickness skin grafting at 5 to 6 days. Immediate open reduction and internal fixation can be undertaken with forefoot fracture–dislocation injuries (Lisfranc fractures). After fasciotomy, delayed reduction and stabilization at 10 to 14 days is recommended for calcaneus fractures.

The primary reported sequelae of an untreated compartment syndrome are claw deformities of the lesser toes. These can affect a variable number of toes. If the deformity decreases with plantarflexion of the ankle, the FDL muscle and deep posterior compartment of the leg are involved. If both the foot and leg are involved, a cavovarus deformity of the foot occurs secondary to contracture of both extrinsic and intrinsic muscles.

Reflex Sympathetic Dystrophy of the Foot and Ankle

Reflex sympathetic dystrophy (RSD), a complex and often progressive disorder, is frequently initiated by trauma to neural structures or soft tissue. The absence of objective pathognomonic markers confounds the diagnosis, which depends on a clinical picture of pain, edema, autonomic dysfunction, functional impairment, and trophic changes. RSD is a common complicating event after lower extremity injury or surgery. Pain syndromes may be either sympathetically maintained or sympathetically independent. The former responds to sympathetic blockade, which decreases reflex sympathetic autonomic dysfunction. RSD is a dynamic process with large variations in intensity and pathologic responses. Transition times from one stage to the next may be variable; some evidence from a large clinical prospective study suggests that three consecutive phases of RSD are not present consistently.

After trauma, alterations in physiology of the injured extremity, associated with abnormal sympathetic discharge and pain, are normal. Painful (nociceptive) experience, when associated with cellular insults produces secondary inflammation with activation of alpha-1 adrenoreceptors (polymodal afferent neurons) with secondary excitation of c-nociceptor fibers, which, in turn, activate peripheral nerve relays through the dorsal horn of the spinal cord to higher cognitive centers. Over time, irreversible events occur in the end-organ anatomy. Therefore, RSD is an abnormal prolongation of an otherwise normal physiologic process. Permanent compromise of the extremity may occur if the dystrophic cycle persists. Prolonged symptoms—hyperpathia (increased pain), allodynia (painful responses to nonpainful stimuli), and thermoregulatory and vasomotor disturbances—may produce functional impairment. The dystrophic process is initiated in the periphery through local responses and neurovascular events, but central processing exacerbates the problem and may predominate over time.

Radiographically, RSD is seen as diffuse patchy osteopenia, which is classically periarticular and involves all joints (Sudek's atrophy). Recent data demonstrate that osteopenia associated with RSD involves both cortical and cancellous bone, and that total mineralization, without regard to treatment, is less in patients with dystrophy than in patients without it. Five bone resorption patterns associated with RSD have been described: (1) irregular metaphyseal trabecular, (2) generalized subperiosteal, (3) intercortical, (4) endosteal, and (5) surface erosions in subchondral and juxtachondral areas.

Three-phase bone scans continue to be used in the diagnosis of RSD in spite of mixed specificity and sensitivity of data and questions concerning their positive predictive value. A positive three-phase scan does not explain the documented physiologic events seen in RSD, and the role of scans in variant forms of dystrophy is not well delineated. Furthermore, three-phase bone scans following successful treatment are identical to those during active disease. Bone scans do not correlate with staging criteria, do not identify recovery, and do not have demonstrable prognostic implications.

Evaluation of peripheral blood flow before, during, and after stress has been shown to provide objective information regarding autonomic function, response to intervention, and outcome. Monitoring techniques include skin temperature, laser Doppler, duplex Doppler ultrasound, and quantitative sensory measurements. Videothermography is not an appropriate tool to use alone for the diagnosis or monitoring of RSD.

The treatment of RSD remains controversial. Early identification and treatment provide the best results. In general, combinations of interventions are necessary (Table 1). Lesions involving peripheral nerves may be identified by continuous sympathetic blockage combined with nerve repair or reconstruction. After the dystrophic process is controlled, surgical reconstruction may be performed.

Foot Drop

Peripheral nerve lesions account for most cases of foot drop (68%); 18% are due to various polyneuropathies and usually are bilateral. Mononeuropathies involve injury to the peroneal nerve alone in 30% and the entire sciatic nerve in 11.5%. The remainder are caused by radiculopathies (20%) and injuries to the cauda equina or conus medullaris. In cases of incomplete sciatic nerve injury, the peroneal component is injured more often because it is in the posterolateral position and contains less connective tissue and fewer but larger funiculi than the tibial component. Peroneal nerve injury also is common distally near the proximal fibula. Neurapraxia at this level usually is caused by compression or traction, but may also result from knee surgery.

Anterior tibial weakness due to peripheral nerve lesions usually does not produce more than a 15° plantarflexion ankle contracture in adults. Pure anterior tibial muscle weakness causes a plantarflexion and eversion deformity. Complete peroneal nerve palsy usually leads to plantarflexion and inversion. Electrodiagnostic studies can help determine the level of injury of the peroneal nerve, diagnose double crush injuries, and differentiate patterns of polyneuropathies. They are essential if surgical reconstruction with tendon transfer is contemplated. High-risk zones have been delineated to avoid damage to the peroneal nerve and its branches during fibular osteotomy or placement of external fixation pins. The first zone, which is the level at which the common peroneal nerve crosses the fibula, begins at the fibular neck (2 cm distal to a line drawn between the prominence of the fibular head and the tibial tubercle) and extends distally 4 cm. The second high-risk interval, in which the innervation of the EHL is vulnerable, begins 8 cm distal to the fibular head and continues for an additional 6 cm. The mainstay of conservative treatment of foot drop is the AFO. Surgery usually is not necessary. Tendon transfers, however, can be helpful in some foot drop cases.

Table 1. Management options in reflex sympathetic dystrophy

Option	Method of Administration
Nonpharmacologic	
Physical (occupational) therapy	
Active/passive range of motion	
Stress loading	
Contrast baths	
Continuous passive motion	
Noninjectable pharmacologic agents	
Amitriptyline hydrochloride (Elavil)	Oral
Phenytoin (Dilantin)	Oral
Phenoxybenzamine hydrochloride (Dibenzyline)	Oral
Nifedipine (Procardia)	Oral
Corticosteroids	Oral
Carbamazepine (Tegretol)	Oral
Clonidine (Catapres-TTS -2, -3)	Patch
Injectable pharmacologic agents	
Guanethidine sulfate	IV regional
Clonidine	Continuous epidural
Phentolamine (Regitine)	IV injection
Cortisone sulfate (usually with lidocaine)	IV injection
Reserpine	IV injection
Brytilium	IV injection
Invasive procedures	
Neurolytic blockade	
Percutaneous ethanol (alcohol)	
Lumbar surgical sympathectomy	
Neurosurgical procedures	
Dorsal column stimulators	
Thalamic stimulators	
Periventricular gray matter stimulators	
Cingulotomy	
Peripheral nerve stimulators	

Foot and Ankle Tumors

Primary and metastatic neoplasms of the foot are rare. A review of 260 foot and ankle tumors found 191 benign, 58 malignant, and 11 metastatic lesions. A predilection existed for the hindfoot (57%) and the forefoot (33%). Osteoid osteoma was the most common benign lesion, and Ewing's sarcoma the most common neoplasm. A similar study of 83 soft-tissue masses in the foot revealed a 13% incidence of malignancy, mostly synovial sarcomas. Appropriate imaging and a multidisciplinary approach should be used to provide optimal care.

Soft-tissue lesions are the most common tumors found in the foot. Plantar fibromatosis is a relatively common benign fibroblastic proliferation of the plantar fascia and may present as an isolated fibroma, juvenile aponeurotic fibroma, or generalized (aggressive) fibromatosis. Associations of plantar fibromatosis with Dupuytren's contracture (palmar fibromatosis) and Peyronie's disease have been reported. However, contractures in the foot are generally not seen because of the usually insignificant extension of the fascia to the phalanges. Treatment is directed at alleviating the symptoms. Pain inadequately relieved by shoe modifications and inserts is the major indication for surgical intervention. Wide excision with skin grafting, if needed, is the recommended surgical procedure. Recurrences are frequent. In some aggressive lesions, a wide margin en block excision is done and a free flap applied. Central ray excisions have also been used when lesions have penetrated the dorsum of the foot, leaving medial and lateral areas free of disease.

Melanomas, the most common malignant neoplasm of the foot and ankle, are skin lesions characterized by asymmetric irregular borders and nonuniform color distribution, with a diameter exceeding 7 mm (although suspicious lesions of any diameter should be biopsied). In noncaucasians, the sole of the foot is the most prevalent site. Of 1,018 patients with melanoma, 282 had primary cutaneous foot melanomas, which have a poorer prognosis than melanomas of other parts of the lower extremity. The discrepancy was felt to be secondary to their more advanced histologic and clinical stage at the time of presentation. When compared to dorsal lesions, plantar and subungual lesions were associated with a particularly poor prognosis.

Amelanotic melanoma of soft parts and clear cell sarcoma of tendon sheaths are tumors with similar histology. These malignant tumors, frequently found in the extremities, especially the foot, appear to have a predilection for young women and not infrequently may present after a long duration of symptoms. Metastases are common and survival poor, especially in lesions greater than 5 cm in diameter at presentation.

The bones of the foot and ankle also can be affected by primary and metastatic disease processes. The ratio of cortical to cancellous bone in the small bones of the foot may make radiographic presentation atypical. As in the hand, benign enchondromas are the most common tumors found. Evaluation and treatment are similar to those for the remainder of the skeleton.

The Diabetic Foot

Approximately 20% of all diabetic hospital admissions are for problems of the foot. The Center for Disease Control estimates that 50% of foot problems and subsequent amputations can be eliminated by educating both patients at risk and their physicians, as well as providing proper prevention and early treatment. The Diabetes Control and Complications Trial (DCCT), a 10-year landmark study sponsored by the National Institutes of Health and completed in 1993, demonstrated that the severity of diabetic complications is related to the control of blood glucose levels rather than to the severity of the disease. This study found that intensive treatment of blood sugar reduced clinically significant neuropathy by 60%. Side effects of the increased glucose control included a threefold increase in the incidence of severe hypoglycemia and weight gain.

Diabetic neuropathy affects the sensory, motor, and autonomic pathways. Sensory neuropathy results in the loss of protective sensibility, making the foot subject to increased mechanical stress that is not modified by the pain avoidance mechanisms present in a healthy foot. Most patients complain of numbness and paresthesia in a stocking distribution; some may have hyperesthesia or even dysesthesia. This painful form of neuropathy often presents as a nocturnal burning sensation and typically will diminish over a period of 1 year.

With motor neuropathy, the intrinsic muscles atrophy, causing claw toes that depress the metatarsal heads. In addition, the plantar fat pad shifts distally. A shortening of the plantar fascia leads to a cavus foot posture, often with plantarflexion of the first ray. These changes result in less plantar protection of bony prominences, which leads to callus formation, pressure necrosis, and ulceration. An isolated motor neuropathy involving a single proximal nerve may also occur. The peroneal nerve is most commonly affected, and the resultant foot drop must be differentiated from a spontaneous rupture of the anterior tibialis tendon.

Changes in blood flow and sweating account for the thick, dry, scaly skin and nail deformities and the increased risk of bacterial invasion seen in diabetic feet. There also is evidence that the autonomic dysfunction in diabetes results in a lack of the normal hyperemic response to infection.

Peripheral vascular disease is present in 8% of adult diabetics at the time of diagnosis and is increased to 45% after 20 years. Vascular changes in the diabetic tend to be diffuse and occur distal to the trifurcation of the popliteal artery. When distal pulses are present and associated with brisk capillary refill, further vascular assessment is not necessary. However, if pedal pulses are absent, noninvasive vascular studies are indicated, particularly in patients with nonhealing ulcers or before surgical intervention. Such studies include determination of ankle-brachial index by Doppler ultrasound, absolute toe pressure, and transcutaneous oxygen measurement. However, the ankle-brachial index is affected by calcification of vessels, and the oxygen level can be falsely lowered in the presence of infection.

When significant ischemia is present on noninvasive testing, arteriography and vascular surgical consultation are recommended. Several studies have demonstrated a 90% distal limb salvage rate with use of aggressive vascular surgery techniques with anastomosis to the arteries of the foot. In addition, before selecting a definitive amputation level, nutritional status should be evaluated by checking total lymphocyte count, total protein, and albumin levels, which are independent predictors of postoperative wound healing.

Imaging of the diabetic foot is used to diagnose osteomyelitis and to differentiate it from neuroarthropathy. Permeative radiolucencies, destructive changes, and/or periosteal new bone formation without reparative response suggest osteomyelitis; however, plain film changes may lag 2 weeks behind the onset of osteomyelitis. The sensitivity and specificity of plain films is about 75%. Three phase bone scans have a 93% sensitivity, but only a 43% specificity and are good for distinguishing cellulitis from osteomyelitis; however, they do not differentiate osteomyelitis from neuroarthropathy. Reports vary as to whether indium-111 white blood cell scans, gallium scans, antibody labeled scans, and MRI scans are helpful in distinguishing osteomyelitis from neuroarthropathy. Some centers rely heavily on the use of simultaneous bone and indium scans to differentiate neuropathic Charcot changes from osteomyelitis. No one test is best in the acute setting, and clinical judgement that weighs all the evidence is the most important factor.

The most widely used classification system for diabetic ulceration is that of Wagner: grade 0, intact skin; grade I, superficial with exposed subcutaneous tissue; grade II, ulcers present with exposed tendons or bone; grade III, ulcers extend to the deep tissue as above and evidence of acute infection or osteomyelitis; and grades IV and V, ulcers involving the dysvascular foot and gangrenous tissue. This system is useful in planning treatment algorithms and for scientific communication, but is limited because it does not include a vascular assessment.

The depth of diabetic ulceration varies according to the early Wagner stages. Diabetic ulcerations are colonized with polymicrobial organisms, but are not necessarily clinically infected. In addition to the development of osteomyelitis, infection may ascend along tendon sheaths and regions of ischemia, with subsequent abscess formation. Subcutaneous emphysema and gas formation may occur in diabetics, but is usually not Clostridial in origin. Unrecognized deep abscess formation may result in acute occlusion of digital arteries, with rapid formation of wet gangrene.

Recent developments in the nonsurgical treatment of the diabetic foot include the new biologic and semipermeable dressings. Plantar neuropathic ulcers result from unprotected forces incurred during normal weightbearing activity, while dorsal ulcers are due to the constant pressure of ill-fitting shoes. Harris mat imprints are a simple way to identify locations of increased pressure. Thermography and force plate analysis systems, although costly, are additional methods of identifying patients at risk. Thermography is based on the principle of hyperemia occurring in areas of increased plantar pressure.

Neuropathic osteoarthropathy or Charcot disease results in fragmentation, destruction, and dislocation of the bones of the foot and ankle. There are two theories of pathogenesis: neurotraumatic and neurovascular. The former involves repetitive trauma sustained by a joint unable to sense pain, whereas the latter refers to a sympathetic dysfunction with persistent hyperemia and active bone resorption. The incidence of Charcot arthropathy is 0.1% to 0.5% in the diabetic population. Although the time between the onset of diabetes and the onset of Charcot averages 16 years, Charcot may also be the first presentation of diabetes. Contrary to common belief, 50% of Charcot feet are actually painful. Crepitance may be present at unstable joints, and most patients have diminished sensation, but bounding pedal pulses. Twenty percent to 25% of patients will develop contralateral involvement. Up to 74% of patients will have associated mal perforans ulcers.

Neuroarthropathy occurs in three clinical stages. The acute stage consists of an acute swollen, warm, erythematous foot. Very early, there may be minimal radiographic changes; therefore, close follow-up is required. The second stage is subacute, in which swelling subsides and new bone formation occurs. The final stage is chronic, in which no warmth or swelling is present, but the foot is deformed. Neuroarthropathy most commonly affects the midfoot, then the hindfoot, and least commonly the ankle joint. Midfoot Charcot tends to become stable with time, but may develop ulceration over medial and plantar bony prominences. Hindfoot and ankle neuroathropathies, however, frequently do not autofuse; they become unstable, painful, and prone to ulceration.

The treatment of Charcot in the acute and subacute stages is total contact casting. This usually needs to be continued for several months. Frequent cast changes may be required because of changes in foot volume. Patients may require lifetime bracing for treatment of Charcot ankle or hindfoot disease, whereas the midfoot can often be managed with a custom shoe and insert alone.

Approximately 50% of cases result in a painless pseudarthrosis, with the goal of treatment being a braceable foot and ankle without ulceration. Due to recalcitrant ulcerations, these feet will occasionally require surgery to decompress a bony prominence. Surgery may also be indicated to fuse and realign the foot or ankle with an unbraceable deformity. Surgery in diabetic patients is arduous with risk of infection and nonunion. After a hindfoot and/or tibiotalar fusion for a Charcot deformity, lifetime bracing is recommended because of the risk of tibial stress fracture.

Annotated Bibliography

Hallux Valgus

Donnelly RE, Saltzman CL, Kile TA, et al: Modified chevron osteotomy for hallux valgus. *Foot Ankle Int* 1994;15:642–645.

This is a retrospective review of 42 feet that underwent a modified chevron osteotomy for hallux valgus deformity. All patients reported some improvement from their preoperative status; there were no malunions, nonunions, or evidence of ON. The authors concluded this modification provides a safe, simple stable fixation for early weightbearing.

Pochatko DJ, Schlehr FJ, Murphey MD, et al: Distal chevron osteotomy with lateral release for treatment of hallux valgus deformity. *Foot Ankle Int* 1994;15:457–461.

In this retrospective review, 17 patients (23 feet) who underwent a chevron osteotomy combined with a modified McBride procedure were evaluated by physical and radiographic examination and subjective questionnaire to determine the clinical outcome and incidence of ON. The average follow-up was 50 months.

Disorders of the Second Metatarsophalangeal Joint

Coughlin MJ: Subluxation and dislocation of the second metatarsophalangeal joint. *Orthop Clin North Am* 1989; 20:535–551.

The author presents a comprehensive review of pathologic conditions that affect the second ray uniquely, as well as conditions that are common to all of the lesser toes. Pertinent anatomy is described and depicted.

Helal B, Gibb P: Freiberg's disease: A suggested pattern of management. *Foot Ankle* 1987;8:94–102.

The authors review their approach to patients with various stages of Freiberg's infraction. Smillies' pathological stating of Freiberg's disease is depicted.

Bunionette

Coughlin MJ: Treatment of bunionette deformity with longitudinal diaphyseal osteotomy with distal soft tissue repair. *Foot Ankle* 1991;11:195–203.

The author describes 20 patients (30 feet) with symptomatic bunionettes who underwent oblique mid diaphyseal osteotomy, lateral condylectomy, and distal MTP realignment. At 31 months average follow-up, 93% noted good or excellent results.

Kitaoka HB, Holiday AD Jr: Lateral condylar resection for bunionette. *Clin Orthop* 1992;278:183–192.

Twenty-one feet in 16 patients underwent simple lateral condylectomy; after follow-up for 6.4 years, 15 were rated as good, three fair, and three poor. Failure was due to inadequate resection, MTP subluxation, and severe forefoot splay.

Tendinitis of the Foot and Ankle

Sangeorzan BJ, Mosca V, Hansen ST Jr: Effect of calcaneal lengthening on relationships among the hindfoot, midfoot, and forefoot. *Foot Ankle* 1993; 14:136–141.

A radiographic analysis of the correction obtained by calcaneal lengthening in adults with symptomatic pes planovalgus is presented.

Trevino S, Baumhauer JF: Tendon injuries of the foot and ankle. *Clin Sports Med* 1992;11:727–739.

This paper is a well-written review of specific tendon disorders of the foot and ankle.

Wapner KL, Pavlock GS, Hecht PJ, et al: Repair of chronic Achilles tendon rupture with flexor hallucis longus tendon transfer. *Foot Ankle* 1993;14:443–449.

A technique for repair of chronic Achilles tendon rupture with flexor hallucis longus tendon is described. All patients had satisfactory return of function.

Wapner KL, Hecht PJ, Shea JR, et al: Anatomy of second muscular layer of the foot: Considerations for tendon selection in transfer for Achilles and posterior tibial tendon reconstruction. *Foot Ankle Int* 1994;15:420–423.

Eighty-five dissections of the second muscular layer of the foot were studied. Based on anatomic findings, the FDL tendon is recommended for transfers in posterior tibial tendon reconstruction while the FHL is recommended for late Achilles tendon reconstruction.

Acquired Flatfoot

O'Malley MJ, Deland JT, Lee KT: Selective hindfoot arthrodesis for the treatment of adult acquired flatfoot deformity: An in vitro study. *Foot Ankle Int* 1995;16:411–417.

This cadaver study demonstrated that talonavicular fusion alone or midtarsal or triple arthrodesis would fully correct severe flatfoot deformity, whereas subtalar or calcaneocuboid fusions alone would not.

Pedowitz WJ, Kovatis P: Flatfoot in the adult. *J Am Acad Orthop Surg* 1995;3:293–302.

The etiologies of flatfoot are summarized and current recommendations for management are given.

Nerve Entrapment Syndromes

Bourke G, Owen J, Machet D: Histological comparison of the third interdigital nerve in patients with Morton's metatarsalgia and control patients. *Aust N Z J Surg* 1994;64:421–424.

Nodule and fibrotic changes were seen in both symptomatic and asymptomatic patients, and demyelination was seen in the asymptomatic group.

Fornage BD: Sonography of peripheral nerves of the extremities. *Radiol Med* 1993;85(suppl 1):162–167.

The virtues of high-resolution sonography are promoted. The authors suggest the technique is particularly useful in diagnosis of nerve tumors at a lower cost than MRI.

Frey C, Kerr R: Magnetic resonance imaging and the evaluation of tarsal tunnel syndrome. *Foot Ankle* 1993; 14:159–164.

MRI showed various lesions in the tarsal tunnel. The lesions were confirmed at surgery.

Kilmartin TE, Wallace WA: Effect of pronation and supination orthosis on Morton's neuroma and lower extremity function. *Foot Ankle Int* 1994;15:256–262.

Repositioning the foot with the use of various orthotics did not alter Morton's neuroma pain.

Pfeiffer WH, Cracchiolo A III: Clinical results after tarsal tunnel decompression. *J Bone Joint Surg* 1994;76A:1222–1230.

Following tarsal tunnel release, 44% excellent results were obtained with 38% dissatisfied patients. There is no correlation between clinical outcome and positive electrodiagnostic studies.

Resch S, Stenström A, Jonsson A, et al: The diagnostic efficacy of magnetic resonance imaging and ultrasonography in Morton's neuroma: A radiological-surgical correlation. *Foot Ankle Int* 1994;15:88–92.

MRI and ultrasonography were not thought to be helpful in diagnosis of Morton's neuroma.

Ruuskanen MM, Niinimäki T, Jalovaara P: Results of the surgical treatment of Morton's neuralgia in 58 operated intermetatarsal spaces followed over 6 (2–12) years. *Arch Orthop Trauma Surg* 1994;113:78–80.

Neurectomy provided improvement in 80% of 45 patients followed up for 6 years.

Sammarco GJ, Chalk DE, Feibel JH: Tarsal tunnel syndrome and additional nerve lesions in the same limb. *Foot Ankle* 1993;14:71–77.

The authors suggested multiple lesions and nerves in the single extremity may account for variable success of tarsal tunnel surgery.

Skalley TC, Schon LC, Hinton RY, et al: Clinical results following revision tibial nerve release. *Foot Ankle Int* 1994;15:360–367.

Clinical history and physical examination were more helpful than electrodiagnositic studies in determining the location of the compression and extent of release required in revision tarsal tunnel surgery.

Cavus Foot

Mann RA: Charcot-Marie-Tooth disease, in Gould JS (ed): *Operative Foot Surgery.* Philadelphia, PA, WB Saunders, 1994, pp 177–183.

The author provides the surgical procedures and technique for correction of the cavus foot in the adult with Charcot-Marie-Tooth etiology.

Thometz JG, Gould JS: Cavus deformity, in Drennan JC (ed): *The Child's Foot and Ankle.* New York, NY, Raven Press, 1992, pp 343–353.

This short chapter describes the pathophysiology related to the cavus foot and recommends a logical surgical sequence to manage the problems. A detailed description of the surgical procedures is given.

Posttraumatic Arthritis of the Hindfoot and Ankle

Bono JV, Jacobs RL: Triple arthrodesis through a single lateral approach: A cadaveric experiment. *Foot Ankle* 1992;13:408–412.

This study demonstrated the difficulty of removing the articular cartilage of the talonavicular joint through a lateral approach. A separate medial incision is recommended for complete removal of the cartilage.

Horton GA, Olney BW: Deformity correction and arthrodesis of the midfoot with a medial plate. *Foot Ankle* 1993;14:493–499.

A method of midfoot arthrodesis is described utilizing a medial one third tubular plate spanning the midfoot joints to be fused. The technique was used on nine feet in eight patients with satisfactory results.

Reconstruction for Complications of Calcaneal Fractures

Myerson M, Quill GE Jr: Late complications of fractures of the calcaneus. *J Bone Joint Surg* 1993;75A:331–341.

A retrospective review is presented of surgical treatment of late complications in 43 calcaneus fractures. Of the patients, 90% received partial pain relief, 83% improved in function, and 76% returned to work or preinjury level of activity.

Romash MM: Reconstructive osteotomy of the calcaneus with subtalar arthrodesis for malunited calcaneal fractures. *Clin Orthop* 1993;290:157–167.

A technique is described to deal with late complications of malunited calcaneus fractures. Satisfactory results were obtained in nine of 14 feet with an average follow up of 14 months.

Ankle and Subtalar Joint Instability

Cass JR, Settles H: Ankle instability: In vitro kinematics in response to axial load. *Foot Ankle Int* 1994;15:134–140.

In this study, an axial load was applied as the foot was rotated and inverted. Tilting of the talus and the mortise occurred only with release of both the anterior talofibular ligament and calcaneofibular ligament. This paper supports the theory that ankle instability can be in the form of axial rotation.

Eiff MP, Smith AT, Smith GE: Early mobilization versus immobilization in the treatment of lateral ankle sprains. *Am J Sports Med* 1994;22:83–88.

This prospective trial concluded that in first-time lateral ankle sprains, early mobilization allowed an earlier return to work, and may be more comfortable for patients.

Hamilton WG, Thompson FM, Snow SW: The modified Broström procedure for lateral ankle instability. *Foot Ankle* 1993;14:1–7.

The authors report 26 excellent results in 28 ankles that had the modified Broström ankle reconstruction for lateral ankle instability. The technique is described in detail.

McCluskey LC, Black KP: Ankle injuries in sports, in Gould JS (ed): *Operative Foot Surgery.* Philadelphia, PA, WB Saunders, 1994, pp 901–936.

A review of the topic that includes indications for nonsurgical and surgical treatment is presented along with descriptions of the techniques used to treat these injuries.

Arthroscopy of the Ankle

Ewing JW: Arthroscopic management of transchondral talar-dome fractures (osteochondritis dissecans) and anterior impingement lesions of the ankle joint. *Clin Sports Med* 1991;10:677–687.

The author presents a brief review of the literature on osteochondral lesions of the talar dome along with a detailed description of the surgical setup to approach these lesions arthroscopically.

Martin DF, Baker CL, Curl WW, et al: Operative ankle arthroscopy: Long-term followup. *Am J Sports Med* 1989;17:16–23.

Fifty-eight ankle arthroscopies with an average follow-up of 25 months are reviewed. The best results occurred in patients with transchondral defects of the talar dome and those with synovitis as the primary diagnosis.

Morgan CD: Arthroscopic tibiotalar arthrodesis, in McGinty JB (ed): *Operative Arthroscopy.* New York, NY, Raven Press, 1991, pp 695–701.

In this chapter, the author presents a detailed description of the surgical procedure for arthroscopic ankle arthrodesis along with preliminary results in 38 patients.

Pritsch M, Horoshovski H, Farine I: Arthroscopic treatment of osteochondral lesions of the talus. *J Bone Joint Surg* 1986;68A:862–865.

Arthroscopy was used to treat 24 ankles with osteochondral lesions of the talar dome. This study documents the poor correlation between routine radiographs and actual arthroscopic examination for predicting the relative intactness of the lesions.

Compartment Syndrome of the Foot

Manoli A II: Compartment syndromes of the foot: Current concepts. *Foot Ankle* 1990;10:340–344.

A comprehensive literature review of compartment syndromes of the foot with particular emphasis on the calcaneal compartment and calcaneus fractures.

Manoli A II, Weber TG: Fasciotomy of the foot: An anatomical study with special reference to release of the calcaneal compartment. *Foot Ankle* 1990;10:267–275.

Nine compartments of the foot are described. The calcaneal compartment is a new compartment. Approaches for surgery and indications discussed. The calcaneal compartment is related to the deep posterior tibial compartment.

Myerson M: Diagnosis and treatment of compartment syndrome of the foot. *Orthopedics* 1990;13:711–717.

A review of anatomy and treatment is presented.

Reflex Sympathetic Dystrophy

Atkins RM, Tindale W, Bickerstaff D, et al: Quantitative bone scintigraphy in reflex sympathetic dystrophy. *Br J Rheumatol* 1993;32:41–45.

Early changes in quantitative bone scintigraphy are demonstrated in RSD after Colles fracture. Posttraumatic RSD (after Colles fracture) is associated with significant loss of trabecular cortical bone compared with uncomplicated fractures.

Bickerstaff DR, Kanis JA: Algodystrophy: An under-recognized complication of minor trauma. *Br J Rheumatol* 1994;33:240–248.

This prospective study of 274 patients with upper extremity fractures demonstrates an incidence far more common than formerly appreciated.

Bickerstaff DR, Charlesworth D, Kanis JA: Changes in cortical and trabecular bone in algodystrophy. *Br J Rheumatol* 1993;32:46–51.

Posttraumatic RSD after Colles fracture is associated with significant loss of trabecular and cortical bone compared with uncomplicated fractures. This study demonstrated that the entire osseous system is involved in RSD, rather than just cortical bone as previously described.

Cooke ED, Steinberg MD, Pearson RM, et al: Reflex sympathetic dystrophy and repetitive strain injury: Temperature and microcirculatory changes following mild cold stress. *J R Soc Med* 1993;86:690–693.

The authors demonstrate altered thermal regulation and hemodynamics in RSD patients.

Jupiter JB, Seiler JG III, Zienowicz R: Sympathetic maintained pain (causalgia) associated with a demonstrable peripheral-nerve lesion: Operative treatment. *J Bone Joint Surg* 1994;76A:1376–1384.

The authors report extremity management of the identifiable nerve lesions using continuous postoperative sympathetic blockade.

Koman LA, Smith BP, Smith TL: Stress testing in the evaluation of upper-extremity perfusion. *Hand Clin* 1993;9:59–83.

Methods and indications for stress evaluation in the upper extremity are discussed. Similar methods are available for the lower extremity.

Mailis A, Meindok H, Papagapiou M, et al: Alterations of the three-phase bone scan after sympathectomy. *Clin J Pain* 1994;10:146–155.

This study demonstrates that alterations in three-phase bone scans after sympathectomy are identical to those reported in an earlier RSD study, and that these alterations do not indicate success of pain relief following intervention.

Pollock FE Jr, Koman LA, Smith BP, et al: Patterns of microvascular response associated with reflex sympathetic dystrophy of the hand and wrist. *J Hand Surg* 1993;18A: 847–852.

This study demonstrates that a positive technetium bone scan does not correlate with vasomotor disturbances in RSD patients.

Sarangi PP, Ward AJ, Smith EJ, et al: Algodystrophy and osteoporosis after tibial fractures. *J Bone Joint Surg* 1993; 75B:450–452.

This prospective study of incidence and natural history of RSD shows that bone mineral density in ankles and feet is related to the development of algodystrophy and that the development of algodystrophy is independent of the type of treatment used.

Sherman RA, Karstetter KW, Damiano M, et al: Stability of temperature asymmetries in reflex sympathetic dystrophy over time and changes in pain. *Clin J Pain* 1994;10:71–77.

This study demonstrates that videothermography alone is not an appropriate tool to use in either single-session diagnosis or multi-session tracking of RSD.

Stanton RP, Malcolm JR, Wesdock KA, et al: Reflex sympathetic dystrophy in children: An orthopedic perspective. *Orthopedics* 1993;16:773–780.

Diagnostic criteria for pediatric RSD patients are presented.

Tu ES, Mailis A, Simons ME: Effect of surgical sympathectomy on arterial blood flow in reflex sympathetic dystrophy: Doppler US assessment. *Radiology* 1994;191:833–834.

The ability of duplex Doppler ultrasound to provide objective reproducible measurements is verified.

Veldman PH, Reynen HM, Arntz IE, et al: Signs and symptoms of reflex sympathetic dystrophy: Prospective study of 829 patients. *Lancet* 1993;342:1012–1016.

This large study found no evidence of the consistent presence of three consecutive phases of the disease. Rather, this study suggests that classic staging criteria may be misleading in many patients.

Foot Drop

Kirgis A, Albrecht S: Palsy of the deep peroneal nerve after proximal tibial osteotomy: An anatomical study. *J Bone Joint Surg* 1992;74A:1180–1185.

The peroneal nerve is dissected in 29 cadavers. The course of the peroneal nerve is described. Areas vulnerable to denervation are discussed.

Diabetic Foot

Gould JS, Erickson JS, Collier BD, et al: Surgical management of ulcers, soft-tissue infections, and osteomyelitis in the diabetic foot, in Heckman JD (ed): *Instructional Course Lectures 42.* Rosemont, IL, American Academy of Orthopaedic Surgeons, 1993, pp 147–158.

This article describes the valuative tools (plain films, MRI, bone and white cell scans) and treatment of the diabetic foot infection from the viewpoints of the multidisciplinary team (diagnostic radiology, nuclear medicine, infectious disease, and orthopaedics).

Myerson MS, Henderson MR, Saxby T, et al: Management of midfoot diabetic neuroarthropathy. *Foot Ankle Int* 1994;15:233–241.

This article is a retrospective review of the results of treatment of a large clinical series of diabetic patients with midfoot neuroarthropathy.

Myerson M, Papa J, Eaton K, et al: The total-contact cast for management of neuropathic plantar ulceration of the foot. *J Bone Joint Surg* 1992;74A:261–269.

The authors review their experience with total contact cast treatment of neuropathic plantar ulceration. They found that 90% of ulcers healed at a mean of 5.5 weeks; 31% of these recurred within 18 months after initial healing, and 86% of these healed after an average of 2 weeks in a second cast.

Papa J, Myerson M, Girard P: Salvage, with arthrodesis, in intractable diabetic neuropathic arthropathy of the foot and ankle. *J Bone Joint Surg* 1993;75A:1056–1066.

This is a retrospective review of the salvage of unbraceable diabetic neuroarthropathic deformities with arthrodesis. The authors review their indications, technique, and outcome.

Smith DG, Stuck RM, Ketner L, et al: Partial calcanectomy for the treatment of large ulcerations of the heel and calcaneal osteomyelitis: An amputation of the back of the foot. *J Bone Joint Surg* 1992;74A:571–576.

Twelve patients with large heel ulcers were managed with partial calcanectomy. The wound went on to heal in 10 of 12 patients. Patients who were mobile before their operation maintained their level of mobility.

Classic Bibliography

Hallux Valgus

Mann RA: Disorders of the first metatarsophalangeal joint. *J Am Acad Orthop Surg* 1995;3:34–43.

Saltzman CL, Brandser EA, Berbaum KS, et al: Reliability of standard foot radiographic measurements. *Foot Ankle Int* 1994;15:661–665.

Thomas RL, Espinosa FJ, Richardson EG: Radiographic changes in the first metatarsal head after distal chevron osteotomy combined with lateral release through a plantar approach. *Foot Ankle Int* 1994;15:285–292.

Shereff MJ, Yang QM, Kummer FJ: Extraosseous and intraosseous arterial supply to the first metarsal and metatarsophalangeal joint. *Foot Ankle Int* 1987;8:81–93.

Hallux Rigidus

Citron N, Neil M: Dorsal wedge osteotomy of the proximal phalanx for hallux rigidus: Long-term results. *J Bone Joint Surg* 1987;69B:835–837.

Holmes GB Jr: Hallux rigidus, in Gould JS (ed): *Operative Foot Surgery.* Philadelphia, PA, WB Saunders, 1994, pp 23–27.

Mann RA, Clanton TO: Hallux rigidus: Treatment by cheilectomy. *J Bone Joint Surg* 1988;70A:400–406.

Moberg E: A simple operation for hallux rigidus. *Clin Orthop* 1979;142:55–56.

Sesamoid Problems of the Hallux

Anderson RB: Sesamoiditis, in Gould JS (ed): *Operative Foot Surgery.* Philadelphia, PA, WB Saunders, 1994, pp 45–53.

McBryde AM Jr, Anderson RB: Sesamoid foot problems in the athlete. *Clin Sports Med* 1988;7:51–60.

Lesser Toe Deformities

Myerson MS, Shereff MJ: The pathological anatomy of claw and hammer toes. *J Bone Joint Surg* 1989;71A:45–49.

Taylor RG: The treatment of claw toes by multiple transfers of flexor into extensor tendons. *J Bone Joint Surg* 1951;33B:539–542

Intractable Plantar Keratosis

Mann RA: Adult forefoot: Part II. Intractable plantar keratosis, in Murray JA (ed): American Academy of Orthopaedic Surgeons *Instructional Course Lectures XXXIII.* St. Louis, MO, CV Mosby, 1984, pp 287–301.

Bunionette

Coughlin MJ: Etiology and treatment of the bunionette deformity, in Greene WB (ed): *Instructional Course Lectures XXXIX.* Park Ridge, IL, American Academy of Orthopaedic Surgeons, 1990, pp 37–48.

Kitaoka HB, Leventen EO: Medial displacement metatarsal osteotomy for treatment of painful bunionette. *Clin Orthop* 1989;243:172–179.

Toenail and Matrix Problems

Cohen PR, Scher RK: Geriatric nail disorders: Diagnosis and treatment. *J Am Acad Dermatol* 1992;26:521–531.

Heifetz CJ: Ingrown toe-nail: A clinical study. *Am J Surg* 1937;38:298–315.

Thompson TC, Terwilliger C: The terminal Syme operation for ingrown toenail. *Surg Clin North Am* 1951;31:575–584.

Zadik FR: Obliteration of the nail bed of the great toe without shortening the terminal phalanx. *J Bone Joint Surg* 1950;32B:66–67.

Nerve Entrapment Syndromes

Andresen BL, Wertsch JJ, Stewart WA: Anterior tarsal tunnel syndrome. *Arch Phys Med Rehabil* 1992;73: 1112–1117.

Erickson SJ, Quinn SF, Kneeland JB, et al: MR imaging of the tarsal tunnel and related spaces: Normal and abnormal findings with anatomic correlation. *Am J Roentgenol* 1990;155:323–328.

Erickson, SJ, Canale PB, Carrera GF, et al: Interdigital (Morton) neuroma: High-resolution MR imaging with a solenoid coil. *Radiology* 1991;181:833–836.

Greenfield J, Rea J Jr, Ilfeld FW: Morton's interdigital neuroma: Indications for treatment by local injections versus surgery. *Clin Orthop* 1984;185:142–144.

Johnson JE, Johnson KA, Unni KK: Persistent pain after excision of an interdigital neuroma: Results of reoperation. *J Bone Joint Surg* 1988;70A:651–657.

Kerr R, Frey C: MR imaging in tarsal tunnel syndrome. *J Comput Assist Tomogr* 1991;15:280–286.

Zongzhao L, Jiansheng Z, Li Z: Anterior tarsal tunnel syndrome. *J Bone Joint Surg* 1991;73B:470–473.

Pollak RA, Bellacosa RA, Dornbluth NC, et al: Sonographic analysis of Morton's neuroma. *J Foot Surg* 1992;31:534–537.

Takakura Y, Kitada C, Sugimoto K, et al: Tarsal tunnel syndrome: Causes and results of operative treatment. *J Bone Joint Surg* 1991;73B:125–128.

Cavus Foot

Coleman SS, Chesnut WJ: A simple test for hindfoot flexibility in the cavovarus foot. *Clin Orthop* 1977;123:60–62.

Gould N: Surgery in advanced Charcot-Marie-Tooth disease. *Foot Ankle* 1984;4:267–273.

Watanabe RS: Metatarsal osteotomy for the cavus foot. *Clin Orthop* 1990;252:217–230.

Wetmore RS, Drennan JC: Long-term results of triple arthrodesis in Charcot-Marie-Tooth disease. *J Bone Joint Surg* 1989;71A:417–422.

Wilcox PG, Weiner DS: The Akron midtarsal dome osteotmy in the treatment of rigid pes cavus: A preliminary review. *J Pediatr Orthop* 1985;5:333–338.

Wukich DK, Bowen JR: A long-term study of triple arthrodesis for correction of pes cavovarus in Charcot-Marie-Tooth disease. *J Pediatr Orthop* 1989;9:433–437.

Ankle and Subtalar Instability

Broström L, Liljedahl SO, Lindvall N: Sprained ankles: II. Arthrographic diagnosis of recent ligament ruptures. *Acta Chir Scand* 1965;129:485–499.

Conlin FD, Johnson PG, Sinning JE Jr: The etiology and repair of rotary ankle instability. *Foot Ankle* 1989;10:152–155.

Edwards GS Jr, DeLee JC: Ankle diastasis without fracture. *Foot Ankle* 1984;4:305–312.

Harper MC, Keller TS: A radiographic evaluation of the tibiofibular syndesmosis. *Foot Ankle* 1989;10:156–160.

Heilman AE, Braly WG, Bishop JO, et al: An anatomic study of subtalar instability. *Foot Ankle* 1990;10:224–228.

Hopkinson WJ, St. Pierre P, Ryan JB, et al: Syndesmosis sprains of the ankle. *Foot Ankle* 1990;10:325–330.

Kannus P, Renström P: Treatment for acute tears of the lateral ligaments of the ankle: Operation, cast, or early controlled mobilization. *J Bone Joint Surg* 1991;73A:305–312.

Karlsson J, Andreasson GO: The effect of external ankle support in chronic lateral ankle joint instability: An electromyographic study. *Am J Sports Med* 1992;20:257–261.

Karlsson J, Bergsten T, Lansinger O, et al: Reconstruction of the lateral ligaments of the ankle for chronic lateral instability. *J Bone Joint Surg* 1988;70A;581–588.

Schon LC, Clanton TO, Baxter DE: Reconstruction for subtalar instability: A review. *Foot Ankle* 1991;11:319–325.

Stormont DM, Morrey BF, An KN, et al: Stability of the loaded ankle: Relation between articular restraint and primary and secondary static restraints. *Am J Sports Med* 1985;13:295–300.

Compartment Syndrome of the Foot

Heckman MM, Grewe SR, Whitesides TE Jr: Compartment syndrome of the foot, in Gould JS (ed): *Operative Foot Surgery.* Philadelphia, PA, WB Saunders, 1994, pp 568–578.

Myerson M, Manoli A: Compartment syndromes of the foot after calcaneal fractures. *Clin Orthop* 1993;290:142–150.

Reflex Sympathetic Dystrophy

Genant HK, Kozin F, Bekerman C, et al: The reflex sympathetic dystrophy syndrome: A comprehensive analysis using fine-detail radiography, photon absorptiometry, and bone and joint scintigraphy. *Radiology* 1975;117:21–32.

Holder LE, Cole LA, Myerson MS: Reflex sympathetic dystrophy in the foot: Clinical and scintigraphic criteria. *Radiology* 1992;184:531–535.

Irazuzta JE, Berde CB, Sethna NF: Laser Doppler measurements of skin blood flow before, during, and after lumbar sympathetic blockade in children and young adults with reflex sympathetic dystrophy syndrome. *J Clin Monit* 1992;8:16–19.

Jadad AR, Carroll D, Glynn CJ, et al: Morphine responsiveness of chronic pain: Double-blind randomised crossover study with patient-controlled analgesia. *Lancet* 1992;339:1367–1371.

Wahren LK, Torebjörk E: Quantitative sensory tests in patients with neuralgia 11 to 25 years after injury. *Pain* 1992;48:237–244.

Wilder RT, Berde CB, Wolohan M, et al: Reflex sympathetic dystrophy in children: Clinical characteristics and follow-up of seventy patients. *J Bone Joint Surg* 1992;74A:910–919.

Foot and Ankle Tumors

Barnes BC, Seigler HF, Saxby TS, et al: Melanoma of the foot. *J Bone Joint Surg* 1994;76A:892–898.

Casadei R, Ferraro A, Ferruzzi A, et al: Bone tumors of the foot: Epidemiology and diagnosis. *Chir Organi Mov* 1991;76:47–62.

Ferreira MC, Besteiro JM, Monteiro AA Jr, et al: Reconstruction of the foot with microvascular free flaps. *Microsurgery* 1994;1:33–36.

Kirby EJ, Shereff MJ, Lewis MM: Soft tissue tumors and tumor like lesions of the foot: An analysis of eighty-three cases. *J Bone Joint Surg* 1989;71A:621–626.

Lee TH, Wapner KL, Heckt PJ: Plantar fibromatosis. *J Bone Joint Surg* 1993;75A:1080–1084.

Lucas DR, Nascimento AG, Sim FH: Clear cell sarcoma of soft tissues: Mayo Clinic experience with 35 cases. *Am J Surg Pathol* 1992;16:1197–1204.

Sara AS, Evans HL, Benjamin RS: Malignant melanoma of soft parts (clear cell sarcoma): A study of 17 cases, with emphasis on prognostic factors. *Cancer* 1990;65:367–374.

Saida T, Ishihara Y, Tokuda Y: Effective detection of plantar malignant melanoma. *Int J Dermatol* 1993;32:722–725.

Selch MT, Kopald KH, Ferreiro GA, et al: Limb salvage therapy for soft tissue sarcomas of the foot. *Int J Radiat Oncol Biol Phys* 1990;19:41–48.

V

Spine

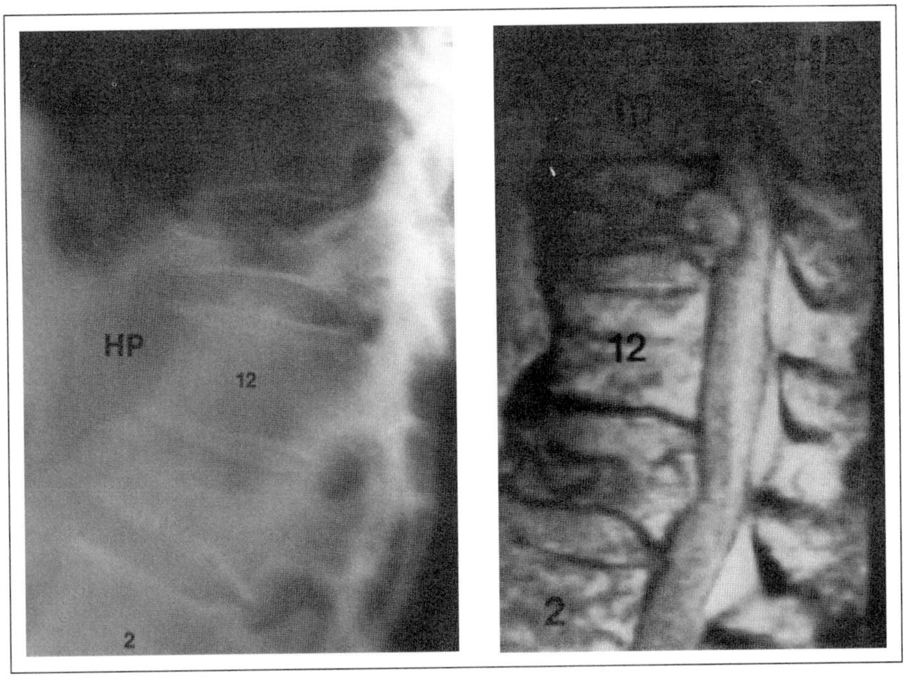

45

Pediatric Spine

Pediatric Spinal Deformity

Congenital Scoliosis

Congenital scoliosis is a developmental curvature of the spine caused by vertebral anomalies that develop in the embryonic period. Although present at birth, clinical deformity may only become evident with growth. The true incidence of congenital scoliosis in the general population is unknown because some vertebral anomalies are well balanced and produce so little deformity that they are never identified. Congenital scoliosis has been categorized on an etiologic basis: defects in segmentation, including block vertebrae, unilateral bar, and unilateral bar with hemivertebrae; defects in formation, including hemivertebra (fully, semi-, and nonsegmented hemivertebra), incarcerated hemivertebra, and wedge vertebra; mixed; and unclassifiable. Because the neural axis and the vertebral column develop concomitantly, there is a risk for spinal cord abnormalities in patients with congenital scoliosis (Fig. 1).

Unilateral unsegmented bar is one of the most common etiologies of congenital scoliosis. The unsegmented bar prevents growth on one side of the vertebral column. As the vertebral bodies on the contralateral side elongate, the bar is incorporated into the concavity of the curve. The unilateral bar with contralateral hemivertebrae must be recognized because the combination leads to the most severe and rapidly progressive of all types of congenital scoliosis. The block vertebra is the result of bilateral failure of segmentation. Depending on the magnitude of angulation of the end plates, its presence may be relatively inconsequential. In failure of segmentation, the bar on the concavity will not produce growth should a contralateral hemiepiphysiodesis be performed. Anterior spinal fusion should be done as soon as the anomaly is recognized; this may be combined with posterior fusion if indicated.

The hemivertebra is a failure of formation in which one of the complements of the sclerotomal tissue, which combine centrally to form the vertebral body, fails to develop normally. Hence, this vertebral level will demonstrate a single pedicle, a wedged vertebra, and a fraction of a lamina. The most common hemivertebra is a fully segmented nonincarcerated vertebra (lateralized, not in full alignment with the spine). The semisegmented vertebra is the next most common, and the nonsegmented or incarcerated vertebra is the least common.

Curve progression parallels the frequency of presentation of the hemivertebrae. Because the fully segmented hemivertebra has an open disk both above and below, there is greater potential for growth, producing angular deformity with age. The semisegmented hemivertebra has a single angled growth plate and tends to progress less rapidly, with curves usually not exceeding 40° at skeletal maturity. Treatment generally is not required. The exception occurs when the semisegmented hemivertebra is at the lumbosacral junction, because the lumbar spine attaches at an oblique angle, causing a more cephalad secondary compensatory curve, which will later become fixed. Nonsegmented hemivertebrae tend not to progress and, in general, are only observed. The incarcerated hemivertebra may result in a slowly progressive scoliosis, which warrants observation.

Three options exist for management of fully segmented hemivertebrae. Anterior and posterior spinal fusion alone may be done to control progression of the spinal deformity. The second option includes hemiepiphysiodesis, in which one third to one half of the vertebral end plates are removed along the convexity of the curve anteriorly and fusion performed. A similar procedure is performed on the posterior aspect of the spine at the same time. The remaining growth on the concavity may be adequate to provide correction of the existing deformity with time. The ideal candidate for a hemiepiphysiodesis is a patient younger than 5 years of age with a short curve of less than 70°. The curve should involve five or fewer segments, with no significant kyphotic deformity.

The third option is hemivertebra excision. This is the procedure of choice for a lumbar hemivertebra, particularly at the L5 level, due to its significant potential for truncal imbalance. The best long-term results following resection of hemivertebrae are achieved if the scoliosis can be nearly completely corrected. Once secondary structural differences are fixed, compensatory curves have developed. Correction by hemivertebrectomy at this time may leave the spine in a decompensated state. Consideration should be made for anterior and posterior hemiepiphysiodeses on the convexity of the curve one level above and below the level of the hemivertebrectomy. With growth, some correction of the spinal deformity may occur.

Although posterior spinal fusion alone can be used in management of congenital scoliosis, it may not be adequate to control progression of the anterior curve. It is often best to perform combined anterior and posterior spinal fusion in the presence of severe growth imbalance. Before undertaking surgical correction of congenital scoliosis, magnetic resonance imaging (MRI) or myelography should be performed to see if there are any associated intraspinal anomalies. Should an anomaly, such as diastematomyelia, be discovered, it should be resected before correction of the scoliotic curve.

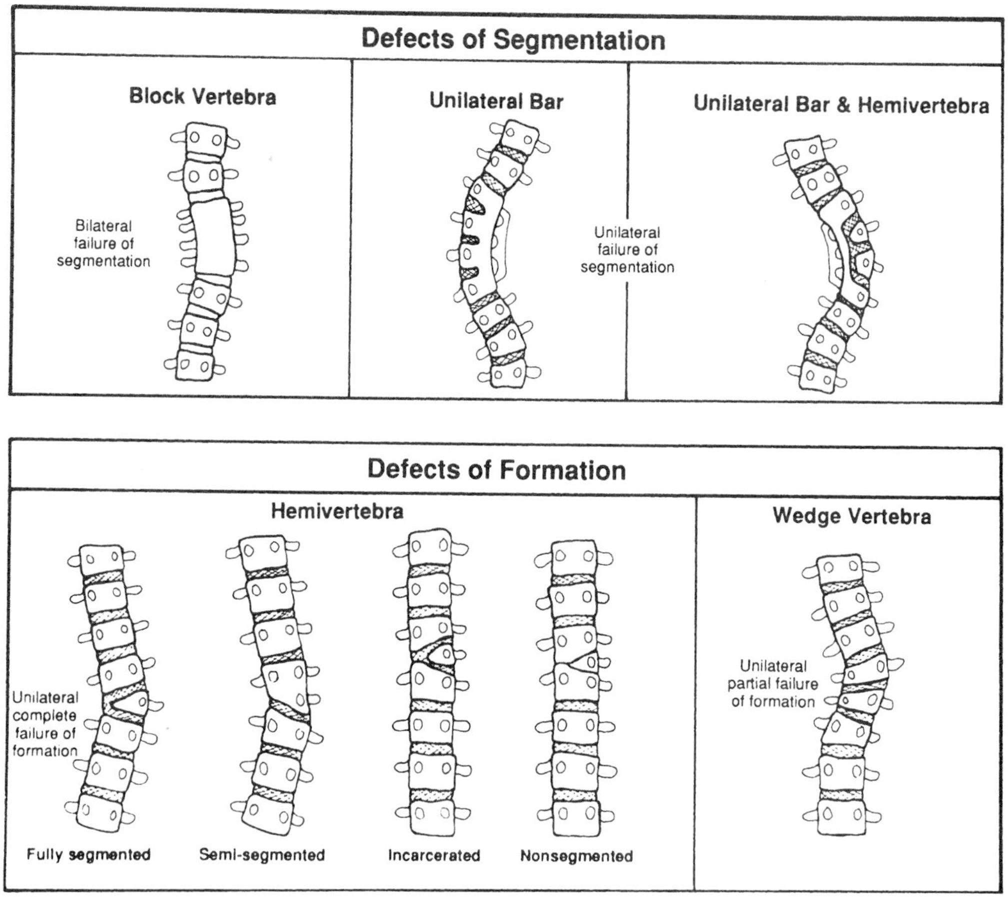

Fig. 1 Congenital scoliosis: A unilateral bar with hemivertebra carries the highest risk of rapid progression. The fully segmented nonincarcerated hemivertebra grows from both the cephalad and caudal growth centers causing progressive scoliosis. The nonsegmented hemivertebra may not be apparent clinically. (Reproduced with permission from McMaster MJ: Congenital scoliosis, in Weinstein SL (ed): *The Pediatric Spine: Principles and Practice.* New York, NY, Raven Press, 1994, pp 227–258.)

Adolescent Idiopathic Scoliosis

Etiology Despite extensive research, the true etiology of adolescent idiopathic scoliosis remains obscure. There are hereditary patterns of idiopathic scoliosis that have been confirmed in the study of mono and dizygotic twins. Affected siblings of patients with idiopathic scoliosis have been seen in approximately 7% of families, and parental scoliosis has been seen in 6% to 14% of the families. A discrete gene as well as mode of inheritance is yet to be identified.

Another factor under consideration is growth, because it is necessary for the development of structural scoliosis. Studies in the 1970s confirmed taller stature in adolescent idiopathic scoliotic patients when compared with healthy nonscoliotic controls. In conjunction with growth, hormonal influence has been studied. An increased sensitivity to growth hormone stimulation testing has been noted in the scoliotic population. Analysis of the connective tissue in scoliotic patients has yet to conclusively shed light on the cause. Analysis of the intervertebral disks has yielded a 25% increase in collagen content with concomitant decrease in glycosaminoglycans in the scoliotic population relative to age-matched controls. Also, analysis of interspinous ligaments in the scoliotic population has yielded a decreased density of fibralin fibers as well as qualitative differences in fiber function in in vitro cultures.

Brain stem function and postural reflexes have also been implicated in the etiology of adolescent idiopathic scoliosis. Equilibrium dysfunction as demonstrated by changes in proprioceptive reflexes as well as in the optic reflex system has been documented. Also, spontaneous and positional nystagmus have been observed in 50% of scoliotic persons, compared with 3% of controls. Multiple tests using vibration sensitivity as an assessment of posterior column function have demonstrated decreased sensitivity in the scoliotic patients compared with normal controls. Many of these observations have been contradicted by studies in other centers, thus their importance remains uncertain.

Prevalence Scoliosis is defined as lateral curvature of the spine that exceeds 10° as measured by the Cobb method on standing radiographs. Spinal curvature below this threshold should be referred to as spinal asymmetry. With a Cobb angle of 10° as the lower threshold for the diagnosis of adolescent idiopathic scoliosis, there is a prevalence of approximately 25 per 1,000 in the population. Increasing the threshold reduces the prevalence. The prevalence drops to approximately three to five per 1,000 for curves > 20° and to one to three per 1,000 for angles > 30°. Curves > 40° have a prevalence of less than one per 1,000. The female to male ratio for the group of curves > 10° reveals a 1.4 to 2 to 1 ratio of females to males. The female to male ratio increases to 5.4 to 1 for curves > 20° and to 10 to 1 for curves > 30°.

Screening Widespread school screening of adolescents has been advocated in the diagnosis and management of scoliosis. Simple methods of screening are available. The most basic method is visual observation, including standing posture and forward bending from the front, back, and side to evaluate for trunk asymmetry. Other methods, such as Moire topography (a photographic technique to analyze and quantify spinal asymmetry), although they have potential, are impractical for widespread usage.

A more practical method of documenting trunk rotation in forward bend is by use of an inclinometer to assess the angular prominence of the ribs at the upper and middle thoracic regions, as well as the lumbar region. The referral rate varies, depending on the threshold of trunk rotation used. With a 5°-referral criterion, up to 12% of students might be sent for further evaluation. This number is reduced to 6% for 6° of trunk rotation and to 3% for 7° of trunk rotation. The cost of underreferral is the false negative of missing a patient with scoliosis. When a 5° angle is used for referral, only 2% of 20° curves are missed. With a 6° threshold, 6% of 20° curves will be missed, and with a 7° threshold, 12% of 20° curves may be missed. The 7° threshold is an acceptable compromise between over-referral and a high false-negative rate.

The cost to society of scoliosis is significant. The estimate for allowing the disease to progress along its natural history and performing only late fusions has been estimated at $186 million to perform 4,800 fusions in the United States. The cost of a screening program and the resultant medical treatment was estimated to be nearly $220 million, resulting from evaluation of 144,000 patients who received 1.6 million office visits, nearly 1 million radiographs, 14,000 braces, and 1,400 spinal fusions. The approximate cost per student referral is $1,500, with each additional 1% of students referred adding $74 million to the total annual cost.

Natural History The management of any disease should be based on the effectiveness of treatment instituted relative to the natural history of the disease left untreated. The natural history of idiopathic scoliosis has been studied at multiple centers. If a child has a thoracic curve of 19° or less with a Risser sign of 0 or 1, the chance for progression is 22%. For a child with a curve of 19° or less with a Risser sign of 2, 3, or 4, it is only 1.6%. If a child has a Risser sign of 0 or 1 with a curve of 20° to 29°, the chance of progression is 68%; but if the Risser sign is 2, 3, or 4, it is only 22%.

Studies have been performed to identify factors that can be used to predict a patient's chance of progression as well as to plan treatment. Nonpredictive factors include family history, thoracic kyphosis, lumbar lordosis, lumbosacral transitional anomalies, and trunk imbalance. Predictive factors include sex (female versus male), growth potential (which can be assessed as the onset of menses), the Risser sign, and the age at diagnosis. Vertebral rotation and trunk rotation have not yet been documented as predictive factors but are probably predictive. In one study of the progression of untreated scoliosis, progression was defined as an initial curve of 19° or less that increased at least 10°, or an initial curve between 20° and 29° that increased by 5° or more. These measurements are based on the Cobb angle, which has been shown to have an interobserver reproducibility of approximately 5° to 7°. It has been demonstrated recently that the Cobb angle obtained on radiographs can be related to the time of day the film was taken, because the curves tend to progress when comparing morning with evening films. The average increase was 5°, but was as high as 10° to 20° in some cases. Use of the Risser sign as a predictor of remaining growth has also been challenged because of the significant variation in skeletal age as compared with the Risser sign in any one patient. This variation leads to significant overlap of skeletal age with Risser categorization. Although these challenges have been raised, the Risser sign continues to be widely used and valued in the evaluation and management of adolescent idiopathic scoliosis. The use of the triradiate cartilage to assess maturation has been suggested.

Clinical Evaluation Evaluation of the patient with idiopathic scoliosis begins with a thorough physical examination with careful attention to the neurologic examination. Thoracic and lumbar prominences on forward bending as viewed from behind are quantitated with an inclinometer. Pelvic obliquity, relative limb lengths, and trunk shift are noted. Initial radiologic evaluation of the scoliotic patient includes a standing posteroanterior (PA) spine film with lateral views if abnormalities are suspected. Only when surgical correction is planned are best bending films to the left and right required to assess curve flexibility. An MRI study is indicated for selected cases, including patients with structural abnormalities found on plain films, with excessive kyphosis on plain film evaluation, with early onset scoliosis, with rapid progression of curve magnitude, with neurologic symptoms or signs, with associated syndromes, and with apex left thoracic or thoracolumbar curves. In this selected population, MRI demonstrated abnormalities in 37% of cases studied. Patients at risk for progression of scoliosis require follow-up radiographic studies. Because the body's absorbed radiation dose is cumulative over the life of the patient, measures should be taken to minimize exposure of the more sensitive tissues to radiation. These include the breast, thyroid, and bone marrow. Such dose-limiting measures include use of PA rather than anteroposterior exposures, high-speed film screen combinations, tube head filters, and beam collimation.

Nonsurgical Management Multiple methods have been used in the nonsurgical management of scoliosis. Exercise programs have not been shown to affect the natural history of the disease. Exercise is encouraged in scoliosis patients to minimize any potential decrease in functional ability over time. However, it is designed to maintain the overall level of fitness and oxygen capacity, not to alter the patient's curve magnitude. In multiple studies of patients treated with various modes of electrical stimulation, researchers have been unable to demonstrate a difference in the experimental group relative to the natural history.

Bracing has been shown to be effective in correctly selected patients. No indication currently exists for bracing curves of 20° (Cobb) or less. Curves that fall between 20° and 29° should be braced in patients who are Risser 0 to 1 and premenarchal. For patients who are Risser 2 to 4 and have a 20° to 29° curve, curve progression of 5° or more should be documented before bracing. For patients with curves in the 30° to 39° range, bracing should be initiated at the first visit if growth remains. If the patient is Risser 4 to 5, bracing is not indicated.

The brace should be designed to fit the patient's specific curve. For patients with a curve apex at the level of T8 or lower, an underarm brace such as the Wilmington or Boston type brace, is appropriate. For patients with curve apex at the level of T7 or higher, either a Milwaukee brace or a Boston underarm brace with a Milwaukee superstructure to control the upper portion of the curve is required. The appropriateness of full-time bracing versus part-time bracing is currently being debated. Advocates of part-time bracing claim that they advise only 16 hour/day wear because patients instructed to wear the brace full time wear it for only 16 hours a day. Unfortunately, patients instructed to wear the brace 16 hours a day often wear the brace only 8 to 9 hours a day. Part-time bracing advocates claim results equal to those for full-time bracing. However, this has not been proven in large, long-term prospective evaluations. The efficacy of full-time bracing has been well demonstrated. Recent studies have concluded that the effectiveness of a brace in idiopathic scoliosis is dose-related (the more the brace is worn each day, the more effective it is).

The brace wear does carry the potential for psychological impact on the child as well as the family. Adolescence is a stressful time in a normal patient's life, let alone in the life of one subjected to bracing in front of his or her peers. While no psychopathology has been attributable to bracing, psychosocial stress is clearly an issue to be considered. Brace wear is continued until skeletal maturity as determined by the Risser sign. Once the patient has stopped growing, the brace is weaned over a 6- to 9-month period.

Surgical Treatment Surgical management of idiopathic scoliosis includes many options, the most widely accepted and standard of which is posterior spinal instrumentation with fusion. There are indications for anterior spinal diskectomy with fusion and instrumentation for lumbar and thoracolumbar curves. The traditional standard for posterior instrumentation has been the Harrington rod system that corrects by simple distraction. More recently designed instrumentation methods include multisegmental hook systems, which provide multiple points of fixation to the spine, allowing compression, rotation, and distraction along the same rod. These systems theoretically allow derotation of the spine in the transverse planes, thereby allowing maintenance of the normal sagittal contours of kyphosis and lordosis of the spine (Fig. 2). This instrumentation has been demonstrated to correct the coronal curve an average of 48%, improve apical translation an average of 60%, and improve vertebral body rotation 11% while maintaining the normal sagittal contour of the spine. Pulmonary parameters improved an average of 20% following such instrumentation.

Regardless of the instrumentation system chosen, the goals are correction of the curve in the sagittal and coronal planes, decrease of the rotation of the vertebral bodies, and fusion of as few segments as possible to allow maximal normal motion. The levels of fusion to be performed are more critical than the instrumentation system chosen. In preoperative planning for scoliosis correction, the King-Moe classification (Fig. 3) proves useful. In the double major King-Moe type I curve the lumbar curve is greater and less flexible than the thoracic curve. The scoliosis can be corrected by isolated posterior instrumentation, although this procedure requires fusion of both the lumbar and thoracic regions. Anterior diskectomy with interbody fusion and anterior instrumentation may allow fusion of only the lumbar curve, with the compensatory thoracic curve decreasing over time. Care must be taken to not create lumbar kyphosis with anterior instrumentation. Use of rib, iliac crest, or allograft as structural intrabody support helps to prevent excessive kyphosis during anterior instrumentation.

In the King-Moe type II curve, the thoracic curve is more severe and less flexible than the lumbar curve, requiring fusion down to the most cephalad stable vertebra of the thoracic curve. In cases with severe lumbar curves (more than 50°), the lumbar curve may also need to be fused. Types III (thoracic) and IV (long thoracolumbar curves) are usually treated by posterior instrumentation and fusion to the stable vertebra caudally. The shorter curves are again amenable to anterior diskectomy with instrumentation and fusion. This procedure allows fusion of

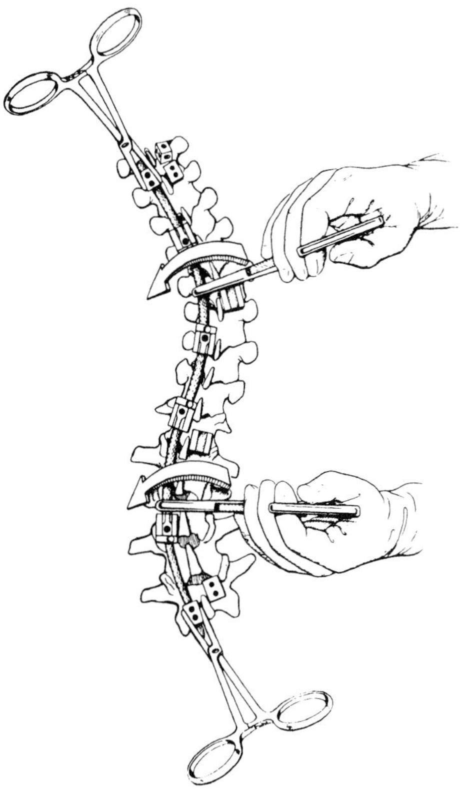

Fig. 2 Spinal instrumentation: Example of the derotation maneuver for idiopathic scoliosis performed with a posterior segmental instrumentation system. The rod is contoured to match the scoliosis, then rotated 90° to provide thoracic kyphosis and lumbar lordosis. (Reproduced with permission from Denis F: Cotrel-Dubousset instrumentation in the treatment of idiopathic scoliosis. *Orthop Clin North Am* 1988;19:291–311.)

fewer levels than would be possible with posterior instrumentation.

The King-Moe type V double thoracic curve requires careful evaluation. The preoperative examination as well as evaluation of the flexibility of the curves on the best bending films are key. If the left shoulder is elevated on presentation or a left trapezius prominence is observed, then the high left curve must be included in the posterior fusion because correction of the right thoracic curve will push the left shoulder into greater elevation. If the patient demonstrates balanced shoulders with a rigid right thoracic curve and a flexible left cervicothoracic curve, then the surgeon may safely fuse the right thoracic curve only. If, however, the patient presents in a balanced state with an upper cervicothoracic curve that is rigid and a more flexible lower right thoracic curve, caution must be taken in that correction of only the right thoracic curve will lead to an unbalanced result with left shoulder elevation. Hence, the high left curve and the right thoracic curve must be incorporated into the fusion. The lumbar curve is not incorporated into the fusion in the King-Moe type V patient because it is a compensatory curve and should partially resolve, following correction of the thoracic curves. The dogma of never ending a fusion at the thoracolumbar junction is unjustified with modern instrumentation systems, and ending a fusion at T11 or T12 is certainly acceptable to preserve motion segments. Also, in all curve types to be treated with posterior corrective instrumentation, the preoperative lateral spine films are evaluated to determine areas of junctional kyphosis, which occur at the upper and lower ends of the frontal plane curve. The levels selected for instrumentation should correct rather than exacerbate this junctional kyphosis.

Spinal cord monitoring during the correction of idiopathic scoliosis is strongly advocated. Cord monitoring most frequently involves the use of somatosensory- and, if available, motor-evoked potentials. If such monitoring is unavailable, the intraoperative Stagnara wake-up test serves as an acceptable substitute. In this test, anesthesia is lightened, and the patient asked to move the lower extremities after spinal correction has been obtained.

Monitoring of somatosensory-evoked potentials (SSEPs) limits the use of halogenated anesthetic agents, which interfere with the monitoring. The SSEPs have been described as sensitive but not specific. The amplitude and latency of the signals are monitored periodically throughout the corrective surgery. Should alterations be encountered, it is prudent to determine at what stage during the procedure this may have occurred and to take corrective action. If alterations occur after installation of the instrumentation with correction of the spinal curve, removal of the instrumentation and re-implantation with a less ambitious correction may be necessary to avoid postoperative neurologic deficit. The false-positive rate with SSEPs is between 10% and 20%. False negatives, ie, normal monitoring throughout surgery followed by postoperative neurologic deficit, are extremely rare but have been reported. One reported deficit was a motor deficit, which is not monitored intraoperatively by the SSEPs. More recently brain stem-evoked potentials have been advocated for routine use because they are not affected by the halogenated anesthetic agents and because SSEPs can be difficult to obtain in patients with a brain injury or cerebral palsy. Brain stem-evoked potentials may be the monitoring treatment of choice in patients with neuromuscular disorders. The monitoring SSEPs have also been shown to be quite sensitive to temperature changes. A drop in core temperature of 1° to 2°C can cause a significant diminution in the amplitude and latency being monitored.

Complications of Surgical Correction Spinal decompensation may occur secondary to improper selection of levels for instrumentation and fusion. This problem is common with use of modern modular corrective instrumentation methods that have great power for correction.

The "crankshaft phenomenon" may occur in the setting of posterior spinal fusion in the skeletally immature child.

The posterior spinal fusion acts as a tether while anterior vertebral body growth continues. With the posterior tether, the anterior growth results in potentially marked increased rotation of the vertebral bodies. To avoid this phenomenon, anterior diskectomy with intrabody fusion should be added to posterior spinal fusion in the immature patient with significant growth remaining, (ie, Risser grade 0 to 1 patients who are girls younger than 11 and boys younger than 13) who has progressive scoliosis in excess of 50°.

Neurologic deficit may follow instrumented correction. SSEPs can be used during surgery to monitor for the occurrence of a neurologic injury. If SSEPs change during surgery, attention should be paid to the relevant stage of the procedure and corrective measures taken as appropriate. The risk of neurologic complication has been estimated by the Scoliosis Research Society to be 0.72% in posterior spinal fusions.

Rib prominence may persist following surgical correction. Harrington rod distraction correction does not address the rotational component of scoliosis; therefore, the rib prominences are not diminished. Use of derotation systems does allow partial correction of rotational deformity of the thoracolumbar spine; however, correction is not complete. Partial thoracoplasty has been advocated in the instance of more significant curves. This group includes patients with a rib prominence angle greater than 15°, curve severity in excess of 60°, flexibility less than 20%, and postoperative correction less than 50% on intraoperative films. The ribs harvested for the thoracoplasty often are adequate to provide the autogenous bone graft necessary for posterior spinal instrumentation and fusion.

Infantile and Juvenile Idiopathic Scoliosis

Infantile scoliosis occurs between birth and 3 years of age. Juvenile scoliosis occurs between the ages of 4 and 10 years. Although this is the classic definition, an alternative grouping has been suggested for juvenile scoliosis, with early onset from 0 to 5 years of age and late onset from 5 to 10 years of age. This distinction is made because the large thoracic deformity that is typical in curves with onset prior to age 5 years will lead to certain cardiopulmonary compromise. Pulmonary function diminishes in curves in excess of 60° with cor pulmonale occurring in severe curves. The onset of scoliosis beyond age 5 years appears to carry a decreased risk of subsequent cardiopulmonary compromise.

The etiology of infantile idiopathic scoliosis is unclear. It may be due to injury during prenatal molding or, alternatively, due to postnatal pressure. In this theory semisupine infants have asymmetric pressure on the chest wall, which induces a curve in the thoracic spine. The incidence is higher in countries where the infant population is kept in a supine or semisupine position when compared with countries where the infants lie prone for sleeping. The rib vertebral angle difference from side to side has been found to be a valuable predictor of curve progression (Fig. 4). When this difference exceeds 20° in the early onset idiopathic scoliosis population, the risk of progression is high. This value decreases to a 10° threshold for progression in the late onset idiopathic scoliosis group.

Another difference between the early and late onset groups is the curve pattern. Approximately three fourths of the thoracic curves in the early onset group are convex

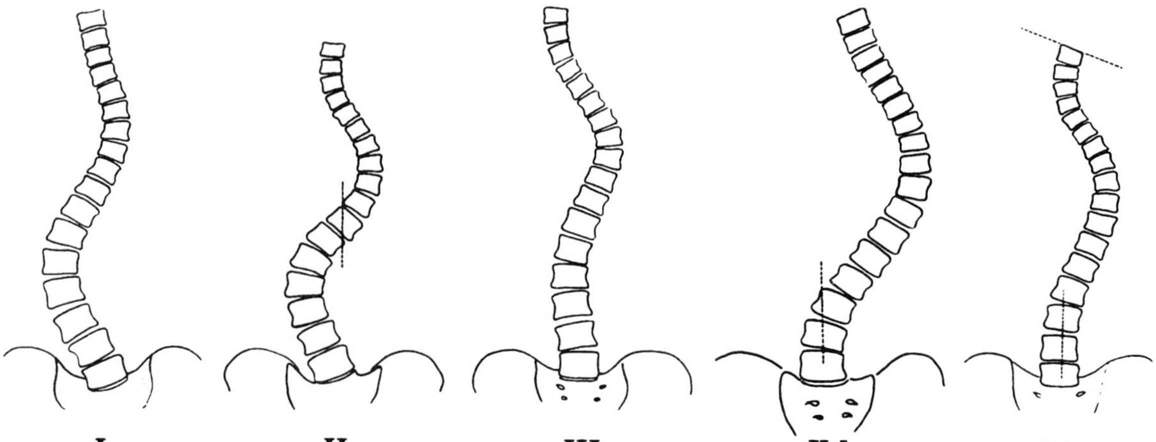

I II III IV V

Fig. 3 King-Moe classification system for idiopathic scoliosis: type I, primary lumbar curve greater than the compensatory thoracic curve; type II, primary thoracic curve with compensatory lumbar curve; type III, short pure thoracic curve; type IV, long C-shaped thoracolumbar curve; type V, double thoracic curve with extension into cervical spine and compensatory lumbar curve. (Adapted with permission from King HA, Moe JH, Bradford DS, et al: The selection of fusion levels in thoracic idiopathic scoliosis. *J Bone Joint Surg* 1983;65A:1302–1313.)

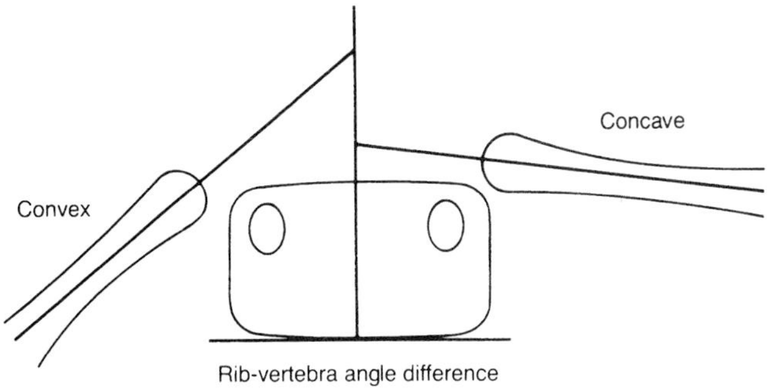

Fig. 4 The rib-vertebra angle difference (RVAD) is calculated by subtracting the angle of the rib on the convex side of the curve relative to a line perpendicular to the vertebral body end plate from the angle on the concave side of the curve. (Reproduced with permission from Koop SE: Infantile and juvenile idiopathic scoliosis. *Orthop Clin North Am* 1988;19:331–337.)

to the left. Females with right-sided thoracic curves appear to have a worse prognosis. Curves in the late onset scoliosis group are most frequently thoracic followed by double thoracic, thoracolumbar, and lumbar. Recent studies have suggested that children with scoliosis onset before the age of 9 to 10 years should routinely have an MRI study. All patients with neurologic findings must undergo MRI imaging to evaluate the spinal cord prior to intervention.

Management of the early onset idiopathic scoliotic patient can begin with careful elongation derotation flexion cast application. The earlier the age at which casting is commenced, the better the outcome. Casting can be continued up to approximately age 4 to 5 years. Beyond 5 years, observation three times a year without casting should be routine. In those patients whose curve progresses relentlessly despite proper casting and/or bracing management, surgical intervention is justified. Anterior and posterior spinal surgery in this instance is mandatory. Anteriorly, the growth plates can be excised completely over the four to five apical segments only. A posterior procedure is then performed in which an "expandable" instrumentation system is used without fusion. Repeat distraction can be performed every year thereafter.

The late onset or juvenile idiopathic scoliosis population is made up primarily of females with right thoracic curves. Approximately 70% of the curves in patients with late onset juvenile idiopathic scoliosis require some form of treatment; approximately one half require bracing and one half surgical intervention.

Management of the patient with juvenile idiopathic scoliosis begins with evaluation and assessment of the curve. Should intervention be required, bracing is the first step, with the Milwaukee thoracolumbar spinal orthosis (TLSO) brace the generally preferred method. Some report excellent prognosis with part-time bracing for curves less than 35° and rib vertebral angle differences less than 20°. Patients with curves of more than 45° or rib vertebral angle difference of more than 20° have a poorer prognosis for the success of brace treatment. Curve progression despite bracing does not necessitate immediate surgical intervention. Continuation of a well-applied brace may slow the progression of the curve, thereby allowing additional spinal growth prior to performing the fusion procedure. Surgery may be delayed until the curve attains a magnitude of 55° to 60°. Combined anterior and posterior fusion is appropriate to reduce the occurrence of the crankshaft phenomenon. The surgeon must use clinical judgment to determine the estimated anterior growth remaining when considering an anterior combined with posterior procedure. An additional temporizing measure is instrumentation posteriorly without fusion. A subcutaneous Harrington rod (Moe rod) can be inserted with distraction applied. As the patient grows, repeat surgery is required to further distract the spine and maintain correction. The newer instrumentation systems have now been modified to allow a more sophisticated variation of the Moe rod concept. The patient must be braced full time while the growth rod is in place to prevent hook and rod dislodgment. Once the patient has attained adequate growth, a formal posterior fusion is performed with instrumentation.

Neuromuscular Scoliosis

Cerebral Palsy Scoliosis is the most common spinal deformity in cerebral palsy (CP) and is ten to 15 times more prevalent in patients with spastic quadriplegia than in those with spastic diplegia. Progression of the scoliosis is variable because the onset of puberty in these patients may occur early or may not occur until the twenties. In addition, scoliosis seen in CP may show progression even into adulthood.

Treatment depends on the severity of the curve. Small curves with no loss of function or larger curves in severely involved patients may require observation alone. Seating support is used for nonambulatory patients. A TLSO may be beneficial in ambulatory patients in whom response to brace treatment is similar to that in idiopathic scoliosis. Bracing may not have a long-term corrective effect.

Surgical indications include curves over 45° to 50°, documented progression of > 10°, or a deterioration of function. Curve patterns in CP have been divided into two types. Group I curves are double thoracic curves with thoracic and lumbar components and little pelvic obliquity. Fusion criteria in ambulatory group I patients are the same as those in idiopathic scoliosis. In group II, there are large lumbar or thoracolumbar curves with marked pelvic obliquity. In these patients fusion should be continued to the pelvis. Even for group I patients who are sitters, fusion should probably be continued to the pelvis. The upper extent of fusion should be T2 to prevent focal kyphosis with upper spine fall-off, which is seen when fusion is stopped in the midthoracic region. Combined anterior and poste-

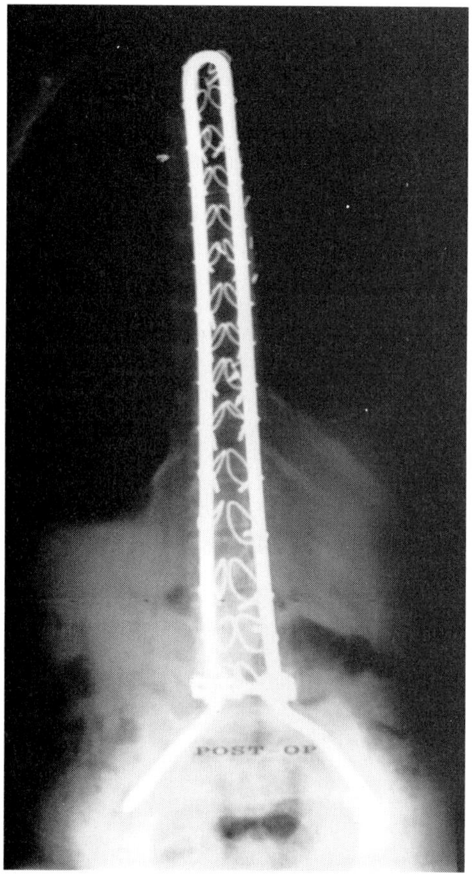

Fig. 5 Radiograph of a 13-year-old boy with cerebral palsy: Luque-Galveston instrumentation and fusion to the sacro-pelvis because of curve severity.

rior fusion is often required for group II curves, particularly in the skeletally immature patient. Posterior fusion alone is often adequate for group I curves.

Luque rods with sublaminar wires and Galveston pelvic fixation (where indicated) are the instrumentation of choice. The "unit rod" concept or Luque rods plus cross-link fixation will provide added stability. Allograft bone is added to autogenous graft to supplement the arthrodesis (Fig. 5).

Although the most common sites for pseudarthrosis are the thoracolumbar and lumbosacral junctions, rates are low with use of Luque segmental instrumentation and Galveston pelvic fixation and anterior fusion when indicated. Preoperative nutritional status is important because malnourished patients have significantly higher infection rates and longer hospitalizations. Patients requiring both anterior and posterior fusions may have fewer complications if both procedures are performed on the same day rather than at 1 to 2 week intervals. The surgeon's skill, speed, and stamina as well as blood loss and other factors determine the wisdom of same day anterior and posterior procedures in neuromuscular scoliosis.

Duchenne and Becker Muscular Dystrophy After age 5, walking gradually becomes more labored for patients with Duchenne muscular dystrophy. These patients usually become wheelchair users by 10 to 12 years of age and subsequently develop a progressive thoracolumbar scoliosis. A relentless progression of spinal deformity and associated decline in pulmonary function contribute directly to early death. Death generally occurs in the late teens or early twenties as a result of cardiopulmonary failure and respiratory infections.

Becker muscular dystrophy is a milder, genetically distinct form of muscular dystrophy, similar to the Duchenne type in clinical symptoms. The onset of symptoms occurs later and the condition is less severe, so the ability to walk often persists into the twenties and beyond. Chromosome analysis as well as the quantity and quality of dystrophin in the muscle can distinguish Duchenne from Becker muscular dystrophy.

The incidence of progressive scoliosis in Duchenne and Becker muscular dystrophy is about 95%. The natural history of these curves is progression to more than 100°. There is an average 10° increase in thoracic scoliosis for each year of life, once the child becomes a wheelchair user. The scoliosis greatly interferes with sitting comfort and proper positioning in the wheelchair, upper-extremity function, caloric ingestion, respiratory function, and cosmesis.

Percent forced vital capacity is the best test for monitoring a Duchenne patient's pulmonary function, which begins to decline rapidly once the patient becomes a wheelchair user (at least 4% a year) and stabilizes around 25% of normal. Tracheostomy and mechanical ventilation are treatment options to be considered in the later stages of the disease.

Braces and spinal support systems slow the rate of progression of the curve but do not halt it. They are not recommended, because further decline in pulmonary function occurs while procrastinating on surgical management of the scoliosis. In countries with adequate economic resources, early surgical correction of scoliosis in muscular dystrophy has become common.

Luque spinal instrumentation and posterior fusion is the treatment of choice once the patients are unable to ambulate. Surgery is indicated to improve quality of life and upright wheelchair positioning. Segmental instrumentation has the advantage of permitting immediate postoperative mobilization without a cast or orthosis. Spinal surgery is performed when the patient's curve reaches 20° and forced vital capacity is still greater than 40%.

It is generally agreed that fusion must be extended into the upper thoracic area so that cephalad progression of the curve due to progressive trunk weakness is avoided. It is also essential to center the patient's head over the midpelvis in both the coronal and sagittal planes so that the

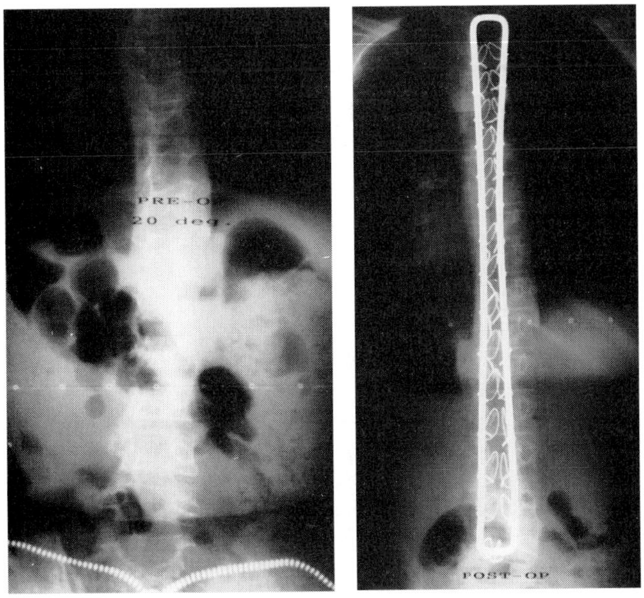

Fig. 6 Twelve-year and 9-month-old boy with Duchenne muscular dystrophy: **Left,** A reoperative sitting anteroposterior radiograph showing a 20° right thoracolumbar curve. **Right,** Posterior spinal fusion and instrumentation from T2 to L5 with Luque box and sublaminar wiring.

upper body weight is prevented from acting as a pendulum, which could lead to loss of head control and extension of the curve cephalad. Because of these concerns, many surgeons have recommended that instrumentation and fusion be carried out to the sacrum to prevent or correct pelvic obliquity. In a controlled study, it has been demonstrated that caudal instrumentation and fusion to L5 are sufficient if treatment is initiated early (Cobb measurement 20 to 30) (Fig. 6). If the preoperative pelvic obliquity is greater than 10° and/or the scoliosis curve greater than 40°, the surgeon should instrument to the pelvis to correct this obliquity and ensure a level pelvis. Use of a unit rod or use of Luque rods plus cross-links will provide additional stability. The intensive-care unit stay is usually 2 days, and the average hospital stay is about 9 days. A lightweight orthoplast body jacket is recommended for 6 months when the patient is upright or being transferred, for both comfort and safety.

Patients with the Becker type have fewer problems, because the scoliosis usually develops after maturity. Once the patient's curve exceeds 30°, treatment is the same as for Duchenne muscular dystrophy. The ultimate goal in the treatment of spinal deformity in muscular dystrophy is the maintenance of upright sitting posture and maximal pain-free function.

Poliomyelitis The incidence of scoliosis in poliomyelitis varies depending on the patient population, with reported ranges from 25% to 68%. The type and severity of the curve depend on the involved musculature. Weakness of the lateral abdominal and quadratus lumborum muscles is felt to be most important in the development of scoliosis, with chest muscle paralysis being responsible for thoracic scoliosis. Double major thoracic-lumbar curves are the most common deformity. Kyphosis in the lumbar spine and lordosis in the thoracic spine are also seen as a result of rotational deformities.

Nonsurgical treatment measures, such as electrical stimulation, brace application, and serial casting, have met with little success in poliomyelitic patients. Luque rod constructs, a combination of Harrington and Luque instrumentation, and modern modular corrective rod systems have been successful in treatment of poliomyelitic scoliosis. For curves less than 60°, posterior instrumentation alone may be sufficient. In curves greater than 60°, combined anterior and posterior surgery with or without anterior instrumentation may be necessary.

Myelomeningocele Spinal deformity in myelomeningocele is so common in high-level patients (L3 and above) that it is rare to see a patient reach adulthood without undergoing spine surgery. Spinal deformities are severe and usually progressive. The most consistent abnormality seen is incomplete posterior arches in the lumbosacral spine. Because central nervous system abnormalities are often the underlying cause, they must be dealt with in association with treatment of the scoliosis. Numerous congenital malformations may be present, including hemivertebrae, diastematomyelia, and unsegmented bars. Infection rates are also very high in this group, secondary to frequent septicemia and poor skin quality over the lumbar spine.

Virtually all patients with thoracic level paraplegia will develop scoliosis, versus approximately 60% with paraplegia at the L4 functional level. Lordosis in the absence of scoliosis most likely results from hip flexion contractures.

Curves $< 20°$ progress slowly, while those $> 40°$ progress quickly, as much as 13° per year. Nonambulatory patients have a higher risk of scoliosis development; thus, regular clinical and radiographic assessments are important in this patient group. Bracing can be used; however, care must be taken to prevent pressure sores and rib cage deformities.

Most patients will eventually require spinal fusion, with the general dictum being to fuse long. Compensatory thoracic curves should be fused because of the high incidence of repeated surgery for progression. The need for fusion to the pelvis is debatable, and pseudarthroses at this level are common due to lack of the posterior vertebral arches. For children with upper lumbar or thoracic levels of paraplegia, fusion should probably be continued to the sacrum. Recent reports on the use of specialized constructs of derotational hook system instrumentation in neuromuscular scoliosis have been promising, but Luque segmental instrumentation and fusion to the sacropelvis is still the standard.

Lumbar kyphosis is seen in 8% to 15% of patients with

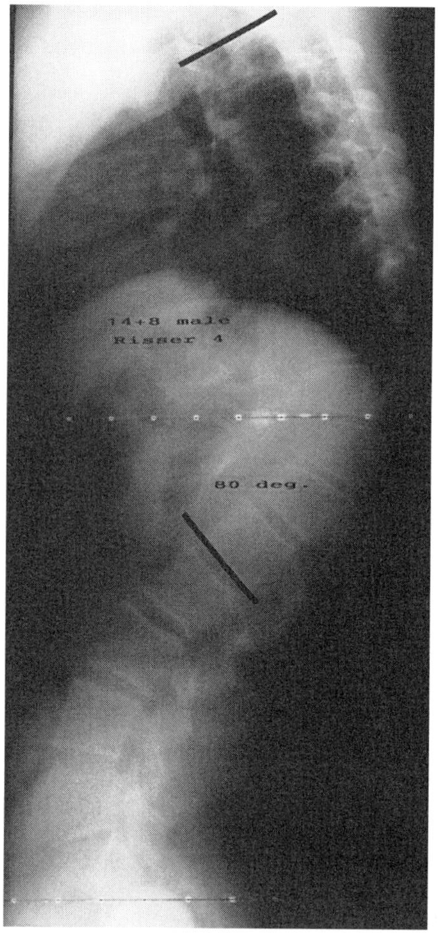

Fig. 7 Radiograph of 14-year and 8-month-old boy, Risser 4, with 80° Scheuermann's kyphosis.

myelomeningocele. It is almost always progressive and can measure up to 80° or more at birth. Brace treatment can be attempted; however, it is usually not successful, with most patients requiring surgical correction. Surgical techniques vary with the age of the patient. Good results have been reported for use of Luque rod instrumentation and various described modifications. A significant decrease in the complication rate was found when Luque instrumentation using a modification of the Dunn technique was compared to traditional Harrington rod instrumentation.

Spinal Muscular Atrophy Scoliosis is the most common spinal deformity found in spinal muscular atrophy. The reported incidence varies from 54% to virtually 100% in patients who survive into adulthood. A major factor associated with the development and progression of scoliosis appears to be the level of retained motor function. Patients with more severe muscle weakness usually present earlier with more involvement, and in one series, only in the ambulatory group of patients were there cases with no spinal involvement. The mean age at onset is reported to be between 5 and 9 years. Patients with the acute infantile form (type I or Werdnig/Hoffmann disease) are more severely affected, and virtually all develop spinal deformities. Kyphosis is frequently associated with scoliosis and usually appears earlier. Scoliosis in spinal muscular atrophy has a typical neuromuscular pattern, with a single large collapsing C-shaped curve involving the thoracolumbar spine. Ninety percent of patients will have single curves, usually right-sided.

Most authors recommend a trial of orthotic use to delay fusion and improve functional performance of the child. Most also recommend posterior spinal fusion in patients with curves between 40° and 60° who are older than age 10 years. The use of Luque instrumentation has been generally successful. The thin iliac bone in these patients usually necessitates the addition of allograft bone. Postoperative immobilization with a TLSO may be required. Complications including rod breakage, failure, painful prominence of the hardware, and pseudarthroses have been reported. Combined anterior and posterior procedures may be necessary for more severe curves, particularly in the skeletally immature patient. Posterior instrumentation should include the entire spine from T2 to the sacrum.

Kyphosis

Scheuermann's Disease The etiology of Scheuermann's disease remains controversial. Theories range from a form of aseptic necrosis of the ring apophysis to a form of osteochondrosis, a form of juvenile osteoporosis, an endocrine abnormality involving growth hormone, and tight hamstring muscles. The incidence of Scheuermann's disease has been reported to be between 0.4% and 8%, predominantly in males. Onset appears to be around age 10 years. Radiographic evidence of Scheuermann's kyphosis has not been demonstrated in patients younger than 10 years.

Two forms have been identified by location. The thoracic Scheuermann's disease is the classic form defined as 5° of wedging of the anterior vertebral body at a minimum of three adjacent vertebral levels (Fig. 7). Associated nonprogressive scoliosis of 10° to 20° is common. The lumbar form of Scheuermann's disease frequently presents as a chronic backache, which is found predominantly in teenage males who perform hard labor or who are very active in sports, and is characterized by irregular vertebral end plates, Schmorl's nodes, and reduction in the disk space height that is not associated with wedging (Fig. 8). Scheuermann's disease may exist in the region of the thoracolumbar junction. In this location it may actually induce a paradox of thoracic lordosis by the presence of extreme kyphosis at the junction level.

Pain is a frequent presenting complaint in the disease. This aspect seems to decrease with skeletal maturation. Occasionally short-term casting or bracing is necessary for relief of pain. Differential diagnosis for Scheuermann's dis-

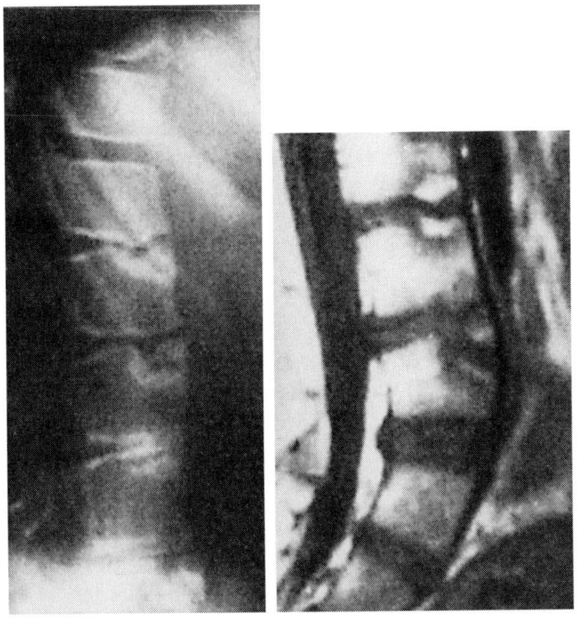

Fig. 8 **Left,** Tomogram of lumbar Scheuermann's kyphosis. **Right,** Magnetic resonance imaging demonstrates the anterior marginal detachment. (Reproduced with permission from Askani E, La Rosa G: Scheuermann's kyphosis, in Weinstein SL (ed): *The Pediatric Spine: Principles and Practice.* New York, NY, Raven Press, 1994, pp 557–584.)

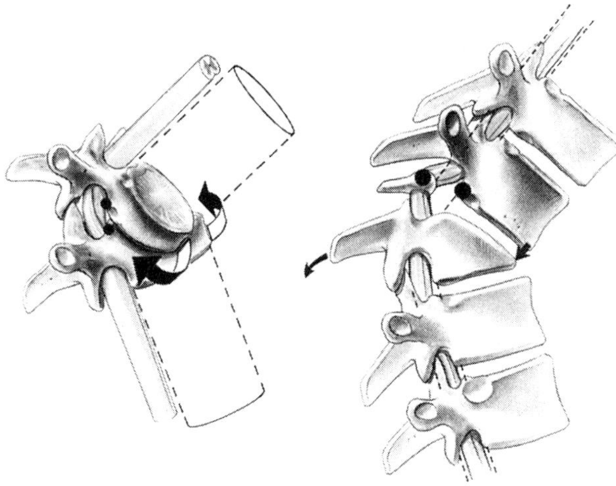

Fig. 9 Congenital kyphosis. Note failure of formation of the vertebral body anteriorly. This is an example of congenital dislocation of the spine with entrapped neural elements. Risk of paraplegia is high with acute correction. (Reproduced with permission from Dubousset J: Congenital kyphosis and lordosis, in Weinstein SL (ed): *The Pediatric Spine: Principles and Practice.* New York, NY, Raven Press, 1994, pp 245–258.)

ease includes postural kyphosis, which does not demonstrate anterior wedging or vertebral end plate irregularities and which corrects well with passive extension. Spondylitic disorders may also be differentiated from Scheuermann's disease based on the lack of sclerotic rim around the vertebral end plate erosions. Additional differentials include spondyloepiphyseal dysplasia and other osteochondral dystrophies, which will affect other joints in the axial skeleton. Congenital kyphosis, which is a failure of segmentation, must be differentiated from Scheuermann's kyphosis.

Management of Scheuermann's disease includes physical therapy for general fitness and strengthening of the trunk and shoulder extensor muscles. Electrical stimulation has not been demonstrated to be useful. Bracing, either with a modified Milwaukee brace for active correction or anti-gravity cast in passive correction, is based on the degree of flexibility. The Milwaukee brace may be used for a kyphotic curve with an apex between T6 and T9. The indications for brace treatment are initial curves less than 70° with a Risser sign less than grade 3. The goal of bracing is to achieve a curve that is near 50° at maturity. Casts can be considered when the kyphosis is quite rigid. Following three casts for 45 days each, adequate mobility should have been obtained to allow application of a Milwaukee brace to maintain the correction.

Surgical intervention in Scheuermann's kyphosis is rarely required, but when necessary it can be performed either by posterior alone or posterior plus anterior corrective fusion techniques. Long posterior fusions may be performed with complete facetectomies of the kyphotic area to improve correction. Instrumentation systems, either Harrington compression rods or modern modular systems, are applied and used in a compression mode. Correction is gained through sequential segmental compression of the hooks. The patient with curves > 75° and with anterior vertebral wedging in excess of 10° tend to lose the surgical correction obtained with posterior instrumentation and fusion alone. For permanent correction, such patients require anterior release and posterior instrumentation.

Congenital Kyphosis Congenital kyphosis may be divided into three types according to basic defect: failure of formation, failure of segmentation, and rotatory dislocation of the spine. In the failure of formation category, two aspects of evaluation are key: the location of the malformed parts and the alignment of the spinal canal. Failure of formation can be subdivided into partial failure of formation with a well-aligned canal, partial failure of formation with a dislocated canal, and total failure of formation of the vertebral bodies. The risk of existing or progressive neurologic deficit with congenital kyphosis is substantial. This risk is highest in failure of formation with dislocated canal and total failure of formation, ie, vertebral agenesis (Fig. 9). The failure of segmentation defect consists of an anteriorly located bar between adjacent vertebral bodies that causes progressive kyphosis with growth. The resulting kyphosis generally has a split shape with no sharp angles and, thus, minimal neurologic risk. The progression may be rapid during the growth spurt near the end of puberty. Rotatory dislocation of the spine is a rare entity in which a kyphotic zone is interposed between two areas of congenital scoliosis. Because the apex is abrupt and the cord may twist within the canal in this region, neurologic complications are common. The progression of this type of kyphosis is variable, depending on the nature of the congenital scoliosis adjacent. Brace treatment is ineffective. Most cases require an in situ surgical stabilization–posterior fusion alone in curves under 50° and combined anterior and posterior fusion for more severe kyphosis.

Miscellaneous Spine Problems

Neurofibromatosis Scoliosis is the most common musculoskeletal complication of neurofibromatosis. The reported incidence of spinal deformity in neurofibromatosis patients varies from 2% to 30%. Conversely, 2% to 3% of all scoliosis patients with significant curves have neurofibromatosis. The scoliosis has typically been described as a short, sharply angulated curve in the thoracic spine. Recent authors, however, question the existence of a consistent pattern of scoliosis in neurofibromatosis. Some cases of so-called idiopathic scoliosis may actually be secondary to neurofibromatosis. Computed tomography (CT) as well as three-dimensional reconstructions have been beneficial in visualizing complex deformities. Myelogram enhanced CT and MRI have been useful in identifying lesions within or about the spinal cord. Routine spinal MRI studies are not required when managing scoliosis in neurofibromatosis but are considered when indicated.

Proposed etiologies of thoracic scoliosis in neurofibromatosis patients include osteomalacia, localized tumor eroding bone, endocrine abnormalities, and mesodermal dysplasia. Prognosis and management depend highly on the presence of dystrophic changes, such as rib rotation, spindling of transverse processes, vertebral scalloping, apical vertebral rotation, foramen enlargement, and adjacent soft-tissue neurofibromas.

Brace treatment has not been effective in dystrophic curves, even in young children. Because the curves are short, early fusion usually does not lead to significant trunk height loss. Because the reported incidence of pseudarthroses ranges from 6% to 38%, many authors recommend the addition of anterior fusion for dystrophic scoliosis. Nondystrophic curves can be managed similarly to idiopathic scoliosis.

The reported incidence of head and neck involvement in neurofibromatosis varies from 20% to 45%, with the usual cervical spine deformity being kyphosis. Atlantoaxial dislocation has been reported in five patients. Other complications include dysphagia and torticollis. If dystrophic changes are noted on the original cervical spine films, oblique views should be obtained to rule out dumbbell lesions in the neural tissue. Flexion and extension views will assess cervical instability. Posterior spinal fusion is recommended for severe cervical spine deformity with instability. Autologous bone graft and halo immobilization usually lead to a solid fusion. Prior laminectomy may necessitate the addition of anterior surgery.

Kyphosis in neurofibromatosis typically has marked acute posterior angulation. Posterior fusion alone is usually insufficient in patients with dystrophic kyphosis. Decompression of the cord with laminectomy is contraindicated because the lesion is usually anterior, and removal of the posterior elements predisposes the patient to further postlaminectomy kyphosis. All decompression procedures should include arthrodesis. Patients presenting with paraplegia must be evaluated to rule out intraspinal lesions as opposed to kyphotic angular cord compression as the cause.

Marfan's Syndrome Spinal involvement occurs in approximately 75% of patients with Marfan's syndrome. Scoliosis is the most common spinal deformity, with the cervical spine almost always normal. Deformities occur early; one half of patients who will develop scoliosis do so by age 6 years. Almost all develop it by 9 years of age. Curve patterns resemble idiopathic scoliosis with frequent progression during adolescence. Despite the patients' generalized ligamentous laxity, many of the curves are quite rigid. These curves also tend to be painful, progressive, and often cause respiratory problems. Curve progression rates have averaged 7° to 10° per year, with the most rapid increase occurring during the early adolescent period.

Controversy exists regarding brace treatment of early curves. Most patients fail brace treatment, but orthotics may be used as a holding device for patients who will eventually undergo fusion. Posterior spinal instrumentation and fusion with autogenous bone graft has been the mainstay of treatment; however, a high rate of pseudarthrosis can be expected. The addition of anterior fusion, massive bone grafting, and postoperative immobilization may lower the incidence of pseudarthrosis. Meticulous preoperative workup is essential because of the high incidence of cardiac abnormalities. If placed in a body jacket, these patients have a higher incidence of superior mesenteric artery syndrome.

The second most common spinal deformity seen in Marfan's patients is thoracic lordosis, which usually is associated with loss of normal lumbar lordosis. Thoracolumbar kyphosis may occasionally occur. Segmental fixation with massive bone grafting is recommended.

Osteogenesis Imperfecta Spinal deformities are found in 20% to 80% of patients with osteogenesis imperfecta (OI). Risk factors include severe disease with nonambulatory status, multiple long bone fractures, and chest deformities. Scoliosis in OI may progress after skeletal maturity and may be related to weakened osteoporotic bone. The increase seen with age has been postulated to be a result of increased axial loading with upright posture.

Bracing in OI has universally led to poor results. Surgical intervention should include instrumentation because of the significant loss of correction and progression of deformity seen with fusion alone. Some authors advocate polymethylmethacrylate augmentation around the hooks to improve purchase in the osteoporotic bone; however, augmentation is generally not required with segmental (Luque) fixation. Associated kyphotic deformities may also complicate instrumentation and must be addressed as part of the surgical correction. A progressive curve that has reached 35° to 40° should be fused regardless of the patient's age because significant correction cannot be expected.

Few reports address cervical spine deformities in osteogenesis imperfecta. One of the most serious abnormalities is basilar impression, with the foramen magnum invaginating into the posterior fossa. This abnormality leads to stenosis with resultant hydrocephalus as well as compression of the cerebellum, brain stem, and cervical cord. Diagnosis of basilar impression is made using plain radiographs. The lateral cervical spine radiograph, in particular, shows the upward migration of the cervical spine into the base of the skull. The deformity may be subtle and requires careful scrutiny of the radiographs. Various descriptions of the characteristic skull shape have been described including the "Tam-O'-Shanter" beret and "Darth Vader" helmet. Treatment is by anterior decompression and posterior fusion.

Postlaminectomy Spine Deformity After removal of spinal cord tumors by a multilevel posterior laminectomy, progressive deformity (particularly kyphosis) can occur. Brace protection and early spinal fusion can minimize progressive deformity. Increasing use of multilevel laminoplasties (maintain and repair lamina, do not discard) by neurosurgeons appears to decrease the risk for marked early development of deformity.

Irradiation-Induced Deformity Vertebral bodies grow axially by endochondral ossification. It has been shown that sufficient radiation exposure inhibits normal endochondral maturation. Children irradiated at age 2 years or younger are most affected. Spinal deformity is the most common side effect of abdominal irradiation. Irradiation of the entire vertebra produces a symmetric hypoplastic vertebral body without significant misalignment. Irradiation of a portion of the body, however, causes segmental loss of growth with resultant scoliotic deformities.

Soft-tissue fibrosis and contracture may be a cause of spinal curvature. One study of Wilm's tumor patients showed a sevenfold increase of scoliosis in patients who underwent radiation treatment. Overall incidence of post-irradiation deformity is reported to be from 10% to 100%. Leg length discrepancy secondary to irradiation of the iliac crest or femoral heads may also result in a nonstructural scoliosis.

Milwaukee brace treatment is indicated in a young child with a flexible curve caused by irradiation. Early posterior fusion and instrumentation is recommended. Repeat bone grafting may be necessary. The duration of postoperative immobilization is longer than in other forms of scoliosis, and several authors recommend a duration of up to 1 year.

Cervical Spine Deformities

Congenital Anomalies: Klippel-Feil Syndrome The term Klippel-Feil syndrome has classically been associated with a clinical triad including short neck, low posterior hairline, and marked limitation in neck range of motion. Most now use the term Klippel-Feil syndrome to denote any congenital failure of segmentation within the cervical spine. The true incidence of Klippel-Feil syndrome or failure of segmentation of the cervical spine is not truly known because many patients with cervical spine anomalies are asymptomatic and never present to a physician. An estimation of 0.2 symptomatic congenital fusions per thousand population, which has been quoted in the literature, is felt to be a minimum estimate. Other studies estimate the incidence to be between six and seven per thousand. The etiology of Klippel-Feil syndrome is only partially understood. Based on the embryologic development of the spine, the failure of segmentation occurs between the third and eighth weeks of gestation. Theories vary from an alteration in vertebral artery development resulting in segmental ischemia and perhaps failure of segmentation to an unknown global fetal insult that may account for the anomalies observed. Primary neural tube abnormalities have been implicated, as well as genetically controlled developmental patterns. Klippel-Feil syndrome is also associated with multiple syndromes, including fetal alcohol syndrome and Goldenhar's syndrome, VATER, and other musculoskeletal anomalies including clubfoot, Sprengel's scapular deformity, developmental dysplasia of the hip, and upper extremity radial defects.

The classical triad that defines Klippel-Feil syndrome is found in only 40% to 50% of the patients (Fig. 10). The most common finding is decreased neck range of motion. Patients with Klippel-Feil syndrome may have a variety of complaints, including abnormal appearance of the head and neck, discomfort, radicular symptoms, and para- or quadriparesis. Also, patients may present indirectly secondary to evaluation of associated genitourinary, cardiovascular, or gastrointestinal anomalies.

The most common musculoskeletal anomaly associated with Klippel-Feil syndrome is typical scoliosis, in the thoracic or lumbar spine, which is found in 60% of patients. There is a high likelihood of curve progression, with over half requiring treatment. There is also a frequent association with congenital scoliosis in the lower spine. Sprengel's deformity has been identified in 20% to 50% of the patients with Klippel-Feil syndrome; hence, investigation of the cervical spine of any patient diagnosed with a Sprengel's deformity is warranted. Rib anomalies occur commonly in association with Klippel-Feil syndrome and are found in

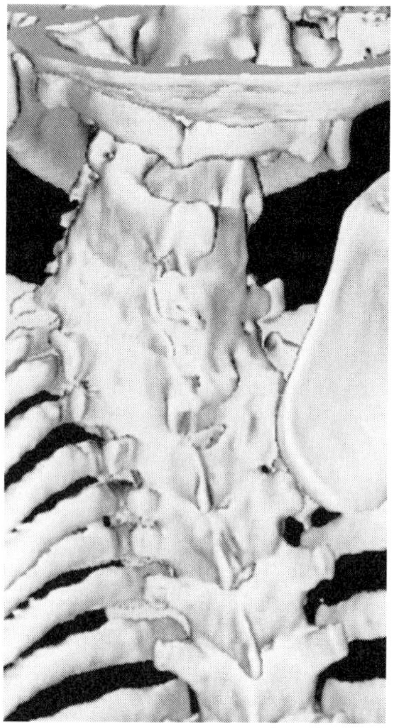

Fig. 10 Klippel-Feil syndrome: three-dimensional CT.

approximately one third of the patients. Cervical ribs occur in approximately 12% to 15% of the patients. Also, a thoracic outlet syndrome may be manifest in association with this syndrome, with or without the finding of cervical ribs.

Genitourinary anomalies are strongly associated with Klippel-Feil syndrome, and significant renal abnormalities are noted in approximately 25% to 35% of the patients. All patients diagnosed with Klippel-Feil syndrome should undergo ultrasound evaluation of their renal anatomy and collecting system. Should abnormalities be identified, an intravenous pyelogram should be performed to further delineate their urologic anatomy. Another strong association with Klippel-Feil syndrome is hearing loss, found in 15% to 35% of Klippel-Feil patients. The majority of the hearing loss is secondary to abnormalities of the inner ear that result in sensory neural hearing loss.

Cardiovascular anomalies are also frequent in patients with Klippel-Feil syndrome; they are estimated to occur in 14% to 29% of the patients. The majority of the cardiac anomalies produce a murmur. Central nervous system anomalies associated with the Klippel-Feil patient include synkinesia (involuntary movements of the extremity contralateral to that moved volitionally), seen in 15% to 20% of patients. Spinal cord anomalies can also be associated; however, these are much less common.

The natural history of Klippel-Feil syndrome is such that the majority of patients lead an active, normal life. Pain in the cervical spine as well as neurologic deficits may be present. Prophylactic management of asymptomatic individuals who have cervical anomalies is controversial. Meticulous evaluation of the asymptomatic patient is paramount. Flexion-extension plain films are warranted to assess stability of the cervical spine. Flexion-extension MRIs may also be of assistance. Care must be taken to evaluate for brain stem abnormalities, such as a Chiari malformation or evidence of congenital or acquired spinal stenosis. Patients with congenital cervical fusions should avoid contact sports as well as occupations and recreational activities that put them at risk for head trauma. Management of the symptomatic patient is less controversial, particularly those with spinal instability that can worsen over time. The not infrequent pattern of occipitalization of the atlas in conjunction with a C2 to C3 fusion is at high risk for instability at the C1-C2 level. These patients should be followed carefully. Cervical fusion is performed as warranted by the patient's development and the progression of symptoms.

Torticollis Torticollis is a clinical diagnosis based on the findings of head tilt in association with a rotatory deviation of the cranium. The differential diagnosis of torticollis is extensive and may be broken down into congenital and acquired etiologies. Congenital torticollis may be further subdivided into occipitocervical anomalies and soft-tissue conditions, such as congenital muscular torticollis and pterygium colli. Acquired torticollis may be divided into multiple categories, including basilar impression, inflammatory etiology, neurogenic etiology, neoplastic etiology, and idiopathic.

Congenital Muscular Torticollis Congenital muscular torticollis is the most common etiology of torticollis in the infant and young child. It has been suggested to be due to a compartment syndrome secondary to compression of the sternocleidomastoid muscle within the birth canal in prolonged labor. The diagnosis is generally made within the first 2 months of life. During the first 4 weeks of life, a palpable mass may be present in the region of the involved sternocleidomastoid muscle. Because developmental dysplasia of the hip is present in up to 20% of the patients with congenital muscular torticollis, the infant's hips should be evaluated at the time of the neck examination.

If the asymmetric position of the head is not addressed at an early age, plagiocephaly may develop within the first year of life. The flattening of the features of the face is secondary to preferential positioning by the infant in response to a lack of normal motion. Prior to instituting formal physical therapy to stretch the sternocleidomastoid, radiographic evaluation of the cervical spine should be performed to rule out congenital cervical anomalies as a cause for the head tilt. Initial management begins with a careful stretching program. Because the head tilts toward the affected sternocleidomastoid muscle and rotates away from that side, the stretching program is designed to reverse these motions and hence stretch the muscle. The ear contralateral to the affected sternocleidomastoid muscle is drawn towards its ipsilateral shoulder while the chin is drawn toward the shoulder ipsilateral to the affected muscle. The exercises are initiated in the neutral position and once adequate motion is gained in this position, they are continued in the extended position to maximize stretching.

Surgical management is withheld until approximately 1 year of age when adequate conservative management has failed. Approximately 90% of the patients will be managed successfully with stretching alone. Because plagiocephaly is a progressive condition, the earlier surgical correction is performed, the better the result. The exact technique for muscle release is somewhat controversial, however, bipolar release (proximal and distal attachments) of the muscle is advocated to minimize the chance of recurrence. The deep fascia on the posterior surface of the distal attachments (clavicular, sternal heads) must be released to assure adequate release. Postoperative management often includes a rigid cervicothoracic orthosis designed to maintain an elongated length of the involved muscle by overcorrecting the position of the neck on a temporary basis. Some surgeons advise only postoperative physical therapy.

Other nonbony etiologies for torticollis include Sandifer's syndrome, in which the abnormal torticollis posture is associated with gastroesophageal reflux. Posterior fossa tumors may first present as torticollis. Ocular dysfunction (superior oblique palsy) may produce torticollis as a compensatory phenomenon. Various inflammatory and infectious conditions of the cervical spine may also lead to the findings of torticollis. Bony etiologies of torticollis include basilar impression, atlanto-occipital anomalies, unilateral absence of the atlas, familial cervical dysplasia, atlantoaxial rotatory displacement, and neoplasms. Because of the eclectic etiologic possibilities, patients who have significant torticollis in early childhood and are being considered for a surgical release (after failed physical therapy) should have neurologic and ophthalmologic consultations before muscle release surgery to be certain that there is not some cause for the torticollis other than muscle contraction.

Basilar Impression Basilar impression is a deformity of the base of the skull in which the occipital condyles invaginate within the vault of the cranium, resulting in the relative migration of the atlas and the dens into the foramen magnum. The occupation of space within the limited dimensions of the foramen magnum may lead to brain stem encroachment. Pressure produced on the brain stem by the tip of the dens may directly cause neurologic impairment or may indirectly cause neurologic deficit secondary to interference with blood supplied to the spinal cord or with the flow of cerebral spinal fluid. Basilar impression may be a primary phenomenon associated with other vertebral anomalies, such as Klippel-Feil syndrome, atlanto-occipital fusion, odontoid abnormalities, and hypoplasia of the atlas. Primary basilar impression is also associated with some skeletal dysplasias, including achondroplasia, spondyloepiphyseal dysplasia, and Morquio syndrome. Secondary basilar impression is a progressive condition that results from softening of the base of the occiput with gradual invagination of the cervical spine into the foramen magnum. Diseases such as Paget disease, renal osteodystrophy, rickets, and osteomalacia may cause this condition as well as osteogenesis imperfecta, rheumatoid arthritis, neurofibromatosis, and trauma. The most common clinical finding is a short neck. This finding is followed closely by asymmetry of the skull and/or face and painful range of motion in the cervical spine. Torticollis is associated with basilar impression in approximately 15% of cases.

MRI scan in sagittal section can demonstrate impingement of the dens on the brain stem. Excessive migration of the dens within the foramen magnum and secondary basilar impression may lead to progressive encroachment on the medulla oblongata. This encroachment causes restriction of cerebral spinal fluid flow in the aqueduct of Sylvius, which results in hydrocephalus.

Management of basilar impression is difficult. Surgical decompression of the impinged neurologic structures is the cornerstone of treatment. Symptoms and MRI findings can be used to identify the structure causing neurologic impingement. The impingement can be addressed directly either anteriorly by excision of the odontoid as necessary or posteriorly through suboccipital decompression and enlargement of the foramen magnum. Posterior stabilization should accompany either procedure.

Odontoid Hypoplasia Hypoplasia of the odontoid can vary anywhere from a small remnant of the dens being present to complete aplasia with the dens being absent. Atlantoaxial instability is present and vascular compromise may also exist from stretching of the vertebral arteries.

Os Odontoideum An os odontoideum, when present, is a separate ossicle from the hypoplastic dens. It is usually seen in place of the normal odontoid process (orthotopic type) or under the tip of the basi-occiput (dystopic type) where it may fuse and move in unison with the clivus. Neurologic compromise is more often seen with the dystopic type.

Differentiation between os odontoideum and odontoid fracture may be difficult. Most authors favor an unrecognized previous fracture of the odontoid as the most common cause of os odontoideum. It has also been seen in Down syndrome, spondyloepiphyseal dysplasia, and Morquio syndrome. Polytomography or flexion-extension MRI may be useful in evaluating patients. Stabilization is warranted in symptomatic patients with evidence of instability; however, the treatment of asymptomatic patients who have routine radiographs that show the presence of an os odontoideum remains unsettled.

Cervical Spine in Down Syndrome Children with Down syndrome have underlying collagen defects and, therefore, often have cervical instabilities at both the occiput-C1 level (60% of patients) and C1-C2 level (15% to 20%). Although these patients have generalized ligamentous laxity, a correlation between the degree of laxity and cervical spine instability has not been established.

Clinical symptoms of neurologic compromise are rare, occurring in only 2% to 3% of patients. Children with atlantoaxial instability also have a higher incidence of cervical spine anomalies. The definition of atlantoaxial instability is made radiographically, based on an atlanto-dens interval of more than 4 or 5 mm on flexion-extension radiographs. A 4-mm posterior subluxation of the atlanto-occipital relationship on a lateral extension view has been postulated as evidence of atlanto-occipital instability.

One recent report showed a high correlation between radiographically documented atlanto-occipital instability and positive neurologic findings in a large population of patients with Down syndrome. Radiographs should also be reviewed for other associated anomalies, such as persistent synchondrosis of C2, spina bifida occult of C1, ossiculum terminale, or os odontoideum. CT and MRI may be beneficial.

All children who wish to participate in sports that involve possible trauma to the head and neck should have lateral radiographs of the cervical spine in neutral, flexion, and extension before beginning training or competition. When the atlanto-dens interval exceeds 4.5 mm or there is an abnormality of the odontoid, there should be restrictions on sports that involve trauma to the head and neck. Such sports include tumbling, diving, gymnastics, soccer, high jumping, football, and skiing. Surgical stabilization of the cervical spine should be considered in Down syndrome patients with atlantoaxial instability (> 6 mm) and neurologic signs or symptoms (neck pain, stiff neck, torticollis, progressive weakness or change in sensation in any extremity, decreasing endurance, loss of bowel or bladder control or a change in bowel habits, increased clumsiness, or change in gait pattern). Complications of posterior arthrodesis in Down syndrome are common. One recent study reported a 100% complication rate in ten patients, including two perioperative deaths. Long-term results are not available.

Back Pain in Children

Back pain in children, unlike that in adults, usually has a defined cause in 50% to 60% of cases. By taking a complete history, performing a careful, detailed physical examination, and utilizing the appropriate laboratory and imaging modalities, a diagnosis can usually be made and treatment instituted.

Spinal Trauma in Children and Adolescents

Cervical Spine

Assessment of the Injury Immediate immobilization of the spine should be performed at the time of the injury. Herzenberg and colleagues, noting the large size of children's heads, recommend transportation to the hospital with either a board with a recessed area for the skull or a double mattress pad under the thoracic spine. If the injury is on the football field, to prevent neck flexion, the helmet should be left in place until the patient is in the hospital setting.

Children with head or facial injuries have a presumed spinal injury until proven otherwise. A brain-injured child who does not have decerebrate posturing may have a spinal cord injury as well. If a child has a cardiopulmonary arrest after trauma without a significant hemodynamic problem, an upper cervical spine injury should be suspected. In awake, cooperative children, neck tenderness, widening of the interspinous space, muscle rigidity, and torticollis can be elicited. A complete neurologic examination (including rectal examination) should be performed in all cases of suspected cervical spine injury.

Radiographic assessment of cervical spine injuries is often difficult because much of the spine is cartilaginous, especially in the young infant. Prior to age 8 years, most of the spinal injuries occur above C4 due to the relatively large size of the child's head combined with the horizontal orientation of the upper cervical facets, which allows hypermobility of the upper cervical spine. Children older than 8 years have adult patterns of injury.

Occipitoatlantal Dislocation This is a common cause of fatal cervical spine injury in the younger child. Those children who survive usually have significant neurologic involvement. In surviving patients, the lateral radiograph demonstrates subluxation of the occiput on C1. It may be evaluated by determining the Powers ratio (Fig. 11) or by constructing a line along the posterior aspect of the sella turcica. This line should intersect the odontoid process on both flexion and extension. If it does not, then subluxation is present. Halo immobilization is recommended as soon as the diagnosis is made. Traction should not be used. Some authors recommend halo immobilization as the final treatment; however, because it is a ligamentous injury with marked instability, other authors recommend a posterior occipitocervical fusion as the treatment of choice.

Atlas Fractures This fracture is secondary to a direct blow on the head with a resultant burst fracture of the C1 ring. In children younger than 7 years of age, the fracture may occur through the neurocentral synchondrosis. Treatment is long term (up to 6 months) in a Minerva cast or halo immobilization (Fig. 12).

Atlantoaxial Instability This injury is extremely uncommon in children; it occurs with a fracture at the synchondrosis at the base of the dens or a transverse ligament rupture. Treatment is warranted if there is greater than a 5 mm atlanto-dens interval. Treatment consists of 8 to 12 weeks of immobilization in a halo jacket. Nontraumatic instability occurs in Down syndrome, Klippel-Feil syndrome, and some skeletal dysplasias. Patients with these

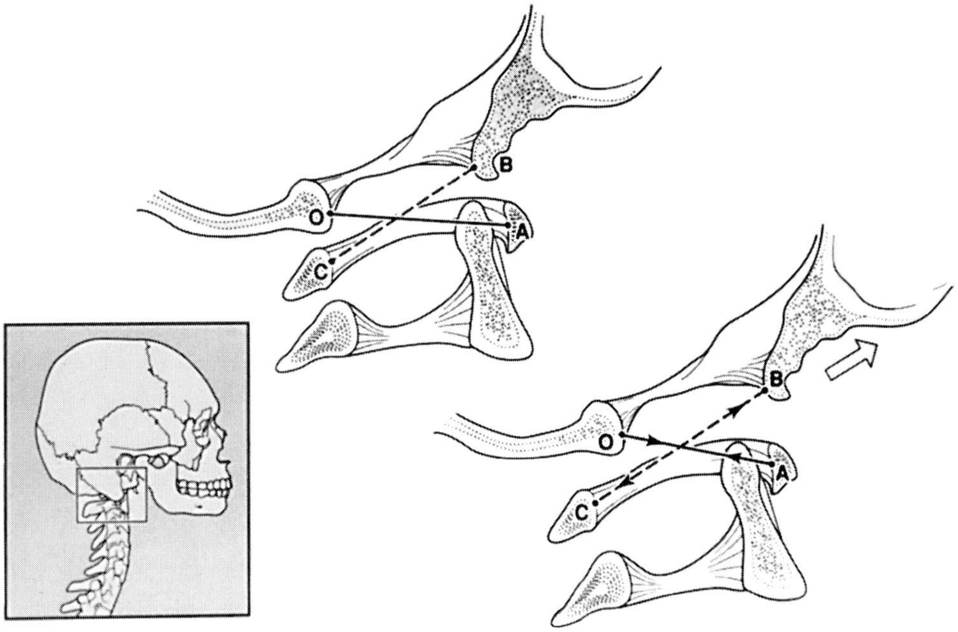

Fig. 11 Power's ratio is determined by drawing a line from the basion (B) to the posterior arch of the atlas (C) and a second line from the opisthion (O) to the anterior arch of the atlas (A). The length of the line BC is divided by the length of the line OA. A ratio greater than 1.0 is diagnostic of anterior occipitoatlantal dislocation. Values less than 0.9 are definitely normal. (Reproduced with permission from Lebwohl N, Eismont F: Cervical spine injuries, in Weinstein SL (ed): *The Pediatric Spine: Principles and Practice.* New York, NY, Raven Press, 1994, pp 725–741.)

conditions should be routinely screened. If the atlanto-dens interval is greater than 10 mm or there are any signs of neurologic involvement, then posterior cervical fusion is advocated. As previously noted, there is a very high complication rate reported in posterior cervical fusion in Down syndrome.

Atlantoaxial Rotatory Subluxation Patients with this entity have painful torticollis, which is thought to be caused by inflammation of the ligaments that support the atlantoaxial complex. Plain radiographs are very difficult to interpret. A CT scan with neutral views as well as views in maximal lateral rotation to both the right and left is the best study to confirm the diagnosis of atlantoaxial rotatory subluxation (Fig. 13). In the first week, bed rest and a soft cervical collar plus nonsteroidal anti-inflammatory drugs may allow reduction of the torticollis. If symptoms remain for more than 1 week, then head-halter traction should be applied. After resolution, a soft cervical collar is worn for 6 weeks. In long-standing torticollis, initial traction with lateral posterior cervical fusion should be performed.

Odontoid Fractures Odontoid fractures in children up to the age of 6 years are almost always fractures through the basal physis. There is often marked (greater than 50%) displacement. Tomograms or CT reconstructions are neces-

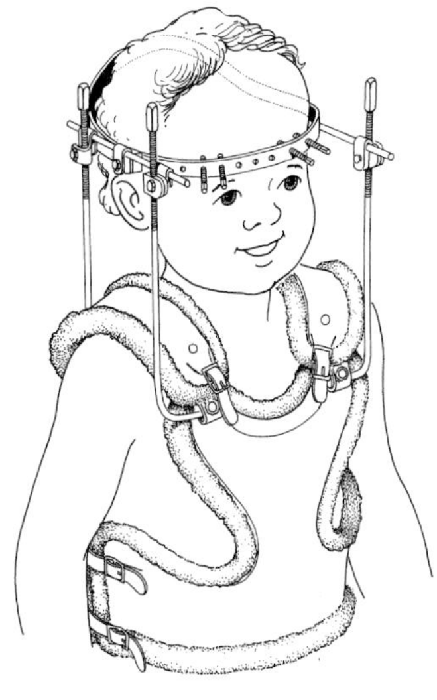

Fig. 12 Custom-made halo vest and lightweight superstructure. There are ten pin placement sites for infant halo ring attachment using a multiple-pin, low-torque technique. Usual pin placement: four anteriorly, avoiding the temporal area, with the remaining six pins in the occipital area. (Reproduced with permission from Mubarak S, Camp J, Vuletich , et al: Halo application in the infant. *J Pediatr Orthop* 1989;9:612–614.)

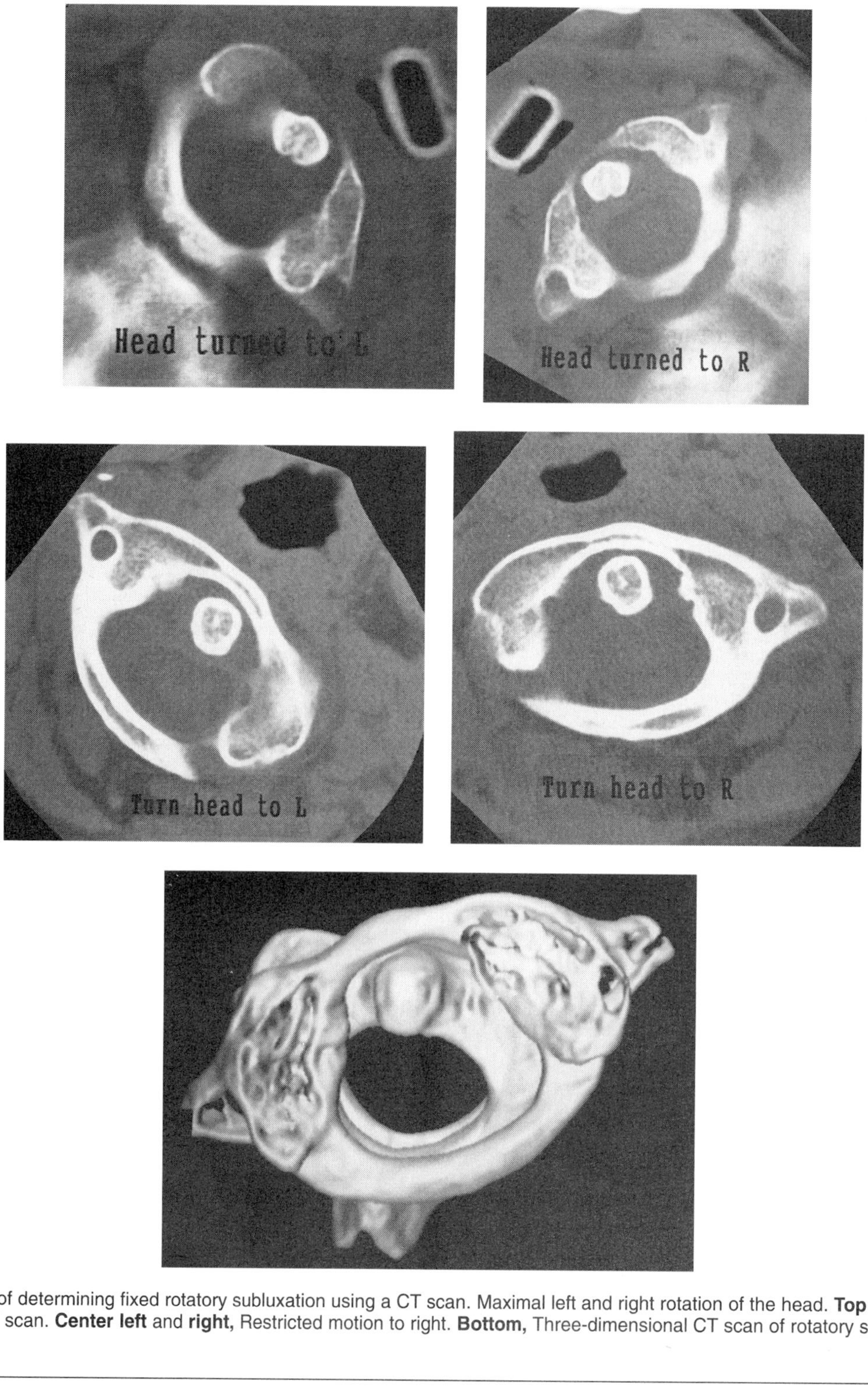

Fig. 13 Method of determining fixed rotatory subluxation using a CT scan. Maximal left and right rotation of the head. **Top left** and **right,** Normal rotation CT scan. **Center left** and **right,** Restricted motion to right. **Bottom,** Three-dimensional CT scan of rotatory subluxation (view from cephalad).

sary to adequately image this area of the spine. Reduction and halo immobilization (or Minerva casting) should be placed for 6 weeks. Failure to diagnose and treat this fracture is the most likely cause of later os odontoideum.

C2 Pedicle Fracture This fracture may be difficult to diagnose because there is difficulty in imaging this area with the physiologic hypermobility of C2-C3. The posterior cervical line (line joining C1, C2, C3 spinous process base) is helpful in determining if there is pseudosubluxation or actual motion at this level. If the posterior line of C2 is greater than 2 mm posterior to the posterior cervical line, a fracture is present. If there is minimal displacement of the fracture, immobilization in a collar for 8 weeks is adequate. If > 3 mm displacement is present, halo immobilization should be used.

Subaxial Injuries Subaxial injuries usually occur in children over the age of 8 years. Flexion injuries are the most common, with compression fractures predominating. Many fractures can be treated with simple neck immobilization. More severe fractures can be treated with posterior spinal fusion. Anterior spinal fusion should be avoided because most of the growth is anterior and kyphosis secondary to growth arrest may occur. Salter-Harris I fractures can occur in infants or younger children, with Salter-Harris III fractures occurring in adolescents. Salter-Harris I fractures are very difficult to diagnose but, if found, should be surgically stabilized because they are very unstable. Type 3 anterior ring apophysis fractures can be treated with a cervical collar for 6 weeks.

Spinal Cord Injury Without Radiographic Abnormalities (SCIWORA)

Approximately 16% to 19% of spinal cord injuries in children have an unknown cause. There is elongation of the spinal cord in flexion and shortening in extension. Infantile spinal canals can be stretched by approximately 2 inches, but the spinal cord can be stretched by only one quarter inch before rupturing. Because of the stretching, there is often a marked discrepancy between the level of neurologic deficits and the vertebral injury.

The etiology of SCIWORA is not known. Longitudinal traction, traumatic infarction, cord rupture, traumatic section of the cord, disk rupture, posterior end plate fractures, and soft-tissue infolding are all causes of SCIWORA. MRI may be of use in delineating the etiology. Although many patients manifest their neurologic symptoms immediately, approximately 50% of patients with SCIWORA have a delayed onset of neurologic symptoms. This predicament necessitates careful and serial neurologic examinations in the patient with a cervical spine injury.

Thoracic, Lumbar, and Sacral Fractures

Approximately 50% of all children's spinal fractures occur in this region. There are two peaks of injury: children younger than 5 years of age, and those older than 10 years of age. The most common cause of fracture is motor vehicle accidents, with falls from heights, sports-related activities, and child abuse as the other common causes.

Vertebral End Plate Fractures

Fracture and displacement of the vertebral apophyseal end plate may contribute to the SCIWORA syndrome. There is often a small, bony fracture fragment attached to the apophysis. These fragments are often found in the lumbar region and may present as a herniated nucleus pulposus (Fig. 14). There is often a late diagnosis of this injury, and CT scanning is the preferred imaging modality. Treatment is determined by the extent of the injury, neurologic involvement, and pain. Laminotomy and removal of bone and cartilage fragments are often necessary.

Major Spinal Fractures

The three-column spine concept of Denis is useful in understanding and predicting the outcome of spinal fractures (Fig. 15). The posterior column consists of the posterior laminar arch, supraspinous ligament, interspinous ligament, posterior lateral capsule, and ligamentum flavum. The middle column includes the posterior longitudinal ligament, the posterior annulus fibrosis, and the posterior wall of the vertebral body. The anterior column consists of the anterior vertebral body, the anterior annulus fibrosis, and the anterior longitudinal ligament. The three-column system permits injuries to be divided into four major types. A compression fracture is failure of the anterior col-

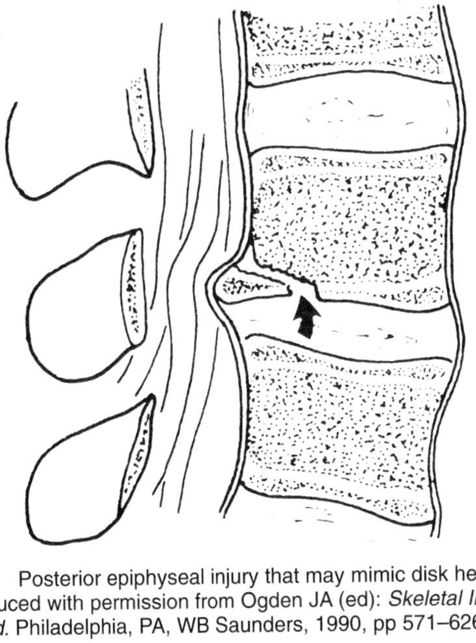

Fig. 14 Posterior epiphyseal injury that may mimic disk herniation. (Reproduced with permission from Ogden JA (ed): *Skeletal Injury in the Child.* Philadelphia, PA, WB Saunders, 1990, pp 571–626.)

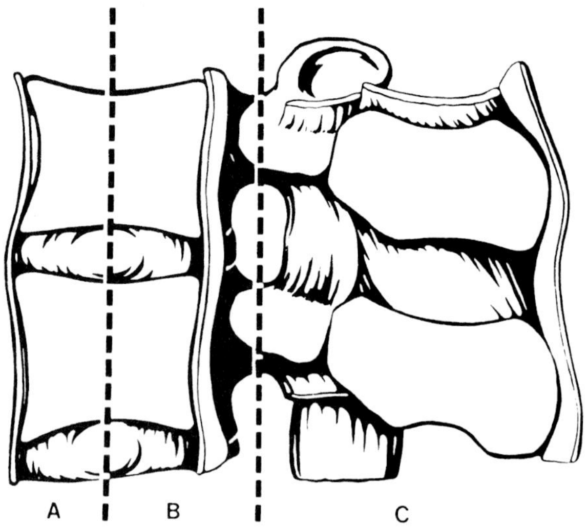

Fig. 15 The three-column concept. Anterior column (**A**), middle column (**B**), and posterior column (**C**). (Reproduced with permission from Chambers H, Akbarnia B: Cervical spine injuries, in Weinstein SL (ed): *The Pediatric Spine: Principles and Practice.* New York, NY, Raven Press, 1994, pp 743–766.)

umn with an intact middle column. A burst fracture is a failure under compression of both the anterior and middle columns. A seat belt fracture is a compression injury of the anterior column with a distraction of the middle and posterior columns through either bony or ligamentous elements. The fourth type of injury is a fracture-dislocation in which all three columns fail in compression, with rotation in shear of the anterior column, distraction with shear of the middle column, and distraction with rotation in shear of the posterior column.

There are three types of spinal instability: first degree instability, which is a mechanical instability with risk of kyphosis; second degree instability, which is a neurologic instability, such as a collapsing "stable" burst fracture; and third degree instability, which is a mechanical and neurologic instability, such as an unstable burst fracture or a fracture-dislocation.

Compression Injury

These are the most common injuries in children. The compression is usually 20% or less and may occur over several levels. The wedging, if only in the sagittal plane, usually reconstitutes the vertebral height if the child is less than 10 years old. If there is no posterior involvement, most are stable and can be treated with external bracing. If the fracture is greater than 50%, then posterior spinal fusion with compression instrumentation should be performed.

Burst Fractures

When an axial compression force is applied to the vertebra, then the vertebral end plate fractures and the nucleus of the disk is forced into the vertebral body, which explodes and shatters. Burst fractures usually occur in the lower thoracic region, thoracolumbar junction, and lumbar region where axial loading is possible. The burst fracture may be either mechanically or neurologically unstable with a middle column retropulsed into the spinal canal and neuroforamina. The extent of bursting should be evaluated with CT scanning. The treatment of burst fractures depends on the amount of canal compromise and neurologic involvement. The fracture must be reduced and, if there is significant loss of anterior body height greater than 60%, anterior grafting from either a posterior eggshell approach or an anterior approach may be required. Either posterior or anterior spinal instrumentation is often used.

Flexion Distraction (Seat Belt Injuries)

A flexion and distraction mechanism of injury is the cause of this fracture. There are three types: Type 1 extends through the spinous process and travels symmetrically forward through all the posterior bony elements to emerge in a variable position in the vertebral body; type 2 is identical except that the fracture line traverses the posterior elements between the spinous processes; and type 3 is asymmetric, involving the posterior elements more on one side than the other. Type 3 is possibly associated with a rotational force occurring around a seat belt strap. An MRI should be obtained in all seat belt injuries because there is a possibility of a bony injury at one level and a disk injury at another level.

If reduction is not achieved by nonsurgical methods of casting or postural reduction, surgery may be indicated. A posterior compression force is required to reduce the fracture. This force can be achieved by wiring in small children, or by using posterior instrumentation in older patients. Instrumentation is usually extended one level above and one level below the injury.

Fracture Dislocation Injuries

These rare fractures usually occur at the thoracolumbar junction. They are often associated with neurologic injuries of either the conus medullaris or nerve roots. This injury is always unstable; it requires surgical stabilization and decompression and should be treated with rigid fixation with long instrumentation levels and multiple anchors. The indications for decompression in neurologically intact patients with spine fractures are controversial.

Sacral Fractures

Sacral fractures are usually associated with pelvic injuries and are not common in children. They may occur in association with more obvious thoracolumbar spinal fractures. Epiphyseal injuries are often mistaken for sacroiliac dislocations.

Annotated Bibliography

Congenital Scoliosis

McMaster MJ, David CV: Hemivertebra as a cause of scoliosis: A study of 104 patients. *J Bone Joint Surg* 1986;68B:588–595.

Fully segmented, non-incarcerated hemivertebra may require prophylactic treatment to prevent significant deformity while semisegmented and incarcerated hemivertebra usually require no treatment.

Terek RM, Wehner J, Lubicky JP: Crankshaft phenomenon in congenital scoliosis: A preliminary report. *J Pediatr Orthop* 1991;11:527–532.

Seven of the 23 curves progressed greater than 10° during the course of follow-up, and six of the seven demonstrated increased rotation, demonstrating the crankshaft phenomenon. No curve that underwent anterior and posterior hemiepiphysiodesis demonstrated the crankshaft phenomenon. The authors suggest that anterior fusion should be performed to prevent crankshaft phenomenon in young children.

Adolescent Idiopathic Scoliosis

Goldberg CJ, Dowling FE, Hall JE, et al: A statistical comparison between natural history of idiopathic scoliosis and brace treatment in skeletally immature adolescent girls. *Spine* 1993;18:902–908.

Thirty-two braced adolescent girls from Boston were compared with 32 matched girls from Ireland. All were Risser 0 at diagnosis. The authors found no statistical difference between the groups on any parameter of curve progression.

US Preventive Services Task Force: Screening for adolescent idiopathic scoliosis: Policy statement and review article. *JAMA* 1993;269:2664–2672.

These two articles concluded, based on the published literature, that the available evidence in support of school screening is generally weak. Routine screening may lead to inconvenience, increased cost, and potential radiation exposure.

Upadhyay SS, Ho EK, Gunawardene WM, et al: Changes in residual volume relative to vital capacity and total lung capacity after arthrodesis of the spine in patients who have adolescent idiopathic scoliosis. *J Bone Joint Surg* 1993;75A:46–52.

Residual volumes were increased at 3-year follow-up corrected for age but vital capacity and forced vital capacity were reduced following spinal fusion for idiopathic scoliosis.

Neuromuscular Scoliosis

Mubarak SJ, Morin WD, Leach J: Spinal fusion in Duchenne muscular dystrophy-fixation and fusion to the sacropelvis? *J Pediatr Orthop* 1993;13:752–757.

In this retrospective study of 22 patients with Duchenne muscular dystrophy who underwent Luque segmental instrumentation and fusion, 12 were instrumented to the sacral pelvis, and 10 were instrumented to L5. There was no difference in the outcome of the two groups. Recommendations were made for surgery to be performed if the curve is greater than 20° and if the forced vital capacity is greater than 40%.

Miscellaneous Spine Problems

Funasaki H, Winter RB, Lonstein JB, et al: Pathophysiology of spinal deformities in neurofibromatosis: An analysis of seventy-one patients who had curves associated with dystrophic changes. *J Bone Joint Surg* 1994;76A:692–700.

Four different patterns of spinal deformities were identified in 71 patients. Two of the patterns had the most severe progression: kyphoscoliosis with angular kyphosis (gibis) and marked dystrophic changes; and kyphosing scoliosis. Risk factors for progression include early age of onset, an abnormal kyphosis, vertebral scalloping, severe rotation at the apex, apex in the mid to lower thoracic area and rib penciling.

Hanscom DA, Winter RB, Lutter L, et al: Osteogenesis imperfecta: Radiographic classification, natural history, and treatment of spinal deformities. *J Bone Joint Surg* 1992;74A:598–616.

Forty-three patients were studied radiographically to classify them based on the shape, dimension, and appearance of the long bones; the presence of a trefoil pelvis and protrusio acetabula; and the shape of the vertebrae. Six distinct types (A–F) were discerned. Based on the radiographic criteria, the natural history and successful treatment regimens could be predicted.

Cervical Spine Disorders

Segal LS, Drummond DS, Zanotti RM, et al: Complications of posterior arthrodesis of the cervical spine in patients who have Down syndrome. *J Bone Joint Surg* 1991;73A:1547–1554.

A retrospective review of patients with Down syndrome who had a posterior arthrodesis of the upper cervical spine. There was 100% complication rate including infection and dehiscence at the site of the wound, incomplete reduction of the atlantoaxial joint, instability of the adjacent motion segment, neurologic sequelae, resorption of the autogenous bone graft, and death in the postoperative period.

Tredwell SJ, Newman DE, Lockitch G: Instability of the upper cervical spine in Down syndrome. *J Pediatr Orthop* 1990;10:602–606.

Pueschel SM, Scola FH, Tupper TB, et al: Skeletal anomalies of the upper cervical spine in children with Down syndrome. *J Pediatr Orthop* 1990;10:607–611.

These two studies demonstrated that there is a greater incidence of ligamentous laxity of the upper cervical spine in children with Down syndrome. Although most of the attention has been focused on the C1-C2 instability, there is very high incidence of instability at more than one location in the cervical spine.

Classic Bibliography

Broom MJ, Banta JV, Renshaw TS: Spinal fusion augmented by Luque-rod segmental instrumentation for neuromuscular scoliosis. *J Bone Joint Surg* 1989;71A: 32–44.

Green NE: Part-time bracing of adolescent idiopathic scoliosis. *J Bone Joint Surg* 1986;68A:738–742.

Hensinger RN: Spondylolysis and spondylolisthesis in children and adolescents. *J Bone Joint Surg* 1989;71A: 1098–1107.

King HA, Moe JH, Bradford DS, et al: The selection of fusion levels in thoracic idiopathic scoliosis. *J Bone Joint Surg* 1983;65A:1302–1313.

Lonstein JE, Carlson JM: The prediction of curve progression in untreated idiopathic scoliosis during growth. *J Bone Joint Surg* 1984;66A:1061–1071.

Mazur J, Menelaus MB, Dickens DR, et al: Efficacy of surgical management for scoliosis in myelomeningocele: Correction of deformity and alteration of functional status. *J Pediatr Orthop* 1986;6:568–575.

Mielke CH, Lonstein JE, Denis F, et al: Surgical treatment of adolescent idiopathic scoliosis: A comparative analysis. *J Bone Joint Surg* 1989;71A: 1170–1177.

Nicol RO, Scott JH: Lytic spondylolysis: Repair by wiring. *Spine* 1986;11:1027–1030.

Weinstein SL, Ponseti IV: Curve progression in idiopathic scoliosis. *J Bone Joint Surg* 1983;65A:447–455.

Wiltse LL: Spondylolisthesis in children. *Clin Orthop* 1961;21:156–163.

46

Spine: Trauma

Introduction

More than a million spinal column injuries occur each year. The vast majority of these injuries are soft-tissue injuries that do not require surgical stabilization or prolonged immobilization. In the United States, there are approximately 50,000 spine fractures each year, 10,000 of which involve injury to the spinal cord with associated neurologic deficit. Although spine fractures are most often secondary to motor vehicle accidents, falls, or diving accidents, recent reports indicate a disturbingly increased incidence of spine injuries related to firearms. Typically, the patient who has sustained a spinal column injury is a young male between the ages of 15 and 35 years. The injury to the spinal column frequently occurs at either the thoracolumbar or the cervicothoracic junction.

An increased vigilance by emergency personnel for early spine stabilization both at the accident site and in the emergency room has contributed to a reduction in the progression of an incomplete spinal cord lesion to a complete spinal cord lesion. Safety improvements in motor vehicles, including the addition of shoulder straps, air bags, and side impact systems, have also led to a reduction in the incidence of serious injury from blunt trauma to the spine.

Despite heightened awareness of cervical spine injuries, both in the field and in the emergency room, a number of cervical spine fractures are missed in the emergency room. Evaluation for spine injury requires taking a complete history from the patient or emergency medical technicians (EMTs), as well as a comprehensive examination.

General Principles of Treatment of Patients With Spine Injury

Initial Care

The important steps of treating patients who have sustained a spine injury are immobilization, medical stabilization, restoration of spinal alignment, surgical decompression, and spine stabilization.

Management of a vertebral column injury begins at the scene of the accident. Immobilization should be performed in the field with placement of a rigid cervical collar as well as a spine board and sandbags. Immobilization should be maintained until the patient has been evaluated and cleared by the treating physician. If the patient has not been stabilized in the field, cervical spine stabilization is one of the first steps taken by the evaluating physician in the emergency room.

In the emergency room, it is often helpful for EMTs to relay information concerning the accident scene. Injury mechanism reconstruction can further heighten awareness for possible types of spine trauma. An initial trauma survey is mandatory because abdominal and musculoskeletal trauma are commonly associated with thoracolumbar spine fractures. Head injuries are also frequently seen with spinal cord injury, and unconscious patients should be treated as if they had a possible cord injury until proven otherwise. Noncontiguous spine injuries occur in 5% to 20% of those with spine fractures. Up to 15% of patients have associated major visceral involvement.

Medical stabilization follows the basic principles of trauma care, which generally require continuous monitoring of the patient's respiratory and cardiovascular status. Monitoring is generally conducted in the emergency room or intensive care unit setting. Patients with spinal cord injuries and neurogenic shock will have hypotension and bradycardia as a result of the traumatic sympathectomy. Spinal shock is different from neurogenic shock and is defined as the absence of spinal reflex activity below a spinal cord injury. The significance of spinal shock is that it limits the ability to predict recovery of spinal cord function. Spinal shock should be considered over by 48 hours or with the return of the bulbocavernosus reflex.

The injured cervical spine is usually realigned with skeletal traction via halo ring or Gardner Wells tongs. Although recently there have been some concerns about the necessity of magnetic resonance imaging (MRI) or myelography before the reduction of a cervical spine dislocation, these generally are not necessary in the setting where a patient is being placed in traction while awake and subjected to repeat neurologic and radiographic evaluation. Skeletal traction for realignment of thoracic or lumbar injury is rarely indicated.

Decompression for spine injury is usually reserved for significant canal compromise following reduction. In general, because of its relative size, decompression of the upper cervical spine is rarely, if ever, indicated. In the lower cervical spine, significant canal compromise by disk or bony fragments following reduction will warrant an anterior decompression along with surgical stabilization. Often, in thoracic and lumbar injuries, the posterior stabilization procedure will provide an indirect decompression of the spinal canal, thereby eliminating the requirement for an anterior decompression. Ultimately, the decision to perform an anterior decompression depends on the specific spine injury.

Spinal Cord Injury

Most spinal cord deficit is attributed to contusion and/or compression, rather than to complete transection. The initial blunt injury leads to a sequence of molecular and cellular as well as macroscopic events that results in ischemia, tissue hypoxia, and secondary tissue degeneration. The extent of tissue damage and resulting neural injury can be related to the magnitude of the initial force. Whether the initial blunt insult or the effect of continued pressure on the damaged neural elements is greater in causing persistence of neural deficit remains a topic of controversy.

The microvasculature can be disrupted by mechanical deformation and propagated by edema, thrombosis, or further vasoconstriction induced by local and circulating factors. Although it is currently not possible to reverse the initial insult to the spinal cord, maintaining perfusion at the cellular level of the spinal cord, if possible, is important to protect the remaining living, healthy tissue, and possibly to improve recovery. Although numerous therapies have been suggested, none have been unequivocally demonstrated to reverse spinal cord injury, especially in complete lesions.

With unstable spinal column injuries, segmental motion must be minimized in order to prevent further trauma to the spinal cord. In these situations, even log rolling has been found to cause motion at the injured level. If possible, the patient should be maintained supine, in a roto-bed.

Certain drugs, such as epinephrine, produce vasoconstriction, which further compromises cord perfusion. If possible, these beta agonists should be avoided in an acute situation or where spinal cord injury is present. Other medications studied experimentally include corticosteroids, thyrotropin releasing hormone (opiate antagonist), and naloxone (opiate receptor blocker). Although beneficial effects have been demonstrated experimentally, clinical efficacy has yet to be proven.

Steroids

Steroids continue to be studied extensively. They are known to contribute to cellular membrane stabilization, to reduce edema, and to counteract sodium and potassium imbalance. A multicenter, randomized, double blind, placebo-controlled trial in patients with acute spinal cord injury used methylprednisolone as a bolus (30 mg/kg body weight) followed by infusion (5.4 mg/kg/hr) for 23 hours. Patients with an acute spinal cord injury treated within the first 8 hours following the accident appear to respond best. Improvement, however, did not always indicate a recovery to "motor function useful" and was often limited to sensory recovery, especially in the complete injury group. Those patients with complete spinal cord injury at presentation did not improve as predictably with this regimen. To better understand the effects of high-dose steroids in acute spinal cord injury, this study continues, using other forms of steroids.

Timing of Surgery

When a progressive neurologic deficit exists in the presence of malalignment and/or spinal canal compromise, emergency decompression is indicated. In all others with spinal cord injuries, the timing of surgery is controversial. Some authors recommend treatment as soon as the patient is medically stable, while others advocate a delay of 4 or more days to allow for posttraumatic swelling to resolve.

Whether early decompression and reduction of neural structures enhances neurologic recovery continues to be debated. Significant functional recovery has been observed as long as 20 years following anterior decompression of the spinal cord. Currently, a reasonable approach would be to treat nonprogressive neurologic deficits on a semiurgent basis, when the patient's systemic condition is medically stable.

History and Physical Examination

A complete and precise history of the patient's injury, in addition to the physical examination, is critical at the time of arrival to the hospital. The examination should include all systems and is repeated over time, to detect occult injuries. The patient is kept rigidly immobilized on a spine board until complete radiographic and physical examinations have been carried out.

A complete neurologic evaluation includes motor and sensory evaluation, as well as assessment of deep tendon and pathologic reflexes (Tables 1–3). The presence of sensory sparing should be documented, because it may indicate a better prognosis. Primitive reflexes, such as the bulbocavernosus reflex or anal wink, which are mediated by the sacral nerve roots, complete the neurologic examination. Their absence in the first 48 hours indicates that neurologic deficit may be related to spinal cord shock or contusion rather than to a complete and permanent spinal cord injury. This information is important prognostically. In the majority of cases, these reflexes return within 48 hours, whereupon complete absence of distal motor or

Table 1. Muscles affected by spinal cord injuries

Root Level	Key Muscles
C3, C4	Diaphragm
C5	Deltoid, elbow flexors, diaphragm
C6	Elbow flexors, wrist extensors
C7	Elbow extensors, wrist flexors
C8	Finger flexors (distal phalanx of middle finger)
T1	Finger abductors (5th digit), intrinsics of hand
T1–T12	Segmental innervation to intercostal muscles, abdominal and paraspinal muscles
(T12) L1, L2, L3	Hip flexors
L2, L3, L4	Quadriceps
L4	Tibialis anterior
L5	Toe extensors, hip abductors
S1	Ankle plantarflexors, peronei

(Reproduced with permission from Connolly P, Yuan HA: Cervical spine fractures, in *Spine Care: Diagnosis and Treatment,* in press.)

Table 2. Muscle grading chart

Grade	Muscle Action
0 = zero	Total paralysis
1 = trace	Visual or palpable contraction
2 = poor	Active movement, gravity eliminated
3 = fair	Active movement against gravity
4 = good	Active movement against resistance
5 = normal	Active movement against full resistance

(Reproduced with permission from Connolly P, Yuan HA: Cervical spine fractures, in *Spine Care: Diagnosis and Treatment,* in press.)

Table 3. Frankel grades

Grade	Function
A	Complete neurologic injury
B	Preserved sensation distal to level of injury
C	Preserved motor nonfunctional
D	Preserved motor functional
E	Normal

sensory function or perianal sensation indicates a complete spinal cord injury.

Imaging Studies

Standard anteroposterior (AP) and lateral radiographs should be obtained once the patient is medically stabilized. Further imaging depends on the need to better evaluate the fracture configuration. Oblique radiographs are sometimes, although rarely, helpful in visualizing facet and pedicle pathology. Flexion–extension views are rarely obtained in the acute situation.

The open-mouth AP view of the spine is essential for evaluation of the upper cervical spine. The standard AP views allow evaluation of lateral mass and sagittal plane fractures, widening of the interpedicular distance, or interlaminar and/or spinous process gaping. Lateral radiographs are an essential part of the evaluation; 85% of significant injuries will be detected with a lateral film (particularly in the cervical region). An injury at the cervicothoracic junction, however, may escape detection unless protocols require full visualization of the body of T1.

Computed tomography (CT) remains the standard for demonstrating fractures and canal compromise in thoracolumbar injuries. Benign appearing compression fractures on plain films should be assessed by CT scanning, particularly in cases associated with high-energy trauma. Other compression fractures diagnosed on a radiograph may, in reality, be burst fractures. Axial CT is excellent in demonstrating the degree of neural compromise and anterior and posterior element involvement. With new spiral CT technology, high-quality sagittal reconstructions that are almost comparable to tomograms are possible; these reconstructions allow detection of subtle, horizontally oriented injuries of the vertebral column. Additionally, CT enhanced by intrathecal metrizamide is superior to myelography in localizing soft-tissue compromise of the spinal cord. A high incidence of dural laceration occurs in patients who have a spinal cord injury and burst fracture associated with a laminar fracture at the same level on the CT scan.

MRI is possibly the best way to evaluate spinal soft tissues, as well as to evaluate the integrity of the disk and the extent of ligamentous disruption posteriorly. The presence of a spinal cord injury without obvious osseous or ligamentous injury may be differentiated on an MRI. However, an MRI may be difficult to obtain in certain situations, including acute trauma victims requiring mechanical ventilation or persons who have ferromagnetic implants or cardiac pacemakers. MRI does not, however, totally replace the CT scan of the spine, which provides greater bone detail and demonstrates fracture pattern and canal compromise from bone or alignment changes. Technetium bone scanning is occasionally helpful in ruling out occult injuries of the cervical spine in patients with prolonged symptoms and negative radiographs.

Cervical Spine Injuries

Classification of Spinal Cord Injury

Spinal cord injury can be broadly classified as complete and incomplete. The diagnosis of complete spinal cord injury cannot be made until spinal cord shock resolves. If the bulbocavernosus reflex is present and there is no motor or sensory function below the injury, by definition, the injury becomes complete. If, following the return of the bulbocavernosus reflex, the patient has some sensation below the level of injury, the injury is considered to be sensory incomplete. If the bulbocavernosus reflex has returned and the patient has some motion and sensation below the level of injury, the injury is sensory and motor incomplete.

There are four incomplete spinal cord injury syndromes (Fig. 1). The anterior cord syndrome is characterized by injury to the anterior horn cells opposite the area of spine injury. The mechanism of injury is usually a compression or flexion type injury. Clinically, there is paralysis or paresis of the upper limbs (all or portions). Deep pressure and position sense are usually preserved in the lower extremities, with no motor function below the area of injury. Anterior cord syndrome has the worst prognosis for recovery of the incomplete injury syndromes. Posterior cord syndrome is rare. In this injury, there is preservation of motor function with loss of sensory function below the level of injury. The central cord syndrome is common. The mechanism of injury is usually an extension injury that occurs in an older patient with a preexisting cervical spondylosis. Clinically, the patients have greater loss of function in the upper extremities than the lower extremities, with perianal sensation usually preserved. This relates to central cord damage directly affecting the cell bodies at the level of injury, with axon/tract compromise to the lower levels. Brown-Séquard syndrome is produced by a penetrating in-

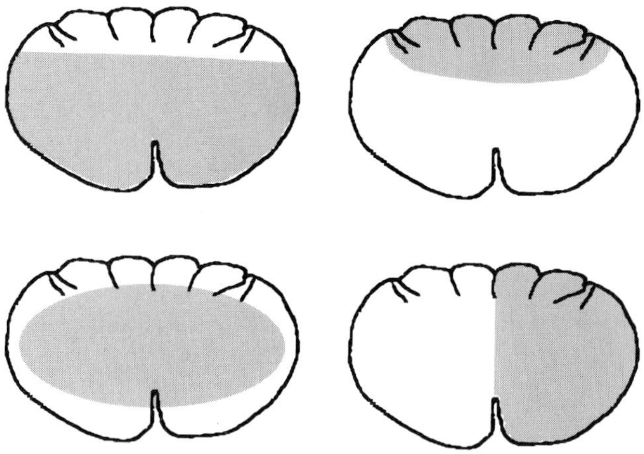

Fig. 1 The four incomplete spinal cord injury syndromes: Anterior cord syndrome (**top left**), posterior cord syndrome (**top right**), central cord syndrome (**bottom left**), and Brown-Séquard syndrome (**bottom right**).

jury to the lateral half of the cord. Motor paralysis is greater on the side of the injury, and sensory loss is greater contralateral to the side of the spinal cord injury. Patients with isolated nerve root injuries should be classified as having neurologic loss without spinal cord injury.

Mechanism of Injury

Most injuries can be classified on the basis of the mechanism of injury. It is important to obtain as much information as possible about the circumstances of the accident when evaluating the patient with a fracture and/or dislocation. Each fracture has a "personality" of its own. The major goal of any classification system is not necessarily to label every injury, but rather to provide the treating physician with a better understanding of the mechanism of specific injuries and to determine the pathologic anatomy based on the bony injury and the relative displacements seen on imaging studies.

Spinal Stabilization

The method of spinal stabilization depends on the personality of the bone and ligamentous damage as well as the abilities of the surgeon. The majority of patients with spinal cord injury are probably best treated with surgical stabilization. Patients who have been realigned with traction and do not have significant canal compromise are most often treated with posterior stabilization and fusion alone. The choice of Roger wire technique versus other wiring techniques or spinal plates affixed with screws is often determined by the number of levels involved and the status of the posterior elements. Generally speaking, simple facet dislocations can be treated with wiring alone. If there are concomitant significant facet fractures, lateral mass plates (not FDA approved for use in this manner) can be considered for greater rotational stability. For injuries that require an anterior decompression procedure, anterior bone grafting alone may not provide immediate stabilization, and the anterior cervical plate or additional posterior fixation is often required.

Role of Anterior Decompression

In upper cervical cord injury, realignment and stabilization of the spine is the most important aspect of treatment. Because of the space available for the cord following realignment, anterior decompression is rarely if ever indicated.

In the lower cervical spine, anterior decompression is indicated when anterior spinal cord compression persists following realignment. In the past, there was concern about further injury and destabilization by anterior procedures, but recent work has shown significant benefit for patients with both complete and incomplete quadriplegia. Although the exact timing of anterior decompression procedures is not entirely clear, recent laboratory and clinical investigations indicate that the effect of spinal cord compression is inversely related to the duration of compression. It appears that patients with both complete and incomplete spinal cord injury should undergo an imaging assessment following their initial stabilization and realignment. If significant anterior cord compression and significant neurologic deficit remain following realignment by traction, then an anterior decompression procedure should be considered to maximize both the recovery of cord function and, perhaps more frequently, root return.

Cervical Orthoses

In treating cervical spine injuries nonsurgically or postoperatively, the surgeon has the choice between a soft collar, a more rigid cervical orthosis, a cervical thoracic orthosis (CTO), and/or a halo vest. A soft collar restricts less than 10% of the total flexion–extension motion, whereas the CTO two-poster orthosis provides the greatest restriction of flexion–extension motion. The halo vest is the only orthosis that provides significant rotational control. Generally speaking, the halo device should be considered when treating highly unstable conditions of the cervical spine.

Atlanto-occipital Dislocation

This devastating injury usually results from high-speed accidents and is usually fatal. The majority of patients have an associated intracranial injury. The injury involves the ligaments that secure the cranium to the cervical spine. Hyperextension, rotation, and distraction are considered the most important mechanisms of injury.

Atlanto-occipital dislocations are classified into three specific types: anterior displacement of the occiput, longitudinal distraction, and posterior dislocations. Radiographically, displacement is determined by Wackenheim's line, which is a line that extends caudally along the posterior surface of the clivus. Normally, this line should be tangential to the posterior tip of the dens. If the occiput is displaced anteriorly, the line will intersect the dens. If the occiput is distracted or displaced posteriorly, the line will be separated from the tip of the dens.

Traction is contraindicated and a halo vest alone will not provide adequate stabilization. Early surgical intervention with posterior occipital cervical fixation and fusion is the treatment of choice.

Occipital Condyle Fractures

Patients are often unconscious following a motor vehicle accident or fall. This diagnosis requires a high index of suspicion. A type 1 occipital condyle fracture is an impaction injury secondary to axial loading. The diagnosis is confirmed by CT scan, which shows comminution of the occipital condyle with minimal displacement of fragments into the foramen magnum. A type 2 injury occurs as part of a basilar skull fracture; the mechanism of injury is a direct blow. The type 3 fracture is an avulsion injury secondary to either a rotation or lateral bending moment that causes the alar ligaments to avulse a portion of the occipital condyle. Types 1 and 2 are stable injuries and can be managed with a rigid cervical orthosis. The type 3 injury is potentially an unstable injury and requires halo immobilization and/or occipitocervical fusion.

Atlas (C1) Fractures

Fractures of the atlas generally are the result of an axial load injury. The C1 ring fracture, which may be isolated to the anterior arch, is felt to be secondary to an axial load with flexion force. Isolated posterior arch fractures are due to an extension force combined with the axial load. The classic Jefferson fracture is a four-part atlas fracture that can potentially be unstable. Stability is determined by measuring the spreading of the lateral masses on the open mouth AP radiograph. If the total radiographic excursion of the lateral masses is greater than 8 mm, the transverse ligament is most likely torn and the fractures deemed unstable.

Stable C1 fractures can be treated with a hard collar to allow bony healing. Unstable C1 fractures require initial treatment with halo vest immobilization for 8 weeks, which is usually followed by an additional 4 weeks in a Philadelphia collar.

Not all patients with stable C1 fractures heal by osseous union. They may develop a fibrous union. If they are asymptomatic, no further treatment is necessary. Patients with a fracture through the facet joint or a comminuted ring pattern are at a higher risk for nonunion, chronic neck pain, and spastic torticollis. These patients may benefit from posterior C1-C2 arthrodesis if they develop chronic pain. A patient that develops an unstable nonunion of C1 will require an occiput-C2 fusion.

C1-C2 Subluxation

Atlantoaxial instability without fracture is an uncommon injury. It is usually an anterior dislocation of the atlas on the axis, which indicates disruption of the transverse ligament. The diagnosis is confirmed by measurement of the atlantodens interval (ADI), which should not be greater than 3.0 mm in the adult or 4.0 mm in the child. Posterior atlantoaxial dislocation is extremely rare and indicates disruption of the apical and alar ligaments with maintenance of the transverse ligament.

These are both unstable injuries. The anterior C1-C2 instability is treated by reduction and posterior C1-C2 fusion. The rare posterior C1-C2 dislocation requires axial skeletal traction for reduction, and then a posterior C1-C2 fusion.

Odontoid Fractures

Fractures of the odontoid may occur with or without displacement. These fractures are most often the result of a flexion force causing anterior displacement of the odontoid process. Odontoid fractures with posterior displacement have a much higher incidence of neurologic injury and are caused by hyperextension force.

A type 1 injury is extremely uncommon. It is an oblique fracture at or above the transverse ligament. This fracture probably represents an avulsion injury in which the alar ligaments attach to the tip of the odontoid process. A type 2 fracture occurs at the junction of the odontoid process and the body of the second cervical vertebra. In the type 3 fracture, the fracture line extends downward into the cancellous portion of the vertebral body. The importance of this classification system is that it enables the prediction of outcomes of treatment. Type 1 fractures can be safely treated with a Philadelphia collar for 6 to 8 weeks. Type 3 odontoid fractures have an 85% to 90% union rate and most often can be successfully treated with a halo vest for 12 weeks. These fractures, however, are not benign lesions, and because they have a high rate of malunion in some series, careful alignment in the halo vest is necessary.

The blood supply to the odontoid is through cephalad and caudad vessels. The mid portion of the odontoid represents a watershed area. Therefore, there is a higher incidence of delayed union and nonunion in type 2 odontoid fractures. A nonunion rate of up to 60% has been reported for these fractures. Displacement greater than 4 mm, angulation greater than 10°, and age greater than 40 years contribute to a higher rate of nonunion.

A significant number of type 2 odontoid fractures will heal with halo vest immobilization if the surgeon is able to obtain and maintain anatomic alignment and avoid overdistraction in the halo vest. Primary posterior C1-C2 fusions or anterior screw fixation are surgical alternatives for treating patients at high risk for nonunion.

Anterior screw fixation of the odontoid process has the advantage of decreasing the nonunion rate while theoretically preserving atlantoaxial rotation. Although this technique was initially used in the treatment of odontoid nonunions, it is currently used to treat type 2 and "shallow" type 3 odontoid fractures. The procedure has a number of relative contraindications, it is technically demanding, and there are a number of potentially serious complications.

However, odontoid screw fixation allows for preservation of atlantoaxial motion and may have an increased union rate over posterior fusion procedures.

Pedicle Fractures of C2 (Hangman's Fracture)

Traumatic spondylolisthesis of the axis (C2) is caused by a hyperextension force in which the occiput is forced into extension against the atlas, producing a fracture of the C2 pedicles. If a flexion component is added to the injury, there may be disruption of disks and ligaments causing a forward subluxation of C2 on C3. A type 1 injury is secondary to hyperextension and axial loading and includes all nondisplaced hangman's fractures as well as all fractures that have no angulation and less than 3 mm of displacement of C2 on C3. Type 2 injuries are due to hyperextension and axial loading and have significant angulation and translation. The type 2A hangman's fracture is caused by flexion as well as posterior distraction force; these fractures have minimal anterior translation but they have severe angulation and appear to be hinging from the anterior longitudinal ligament. Type 3 injuries are secondary to a flexion as well as a posterior distraction force. They have both severe angulation and displacement along with a unilateral or bilateral C2–C3 facet dislocation.

Unlike the type 1 and 2 hangman's fractures, the atypical hangman's fracture (Fig. 2) occurs through the posterior aspect of the vertebral body. The atypical hangman's fracture produces canal compromise and is associated with a much higher rate of neurologic injury than the other forms of C2 traumatic spondylolisthesis.

The traumatic C2 spondylolisthesis can be successfully treated with initial traction for reduction and then halo immobilization. Because there often is an increase in deformity with traction of the type 2 injury, it is best treated with reduction under fluoroscopy followed by halo vest immobilization. The type 3 hangman's fracture usually requires open reduction of the unilateral and/or bilateral facet dislocation and fusion at this level.

Anterior Wedge Compression Fractures

Anterior wedge compression fractures occur most often at the C4-C5 and C5-C6 levels. The wedge is formed by depression of the superior end plate. The degree of depression depends on the severity of the forces. These injuries can be subtle; if the anterior height of the vertebral body is 3 mm or greater than the posterior height, a fracture should be suspected. These fractures do not involve compromise of the spinal canal but there is a risk of posttraumatic kyphotic deformity. Treatment consists of a rigid cervical orthosis for 8 to 12 weeks.

Fractures of the Vertebral Body With Canal Compromise

Fractures with marked anterior wedging or comminution of the vertebral body are often associated with canal compromise and neurologic injury. These injuries are caused by compression–flexion or vertical compression forces. Before deciding on appropriate treatment for these fractures, the surgeon must know the patient's neurologic status, the amount of canal compromise, and the status of the posterior elements.

Patients with neurologic deficit and significant canal compromise may benefit from anterior corpectomy and strut graft reconstruction. If the patient has no disruption of the posterior elements, then an anterior strut graft supported by an anterior cervical plate is usually sufficient. If the patient has posterior element injury, then supplemental posterior fusion and instrumentation should be considered. If patients with cervical burst fractures are treated with anterior strut graft alone without supplemental pos-

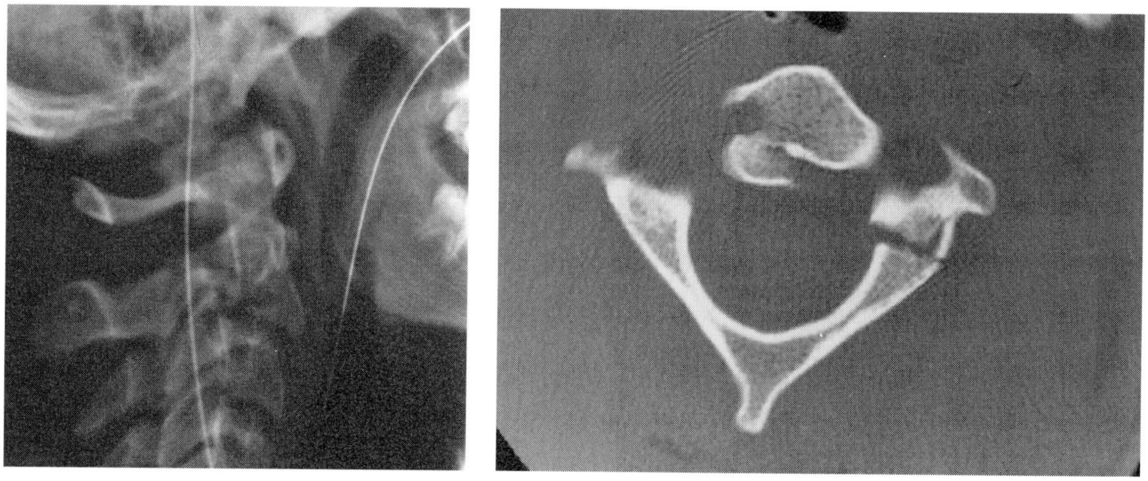

Fig. 2 **Left,** Lateral cervical spine radiograph of patient with atypical hangman's fracture. **Right,** Computed tomography scan of fracture. Patient was neurologically intact. Patient healed with 12 weeks of halo immobilization.

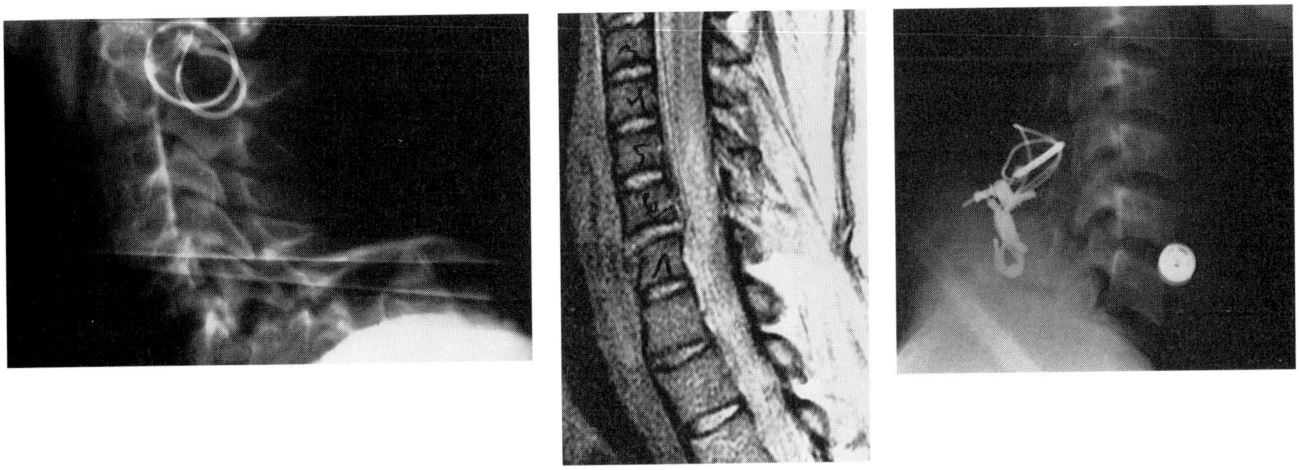

Fig. 3 **Left,** Distraction flexion injury with complete dislocation of C6–C7 and C6 quadriplegia. **Center,** Sagittal magnetic resonance imaging scan following closed reduction with halo skeletal traction. **Right,** Lateral radiograph following posterior stabilization and fusion C5 to C7 using Dewar technique.

terior stabilization and fusion or anterior cervical plate fixation, there is an increased risk of graft displacement or settling with development of a late kyphotic deformity.

Facet Joint Injuries

Injuries to the facet joints of the cervical spine are among the most common injury patterns seen in patients with cervical spine injury. They are often associated with motor vehicle accidents or falls from heights, and the injury is usually at the C5–C6 or C6–C7 level. The mechanism is that of distractive flexion. The injuries include facet joint subluxation, perched facets, unilateral facet dislocation, bilateral facet dislocation, and facet subluxation/dislocation associated with facet fracture. These injuries are often associated with neurologic deficit in the form of nerve root and/or spinal cord injury. These injuries are best treated with closed reduction via halo skeletal traction followed by posterior stabilization and fusion (Fig. 3).

Recent reports of catastrophic neurologic damage following closed reductions have brought this classic approach to the treatment of this injury into question. This injury pattern almost always involves some injury to the disk, and the issue of whether all patients should have an MRI prior to attempt at reduction has not been totally resolved. If the patient is awake and alert, it is reasonable to attempt closed reduction via skeletal traction before MRI. However, if closed reduction cannot be obtained, before the patient goes to the operating room for reduction and stabilization, an MRI should be obtained. If a large protruding disk is noted, an anterior approach for diskectomy, reduction, anterior fusion, and plate stabilization should be performed.

Following reduction of the facet dislocation, surgical treatment is posterior stabilization and fusion using wiring techniques or posterior cervical plates. These injuries can be treated with halo immobilization without surgical intervention, but run the risk of upwards of 60% loss of reduction as well as potential long-term instability and pain. Associated facet fractures need to be addressed at the time of surgery. They often require a limited foraminotomy for removal of bony fragments. Ignoring these facet fragments can lead to chronic nerve root irritation.

Fractures of the Posterior Elements

These injuries occur most often from motor vehicle accidents or falls and are associated with injuries to the upper cervical spine. The mechanism of injury is a compressive or a distractive extension injury. One or more levels may be involved. These injuries are treated with 8 to 12 weeks of rigid cervical immobilization. The more severe fractures involve injury to the disk and have a tendency toward delayed forward subluxation. For this reason, they should be observed carefully during nonsurgical treatment.

Lateral Mass Fracture

The floating lateral mass fracture involves a pedicle fracture and an ipsilateral lamina fracture, which cause a complete detachment of the entire lateral mass from the vertebral body. This fracture pattern may be isolated, as a result of a lateral flexion type of injury, or may be a component of a more severe hyperextension injury. Treatment consists of a rigid cervical orthosis for 8 to 12 weeks. If there is an associated disk injury or anterior column disruption, there is a tendency for forward subluxation, and surgical stabilization may be indicated. The presence of nerve root compression may suggest the need for a limited posterior foraminotomy and posterior fusion.

Posterior Element Fracture Associated With Vertebral Body Dislocation

This is the most severe form of the compressive extension injuries and should not be confused with fracture-dislocation associated with facet dislocation. It involves a fracture of the vertebral arch along with anterior displacement of the vertebral body. This injury is quite unstable and is best treated with both anterior and posterior stabilization.

Hyperextension Injuries of the Cervical Spine

The mechanism of injury is one of distractive extension and is associated with blows to the head and face. The milder form is the teardrop avulsion fracture, which is a small bony avulsion off the anteroinferior portion of the vertebral body. Patients with this injury can be treated with a rigid cervical orthosis for 8 weeks. If the injury force is severe enough, there can be a posterior dislocation of the vertebral body up to 25%. This dislocation is a very unstable injury that is best treated with reduction and anterior cervical fusion with anterior plate stabilization.

Transient Quadriplegia

This syndrome of neurapraxia of the cervical spinal cord is seen clinically after an athlete has sustained a forced hyperextension, hyperflexion, or axial load injury to the cervical spine. This syndrome manifests as a bilateral burning paresthesia associated with varying degrees of bilateral extremity weakness or paralysis. It is associated with developmental stenosis of the cervical spine, congenital fusion, cervical instability, or cervical disk protrusion. The ratio of the spinal canal size to vertebral body size (torg ratio = canal size/vertebral body size) is sensitive in detecting significant stenosis (torg ratio of 0.8 or less) of the cervical spine, but unfortunately has a low positive predictive value and, therefore, cannot be relied on as a screening method for the diagnosis of cervical spinal stenosis.

Currently, there is no evidence that the occurrence of neurapraxia of the cervical spinal cord predisposes an individual to permanent neurologic injury. Patients who have associated instability of the cervical spine or acute or chronic degenerative changes should, however, be precluded from further participation in contact sports.

Thoracic, Thoracolumbar, and Lumbar Spine Injuries

Mechanisms of Injury

Although there are often complex forces occurring at the time of injury to the spine, only a few account for most bone and/or ligamentous damage. The forces most commonly associated with thoracolumbar injuries include axial compression, flexion, lateral compression, flexion–rotation, shear, flexion–distraction, and extension.

Axial Compression In the presence of thoracic kyphosis, an axial compression load in the thoracic spine will usually result in an anterior flexion load to the vertebral body. Lower in the thoracolumbar region, a similar load results in a more uniform compression of the vertebra(e). The resulting injury may be end-plate failure followed by a vertebral-body compression (wedge fracture). As force increases, fractures occur through the vertebral body, producing a burst injury. When there is even more loading, centripetal displacement of the bone occurs, often with disk fragmentation and posterior disruption. If the force is centripetal, fractures at the pedicle–vertebral body junction result in widening of the interpedicular distance and, often, in fracture of the lamina. With an additional flexion component, there may be significant posterior element disruption.

Flexion Flexion forces cause anterior compression and posterior tension. With rapid loading rates, the posterior ligaments usually do not fail immediately, but posterior avulsion fractures may develop. Anteriorly, as the bone fails and angulation increases, the force is dissipated. If the posterior ligaments remain intact, a stable fracture configuration most often results. If anterior wedging is excessive, usually more than 50%, the posterior ligament may also fail, leading to late instability.

Lateral Compression Lateral compression force creates damage similar to that caused by anterior wedge compression, except that the force is applied laterally. The resultant deformity is asymmetric, involving compression on one side and, with severe forces, ligament failure on the contralateral side. This combination may lead to a chronically unstable and painful deformity that develops into a focal scoliosis.

Flexion–Rotation This combination of forces produces an injury similar to that described for pure flexion; however, the addition of rotational forces leads to failure of the ligaments and facet capsules, with disruption of both anterior and posterior columns as rotation increases (shear injuries). In the thoracic or lumbar spine, pure dislocations are rare because the size and orientation of the posterior facets require a high degree of flexion for dislocations to occur. Fracture dislocations indicate a grossly unstable injury.

Flexion–Distraction Flexion–distraction forces across the thoracolumbar spine often produce the typical seat belt injury. The axis of flexion is moved anteriorly, close to the anterior abdominal wall, leading to significant tensile force distribution through the posterior elements, as well as anteriorly through the vertebral bodies and/or disks. If the axis of rotation is moved posteriorly into the vertebral body, it is possible to have associated compressive forces across the vertebral body. Thus, compression fractures that are components of a more significant flexion–distraction lesion may be deceptively unstable injuries.

These forces can produce a pure osseous lesion, a mixed osteoligamentous lesion, or pure soft-tissue damage. Osseous injuries often heal with solid bony union, whereas pure ligamentous and mixed lesions are at risk for late instability and pain.

Extension With the head or upper trunk thrust posteriorly, extension forces are created. This produces a pattern that is the reverse of that of pure flexion. Tension is applied anteriorly to the anterior longitudinal ligaments and anterior portion of the disk, while compression forces are transmitted to the posterior elements. Fractures (compression) of the posterior elements may result, and avulsion fractures of the anteroinferior portions of the vertebral bodies may occur.

Spinal Stability

The concept of thoracolumbar stability following traumatic injury continues to evolve. Initially, the posterior ligamentous complex was thought to be the major determinant of spinal stability. Only fracture dislocations and severe shear injuries with complete disruption of the posterior ligamentous complex were thought to be unstable; most others were thought to be stable. Later, as various ideas were merged, a two-column (anterior and posterior) concept of spinal stability was proposed. The destruction of either of these columns would be enough to produce instability. This model helped to explain the chronic instability often seen after spine injuries, particularly those resulting in a kyphotic deformity. It fell short, however, of fully explaining acute unstable fracture patterns.

With the advent of CT, Denis defined a three-column system, which allows a better understanding of acute unstable patterns. In this classification system, the posterior column is composed of the posterior elements including the spinous process, laminae, facets, and pedicles, as well as posterior ligamentous structures. The middle column is composed of the posterior aspects of the vertebral body, the posterior anulus fibrosis, and posterior longitudinal ligament. The anterior column includes the anterior longitudinal ligament, the anterior anulus fibrosis, and the anterior vertebral body. This classification, although useful in defining vertebral column instability, does not include the neural elements, which should not be ignored when considering segmental stability.

Denis proposed four categories based on the presence and type of instability. Stable injuries include minimal and moderate compression fractures associated with an intact posterior column. Injuries associated with mechanical instability include those in which two of the three columns are injured, for example, a flexion–distraction injury with disruption of the posterior and middle columns. A third category refers specifically to a burst fracture that is potentially neurologically unstable as a result of middle column failure and protrusion of bone into the spinal canal. Finally, mechanical and neurologic instability may be seen following a fracture dislocation with disruption of all three columns and either a neurologic deficit or an impending neurologic deterioration. Although some believe that the integrity of the middle column is the key anatomic determinant of stability, this belief is not universally accepted. Therefore, other classifications have been described, but they will not be discussed here.

Decompression

Decompression of the neural elements can be achieved directly by an anterior or posterolateral approach or indirectly with the use of posterior instrumentation. The indirect method usually depends on distraction instrumentation, ideally using three- or four-point bending forces to realign the spine. Contouring the rods or adding sleeves to the distraction rods provides an anterior force across the fracture, which may improve reduction of the retropulsed bone from the canal. The reduction of the fragment causing compression of the spinal cord depends on minimal comminution and limited rotation of the fragments, as well as a relatively intact anulus fibrosis, which when stretched, pulls the bone out of the canal. If there is significant comminution or rotation, the surgeon may need to depend on alternative methods of decompression.

A posterolateral decompression may be performed through a posterior midline incision. The reduction of the fragment(s) is accomplished through a laminectomy with the help of an initial reduction using contralateral hooks and rods. Removal of parts of the pedicle may be necessary to gain access to the fragments. With angled instruments, the fragments of bone can be impacted back into the vertebral body. Promising results have been shown using this technique; however, greater caution must be exercised when performing posterolateral decompressions above the thoracolumbar junction where less room is available for the spinal cord.

The extent of decompression is difficult to assess intraoperatively from the posterior aspect. Intraoperative ultrasonography has been shown to be beneficial in demonstrating the extent of decompression. This procedure uses a sterile transducer head and requires creation of a laminotomy. Intraoperative myelography has been used in the past, but is less commonly used today because of its lack of resolution.

The most direct approach for decompression is anterior. This technique allows for complete removal of bone from the spinal canal. It is particularly useful in spinal column injuries treated after a delay of more than 2 to 3 weeks in which posterior instrumentation alone would be of limited benefit to realign the fracture or allow for indirect decompression of the spinal cord. The use of modern facilities has minimized the potential morbidity of this approach. Modern anterior internal fixation devices have been developed and others are currently being developed that can be used to rigidly stabilize the spine through the anterior column, thus avoiding further additional posterior surgery. However, if there is extensive damage of the posterior elements, further posterior stabilization surgery

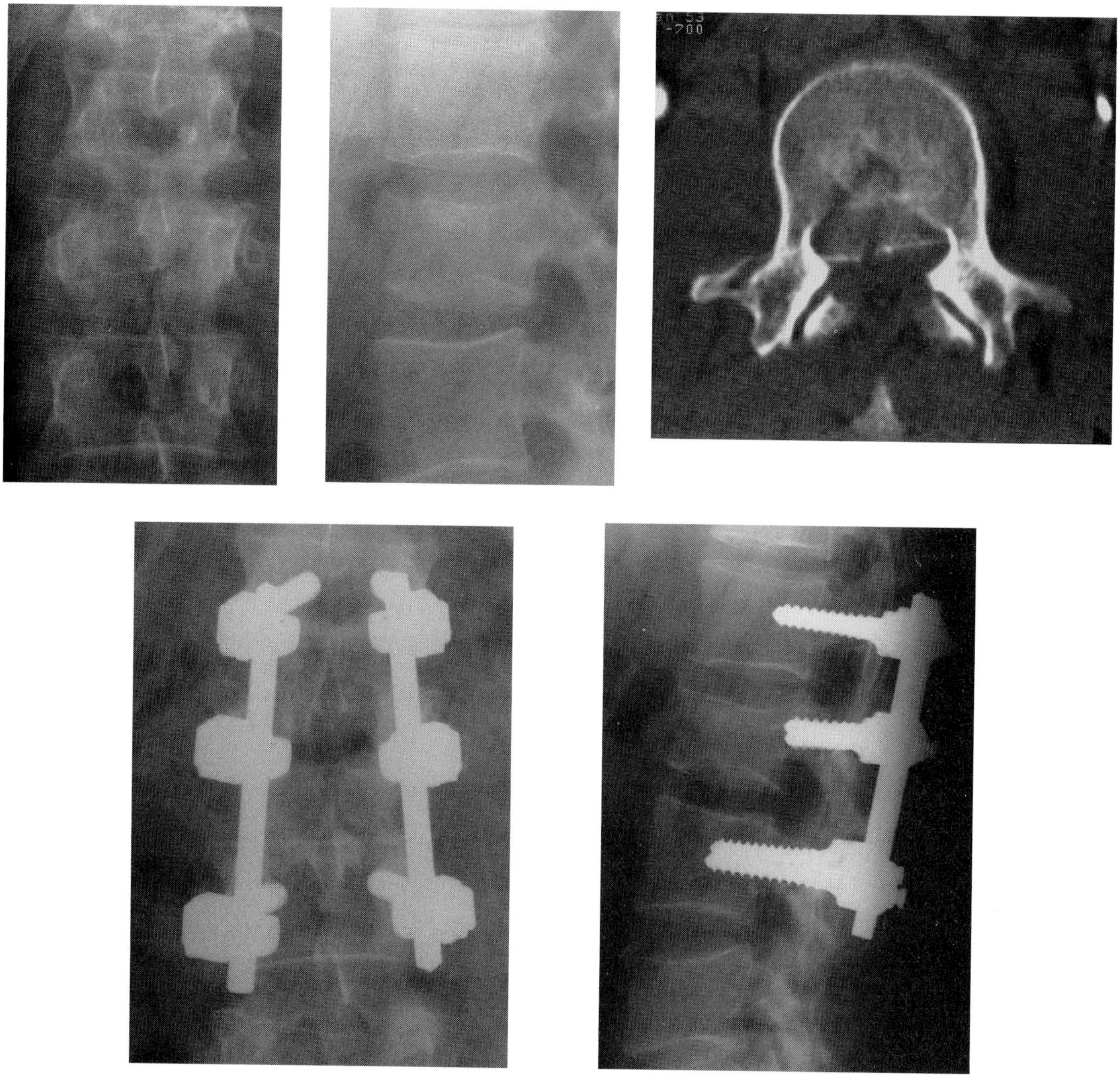

Fig. 4 **Top left,** Anteroposterior lumbar radiograph of a 37-year-old male who became paraparetic with this burst fracture of L2. Collapse of the L2 vertebral body and widening of the interarticular distance as compared to the level above and below can be seen. A laminar fracture of L2 is also present. **Top center,** Lateral radiograph showing collapse of the L2 vertebral body. Note the rotation of the posterior superior corner at the level of the pedicle leading to the intracanal fragment. **Top right,** Computed tomography scan through the body of L2 at the level of the pedicles. There are large retropulsed fragments causing severe canal narrowing. **Bottom,** At surgery, this patient initially had unilateral distraction rodding on the right side with a posterior lateral decompression performed through a laminectomy site. A pedicle screw fixation device was placed on the opposite side from the distraction rodding. The latter was subsequently removed and replaced with a rigid segmental pedicle screw and rod system. Note the restoration of lordosis on the lateral radiograph with the reduction of the posterior superior corner at L2.

may be required, even in the presence of anterior instrumentation.

Laminectomy alone has been shown repeatedly to be ineffective in decompressing the spinal cord or cauda equina after anterior pathology and often leads to increased late deformity, pain, and further neurologic demise. If, after posterior instrumentation and/or posterolateral decompression, significant bone remains within the spinal canal, particularly in the presence of neurologic symptoms, an anterior decompression and fusion may be performed.

Treatment of Specific Injuries

Compression Fractures By definition, compression fractures include disruption of the anterior column with an intact middle column. The treatment of these injuries depends on the status of the posterior elements. If the anterior column is compressed 40% or more, or if kyphosis exceeds 30°, it is probable that the posterior ligaments are either attenuated or disrupted.

Nonsurgical treatment is preferred in those compression fractures with less than 40% anterior compression and less than 30° kyphosis. A hyperextension brace or thoracolumbosacral orthosis (TLSO) is effective in restricting motion while the injury heals and is worn for approximately 3 months.

Initial surgical treatment may be recommended if the anterior column is compressed more than 40% or kyphosis exceeds 30°. A posterior surgical approach is usually effective. A distraction system can be used with three-point fixation (eg, contoured distraction rods or a rod and sleeve system). If the middle column is intact, a compression system could be used, but overcompression must be avoided to prevent posterior protrusion of an already injured disk leading to possible neurologic deterioration.

Burst Fractures Effective management of burst fractures depends on the extent of spinal canal compromise, the degree of angulation present at the site of injury, and the presence or absence of a neurologic deficit. By definition, every burst fracture includes disruption of the anterior and middle columns and possibly the posterior column (Fig. 4). If angulation is minimal, with less than 40% canal compromise and an absence of a neurologic deficit, these patients may be treated in a total contact orthosis such as a TLSO following a brief period of bed rest. It is possible for intracanal fragments to gradually resorb after fracture healing. Resorption depends on the fragment size, position, and amount of comminution.

In those patients with greater than 40% to 50% canal compromise, significant kyphosis, and/or neurologic deficit, surgery appears to be a preferable alternative. Most stabilization procedures can be carried out from a posterior approach using a system allowing for distraction and three- or four-point fixation. Adequate canal decompression can often be achieved posteriorly with distraction instrumentation with or without posterolateral decompression. Intraoperative ultrasound may be useful in assessing the extent of canal clearance. Alternatively, a repeat CT scan can be performed following surgery to determine the adequacy of canal decompression. If significant neural compression remains, especially in the presence of a neurologic deficit, a second-stage anterior procedure can be performed. Radiologic decompression following surgery does not always correlate with neurologic outcome.

Low lumbar injuries present a unique problem. Because of the large disks and lordosis, the facet joints and disks support high physiologic loads. Long-term pain and deformity are significant considerations in treating these injuries. Attempts must be made to restore both vertebral height and lordosis (Fig. 5). Conventional hook-rod instrumentation systems often lead to flat-back deformities, if the hooks can even be inserted at L4 or caudally. Hook fixation in the low lumbar spine (L4 and L5) and sacrum has a 5% and 20% failure rate, respectively. In the mid and low lumbar spine, devices that offer the ability to instrument only one to two levels above and one below the level of injury are more desirable. Posterior distraction instrumentation with hooks should be avoided, if possible, below L3 to avoid creating or exacerbating sagittal plane imbalance (kyphosis). It is preferable to use pedicle screw systems at these levels.

Anterior decompression and fusion may be performed to treat burst fractures in those patients with significant neural compression and neurologic deficits, particularly if a minimal kyphotic deformity exists. This procedure should be routinely considered if the injury occurred 2 or more weeks earlier. It assures adequate neural decompression. With the use of current anterior instrumentation, correction of deformity and decompression and stabilization are possible. Alternatively, anterior decompression and strut grafting can be followed by posterior compression instrumentation to help lock the graft in the position and stabilize and realign the spine.

Laminectomy by itself is never indicated in the treatment of burst fractures. It does not relieve the anterior neural compression and further destabilizes the spine, possibly contributing to further neurologic demise.

Flexion–Distraction Injuries Flexion–distraction injuries can occur through bone, soft tissue, or a combination of both. The decision for nonsurgical treatment depends primarily on whether the injury is completely through bone, as originally described by Chance, or whether it also involves significant soft-tissue (ligament and/or disk) injuries. A Chance fracture extending only through bone has an excellent prognosis for healing. Injuries with significant ligamentous disruption tend to heal in a less predictable fashion and should be considered unstable, both acutely and long-term.

Nonsurgical treatment when injury occurs through bone may consist of bed rest followed by immobilization in an extension cast or a total contact TLSO or body cast in hyperextension. Frequent follow-up radiographs should be taken in a standing position in order to rule out progressive deformity. After 3 or 4 months, flexion–extension radiographs are obtained with the patient out of the brace to assess for excessive motion. Late surgical treatment may be performed in the presence of instability.

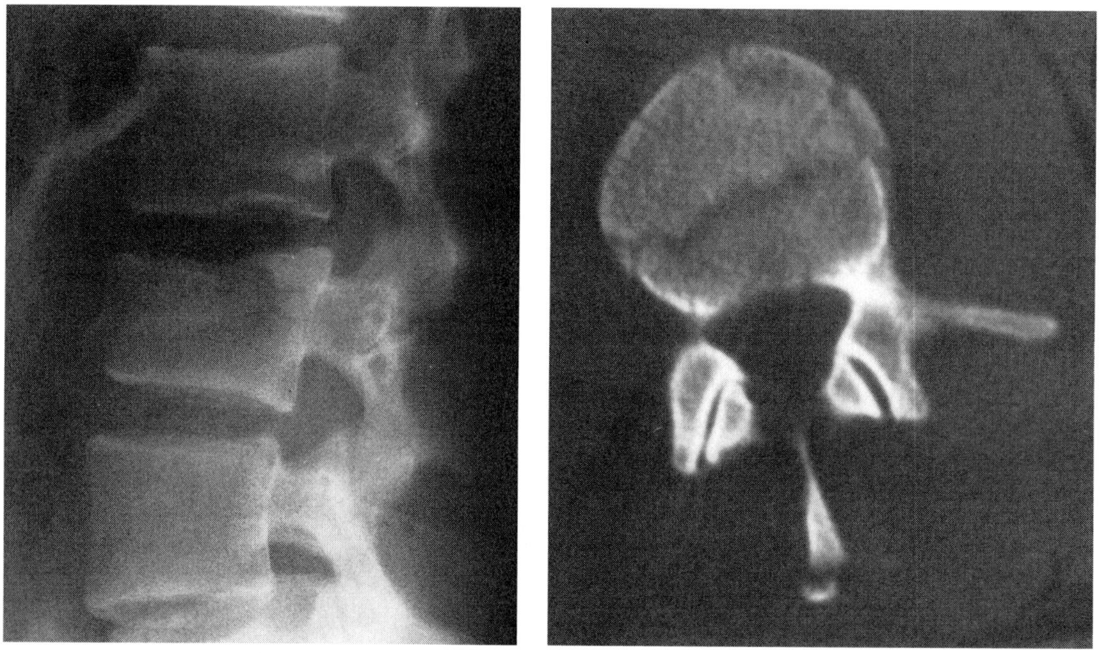

Fig. 5 **Left,** Lateral radiograph of a 19-year-old male with collapse of the anterior portion of the vertebral body of L3 and lumbar kyphosis at the injured level. **Right,** Computed tomography scan through L3 demonstrates extensive comminution extending to the posterior vertebral cortex, although minimal collapse of the middle column was apparent on the lateral radiograph. Restoration of lordosis is important for a good long-term outcome when treating these injuries with either a brace, a cast, or surgery.

Early surgical intervention using posterior compression instrumentation should be considered in the presence of significant ligamentous disruption. This instrumentation often needs to extend only one level above and below the posterior element disruption (Fig. 6).

Fracture-Dislocations Fracture-dislocations have the highest incidence of neurologic deficit. The majority of patients with these injuries require surgical treatment. When there is no neurologic deficit, surgery is performed to stabilize the spine and prevent the occurrence of neurologic injury by allowing for early mobilization. In the presence of a neurologic deficit, surgery is performed to stabilize the spine and to decompress the neural elements if there is an incomplete spinal cord injury. This surgery allows for earlier mobilization and a shortened hospital stay, and it hastens the patient's potential for rehabilitation. Rigid fixation also reduces the need for prolonged external immobilization postoperatively. These injuries are usually treated using a rigid segmental instrumentation device via the posterior approach. There is rarely a role for primary acute anterior decompression in fracture-dislocations because the main problem in these injuries is usually pain, significant motion segment instability, and gross malalignment. Realignment by itself frequently decompresses the compromised neural elements. An anterior decompression may be used in conjunction with posterior instrumentation if an adequate decompression cannot be achieved from reduction of the fracture-dislocation. This step is especially important in a patient with a partial neurologic deficit.

Minor Fractures Fractures of the transverse processes usually occur from direct trauma or as a result of a violent muscular contraction in response to injury. Similarly, isolated fractures of the spinous processes may occur as a result of a direct blow, as may a fracture of an articular process. Further evaluation is necessary to make sure that there are no associated spine injuries. This is easily accomplished using a CT scan or AP and lateral tomograms through the vertebrae in question, as well as the adjacent vertebral column. If the CT scan and/or tomograms are negative, then flexion–extension radiographs should be obtained to make sure that there is no dynamic instability. Usually, these patients can be mobilized with no special brace or activity restrictions other than those needed for symptomatic relief.

A fracture of the pars interarticularis in the thoracolumbar or upper lumbar spine is often seen in combination with a history of severe trauma, which suggests a major injury, such as a seat belt injury. CT scans and tomograms may be useful to visualize these injuries, which may be missed on plain films, and to differentiate acute from chronic injuries. In the case of an isolated, unilateral injury, a total contact TLSO is appropriate treatment.

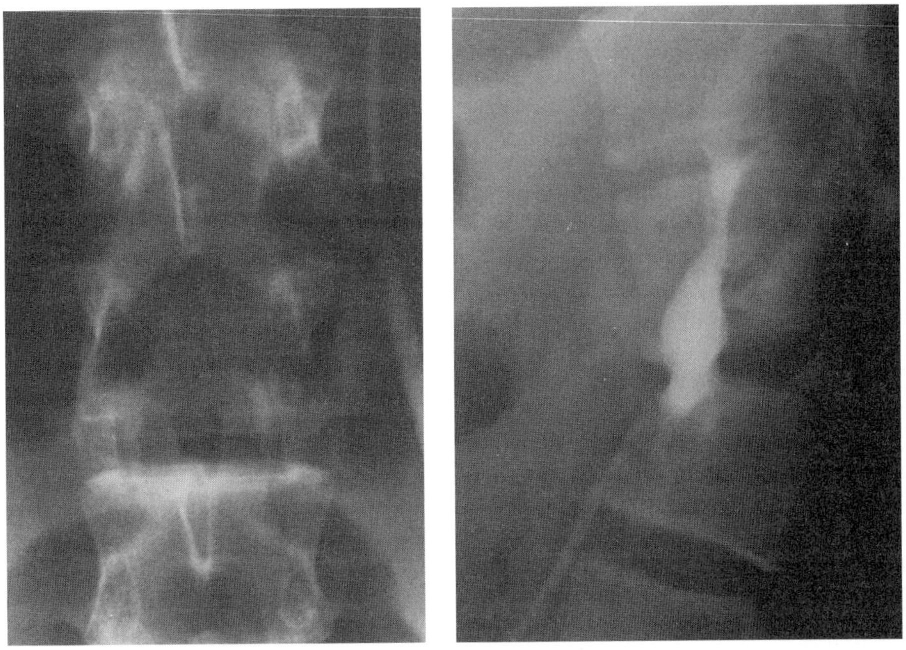

Fig. 6 **Left,** Anteroposterior radiograph of a 15-year-old female who sustained a flexion–distraction injury at L2–L3. She was neurologically intact. Note the significant interspinous process widening as well as fractures through both pedicles. **Right,** Lateral radiograph highlighting the flexion–distraction nature of this injury, with distraction through the pedicles of L2. There is minimal compression of the anterosuperior corner of the body of L2. Severe kyphosis through the injured level is also apparent. Residual dye from the intravenous pyelogram overlies the injured level. Open reduction was necessary to restore the sagittal alignment using compression molding across the injured level.

Gunshot Wounds In the past two decades, most authors reporting on civilian gunshot wounds to the thoracic or thoracolumbar spine have recommended avoidance of surgery regardless of associated neurologic injury. However, in the presence of progressive neurologic deterioration and with proven neural compression by bone, disk, or bullet fragments and/or hematoma, surgical decompression is indicated. Additionally, gunshot wounds that perforate the colon and then transverse the spine should be treated with surgical debridement and/or with coverage by broad spectrum parenteral antibiotics for the organisms discovered at the time of intestine repair. Because ligaments are often spared in civilian gunshot wounds, most of these patients can be mobilized immediately, using either no brace or occasionally a total contact orthosis, if significant damage to one to two columns is apparent.

Osteoporotic Compression Fractures

One of the most frequent areas for manifestation of osteoporosis is in the spinal column. Osteoporosis occurs in elderly people and younger, postmenopausal (naturally or surgically/medically induced) females. Most often it is detected radiographically; it is frequently asymptomatic. Subtle compression fractures can occur without the patient being aware of the fracture or complaining of episodes of severe, increasing pain. Osteoporosis affects 15 to 20 million people in the United States.

Patients (most often elderly) may come to the orthopaedist complaining of severe pain and/or the patients or their families may note an increasing back roundness or deformity. Radiographs may demonstrate a compression fracture, which may progress over time. Fortunately, most of these osteoporotic vertebral compression fractures, even with a burst component, do not lead to neurologic dysfunction. The acute pain can last weeks to months, but usually subsides over time.

Spine fractures may occur during normal activity, as well as from minimal to moderate trauma. Acute spine fractures can be associated with severe pain. Usually, the pain distribution is over the affected area. It does not typically radiate down the legs. Leg symptoms could suggest involvement of the spinal cord or cauda equina following collapse of the vertebral body, either acutely or chronically, with spinal canal compromise. Although the acute pain usually improves as the fracture heals, patients may have chronic complaints of pain, either at the fracture site or below.

In the thoracic spine, the fracture configuration typically takes on a wedge shape appearance due to the normal kyphosis of this region and the concentration of forces to the anterior aspect of the vertebrae. In contrast, in the lumbar region, the forces are distributed more equally throughout the vertebral body, creating a compression or possibly burst type injury of the vertebrae. This injury may occur either acutely or progressively over time.

The differential diagnosis of all osteoporotic compression fractures includes tumors, metastatic disease, and/or infection. The initial workup should include a medical examination to ensure there are no underlying medical conditions leading to the fracture or the osteoporosis and laboratory studies that include complete blood count with differential, erythrocyte sedimentation rate, chemistry panel with calcium and phosphorus, renal, liver, and thyroid function, serum protein electrophoresis (for evaluation of myeloma), and a urinalysis. Additionally, a CT scan may be helpful in separating malignant disease from an osteoporotic fracture, as well as determining the amount of retropulsed bone within the canal. The latter, however, does not by itself suggest the need for surgical intervention.

The treatment, in general, is directed toward the symptoms. If the patient is asymptomatic at the time of detection of the fracture, the treatment involves appropriate medications for osteoporosis and an attempt to institute low impact loading and/or aerobic exercises to help increase the stresses applied to the bone. If the patient has deformity and acute pain, a balance must be reached between rest (to reduce the pain) and activity (to decrease ongoing osteoporosis that would occur with bed rest). External bracing is helpful to reduce the pain, but rigid orthotics are often poorly tolerated by elderly patients. Therefore, soft braces, such as corsets, or semirigid orthotics, such as a Jewett brace or dorsolumbar corset, are better tolerated and provide some relief while maintaining the patients in a semiactive condition. Analgesic medication is often necessary, and a discussion with the patient and the family of the importance of at least limited activity, as opposed to strict bed rest, is helpful.

Occasionally, neurologic deficits do occur. These can include leg pain or symptoms related to bowel or bladder dysfunction. Although the injury is acute, the bone is often too soft to support posterior instrumentation. In general, because of the acute deformity and bone retropulsion, anterior decompressions and strut fusions are more useful and direct. If anterior instrumentation can be inserted at this time to support and supplement the graft, that step is helpful. If not, and the bone is soft, posterior instrumentation either through bone screws placed in the pedicle or a claw type configuration with laminar hooks may be used to supplement and support the fusion. Surgical intervention, however, is rarely necessary.

Annotated Bibliography

Cervical Spine

Anderson PA, Bohlman HH: Anterior decompression and arthrodesis of the cervical spine: Long-term motor improvement: Part II. Improvement in complete traumatic quadriplegia. *J Bone Joint Surg* 1992;74A:683–692.

The authors demonstrated long-term improvement of motor root function in 31 of the 51 patients who underwent anterior decompression following complete traumatic quadriplegia. They conclude that patients with traumatic quadriplegia, who continue to have a compressive lesion from displaced fragments of bone or disk, should undergo an anterior decompression procedure to maximize root return.

Bohlman HH, Anderson PA: Anterior decompression and arthrodesis of the cervical spine: Long-term motor improvement: Part I. Improvement in incomplete traumatic quadriparesis. *J Bone Joint Surg* 1992;74A: 671–682.

Twenty-nine of 58 patients with incomplete traumatic quadriparesis became functional ambulators following anterior decompression. No patients lost neurologic function. Improvement is best when the procedure is done within 12 months from injury.

Bracken MB, Shepard MJ, Collins WF, et al: A randomized, controlled trial of methylprednisolone or naloxone in the treatment of acute spinal-cord injury: Results of the Second National Acute Spinal Cord Injury Study. *N Engl J Med* 1990;322:1405–1411.

This multi-center study demonstrated the improvement of neurologic recovery following the use of high dose methylprednisolone.

Eismont FJ, Arena MJ, Green BA: Extrusion of an intervertebral disc associated with traumatic subluxation or dislocation of cervical facets: Case report. *J Bone Joint Surg* 1991;73A:1555–1560.

The authors discuss potential catastrophic results from doing closed reductions under general anesthetic for dislocated cervical facet fractures. The article raises the question of the role of preoperative MRI in evaluation of patients with facet dislocations. None of the patients in this small series had increasing neurologic deficit secondary to reduction with cervical traction while awake.

Geisler FH, Dorsey FC, Coleman WP: Recovery of motor function after spinal-cord injury: A randomized, placebo-controlled trial with GM-1 ganglioside. *N Engl J Med* 1991;324:1829–1838.

A small pilot study demonstrated improved recovery of motor function with the administration of neuroganglioside GM-1 (Sygen).

Jeanneret B, Magerl F: Primary posterior fusion C1/C2 in odontoid fractures: Indications, technique, and results of transarticular screw fixation. *J Spin Disord* 1992;5:464–475.

This is an excellent review of the indications, techniques, and results of posterior transarticular screw fixation. Authors demonstrate safety and efficacy of this demanding technique.

Ripa DR, Kowall MG, Meyer PR Jr, et al: Series of ninety-two traumatic cervical spine injuries stabilized with anterior ASIF plate fusion technique. *Spine* 1991;16(suppl 3):S46-S55.

Authors demonstrate the safety and efficacy of an anterior cervical plate technique in the treatment of cervical spine fractures. There was a minimal complication rate and an excellent fusion rate.

Star AM, Jones AA, Cotler JM, et al: Immediate closed reduction of cervical spine dislocations using traction. *Spine* 1990;15:1068–1072.

Closed reduction of facet dislocation via axial cervical traction and Gardner Wells tongs is a safe and effective method. None of a series of 57 patients had worsening of the neurologic injury.

Torg JS, Glasgow SG: Criteria for return to contact activities after cervical spine injury, in Torg JS (ed): *Athletic Injuries to the Head, Neck, and Face,* ed 2. St. Louis, MO, Mosby Year Book, 1991, pp 589–608.

This excellent chapter discusses the criteria to determine return to sports participation following cervical spine injury.

Waters RL, Adkins RH: The effects of removal of bullet fragments retained in the spinal canal: A collaborative study by the National Spinal Cord Injury Model Systems. *Spine* 1991;16:934–939.

Removal of bullet fragments made no difference with regard to reducing pain or improving recovery of sensory and motor function in patients who had sustained injury between T12 and L4. The cervical spine region, due to small sample size and the high mortality rate for gunshot wounds to the neck, was not addressed.

Thoracic, Thoracolumbar, and Lumbar Injuries

Braakman R, Fontijne WP, Zeegers R, et al: Neurological deficit in injuries of the thoracic and lumbar spine: A consecutive series of 70 patients. *Acta Neurochir* 1991;111: 11–17.

Seventy consecutive patients with injuries of the thoracolumbar spine accompanied by neurologic deficits were prospectively studied and followed. The correlation of neurologic recovery with spinal canal compromise, as well as surgical decompression and stabilization, was reviewed.

Cammisa FP Jr, Eismont FJ, Green BA: Dural laceration occurring with burst fractures and associated laminar fractures. *J Bone Joint Surg* 1989;71A;1044–1052.

The presence of preoperative neurologic deficit in patients with burst fractures and associated laminar fractures was an excellent predictor of dural lacerations. This pattern also predicted the risk of entrapped neural elements within the laminar fracture.

Gardner VO, Armstrong GW: Long-term lumbar facet joint changes in spinal fracture patients treated with Harrington rods. *Spine* 1990;15:479–484.

The authors retrospectively studied the effects of Harrington distraction rods spanning unfused spinal segments in thoracolumbar fractures to determine the long-term incidence of facet joint osteoarthritis. Eighty-five percent of patients were found to have good to excellent results regarding back pain, with 90% returning to their preinjury occupations.

Itoi E, Sakurai M, Mizunashi K, et al: Long-term observations of vertebral fractures in spinal osteoporotics. *Calcif Tissue Int* 1990;47:202–208.

A profile on the long-term observations of vertebral fractures occurring in 21 spinal osteoporotic patients is presented.

Keene JS, Fischer SP, Vanderby R Jr, et al: Significance of acute posttraumatic bony encroachment of the neural canal. *Spine* 1989;14:799–802.

The authors studied 80 consecutive patients with acute fractures at the thoracolumbar spine and correlated the amount of neural canal impingement with neurologic status. The posttraumatic neurologic status did not directly correlate with the percent of neural impingement demonstrated on CT scans.

Kostuik JP, Matsusaki H: Anterior stabilization, instrumentation, and decompression for post-traumatic kyphosis. *Spine* 1989;14:379–386.

The authors present the results of 37 patients undergoing surgery for late posttraumatic kyphosis in the thoracolumbar region. The indications for surgery included increasing deformity, pain, and persistent neurologic deficit.

Mann KA, McGowan DP, Fredrickson BE, et al: A biomechanical investigation of short segment spinal fixation for burst fractures with varying degrees of posterior disruption. *Spine* 1990;15:470–478.

A Fixateur Interne pedicle screw system and the Syracuse I-Plate anterior fixation system were compared by mechanically determining their effectiveness using human cadaver spines. The Fixateur Interne provided much better stabilization than the anterior I-Plate for those cases in which there was a large amount of posterior disruption in addition to an anterior burst injury. Neither device provides extensive support in axial rotation loading.

Shikata J, Yamamuro T, Iida H, et al: Surgical treatment for paraplegia resulting from vertebral fractures in senile osteoporosis. *Spine* 1990;15:485–489.

The authors discuss cases of paraplegia secondary to senile osteoporotic vertebral compression fractures treated by posterior decompression and Harrington rod stabilization. This report demonstrates that osteoporotic vertebral body fractures can go on to neurologic demise.

Vincent KA, Benson DR, McGahan JP: Intraoperative ultrasonography for reduction of thoracolumbar burst fractures. *Spine* 1989;14:387–390.

The authors review the efficacy of intraoperative ultrasound monitoring in the reduction and stabilization of thoracolumbar burst fractures of the spine. Ultrasonography is recommended as a safe and accurate method of intraoperatively evaluating reduction of the culprit fragment in burst fractures from the posterior approach.

Whitecloud TS III, Butler JC, Cohen JL, et al: Complications with the variable spinal plating system. *Spine* 1989;14:472–476.

The results of 40 patients undergoing transpedicle fixation and fusion using the variable spinal plate for various diseases of the thoracolumbar spine are presented. The overall complication rate was 45%. Most complications were minor in nature and resolved before discharge. Indications for plating are presented.

Classic Bibliography

Cervical Spine Injuries

Allen BL Jr, Ferguson RL, Lehmann TR, et al: A mechanistic classification of closed, indirect fractures and dislocations of the lower cervical spine. *Spine* 1982;7:1–27.

Anderson LD, D'Alonzo RT: Fractures of the odontoid process of the axis. *J Bone Joint Surg* 1974;56A:1663–1674.

Bohler J: Anterior stabilization for acute fractures and non-unions of the dens. *J Bone Joint Surg* 1982;64A:18–27.

Bohler J, Gaudernak T: Anterior plate stabilization for fracture-dislocations of the lower cervical spine. *J Trauma* 1980;20:203–205.

Bohlman HH: Acute fractures and dislocations of the cervical spine: An analysis of three hundred hospitalized patients and review of the literature. *J Bone Joint Surg* 1979;61A:1119–1142.

Clark CR, White AA III: Fractures of the dens: A multicenter study. *J Bone Joint Surg* 1985;67A:1340–1348.

Levine AM, Edwards CC: The management of traumatic spondylolisthesis of the axis. *J Bone Joint Surg* 1985;67A:217–226.

Rogers WA: Fractures and dislocations of the cervical spine: An end-result study. *J Bone Joint Surg* 1957;39A:341–376.

Stauffer ES, Kelly EG: Fracture-dislocations of the cervical spine: Instability and recurrent deformity following treatment by anterior interbody fusion. *J Bone Joint Surg* 1977;59A:45–48.

Torg JS, Pavlov H, Genuario SE, et al: Neurapraxia of the cervical spinal cord with transient quadriplegia. *J Bone Joint Surg* 1986;68A:1354–1370.

Thoracic, Thoracolumbar, and Lumbar Injuries

Bohlman HH: Treatment of fractures and dislocations of the thoracic and lumbar spine. *J Bone Joint Surg* 1985;67A:165–169.

Bohlman HH, Freehafer A, Dejak J: The results of treatment of acute injuries of the upper thoracic spine with paralysis. *J Bone Joint Surg* 1985;67A:360–369.

Bradford DS, McBride GG: Surgical management of thoracolumbar spine fractures with incomplete neurologic deficits. *Clin Orthop* 1987;218:201–216.

Denis F: The three column spine and its significance in the classification of acute thoracolumbar spinal injuries. *Spine* 1983;8:817–831.

Dickson JH, Harrington PR, Erwin WD: Results of reduction and stabilization of the severely fractured thoracic and lumbar spine. *J Bone Joint Surg* 1978;60A:799–805.

Dommisse GF: The blood supply of the spinal cord: A critical vascular zone in spinal surgery. *J Bone Joint Surg* 1974;56B:225–235.

Edwards CC, Levine AM: Complications associated with posterior instrumentation in the treatment of thoracic and lumbar injuries, in Garfin SR (ed): *Complications of Spine Surgery.* Baltimore, MD, Williams & Wilkins, 1989, pp 164–199.

Edwards CC, Rosenthal MS, Gellad F, et al: The fate of retropulsed bone following thoracolumbar burst fractures: Late stenosis or resorption? *Orthop Trans* 1989;13:32–33.

Eismont FJ, Green BA, Berkowitz BM, et al: The role of intraoperative ultrasonography in the treatment of thoracic and lumbar spine fractures. *Spine* 1984;9:782–787.

Fredrickson BE, Mann KA, Yuan HA, et al: Reduction of the intracanal fragment in experimental burst fractures. *Spine* 1988;13:267–271.

Garfin SR, Mowery CA, Guerra J Jr, et al: Confirmation of the posterolateral technique to decompress and fuse thoracolumbar spine burst fractures. *Spine* 1985;10:218–223.

Gertzbein SD, Court-Brown CM: Flexion-distraction injuries of the lumbar spine: Mechanisms of injury and classification. *Clin Orthop* 1988;227:52–60.

Levine AM, Edwards CC: Lumbar spine trauma, in Camins MB, O'Leary PF (eds): *The Lumbar Spine.* New York, NY, Raven Press, 1987, pp 183–212.

McAfee PC, Bohlman HH, Yuan HA: Anterior decompression of traumatic thoracolumbar fractures with incomplete neurological deficit using a retroperitoneal approach. *J Bone Joint Surg* 1985;67A:89–104.

Wenger DR, Carollo JJ: The mechanics of thoracolumbar fractures stabilized by segmental fixation. *Clin Orthop* 1984;189:89–96.

47

Spondylosis: Degenerative Process of the Aging Spine

Spondylosis, a generalized process that affects all levels of the spine, encompasses a sequence of progressive degenerative changes in the intervertebral disks, vertebral bodies, facet joints, and ligamentous structures. Spondylosis occurs in a sequential fashion as the body and spine age. In any individual, symptoms due to senescent versus pathologic processes can be very difficult to differentiate.

Clinicians dealing with the clinical signs and symptoms of the aging process must also consider superimposed pathophysiology. The changes seen in the normal aging spine grossly, radiographically, biochemically, and biomechanically are within the spectrum of changes seen in a pathologic and symptomatic spine. Thus, it is extremely difficult to predict or identify at what point along the continuum of degenerative changes symptoms may arise. It is, however, useful to describe the changes that occur in the normal aging spine as well as the abnormalities seen within the basic pathologic entities of disk protrusion and spinal stenosis.

Morphologic Changes

For the first two decades of life, very few morphologic changes occur in the spine. The intervertebral disk is a hydrostatic load-bearing structure between the vertebral bodies. The nucleus pulposus, which acts as a confined fluid within the annulus fibrosis, is able to convert axial loads into tensile strain on the annular fibers and the vertebral endplates. The disks maintain their full height, vertebra are square in shape, and the facet joints are well defined, with smooth capsules and healthy articular cartilage. The ligamentum flavum is only a few millimeters thick, and ample space exists for the neural elements within the spinal canal. In these first 20 years, disk protrusion through the cartilaginous endplates (Schmorl's node) and facet tropism (asymmetric facet origination at the same level) may be seen, but are not felt to be responsible for any set of well-defined symptoms. Traumatic, infectious, and neoplastic conditions account for the majority of clinically significant pathologic entities.

Over the third through the fifth decades of life, progressive degenerative changes occur in the spine that may be quite dramatic. In general, the first manifestations of aging are seen in the intervertebral disks, with subsequent changes in the bones and articular processes becoming evident. Diffuse bulging or focal extrusion of disk material will result in narrowing of the intervertebral disk space. The loss of disk height allows close approximation of adjacent vertebral bodies that may lead to osteophyte formation, facet joint arthritis with hypertrophic changes, and encroachment of the neural elements in the foramina or within the spinal canal itself. These findings may also be manifest in the older spine as end-stage changes of the general aging process. In addition, the facet joint capsule thickens and the ligamentum flavum hypertrophies.

Loss of disk space height is commonly felt to be part of the degenerative changes that occur in both the cervical and the lumbar spine. Although reduction of stature in old age has been attributed to loss of disk height, measurements of average disk heights in cadaveric lumbar spines have shown that only a minority of lower lumbar disks show significant thinning. Thus, loss of stature in the elderly spine is likely due to diminished vertebral body height rather than loss of disk height.

The previously discussed changes in the intervertebral disk and facet joint are generally associated with decreased movement in each motion segment. An olisthesis, or slip (forward or backward), of one vertebra on another may occur as a result of disk incompetence followed by facet subluxation. Such slips are noteworthy but rarely show significant motion on flexion-extension films. Anterior osteophytes, sometimes called traction spurs, are frequently indicative of abnormal motion at a spinal segment.

As the spine ages, postural alterations are also common. In the lumbar spine, a reduction in lordosis can be seen as an attempt to unload the degenerative articular facets by maintaining a more flexed rather than extended posture. A flexed position can also provide more room for the susceptible neural elements within the canal and foramina, which are dynamically compromised in extension.

Intervertebral disk degeneration is closely associated with aging as shown in many cadaveric and radiologic surveys. In the cervical region, the majority of spines show implications of degeneration in one or more disks after the fourth decade, and after the fifth decade, there is a sharp rise in the severity of the degenerative process. In specimens from patients over the age of 70 years, 72% showed severe cervical abnormalities with the C5–6 and C6–7 levels most frequently involved. In the lumbar spine, degenerative changes are almost universal after age 60 years and the most frequently involved levels are L4–5 and L5–S1.

Biochemical Changes

Perhaps the major consequence of disk degeneration is the loss of its hydrostatic properties. In a young adult disk, the nucleus pulposus is 85% water and the annulus, 78% water. The water content in both tissues falls to about 70% with aging. There is a gradual decrease in the osmotic swelling pressure of the intervertebral disk and a twofold increase in creep under compression from age 30 years to 80 years. The ability of the disk to imbibe water and evenly distribute load deteriorates with age, largely owing to changes in the molecular meshwork of proteoglycans and collagen.

The major structural components of the intervertebral disk, aside from water, are collagen and proteoglycans. The nucleus pulposus is able to hold its fluid pressure largely because of the presence of negatively charged groups of glycosaminoglycan chains. The crossing collagen fibril arrangement in the layers of the annulus is ideally suited to accommodate the complex stresses caused by compression of the nucleus. The collagen in the nucleus is largely type II, that seen in hyaline cartilage, whereas the collagen in the annulus is mostly type I, which provides increased tensile strength as in tendons.

The biochemical changes in the aging nucleus pulposus can be summarized as follows: (1) loss of clear distinction between nucleus and annulus; (2) gradual increase in collagen content within the disk; (3) loss of negatively charged proteoglycan side chains, decreasing the imbibing capability of the nucleus; and (4) greatly reduced numbers of proteoglycan aggregates. Similar changes have been seen in herniated intervertebral disks. The initiating event, if one exists, remains unknown. Evidence has demonstrated that normal disks do contain collagenase enzymes capable of degrading their extracellular macromolecular matrix.

Changes in the annulus fibrosis have also been noted with aging. The number of cells per unit of tissue surface decreases progressively, along with a gradual reduction in cellular metabolic activity. The major biochemical change in the aging annulus seems to be a decrease in the total content of proteoglycans. Larger collagen fibrils also appear, which may increase the likelihood of failure of an over-stressed region of the annulus. Localized biochemical changes may predispose certain areas of the annulus to tearing. Focal decrease in collagen content and increase in type III collagen have been associated with annular tears. Unfortunately, significant healing of the torn annulus does not appear to occur.

In addition to changes in the nucleus and annulus with aging, there are associated changes in the vertebral endplates and adjacent bone marrow. Such changes can affect the nutrition of the avascular disk, which depends on diffusion of nutrients through the cartilaginous vertebral endplates. Calcification of the endplate cartilage and vascular changes seen in older vertebra probably impede the delivery of disk nutrients from the blood. It is possible that these adverse alterations in the nutrient delivery system to the intervertebral disk initiate or at least potentiate the undesirable biochemical changes in the degenerating disk.

Biomechanical Changes

Initially, the liquid and elastic properties of the intervertebral disk allow it to withstand virtually all physiologic moments applied to it. In compression, the disk can withstand a variety of deforming forces. The annulus receives most of the forces dispersed by the nucleus. Compressive forces are redirected into a radial direction, in which they are resisted by the lamellar configuration of the annulus. Although the annulus has virtually no elastic fibers, the relative movement of neighboring sheets of fibrous tissue permits increased girth.

With normal aging, this time-dependent deformability, or creep, of the disk increases twofold. This increase leads to diffuse bulging of the intervertebral disk with a resultant narrowing of the disk space. Simultaneously, age-related degenerative changes are occurring in the facet joints. Subchondral sclerosis, osteophyte formation, and loss of articular cartilage occur. Laxity is introduced into each mobile segment. The early rolling motion at each segment becomes uneven, and sliding of one vertebral body on another can occur. This change in the center of motion can lead to segmental instability.

Clinical Sequelae of the Aging Spine

In the majority of patients, many of the described structural, biochemical, and biomechanical changes occur generally over time without resulting symptoms. In others, perhaps those with smaller (less tolerant) spinal canals, or faster rates of degeneration, symptoms may become severe. It is often difficult to differentiate normal aging from pathophysiologic changes.

Disk Protrusion

With aging, the annulus fibrosis fibrillates and weakens. Radial cracks develop centrally and extend outward toward the periphery. These radiating clefts in the annulus reduce its resistance, and nuclear herniation or annular protrusion ensues.

If herniation does not occur early in the process, disk degeneration continues with a subsequent decrease in proteoglycans and increase in collagen. The higher collagen content replaces the previously gelatinous nucleus, and the boundary distinguishing nucleus from annulus, once clearly defined, becomes blurred. The results are disk fibrosis, loss of disk height, and annular weakening, which results in annular protrusion or bulging. In the cervical spine, secondary osteophytes forming a "hard disk" can result in the gradual onset of symptoms. Bony hypertrophy can occur at the uncovertebral joints in addition to the facet joints, as in the lumbar spine.

Nuclear disk material can herniate anterior, posterior, or lateral to the disk space. The weakest portion of the posterior annulus is on either side of the midline where it lacks reinforcement by the strong, central fibers of the posterior longitudinal ligament (PLL). Thus, it is not surprising that posterolateral disk protrusions are the most common. Posterior disk herniations can be further distinguished by the structures through which the nuclear material has herniated. If the nuclear material herniates through the annulus but not the PLL, it is called a constrained herniation. If the nuclear material also violates the PLL, the herniation is not constrained, and free sequestered fragments may be present in the spinal canal or neural foramen. A true midline posterior protrusion is usually contained within the PLL, but it may dissect cephalad or caudad, shift laterally, or even stretch the PLL to the point of rupture.

The clinical symptoms of disk protrusions are likely the result of more than just mechanical forces acting on the neural elements. Large protrusions, in addition to generating tension on the neural roots, compress the nerve against bone or hypertrophied ligamentum flavum. Because of the lack of elasticity of the roots, minimal tension may generate secondary local inflammatory changes and, eventually, fibrosis around the nerve root. The root responds to the abnormal situation by becoming edematous and cordlike. The neurologic deficits from this process may be permanent.

Spinal Stenosis

The secondary alterations that occur in the wake of intervertebral disk degeneration involve all the elements making up the spinal motion segment. With the loss of the hydrostatic mechanism between the vertebrae, the anterior portions of the vertebral bodies are in closer proximity and may be subjected to direct compressive forces. As a result, beak-shaped osteophytes may form along the vertebral body rims. There is telescoping of the articular facets of the posterior joints (and the uncovertebral joints in the cervical spine) and stretching of their capsules. Continuous stretch of the posterior joint capsule and ligaments results in a profound thickening of these structures. Compression of the intervertebral joints results in hypertrophic osteophyte formation, which may encroach on the neural foramen or the canal itself.

Ultimately, these degenerative changes result in a narrowing of the spinal canal diameter and a decrease in the size of the neural foramina. The decrease in disk height results in foraminal encroachment from facet hypertrophy posteriorly, the relative descent of the pedicle superiorly, and disk bulging anterior to the foramen. These changes occur gradually, and the patient may remain asymptomatic until late in the degenerative process. In some instances, the patients never become symptomatic.

Annotated Bibliography

Hukins DW, Kirby MC, Sikoryn TA, et al: Comparison of structure, mechanical properties, and functions of lumbar spinal ligaments. *Spine* 1990;15:787–795.

Different lumbar spinal ligaments were tested to evaluate their functional contribution to the stability of the lumbar spine.

Keller TS, Holm SH, Hansson TH, et al: 1990 Volvo Award in experimental studies: The dependence of intervertebral disc mechanical properties on physiologic conditions. *Spine* 1990;15:751–761.

The authors evaluated the interrelationship between different physiologic conditions and the mechanical properties of the intervertebral disk.

Lipson SJ: Aging versus degeneration of the intervertebral disc, in Weinstein JN, Wiesel SW (eds): *The Lumbar Spine.* Philadelphia, PA, WB Saunders, 1990, pp 261–265.

This is a review of aging changes that take place in the intervertebral disk.

Pope MH, Frymoyer JW, Lehmann TR: Structure and function of the lumbar spine, in Pope MH, Andersson GBJ, Frymoyer JW, et al (eds): *Occupational Low Back Pain: Assessment, Treatment and Prevention.* St. Louis, MO, Mosby Year Book, 1991, pp 3–19.

This is an excellent update of the biomechanical properties of the lumbar spine.

Simon SR, Alaranta H, An KN, et al: Kinesiology, in Simon SR (ed): *Orthopaedic Basic Science.* Rosemont, IL, American Academy of Orthopaedic Surgeons, 1994, pp 519–622.

This is an up-to-date overview of the structure and function of the cervical and lumbar spine.

White AA III, Panjabi MM (eds): *Clinical Biomechanics of the Spine,* ed 2. Philadelphia, PA, JB Lippincott, 1991, pp 85–125.

This is a straightforward review of the biomechanics of the spine with appropriate clinical correlation.

Wilder DG, Pope MH, Frymoyer JW: The biomechanics of lumbar disc herniation and the effect of overload and instability. *J Spinal Disord* 1988;1:16–32.

The authors describe mechanical properties that contribute to lumbar disk herniation.

Classic Bibliography

Brickley-Parsons D, Glimcher MJ: Is the chemistry of collagen in intervertebtal discs an expression of Wolff's Law? A study of the human lumbar spine. *Spine* 1984; 9:148–163.

Buckwalter JA, Pedrini-Mille A, Pedrini V, et al: Proteoglycans of human infant intervertebral disc: Electron microscopic and biochemical studies. *J Bone Joint Surg* 1985;67A:284–294.

Coventry MB, Ghormley RK, Kernohan JW: The intervertebral disc: Its microscopic anatomy and pathology. Part II: Changes in the intervertebral disc concomitant with age. *J Bone Joint Surg* 1945;27:233–247.

Coventry MB, Ghormley RK, Kernohan JW: The intervertebral disc: Its microscopic anatomy and pathology. Part III: Pathological changes in the intervertebral disc. *J Bone Joint Surg* 1945;27:460–474.

Gower WE, Pedrini V: Age-related variations in protein-polysaccharides from human nucleus pulposus, annulus fibrosus, and costal cartilage. *J Bone Joint Surg* 1969; 51A:1154–1162.

Lipson SJ, Muir H: Experimental intervertebral disc degeneration: Morphologic and proteoglycan changes over time. *Arthritis Rheum* 1981;24:12–21.

Miller JA, Schmatz C, Schultz AB: Lumbar disc degeneration: Correlation with age, sex, and spine level in 600 autopsy specimens. *Spine* 1988;13:173–178.

Pearce RH, Grimmer BJ, Adams ME: Degeneration and the chemical composition of the human lumbar intervertebral disc. *J Orthop Res* 1987;5:198–205.

Pritzker KP: Aging and degeneration in the lumbar intervertebral disc. *Orthop Clin North Am* 1977;8:66–77.

Urban JP, McMullin JF: Swelling pressure of the lumbar intervertebral discs: Influence of age, spinal level, composition, and degeneration. *Spine* 1988;13:179–187.

48

Cervical Degenerative Disk Disorders

Natural History

The natural history of cervical radiculopathy was investigated by Lees and Turner in 1963. They reported 51 patients with initial symptoms of cervical radiculopathy who were followed up for as long as 19 years. Of the study group, 45% had only one episode of radicular pain without recurrence, 30% had mild symptoms, and 25% had persistent or worsening symptoms. No patient developed myelopathy if it was absent initially. The authors concluded that wearing a collar often relieved symptoms, but that any or no treatment will often give the same final result.

These authors also reported on 44 patients with symptoms of a cervical myelopathy. Those patients who initially had a mild disability had the best prognosis. Of the 15 patients who initially had a severe disability, 14 remained moderately or severely disabled after long-term follow-up. The authors concluded that the course of cervical spondylitic myelopathy is usually prolonged and that the disorder is characterized by long periods of nonprogressive disability, with rare instances of progressive deterioration.

The natural history of cervical myelopathy was also examined by Nurick who reported on 36 patients treated nonsurgically over a 20-year period. Of the 27 patients who initially had a mild disability, 18 were still graded as mild at final assessment. Six of the nine patients who initially had moderate to severe symptoms continued to have moderate to severe symptoms at the final follow-up. The feature most often associated with deterioration was the age of the patient at the time of the initial presentation, with patients over the age of 60 years having a poor prognosis.

History and Physical Examination

Patients with cervical degenerative disk disease may present with neck pain, radiculopathy, and/or myelopathy. Neck pain alone, without radicular pain or a neurologic deficit, is a common finding. The neck pain frequently is referred cranially towards the occiput and may be associated with headaches as well as bilateral or unilateral shoulder and arm pain. Studies to locate the pain generator may include provocative injections in either the facet joints or the cervical disk. Unfortunately, there has been little, if any, evaluation of the utility of these procedures using a controlled randomized study. The relief of neck pain following cervical fusion is usually within the expected improvement rate of the natural history of the disease process. Therefore, surgical intervention for neck pain alone is, in general, discouraged.

Nerve root compression may occur with soft-disk herniation or spondylosis secondary to uncovertebral joint osteophytes. Nerve root compression at a specific level in the cervical spine may cause the classic symptoms of motor, sensory, and reflex deficits. The classic findings described in numerous textbooks (Table 1) are not often seen because of the fairly high degree of functional overlap among the spinal nerve roots.

Spurling's test is performed by having the patient rotate and laterally bend the head towards the affected side. The examiner then applies a vertical compressive force to the top of the patient's head. A positive test causes exacerbation of radicular symptoms. Extension of the head and neck may also recreate radicular symptoms if this position is held for 15 to 25 seconds. The shoulder abduction relief sign is performed by placing the painful extremity in the abducted position with the palm of the hand resting on top of the head. This maneuver will frequently reduce radicular pain.

Cervical myelopathy can be precipitated by either a large central disk herniation or, more commonly, by severe spondylitic changes with or without a congenitally narrow spinal canal. The spondylitic changes may occur at numerous levels throughout the cervical spine and can produce a combination of both myelopathy and radiculopathy. Although minor trauma may precipitate the onset of symptoms, most patients are usually unaware of the precise time of onset. Symptoms vary widely, but frequently include a deterioration in gait and manual dexterity, generalized weakness, and/or urinary urgency or frequency.

An understanding of the anatomy of the cervical spinal cord is helpful to fully evaluate the patient with cervical spondylitic myelopathy (Fig. 1). The posterior columns of the spinal cord convey information regarding vibration

Table 1. Neurologic testing of the upper extremity

Nerve Root	Reflex	Sensation	Muscle
C4	None	Back of neck, scapula	None
C5	Biceps	Lateral arm	Deltoid Biceps
C6	Brachioradialis	Lateral forearm, thumb, index finger	Wrist extensors Biceps
C7	Triceps	Middle finger	Triceps Wrist flexors Finger extensors
C8	None	Ring, little finger	Finger flexors Intrinsics

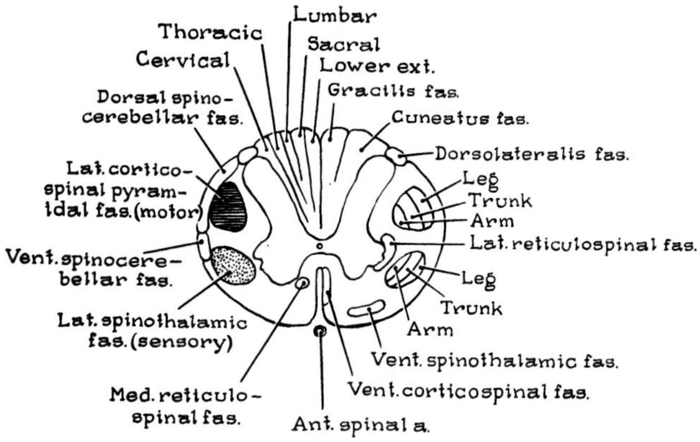

Fig. 1 The cervical spinal cord. The ascending tracts include: fasciculus gracilis and cuneatus convey proprioception, vibration, and pressure. The lateral spinothalamic tract is the predominant pathway for somatic pain and thermal sensibilities. The descending tracts include the anterior corticospinal tract, which contains uncrossed pyramidal motor fibers, and the lateral corticospinal tract, which has fibers from the cortical motor cells. (Reproduced with permission from Bohlman HH, Ducker TB: Spine and spinal cord injuries, in Rothman RH, Simeone FA (eds): *The Spine*. Philadelphia, PA, WB Saunders, 1992, pp 973–1104.)

and extremity position sense. Motor impulses are transmitted through the foraminal tracts, which are found anteriorly. Compression of these foraminal tracts causes upper motor neuron signs, such as hyperreflexia, spasticity, muscle weakness, and Babinski reflexes. The lateral spinal thalamic tracts are responsible for transmission of pain, temperature, and touch sensations.

A common complaint in myelopathy is lower extremity weakness, which results from involvement of the corticospinal tracts early in the disease process. As the disease progresses, the posterior tracts are affected, resulting in loss of proprioception. The combination of muscle weakness and loss of proprioception results in the characteristic wide-based myelopathic gait. Although not as common, upper extremity dysfunction frequently occurs in patients with cervical spondylitic myelopathy. Additionally, patients frequently are unable to rapidly open and close the fist. Long tract findings of spasticity and hyperreflexia in the arms are typically accompanied by lower motor neuron findings at the level of the lesion, resulting in muscle wasting and fasciculations. The finger escape sign, which is seen in patients with myelopathy, is characterized by deficient adduction and/or extension of the ulnar digits of the affected hand.

Multiple root sensory findings in the upper extremities are common in myelopathy. Patients often complain of pain and paresthesias in the upper extremities. If there are complaints of pain in the lower extremities, the clinician should be aware of the possibility of coexistent lumbar radiculopathy or spinal stenosis secondary to lumbar degenerative disk disease.

Reflex changes are important in the evaluation of patients with cervical spondylitic myelopathy. Generally, the lower extremities are hyperreflexic. Upper extremity reflexes may either be hypo- or hyperreflexic, depending on the level of the lesion in the spinal cord. A positive Hoffman sign is indicative of upper motor neuron disease and is found by flicking the nail of the middle finger toward the palm and observing an abnormal reflex contraction of the thumb and/or index finger. Compression at the C5 level may cause an inverted radial reflex. This reflex is demonstrated by tapping the brachioradialis tendon and noting a diminished response as well as reflex contraction of the (spastic) finger flexors. Assessment of the jaw jerk reflex is important in those patients who have global hyperreflexia. This reflex is a stretch reflex involving both the masseter and temporalis muscles, with innervation through the fifth cranial nerve (trigeminal). An absent or diminished reflex is indicative of pathology along the course of the nerve. A normal jaw jerk reflex will exclude pathology above the foramen magnum, whereas a hyperreflexic reflex indicates intracranial pathology or systemic disease.

Numerous classification systems have been developed regarding cervical myelopathy. The system most commonly used is based on the differential susceptibility of various spinal cord tracts. The most common syndrome, the transverse lesion syndrome, includes involvement of the posterior columns, spinothalamic, and corticospinal tracts and is characterized by motor/sensory findings and dysfunction below the level of pathology. The motor system syndrome involves corticospinal tract involvement only and is characterized by upper and lower extremity weakness, gait disturbance, and spasticity. In the central cord syndrome, upper extremities are typically weaker than lower extremities, and hand weakness is often profound.

Brown-Séquard syndrome is a classic presentation of unilateral spinal cord compression. The corticospinal tract compression leads to ipsilateral hemiparesis with contralateral loss of pain and temperature sensation resulting from spinothalamic tract compression. Finally, the brachialgia cord syndrome combines upper extremity root compression with long tract findings due to cord compression. This syndrome is characterized by radicular pain, paresthesias, and hyperreflexia, as well as long tract signs, weakness, and gait disturbances, and it has the best prognosis following decompression.

Pathologic studies of cervical spondylitic myelopathy demonstrate that the spinal cord pathology correlates with the clinical severity of the disease. Findings include atherosclerotic changes in the major spinal arteries and intimal fibrosis. Compression of the spinal cord usually is associated with extensive destruction of both grey and white matter and with demyelinization ascending and descending from the compression. The anterior-posterior compression ratio (the ratio of the anterior-posterior diameter to the lateral diameter) correlates with the degree of pathology in the spinal cord.

Demyelinating diseases of the central nervous system, such as multiple sclerosis, can also cause both motor and sensory abnormalities in the upper and lower extremities. However, cervical myelopathy usually does not occur in an episodic fashion as does multiple sclerosis. Multiple sclerosis usually presents with cranial nerve dysfunction (and an abnormal jaw jerk reflex).

Amyotrophic lateral sclerosis (ALS) is a pure motor neuron disease, unlike cervical myelopathy. There is no alteration in superficial or deep sensation. Tumors of the spinal cord, as well as a syrinx, can cause symptoms identical to those of cervical myelopathy. However, the two disease processes can be distinguished by radiographic evaluation, such as magnetic resonance imaging (MRI).

Radiographic Evaluation

Degenerative changes of the cervical spine (cervical spondylosis) include intervertebral osteochondrosis, spondylosis deformans, osteoarthritis of the apophyseal joints, and uncovertebral arthrosis.

The standard radiographic evaluation of cervical spondylosis includes obtaining lateral and anteroposterior (AP) views. The lateral view allows evaluation of the intervertebral disk space height, assessment of osteophytosis, and overall alignment of the cervical bodies and apophyseal joints. In the AP view, the disk spaces, uncinate processes, and uncovertebral joints are seen. Oblique views evaluate the intervertebral foramina, pedicles, articular masses, and apophyseal joints. They frequently do not help in the clinical management of the patient, and should not be a routine part of every assessment. Flexion and extension views of the cervical spine may be obtained if subluxation is suspected.

Radiographic findings in the degenerative cervical spine must be interpreted with caution. Degenerative changes in the disk spaces of the cervical spine are common after the age of 40 years and affect more than 70% of the population by the age of 70 years. These changes often are found in individuals who are asymptomatic and frequently do not correlate with clinical symptoms.

Disk space narrowing is the most common finding in cervical spondylosis and can lead to a relative loss of lordosis. Anterior osteophytes are generally larger than posterior, but are usually asymptomatic, unless esophageal compromise occurs. Large anterior osteophytes at multiple levels may be indicative of diffuse idiopathic skeletal hyperostosis. Posterior osteophytes are generally smaller, but are more important clinically due to neural compression. The space available for the spinal cord is generally measured from a point along the posterior cortex of the vertebral body to the corresponding laminar line. In the normal adult, this should measure approximately 17 mm. However, if narrowed by a posterior osteophyte, impingement can begin if the space approaches 13 mm, and a space of less than 10 mm correlates highly with clinical evidence of spinal cord compression.

Plain radiographs do not visualize the neural elements either directly or indirectly. Other imaging tests are necessary to determine the amount of neural compression and should be ordered when this information affects treatment. Although myelography will not directly visualize the compressing structures, it can be used to diagnose both intradural and extradural neural compression. This compression can be inferred by changes in the contour of the normal contrast-filled thecal sac. Currently used water soluble nonionic agents have eliminated the need for overnight hospital admissions and decreased the incidence of side effects associated with myelography.

The major advantage of myelography is that it can provide visualization of the entire spinal canal from the occiput to the sacrum. The major disadvantage is that it is invasive and somewhat nonspecific. Central compression at the level of the disk space may be due either to a soft disk herniation or to compression by a marginal osteophyte. Nerve root sleeve cut off can be due either to a lateral disk herniation or to foraminal narrowing. Accuracy rates for myelography are similar to those for unenhanced cervical computed tomography (CT) scans and range from 70% to 90%. Myelography, as well as CT scans and MRI scans, often demonstrates radiographic abnormalities in patients who are asymptomatic. Therefore, it is important to correlate the patient's symptoms with the test findings in order to make the appropriate treatment recommendations.

Myelogram accuracy can be greatly enhanced through the use of a postcontrast CT scan. A CT scan permits more direct visualization of the neural compression and allows better visualization of lateral pathology, such as foraminal stenosis. High quality scanners are also potentially able to distinguish hard from soft disk herniations.

MRI of the cervical spine is noninvasive, involves no radiation exposure, and provides excellent resolution of the cervical disk and the neural elements (Fig. 2). MRI scans must be interpreted with caution, however, because there is a fairly high incidence of asymptomatic findings. Nineteen percent of asymptomatic subjects have major abnormalities on their cervical spine MRI scans. Of those younger than 40 years of age, 14% have either a herniated nucleus pulposus or foraminal stenosis; this increases to 25% in patients over the age of 40 years.

Electrodiagnosis

Electromyography (EMG), nerve conduction velocity (NCV), and somatosensory evoked potentials (SSEP) are useful adjuncts to the history and physical examination, but should not be used alone for diagnoses. Electrodiagnostic studies are useful for confirmation of abnormalities observed on physical examination, assistance in defining the anatomic localization of a lesion, and distinguishing between overlapping pathologic conditions.

EMGs are usually highly sensitive, but fairly nonspecific. Electrodiagnostic abnormalities may be noted as

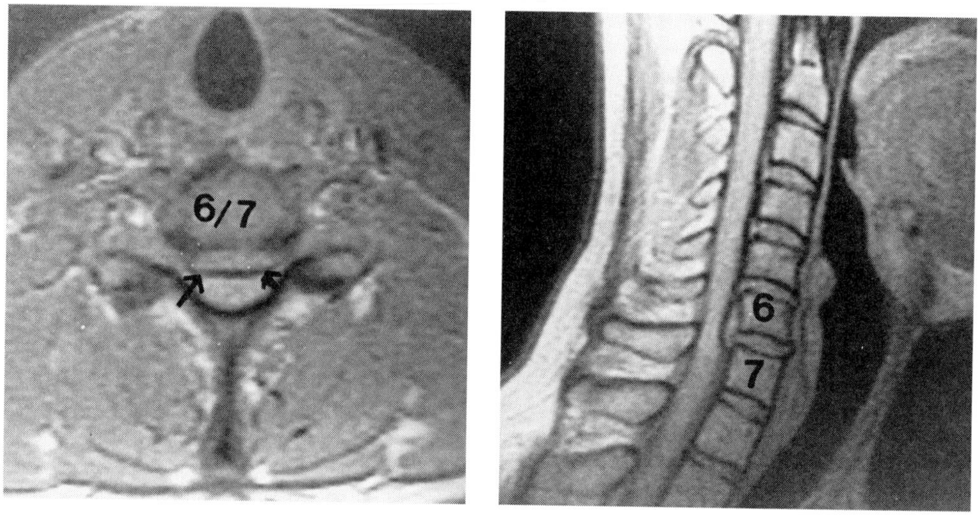

Fig. 2 Magnetic resonance images demonstrating a central disk herniation at C6–7. **Left,** cross section; **right,** sagittal.

early as 7 days after a specific injury, and abnormalities are usually found in the paraspinal muscles as well as the limb muscles. In addition, EMG and NCV can help distinguish between a cervical radiculopathy and a peripheral nerve entrapment or brachial plexus injury.

Treatment

Nonsurgical Treatment

There are numerous treatment options for patients who present with either neck pain, cervical radiculopathy, or cervical myelopathy. Surgical treatment is rarely considered initially. The majority of patients will respond well to either medication and/or physical therapy programs unless a severe fixed or a rapidly progressive neurologic deficit is present.

The most common medication used in the management of degenerative disorders and painful syndromes involving the cervical spine are nonsteroidal anti-inflammatory agents (NSAIDs). There are five classes of these drugs with individual variations, costs, action, and side effects. Mechanical compression of nerve roots can lead to an inflammatory response, which produces radicular symptoms. Decreasing inflammation will usually cause pain to subside.

Physical therapy modalities include both active exercise and a passive program for pain modulation. The passive modalities may be used initially during the acute phase of the patient's care. After the patient's acute symptoms have subsided, passive treatment should be altered in favor of a more active program. Active modalities include isometric neck strengthening, neck and shoulder stretching, and aerobic exercises.

Surgical Treatment

Anterior Approach Smith and Robinson popularized the anterior approach for the surgical treatment of cervical disk disease in 1958 (Fig. 3). They reported that surgery was indicated if nonsurgical treatment failed to relieve upper extremity radicular symptoms or if the pain became excessive. Current indications for surgery in cervical radiculopathy include confirmatory imaging studies consistent with clinical findings and (1) persistent or recurrent arm pain unresponsive to a trial of nonsurgical treatment (3 months), (2) progressive neurologic deficit, or (3) static neurologic deficit associated with significant radicular pain. Surgical treatment of cervical myelopathy by an anterior approach is recommended in patients who have progressive impairment of function without sustained remission. In addition, the following criteria should be met: (1) one, two, or three level pathology; (2) pathology primarily at the disk level; and (3) anterior cord compression.

The Smith and Robinson technique of anterior cervical diskectomy and fusion becomes increasingly difficult over multiple levels, and the rate of successful fusion decreases as the number of attempted fusion levels increases. For these reasons, it is recommended that corpectomies be considered for multiple-level spondylitic myelopathy and myeloradiculopathy (Fig. 4). Stabilization is then performed with a strut graft. This technique allows more complete anterior decompression over numerous motion segments.

Results The first large series of patients treated with anterior interbody fusion for cervical degenerative disk disease was reported in 1962. Overall, 73% of the patients had either an excellent or good result. Patients who had

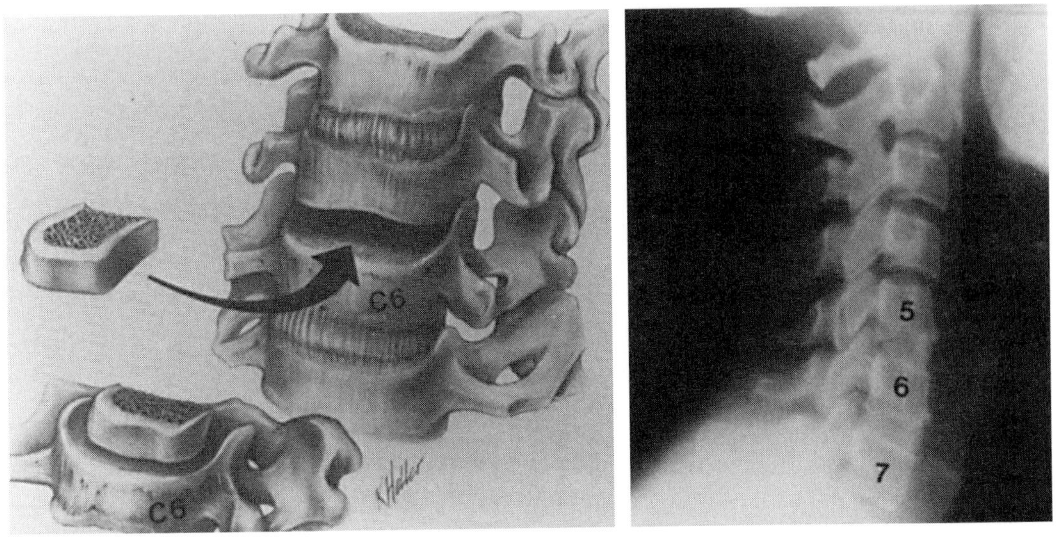

Fig. 3 Anterior cervical diskectomy and fusion. **Left,** Insertion of graft. **Right,** postoperative lateral.(Reproduced with permission from Herkowitz HN: Surgical management of cervical radiculopathy, in Rothman RH, Simeone FA (eds): *The Spine.* Philadelphia, PA, WB Saunders, 1992, pp 597–608.)

multiple level fusions had worse results than those who had single level disease, and the author postulated that the poor results may be due to greater disease severity.

The largest reported series of anterior interbody fusions included 229 patients with 442 disk levels that were fused using the Robinson technique. After a mean follow-up of 57 months, 63% of the patients were considered to have satisfactory results. Pseudarthrosis was noted to occur in 12% of the patients; however, it failed to affect the quality of the result. The lack of correlation between a successful fusion and patient outcome can be explained by the fact that even though bone union does not occur, a stable fibrous union does. In addition, removal of the degenerative disk alleviates some of the mechanical pressure on the nerve root. Finally, distraction of the disk space and neuroforamen occurs although much of the initial height of the interspace gained by the bone graft is lost.

Surgical treatment of myelopathy generally involves a more extensive anterior decompression. Bohlman reported in 1977 on 17 patients who were treated for cervical myelopathy with a Robinson type anterior cervical diskectomy and fusion at one or more levels. Fourteen of the 17 patients were noted to have increased strength in the upper extremities after the surgery, and most patients had significant gains in ambulation. These excellent results occurred in spite of the fact that Bohlman made no attempt to remove the posterior osteophytes. If, however, osteophytes are significantly impinging upon the spinal cord and/or cervical stenosis exists behind the vertebral body, a more thorough decompression is recommended. This involves either a complete or partial corpectomy with an iliac or fibular strut graft placed following decompression. Generally, an iliac graft can be used for up to three vertebral levels, whereas a fibular graft or allograft can be used for more levels.

Neurologic recovery following surgery for cervical myelopathy depends on the degree of spinal cord compression. Surgical results are generally poor when there is less than 30 mm^2 of spinal cord area preoperatively. Additionally, atrophy of the spinal cord as seen on MRI is often predictive of an unsatisfactory result.

Posterior Surgical Procedures The most common posterior cervical procedures performed for cervical radiculopathy and myelopathy are laminotomy with foramino-

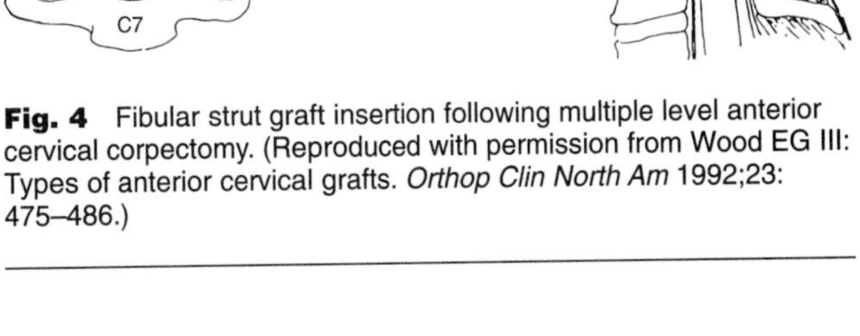

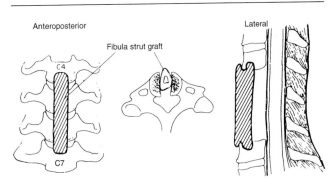

Fig. 4 Fibular strut graft insertion following multiple level anterior cervical corpectomy. (Reproduced with permission from Wood EG III: Types of anterior cervical grafts. *Orthop Clin North Am* 1992;23: 475–486.)

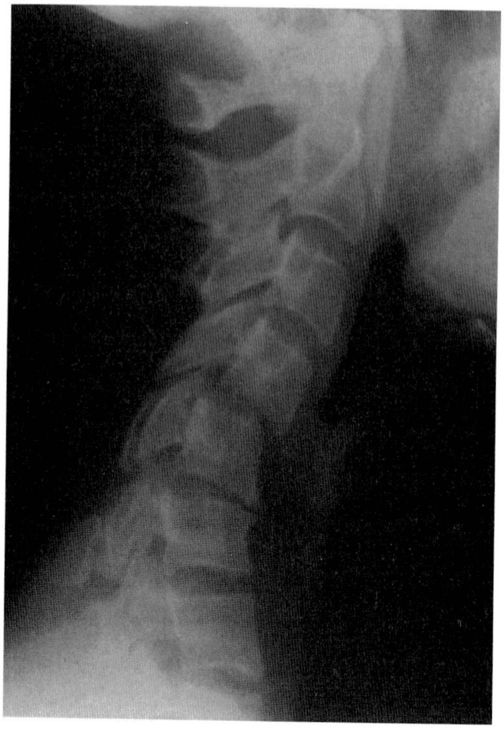

Fig. 5 Cervical kyphosis following multi-level laminectomy.

tomy, laminectomy, and laminoplasty. These three procedures vary in the amount of neural element decompression achieved. It is generally recommended that these procedures be performed with the patient prone to allow for collapse of the epidural veins to minimize the risk of embolism.

Laminotomy and foraminotomy require only a minimal amount of lamina resection to expose the lateral edge of the dura. The best results are usually achieved in patients with one level unilateral radicular pain due to a soft disk herniation. Resection of the medial aspect of the facet joint allows visualization of the exiting nerve root in the foramen. This procedure does not decompress the spinal cord and has minimal effect on cervical spine stability.

Laminectomy may be considered in patients with myelopathy due to multiple level cervical spondyloses. Isolated laminectomies are contraindicated in patients with preexistent cervical kyphosis or fractures and in children unless fusion is performed at the same time. A common concern regarding cervical laminectomy is the development of postoperative cervical kyphosis or instability (Fig. 5). Postoperative cervical kyphosis following laminectomy is directly related to the amount of intraoperative facet joint resection. A 50% facetectomy allows visualization of 3 to 5 mm of nerve root, while 70% resection allows visualization of 8 to 10 mm. Resection of greater than 50% of the facet joint, however, significantly compromises facet strength, with resulting segmental hypermobility.

Patients undergoing laminectomy for spondylitic myelopathy and/or radiculopathy usually have multiple level involvement and require multiple level procedures. As little as 25% facetectomy significantly increases all dominant motions (flexion, extension, right and left axial rotation, and lateral bending), and the development of postlaminectomy kyphosis alters the normal alignment and biomechanics of the cervical spine. Additionally, if the laminectomy was initially performed to relieve cord compression from anterior structures, lordosis is necessary to allow the cord to fall away from the impinging anterior elements. If postlaminectomy kyphosis does occur, extensive surgical intervention may then be indicated to salvage these patients.

For the patient with multiple level, bilateral myeloradiculopathy, extensive neurologic decompression is often necessary at multiple levels. This extensive resection obviously increases the chances of postoperative instability. Another option would be an anterior procedure. This procedure could be either multiple-level diskectomy and fusion, or a multilevel cervical corpectomy. For patients with three- to four-level nerve root compression, an anterior procedure may lead to a long operating time under general anesthesia, as well as being a potential risk to both the carotid artery and esophagus from prolonged retraction. In addition, the pseudarthrosis rate is directly related to the number of fused levels (unless a strut graft is used).

Cervical laminoplasty was developed in response to the high incidence of postlaminectomy deformity seen after extensive cervical laminectomy. The advantage of laminoplasty is that it does not violate the facet joints while maintaining additional stability on the hinged side of the procedure (Fig. 6).

Comparative Studies Unlike the surgical management of lumbar disk herniations, the surgical approach to cervical soft disk herniations has remained controversial. Excellent results have been reported for use of either the posterior or anterior approach.

Henderson reported on 736 patients who had a posterior lateral foraminotomy for simple cervical radiculopathy. There was no distinction made between soft disk herniations, hard disk herniations, or spondylitic spurring. Overall, the author reported an excellent or good result in 91% of cases. However, recurrent signs of radiculopathy were present in 20%, and 14% required a second posterior surgical procedure.

Herkowitz's prospective study evaluated the results of anterior cervical diskectomy and fusion compared to those of laminotomy and foraminotomy in patients with a diagnosis of cervical disk herniation. Thirty-three patients with a soft posterolateral disk herniation underwent either anterior cervical diskectomy and fusion or posterior cervical laminotomy and foraminotomy. At follow-up of over 4 years, the excellent or good rate following an anterior procedure was 94%, and was only 75% in patients who had a posterior procedure. Based on this study, anterior

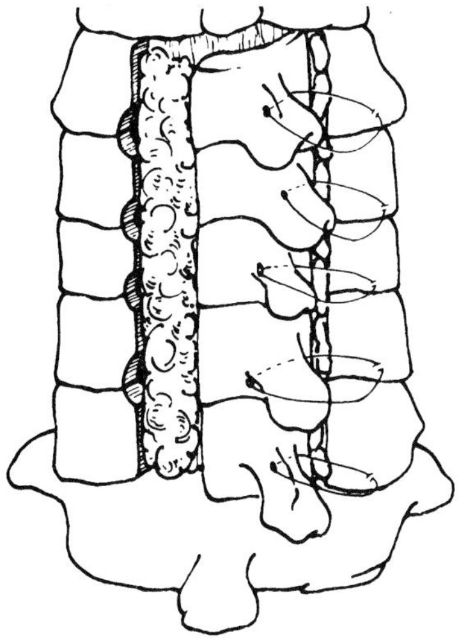

Fig. 6 Diagram demonstrating a cervical laminoplasty. (Reproduced with permission from Herkowitz HN: Cervical laminoplasty, in Rothman RH, Simeone FA (eds): *The Spine.* Philadelphia, PA, WB Saunders, 1992, pp 631–638.)

cervical diskectomy and fusion has the best long-term results in the surgical management of posterolateral disk herniations. Posterior laminectomy and foraminotomy may be considered in the following situations: (1) technical limitations of the anterior approach (eg, short, thick neck, particularly with C2–C3 or C7–T1 disks; marked kyphotic or spondylolisthetic deformation), and (2) prior anterior surgery restricting access to the surgical level.

Forty-five patients with nerve root compression at three or more levels due to spondylosis were also reviewed. Excellent or good results were seen in 92% of the patients who had an anterior procedure, while only 66% of the laminectomy group had similar results. In addition, 15 patients had a cervical laminoplasty with excellent or good results occurring in 86% of the patients. Based on the results of this study, the following conclusions were drawn: (1) anterior cervical diskectomy and fusion is the procedure of choice for multiple level spondylitic radiculopathy; (2) laminoplasty is preferred for patients with developmental stenosis, failure of anterior fusion, or patients with prior anterior neck surgery; and (3) cervical laminectomy may be considered for patients with failed laminoplasty or patients with anterior bony ankylosis due to degenerative or inflammatory disorders.

There are currently no available reports of prospective, randomized studies set up to compare surgical approaches and results for cervical myelopathy. Many studies are retrospective reviews of different procedures that have been performed at the same institution. In general, for two or three level decompression, the results of corpectomies are significantly better than those of anterior diskectomies and fusions. Moreover, two or three level anterior decompressions generally have more favorable neurologic recovery rates when compared to laminectomies.

Complications Complications of surgery for cervical disk disease can be divided into those occurring at the graft site and those occurring in the neck. Donor site pain is the most common patient complaint following spinal arthrodesis with autogenous bone grafting. The ilium is the most common area from which bone graft is harvested. Additional complications include cosmetic deformity, infection, hematoma, gait disturbance, ilium fracture, peritoneal perforation, hernia, and injuries to the lateral femoral cutaneous, superior cluneal, and ilioinguinal nerves. When approaching the posterior ilium, a limited incision within 8 cm of the posterior superior iliac spine should be used to avoid the superior cluneal nerves and prevent the formation of painful neuromas. When approaching the anterior ilium, the incision should end 2 cm lateral to the anterior superior iliac spine to avoid the lateral femoral cutaneous nerve.

The most common problem seen in the neck following anterior cervical surgery is a transient sore throat or difficulty swallowing. Unilateral vocal cord paralysis is due to injury to the recurrent laryngeal nerve during surgery. This complication is more common when using a right-sided approach, because the nerve may leave the carotid sheath at a variable higher level and is, thus, more susceptible to injury. Therefore, it is recommended that the approach be performed on the left side where the nerve constantly enters the thorax within the carotid sheath and then loops under the aortic arch. The risk of injury to the trachea and esophagus can be decreased by using hand-held retractors rather than self-retaining retractors. Although perforating injuries of the esophagus are rare, when they do occur they can be life threatening. Intraoperative perforations of the esophagus are usually secondary to inadvertent puncture by either sharp or motorized instruments. Late perforation by graft dislodgment or metal implants can also occur.

The most feared neurologic complication is that of iatrogenic spinal cord injury. Flynn compiled the results of over 700 neurosurgeons who described over 30,000 anterior cervical interbody fusions. In this large series, there were 100 cases of significant permanent myelopathy or myeloradiculopathy after surgery. Seventy-five percent of these patients were noted to have a deficit immediately after surgery, while 25% developed a neurologic deficit during the initial postoperative recovery phase. Regardless of the etiology of the myelopathy, additional surgery had little effect on the ultimate status of the neurologic deficit. Most surgeons were unable to determine the exact etiology of the neurologic deterioration.

Controversies Anterior cervical diskectomy without fusion was developed as an alternative to cervical fusion based on the premise that if successful results of anterior fusions occur with pseudarthrosis, then diskectomy can be performed without fusion. Most authors who advocate this procedure have reported good early results, with the majority of patients developing a spontaneous fusion at the diskectomy level as well as some degree of postoperative kyphosis. Unfortunately many studies examined only the neurologic recovery rate and failed to mention the significant problem of postoperative neck pain. Most longer-term studies of anterior cervical diskectomy without fusion have noted a very high rate of postoperative cervical and/or intrascapular pain (not evident as preoperative symptoms) in up to 50% of the patients.

This procedure, unlike anterior fusions, does not decrease nerve root irritation by neuroforamen distraction or reduce buckling of the ligamentum flavum. The results for radicular pain due to soft disk herniation are better than those for spondylosis. This procedure cannot be recommended until better long-term follow-up studies are available.

In an attempt to eliminate donor site problems while maintaining acceptable fusion rates, several authors have recommended substituting allograft for autogenous bone in cervical fusions. For one-level anterior cervical diskectomy and fusion, the union rate is comparable for allograft and autograft fusions. For multilevel anterior cervical procedures, the nonunion rate using freeze-dried allograft bone is significantly higher and is associated with graft collapse.

In an attempt to increase the fusion rate for anterior cervical fusion, anterior cervical instrumentation has been used. The anterior cervical plate theoretically provides increased stability postoperatively following anterior cervical decompression and can act as a buttress to prevent graft extrusion. However, the anterior cervical plate adds additional time and expense to the surgical procedure. Improper use of the anterior cervical plate can lead to postoperative dislodgment with subsequent esophageal irritation or perforation. However, in the case of multiple level cervical fusions in which the fusion rate is known to be lower, or multiple level cervical corpectomies in which cervical stability is in question, the use of an anterior cervical plate may increase the chance of successful fusion and decrease the need for postoperative stabilization, such as a halo brace.

Annotated Bibliography

Bohlman HH, Emery SE, Goodfellow DB, et al: Robinson anterior cervical discectomy and arthrodesis for cervical radiculopathy: Long-term follow-up of one hundred and twenty-two patients. *J Bone Joint Surg* 1993;75A:1298–1307.

This study evaluated the results of 122 patients with a mean 6-year follow-up undergoing anterior Robinson fusion for cervical radiculopathy. Neck and arm pain relief occurred in the majority of patients. Motor strength improved in 53 of 55 patients. The occurrence of a pseudarthrosis did not preclude a satisfactory outcome.

Emery SE, Smith MD, Bohlman HH: Upper-airway obstruction after multilevel cervical corpectomy for myelopathy. *J Bone Joint Surg* 1991;73A:544–551.

Seven patients who had undergone multiple level cervical corpectomy with strut graft developed postoperative airway obstruction. This was felt to be due to edema. Risk factors included smoking and asthma. The authors recommend intubation for 24 to 72 hours after surgery.

Farey ID, McAfee PC, Davis RF, et al: Pseudarthrosis of the cervical spine after anterior arthrodesis: Treatment by posterior nerve-root decompression, stabilization, and arthrodesis. *J Bone Joint Surg* 1990;72A:1171–1177.

Nineteen patients with persistent radiculopathy following anterior fusion with pseudarthrosis were treated with posterior nerve root decompression and fusion. All patients went on to solid fusion. Eighteen of 19 had relief of radiculopathy.

Fernyhough JC, White JI, LaRocca H: Fusion rates in multilevel cervical spondylosis comparing allograft fibula with autograft fibula in 126 patients. *Spine* 1991;16(suppl 10):S561-S564.

This study compared the nonunion rate of 126 patients undergoing allograft versus autograft fibula fusion. The nonunion rate was 27% for autograft versus 47% for allograft. The proximal insertion site had a much higher nonunion rate than the lower site.

Herkowitz HN, Kurz LT, Overholt DP: Surgical management of cervical soft disc herniation: A comparison between the anterior and posterior approach. *Spine* 1990;15:1026–1030.

This reports a prospective study of 44 patients with cervical disk herniation in which anterior fusion was compared to posterior foraminotomy. Anterior fusion has a better outcome for posterolateral soft disk herniations than foraminotomy and is the treatment of choice for central disk herniation in the cervical spine.

Jones AA, Dougherty PJ, Sharkey NA, et al: Iliac crest bone graft: Osteotome versus saw. *Spine* 1993;18:2048–2052.

This biomechanical study compared osteotome versus saw-harvested horseshoe shaped iliac crest bone grafts. The saw-harvested grafts were strongest, with the middle third of the iliac crest being the optimal location.

Okada K, Shirasaki N, Hayashi H, et al: Treatment of cervical spondylotic myelopathy by enlargement of the spinal canal anteriorly, followed by arthrodesis. *J Bone Joint Surg* 1991;73A:352–364.

Thirty-seven patients underwent diskectomy and varying degrees of corpectomy stabilized with either iliac or fibular strut graft for cervical spondylotic myelopathy. Improvement in neurologic status occurred in 29 of 37 patients. Atrophy of the spinal cord was a poor prognostic sign.

Satomi K, Nishu Y, Kohno T, et al: Long-term follow-up studies of open-door expansive laminoplasty for cervical stenotic myelopathy. *Spine* 1994;19:507–510.

Fifty-one patients with cervical myelopathy were followed up for a mean of 7.8 years after laminoplasty. The average spinal canal diameter did not decrease over the follow-up period. Factors which led to less than optimal outcome were age over 60 years, loss of sagittal canal diameter, progression of ossification of the posterior longitudinal ligament, and trauma.

Yonenobu K, Hosono N, Iwasaki M, et al: Neurologic complications of surgery for cervical compression myelopathy. *Spine* 1991;16:1277–1282.

In 384 cases of cervical myelopathy treated by anterior or posterior procedures, 21 patients (5.5%) sustained neurologic deterioration.

Zdeblick TA, Ducker TB: The use of freeze-dried allograft bone for anterior cervical fusions. *Spine* 1991;16:726–729.

Eighty-seven patients undergoing anterior cervical horseshoe autografts or allografts were compared for union rate. Nonunion rates for one-level fusion were similar in both groups. Significantly more nonunions occurred with the freeze-dried allograft for two- and three-level fusions.

Classic Bibliography

Bernard TN Jr, Whitecloud TS III: Cervical spondylotic myelopathy and myeloradiculopathy: Anterior decompression and stabilization with autogenous fibula strut graft. *Clin Orthop* 1987;221:149–160.

Bohlman HH: Cervical spondylosis with moderate to severe myelopathy: A report of seventeen cases treated by Robinson anterior cervical discectomy and fusion. *Spine* 1977;2:151–162.

DePalma AF, Rothman RH, Lewinnek GE, et al: Anterior interbody fusion for severe cervical disk degeneration. *Surg Gynecol Obstet* 1972;134:755–758.

Flynn TB: Neurologic complications of anterior cervical interbody fusion. *Spine* 1982;7:536–539.

Gore DR, Sepic SB, Gardner GM, et al: Neck pain: A long-term follow-up of 205 patients. *Spine* 1987;12:1–5.

Henderson CM, Hennessy RG, Shuey HM Jr, et al: Posterior-lateral foraminotomy as an exclusive operative technique for cervical radiculopathy: A review of 846 consecutively operated cases. *Neurosurg* 1983;13:504–512.

Herkowitz HN: A comparison of anterior cervical fusion, cervical laminectomy, and cervical laminoplasty for the surgical management of multiple level spondylotic radiculopathy. *Spine* 1988;13:774–780.

Hirabayashi K, Watanabe K, Wakano K, et al: Expansive open-door laminoplasty for cervical spinal stenotic myelopathy. *Spine* 1983;8:693–699.

Lees F, Aldren Turner JW: Natural history and prognosis of cervical spondylosis. *Br Med J* 1963;5373:1607–1610.

Nurick S: The natural history and the results of surgical treatment of the spinal cord disorder associated with cervical spondylosis. *Brain* 1972;95:101–108.

Raynor RB, Pugh J, Shapiro I: Cervical facetectomy and its effect on spine strength. *J Neurosurg* 1985;63:278–282.

Smith GW, Robinson RA: The treatment of certain cervical-spine disorders by anterior removal of the intervertebral disc and interbody fusion. *J Bone Joint Surg* 1958;40A:607–624.

49

Thoracic Disk Herniation

Incidence

The true incidence of thoracic disk herniations (TDH) is unknown. An approximate incidence of 11% to 15% has been proposed. The prevalence of patients with objective neurologic findings secondary to a disk herniation is one per million per year. Thoracic diskectomies for clinically significant thoracic disk herniations account for 0.2% to 2% of all diskectomy operations.

Classification

Thoracic disk herniations are classified according to level and location. This classification is helpful in determining the surgical approach. Location may be central, centrolateral, lateral, or intradural. Patients with central herniations may have symptoms of myelopathy, whereas lateral protrusions commonly elicit radicular symptoms. Intradural herniations are rare. Seventy percent of thoracic disk herniations are either central or centrolateral. The most commonly involved level is T11–12 at which 25% of all herniations occur; 75% of herniations occur between T8 and T12. Differentiation between soft and hard disk herniations should be made because this difference also influences the surgical approach.

Etiology

Trauma involving the thoracic spine is reported to be a precipitating event in about 25% to 50% of cases. Torsional or twisting movements or lifting of heavy objects are the most commonly described events; falls are rarely implicated. Scheuermann disease with myelopathy due to thoracic disk calcification can occur in younger patients. In the elderly, thoracic spondylosis with associated posterior hypertrophic changes in the facet joints and ligamentum flavum may produce stenosis and myelopathy.

In contrast to cervical and lumbar disk herniations, a significant percentage of TDH undergo calcification; a helpful radiographic feature. The smaller cross sectional diameter of the thoracic spine and the close proximity of the spinal cord to the posterior margin of the vertebral bodies can lead to the commonly seen progressive spinal cord compression associated with TDH.

Clinical Presentation

Eighty percent of patients are in their fourth to sixth decades with a 1.5 to 1 male to female ratio; 33% seek medical attention when in their 50s. Pain, the most frequent initial symptom, may be constant, intermittent, dull, sharp, or shooting in nature. Depending on the disk location, pain distribution may be axial, unilateral, or bilateral. Patients may also complain of pseudoradicular, unilateral lower limb pain, which mimics that of a lumbar disk herniation. Circumferential radiating pain around the chest wall is also commonly described. Symptoms may be aggravated with coughing, sneezing, or increased activities and frequently are improved with rest. Atypical radiating pains also occur. Groin pain may simulate degenerative hip and renal disease. Patients with midthoracic disk herniations may have chest and abdominal pain. Neck pain, upper extremity pain, and Horner's syndrome secondary to a T1 or T2 disk herniation can mistakenly be attributed to degenerative cervical disease. Sensory changes, especially numbness, are the second most common initial symptom (Table 1). Paresthesias and dysesthesias have also been reported. In the absence of pain, these symptoms may be the only clue in the diagnosis of TDH. Pain, motor weakness, or bladder dysfunction are usually the first symptoms recalled by patients (Table 2).

At the time of presentation to a physician, however, 30% of cases will have bladder dysfunction, whereas 18% will manifest with both bowel and bladder disturbances. Motor and sensory involvement has been reported in 60% of symptomatic patients.

Given the nonspecific and varied presentation, delay in diagnosis and misdiagnosis are common. Other neurologic disorders, such as multiple sclerosis, amyotrophic lateral

Table 1. Initial symptoms of Thoracic Disk Herniations

Initial Symptoms	Occurrence
Pain	57%
Sensory	24%
Motor	17%
Bladder	2%

(Reproduced with permission from Arce CA, Dohrmann GJ: Herniated thoracic discs. *Neuro Clin* 1985;3:383–392.)

Table 2. Symptoms when patients present to a physician

Symptoms	Occurrence
Motor and sensory	61%
Motor only	6%
Sensory only	15% to 39%
Weakness	59%
Bladder	30%
Bowel and Bladder	18%
Radicular Pain	9% to 16%

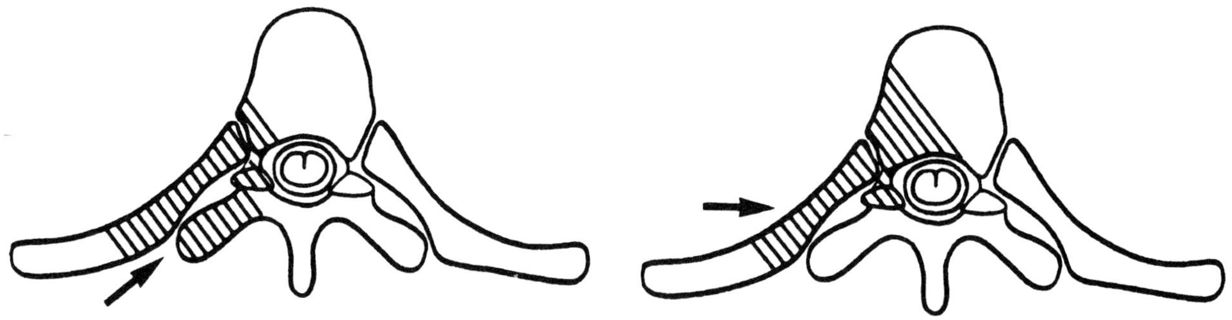

Fig. 1 Extent of bony resection (cross-hatch) and angle of approach (arrows) to disk space with costotransversectomy (**left**) and lateral extracavitary (**right**) procedures.

sclerosis, and transverse myelitis, should be considered in the differential diagnosis.

Physical Examination

Early in the course of TDH, there are few physical findings. Decreased dermatomal light touch or pinprick sensation may be found with thoracic radiculopathy. Spinal cord compression secondary to TDH produces typical signs of weakness, spasticity (hyperreflexia, Babinski signs), gait disturbances, and decreased sensory reaction to pinprick or light touch. Incomplete spinal cord syndromes, such as Brown-Séquard syndrome secondary to centrolateral TDH, are also associated with myelopathy.

Imaging Studies

Magnetic resonance imaging (MRI) is the screening study of choice for suspected TDH. Imaging studies must be interpreted with the awareness of the high asymptomatic prevalence of TDH. Saggital T1-weighted MRI of the thoracic spine provides visualization of thoracic disk degeneration that is unsurpassed by other radiographic techniques (eg, computed tomographic [CT] scanning myelography). The sensitivity of MRI of the thoracic spine has increased the diagnosis of TDH and thus will allow follow-up of smaller TDH. The key features of TDH on sagittal T1-weighted images are extension of disk material beyond the posterior margin of the adjacent vertebral bodies and indentation of the spinal cord. Herniated disk material or posterior osteophytes may be of low signal intensity on T1-weighted images and, therefore, difficult to distinguish from the spinal cord. In those cases, sagittal or axial T2-weighted images produce the myelogram effect in which the cerebrospinal fluid is brighter than the spinal cord and low intensity disk or osteophytes. In cases of lateral foraminal TDH, conventional myelography with postmyelographic CT scanning may still be helpful.

Differential Diagnosis

Given the wide variety of presenting complaints, both a spinal and nonspinal pain origin should be considered.

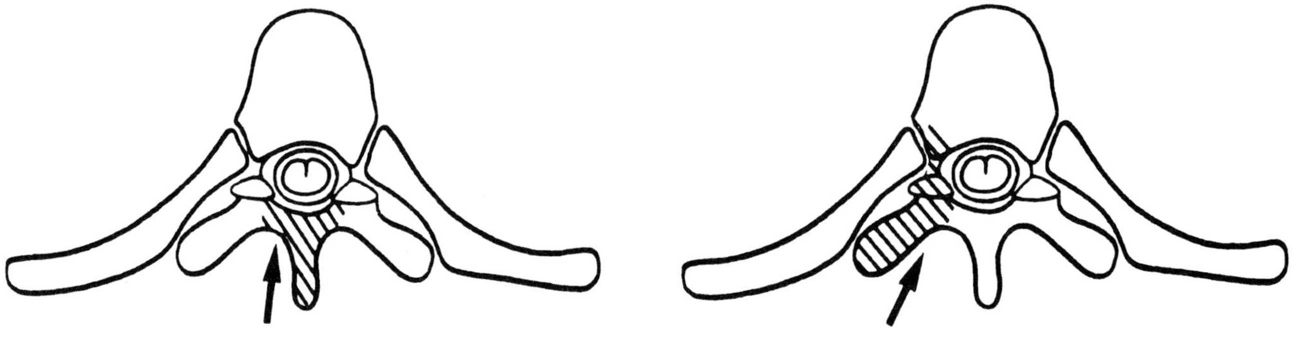

Fig. 2 Extent of bony resection (cross-hatch) and angle of approach (arrows) to disk space with laminectomy (**left**) and facetectomy/pediculectomy (**right**) procedures.

Other spinal disorders with similar initial symptoms include amyotrophic lateral sclerosis, transverse myelitis, spinal cord tumors, and arteriovenous malformations. Nonspinal disorders with referred symptoms that mimic those of TDH include cholecystitis, aneurisms, retroperitoneal neoplasms, and other intra-abdominal and intrathoracic disorders.

Natural History

The natural history is variable. Thoracic pain associated with acute traumatic disk herniations in younger patients may precede progressive myelopathy. In the middle-aged population with degenerative disk herniations, the onset of symptoms secondary to spinal cord compression tends to be more gradual. In the absence of myelopathy, nonsurgical treatment and activity modifications may be warranted. Approximately 80% of patients in the nonsurgical group may return to their previous activity level. Patients with unrelenting pain and lower extremity complaints are more likely to require surgery.

Nonsurgical Treatment

Nonsurgical treatment should be considered for patients without long tract signs or major neurologic deficits. A short trial regimen of bed rest with gradual mobilization and limitation of activities involving axial loading and repetitive flexion and extension can be beneficial. Thoracolumbosacral orthosis (TLSO) bracing may be effective. Pain is managed symptomatically with nonsteroidal anti-inflammatories (NSAIDs), acetaminophen, and the judicious use of narcotics. Physical therapy involving postural training, hyperextension strengthening, back school, and cardiovascular conditioning should also be attempted.

Surgical Treatment

Costotransversectomy (Fig. 1)

In order to gain access to central, centrolateral, and lateral TDH posteriorly, an oblique approach, which requires a more lateral exposure, must be used. This approach entails resecting the posterior portion of the rib as it articulates with the transverse process and the vertebral body. Costotransversectomy has the disadvantage of requiring a more extensive resection of bone. However, it facilitates visualization of centrolateral and lateral disk herniations without the need to enter the pulmonary cavity.

Transpedicular Approach (Fig. 2)

The advantage of this approach is that it involves a less extensive dissection in which potentially decreased bleeding and surgery time minimize complications. The main disadvantage is limited visualization, which renders management of central and centrolateral fragments, as well as osteophytes and calcified disks, difficult and hazardous. Access to dural fistulas and intradural pathology is limited. Furthermore, segmental stability may be compromised following facet, pedicle, and disk removal. This approach is indicated for soft lateral disk herniations in a medically compromised individual. Complications mainly arise secondary to limited visualization.

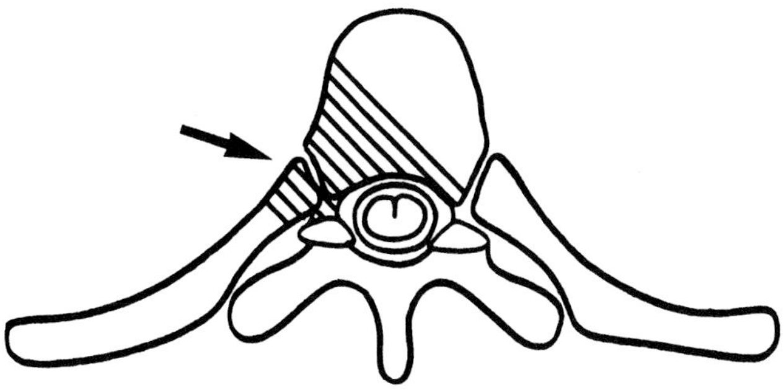

Fig. 3 Extent of bony resection (cross-hatch) and angle of approach (arrow) with transthoracic approach.

Transthoracic Approach (Fig. 3)

The transthoracic approach is the most versatile, allowing excellent central and centrolateral exposure from T4 to the thoracolumbar junction. The advantages include excellent visualization, anteriorly and anterolaterally, which permits safe decompression and dural manipulation. This approach is the safest and best choice for calcified disks in the presence of large osteophytes and TDH located behind the vertebral body. It entails limited bone removal, thereby diminishing the likelihood of destabilization while optimizing anterior interbody graft placement. The intercostal nerves are minimally traumatized. Disadvantages relate mainly to the thoracotomy, which requires chest tube placement, and possible pulmonary complications. Disk herniations at the thoracolumbar level, the location of the majority of thoracic disk herniations, may require take down of the diaphragm. Depending on the extent of bone removal, a transthoracic approach is indicated from T3 to T12. A rib graft fusion may be performed.

Lateral (Extracavitary) Approach (Fig. 1)

The lateral (extracavitary) approach for TDH is applicable to any level of the thoracic spine and is particularly well suited for centrolateral and lateral soft disk and lateral calcified disk herniations. The exposure is entirely extrapleural, requiring removal of portions of the costotransverse joint, facet, and/or pedicle. Additional rib resection allows wider access lateral to the spinal cord, permitting direct visualization of the nerve root and disk space without retraction of the cord. Multiple levels are easily ex-

Table 3. Surgical approaches for varying pathologies

Levels	Disk Herniation	Approaches
Soft Disks		
T1 to T4	Central, centrolateral	Transternal
		Medial clavisectomy
	Central, centrolateral, lateral	Costotransversectomy
T4 to T12	Central, centrolateral, lateral	Transthoracic
	Centrolateral, lateral	Lateral
	Central, centrolateral, lateral	Costotransversectomy
	Lateral	Transpedicular
Calcified Disks		
T1 to T4	Central, centrolateral	Transternal
		Medial clavisectomy
	Lateral	Costotransversectomy
T4 to T12	Central, centrolateral, lateral	Transthoracic
	Lateral	Lateral
	Lateral, centrolateral	Costotransversectomy

posed as is the thoracolumbar junction. Shoulder traction facilitates approaches to the thoracic spine at T1 through T7 by mobilizing the scapula away from the midline. The main drawback is the paraspinal muscle disruption, which usually does not cause long-term sequelae, and the significant removal of bone. These factors may increase blood loss and time of surgery.

Laminectomy (Fig. 2)

Retraction of the thoracic spinal cord through a conventional laminectomy is limited because of the tethering effect of the intact intradural dentate ligaments. Consequently, this often inadequate exposure compromises the anterolateral access for removing disk material. Poor results for treatment of herniated thoracic disks by laminectomy occur in more than 50% of cases and include a high rate of paraplegia. For the majority of patients, this approach should be avoided.

Transternal/Medial Clavisectomy (Table 3)

The approach to upper TDH (T1 to T4) is difficult posterolaterally because the scapula limits the costotransversectomy approach. A direct anterior approach can be considered and is indicated in the presence of calcified disk herniations. A transternal approach or a medial clavisectomy extending distally from a cervical Smith-Robinson approach leaving the sternum intact can be used.

Thoracoscopy

Thoracoscopic diskectomy is an evolving technique. Advantages include decreased postthoracotamy complications, diminished surgical trauma, early rehabilitation, and decreased cost.

Annotated Bibliography

Awwad EE, Martin DS, Smith KR Jr, et al: Asymptomatic versus symptomatic herniated thoracic discs: Their frequency and characteristics as detected by computed tomography after myelography. *Neurosurgery* 1991;28:180–186.

The authors determined a 11% incidence of asymptomatic thoracic disk herniations with CT myelography. This study emphasizes the need for clinical correlation when making surgical decisions.

Brown CW, Deffer PA Jr, Akmakjian J, et al: The natural history of thoracic disc herniation. *Spine* 1992;17(suppl 6): S97–S102.

An important study delineating the natural history of thoracic disk herniations in 55 patients. This study emphasizes that thoracic disk herniations do not always lead to major neurologic compromise, and, therefore, a less aggressive surgical approach should be considered.

Currier BL, Eismont FJ, Green BA: Transthoracic disc excision and fusion for herniated thoracic disks. *Spine* 1994;19:323–328.

Nineteen patients underwent transthoracic diskectomy (22 thoracic disks) and fusion for central or central lateral disk herniation. Unsatisfactory results were noted in three patients with a previous laminectomy and two patients with coexistent multiple sclerosis. Results were "excellent" to "good" in 12 of the 14 patients with uncomplicated thoracic disk herniations.

el-Kalliny M, Tew JM Jr, van Loveren H, et al: Surgical approaches to thoracic disc herniations. *Acta Neurochir (Wien)* 1991;111:22–32.

Various surgical approaches in the treatment of thoracic disk herniations are reviewed, and important factors in choosing a surgical approach are discussed, as well as indications and contraindications for each approach.

Kurz LT, Pursel SE, Herkowitz HN: Modified anterior approach to the cervicothoracic junction. *Spine* 1991; 16(suppl 10):S542-S547.

The authors describe an alternative approach to the upper thoracic spine allowing decompression, reconstruction, and stabilization.

Le Roux PD, Haglund MM, Harris AB: Thoracic disk disease: Experience with the transpedicular approach in twenty consecutive patients. *Neurosurgery* 1993;33:58–66.

A series of 20 patients, with 14 lateral and nine central thoracic disk herniations, treated via a transthoracic approach using a microscope are presented. Forty percent of patients were asymptomatic at 1-year follow-up.

Rosenthal D, Rosenthal R, de Simone A: Removal of a protruded thoracic disk using microsurgical endoscopy: A new technique. *Spine* 1994;19:1087–1091.

A new thoracoscopy assisted transthoracic diskectomy approach is presented. The potential advantages include decreased morbidity and earlier return to activities.

Simpson JM, Silveri CP, Simeone FA, et al: Thoracic disk herniation: Re-evaluation of the posterior approach using a modified costotransversectomy. *Spine* 1993;18:1872–1877.

Twenty-one consecutive patients (23 thoracic disk herniations) were decompressed posteriorly using either the costotransversectomy (16 patients) or the transpedicular (five patients) approach. Eighty-four point two percent "excellent" to "good" results are reported.

Singounas EG, Kypriades EM, Kellerman AJ, et al: Thoracic disc herniation: Analysis of 14 cases and review of the literature. *Acta Neurochir (Wien)* 1992;116:49–52.

Fourteen cases treated by a costotransversectomy approach are presented.

Stillerman CB, Weiss MH: Management of thoracic disc disease. *Clin Neurosurg* 1992;38:325–352.

An excellent comprehensive review of the subject, including surgical options and indications is presented.

Classic Bibliography

Arce CA, Dohrmann GJ: Herniated thoracic disks. *Neurol Clin* 1985;3:383–392.

Bohlman HH, Zdeblick TA: Anterior excision of herniated thoracic discs. *J Bone Joint Surg* 1988;70A: 1038–1047.

Hulme A: The surgical approach to thoracic intervertebral disc protrusions. *J Neurol Neurosurg Psychiatry* 1960;23: 133–137.

Lesoin F, Rousseaux M, Autricque A, et al: Thoracic disc herniations: Evolution in the approach and indications. *Acta Neurochir (Wien)* 1986;80:30–34.

Love JG, Schorn VG: Thoracic-disk protrusions. *JAMA* 1965;191:627–631.

Maiman DJ, Larson SJ, Luck E, et al: Lateral extracavitary approach to the spine for thoracic disc herniation: Report of 23 cases. *Neurosurgery* 1984;14: 178–182.

Patterson RH Jr, Arbit E: A surgical approach through the pedicle to protruded thoracic discs. *J Neurosurg* 1978;48:768–772.

Perot PL Jr, Munro DD: Transthoracic removal of midline thoracic disc protrusions causing spinal cord compression. *J Neurosurg* 1969;31:452–458.

Williams MP, Cherryman GR, Husband JE: Significance of thoracic disc herniation demonstrated by MR imaging. *J Comput Assist Tomogr* 1989;13:211–214.

50

Lumbar Degenerative Disease

Low Back Pain

The consequences of normal aging of the spine include progressive disk dehydration, chemical alterations, and subsequent mechanical "incompetence," which may be manifested in low back pain, although an exact correlation between disk degeneration and low back pain has not yet been established. Nevertheless, many believe that the predominant cause of persistent low back pain is incompetence of the disk. Other attributed causes, particularly for transient or diffuse back pain, are muscular strains or ligamentous sprains. At this point, these etiologies are difficult to differentiate, and they probably will be for some time to come.

It is estimated that 60% to 80% of the adult population have experienced low back pain, with 2% to 5% affected on a yearly basis. People whose work involves repetitive bending or prolonged exposure to stooping, sitting, or vibrational stresses appear to have a higher frequency of occurrence. However, job dissatisfaction, previous low back disorders, or personal problems are at least as important in contributing to low back pain disability. Low back pain impairments rank among the leading causes of time lost from work and permanent disability in North America, and they cost an estimated $50 to $100 billion a year. Remarkably, only about 10% of those affected with low back pain account for the vast majority of the cost (about 90%). This factor is likely due to poorly understood medical and personal problems that still are not accurately diagnosed and treated.

The prognosis of acute low back pain is predominantly spontaneous improvement over a 4-week period, regardless of treatment. The physician should not assume that low back afflictions do not need treatment; however, he or she should be familiar with the natural history of low back pain, what can and what cannot be diagnosed, and the efficacy and safety of various treatment options. Moreover, low back pain should not be confused with the relatively easily diagnosed conditions of lumbar radiculopathy and spinal stenosis, nor should there be confusion among the outcomes of any treatment of these conditions.

Low back pain is discussed in the recently published Agency for Health Care Policy and Research Clinical Practice Guideline on "Acute Low Back Pain Problems in Adults." This publication contains a compilation of a systematic review and analysis of the scientific literature and medical and lay input on the assessment and treatment of low back pain. This study, although admittedly flawed, found that initially a focused physical examination was sufficient to assess a patient with acute or recurrent low back pain of less than 4 weeks' duration, but that clinicians should be aware of findings that might indicate an underlying tumorous, infectious, or traumatic condition or a major neurologic syndrome. For a possible tumor or infection, such findings include age over 50 or under 20, a history of cancer, constitutional symptoms, rest or night pain, and a history of recent bacterial infection or immune suppression. Potential indicators for a spinal fracture are a history of a fall or vehicular trauma or of an energetic insult in older individuals. Saddle anesthesia, sphincter dysfunction, and a lower extremity neurologic deficit indicate at least the potential for a major neurocompressive lesion, which should be treated more expeditiously.

If findings do not indicate one of the underlying conditions described above, appropriate treatment of a patient with an acute low back pain syndrome includes education, assurance, and measures to make the patient comfortable. These measures include brief periods of rest (less than 5 days), nonsteroidal anti-inflammatory drugs (NSAIDs), aerobic exercises, and physical measures, which may include activity modifications. Muscle relaxants and opioid medications appear no more beneficial than nonsteroidal anti-inflammatory medications and may be associated with untoward side effects including drowsiness and dependence. Surgery is not indicated for individuals with acute low back pain problems who have no evidence of neural compression, but this option may be considered for individuals with chronic, clearly definable conditions, as will be discussed subsequently.

Treatments for acute low back pain that are sometimes used, but have not yet been scientifically validated or invalidated, include oral steroids, colchicine, antidepressants, such modalities as ultrasound and transcutaneous electrical nerve stimulation, lumbar supports, traction, biofeedback, trigger point injections, sclerosants, facet joint injections, and acupuncture.

Diagnostic tests of potential benefit when clinical symptoms and findings warrant include electrophysiologic tests, such as electromyography (EMG) and sensory evoked potentials (SEP), and bone scans. Thermography has not been shown to be of benefit. Plain radiographs, although not indicated early on without suspicion of an invasive or neurocompressive disorder, may be appropriate after failure of initial measures. As will be discussed later, computed tomography (CT), magnetic resonance imaging (MRI), and/or myelography may be appropriate when neurologic problems are suspected. Diskography, a highly controversial diagnostic test, also is not appropriate early on.

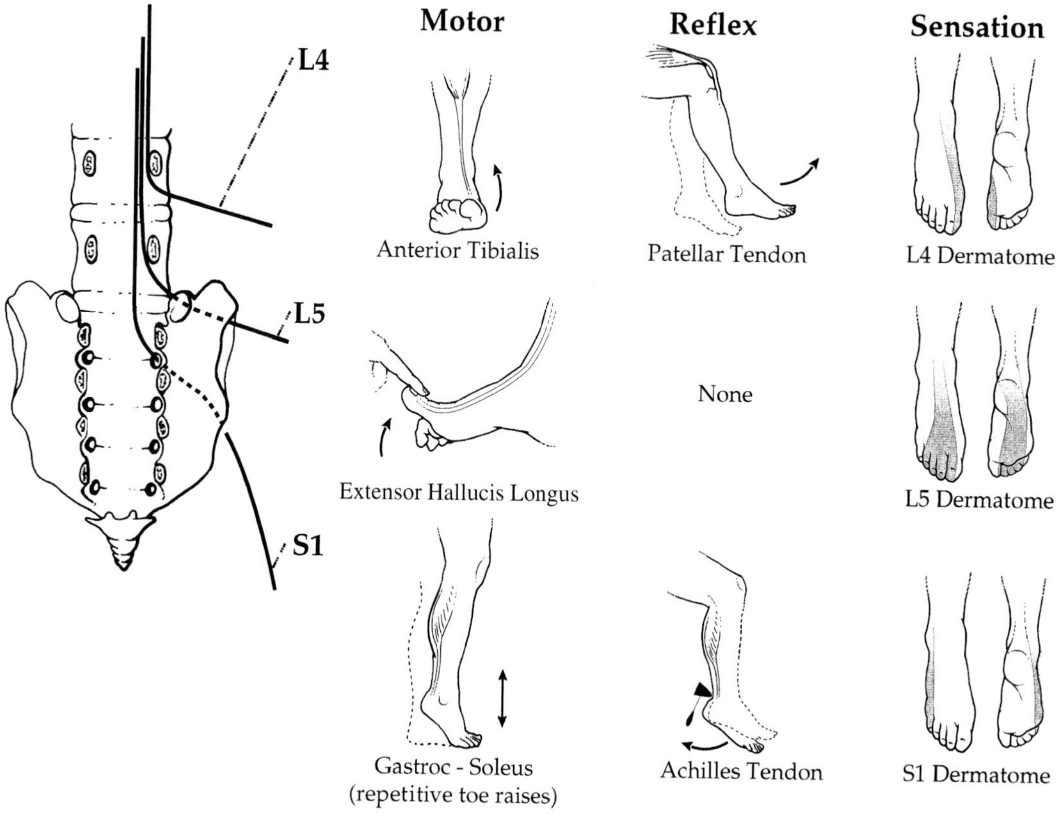

Fig. 1 Lower extremity findings with lumbar radicular symptoms.

Lumbar Radiculopathy: Herniated Disk

Epidemiology, Prognosis, Treatment Indications

Although frequently grouped together in discussions and analyses, there are vast differences between the problems of low back pain and those of sciatica. The magnitude of low back pain in terms of prevalence, diagnosis, treatment perplexity, disability, and cost to society towers over that of the reasonably well-defined entity of sciatica resulting from a herniated intervertebral disk. Apparently a symptomatic herniated disk occurs during the lifetime of approximately 2% of the population. Its prevalence is a small fraction of that of low back pain. The costs related to herniated disks are difficult to determine, but it is reasonable to assume that at least some of them are included in the enormous expenditures attributed to low back conditions.

In most cases, sciatica improves spontaneously. When the prevalence of sciatica (approximately 2%) and the patients who have persistent radiculopathy (10% to 25%) are considered, it is clear that surgical treatment should be entertained for fewer than 0.5% of the population. In the United States, however, the lifetime prevalence for lumbar disk surgery appears to be 3% to 4%, whereas it is only 1% in Scandinavia. Additionally, there are numerous regional variations in rates of disk surgery in the United States.

The intervertebral disk ages naturally from nuclear dehydration through a series of inevitable changes, which may be accentuated in predisposed individuals. With progressive degeneration, disk material may herniate, causing nerve root compression. Herniation generally occurs between the ages of 30 and 50 years. If this occurrence is severe enough and persistent enough to cause distress, the patient may seek medical attention. The exact cause of pain radiating down the leg is controversial. However, it appears that symptomatic lumbar radiculopathy is a result of mechanical contact between the disk and one or more nerve roots or a result of a combination of this contact and yet undetermined biochemical and vascular factors.

Terms used to describe the various distortions of a disk due to herniation are contained and noncontained. In a contained disk abnormality, the annular fibers are intact and contain the protruded disk material. In a noncontained abnormality, disk material has herniated through the annulus: the extruded disk material may be subligamentous or transligamentous, or there may be a sequestered fragment of disk material in the spinal canal.

The effect of a disk herniation on a nerve root can be magnified by lateral recess stenosis. The nerve root then becomes pinched between the disk herniation anteriorly and the hypertrophic stenotic changes laterally and posteriorly.

The symptoms of nerve root encroachment are variable. They depend on the patient's age and medical condition, the degree of root compression, the place on the nerve root or dorsal root ganglion at which the pressure is occurring, and the types of resultant inflammation and/or pathologic changes around and within the nerve root (Fig. 1).

A review of the course of symptomatic lumbar disk herniation reveals that surgery plays mainly a palliative role in its management. Results of long-term comparisons of surgical and nonsurgical treatment groups of patients with herniated disks show no statistically significant differences in outcome. In one study there were no differences between the groups at 4-year follow-up. Results after 1 year were initially better in the surgical group, but this difference diminished with time. Initial results were similar in another study, but by 6 months there was no significant clinical difference. Although the nonsurgical group in the second study was noted to have more back pain than the surgical group at 7 years, there were no clinical differences between groups in the first study with regards to back pain at 10-year follow-up.

The major benefit of surgical treatment for a herniated lumbar disk appears to be more rapid relief from sciatic pain than is provided by nonsurgical treatment. It is the clinician's task to select for surgery patients whose symptoms can be relieved with limited risk and the least possible expense.

In the past, five clinical criteria were used to determine surgical candidates: (1) impairment of bowel or bladder function, (2) gross motor weakness, (3) evidence of increasing impairment of nerve root conduction, (4) severe sciatic pain persisting or increasing despite 4 weeks of treatment, and (5) recurrent incapacitating episodes of sciatic pain. With correct knowledge of sciatica, the majority of these indications are now considered to be "relative."

The acute massive disk herniation that causes bladder and bowel paralysis appears to be best managed by emergent surgical excision (Fig. 2). In the face of progressing motor weakness, it is best to intervene early with surgical excision of the disk herniation. It has been shown that patients with a major neurologic deficit eventually made as much recovery with nonsurgical treatment as they did with surgical treatment. However, many surgeons believe that earlier surgery may accelerate neurologic improvement. Failure of nonsurgical treatment is the most common reason for surgical intervention. Optimal nonsurgical treatment occurs over at least 4 to 6 weeks and not more than 3 to 6 months, and it results in improvement in the patient's symptoms and signs. Current treatment measures consist of limited periods of bed rest (3 to 5 days), NSAIDs, patient education, and various exercise regimens. Epidural steroids may be of benefit. When incapacitating symptoms continue for more than 4 to 6 weeks, are substantiated by appropriate findings (tension signs with or without neurologic deficit), and are verified by collaborative imaging studies (myelogram, CT, MRI), surgery may be appropriate, depending on the patient's desires and needs.

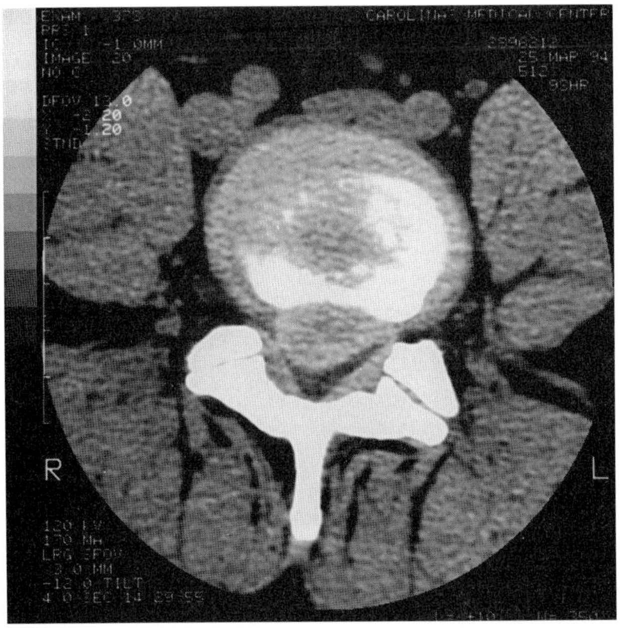

Fig. 2 Massive lumbar disk herniation at L4–5. This patient presented with an acute cauda equina syndrome. Emergent surgery resulted in improvement of the patient's symptoms.

Disabilities with generalized systemic or major nonorganic components may be a contra-indication to surgical intervention. For example, diabetes mellitus, with its systemic effects and known association with neuropathy, negatively influences the outcome of lumbar spine surgery.

Preoperative Investigations

Historically, myelography has been the radiographic study of choice for the diagnosis of a herniated disk. In recent years, CT and MRI have become the primary imaging modalities for this condition. These tests, however, are not without pitfalls or problems in interpretation. It is known that approximately 35% of asymptomatic individuals have evidence of a disk abnormality by myelogram, CT, or MRI, with 20% of those under age 60 years having imaging evidence of a disk herniation. In asymptomatic individuals over 60 years of age, over 50% will have abnormalities, with 36% exhibiting evidence of disk herniation and 21% demonstrating spinal stenosis. Bulging of a disk on an imaging study is probably a normal finding. EMG examination and diskographic radiographic assessment play little, if any, role in the evaluation of the patient with a herniated disk. An exception would be the patient with potential peripheral neuropathy in whom an EMG might be useful.

Surgical Options

The principal goals of surgical intervention are to relieve neural compression and the consequent radiculopathy, while minimizing complications. The most common currently used approach is a limited laminotomy with disk fragment excision. This surgery yields similar results whether it is performed using standard techniques, loupe magnification, or a surgical microscope. More recently, less invasive percutaneous approaches, in which suction, laser, or arthroscopic techniques are used, have been advocated.

Limited excision of a herniated disk for relief of sciatica should provide relief of symptoms in over 90% of properly selected patients. Results of surgery appear to correlate directly with the degree of disk herniation, with over 90% complete relief of sciatica when a free (sequestered) disk fragment is found at surgery, approximately 80% when an incomplete herniation is present, and 60% to 70% when there is only a protruding disk.

These results emphasize the importance of appropriate patient selection. The relief of back pain as the predominant symptom is unpredictable and usually is not obtained at surgery. Even when back pain is not a major component of the patient's symptoms before surgery, it can develop postoperatively. Factors leading to surgical failure as a result of back pain include worker's compensation issues, cigarette smoking, and age over 40 years.

The most common complications associated with lumbar disk excision are missed pathology, dural tears, and disk-space infection. Some believe these to be more common with the use of the microscope, but many think these problems are related primarily to the surgeon's level of experience or to underlying medical problems.

Percutaneous Lumbar Diskectomy Although chymopapain chemonucleolysis remains relatively popular in Europe and other parts of the world, its use as a noninvasive tool for the treatment of lumbar disk herniation diminished dramatically in North America in the mid 1980s after a series of adverse events and serious complications. These occurrences, along with technologic advances related to arthroscopic surgery and a persistent desire to avoid the problems of open disk excision surgery, led to the development of other percutaneous techniques for the treatment of this disease. These newer procedures include automated percutaneous suction lumbar diskectomy (APLD), percutaneous laser disk decompression, and percutaneous arthroscopic disk excision. Although initial reports by the developers and/or early proponents of these procedures showed results close to those of open diskectomy or open microdiskectomy, more current experiences by others indicate much lower success rates. The reasons proposed for these poorer outcomes include difficulties in patient selection (degenerated but not herniated disks, noncontained disk herniations), inherent fallacies of indirect decompressions (removal or ablation of disk material remote from the site of herniation), and technical problems related to the equipment or the surgeon (problems entering L5–S1, skill necessary for arthroscopic disk excision).

Percutaneous Suction Diskectomy In APLD, an aspiration type probe and rotary cutting device are used to remove material from the central portion of the disk, theoretically permitting a contained disk herniation to collapse and, thus, relieve pressure on the affected nerve root. Although excellent results have been reported by some, more recent scientifically designed studies show many fewer successes when randomized patients were treated using either chymopapain (approximately 61% success) or microdiskectomy (approximately 80% success) versus APLD (27% to 44% success). Moreover, success rates for patients who were failures of APLD and who underwent subsequent open surgery were not as good as those for patients primarily treated by open disk excision. Imaging studies performed after percutaneous diskectomy show little, if any, change in the size or configuration of the disk herniation and no correlation with clinical outcome.

Percutaneous Laser Diskectomy In percutaneous laser diskectomy, ablative laser energy is delivered through an optical fiber to the interior of the disk space. Disk material is removed by vaporization rather than by mechanical means as in APLD. The volume of disk material removed depends on the wavelength of laser energy and the amount of energy used. A variety of laser types can be used (CO_2, Holmium: YAG, Neodymium:YAG, Argon). Two types of lasers (KTP and Holmium:YAG) have been approved by the US Food and Drug Administration for lumbar disk applications. Imaging of the disk interior through the endoscope, deflection of the laser beam, and flexible diskoscopy to gain access to peripheral areas of the disk are now possible.

Initial clinical experience with laser disk ablation/decompression showed quite good results. As with APLD, however, as more reports emerge, the enthusiasm for this technique has diminished somewhat. Reported longer-term success rates are in the 55% to 70% range. Difficulty with appropriately selecting patients for the procedure is noted to be a major suspected reason for failure.

Percutaneous Arthroscopic Diskectomy The percutaneous technique that has generated the most interest in the last few years is that based on arthroscopy. With use of multiple "ports" and maneuverable instruments, access to the outer reaches of the disk and even to extruded material within the spinal canal is at least theoretically possible. An 87% success rate with this procedure has been reported for one series. Whether or not the nuances of this procedure are transferrable to other surgeons remains to be seen.

Special Situations With a Herniated Disk

Foraminal Disk Herniation Due to development and refinements in CT and MRI, foraminal and "far lateral" disk herniation syndromes can now be recognized. Most foraminal disk herniations occur in older patients (average age 65 years) at the L4–5 interspace encroaching on the fourth lumbar nerve root. A posterolateral extraforaminal approach has been advocated by some and has a success rate in the vicinity of 70%.

Disk Herniation with Spondylolisthesis Patients with spondylolisthesis may suffer from a disk rupture that causes acute radicular symptoms. The vast majority of these herniations occur at the level above the spondylolisthesis; commonly, an L4–5 disk herniation occurs above an L5–S1 isthmic spondylolisthesis. On rare occasions a true disk herniation may occur at the same level as the slip. For the former situation, a simple disk excision is all that is needed; for disk herniation at the slip level, diskectomy should be accompanied by a stabilization procedure.

Herniated Disk in Spinal Stenosis Patients with underlying spinal stenosis syndromes may occasionally suffer from a herniated disk. Investigation of these patients can be confusing, but an acute increase in leg pain in association with neurologic tension signs is an indicator that this diagnosis is a possibility. For patients with documented asymptomatic spinal canal stenosis, simple removal of the disk herniation is appropriate. If the spinal stenosis component was symptomatic before the occurrence of the herniated disk, surgery should also include a formal, more extensive, decompression procedure.

Recurrent Disk Herniation

With currently used techniques for open disk excision, a 5% to 10% rate of recurrent disk herniation is noted, and individuals with this problem may sometimes be candidates for further interventional treatment. The treatment approach for patients with recurrent disk herniation depends on the characteristics of the complaints, the physical findings, results of imaging studies, and the period of time elapsed and pain-free interval, if any, since the primary procedure. Those patients with minor residual lower extremity pain and/or low back pain that is bothersome, but not incapacitating, are best managed by accepted nonsurgical measures. For individuals with persistent radicular pain, further evaluation and possibly more aggressive intervention may be indicated. The two broad categories into which such patients can be divided are those with radiculopathy only and those with a combination of radiculopathy and low back pain (Fig. 3). Those patients with radiculopathy only, along with imaging studies demonstrating a recurrent disk herniation, can be treated successfully with repeat disk excision. However, patients whose symptoms do not correlate with imaging findings, or those in whom only epidural scar is noted on imaging, should be managed without surgical intervention.

A. RADICULOPATHY ONLY

PE: Tension Signs

Studies: X-Ray; Enhanced CT/MRI

	↙	↓	↘
DX:	Recurrent HNP L4-5	Recurrent HNP L5-S1	Scar
RX:	Disc Excision + In Situ Fusion	Disc Excision	No Surgery

B. RADICULOPATHY AND LOW BACK PAIN

PE: Tension Signs + LBP

Studies: X-Ray + Flexion-Extension; MRI ± Discography

	↙	↓	↘
DX:	Recurrent HNP "Disc Insufficiency"	Recurrent HNP "Instability"	Scar
RX:	Disc Excision + In Situ Fusion	Disc Excision + Instrumentation + Fusion	No Surgery

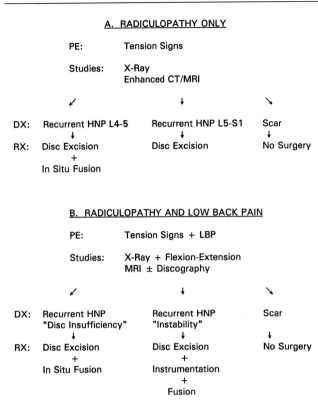

Fig. 3 Algorithmic approach to recurrent disk herniation. Patients can be divided into those with radiculopathy only (A) and those with radiculopathy and low back pain (B). (Reproduced with permission from Hanley EN Jr, Spengler DM, Wiesel S, et al: Controversies in low back pain: The surgical approach, in Schafer M (ed): *Instructional Course Lectures 43.* Rosemont, IL, American Academy of Orthopaedic Surgeons, 1994, pp 415–423.)

Patients with recurrent radiculopathy and low back pain present more of a challenge. Here the major debate is whether back pain symptoms are related to mechanical insufficiency of the disk or to definable instability. Plain radiographs and lateral flexion-extension views may reveal instability caused by degenerative change or iatrogenic spinal destabilization from facet removal, pars interarticularis excision, or fracture. MRI may show disk degeneration/dehydration, but this is insufficient evidence to discern diskogenic pain from insufficiency. Provocative diskography, although controversial, may be useful in such circumstances.

Although numerous criteria have been proposed for instability or hypermobility, most are either vague or incomprehensible. Probably the most reasonable objective measure of hypermobility is greater than 4 mm of translation and/or more than 10° of angular change on lateral flexion-extension radiographs.

If no hypermobility pattern is present, repeat surgery with disk excision and posterolateral fusion may be appropriate. Although it has been suggested that the addition of instrumentation or combined anterior disk excision and fusion may be indicated here, surgery of this magnitude is rarely necessary. The expected outcome in more than 75% of cases should be relief of radicular pain with mild residual low back pain. If the level of recurrence demonstrates frank translational or angular instability, then supplementary fixation/instrumentation may help hold the spine in a stable anatomic position while fusion consolidation occurs. The rate of arthrodesis consolidation may be improved with such techniques.

Degenerative Lumbar Spinal Stenosis

Degenerative lumbar spinal stenosis is the result of chronic disk degeneration, secondary spinal instability, and the body's attempts to control these phenomena. Symptoms may arise during any stage of the degenerative process and depend on mechanical and neurologic factors. These symptoms range from back discomfort to isolated nerve root irritation to frank neurogenic claudication. Successful treatment of the conditions that fall under the heading of lumbar spinal stenosis depends on an understanding of the pathogenesis and pathomechanics of the disease process, as manifested at the time of presentation.

The disease originates with changes in the functional spinal unit, which consists of two adjacent vertebrae and the interconnecting three-joint complex made up of the disk and facet joints. With normal aging of the disk, the water-binding capacity of the nucleus pulposus is dissipated, diminishing its ability to withstand normal compressive and rotational forces. This process may result in the production of degenerative annular tears of the disk. In some individuals, as a result of repeated stress or acute loading, an annular tear may be completed, resulting in disk herniation of the nucleus pulposus. The majority of people, however, progress through this early stage of disk degeneration free of symptoms or with only episodic low back pain. With progressive degeneration of the disk, collapse occurs. This collapse results in overriding of the facet joints and relative lengthening of adjacent capsular and ligamentous structures. At this stage, segmental instability may be manifested as motion-related back pain. Continued instability, which may be multidirectional, results in hypertrophic changes about the periphery of the vertebral body at its annular attachments. Radiologically, these are seen as traction osteophytes. Similarly, with pathologic hypermobility and subluxation, osteophytes form about the facet joints, presumably as an attempt to stabilize the abnormal motion. This facet enlargement may also compromise the size of the neural canal. In some instances instability may persist and predominate, leading to frank rotational and/or translational subluxation, which produce a degenerative spondylolisthesis or scoliosis pattern. This deformity may further compromise canal dimensions. These changes may occur at one level or involve several levels of the lumbar spine. At any time, the patient may complain of back pain and/or lower extremity pain.

With disease progression, hypertrophic changes predominate, leading to ankylosis and autostabilization. At this time, with decreased motion, back pain often diminishes. If the neural canal is of sufficient size, neurologic symptoms and signs may be absent; however, in individuals with less than optimal canal configurations or dimensions or in those with excessive hypertrophic degenerative changes, narrowing of the spinal canal, lateral recesses, and neuroforaminae may result in neurogenic symptoms and signs. These symptoms may be related to direct compression, arterial insufficiency, or impaired venous drainage of the neural elements of the cauda equina.

Diagnosis

Patients presenting with lumbar spinal stenosis are generally middle-aged or older. Depending on the stage of the disease process, low back or lower extremity symptoms may dominate the clinical findings. Often, a long history of nonincapacitating low back pain is given. The onset of radicular or claudicant symptoms usually causes the patient to seek medical help. Symptoms may involve one or multiple roots or may be described as a feeling of fatigue or weakness of the lower extremities with activity, particularly ambulation. This feeling may be relieved by sitting or squatting maneuvers that optimize lumbar spinal canal dimensions.

Symptoms are frequently vague and may be disregarded or attributed to other factors. Because these patients are usually elderly and often have multiple-system diseases, it is essential not to overlook the possibility of claudication-producing vascular disease, peripheral neuropathy, or an occult neoplasm as the source of pain or dysfunction.

Physical findings may be minimal or reveal profound neurologic abnormalities. Spinal alignment may be normal, although in some individuals a step-off deformity (degenerative spondylolisthesis) or scoliosis may be apparent. Lumbar lordosis is often diminished and, with the exception of individuals with persistent instability patterns and predominant back pain, spinal motion may be well preserved. Tension signs may be absent or present only to a mild degree. The neurologic examination may range from normal to the finding of profound sensory, motor, and reflex abnormalities in one or both extremities, which may be referable to one or more spinal levels.

Complete physical evaluation of the patient should include an abdominal exam to exclude an abdominal aortic aneurysm or visceral abnormalities, a rectal exam to rule out prostate and rectal pathology and assess sphincter tone, and palpation of lower extremity pulses. Efforts should be made to distinguish between vascular and neurogenic claudication and to assess the possibility of peripheral neuropathy due to other disease processes.

Ancillary laboratory, radiographic, and electrodiagnostic examinations may aid in the elimination of disease processes that may mimic spinal stenosis and may serve to help in the classification and treatment scheme of spinal stenosis syndromes. Laboratory studies for elderly patients who have symptoms of lumbar spinal stenosis may, when appropriately indicated (inconsistencies in the history, physical examination, radiographs, response to treatment), help exclude infectious, inflammatory, or neoplastic diseases. These studies may include a complete blood count with differential, erythrocyte sedimentation rate, serum protein electrophoresis, and, in male patients over 50 years of age, a prostate specific antigen determination. A whole-body bone scan may be useful in eliminating the possibility of an occult neoplastic or inflammatory process with osseous involvement.

Appropriate radiographic studies of good quality should be obtained and include anteroposterior (AP) and lateral flexion and extension views. The latter are used to aid in assessing instability patterns. Although electrical studies (EMG, nerve conduction velocity, SEP) may be helpful in patients with gross neurologic involvement, these studies may also be normal or fail to implicate all symptomatic levels. Electrical studies are, however, quite useful in excluding peripheral neuropathy, particularly in diabetics; they should be obtained when the diagnosis is in doubt, particularly if surgery is considered and the MRI is nondiagnostic or the medical history suggests concomitant diagnoses.

Treatment

Nonsurgical management is often sufficient to control symptoms and generally consists of a physical therapy regimen (gentle conditioning exercises, aerobic conditioning), judicious activity change, anti-inflammatory medication, and, sometimes, spinal support with a corset or lightweight brace. Epidural steroid injection may be helpful for lower extremity symptoms.

In patients with persistent functional incapacity, indications for surgical consideration include neurologic deficit; severe, intractable pain recalcitrant to nonsurgical treatment; and concomitant impairment of lifestyle. The purpose of the procedure is to improve function and decrease pain and, hopefully, to improve or halt progression of any neurologic deficits.

Surgical procedures in this group of middle-aged and elderly individuals, often with other medical problems, are of significant magnitude. The risks and benefits, as well as the limitations and possible complications of the proposed surgical procedure, should be discussed thoroughly with the patient. Although age is not a contraindication to surgery, there are some individuals whose general medical condition precludes the undertaking of a major surgical procedure without significant risk.

Surgical treatment usually consists of an adequate decompression of the involved neural elements and may, in certain instances, need to be combined with a spinal stabilization and arthrodesis. The surgeon should be comfortable with the techniques of decompression and fusion and able to deal with any complications that may arise during or after the procedure. Good lighting, magnification, microcautery, and a full array of spinal surgery instruments facilitate the procedure. Drains minimize the complication of epidural hematoma. Early postoperative mobilization of the patient should be used to minimize problems related to bed rest.

Classification

Individuals may present at any time during the degenerative process and exhibit any combination of back or lower extremity symptoms from single or multiple level involvement. Most patients with disease entities falling into the category of degenerative lumbar spinal stenosis may be included in one of four basic groups. This classification is based on extent of involvement and characteristics of stability (Fig. 4).

Unisegmental disease may be considered stable (lateral recess stenosis) or unstable (degenerative spondylolisthesis). Similarly, multisegmental spinal stenosis may be stable (ankylosing stenosis) or unstable (degenerative scoliosis). This classification scheme forms the basis for a rational approach to treatment.

Lateral Recess Stenosis The patient with stable unisegmental lumbar spinal stenosis is usually middle-aged with a history of chronic intermittent back pain and radicular symptoms of recent onset. Symptoms are usually unilateral in nature but on occasion may be bilateral. The L4–5 level is the predominant site of involvement, with the L5 nerve root being affected. Although less common, the disease may occur at the L5–S1 level. This level is usually protected from the disease process by the anatomy of the region: recession of the L5 body within the pelvis, and long transverse processes with stabilizing iliotransverse ligaments. In this condition, radiographs reveal isolated disk space narrowing with hypertrophic changes of the facets. CT or MRI reveal prominent facet joint(s) and lateral recess encroachment.

Successful treatment of stable unisegmental lumbar spinal stenosis is based on adequate neural decompression while maintaining spinal stability. Because the disease pro-

	STABLE	UNSTABLE
UNISEGMENTAL	LATERAL RECESS STENOSIS	DEGENERATIVE SPONDYLOLISTHESIS
MULTI-SEGMENTAL	ANKYLOSING STENOSIS	DEGENERATIVE SCOLIOSIS

Fig. 4 Classification of degenerative lumbar spinal stenosis based on levels of involvement and stability. Patients with stable stenosis may be treated with decompression alone. Those with unstable forms are best managed by decompression combined with a stabilization procedure.

cess involves all components of the functional spinal unit, unilateral surgery should be avoided. The patient who is treated with only unilateral decompression often presents at a later date with similar symptoms on the opposite side.

The surgical procedure should encompass adequate lateral canal decompression while maintaining the integrity of the facet joints. The facet joint capsules and pars interarticularis should be preserved, if possible. Preservation may be accomplished by undercutting the medial facets and is technically facilitated by using angled instruments from the opposite side of the operating table. In most instances, excision of the disk is not necessary and can possibly precipitate instability. Stabilization and fusion are not indicated in this stable disease.

Ankylosing Spinal Stenosis Stable multisegmental lumbar spinal stenosis generally affects an older group of patients. This subset appears to include a larger number of smokers and patients with peripheral vascular disease. At presentation, the low back pain may have diminished in intensity, and it is rarely incapacitating. The lower extremity symptoms, often insidious in onset, prompt the patient to seek medical attention. Lower extremity fatigue with activity is relieved by sitting or squatting positions that maximize canal dimensions. Neurologic findings may include motor, sensory, and reflex deficits at multiple root levels.

Radiographs reveal disk space narrowing at more than one level, claw osteophytes and traction spurs are present in combination, and facet joints at multiple levels are hypertrophic and sclerotic. A higher incidence of hip joint arthritis appears to occur in these patients as well.

It is important not to underestimate the number of involved segments. Neural relief with preservation of the facets may be provided with undercutting of the medial facets and foraminal decompression. Multiple levels, often from L2 to the sacrum, are affected, and all should be addressed at the time of surgery to avoid the need for, and risks of, additional procedures. In this disease subset, a mechanically stable situation exists and, therefore, arthrodesis usually is not necessary. The patient may be mobilized early in the postoperative course, but use of a support device may provide some comfort and security.

Degenerative Spondylolisthesis Degenerative spondylolisthesis is an acquired condition thought to be caused by chronic disk degeneration and long-standing segmental instability. Facet changes and rotational instability characterize the pathologic process. Slippage occurs most often at L4–L5, although it may be present at adjacent levels. It rarely progresses to more than 25% to 30% of vertebral body width. As the olisthesis progresses, patients may present with sciatica and/or claudication. Back pain is a frequent complaint, but usually is less than the neural symptomatology. This problem is common in the elderly population (average age 60 years) and more frequent in females.

Physical examination usually reveals minimal findings. In some cases, symptoms may be reproduced by having the patient walk during the physical examination. The L5 nerve root is most commonly affected; this effect may be demonstrated by finding of weakness in the extensor hallucis longus. Plain radiographs demonstrate narrowing of the disk space, facet joint arthropathy, and forward translation of a vertebra on the inferior vertebra. Flexion-extension radiographs may demonstrate some motion, although the gross translational and angular instability is usually minimal to moderate.

Surgical treatment may be considered when the disease becomes functionally incapacitating. Such treatment generally consists of decompression, arthrodesis, or a combination of both. Until recently, reports have not shown objective information to support one approach over the other. Some surgeons have tended to be selective and fuse only younger patients or those who required extensive decompressive procedures. Others have suggested an initial decompressive procedure followed by selective arthrodesis if the initial procedure fails. More recent uncontrolled surgical reports suggest that arthrodesis provides long-term stability, resists torsional and translational forces, and results in successful outcomes in approximately 85% of patients.

The most objective information on the treatment of this disease was reported in 1991 by Herkowitz and Kurz, who prospectively studied 50 patients with spinal stenosis from degenerative spondylolisthesis. They performed decompression alone in 25 patients and decompression and intertransverse fusion in the other 25. The patients in the two groups were similar in characteristics and mimicked those reported in the previous literature. At a follow-up of 3 years, results were significantly better with respect to pain in the back and lower extremities in those patients who had a concomitant arthrodesis. Spondylolisthesis increased postoperatively in 96% of patients without an arthrodesis and in only 28% of those with an arthrodesis. Although the radiographic pseudarthrosis rate was 36% in patients who had undergone fusion, this did not appear to affect the clinical results.

Although this report seems to settle the issue of whether or not to fuse patients with degenerative spondylolisthesis, it does not provide insight into whether or not to stabilize the spine with instrumentation during the procedure. The best available evidence concerning spinal stabilization has recently been published. In a meta-analysis of the literature from 1970 through 1993, Mardjetko and associates presented the results of a review of 25 acceptable papers (889 patients) on degenerative spondylolisthesis. Five of these studies (101 patients) included patients with decompression and fusion with pedicle screw instrumentation, while four (138 patients) detailed results of patients treated with control devices, such as Harrington rods, compression rods, and Luque rectangles with sublaminar wire fixation. They found that posterolateral spinal fusion rates were enhanced by use of spinal instrumentation and that there were no significant differences between control and pedicle screw devices. Device-related complications were similar, while specific types of complications were unique to each device.

In their cohort study of pedicle screw fixation, Yuan and associates detailed a retrospective outcomes analysis of patients treated with pedicle screw fixation for degenerative spondylolisthesis. They compared these outcomes with those of patients who did not undergo pedicle instrumentation at the time of surgical treatment for this condition. There were 2,684 patients in the study, with 2,177 (81%) in a pedicle screw fixation treatment group. Of the two control groups, 456 underwent noninstrumented fusion procedures, and 51 had instrumentation with control devices. The authors found that intraoperative complications related to pedicle screw fixation occurred infrequently, with a low rate (0.2%) of implant breakage. Rates of nerve root, spinal cord, and vascular injuries were also low (< 0.5%). Dural tears related to screw insertion were rare (0.1%), and other dural tears were comparable between instrumented and noninstrumented groups. The reoperation rate was higher in the pedicle screw group than in the noninstrumented treatment group (17.6% versus 15.0%). The majority of these procedures were related to device removal and/or reinstrumentation; the rate of surgery for repeat fusion was similar in instrumented and noninstrumented patient populations. The pedicle screw treatment group had a higher rate of fusion than the noninstrumented control group (89.1% versus 70.4%) as well as a tendency for more rapid fusion consolidation and better maintenance of spinal alignment. Additionally, patients treated with pedicle screw systems had better clinical outcomes related to pain, function, and neurologic recovery than the control, noninstrumented fusion patients. The risks of pedicle screw fixation were manifested mainly as implant breakages. The rates of nondevice-related events, repeated surgery, and deaths were similar between the two treatment groups. The authors concluded that the benefits of pedicle screw usage were substantially greater than the potential risk.

The decision as to whether or not to instrument a patient with degenerative spondylolisthesis should be based on flexion-extension radiographs. For the typical patient with degenerative spondylolisthesis with spinal stenosis and evidence of no additional motion on flexion-extension radiographs, a decompression procedure is advocated in conjunction with a lateral arthrodesis. For patients with objective instability (defined as translational excursion of more than 4 mm, or angular change of more than 10° on motion radiographs), the addition of segmental instrumentation may be appropriate.

Degenerative Scoliosis Degenerative scoliosis can be defined as scoliosis in the thoracolumbar spine developing after the age of 60 years. It is associated with disk degeneration and facet joint arthrosis. The curve is generally not greater than 40°. The overall result of the scoliosis and the degenerative processes is to reduce the volume of the spinal canal. Depending on the degree of canal size reduction, symptomatic spinal stenosis may occur.

The evaluation and treatment of patients with adult scoliosis is challenging. Expectations of treatment outcome should not mirror those reported for younger patients with scoliosis. Adult scoliosis can be divided into two major categories: that which is present before skeletal maturity (preexistent scoliosis) and that which arises later in life as a result of degenerative change and osteoporosis (degenerative scoliosis). Preexistent scoliosis follows the patterns seen in adolescent patients and may be associated with pain, curve progression, cosmetic concerns, and, on occasion, pulmonary decompensation or neurologic compromise. Degenerative scoliosis primarily affects the lumbar spine, and presentation is related to mechanical insufficiency of the spine (low back pain) with or without neurologic symptoms (claudication/radiculopathy).

Patients with degenerative scoliosis may have nonspecific symptoms. These patients have a combination of lower back pain and spinal stenosis; however, they often fail to obtain relief of their stenosis symptoms while sitting. Lack of relief appears to be related to spinal collapse caused by disk degeneration, osteoporosis, facet degenerative change, and rotational abnormality. These abnormalities result in both absolute stenosis from decrease in spinal canal volume and relative stenosis caused by collapse and translational and rotational shift of the spine. Although it is commonly believed that radicular symptoms will predominate on the side of collapse (concavity), neural symptoms may occur as a result of traction and shift on the convexity of the curve.

Symptoms and signs may be nonspecific. Pain is generally of gradual onset and can be localized to the back or legs or, more commonly, a combination of both. Physical findings range from objective neurologic findings of the involved nerve roots to vague tenderness in the lumbosacral area. Tension signs usually are not present or only mildly positive.

Plain radiographs are diagnostic and will demonstrate the level of scoliosis as well as the degenerative pathology. Should surgery be contemplated, a myelogram followed by a CT scan is preferred; although, in less severe deformities, MRI may be sufficient.

Nonsurgical treatment, NSAIDs, patient education and rest, and epidural steroids may be of benefit. Lumbar supports may provide some relief, but more rigid braces are often poorly tolerated by this elderly patient population. Patients with persistent symptoms may be considered for surgery.

Although decompression procedures alone have been proposed as an acceptable method of treatment, this treatment can lead to failure of back pain relief, progressive spinal collapse, and exacerbation of neural symptoms. Recent experience has emphasized the benefits of a more comprehensive surgical approach in which decompression is combined with deformity correction and stabilization

A. LBP

PE: Deformity, Imbalance, LBP
↓
Studies: X-Ray, Bend X-Ray, Hip X-Ray
Myelo/CT
↓
DX: Degenerative Scoliosis

Sx: mild-moderate ↙ ↘ Sx: severe

Nonop Rx
Brace
NSAI

Surgical Rx
Segmental Instrumentation
Fusion
± Anterior Surgery
Brace

B. LBP + CLAUDICATION/RADICULOPATHY

PE: Deformity, Imbalance, LBP, Neuro
↓
Studies: X-Ray, Bend X-Ray, Hip X-ray
Myelo/CT, EMG
↓
DX: Degenerative Scoliosis + Stenosis

Sx: mild-moderate ↙ ↘ Sx: severe

Nonop Rx:
Brace
NSAI
± Epidural Steroids

Surgical Rx:
Decompression
Segmental Instr.
Fusion
Brace

Fig. 5 Algorithmic approach to degenerative scoliosis. Patients with this condition are best divided into those with acute low back pain (LBP) only (A) and those with low back pain with claudication and/or radiculopathy (B). (Reproduced with permission from Hanley EN Jr, Spengler DM, Wiesel S, et al: Controversies in low back pain: The surgical approach, in Schafer M (ed): *Instructional Course Lectures 43.* Rosemont, IL, American Academy of Orthopaedic Surgeons, 1994, pp 415–423.)

with segmental instrumentation and fusion. Thus, decompression and fusion, with or without segmental correction with instrumentation, are recommended for patients whose incapacitating spinal stenosis symptoms and back pain are caused by degenerative scoliosis and who have failed nonsurgical treatment measures (Fig. 5). For the occasional patient with single nerve root involvement and no major back pain, unilateral root decompression may be indicated. For the rare presentation of painful, collapsing, degenerative scoliosis with back pain only, there may be a role for corrective instrumentation and fusion alone. Despite reports of the apparent success of such approaches, the surgeon must keep in mind that other health factors may preclude surgical treatment in some elderly patients, regardless of the severity of their symptoms and the functional disability caused by them.

Instability

Degenerative Segmental Instability

The indications for spinal fusion in the treatment of disk disease are controversial, primarily because of the difficulty in defining degenerative instability. Many theories attempt to correlate both radiographic and biomechanical criteria with instability; however, the typical consistent symptoms of abnormal motion segment behavior have yet to be clearly defined. A key premise is that selective fusion of an unstable motion segment must have a high probability of relieving symptoms, if a diagnosis can be made with certainty. To meet this definition, many classifications have been proposed, including biomechanical, clinical, and radiographic criteria; however, none have withstood the test of time or clinical experience.

Despite these concerns, there is a widely held belief that there are patients with degenerative instabilities who may be amenable to surgical stabilization. Radiographic signs, such as the traction spur and abnormal translational and angulatory motions, continue to be used as clinical criteria for the diagnosis. Additional attempts have been made to quantify more precisely the type and magnitude of motion that occurs or to define the source of pain through facet blocks or diskometry. Most recently, trials of short-term external fixation have shown promise in determining which patients will benefit from fusion. This technique is impractical in most situations and has not gained widespread acceptance. Most individuals use the findings on controlled flexion-extension radiographs of either 10° of angular motion or 4 mm of translation as the criteria for segmental instability and, hence, surgical arthrodesis. Another prerequisite is the presence of a stable psychological state, the absence of confounding work-related problems, and the potential attainment of functionally oriented goals. Despite the use of these criteria, results remain less than optimal as well as variable with reported success rates of 30% to 90% (Fig. 6 and Outline 1).

Iatrogenic Instability

An easier problem to deal with than the primary diagnosis of segmental degenerative instability is the intraoperative definition that decompression has produced an unstable motion segment. Recent biomechanical analyses have shown that sacrifice of more than 50% of both facets or the removal of one entire facet will produce significant loss of mechanical integrity of the spine. This research has tended to confirm the clinical experience of many.

However, other factors may influence the long-term clinical result. The presence of advanced age, marked disk space narrowing, and osteophytes are thought to reduce the need for fusion because they produce additional stabilizing effects on the motion segment. Conversely, surgery on a younger patient, particularly when facet resections are performed, may lead to a dramatically unstable spine. If disk excision is performed in conjunction with the de-

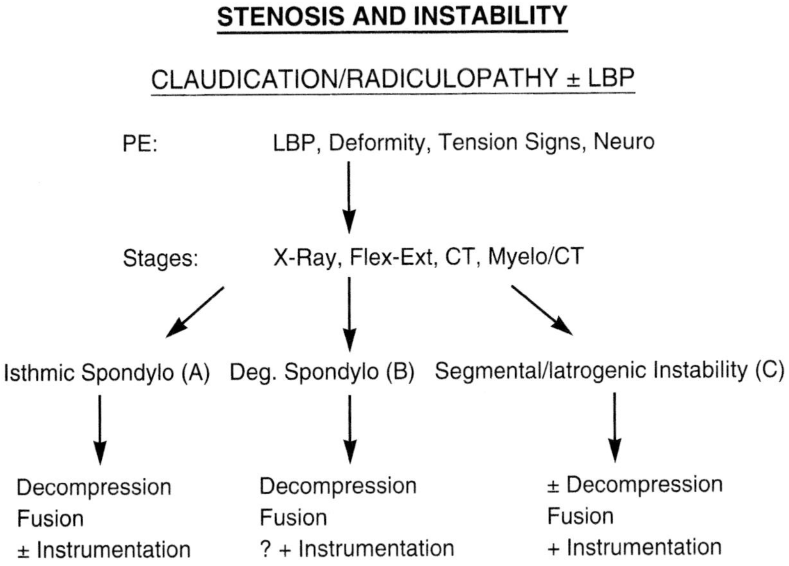

Fig. 6 Algorithmic approach for stenosis and instability. Patients present with a combination of back pain and lower extremity pain. (Reproduced with permission from Hanley EN Jr, Spengler DM, Wiesel S, et al: Controversies in low back pain: The surgical approach, in Schafer M (ed): *Instructional Course Lectures 43.* Rosemont, IL, American Academy of Orthopaedic Surgeons, 1994, pp 415–423.)

compression, this may further increase the instability potential.

With more than 50% removal of both facets or with complete removal of one facet, particularly at more than one level, prophylactic fusion should be considered. No definitive information is available on when instrumentation is appropriate, but it should probably be considered in younger patients when multiple levels are affected or when there is an underlying spinal deformity.

Disk-Related Low Back Pain

The greatest debate with regard to lumbar spine surgery exists for the diagnosis of diskogenic low back pain, now commonly referred to as internal disk disruption and diagnosed by the use of provocative diskography. Recent evidence suggests that diskography is a reliable means to assess pain originating from the intervertebral disk. Some studies have shown that the early hope that MRI would illustrate morphologic aberrations in the disk and lead to accurate clinical diagnoses predictive of surgical fusion outcome has proven to be unfounded. However, there are indications that a morphologic abnormality demonstrated by MRI in conjunction with a provocative pain response by diskography may predict who might benefit from a stabilization procedure.

Just as controversial is the question of what procedure to perform when a diagnosis of symptomatic internal disk disruption is present. A moderate amount of experience has been accumulated with isolated posterior fusion with and without instrumentation, anterior disk excision and interbody fusion, posterior lumbar disk excision and interbody fusion, and, most recently, circumferential stabilization procedures. Success rates for all of these procedures vary widely, ranging from approximately 30% to 90%, with most falling approximately in the middle. Unfortunately, most series include patients who have a wide variety of personal problems and variable outcome parameters, and these variables make the true success of these operations difficult to ascertain.

Also lacking, until recently, has been any information concerning the natural history of accurately diagnosed diskogenic low back pain. A recent study was reported on patients with diskogram concordant severe low back pain

Outline 1. Standardized diagnostic and treatment approach to patients with stenosis and instability

History	Back and/or leg pain with increased leg pain on ambulation
Physical examination	± neurologic deficit or tension sign Positive stress test
Diagnostic study	Dynamic lateral weightbearing radiographs Myelogram/computed tomography scan before surgery
Treatment	Initially, anti-inflammatory medication, controlled physical activity, and a corset Epidural Steroids Surgery Decompression with adequate removal of ligamentum flavum-open foramen Bilateral lateral fusion Only time to consider instrumentation is with motion > 4 mm Do not remove disk or this will lead to progression and increased symptoms

(Adapted with permission from Hanley EN, Spengler DM, Wiesel S, et al: Controversies in low back pain: The surgical approach, in Schafer M (ed): *Instructional Course Lectures 43.* Rosemont, IL, American Academy of Orthopaedic Surgeons, 1994, pp 415–423.)

who for a variety of reasons did not undergo an offered surgical fusion. Although criticized as being flawed, this report indicates that over a period of time a majority of patients with this diagnosis improve (65%) and resume a fairly functional lifestyle. Surgery for this condition should be approached with caution and with realistic expectations on behalf of both the patient and the surgeon.

Failed Prior Surgery

Extensive information is available on the surgical treatment of individuals with failed prior surgery. Analysis reveals that, except for situations in which obvious measurable instability exists, with or without residual neurologic compression, results of repeat surgical procedures are less than optimal, with reported successful outcomes in the 50% range. It appears that most often the source of failure is not a technical or physiologic one, but rather an inability to accurately define the indications for the primary or preceding procedures.

If the variable of a compensable work situation is present in a situation of failed initial surgery, the prognosis is poor (even worse) for a second procedure. In this setting, the chances of being made worse by surgery exceed the success rate.

Recent reports have examined the results of combined anterior and posterior lumbar fusions in patients who have had previous surgery for a wide variety of diagnoses and reveal a better outcome than with other types of surgery. The authors viewed this type of operation as a salvage procedure.

Several factors may lead to failed lumbar surgery. Failure of the initial procedure is frequently related to inappropriate patient selection, inappropriate treatment, or a technical error at surgery. Factors positively influencing repeat surgery include recurrent surgery after a long asymptomatic interval, a new herniation at a new location, and/or a separate identifiable and correctable pathologic condition. Negative factors include chronic radiculopathy, a failed previous surgical fusion, and negative psychosocial characteristics. The number of surgical successes diminishes proportional to the number of procedures performed. The type or magnitude of the procedure, including various instrumentation procedures, appears to have little influence on outcome.

Annotated Bibliography

Low Back Pain

Bigos S, Boyer O, Braen G, et al: *Acute Low Back Pain Problems in Adults: Clinical Practice Guideline No 14.* AHCPR Publication No 95-0642. Rockville, MD, Agency for Health Care Policy and Research, Public Health Service, U.S. Department of Health and Human Services, December, 1994.

Findings and recommendations on the assessment and treatment of adults with acute low back pain problems of less than three months' duration are presented in this AHCPR guideline. This government sponsored statement was developed by a 23-member multidisciplinary panel and was based on the published scientific literature and the opinions of panel members and consultants. An excellent but controversial review of the knowledge about low back pain problems is presented.

Frymoyer JW: Back pain and sciatica. *N Engl J Med* 1988;318:291–300.

This excellent review of the epidemiology, natural history, and treatment of low back conditions includes important references.

Taylor VM, Deyo RA, Cherkin DC, et al: Low back pain hospitalization: Recent United States trends and regional variations. *Spine* 1994;19:1207–1212.

Based on National Hospital Discharge Survey Data from 1979 through 1990, this study noted that while nonsurgical hospitalizations for low back pain decreased dramatically, low back surgery rates increased substantially with great regional variation.

Imaging

Boden SD, Davis DO, Dina TS, et al: Abnormal magnetic-resonance scans of the lumbar spine in asymptomatic subjects: A prospective investigation. *J Bone Joint Surg* 1990;72A:403–408.

Sixty-seven asymptomatic subjects underwent lumbar MRI, with approximately one third having a substantial abnormality. Of individuals under 60 years of age, 20% had a disk herniation. Abnormal scans were seen in 50% of older subjects, with 36% having a disk herniation or bulging and 21% having spinal stenosis.

Lumbar Disk Herniation

Choy DS, Ascher PW, Ranu HS, et al: Percutaneous laser disc decompression: A new therapeutic modality. *Spine* 1992;17:949–956.

Three hundred and thirty-three patients with 377 herniated disks were treated as outpatients with percutaneous Nd:YAG laser partial disk vaporization. Good to fair results were reported in 78%. The authors advocate this treatment for contained, nonsequestrated herniated disks in carefully selected patients.

Donaldson WF III, Star MJ, Thorne RP: Surgical treatment for the far lateral herniated lumbar disc. *Spine* 1993;18:1263–1267.

Far lateral disk herniations were operated on in 29 patients with a 72% satisfactory outcome. Average patient age was 65 years and the L4–5 level was most often affected. A posterolateral approach is described.

Herron L: Recurrent lumbar disc herniation: Results of repeat laminectomy and discectomy. *J Spinal Disord* 1994;7:161–166.

Forty-six patients who had previously undergone laminectomy and diskectomy for lumbar disk herniation were treated for recurrent disk herniation after an average of 7 years. No patients underwent concomitant fusion, and 69% were rated as good results.

Nordby EJ, Wright PH, Schofield SR: Safety of chemonucleolysis: Adverse events reported in the United States, 1982–1991. *Clin Orthop* 1993;293:122–134.

One hundred and twenty-one serious and unexpected adverse events after chymopapain injection are reported after approximately 135,000 underwent this treatment. They included fatal anaphylaxis (seven cases), infection, (24 cases), hemorrhage (32 cases), neurologic events (24 cases), and miscellaneous (15 cases) events, with a reported mortality estimate of 0.019%.

Pople IK, Griffith HB: Prediction of an extruded fragment in lumbar disc patients from clinical presentations. *Spine* 1994;19:156–158.

Back and leg pain proportion were compared with surgical findings in a prospective observational study of 100 diskectomy patients. Patients with an extruded disk fragment had a significantly higher proportion of leg pain than those with a disk protrusion.

Revel M, Payan C, Vallee C, et al: Automated percutaneous lumbar discectomy versus chemonucleolysis in the treatment of sciatica: A randomized multicenter trial. *Spine* 1993;18:1–7.

Of 141 randomized patients with sciatica due to a lumbar disk herniation, 69 underwent automated percutaneous diskectomy and 72 chemonucleolysis. At 1-year follow-up the success rate for chemonucleolysis was 66% and for automated diskectomy 37%. Reoperation rates were higher in the automated percutaneous diskectomy group (33% vs 7%), but back pain was more common in those treated with chemonucleolysis.

Shapiro S: Cauda equina syndrome secondary to lumbar disc herniation. *Neurosurgery* 1993;32:743–746.

Fourteen patients with acute cauda equina syndrome due to a herniated lumbar disk (100% bilateral sciatica and weakness, 93% sphincter dysfunction) were operated on from less than 1 day to more than 30 days. Emergent diagnosis and surgery within 48 hours appeared to improve outcome. The L4–5 level was most commonly affected.

Tullberg T, Isacson J, Weidenheilm L: Does microscopic removal of lumbar disc herniation lead to better results than the standard procedure? Results of a one-year randomized study. *Spine* 1993;18:24–27.

This randomized prospective study of surgery performed by the same surgeon showed no differences between the groups regarding bleeding, complications, hospital stay, time away from work, or end result. The authors concluded that the decision to use the operating microscope should be left up to the surgeon.

Surgery

Cherkin DC, Deyo RA, Loeser JD, et al: An international comparison of back surgery rates. *Spine* 1994;19:1201–1206.

The rate of back surgery in the United States was at least 40% higher than in any other country and more than five times those in England and Scotland. Back surgery rates increased almost linearly with the per capita supply of orthopaedic and neurosurgeons in the country.

Davis H: Increasing rates of cervical and lumbar spine surgery in the United States, 1979–1990. *Spine* 1994;19: 1117–1123.

Analysis of national surgery data indicated that over this time period hospitalizations for spine surgery and particularly lumbar spine fusion increased markedly.

Spinal Stenosis

Johnsson KE, Rosen I, Uden A: The natural course of lumbar spinal stenosis. *Clin Orthop* 1992;279:82–86.

Thirty-two untreated patients with spinal stenosis were followed up for a mean of 4 years. Symptoms in 70% were unchanged, 15% showed improvement, and 15% worsened. No severe neurologic deteriorations were noted.

Katz JN, Lipson SJ, Larson MG, et al: The outcome of decompressive laminectomy for degenerative lumbar stenosis. *J Bone Joint Surg* 1991;73A:809–816.

Older patients and those with concomitant medical conditions had less favorable results at follow-up. Repeat surgery was performed in 17% of patients for recurrent stenosis or instability.

LaBan MM, Viola SL, Femminineo AF, et al: Restless legs syndrome associated with diminished cardiopulmonary compliance and lumbar spinal stenosis: A motor concomitant of Vasper's curse. *Arch Phys Med Rehabil* 1990;71:384–388.

Cases of nocturnal lumbosacral and lower extremity cramps and fasciculations in association with decreased cardiopulmonary reserve and spinal stenosis are described. The authors attribute the condition to paravertebral venous congestion.

Postacchini F, Cinott G: Bone regrowth after surgical decompression for lumbar spinal stenosis. *J Bone Joint Surg* 1992;74B:862–869.

Bone regrowth after spinal decompression occurred in 88% of 40 patients who had undergone decompressive procedures for spinal stenosis. In patients with degenerative spondylolisthesis the rate of bone regrowth was higher, particularly in those who had not had a fusion. The amount of bone regrowth was inversely correlated with clinical outcome.

Sanderson PL, Wood PL: Surgery for lumbar spinal stenosis in old people. *J Bone Joint Surg* 1993;75B: 393–397.

Results of decompression surgery for spinal stenosis in patients over age 65 years were 64% excellent, 17% good, and 19% poor. The authors concluded that the long-term outcome of decompressive surgery is as good as that reported for younger patients.

Simpson JM, Silveri CP, Balderston RA, et al: The results of operations on the lumbar spine in patients who have diabetes mellitus. *J Bone Joint Surg* 1993;75A:1823–1829.

Higher rates of postoperative infection and prolonged hospitalization were noted in decompressive procedures on diabetic patients when compared to matched nondiabetic patients. Similarly, long-term satisfactory outcomes were found in only 39% of diabetics. The poorer results may be related to peripheral neuropathy and microvascular disease.

Degenerative Spondylolisthesis

Bridwell KH, Sedgenick TA, O'Brien MF, et al: The role of fusion and instrumentation in the treatment of degenerative spondylolisthesis with spinal stenosis. *J Spinal Disord* 1993;6:461–472.

Forty-four patients with degenerative spondylolisthesis were treated with either decompression without fusion; with decompression and fusion; or with decompression, fusion, and segmental instrumentation. More spondylolisthesis progression and persistent symptoms occurred in those without instrumented fusions.

Groebler LJ, Anderson PA, Novotny JE, et al: Etiology of spondylolisthesis: Assessment of the role played by lumbar facet joint morphology. *Spine* 1993;18:80–91.

Computed tomography scans revealed more sagittal plane facet orientation in patients with degenerative spondylolisthesis compared to the normal population and spinal stenosis patients.

Herkowitz HN, Kurz LT: Degenerative lumbar spondylolisthesis with spinal stenosis: A prospective study comparing decompression with decompression and intertransverse process arthrodesis. *J Bone Joint Surg* 1991;73A:802–808.

Fifty patients with spinal stenosis and degenerative spondylolisthesis underwent surgery with better results in those having combined decompression and fusion (96% versus 44%).

Mardjetko SM, Connolly PJ, Shott S: Degenerative lumbar spondylolisthesis: A meta-analysis of literature 1970–1993. *Spine* 1994;19(suppl 20):2256S–2265S.

This study conducted as part of a presentation to the FDA Orthopaedic and Rehabilitation Devices Advisory Panel reviewed 25 acceptable papers on the subject of degenerative spondylolisthesis. It reports that fusion significantly improves patient satisfaction and adjunctive spinal instrumentation enhances fusion rates.

Yuan HA, Garfin SR, Dickman CA, et al: A historical cohort study of pedicle screw fixation in thoracic, lumbar, and sacral spinal fusions. *Spine* 1994;19(suppl 20):2279S–2296S.

This cohort study analyzed retrospectively information on patients who had undergone spinal fusions using pedicle screw instrumentation for the treatment of degenerative lumbar spondylolisthesis or fractures during 1990 and 1991. The authors presented these data to the FDA Orthopaedic and Rehabilitation Devices Advisory Panel.

Degenerative Scoliosis

Grubb SA, Lipscomb HJ, Suh PB: Results of surgical treatment of painful adult scoliosis. *Spine* 1994;19:1619–1627.

Results of surgery performed on adults with degenerative scoliosis and idiopathic scoliosis were assessed. Reported pain reduction was 80% among patients with idiopathic scoliosis and 70% among patients with degenerative scoliosis. Improved functional tolerances were seen postoperatively.

Marchesi DG, Aebi M: Pedicle fixation devices in the treatment of adult lumbar scoliosis. *Spine* 1992;17(suppl 8):S304-S309.

Curve correction of better than 50%, pain relief, and improved walking distance were noted in 86% of patients. The pseudarthrosis rate was 4%. Neurologic deficits were treated with concomitant decompression procedures.

Perennou D, Marcelli C, Herisson C, et al: Adult lumbar scoliosis: Epidemiologic aspects in a low-back pain population. *Spine* 1994;19:123–128.

Of 671 patients with low-back pain, lumbar scoliosis was present in 7.5% and increased with age: 2% before 45 years; 15% after 60 years. Scoliosis was manifested in low-back pain in 86% of the cases and averaged 21°. Females had more severe deformities.

Simmons ED Jr, Simmons EH: Spinal stenosis with scoliosis. *Spine* 1992;17(suppl 6):S117-S120.

Forty patients with low-back pain and lower extremity pain from adult lumbar scoliosis underwent spine fusion surgery with segmental instrumentation. Major pain improvement was seen in 93%, with 50% correction in deformity. The value of indirect decompression of the spinal canal with curve reduction is noted.

Lumbar Spine Fusion

Deyo RA, Ciol MA, Cherkin DC, et al: Lumbar spinal fusion: A cohort study of complications, reoperations and resource use in the Medicare population. *Spine* 1993;18: 1463–1470.

An analysis of elderly Medicare patients undergoing surgery with spinal fusion revealed the complication rate to be 1.9 times greater than in those who had surgery without fusion, with higher blood transfusion rates, nursing home placement rates, and hospital charges.

Gill K, Blumenthal SL: Functional results after anterior lumbar fusion at L5-S1 in patients with normal and abnormal MRI scans. *Spine* 1992;17:940–942.

Patients with abnormal magnetic resonance imaging (MRI) scans and abnormal diskography had a 75% success rate versus a 50% success rate in those with normal MRI findings.

Knox BD, Chapman TM: Anterior lumbar interbody fusion for discogram concordant pain. *J Spinal Disord* 1993;6:242–244.

Single-level fusions for diskogram concordant low-back pain achieved 35% good, 18% fair, and 47% poor results. All two-level fusion results were poor. Patients with previous surgery or workers' compensation did poorly.

Turner JA, Ersek M, Herron L, et al: Patient outcomes after lumbar spinal fusions. *JAMA* 1992;268:907–911.

This literature review found 68% of patients had a satisfactory outcome after fusion, but the range was wide (16% to 95%) and the satisfactory rate was lower in prospective than in retrospective studies. Most frequently reported complications were pseudarthrosis (14%) and chronic pain at the bone graft donor site (9%). Results were worse with reoperation.

Wetzel FT, LaRocca HS, Lowery GL, et al: The treatment of lumbar spinal pain syndromes diagnosed by discography: Lumbar arthrodesis. *Spine* 1994;19:792–800.

Forty-eight patients with low back pain positive diskography underwent lumbar spinal fusion. Forty-six percent had a satisfactory clinical outcome and 48% a solid arthrodesis.

Whitecloud TS III, Davis JM, Olive PM: Operative treatment of degenerated segments adjacent to a lumbar fusion. *Spine* 1994;19:531–536.

Fourteen patients with a degenerative adjacent motion segment underwent decompression and fusion. The most commonly involved level was L3–4 and the average time from the first fusion 11.5 years. Results were: excellent, none; good, 3; fair, 6; and poor, 3. Only one of five uninstrumented fusions obtained a solid arthrodesis.

Zdeblick TA: A prospective, randomized study of lumbar fusion: Preliminary results. *Spine* 1993;18:983–991.

For 124 patients who underwent lumbar fusion for degenerative conditions by either posterolateral fusion alone, posterolateral fusion supplemented by a segmental device, or posterolateral fusion with a rigid segmental fixation system, results were better with the rigid device.

Classic Bibliography

Frymoyer JW, Hanley E, Howe J, et al: Disc excision and spine fusion in the management of lumbar disc disease: A minimum ten-year follow-up. *Spine* 1978;3:1–6.

Hakelius A: Prognosis in sciatica: A clinical follow-up of surgical and non-surgical treatment. *Acta Orthop Scand Suppl* 1970;129(suppl):1–76.

Kirkaldy-Willis WH, Wedge JH, Yong-Hing K, et al: Pathology and pathogenesis of lumbar spondylosis and stenosis. *Spine* 1978;3:319–328.

MacNab I: Spondylolisthesis with an intact neural arch: The so-called pseudo-spondylolisthesis. *J Bone Joint Surg* 1950;32B:325–333.

Mixter WJ, Barr JS: Rupture of intervertebral disc with involvement of spinal canal. *N Engl J Med* 1934;211: 210–215.

Spangfort EV: The lumbar disc herniation: A computer-aided analysis of 2,504 operations. *Acta Orthop Scand* 1972;142(suppl):1–95.

Spengler DM, Freeman CW: Patient selection for lumbar discectomy: An objective approach. *Spine* 1979;4:129–134.

Verbiest H: A radicular syndrome from developmental narrowing of the lumbar vertebral canal. *J Bone Joint Surg* 1954;36B:230–237.

Waddell G, McCulloch JA, Kummel E, et al: Nonorganic physical signs in low-back pain. *Spine* 1980;5:117–125.

Weber H: Lumbar disc herniation: A controlled, prospective study with ten years of observation. *Spine* 1983;8:131–140.

51

Evidence-Based Recommendations for Patients With Acute Activity Intolerance Due to Low Back Symptoms

Back problems are common, almost unavoidable, and have become the most expensive musculoskeletal entity and industrial injury. Back problems are the most common cause of disability under age 45 in the United States. Treatment recommendations are variable. As much as ninefold variation has been recorded in the use of treatment and evaluation methods in different parts of the United States. Determining what medical science supports involves determining whether sufficient evidence exists to make a definitive statement. Knowledge about what is predictable can have an impact not only on the decisions made by patients, but on those made by physicians and researchers.

The following recommendations have been formulated by applying scientific rigors to a National Library of Medicine search that provided over 10,000 abstracts of published articles related to low back problems. The abstracts were reviewed independently by two clinicians (orthopaedic surgeon and occupational medicine specialists). This process, along with contributions from an open forum, provided over 4,600 articles that were classified and evaluated according to specific scientific/methodologic criteria for possible entry on evidence tables. A 30-member multidisciplinary panel appointed through the United States Agency for Health Care Policy and Research participated in the process. Evidence tables were created to guide the care and understanding of patients limited by low back symptoms for *less than 3 months* (acute low back problems).

Methodology

A standard methodology is intended to minimize bias in differentiating a hypothesis (generated by review articles and editorial comments) from evidence (adequate scientific scrutiny of a hypothesis through clinical trials or cohort studies) of predictable benefit as a sound basis for recommending actions.

Before a "Finding and Recommendation" statement can be made, the evidence is evaluated from review of the articles and placed on an evidence table according to preestablished criteria. The quality and amount of evidence about benefit is provided through formation of evidence tables by methodologically scrutinizing the scientific literature. The stated strength of effects of treatment and assessment methods is weighed. The consistency of findings between studies is evaluated. The clinical applicability to the population is contemplated. Potential harms and costs relative to the above evidence are considered.

Additionally, the following questions were considered before formulating a clear statement: (1) Does the net potential benefit (effect) outweigh the net potential harm (risks) and, if so, does the net benefit justify the cost for this method? This question provides the basis for each "Finding and Recommendation" statement in Table 1. (2) What amount of evidence justifies the statement concerning the potential benefit to the patient (effect) and the potential harm to the patient (risk)? Finding and Recommendation statements provide a collective judgment of available evidence with relevance (to the population) and specificity (to the method addressed). The Finding and Recommendation statements fall into one of three categories: (1) recommendations for: If the available evidence (amount A, B, C, D) indicated potential benefit outweighed potential harms; (2) options: If the available evidence (amount A, B, C, D) of potential benefit is weak or equivocal (some studies for and some against) but potential harms and costs appear small; and (3) recommendations against: If the available evidence (amount A, B, C, D) indicated either lack of benefit, or that potential harms and costs outweighed potential benefits.

Each statement is aimed at patient understanding with the amount of supporting scientific evidence rated according to the scale in the second footnote to Table 1. The criteria for evidence required at least one adequate scientific study that meets minimal criteria for formal scientific methodology, relevance (to the population), and specificity (to the action being addressed).

These guideline statements of 1994 are intended to be altered by future scientific efforts and are not to be considered a standard or definitive effort. Current unproven entities can be added to the proven "Recommend" category in the future, if efforts find the measurable benefit outweighs the risk and cost. The "Finding and Recommendation" statements in Table 1 are the guidelines developed by the panel. The amount of scientific evidence is provided for each statement.

Table 1. Guideline statements of 1994 for patient understanding of what medical science can or cannot support as predictable

Areas of consideration*	Finding and recommendation statements	Amount of evidence†
	Assessment	
History/physical examination	Information about the patient's age, duration and description of symptoms including impact on activity, and response to previous therapy is important in the care of back problems.	B
	Inquiries about history of cancer, unexplained weight loss, immunosuppression, intravenous drug use, history of urinary infection, pain increased by rest, and fever provide appropriate RED FLAGS of possible cancer and infection, which are especially important in patients older than 50 years of age.	B
	Inquiries about signs and symptoms of cauda equina syndrome, such as a bladder dysfunction and saddle anesthesia in addition to major limb motor weakness, provide appropriate RED FLAGS of severe neurologic risk to the patient.	C
	Inquiries about history of significant trauma relative to age (eg, fall from height or motor vehicle accident in a young adult versus a minor fall or heavy lift in a potentially osteoporotic or older patient) may avoid delays in diagnosing fracture.	C
	Instruments like a pain drawing and Visual Analog Scale may be an option to augment the history.	D
	Recording the results of straight leg raising is of benefit in the assessment of the severity of sciatica in young adults. In older patients with spinal stenosis, the test may be normal.	B
	A neurologic examination emphasizing ankle and knee reflexes, ankle and great toe dorsiflexion strength, and distribution of sensory complaints helps to document the presence of neurologic deficits.	B
Physiologic measures		
Electrophysiologic tests	Needle electromyography (EMG) and H-reflex tests of the lower limb may be useful in assessing suspected nerve root dysfunction in patients with leg symptoms lasting longer than 3 to 4 weeks (regardless of whether they also have back pain).	C
	Sensory evoked potentials (SEPs) may be useful in assessing suspected spinal stenosis and spinal cord myelopathy.	D
	If the diagnosis of radiculopathy is obvious and specific on clinical examination, electrophysiologic tests are seldom necessary.	D
	Surface EMG and F-wave tests are not useful for assessing patients with acute low back problems.	C
Bone scan	A bone scan is an appropriate test for patients with acute low back problems when spinal tumor, infection, or occult fracture is suspected because of RED FLAGS on history, physical examination, or collaborative laboratory test or plain radiograph findings (except in pregnant women).	C
Thermography	There is no evidence to support the use of thermography for assessing patients with acute low back problems.	B
Anatomic images		
Plain radiographs	Plain radiographs are not recommended for the routine evaluation of patients with acute low back problems unless a RED FLAG is noted on clinical examination (as in the next two statements).	B
	Plain radiographs of the lumbar spine are useful for ruling out fractures in patients with acute low back problems when any of the following RED FLAGS are present: recent significant trauma (any age); recent mild trauma (patients older than 50 years); history of prolonged steroid use; osteoporosis; and patients older than 70 years.	C
	Plain radiographs in combination with complete blood count and erythrocyte sedimentation rate may be useful for ruling out tumor or infection in patients with acute low back problems when any of the following RED FLAGS are present: prior cancer or recent infection; fever (over 100°F); intravenous drug use; prolonged steroid use; low back pain worse with rest; and unexplained weight loss.	C
	In the presence of RED FLAGS, especially for tumor or infection, clinical judgment may necessitate the use of other imaging studies, such as bone scan, CT, or MRI, if radiographs are negative.	C

*CT, computed tomography; MRI, magnetic resonance imaging; NSAID, nonsteroidal anti-inflammatory drug; TENS, transcutaneous electrical nerve stimulation.
†A, Strong research-based evidence (multiple specific and relevant high-quality scientific studies); B, Moderate research-based evidence (multiple adequate or one specific and relevant high-quality scientific study); C, Limited research-based evidence (at least one adequate scientific study); D, Some helpful information that did not meet the inclusion trial criteria on evidence tables.

Table 1. (*Continued*)

Areas of consideration*	Finding and recommendation statements	Amount of evidence†
	The routine use of oblique lumbar radiographs is not indicated for adults especially in light of the increased radiation exposure.	B
CT, MRI, myelography, and CT-myelography	RED FLAGS suggesting cauda equina syndrome or progressive major motor weakness are an indication for prompt use of CT, MRI, myelography, or CT-myelography. Because these serious problems may require prompt surgical intervention, it is most beneficial that such imaging studies be discussed with a surgical consultant.	C
	CT, MRI, myelography, or CT-myelography and/or consultation with an appropriate specialist are indicated for clinical findings strongly suggesting tumor, infection, fracture, or other space-occupying lesions of the spine.	C
	Routine spinal imaging tests are generally not indicated in the first month of symptoms except in the presence of RED FLAGS of serious conditions. After 1 month of symptoms, an imaging test is acceptable when surgery is being considered (or to rule out a suspected serious condition).	B
	For patients with acute low back problems who have had prior back surgery, MRI with contrast may be the imaging test of choice, because it is more effective than other tests in distinguishing disk herniation from scar tissue associated with prior surgery.	C
	CT-myelography and myelography are invasive, have an increased risk of complications, and are indicated only in special situations for preoperative planning.	C
	The following are minimal quality criteria for imaging studies of the lumbar spine: CT and MRI cuts to be made no wider than 0.5 cm and parallel to the vertebral end plates; MRI scans to use a magnetic field strength no less than 0.5 T (Tesla) with an adequate scanning time; myelography and CT-myelography to use water-based contrast media; and the technical protocols for these imaging tests to be described on radiologist reports.	B
Diskography	Diskography is invasive and the evidence does not support its use for assessing patients with acute low back pain because the interpretation is equivocal and complications can be avoided with other noninvasive techniques.	C
	Treatment	
Patient education	Accurate information about the following aspects of low back symptoms benefits patients with acute low back problems: expectations for both rapid recovery and recurrence of symptoms based on natural history of low back symptoms; safe and effective methods of symptom control; safe and reasonable activity modifications; best means of limiting recurrent low back problems; the lack of a need for special investigations unless RED FLAGS are present; and effectiveness and risks of commonly available diagnostic and further treatment measures for patients with persistent symptoms.	B
Back school	In the workplace, back school including specific work-site directions may be an effective adjunct to patient education by the clinician in the treatment of patients with acute low back problems.	C
	The efficacy of back schools in nonoccupational settings has yet to be demonstrated.	C
Medications Acetaminophen and NSAIDs	Acetaminophen is reasonably safe and is acceptable for treating patients with acute low back problems.	C
	NSAIDs (including aspirin) are acceptable for treating patients with acute low back problems.	B
	NSAIDs have a number of potential side effects. The most frequent complication is gastrointestinal irritation. The decisions on whether to use these medications can be guided by comorbidity, side effects, cost, and patient/provider preference.	C
	Phenylbutazone is not recommended based on an increased risk for bone marrow suppression.	C
Muscle relaxants	Muscle relaxants as an option may be more effective than placebo, but no more effective than NSAIDs, in the treatment of patients with acute low back problems.	C

*CT, computed tomography; MRI, magnetic resonance imaging; NSAID, nonsteroidal anti-inflammatory drug; TENS, transcutaneous electrical nerve stimulation.
†A, Strong research-based evidence (multiple specific and relevant high-quality scientific studies); B, Moderate research-based evidence (multiple adequate or one specific and relevant high-quality scientific study); C, Limited research-based evidence (at least one adequate scientific study); D, Some helpful information that did not meet the inclusion trial criteria on evidence tables.

Table 1. (*Continued*)

Areas of consideration*	Finding and recommendation statements	Amount of evidence†
	There seems to be no additional benefit of using muscle relaxants in combination with NSAIDs over using NSAIDs alone.	C
	Muscle relaxants have potential side effects, including drowsiness in up to 30% of patients. The use of muscle relaxants as an option should balance the potential for drowsiness against a patient's intolerance of other agents.	C
Opioid analgesics	Opioids appear no more effective in relieving low back symptoms than safer analgesics (ie, acetaminophen, aspirin, or other NSAIDs).	C
	Decreased reaction time, clouded judgment, drowsiness, and other complications lead to early discontinuation in as high as 35% of patients using opioids.	C
	Patients should be warned about potential physical dependence and problems associated with the use of opioids while operating dangerous equipment or driving.	C
	The use of opioid analgesics is an option for management of patients with acute low back problems only for a time-limited course, guided by consideration of potential complications relative to other options.	C
Oral steroids	There is no evidence oral steroids are effective for acute low back problems.	C
	There is potential for severe side effects from extended use of oral steroids or short-term use of high-dose steroids.	B
Colchicine	There is no evidence colchicine is effective for treating patients with acute low back problems. Colchicine has potential serious complications.	C
Physical		
Manipulation	Manipulation seems helpful for patients with acute low back problems without radiculopathy when used within the first month of symptoms.	B
	With findings suggesting progressive or severe neurologic deficits, an appropriate diagnostic assessment to rule out serious neurologic conditions is indicated prior to considering manipulation.	D
	No evidence indicates that manipulation is efficacious for patients with radiculopathy.	C
	A trial of manipulation in patients without radiculopathy with symptoms longer than a month is probably safe but efficacy is unproven.	C
	If manipulation has not resulted in symptomatic and functional improvement after 1 month of treatment, manipulation therapy should be stopped and the patient reevaluated.	D
Physical agents/modalities	There is no evidence that the benefits of physical agents/modalities outweigh costs sufficiently to justify their use other than to teach patients how to use heat or cold options at home.	D
TENS	The literature does not support TENS as a treatment for patients with acute low back problems.	C
Lumbar corsets and back belts	Lumbar corsets and support belts have not been proven beneficial for treating patients with acute low back problems.	D
	There is limited evidence that the use of lumbar corsets (which provide abdominal support) may reduce time lost from work due to low back problems in individuals who do frequent lifting at work.	C
	There is limited evidence that lumbar support belts (which do not provide abdominal support) are not beneficial in reducing time lost from work or the frequency of low back problems.	C
Traction	Traction is not effective in the treatment of patients with acute low back problems.	B
Biofeedback	The panel found no evidence to support the use of biofeedback in the treatment of patients with acute low back problems.	D

*CT, computed tomography; MRI, magnetic resonance imaging; NSAID, nonsteroidal anti-inflammatory drug; TENS, transcutaneous electrical nerve stimulation.
†A, Strong research-based evidence (multiple specific and relevant high-quality scientific studies); B, Moderate research-based evidence (multiple adequate or one specific and relevant high-quality scientific study); C, Limited research-based evidence (at least one adequate scientific study); D, Some helpful information that did not meet the inclusion trial criteria on evidence tables.

Table 1. (*Continued*)

Areas of consideration*	Finding and recommendation statements	Amount of evidence†
Injections		
Trigger point and ligamentous	Trigger point injections are invasive and evidence does not support their use for patients with acute low back problems.	C
	Ligamentous (or sclerosant) injections are invasive and evidence does not support their use for patients with acute low back problems.	C
Epidural (steroids, lidocaine, narcotics)	Epidural injections of steroids, local anesthetics, and/or opioids are invasive, and evidence does not support their use as a treatment for acute low back pain without radiculopathy.	C
	Epidural steroid injections may be useful for short-term relief of radicular pain after failure of conservative treatment as an attempt to avoid surgery.	D
Acupuncture	There is no evidence that invasive needle acupuncture or other dry needling techniques are effective for treating acute low back problems.	C
Surgery		
Disk herniation	After approximately 1 month, the treating clinician should discuss the further available options with the patient who has sciatica. One option is referral to a specialist when all of the following conditions are met: (1) sciatica is both severe and disabling, (2) symptoms of sciatica persist without improvement or with progression, and (3) there is clinical evidence of nerve root compromise.	B
	Standard diskectomy and microdiskectomy are of similar efficacy and appropriate for selected patients with herniated disks and nerve root dysfunction.	C
	Chymopapain is an acceptable treatment for such patients, but less efficacious than standard or microdiskectomy. If chymopapain is being considered, testing patients for allergic sensitivity to this substance can reduce incidence of anaphylaxis.	C
	Percutaneous diskectomy is significantly less efficacious than chymopapain in treating patients with lumbar disk herniation; it is recommended that this and other new methods of lumbar disk surgery not be used routinely until proven efficacious in controlled trials.	C
	Patients with acute low back pain alone, who have neither suspicious findings for a significant nerve root compression nor any positive RED FLAGS, do not need surgical consultation for possible herniated lumbar disk.	D
Spinal Stenosis	Elderly patients with spinal stenosis who can adequately function in the activities of daily living can be managed with conservative treatments. Surgery for spinal stenosis usually is not considered in the first 3 months of symptoms. Decisions on treatment should take into account the patient's lifestyle, preference, other medical problems, and risks of surgery.	C
	Surgical decisions for patients with spinal stenosis must not be based solely on imaging tests, but must also consider the degree of persistent neurogenic claudication symptoms, associated limitations, and detectable neurologic compromise.	C
	Evidence does indicate that spinal fusion is a reasonable consideration following decompression at a level of increased motion due to degenerative spondylolisthesis.	C
Activity recommendations		
Bed rest	A gradual return to normal activities is more effective than prolonged bed rest for treating acute low back problems.	B
	Prolonged bed rest for more than 4 days may lead to debilitation and is not appropriate for treating acute low back problems.	B
	The majority of low back patients will not require bed rest. Bed rest for 2 to 4 days may be an option for patients with severe initial symptoms of primarily leg pain.	D
Exercise	Low-stress aerobic exercises can prevent debilitation due to inactivity during the first month of symptoms and thereafter may help to return patients to the highest level of functioning appropriate to their circumstances.	C

*CT, computed tomography; MRI, magnetic resonance imaging; NSAID, nonsteroidal anti-inflammatory drug; TENS, transcutaneous electrical nerve stimulation.
†A, Strong research-based evidence (multiple specific and relevant high-quality scientific studies); B, Moderate research-based evidence (multiple adequate or one specific and relevant high-quality scientific study); C, Limited research-based evidence (at least one adequate scientific study); D, Some helpful information that did not meet the inclusion trial criteria on evidence tables.

Table 1. (*Continued*)

Areas of consideration*	Finding and recommendation statements	Amount of evidence†
	Aerobic (endurance) exercise programs, which minimally stress the back (walking, biking, or swimming), can be started during the first 2 weeks for most patients with acute low back problems.	D
	Conditioning exercises for trunk muscles (especially back extensors), which are gradually increased, are helpful for patients with acute low back problems, especially if symptoms persist. During the first 2 weeks, these exercises may aggravate symptoms because they mechanically stress the back more than endurance exercise.	C
	There is no evidence that the use of back-specific exercise machines is effective in treating acute low back problems.	D
	No evidence supports the use of stretching as effective in treating acute low back problems.	D
	Recommended exercise quotas that are gradually increased result in better outcomes than telling patients to stop exercising if pain occurs.	C

*CT, computed tomography; MRI, magnetic resonance imaging; NSAID, nonsteroidal anti-inflammatory drug; TENS, transcutaneous electrical nerve stimulation.
†A, Strong research-based evidence (multiple specific and relevant high-quality scientific studies); B, Moderate research-based evidence (multiple adequate or one specific and relevant high-quality scientific study); C, Limited research-based evidence (at least one adequate scientific study); D, Some helpful information that did not meet the inclusion trial criteria on evidence tables.

Annotated Bibliography

Anderson R, Meeker WC, Wirick BE, et al: A meta-analysis of clinical trials of spinal manipulation. *J Manipulative Physiol Ther* 1992;15:181–194.

This article provides reviews of manipulation literature.

Bigos SJ, Battie MC, Spengler DM, et al: A longitudinal, prospective study of industrial back injury reporting. *Clin Orthop* 1992;279:21–34.

Nonphysical factors, socioeconomic and psychological factors, are more important than physical factors in affecting report of symptoms interfering with work.

Bigos SJ, Bowyer OR, Braen GR, et al: *Acute Low Back Problems in Adults.* Rockville, MD, U.S. Department of Health and Human Services, Public Health Service, Agency for Health Care Policy and Research, December 1994, AHCPR Publication No 95-0642.

Bigos SJ, Hansson T, Castillo RN, et al: The value of preemployment roentgenographs for predicting acute back injury claims and chronic back pain disability. *Clin Orthop* 1992;283:124–129.

No difference was found in the incidence of spondylolisthesis or other abnormalities in an evaluation of age-matched males who were symptomatic job applicants, back injury claimants, or patients disabled for more than 6 months.

Deeb ZL, Schimel S, Daffner RH, et al: Intervertebral disk-space infection after chymopapain injection. *Am J Neuroradiol* 1985;6:55–58.

Chymopapain injection was found superior to percutaneous diskectomy.

Deyo RA, Cherkin DC, Loeser JD, et al: Morbidity and mortality in association with operations on the lumbar spine: The influence of age, diagnosis, and procedure. *J Bone Joint Surg* 1992;74A:536–543.

This is a literature analysis for morbidity and mortality related to surgery of the lumbar spine.

Gogan WJ, Fraser RD: Chymopapain: A 10-year, double-blind study. *Spine* 1992;17:388–394.

This randomized clinical trial evaluating chymopapain injection versus saline injection favored chymopapain.

Gundewall B, Liljeqvist M, Hansson T: Primary prevention of back symptoms and absence from work: A prospective randomized study among hospital employees. *Spine* 1993;18:587–594.

Conditioning erector-spinae muscles reduced the impact of low back problems in nurses whose jobs require frequent lifting.

Haldeman S, Chapman-Smith D, Petersen DM (eds): Guidelines for Chiropractic Quality Assurance and Practice Parameters: *Proceedings of the Mercy Center Consensus Conference: 1993.* Gaithersburg, MD, Aspen Publishers, 1993.

This article provides reviews of manipulation literature.

Hoffman RM, Wheeler KJ, Deyo RA: Surgery for herniated lumbar discs: A literature synthesis. *J Gen Intern Med* 1993;8:487–496.

This meta-analysis is a review of only two randomized clinical trials on herniated lumbar disk surgery.

Kent DL, Haynor DR, Larson EB, et al: Diagnosis of lumbar spinal stenosis in adults: A metaanalysis of the accuracy of CT, MR, and myelography. *Am J Roentgenol* 1992;158:1135–1144.

The authors describe significant technological advances in imaging modalities over the past several years.

Koes BW, Bouter LM, van Mameren H, et al: A blinded randomized clinical trial of manual therapy and physiotherapy for chronic back and neck complaints: Physical outcome measures. *J Manipulative Physiol Ther* 1992;15:16–23.

There was no significant difference in patient-reported outcome measures between different physical therapy modalities and placebo.

Koes BW, Bouter LM, van Mameren H, et al: The effectiveness of manual therapy, physiotherapy, and treatment by the general practitioner for nonspecific back and neck complaints: A randomized clinical trial. *Spine* 1992;17:28–35.

There was no significant difference in patient-reported outcome measures between different physical therapy modalities and placebo.

Lindstrom I, Ohlund C, Eek C, et al: The effect of graded activity on patients with subacute low back pain: A randomized prospective clinical study with an operant-conditioning behavioral approach. *Phys Ther* 1992;72: 279–293.

A program of gradual increased aerobic activity and back conditioning exercise for patients with acute low back problems was superior to doing no exercise at all before returning to work.

Lowery WD Jr, Horn TJ, Boden SD, et al: Impairment evaluation based on spinal range of motion in normal subjects. *J Spinal Disord* 1992;5:398–402.

Spinal range of motion was found to be of limited diagnostic value, specifically when related to the presence of symptoms.

Malmivaara A, Häkkinen U, Aro T, et al: The treatment of acute low back pain—bed rest, exercises, or ordinary activity? *N Engl J Med* 1995;332:351–355.

This excellent study provides a new standard of care for patients with acute limitations at work by assuring safety and recommending continuing normal activities, versus McKinsey-like exercise and rest.

Marks RC, Houston T, Thulbourne T: Facet joint injection and facet nerve block: A randomised comparison in 86 patients with chronic low back pain. *Pain* 1992;49: 325–328.

In an evaluation of facet injections in chronic back pain, no difference was found between steroids and local anesthesia.

National Institute for Occupational Safety and Health: *Work Practices Guide for Manual Lifting,* Cincinnati, OH, U.S. Department of Health and Human Services, National Institute for Occupational Safety and Health, March 1981, NIOSH Technical Report No 81–122.

This is a consensus update of the 1980 Lifting Guide.

Reddell CR, Congleton JJ, Huchingson RD, et al: An evaluation of a weightlifting belt and back injury prevention training class for airline baggage handlers. *Appl Ergonom* 1992;235:319–329.

Lifting belts were not found to help baggage handlers.

Sachs BL, Ahmad SS, LaCroix M, et al: Objective assessment for exercise treatment on the B-200 isostation as part of work tolerance rehabilitation: A random prospective blind evaluation with comparison control population. *Spine* 1994;19:49–52.

The authors found a back-specific exercise machine (B-220) did not provide added benefit over traditional exercise in improving lifting back strength and flexibility.

Skovron ML, Szpalski M, Nordin M, et al: Sociocultural factors and back pain: A population-based study in Belgian adults. *Spine* 1994;19:129–137.

Authors of this population-based study suggest psychosocial issues affect how individuals with low back symptoms make decisions about work.

Tullberg T, Isacson J, Weidenhielm L: Does microscopic removal of lumbar disc herniation lead to better results than the standard procedure? Results of a one-year randomized study. *Spine* 1993;18:24–27.

No significant difference was found in this comparison of standard diskectomy to microdiskectomy.

Turner JA, Ersek M, Herron L, et al: Surgery for lumbar spinal stenosis: Attempted meta-analysis of the literature. *Spine* 1992;17:1–8.

Another attempted meta-analysis shows more improvement with surgery, but conservative management may be a reasonable alternative for spinal stenosis.

Turner JA, Ersek M, Herron L, et al: Patient outcomes after lumbar spinal fusions. *JAMA* 1992;268:907–911.

An attempted meta-analysis on spinal fusion is reported.

Volinn E, Mayer J, Diehr P, et al: Small area analysis of surgery for low-back pain. *Spine* 1992:17:575–81.

Rates for hospitalization and surgery for low back problems vary substantially among small areas within the state of Washington.

Waddell G: Biopsychosocial analysis of low back pain. *Baillieres Clin Rheumatol* 1992;6:523–557.

Social, economic, and psychosocial factors are more important than physical factors in affecting symptoms, response to treatment, and long-term outcome of patients with chronic low back problems.

Classic Bibliography

Bigos SJ, Battie MC, Spengler DM, et al: A prospective study of work perceptions and psychosocial factors affecting the report of back injury. *Spine* 1991;16:1–6.

Deyo, RA, Rainville J, Kent DL: What can the history and physical examination tell us about low back pain? *JAMA* 1992;12:760–765.

Hadler NM, Curtis P, Gillings DB, et al: A benefit of spinal manipulation as adjunctive therapy for acute low-back pain: A stratified controlled trial. *Spine* 1987;12: 702–706.

Herkowitz HN, Kurz LT: Degenerative lumbar spondylolisthesis with spinal stenosis: A prospective study comparing decompression with decompression and intertransverse process arthrodesis. *J Bone Joint Surg* 1991;73A:802–808.

MacDonald RS, Bell CM: An open controlled assessment of osteopathic manipulation in nonspecific low-back pain. *Spine* 1990;15:364–370.

Roland M, Dixon M: Randomized controlled trial of an educational booklet for patients presenting with back pain in general practice. *J R Coll Gen Pract* 1989;39:244–246.

Waddell G, Main CJ, Morris EW, et al: Normality and reliability in the clinical assessment of backache. *Br Med J (Clin Res Ed)* 1982;22:1519–1523.

Weber H: Lumbar disc herniation: A controlled, prospective study with ten years of observation. *Spine* 1983;8:131–140.

52

Spondylolysis and Spondylolisthesis: Congenital and Isthmic

Natural History

The incidence of spondylolysis and spondylolisthesis is approximately 5% in the general population. Spondylolysis generally does not occur in nonambulators. There has been a report of one case of spondylolysis in an infant. The lesion develops in children around 5 to 6 years of age, with an incidence of 3.3%. A second peak occurs in the adolescent population. The highest incidence is in white males (6.4%), and the lowest incidence is in African-American females (1.1%). It is also associated with thoracolumbar Scheuermann disease, and there is an increased incidence in gymnasts and football linemen. There is also a familial predisposition, with reported rates of 27% to 69% in close relatives. Six types of spondylolysis and spondylolisthesis have been described; congenital and isthmic will be discussed in this section. Degenerative and pathologic lesions are covered in the lumbar spine section. Congenital (type 1) lesions are associated with deficient superior sacral and/or inferior lumbar facets, spina bifida occulta, and abnormalities of the proximal sacrum. When a slip occurs, there is an elongation of the pars interarticularis without fracture. There are three types of isthmic lesions (types 2A, 2B, and 2C). Type 2A results in a defect in the pars interarticularis, with or without slippage; type 2B resembles type 1, with pars elongation occurring as a result of cyclic healing of microfractures; and type 2C refers to an acute pars fracture.

The development of spondylolisthesis is multifactorial and is associated with female gender and the congenital form of spondylolysis. Females appear to have worse slips, deformity at a younger age (secondary to the earlier onset of puberty), and a higher incidence of surgery. A recent long-term follow-up study of spondylolisthesis found that 90% of the slip had occurred by the first visit to a physician. Multifactorial analysis of radiographic parameters, age, gender, and treatment modality showed the only radiographic predictor to be initial percentage of slip; higher slips had a greater chance of progression. Spondylolisthesis tends to progress during the initial growth spurt in a manner similar to idiopathic scoliosis. Progression of a lytic spondylolysis to spondylolisthesis in adulthood has been reported; however, this is exceedingly rare.

Workup

History and Physical Examination

Patients usually come to a physician's office with one or more of the following complaints: back and/or leg pain, an abnormal gait, abnormal posture or appearance of the trunk, a history of trauma, or a change in bowel or bladder habits. There may be a history of minor or repetitive trauma, which is generally sports related, or the patient may be able to pinpoint the time at which the pain began. Younger patients may complain of insidious back pain, or the lesion may be an incidental finding on a radiograph. Patients with an obvious deformity may have noted the gradual onset of a change in the appearance of the trunk. It is exceedingly important to ask both the parents and the child about any change in bowel or bladder habits. The family history may also reveal similarly affected relatives.

Adults may come to the physician with a remote history of back pain during adolescence, or may have a new onset of low back pain following a minor injury. The pain may be localized to the low back and thigh area, similar to mechanical low back pain, or there may be a component of sciatica. However, acute low back pain or L5 radiculopathy is not necessarily due to a spondylolysis seen on a radiograph. The most common cause of these symptoms is still an L4–5 disk herniation, which is clinically indistinguishable from a symptomatic spondylolysis. In both cases, the symptoms are due to compression of the L5 nerve root. The patients complain of numbness or pain along the dorsum of the foot or weakness of the extensor hallucis longus. In spondylolysis, this symptom is due to tenting of the nerve root beneath the pars defect or to a neurapraxia caused by a mild slip.

The physical examination should consist of observation of the patient's stance. Viewing the patient from the side and rear may reveal scoliosis. Scoliosis may be olisthetic, due to rotation at the lumbosacral junction; it may be sciatic and due to pain; or it may be coexistent and unrelated to the spondylolisthesis. Curve severity is related to the presence of a congenital slip, slip severity, and lumbar rotation. The range of motion of the lumbar spine should be assessed. In symptomatic spondylolysis, extension and rotation of the lumbar spine causes significant back pain. In severe spondylolisthesis, the patient may stand with the hips and knees flexed and the pelvis flexed forward. The hamstrings may be quite tight, contributing to the abnormal posture. There may be flattening of the buttocks and an abdominal crease. A thorough neurologic examination of the lower extremities should be performed, including a rectal examination to check for sensation and tone. A cystometrogram should be performed preoperatively in all patients with congenital slips, patients with bowel and bladder symptoms, or patients in whom there is an abnormal rectal examination.

Radiographs

Plain radiographs of the lumbar spine should be obtained with the patient standing. In general, spondylolysis occurs at the lumbosacral junction, but it may occur at any lumbar level. When spondylolysis occurs at L4, it is generally associated with partial or complete sacralization of L5. Initial radiographs should include an anteroposterior (AP) and lateral of the lumbar spine. Oblique radiographs are helpful if the diagnosis of spondylolysis is in question. A standing lateral view of the lumbar spine is generally sufficient to follow the slip. In cases with a scoliotic component, an AP radiograph should be obtained. The slip percentage is expressed as the ratio of the distance between the posterior aspect of the sacrum and L5 divided by the width of the L5 vertebra. Grade I slips are < 25%, grade II, 25% to 50%; grade III, 51% to 75%; and grade IV, 76% to 100%. Grade V, or spondyloptosis, indicates the complete displacement of the L5 vertebra anterior to the sacrum. The slip angle measures lumbosacral kyphosis and generally is not significant in milder grades of slips (grades I and II). Various methods have been described to measure the slip angle (Fig. 1); however, the most reproducible method measures the angle between a line drawn orthogonal to the posterior body of the sacrum (representing the endplate of S1) and the superior endplate of L5 (Fig. 1, *center*).

Technetium bone scans using single photon emission computed tomography (SPECT scans) have been shown to be an effective method for identifying occult and acute spondylolysis. They may also help in deciding the course of treatment. Magnetic resonance imaging (MRI) scanning has also been shown to be useful in evaluating the disk proximal to the slip, particularly in adolescents and young adults. T1 and T2 signal changes consistent with disk degeneration are generally seen in the lumbosacral disk, and are always present in the case of a slip. It is important not to overread the MRI results and assume the patient's leg pain is due to a disk herniation. In slips with a rotatory olisthesis, a pseudodisk herniation may be apparent on MRI; this herniation is the result of the slip itself. If the MRI is positive, it is essential to look for other causes of pain. The presence of degenerative changes or herniation in a proximal disk with a painful spondylolysis may influence the treatment decision in an adolescent or young adult. Diskography may be used to evaluate proximal disks, because abnormal MRI signals do not correlate well with the presence of symptoms. However, diskography at the level of the spondylolisthesis provides no useful information and should be condemned.

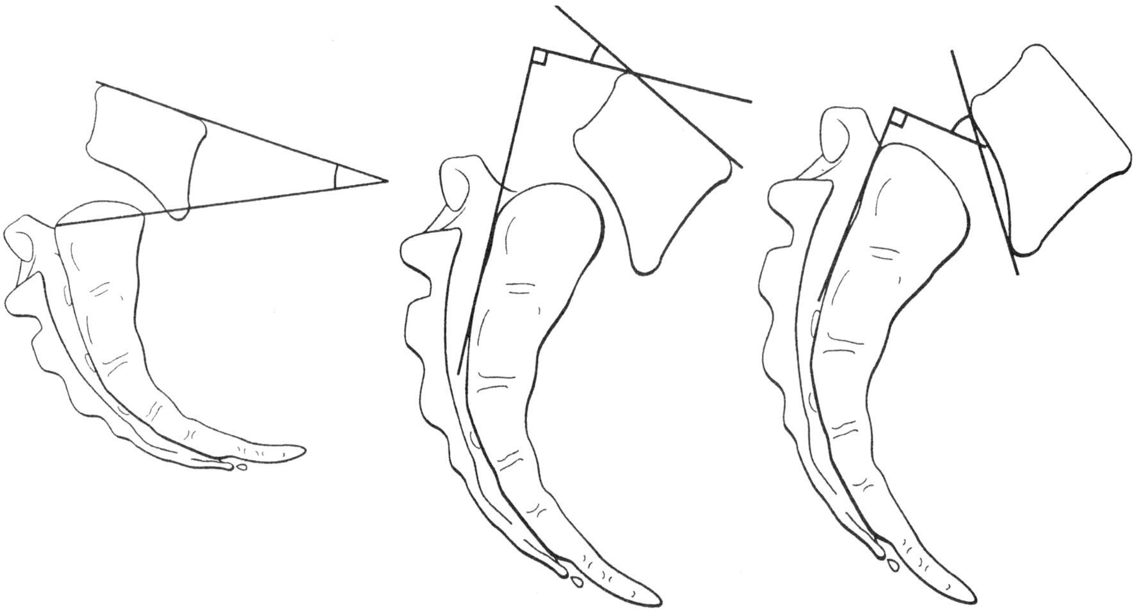

Fig. 1 **Left,** Lumbosacral kyphosis is represented by the angle between the superior end plate of L5 and the superior end plate of S1. **Center,** It is difficult to establish a reference line for the superior end plate of a dome-shaped sacrum. The end plate can be approximated by a line drawn orthogonal to the posterior cortex of the sacrum. **Right,** The inferior end plate of L5 undergoes remodeling changes during slip progression and is not a reliable reference point. The superior end plate of L5 does not undergo these changes and should be used to measure the lumbosacral kyphosis. (Reproduced with permission from Burkus JK, Lonstein JE, Winter RB, et al: Long-term evaluation of adolescents treated operatively for spondylolisthesis. *J Bone Joint Surg* 1992;74A:693–704.)

Treatment

Nonsurgical Treatment

Asymptomatic children and adolescents with spondylolysis or low-grade spondylolisthesis do not require activity restriction. Symptomatic patients should have sports activities restricted. If this restriction fails to alleviate the symptoms, the patient should be braced with the lumbar spine in lordosis for 2 to 6 months. Hamstring stretches, abdominal strengthening exercises, and pelvic tilts should be performed. Exercises should be initiated when the patient is asymptomatic in the brace. The brace may be weaned when extension and rotation of the spine are pain free. Children and adolescents should have radiographs obtained every 6 months until growth is complete. Thereafter, they may be followed up on an as-needed basis. Spondylolysis and low-grade spondylolisthesis in adults should be treated in the same way as other episodes of low back pain. Immobilization of the spine in adults with the use of a body cast or thoracolumbosacral orthosis (TLSO) may help predict those patients who will respond to a fusion.

Surgical Treatment

Indications for the surgical treatment of spondylolysis or grade I spondylolisthesis in children and adolescents include slip progression or back and/or leg pain that is unresponsive to 6 to 12 months of nonsurgical therapy. A direct repair of the pars may be considered in order to save motion segments in the lumbar spine. For older adolescents and adults, direct repair of the defect has been less successful because of degenerative disk changes occurring below the pars defect. These patients would be better served by an in situ L5 to S1 fusion. The most reliable results have been shown with a posterolateral fusion using autogenous iliac crest bone graft and a paraspinous muscle-splitting approach in children and adults. No cast or brace is necessary postoperatively. A decompression should be included for patients with congenital slips and considered in adolescents with slips associated with severe leg symptoms and neurologic signs. Resolution of leg pain in adolescents, however, frequently occurs with a successful fusion, without decompression or reduction. In the child and adolescent, decompression alone often leads to further slippage and should not be performed without a fusion. Supplemental segmental fixation has been used in older patients, but has very little, if any, role in the treatment of children and adolescents with minimal slips. Grade II slips with normal sagittal alignment may also be treated with an in situ L5 to S1 fusion.

Children and young adolescents with grade III and IV slips or a high grade II slip with lumbosacral kyphosis should have the fusion extended to L4 from S1. If the neurologic examination is abnormal, nerve root decompression should also be performed, particularly in congenital slips. Reduction of the lumbosacral kyphosis should be attempted if sagittal alignment compromises function or if the lumbosacral kyphosis is > 55° to 60°. Instrumentation in children and adolescents is generally not indicated, and reduction of the slip angle is best performed postoperatively with the patient awake on a traction table. A single or double pantaloon spica cast is the most effective form of immobilization; however, a TLSO with a thigh extension may also be used. The reduction of grade IV and V slips has been debated in the literature; however, with growth potential remaining, significant remodeling can occur, making an in situ fusion the safest and most reliable method. The need for an anterior fusion is less clear; however, the added stability afforded by an anterior strut may decrease the chance for slip progression. It should be noted, however, that postoperative cauda equina syndromes have been reported in young patients undergoing in situ posterolateral fusions for high-grade slips.

Indications for fusion in the adult include back and/or leg pain unresponsive to nonsurgical therapy or the presence of a functionally significant neurologic deficit. Decompression should be performed when leg pain is a significant symptom. Unless there is a concurrent herniation at the same level, diskectomy should not be performed, because it leads to instability of the motion segment. A posterolateral fusion from L5 to S1 should be performed unless significant degenerative changes are present in the adjacent disk. If this is the case, the fusion should be extended to include the symptomatic disks. Segmental instrumentation may be added in the adult population, but reduction is not always necessary.

The indications for surgical treatment of high-grade slips in adults is back and or leg pain unresponsive to nonsurgical treatment. The use of internal fixation has been described, particularly in salvage cases, but the choice of a staged fusion with reduction, vertebral resection, or in situ fusion is less clear. In general, instrumentation and anterior fusion should be reserved for patients with high-grade slips, salvage procedures, and after decompressions. If a reduction is performed intraoperatively, L5 root neurapraxias may result, and somatosensory evoked potential (SSEP) monitoring of both the posterior tibial and peroneal nerves or root-specific dermatomal sensory monitoring should be used. Patients with staged anterior and posterior fusions should be kept at bed rest between procedures.

Results

The results of in situ fusion for spondylolysis and spondylolisthesis have held up well in long-term follow-up studies of adolescents and children. In a comparison of in situ fusion with and without spica cast immobilization, patients treated with an awake postoperative reduction showed improvement in both slip percentage and angle. Surgical reduction and instrumentation have led to increased complications, surgical time, and blood loss. A well-matched comparison of severe slips treated with in situ fusion or instrumented reduction led to the conclusion

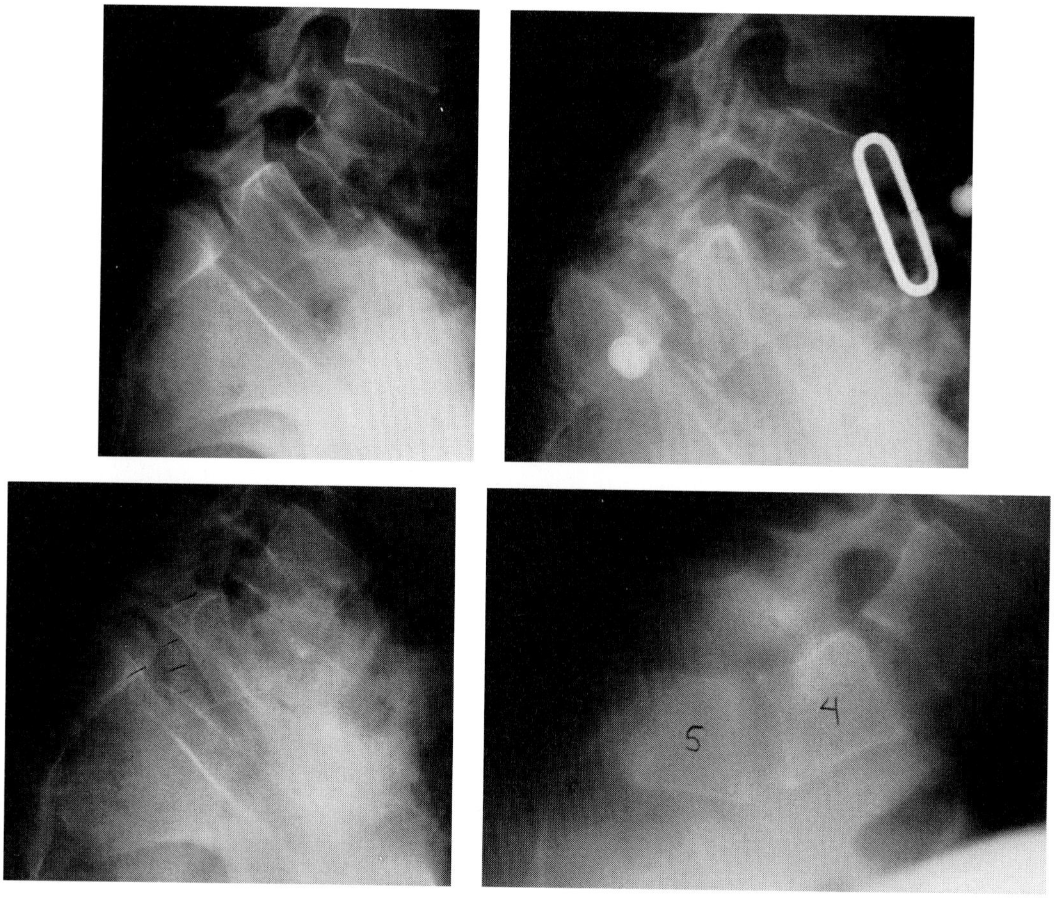

Fig. 2 **Top left,** Standing lateral radiograph of a postmenarchal 14-year-old female with a 4-month history of low back and right leg pain and occasional right foot numbness. The radiograph demonstrates a grade III congenital spondylolisthesis. A posterolateral L4 to S1 fusion with decompression was recommended. **Top right,** Standing lateral radiograph taken 7 days after an L4 to S1 fusion with a right L5 and S1 foraminotomy and hemilaminectomy. Postoperatively, she was placed in a thoracolumbarsacral orthosis with a thigh extension. Reduction was not attempted. **Bottom left,** Lateral radiograph taken 1 year postoperatively. She was fully active in sports. The patient complained of pain in the area of the sacrum, and her kyphosis was more clinically pronounced. There has been a radiographic increase in the lumbosacral kyphosis and a slip progression to grade IV. A pseudarthrosis appears to be present at L5 to S1. Further workup was recommended. **Bottom right,** Lateral tomogram obtained 8 months later demonstrates further worsening of the lumbosacral kyphosis and slip progression. Anteroposterior and lateral tomograms and a computed tomography (CT) scan were performed. The CT scan demonstrated a pseudarthrosis at L5 to S1. Further surgery to include an anterior fusion and possible instrumentation has been recommended.

that in situ fusion is preferable, even in severe slips. In several studies there has been slip progression despite the apparent presence of a solid fusion (Fig. 2); however, critical analysis of the lumbosacral junction using the Ferguson view has revealed a poor quality fusion mass that was not readily apparent on the AP radiograph and was confirmed by computed tomography (CT) scan.

The surgical treatment of adult isthmic spondylolisthesis has received much attention in the past several years. A small series of patients with severe slips and sciatica, who were treated with an in situ fusion without decompression, showed excellent results in terms of pain relief and return to work. This sample excluded workmen's compensation and litigation cases. A second small series of patients with severe slips and neurologic compromise, including cauda equina syndrome, were treated with a single-stage decompression, posterolateral fusion, and anterior fusion. Anterior remodeling did occur, but the technique is quite challenging.

Instrumented reductions for low-grade slips are often not necessary, and decompression should precede any attempt to reduce a high-grade slip. A series of patients treated with a staged anterior-posterior fusion and halo skeletal traction showed improvement in lumbosacral kyphosis, but not in slip percentage. Recommendations for staged reduction and fusion with pedicular fixation should be reserved for salvage cases and following vertebral resection. A consecutive series of patients treated with pedicular fixation showed a 25% failure rate, which may have been due to implant design or inadequate anterior support. Anterior fusion for severe slips has been recommended. The choice of instrumentation is less important than the indications for its use, recognizing that high complication rates have been reported with instrumented reductions.

Annotated Bibliography

Blanda J, Bethem D, Moats W, et al: Defects of pars interarticularis in athletes: A protocol for nonoperative treatment. *J Spinal Disord* 1993;6:406–411.

This article provides a concise treatment protocol for symptomatic spondylolysis: immobilization in a TLSO with normal lumbar lordosis to appose the pars defect, exercises, and physical therapy. When extension and rotation of the spine are pain free, the brace may be weaned.

Boos N, Marchesi D, Aebi M: Treatment of spondylolysis and spondylolisthesis with Cotrel-Dubousset instrumentation: A preliminary report. *J Spinal Disord* 1991;4:472–479.

Fifty consecutive adults and children with a variety of slips were treated with Cotrel-Dubousset pedicular instrumentation. Hardware failure occurred in 25%; two were due to pseudoarthrosis. The authors do not recommend reduction of low-grade slips when back pain is the sole complaint. Anterior–posterior fusion should be done if reduction is desired. There is a high implant failure rate. Instrumentation in children is perhaps unnecessary except in high-grade slips.

Boxall D, Bradford DS, Winter RB, et al: Management of severe spondylolisthesis in children and adolescents. *J Bone Joint Surg* 1979;61A:479–495.

This is a classic review article of 43 patients with >50% slips treated surgically. The authors recommend spica casting after fusion for a slip angle above 55°. Progression was shown after fusion; it was associated with a high slip angle or degree, a midline fusion, or lack of immobilization.

Bradford DS, Boachie-Adjei O: Treatment of severe spondylolisthesis by anterior and posterior reduction and stabilization: A long-term follow-up study. *J Bone Joint Surg* 1990;72A:1060–1066.

This retrospective study reviews the results of 22 patients treated with a staged Gill procedure and posterolateral fusion followed by halo skeletal traction and an anterior fusion and casting. No appreciable change in the slip percentage occurred, but the lumbosacral kyphosis improved. The authors stress the need for decompression prior to any attempt at reduction and believe that a combined anterior–posterior approach with pedicular screws should be used in salvage cases or with vertebral resection.

Burkus JK, Lonstein JE, Winter RB, et al: Long-term evaluation of adolescents treated operatively for spondylolisthesis: A comparison of in situ arthrodesis only with in situ arthrodesis and reduction followed by immobilization in a cast. *J Bone Joint Surg* 1992;74A:693–704.

This study is a retrospective comparison of 42 patients treated with a posterolateral fusion via a paraspinous approach. Twenty-four had reduction and spica casting performed on a Cotrel table 5 to 14 days postoperatively. Patients with spica casting had improvement in the slip percentage and angle. Anterior remodeling occurred in younger patients. The authors recommend in situ fusion (L5 to S1 for mild slips, L4 to S1 for severe slips) with decompression as necessary, followed by spica casting.

Frennerd AK, Danielson BI, and Nachemson AL: Natural history of symptomatic isthmic low-grade spondylolisthesis in children and adolescents: A seven-year follow-up study. *J Pediatr Orthop* 1991;11:209–213.

This is a retrospective study of children younger than 16 years of age with < 50% slips. Average follow-up was 7 years. Thirty percent of patients ultimately required surgery; 83% of conservatively treated patients had excellent or good results. A small (4%) chance of slip progression occurred during the follow-up period, but there was no single finding to predict slip progression.

Harris IE, Weinstein SL: Long-term follow-up of patients with grade-III and IV spondylolisthesis: Treatment with and without posterior fusion. *J Bone Joint Surg* 1987;69A:960–969.

This article reports the long-term follow-up (average 18 years) of patients treated with posterior interlaminar fusion compared with those treated conservatively. Patients with fusions fared slightly better at follow-up, but conservative treatment did not significantly alter the patient's lifestyle. The authors recommend in situ fusion for symptomatic skeletally immature patients.

Hensinger RN: Spondylolysis and spondylolisthesis in children and adolescents. *J Bone Joint Surg* 1989;71A:1098–1107.

This is a comprehensive review of the subject, although the roles of MRI and diskography are not discussed. The surgical recommendations are still valid.

Johnson GV, Thompson AG: The Scott wiring technique for direct repair of lumbar spondylolysis. *J Bone Joint Surg* 1992;74B:426–430.

Twenty-two patients underwent direct repair of a spondylolysis or grade I slip using a modified wiring technique described in the paper. All patients younger than 25 years old had good results. Two thirds of patients older than 25 years had poor results. The results suggest that the pseudoarthrosis defect is the source of pain in younger patients, and disk degeneration may be the source in older patients.

Lindholm TS, Ragni P, Ylikoski M, et al: Lumbar isthmic spondylolisthesis in children and adolescents: Radiologic evaluation and results of operative treatment. *Spine* 1990; 15:1350–1355.

This is a study of 75 patients treated with a variety of surgical procedures. If scoliosis was present, it tended to correlate with slip severity. The authors recommend that patients with low-grade slips have a posterolateral fusion with autogenous iliac crest bone graft; those with high-grade slips should have an interbody fusion.

Lusins JO, Elting JJ, Cicoria AD, et al: SPECT evaluation of lumbar spondylolysis and spondylolisthesis. *Spine* 1994; 19:608–612.

SPECT scanning of spondylolysis and spondylolisthesis shows a pattern change with symptom resolution or slip progression. Spondylolysis and spondylolisthesis have different patterns that vary with time. The authors conclude that SPECT scanning is not positive or negative but varies with time and stability of the spine.

Peek RD, Wiltse LL, Reynolds JB, et al: In situ arthrodesis without decompression for grade-III or IV isthmic spondylolisthesis in adults who have severe sciatica. *J Bone Joint Surg* 1989;71A:62–68.

Eight adults with severe spondylolisthesis (average 82%) and sciatica were treated with an in situ posterolateral L5 to S1 fusion. All patients had resolution of their pain and neurologic symptoms. No immobilization was used. No patients were in litigation or workmen's compensation and all patients returned to work. No patient required decompression at a later date. The results were excellent in this small group of carefully selected patients.

Poussa M, Schlenzka D, Seitsalo S, et al: Surgical treatment of severe isthmic spondylolisthesis in adolescents: Reduction or fusion in situ. *Spine* 1993; 18:894–901.

In this small study of well-matched patients, the results were compared of instrumented reduction and in situ fusion without instrumentation. Patients with instrumented reduction had longer surgical times and more blood loss. In situ fusion led to further slippage; however, the kyphotic deformity worsened in both groups. The uninstrumented patients had no complaints of poor cosmesis, but several instrumented patients had complaints. The authors recommend fusion in situ for severe slips.

Schlenzka D, Poussa M, Seitsalo S, et al: Intervertebral disk changes in adolescents with isthmic spondylolisthesis. *J Spinal Disord* 1991;4:344–352.

In this preoperative radiographic study of 27 patients considered candidates for lysis repair, MRI, diskography, and radiographs were compared. Twelve patients had all three tests. Degenerative changes on diskography and MRI made authors less likely to recommend defect repair.

Schoenecker PL, Cole HO, Herring JA, et al: Cauda equina syndrome after in situ arthrodesis for severe spondylolisthesis at the lumbosacral junction. *J Bone Joint Surg* 1990;72A:369–377.

The authors of this review of 12 patients who developed cauda equina syndrome after in situ fusion recommend a cystometrogram, myelogram, or MRI in patients with congenital slips. If cauda equina syndrome develops, immediate decompression by resecting the posterosuperior lip of the sacral dome should be performed. The need for internal fixation should also be considered.

Seitsalo S, Osterman K, Poussa M, et al: Spondylolisthesis in children under 12 years of age: Long-term results of 56 patients treated conservatively or operatively. *J Pediatr Orthop* 1988;8:516–521.

This study followed 56 children to skeletal maturity. Thirty-two patients had surgery. No correlation was found between slip progression and pseudoarthrosis. Risk factors for early progression and severe symptoms included females and those with the congenital form. Authors recommended frequent checks during the growth spurt.

Seitsalo S, Osterman K, Hyvarinen H, et al: Severe spondylolisthesis in children and adolescents: A long-term review of fusion in situ. *J Bone Joint Surg* 1990;72B: 259–265.

This a retrospective study of 93 children with > 50% slips who underwent an in situ fusion. Average follow-up was 14.8 years. Preoperative pain correlated with lumbosacral kyphosis, and slip progression was worse in decompressed patients. In patients with severe lumbosacral kyphosis, the authors recommend immobilization in a cast or brace for 8 to 16 weeks.

Seitsalo S, Osterman K, Hyvarinen H, et al: Progression of spondylolisthesis in children and adolescents: A long-term follow-up of 272 patients. *Spine* 1991;16:417–421.

The authors of a long-term retrospective radiographic study of conservatively and surgically treated patients found that 90% of the slip occurred by the first visit. Spina bifida and female gender were associated with more severe slips. Early puberty lead to progression, and fusion had no effect on slip progression. Authors suggest that severe slips be treated by a combined anterior–posterior approach.

Seitsalo S: Operative and conservative treatment of moderate spondylolisthesis in young patients. *J Bone Joint Surg* 1990;72B:908–913.

In this retrospective study of 149 children treated surgically and conservatively for slips < 30%, average follow-up was 13.8 years. At follow-up, children treated surgically had less pain and better clinical results, but slip progression was equivalent in both groups. The results suggests that spontaneous segmental degeneration occurs as a result of disk degeneration at the level of the slip. The authors recommend diskography or MRI after adolescence.

Smith MD, Bohlman HH: Spondylolisthesis treated by a single-stage operation combining decompression with in situ posterolateral and anterior fusion: An analysis of eleven patients who had long-term follow-up. *J Bone Joint Surg* 1990;72A:415–421.

Eleven adults with high grade spondylolisthesis and severe back and leg pain were treated by a single-stage decompression, posterolateral fusion, and anterior fusion with a fibular strut graft placed from the rear. Five patients had a preoperative cauda equina syndrome; at follow-up all patients had major or complete neurologic recovery and remodeling had occurred as manifest by a change in the slip angle. No postoperative immobilization was used. The authors believe that instrumentation and reduction are unnecessary.

53

Adult Scoliosis

The natural history, spectrum, host physiology, and clinical outcomes in adult scoliosis are quite different from those of adolescent scoliosis. The biologic, biochemical, and mechanical changes that occur with aging require careful analysis in the management of these patients. There are two broad categories of adult scoliosis. The scoliosis may be present at the onset of adulthood and may be due to any of the known causes of scoliosis (most commonly, idiopathic) or the scoliosis may develop during adulthood in a previously straight spine (degenerative, senescent, or de novo). Metabolic bone disease has been implicated as a cause for adult scoliosis but there is as yet no evidence that associates bone demineralizing disorders in adults with scoliosis.

The number of adults in the United States with a scoliosis of greater than 30° has been estimated to be approximately 500,000. The figure may be higher if de novo cases are included. In a study of 5,000 adult patients having intravenous pyelograms, 3.9% were found to have lumbar curves greater than 10°. Only a small number of these present with clinical complaints.

The adult patient with scoliosis may present with pain, curve progression, spinal and truncal imbalance, spinal stenosis, or cardiorespiratory problems. Although pain is extremely rare in adolescent idiopathic scoliosis, pain develops in 25% to 80% of adults with scoliosis. The pain is frequently resistant to conventional treatments; it tends to increase with age and with the degree of deformity. Pain tends to be more common in the lumbar area than in the thoracic spine. Pain may be a frequent cause for surgical intervention. The workup should exclude other causes of pain. Spine pain may be localized to the curve or to lumbar segments outside the curve; it may be radicular or combined. Localized spine pain occurring on the convexity of the curve, exacerbated by exertion, is usually due to muscular fatigue. Disk or facet degeneration perhaps related to uneven loading more commonly produces pain on the concavity of the curve. Localized pain may be associated with facet sclerosis and disk degeneration. Facet injections and diskography may help to localize the pain. There are no controlled studies conclusively demonstrating the validity of diskography in localizing pain or determining the surgical outcome in adult patients with back pain and scoliosis. Magnetic resonance (MR) images may show disk degeneration and computed tomography (CT) scans may show facet arthrosis, but clinical correlation of symptoms, radiographic abnormalities, and outcome is variable and unpredictable. Radicular pain is often due to root entrapment in the concavity of lumbar or lumbosacral curves. Contributing factors to radicular pain include facet hypertrophy, radicular kinking, foraminal narrowing, osteophytes, and/or hypertrophy of the ligamentum flavum. Adult patients with the idiopathic variety of scoliosis have mechanical low back pain (83%), stenotic (neurogenic) symptoms with low back pain (13%), or low back pain with radicular symptoms (4%). Most patients with painful degenerative adult scoliosis have stenotic symptoms. Less than one half also have mechanical low back pain. The diskogenic pain associated with idiopathic scoliosis may influence the fusion level, although it is the stenotic symptoms that will frequently determine the nature of surgery in patients with degenerative scoliosis.

Scoliosis progression occurs in adults. It may increase 15% to 32% over a 10-year period, given 60- or 70-year-old patients. Studies with 35- to 40-year follow-up from adolescence into adulthood have shown an average progression of 13° to 15°. Risks for progression include thoracic curves greater than 60°, lumbar curves greater than 50°, and the lumbar portions of double major curves. The average progression of the scoliosis in adults is 1° per year. Curves less than 30° are unlikely to progress. Progression of scoliosis may lead to increased pain, pulmonary compromise, cor pulmonale, and poor body image. The risk of curve progression is 65% for progression greater than 5° in patients with adolescent onset scoliosis. However, the risk of progression of de novo lumbar curves is lower. Although pregnancy has been implicated as a risk factor for progression during adulthood, most studies show that curves progressing during pregnancy correlate with a progression prior to the pregnancy. Progression during pregnancy is associated with multiple pregnancies occurring before age 23. Although these natural history studies indicate low risks and rates of progression, they should not create complacency. Regular evaluation is advised. For each patient, curve progression should be established with follow-up at 1- to 2-year intervals.

Scoliosis can be noted by the lateral curve of the spine, paravertebral prominence, rib hump (due in part to vertebral rotation), asymmetric waist folds, trunk shift when standing, shoulder elevation, breast/rib or costal margin asymmetry, and/or hip prominence.

Spinal deformity may be noted incidentally in a patient complaining of pain, but frequently patients present because they or someone else has noted deformity progression. They may have no other symptoms. Patients may also note differences in the way their clothes fit, a loss of height, or a change in posture or gait. Spinal imbalance or decompensation may occur in either the sagittal or coronal planes, exaggerating the cosmetic deformity. This imbalance often requires more energy to remain in an erect position and results in greater muscle fatigue and pain.

Cardiopulmonary symptoms occur more frequently in patients with scoliosis greater than 100°. Progressive pulmonary function deterioration may result in pulmonary hypertension and cor pulmonale. Pulmonary function tests are seldom abnormal in thoracic deformities less than 60°. Parenchymal dysfunction is usually present only in curves greater than 100°. Scoliosis patients may have decreased maximal inspiratory pressures, but normal expiratory pressures. They frequently require increased effort for breathing, related to an increase in chest wall compliance. While large thoracic curves are associated with decreased vital capacity and oxygen transport, subjective dyspnea is experienced only by those patients with 90° to 100° curves. Other causes for cardiorespiratory problems such as smoking, asthma, chronic obstructive pulmonary disease, or occupational lung disease should also be considered in the adult patient with scoliosis.

The complexity of the deformity and host considerations make management of adult deformities difficult. These patients should be carefully evaluated with attention to pain and its source and characteristics, curve progression, cardiopulmonary and neurologic symptoms/signs, and cosmetic and psychologic considerations. Radiographs should include standing, full length anteroposterior (AP), and lateral radiographs, as well as supine, side bending films. CT, myelography, or MR imaging (MRI) are indicated if neurologic symptoms and signs are present. CT-myelography is more helpful in identifying the cause of compression and in operative planning. Tests of pulmonary function and arterial blood gases are indicated if there are cardiorespiratory symptoms or to establish base line data for patients with large thoracic curves. Diskography may be considered to evaluate the source of back pain prior to surgery. There are no controlled studies to support the validity of this in planning surgery. Competent medical consultation is necessary in patients with abnormal medical histories.

The treatment of back pain is the same for patients with and without scoliosis, and includes nonsteroidal antiinflammatories, physical therapy, and appropriate injections. For patients in their sixth and seventh decades, orthoses may be helpful in controlling pain and increasing mobility and function. Orthoses should be worn while the patient is ambulatory. The orthosis should be taken off on a regular basis and patients should participate in an exercise program so that they do not become dependent on the orthosis and develop muscular atrophy. Orthoses do not prevent curve progression or improve deformities. If localized pain is associated with degeneration in a mild deformity, an off-the-shelf orthosis may be satisfactory. For moderate and severe deformities, a custom fit thoracolumbosacral orthosis (TLSO) is better tolerated.

The main indications for surgery include progressive deformity and pain. Deterioration of pulmonary function as well as cosmesis are rare indications. The evaluation of the adult patient is more complex than that of the adolescent. The precise localization of the pain is difficult. Objective demonstration of curve progression is frequently lacking. Deterioration of pulmonary function in the patient with respiratory disease, or who is smoking, is difficult to assess. The complication rate in adult patients undergoing such major reconstructive surgery is high (Table 1). The surgical procedures compared to those for adolescent scoliosis are frequently prolonged with greater blood loss. Instrumentation related problems frequently occur, particularly with coexistent osteoporosis. Recovery time is also considerably prolonged.

The type of procedure undertaken depends on the surgical indications. If the indication for the surgery is pain, then the source of the pain should be localized before embarking on surgery. In the AP and lateral radiographs of the full spine curve, flexibility and coronal and sagittal balance should be considered in determining the levels for instrumentation and fusion. If the patient has disk degeneration with segmental instability, and low back pain associated with the scoliosis, it may be necessary to fuse and instrument.

If the indication for surgery is spinal stenosis, localizing the source of the stenotic symptoms is necessary. If the patient has a general neurogenic claudication associated with central stenosis, laminectomies should be performed. If the patient has evidence for single-level nerve root impingement, an appropriate, limited decompression can be considered. The need to augment such a decompressive procedure with fusion and stabilization depends on the extent of the decompression and instability produced. If the patient's symptoms are purely related to the stenosis, then it may not be necessary to instrument and fuse the entire scoliosis, but only to address the problem of focal stenosis with local decompression and possible stabilization and fusion. These patients frequently do not have severe neurologic deficits and only single (or few) roots can be identified as the source of the radicular pain. Indications for surgery are based on the patient's interpretation of disability. If the decompression involves multiple segments, instrumenting and fusing the entire curve is frequently necessary.

Decompressive procedures for stenosis are more commonly performed in patients with degenerative scoliosis, whereas patients with adolescent onset idiopathic scoliosis frequently have surgery related to the structural deformity of the scoliosis. However, progression of scoliosis may oc-

Table 1. Complications of surgery in adult scoliosis

Complication	Occurrence
Pseudarthrosis	5% to 27%
Residual pain	5% to 15%
Mortality	<1% to 5%
Neurologic	<1% to 5%
Infection	0.5% to 5%
Pulmonary embolism	1% to 20%

cur in all groups, and the principles of treatment of the curves are the same. The goals of surgery in treating patients for progressive spinal deformity are to produce a painless, stable, balanced spine. The challenge is to incorporate a sufficient number of motion segments to improve the balance and perhaps provide some correction, without producing a secondary deformity or incorporating more lumbar segments than necessary. The major contraindications to surgery are cor pulmonale, poor medical health, psychiatric disturbances including depression and neuroses, and unrealistic expectations. Useful adjuncts in the surgery for adult scoliosis include autologous blood transfusion, the use of a cell saver, intraoperative hypotension, banked bone, skilled anesthesiologists, and intra-operative neurophysiologic monitoring.

Indications for surgery in treating the deformity include: (1) a thoracic curve greater than 55° with disabling curve pain; (2) thoracic and lumbar curves that have demonstrated progression; (3) lumbar curves associated with symptoms and signs of spinal stenosis; and (4) thoracic curves greater than 90° with decreased pulmonary function.

The usual primary procedure in scoliosis surgery is arthrodesis to prevent curve progression. The role of instrumentation is to produce stabilization, but it can also be used to improve balance and provide spinal deformity correction. Where the spine has collapsed, and the ribs are impinging against the pelvis, resulting in loss of pulmonary function and pain, straightening the lumbar spine with instrumentation and fusion may secondarily improve pulmonary function. As discussed, nerve root decompression may also be a primary procedure. Ancillary procedures include a thoracoplasty that serves the purpose of decreasing the cosmetic deformity and simultaneously providing a source of bone graft.

The fusion may be performed from posterior, anterior, or both. Posterior approaches are generally indicated in single thoracic curves less than 70° to 80°, and thoracic and lumbar double curves less than 60° with a balanced or flexible spine. The extent of the fusion superiorly should include the entire thoracic curve, and it should extend at least two to three segments above the apex of the thoracic kyphosis (sagittal plane). The risk of junctional kyphosis is greater if the superior end of the fusion ends at the apex of the kyphosis. An anterior approach with instrumentation is indicated in single lumbar or thoracolumbar curves when fusion to the sacrum is not needed and there is a flexible fractional curve below. If the anterior approach does not save segmental levels, it may not have any advantage. A combined anterior and posterior approach is indicated in rigid single thoracic curves greater than 70° and double curves if greater than 70° with an unbalanced spine in which the lumbar curve is considerably more rigid than the thoracic curve. Combining an anterior diskectomy and interbody cancellous graft fusions with posterior instrumentation and fusion provides greater correction and improves the success rate. It is better to perform combined procedures under one anesthetic if the patient's medical condition allows. If staged procedures are performed, careful attention to the patient's nutritional status between steps is recommended, with parenteral hyperalimentation, if necessary.

Derotation maneuvers are not recommended in adults, but segmental correction using any of the numerous methods of segmental spinal translation to a rod (including sublaminar wires) can be used to improve correction and stabilization. If the curve is greater than 100°, anterior resection of the apical vertebra is helpful. An anterior thoracoplasty on the convex side should be considered at the same time. If, after extensive release, the spinal curves remain fairly rigid and large, multiple rods in the concavity of the scoliosis should be used and connected with transverse cross-connecting devices. It is important to avoid distraction maneuvers in the lumbar spine below L2 because they may produce a loss of lordosis and a "flatback."

Indications for fusion to the sacrum include: (1) lumbar curves with a fixed lumbosacral obliquity greater than 15°; (2) loss of coronal and sagittal balance; and (3) lumbosacral degeneration with segmental instability and pain. A combined anterior and posterior procedure is indicated in these patients. There is a high incidence of pseudoarthrosis and/or implant failure if only a posterior approach with instrumentation and fusion is performed. The anterior procedure should include anterior strut grafting. It is important also to produce, or maintain, appropriate sagittal plane balance, as well as lumbar lordosis. Posterior fixation to the sacrum or pelvis can be done by using the Galveston technique or multiple sacral screws.

Annotated Bibliography

Bradford DS: Adult scoliosis, in Moe JH, Lonstein JE (eds): *Moe's Textbook of Scoliosis and Other Spinal Deformities,* ed 3. Philadelphia, PA, WB Saunders, 1995, pp 369–386.

This excellent book chapter is devoted to discussion of the management of the adult patient with spinal deformity. Specific sections of the chapter explore in detail issues of prevalence, presentation, evaluation, and treatment for these patients.

Grubb SA, Lipscomb HJ: Diagnostic findings in painful adult scoliosis. *Spine* 1992;17:518–527.

Diagnostic findings in a group of 55 adult patients with both scoliosis (49% degenerative onset, 44% idiopathic onset) and pain were documented. Patients with degenerative onset scoliosis had myelographic defects most commonly within the primary curve, and on diskography, multiple abnormal, not necessarily painful, disks were seen throughout the lumbar spine. Patients with idiopathic onset scoliosis had myelographic defects most commonly in a compensatory lumbar or lumbosacral curve, and all patients had at least one abnormal, painful disk (88% with pain reproduction). Pain-producing pathology was frequently identified in areas that would not have been included in the fusion area according to accepted rules for treatment of idiopathic scoliosis.

Grubb SA, Lipscomb HJ, Suh PB: Results of surgical treatment of painful adult scoliosis. *Spine* 1994;19: 1619–1627.

Twenty-eight adults with idiopathic scoliosis and 25 adults with degenerative scoliosis treated with spinal fusion were followed prospectively for 2 to 7 years. Pain relief was associated with solid fusion ($p = 0.02$). Reported pain reproduction was 80% among patients with idiopathic scoliosis and 70% among patients with degenerative scoliosis. Sitting and walking tolerances were improved in patients with idiopathic scoliosis, and standing and walking were improved in patients with degenerative scoliosis.

Ogilvie JW: Adult scoliosis: Evaluation and nonsurgical treatment, in Eilert RE (ed): *Instructional Course Lectures XLI.* Park Ridge, IL, American Academy of Orthopaedic Surgeons, 1992, pp 251–255.

This article states that it is incumbent on the surgeon to understand the pathology involved in painful adult spinal deformities and to have a reasonable understanding of the prognosis before attempting invasive therapy. The decision to proceed with surgical treatment is justified in many cases, but it must be based on a thorough understanding of the anticipated benefits and of the risk of serious complications.

Simmons ED Jr, Kowalski JM, Simmons EH: The results of surgical treatment for adult scoliosis. *Spine* 1993;18: 718–724.

The authors found that the relative incidence of pain and progression as indications for surgery were found to vary with respect to age. In the younger groups, progression was more often the indication for surgery, and these patients also had greater deformity. The degree of pain was not found to correlate with the magnitude of the deformity. Surgical treatment can be done with a relatively low serious complication rate and good results in terms of pain relief and reasonable correction of the deformity.

Classic Bibliography

Ascani E, Bartolozzi P, Logroscino CA, et al: Natural history of untreated idiopathic scoliosis after skeletal maturity. *Spine* 1986;11:784–789.

Balderston RA, Winter RB, Moe JH, et al: Fusion to the sacrum for nonparalytic scoliosis in the adult. *Spine* 1986;11:824–829.

Bradford DS: Adult scoliosis: Current concepts of treatment. *Clin Orthop* 1988;229:70–87.

Bradford DS, Lauerman WC: Fusion techniques for adult spine deformity, in Cotler JM, Cotler HB (eds): *Spinal Fusion: Science and Technique.* New York, NY, Springer-Verlag, 1990.

Edgar MA, Mehta MH: Long-term follow-up of fused and unfused idiopathic scoliosis. *J Bone Joint Surg* 1988;70B:712–716.

Fowles JV, Drummond DS, L'Ecuyer S, et al: Untreated scoliosis in the adult. *Clin Orthop* 1978;134:212–217.

Grubb SA, Lipscomb HJ, Coonrad RW: Degenerative adult onset scoliosis. *Spine* 1988;13:241–245.

Hall JE: Dwyer Instrumentation in anterior fusion of the spine. *J Bone Joint Surg* 1981;63A:1188–1190.

Jackson RP, Simmons EH, Stripinis D: Coronal and sagittal plane spinal deformities correlating with back pain and pulmonary function in adult idiopathic scoliosis. *Spine* 1989;14:1391–1397.

Kostuik JP: Operative treatment of idiopathic scoliosis. *J Bone Joint Surg* 1990;72A:1108–1113.

Kostuik JP: Treatment of scoliosis in the adult thoracolumbar spine with special reference to the sacrum. *Orthop Clin North Am* 1988;19:371–381.

Nachemson A: Adult scoliosis and back pain. *Spine* 1979;4:513–517.

Robin GC, Span Y, Steinberg R, et al: Scoliosis in the elderly: A follow-up study. *Spine* 1982;7:355–359.

Simmons EH, Jackson RP: The management of nerve root entrapment syndromes associated with the collapsing scoliosis of idiopathic lumbar and thoracolumbar curves. *Spine* 1979;4:533–541.

Weinstein SL, Ponseti IV: Curve progression in idiopathic scoliosis. *J Bone Joint Surg* 1983;65A:447–455.

Winter RB, Lonstein JE, Denis F: Pain patterns in adult scoliosis. *Orthop Clin North Am* 1988;19:339–345.

54

Spinal Infections

Introduction

Spinal infections affect the bony elements, intervertebral disks, and neural elements to varying degrees. The spectrum of causative organisms is vast and changes with time. In the pre-antibiotic era, the mortality rate associated with these diseases approached 70%. Modern diagnostic and treatment techniques have reduced the mortality rate to 5% or less. Successful treatment begins with timely diagnosis. Careful attention to the patient's history, assessment of host risk factors, and judicious use of imaging and laboratory technology should establish the diagnosis. Treatment then rests on obtaining confirmatory bacteriologic evidence of infection and the decision to proceed with either nonsurgical or surgical management. The goals of treatment are to eradicate the infection while preserving or restoring neurologic function and the structural integrity of the spine.

Pyogenic Vertebral Osteomyelitis

Vertebral osteomyelitis is analogous to the process occurring in the metaphyses of long bones. Endarteriolar circulation at the vertebral end plates is an area predisposed to hematogenous seeding. Information available favors an arterial, rather than venous, mechanism for hematogenous spread. The role of Batson's venous plexus has been overstated. Septic emboli in the endarteriolar loops are thought to establish a local infection. The process then may spread to the contiguous intervertebral disks, or along fascial planes, such as the anterior longitudinal ligament, to involve adjacent vertebral levels. The infection may also invade the spinal canal, giving rise to spinal cord and/or nerve root compromise. Paraspinal abscess formation is common, especially with granulomatous infections. These abscesses may develop in various extraspinal locations. Paralumbar abscesses may point in the flank at Petit's triangle, in the groin, the buttock, the popliteal fossa, or as a perirectal abscess. Abscesses associated with cervical osteomyelitis may obstruct the airway or point in the posterior triangle of the neck or the supraclavicular fossa or may extend into the mediastinum as a life-threatening infection. Pyogenic osteomyelitis occurs most frequently in the lumbar spine followed by the thoracic spine. Cervical spine involvement is seen in less than 10% of cases.

A number of factors have been identified that place a host at risk. Most are conditions that give rise to bacteremias, such as remote sites of infections (eg, skin, genitourinary tract, lungs, and heart), invasive procedures, and intravenous drug abuse. Patients with spinal cord injury are also at risk, presumably because of chronic urinary tract infections and skin ulcers. The very old and the very young are at higher risk, as are immunocompromised hosts. Direct inoculation of the spine through penetrating trauma, recent spinal surgery, or extension from a contiguous focus visceral infection are also risk factors. Diabetes, rheumatoid arthritis, long-term steroid use, advanced age, *Staphylococcus aureus* infections, and more cephalad levels of infection are factors in the development of neurologic deficits. The bacteriology of vertebral osteomyelitis is changing. *S aureus,* once almost always the cause, is now responsible for only 50% of culture-positive cases. An increasing proportion of cases are due to gram-negative and anaerobic organisms. The most common gram-negative organisms identified are *Escherichia coli* and *Pseudomonas* and *Proteus* species. Pseudomonads appear to be particularly common among intravenous drug abusers. Indolent infections may also be seen with *S epidermidis* and some anaerobic organisms. Polymicrobial infections may occur. Pyogenic infections may superinfect underlying granulomatous infections, especially following attempts at biopsy. As the prevalence of acquired immunodeficiency syndrome (AIDS) increases, increasing frequency of opportunistic infections in the spine and continuing evolution of the spectrum of causative organisms can be anticipated.

The diagnosis of spinal infection begins with an awareness of the disease. The primary complaint is pain, not unlike most degenerative spinal conditions. However, the pain associated with infections tends to be relentless, not proportional to activity. Nocturnal pain is a hallmark of infection or tumor. Fevers are noted in less than half of patients. Florid sepsis is uncommon. Neurologic complaints are seen in fewer than 10% of patients at the time of presentation. A paucity of findings is present on physical examination. Local pain, tenderness to palpation and percussion, and muscle spasm may be noted. Late in the course of an infection, vertebral destruction may give rise to a gibbous deformity. Careful neurologic examination should be undertaken to identify neurologic deficits. Meningeal signs should also be sought, because a small percentage have an associated meningitis.

Laboratory studies may be suggestive. The white blood cell (WBC) count is helpful when elevated, but is often normal. The erythrocyte sedimentation rate (ESR) and C-reactive protein (CRP) are elevated in over 90% of patients. Although nonspecific, the ESR and/or CRP may be useful in monitoring response to treatment. No other laboratory tests are useful diagnostically, except for bacte-

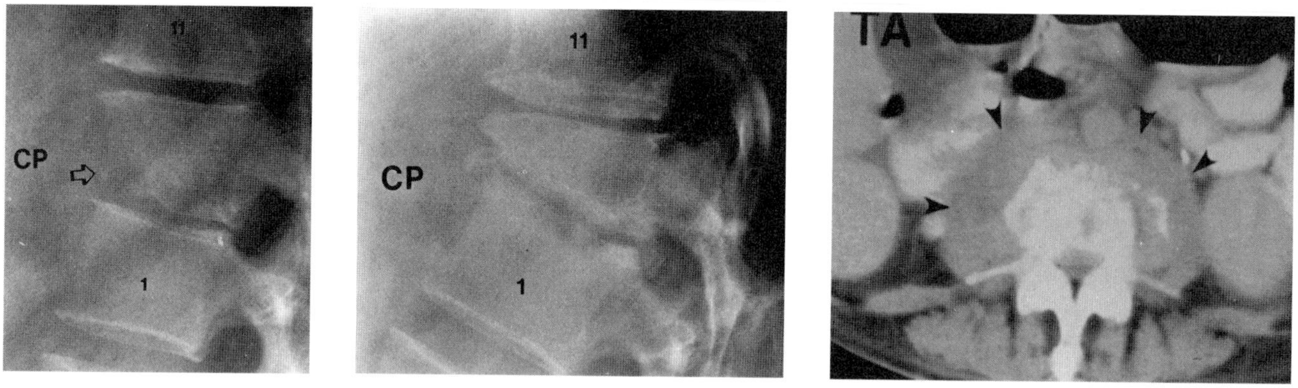

Fig. 1 A previously healthy 49-year-old man awoke one morning with severe back pain. A lateral radiograph taken 1 month after the onset of symptoms (**left**) demonstrates the early radiographic manifestations of vertebral osteomyelitis (open arrow). Medical management failed. Another lateral radiograph taken 6 months later (**center**) reveals progression of the disease across the T12–L1 disk space into the L1 vertebral body. Bone destruction is nearly complete at T12, with associated fracture, collapse, kyphosis, and paraspinal abscess formation (**right,** arrowheads).

riologic information. Biopsy and culture must be done to obtain tissue for bacteriologic processing as well as to exclude the possibility of neoplasm. A positive blood culture may confirm the diagnosis. However, blood cultures are positive in less than one fourth of adults with vertebral osteomyelitis. Needle biopsies guided by computed tomography (CT) or fluoroscopy are usually necessary. Cultures are positive in 68% to 86% of cases. When negative, open biopsy, positive in greater than 80% of cases, may be necessary. All samples should be sent for pathologic examination to exclude malignancy. Stains should be done for acid-fast bacilli, fungal organisms, and pyogens. In addition, the differential diagnosis includes a variety of sterile inflammatory processes as well as metabolic disease that gives rise to fractures.

Imaging is essential; radiographs are often the first line of evaluation. The findings lag 2 to 3 weeks behind the onset of symptoms. Films may show evidence of osteolysis in the anterior vertebral metaphyseal region, loss of disk space height, end plate blurring, and subchondral reactive bone formation (Fig. 1, *left*). Long-standing disease causes vertebral destruction, leading to collapse, kyphosis, and abscess formation (Fig. 1, *center* and *right*). Infection often crosses the disk space to involve adjacent vertebrae. The paravertebral soft tissues should be carefully examined on the lateral cervical spine film as well as on the posteroanterior thoracic and lumbar views. Retropharyngeal edema, a widened mediastinal shadow, or distortion of the psoas contours are important clues.

Technetium bone scans and gallium scans have a relative accuracy of 86% in diagnosing vertebral osteomyelitis. When the two tests are combined, they are 94% accurate. Indium 111 WBC scans are not recommended for the diagnosis of vertebral osteomyelitis because they are only 31% accurate. Antibiotic administration prior to scanning decreases the accuracy of gallium and indium scans in the diagnosis of vertebral osteomyelitis.

CT scans provide excellent detail of local bone anatomy with relatively good definition of soft-tissue structures. Multiple lytic areas surrounded by reactive bone adjacent to a narrowed disk space and paravertebral soft-tissue thickening distinguish infection from malignant destruction. When combined with myelography, enhanced CT scans provide a useful view of the spinal canal, identifying areas of local neurologic compromise. In addition, cerebrospinal fluid (CSF) samples may be obtained at the time of lumbar puncture for a myelogram. Analysis of CSF can

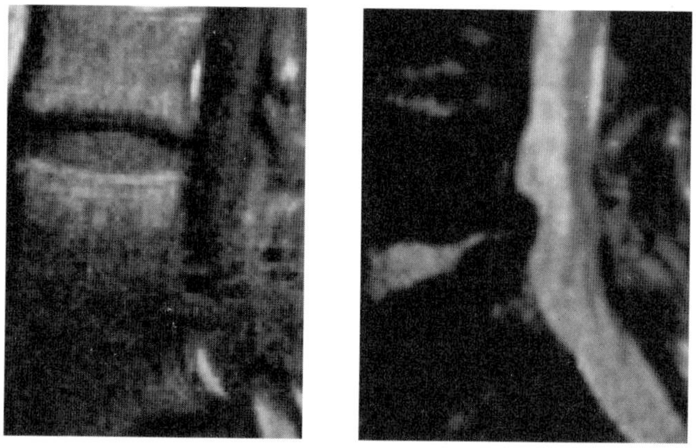

Fig. 2 Sagittal T1 (**left**) and T2 (**right**) magnetic resonance images illustrating the features diagnostic of intervertebral disk space infection. (Reproduced with permission from Heller JG: Postoperative infection of the spine, in Rothman RH, Simeone FA (eds): *The Spine,* ed 3. Philadelphia, PA, WB Saunders, 1992, pp 1817–1837.)

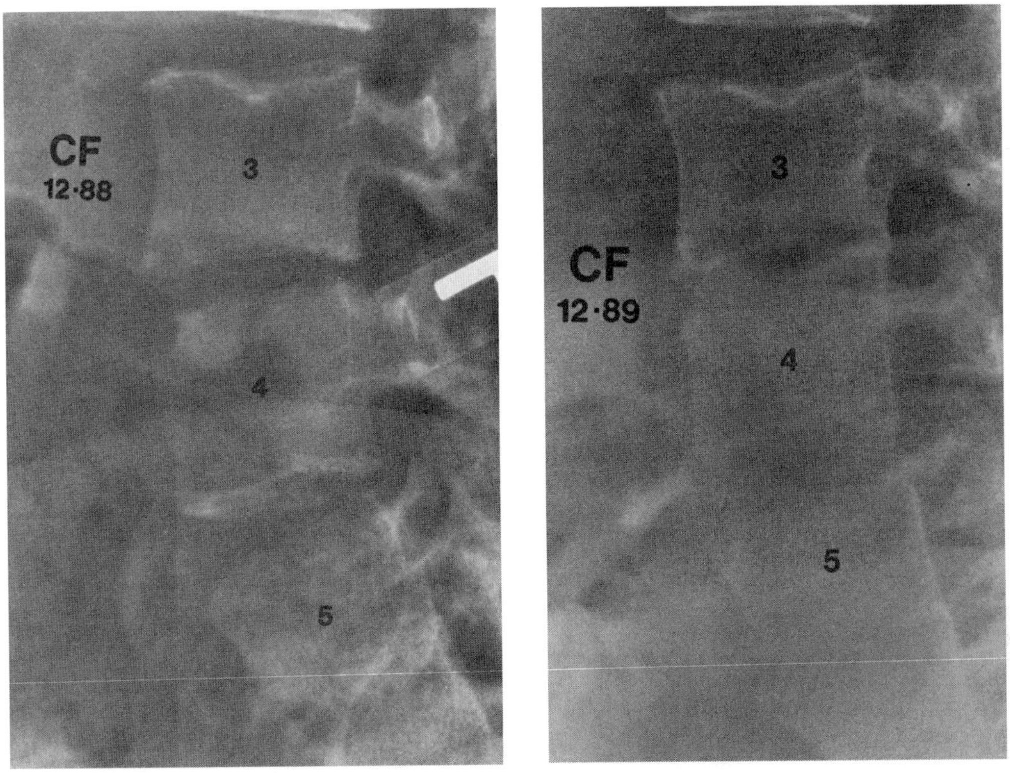

Fig. 3 HIV positive male with progressive low back pain. A radiograph (**left**) taken a few months after the onset of symptoms illustrates two different phases of intervertebral diskitis. Early changes of disk height loss, marginal osseous erosion, and end-plate blurring are present at L3–4. At L5-S1, the changes are more advanced, with virtually complete destruction of the disk space and possible ankylosis. Following medical treatment with intravenous antibiotics and spica cast immobilization, another lateral radiograph (**right**) reveals complete ankylosis at L5-S1 and virtually complete ankylosis at L3–4. (Reproduced with permission from Heller JG: Postoperative infection of the spine, in Rothman RH, Simeone FA (eds): *The Spine,* ed 3. Philadelphia, PA, WB Saunders, 1992, pp 1817–1837.)

exclude the possibility of concurrent meningitis. In general, CT scanning provides useful and complementary information to magnetic resonance (MR) images.

MR is the imaging modality of choice for spinal infections. The imaging characteristics of pyogenic diskitis and vertebral osteomyelitis are virtually pathognomonic (Fig. 2). T1-weighted images show loss of the normal anatomic detail of the nucleus pulposus, the vertebral end plates, and the associated metaphyseal region. The normal intranuclear cleft of the disk is lost. The complementary T2-weighted images show hyperintensity of the disk space and possibly associated epidural abscesses. These findings are more characteristic for pyogenic infections. Granulomatous infections are less easily diagnosed. The false-negative rate may be further reduced with the addition of gadolinium enhancement. The 95% accuracy of MR imaging (MRI) surpasses that of any single radionuclide study and compares favorably with that of the combined technetium and gallium scans. MRI has the added benefit of providing regional anatomic information, especially neuroanatomic features. In combination with CT scanning, MRI provides excellent diagnostic accuracy and anatomic detail.

The goals of treatment in vertebral osteomyelitis are: (1) to identify the pathogen; (2) to eradicate the infection with minimal chance of recurrence; (3) to preserve or restore neurologic function; (4) to insure adequate spinal alignment and stability; and (5) to relieve pain. All of this must be undertaken while attending to any host risk factors that may have predisposed to infection. Medical treatment of vertebral osteomyelitis may be successful in many cases (Fig. 3). The choice of antibiotics is guided by the culture and sensitivities. Current recommendations are for 6 weeks of intravenous antibiotics, possibly supplemented by oral antibiotics thereafter. Shorter lengths of parenteral treatment have been associated with increasing rates of recurrence. In addition to antimicrobial therapy, successful treatment includes appropriate immobilization of the spine. Suitable bracing with or without bed rest is usually sufficient. Molded total contact braces are recommended for the lumbar and low thoracic spine. If cervical osteomyelitis is to be treated nonsurgically, a halo vest should be considered. Finally, while embarking on a course of medical management, patients should be observed for change in neurologic status, radiographic progression of the disease, or failure to show adequate clinical response. If the patient does not demonstrate favorable response to treatment by improvement of temperature, symptoms, and sedimentation rate within 1 to 2 weeks of treatment, medical therapy can be considered to have failed.

Indications for surgical treatment include: (1) a need for open biopsy; (2) significant and/or progressive neurologic deficit; (3) vertebral collapse with or without spinal deformity, especially in the cervical spine; (4) significant intraosseous or paraspinal abscesses, especially with a septic course; and (5) failure of clinical response to medical treatment. The surgical objective is removal of all infected or necrotic tissues. This procedure should produce surgically clean margins with decompression of the spinal canal, restoration of normal spinal alignment, and reconstruction by applicable techniques. The approach is dictated by anatomy and by the location of the infection. Most often the pathology is located within the vertebral body and intervertebral disks; therefore, the approach is generally anterior. Anterior approaches permit direct access to the pathology and facilitate reconstructive measures. These include the extrapharyngeal (upper cervical), the standard anterior Smith-Robinson (subaxial cervical), transthoracic (thoracic), and retroperitoneal (lumbar). Infections confined to the lumbosacral junction are best approached from an anterior retroperitoneal approach. Consideration can be given to a costotransversectomy or lateral extracavitary approach in the thoracic spine under certain circumstances, but visibility of the anterior aspect of the thecal sac is limited, and anterior reconstruction is technically more difficult.

Anterior decompression should include removal of all accessible infected and/or necrotic tissue. If significant reactive bone formation is present adjacent to the disk spaces, then portions of the remaining vertebral bodies should be resected back to healthy bleeding bone. Paraspinal abscesses should be debrided aggressively. To the extent possible, the wound should be rendered surgically clean. Tissue should be sent for both bacteriologic processing and pathologic review. Stains should be done to look for atypical organisms.

Corpectomy defects are reconstructed with bone graft. Tricortical iliac grafts are favored for one-level corpectomies. Corpectomies of two or more levels require other grafting methods, such as multiple fibular autograft struts supplemented by morcellized local rib graft, or fresh frozen allografts. Multiple rib grafts alone and/or vascular rib grafts are prone to fracture and dislodgement. They are mechanically unsatisfactory by themselves. Supplemental segmental posterior instrumentation and fusion should be considered with anterior resections of two or more vertebral bodies. Patients should be adequately protected with orthoses postoperatively; thoracolumbosacral orthoses should be used for pathology from the midthoracic spine to the sacrum. Cervicothoracic orthoses or halo vests are recommended for cervical reconstructions. Adjunctive posterior procedures may obviate the need for long-term, rigid external immobilization.

Tuberculosis

Although endemic in many third world countries, tuberculosis had become relatively uncommon in the United States. Recent resurgence of the disease has accompanied more aggressive medical management of chronic illness as well as the emergence of immunocompromised states, particularly AIDS. This diagnosis must be considered when evaluating destructive lesions of the spine. Approximately 10% of patients with tuberculosis will manifest bone or joint disease; half of them will have lesions in the spine. As with other spinal infections, the principal mode of spread is hematogenous. Occasionally, direct extension from a visceral focus will occur, such as from the lung, kidney, or mesenteric lymph nodes.

Tuberculosis is the paradigm for a number of granulomatous infectious processes. The pathologic hallmarks are caseating granulomata in association with Langhans giant cells. Acid-fast stains can identify the organisms; however, immunofluorescent techniques are more sensitive. The primary focus (eg, lung, gastrointestinal, or genitourinary tracts) may be either active or inactive. The spine is usually a secondary focus of disease. The early stages of the process are analogous to those described for pyogenic osteomyelitis. The initiating event is deposition of septic microemboli within the endarteriolar circulation of the vertebral metaphysis. Once established, these microabscesses may progress. The thoracic spine is most frequently involved, followed by the lumbar spine. Cervical spine involvement is rare. Primary involvement of the posterior arches is exceedingly rare, occurring in $< 0.5\%$ of cases. There is a greater incidence of multilevel involvement than in pyogenic vertebral osteomyelitis. Paraspinal abscess formation is more common and more extensive with tuberculosis, and it is more likely in children than in adults. Epidural extension is common, particularly following pathologic fracture. Neural compression is usually anterior. Transdural penetration has been reported, but is unusual.

The clinical presentation is nonspecific and can be deceptive. The typical complaint is that of slowly progressive spinal pain localized to a particular region of the spine. Symptoms of a chronic illness, fever, malaise, weight loss, and anorexia are common. A history suggesting compromised immune defenses should be sought. Late in the disease process, patients may present with obvious spinal deformity and neurologic deficits. The latter are more common with thoracic and cervical involvement. Age appears to have a significant influence on the risk of paralysis. Cervical tuberculosis in children younger than 10 years of age carries little risk (17%) of spinal cord injury. Cervical involvement has a risk of significant paralysis in up to 81% of patients older than 10 years of age. As with other cases of osteomyelitis, the evaluation begins by considering tuberculosis in the differential diagnosis of spinal pain and destructive lesions. Laboratory findings are nonspecific. Most patients have an elevated ESR; the WBC count is highly variable, and might be subnormal; septicemia is relatively rare. The chest radiograph should be scrutinized for the presence of active lung disease as well as paraspinal soft-tissue shadows that indicate abscess formation. A purified protein derivative (tuberculin) test (PPD) with anergy screens should be applied and is most often positive. However, anergy is a distinct possibility as immunocompromised states increase in prevalence. Although frequently slow to grow, cultures of sputum, gastric washings, and morning urine samples may yield the organism. The most rapid identification of the pathologic process, as well as differentiation from other potential causes, usually rests on biopsy.

Radiographs may be of help, although the features are similar to those of pyogenic vertebral osteomyelitis (Fig. 4, *top left*). Extensive destruction, which appears out of proportion to the amount of pain, and a prolonged onset of symptoms favor a tuberculous etiology. There is also a tendency towards preservation of the intervertebral disks until late in the disease. Tuberculosis tends to involve more levels of the spine than pyogenic processes, and the abscesses tend to be more extensive. Radiographs may fail to distinguish focal tuberculosis, especially the central vertebral body pattern or posterior arch involvement, from primary or metastatic disease of the spine. Radionuclide imaging tends to be of little help. There is a high false-negative rate for technetium bone scans (33%) and gallium scans (70%). If the plain radiographs identify a destructive process and/or paraspinal soft-tissue masses, the orthopaedist should proceed to more direct imaging techniques.

CT scans of the involved areas are helpful in identifying the nature and extent of vertebral involvement as well as the associated soft-tissue masses (Fig. 4, *top right*). Intrathecal contrast is required to image the spinal canal. CT scans cannot distinguish granulation tissue from frank abscess formation. MRI scans are probably the imaging modality of choice. They provide excellent definition of the extent of vertebral involvement, spinal canal compromise, and abscess formation (Fig. 4, *bottom left*). MRI may be able to distinguish abscesses from granulation tissue. Unfortunately, the ability to distinguish an infectious process from a neoplastic process may not be that reliable with MRI. The hyperintensity seen on T2-weighted images in pyogenic infections is not as prevalent with tuberculous processes, and the degree of bone destruction is not well illustrated with MRI. Complementary noncontrasted CT scans are recommended in planning treatment, especially when surgical intervention is contemplated.

The differential diagnosis is extensive. Spinal neoplasms, primary or metastatic, need to be considered and their possibility excluded. This can usually be done on the basis of pathologic examination. Pyogenic organisms are infectious possibilities that must be considered when acute inflammation is noted. Chronic infection and granulomatous reaction could be caused by bacteria such as *Actinomyces, Nocardia,* and *Brucella.* These opportunistic infections are occurring with greater frequency. In addition to *Mycobacterium tuberculosis,* nontuberculous opportunistic infection should also be considered. Atypical mycobacteria may ultimately be identified with cultures. Fungal infections, such as coccidioidomycosis, blastomycosis, cryptococcosis, candidiasis, and aspergillosis, are possibilities. Although many of the pathogens on this list are rare, in certain geographic and clinical settings, they do occur. Dialogue with infectious disease associates, microbiology laboratory personnel, and pathology personnel helps ensure proper examination of specimens.

The management of spinal tuberculosis must be individualized to each patient's needs. In the United States, the presence of fracture, collapse, spinal deformity, significant neurologic deficits, or large abscesses are indications for surgical as well as medical management. More aggressive management will ensure lower rates of complications in spinal disease and more rapid return to normal activities. The surgical principles are as described for pyogenic vertebral osteomyelitis. Because the disease is usually anterior, debridement and reconstruction can require anterior procedures. If the disease involves two or more levels of reconstruction, especially in the lumbar and cervical spine, supplementary posterior stabilization and fusion are advisable (Fig. 4, *bottom right*). Isolated posterior procedures are rarely indicated. If laminectomy is performed for isolated posterior arch disease or a dorsolateral epidural abscess, supplemental fusion is recommended.

Surgery should be considered an adjunct to medical management. Because eradication of the disease is the primary goal, drug therapy is indispensable. With emergence of resistant strains, close cooperation with infectious disease colleagues is essential. The current pharmaceutical armamentarium includes isoniazid, rifampin, ethambutol hydrochloride, pyrazinamide, streptomycin, and para-aminosalicylic acid. The number, combination, sequence, and duration of treatment with these drugs depend on clinical circumstances. Current recommendations favor treatment for at least 6 months, and more commonly for 9 months. In the absence of a substantially immunocompromised host, the mortality rate for spinal tuberculosis should be less than 5% with relapse rate of 10% to 20%. In those with severely impaired immune systems, suppression of the disease may be the primary goal of treatment.

Intervertebral Diskitis and Osteomyelitis in Childhood

Diskitis and vertebral osteomyelitis do not appear to be distinct clinical entities but points on a continuum of disease. The current hypothesis is that diskitis or peridiskal metaphyseal infection is a primary event. If it is unrecognized and untreated, the clinical picture of osteomyelitis with its attendant features will evolve. Increased awareness of spinal infections has contributed to earlier diagnosis, more aggressive treatment, and a decrease in the reported incidence of childhood vertebral osteomyelitis with a reciprocal rise in the number of cases of diskitis in recent years. Early treatment of otitis media and other common

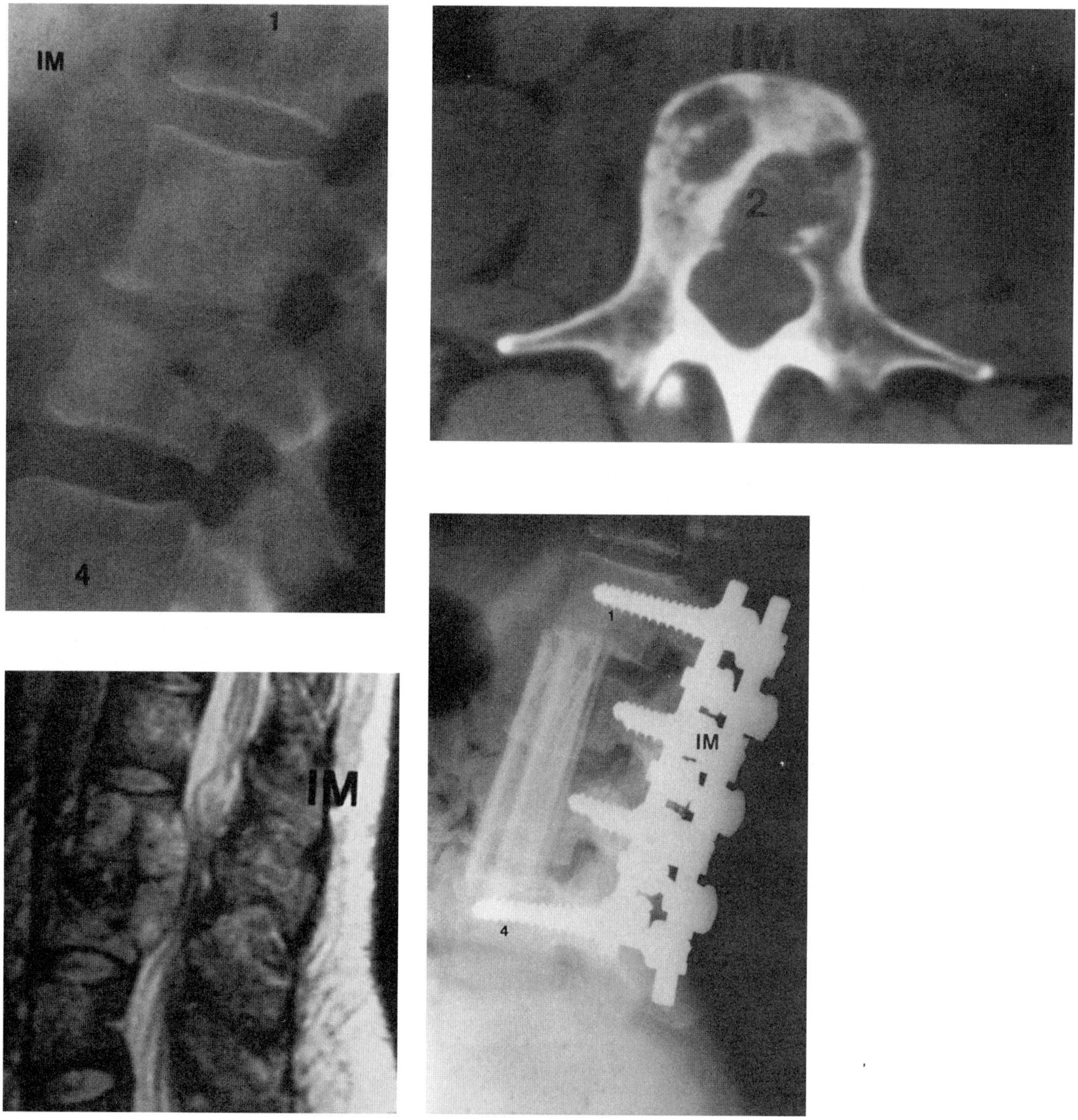

Fig. 4 A 47-year-old black woman presented with 3 months of progressive low back pain, malaise, and weight loss, followed by acute severe worsening of her pain. The initial radiograph (**top left**) revealed a fracture of L3 associated with disk height loss at L2–3. A computed tomography scan (**top right**) depicts extensive intraosseous extension of the destructive process into the L2 vertebral body. Note the marked reactive bone formation around the lytic regions and the paraspinal soft-tissue thickening. The magnetic resonance image (**bottom left**) demonstrates profound soft-tissue compromise. Biopsy established a diagnosis of tuberculosis. The patient underwent L2 and L3 corpectomies with autogenous fibular reconstruction, followed by posterior segmental instrumentation and fusion from L1–L4 (**bottom right**).

childhood infections may have further reduced the risk of bacteremia and vertebral column infection. *S aureus* remains the most common pathogen, growing in 80% to 90% of culture-positive cases. However, a significant number of cases remain culture negative. Positive blood cultures are obtained in half of the children with signs of systemic illness and symptoms of spinal infection. Needle biopsies of the intervertebral disks are reported positive in two out of three cases. Whether the high incidence of negative cultures supports a nonbacterial etiology or faulty culture technique is unclear. However, the rapid response to intravenous antibiotics provides circumstantial evidence in favor of a bacterial process. It should be remembered that children with clinically proven suppurative septic arthritis have only a 60% positive culture rate from joint aspirates. The biopsy technique must also be considered, because aspiration of the disk may not be diagnostic if the patient has a peridiskal metaphyseal process.

The clinical presentation varies with age. Children younger than 3 years, unable to articulate their symptoms, present with abnormalities of gait or refusal to walk. Such presentations may be confused with the more common septic arthritis or toxic synovitis of the hip, injury, abdominal pathology, or even suspicion of progressive neurologic syndromes. Children aged 3 to 8 years may complain of truncal pain, especially in the abdomen. Lumbar or low thoracic infections will refer pain to the abdominal wall and groin. The initial presentation may be suggestive of acute abdominal processes, such as appendicitis, mesenteric adenitis, and other inflammatory bowel disorders. Consideration may also be given to genitourinary pathology, such as acute pyelonephritis, nephrolithiasis, or obstructive neuropathies. In adolescents, symptoms often evolve more fully prior to presentation. Teenagers may present with complaints of back pain, radicular pain, and spinal deformity. In this case, the differential diagnosis of spontaneous spinal pain, although broad, mandates aggressive workup. The possibility of spinal tumor, benign or malignant, must be excluded along with that of infection, herniated disk, spondylolisthesis, Scheuermann's disease, and so forth. In the setting of an elevated sedimentation rate, fever, and appropriate imaging, the diagnosis can be established.

Physical examination can be of considerable help in guiding the workup of the patient. In the early childhood years, when the pediatrician is more than likely to consider intra-abdominal processes or infections of the weightbearing joints, careful attention to the musculoskeletal examination is essential. The physician will note painless gliding of the weightbearing joints within a limited arch of motion. It may be difficult to distinguish between a psoas sign and signs of septic arthritis of the hip. Joint aspiration and appropriate imaging will usually make this distinction. In the older child, the observance of normal spinal motion or a loss of spinal rhythm should be sought. Pain can usually be elicited with local palpation or percussion of the spine. Deep palpation of the abdomen may yield tenderness along the vertebral column in the midline, which is to be distinguished from pain in the region of the appendix, the spleen, or the liver. Neurologic deficits, tension signs, such as a positive straight leg raise, and tight hamstrings may be noted.

Laboratory investigations are of limited help. The ESR and CRP levels are usually elevated. The WBC count and differential WBC count are variable. At least half of children are febrile; fewer are systemically ill. Blood cultures are positive in approximately half of patients with proven diagnoses. Urinalyses and joint aspirates may be appropriate in certain clinical settings to exclude other likely diagnoses. Radiologic imaging confirms the diagnosis. Plain radiographic findings are subtle and slow to evolve. Unless the child presents 2 to 3 weeks after the onset of symptoms, radiographs are of little use. If the infection has progressed to vertebral osteomyelitis, evidence of intervertebral destruction and collapse may be seen and must be distinguished from similar-looking neoplastic processes, especially vertebra plana. Radionuclide imaging may be quite useful. Whereas gallium scans engender significant delay in obtaining images, technetium bone scans are readily available and yield information within 4 to 6 hours. Their overall accuracy is rather high, but they lack in local anatomic detail, especially of the neural elements. These scans are not necessarily able to distinguish involvement of the disk and vertebral body.

CT scans provide far greater detail of local bone and soft-tissue anatomy. As with the adult, in the absence of intrathecal contrast, CT scans do not yield useful information regarding the spinal canal and neural elements. However, the rendering of local osseous anatomy and paravertebral soft tissues is excellent. MRI is the imaging modality of choice (Fig. 5). As in adults, the findings of intervertebral diskitis or vertebral osteomyelitis are virtually pathognomonic. MRI also can distinguish these infectious processes from many spinal tumors. The MRI findings might also influence the biopsy location (ie, disk versus metaphysis).

The differential diagnosis of spinal infections in children is extensive. First, the physician must rule out the possibility of a spinal neoplasm. (See "Tumors of the Spine.") Appropriate imaging studies are useful in this regard. Various other infections may be confused with diskitis and intervertebral osteomyelitis. Consideration should be given to epidural abscesses, retrocaecal appendicitis, pyelonephritis, mesenteric adenitis, and sacroiliac joint infections, as well as septic arthritis. Sterile inflammatory conditions such as Scheuermann's disease must also be considered. Finally, the possibility of nonpyogenic infections of the spine must be evaluated. Tuberculosis and other granulomatous diseases appear to be increasing in frequency. Patients suspected of pyogenic vertebral column infections should be given a PPD.

The goals of treatment include early diagnosis, eradication of infection, and prevention of the late sequelae of spinal infections. Neurologic loss may also be caused by

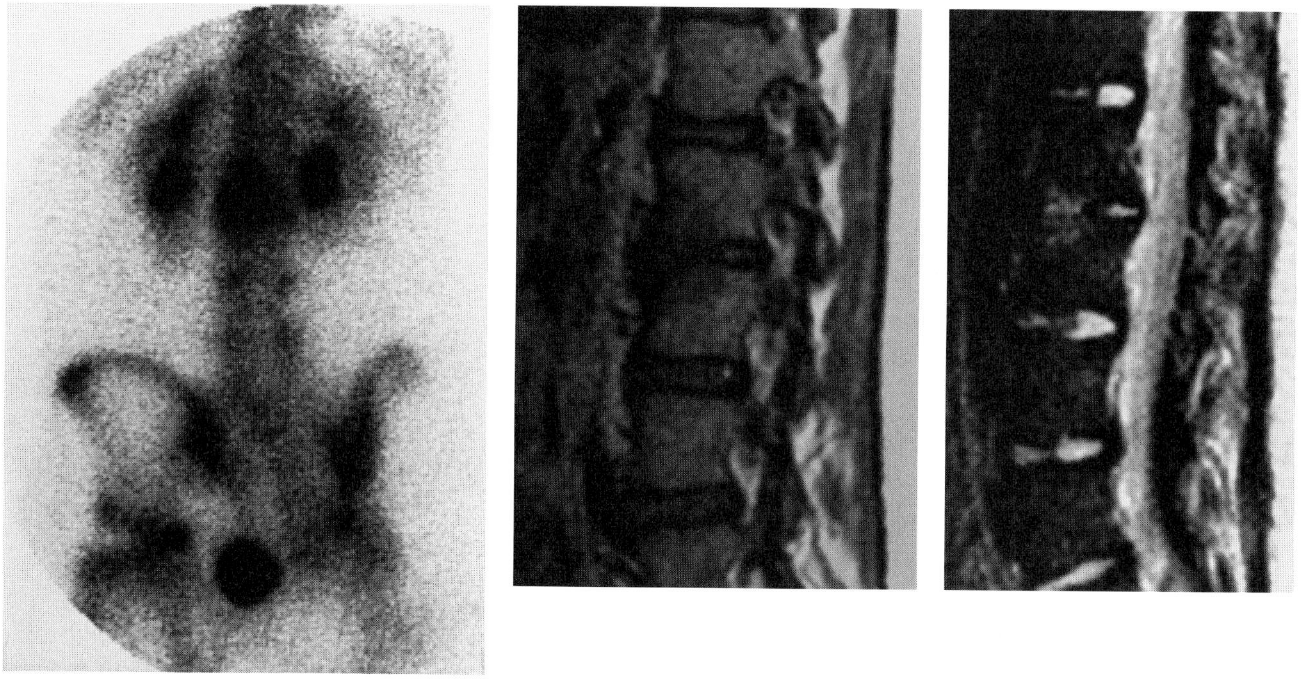

Fig. 5 Childhood diskitis. **Left,** Technetium bone scan of a child suspected of having intervertebral diskitis at L2–3. T1 (**center**) and T2 (**right**) magnetic resonance images of the same child showing the characteristic signal changes of diskitis at L2–3.

associated epidural abscesses. The process should be treated early enough to avoid systemic sepsis. Diagnosis begins with awareness of the disease and a low threshold of suspicion. If the clinical presentation, physical examination, and ESR are suggestive, the physician should begin imaging with the best available technology. Confirmation of the diagnosis may then be obtained through either blood cultures or direct aspiration and biopsy. Treatment is medical in the majority of pediatric patients. The possibility of tuberculous infection must be excluded with a PPD. Empiric intravenous antibiotics are initiated to treat presumptive staphylococcal infections. Oral antibiotics may be substituted after clear clinical improvement is apparent, usually within 4 to 7 days. Generally treatment is continued for 4 weeks. The patient is placed at bed rest until comfortable, then allowed up to ambulate as tolerated. Bracing is not usually necessary in childhood, except in cases of significant pain. The requirements for external immobilization tend to increase with age. Patients should be observed on a long-term basis for the possibility of growth arrest and progressive deformity. If the infection is treated early and aggressively, this possibility is unlikely. Surgery is reserved for patients who present with advanced disease, including vertebral collapse, deformity, neurologic deficit, epidural abscesses, or significant psoas abscesses. Surgery also may be indicated in patients who fail to respond to appropriate medical management as described above. The principles of surgical intervention are as described for vertebral osteomyelitis in adults.

Epidural Abscesses

Epidural abscesses are uncommon, but important in the differential diagnosis of acute spinal pain. The frequency of occurrence has risen from 0.2 to 1.2 cases per 10,000 hospital admissions to at least 2.8 cases per 10,000. The rising incidence may reflect changes in the population at risk, aggressive medical treatment of chronic illness, or increased diagnostic acumen. Known risk factors include diabetes mellitus, malignancy, immunosuppression, blunt trauma, vertebral fractures, alcohol abuse, remote infectious foci, and invasive procedures, such as diskography, epidural catheterization, or spinal surgery. Most of the historic features overlap with those of known risk factors for other spinal infections. An epidural process should be kept in mind when evaluating patients suspected of spinal infections and/or tumors. The clinical presentation can be misleading. The initial complaint is usually axial pain. Other constitutional symptoms and signs of infection are present in approximately one half of cases. If not diagnosed and treated, the progression of the disease is rather predictable. Axial pain intensifies, progressing to radicular and, ultimately, spinal cord deficits, often over 72 to 96 hours. For

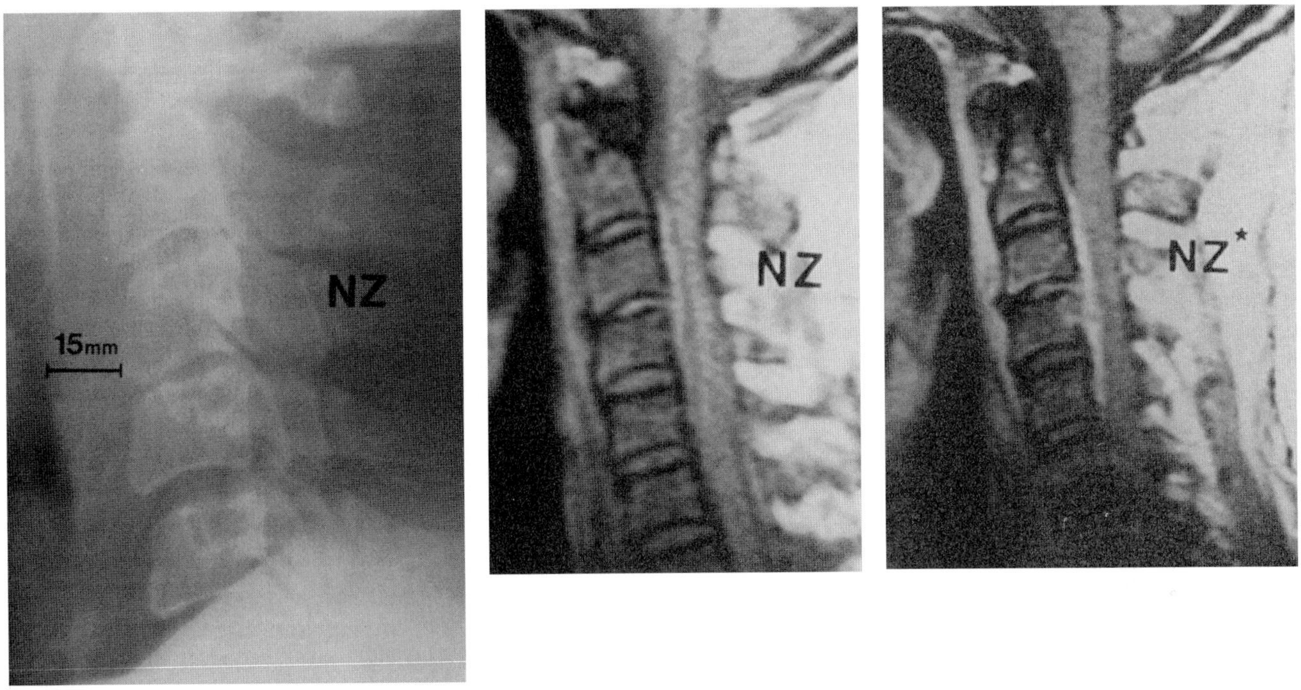

Fig. 6 Lateral cervical radiograph (**left**) illustrating subtle anterior retropharyngeal soft-tissue thickening in association with C3–4 disk height loss in a young man complaining of severe neck pain. The subsequent magnetic resonance (MR) images (**center** and **right**) diagnosed an epidural abscess associated with a disk space infection. Note that abscess signal is hyperintense on the post-gadolinium image (**right**). (Reproduced with permission from Heller JG: Infections of the cervical spine, in An HS, Simpson JM (eds): *Surgery of the Cervical Spine.* London, UK, Martin Dunitz, 1994, pp 335–356.)

those progressing to complete paralysis, the prognosis is bleak. The mortality rate is in excess of 12%.

Optimal outcome depends on early diagnosis. Unfortunately, accurate diagnosis at the time of admission is the exception rather than the rule. Only 20% of epidural abscesses are recognized at the time of hospital admission. Heightened awareness of the diagnostic possibility is essential. The presence of fever, leukocytosis, an elevated ESR, and sepsis are highly suggestive in the presence of acute spinal pain. However, the same findings may be present with intervertebral diskitis or acute vertebral osteomyelitis. Because remote sites of infection are present in up to one half of these patients, these laboratory findings may be incorrectly attributed to the other site of infection.

When no explanation for the patient's acute spinal pain is readily apparent and one or more of the clinical risk factors are present, consideration should be given to urgent and appropriate imaging studies. Plain radiographs may identify areas of soft-tissue swelling or vertebral destruction, which suggest a vertebral column infection (Fig. 6, *left*). Epidural abscesses often occur in conjunction with intervertebral diskitis and/or osteomyelitis; however, the absence of such findings does not exclude the diagnosis of an intraspinal infection. Radionuclide studies are of no value. Myelography with postmyelography CT may be diagnostic. Although it is invasive, myelography has the advantage of providing cerebrospinal fluid (CSF) for analysis. CSF samples should be sent for Gram stain, culture and sensitivity, cytology, WBC count and differential, glucose, and protein levels. Concurrent meningitis is present in up to 13% of patients. The myelographic images will identify the extent of the myelographic block. Frequently, a second injection (lateral C1–2 for contrast above the block, and lumbar below the block) may be required to define the cranial and caudal limits of the abscess. Postmyelography CT scanning will locate the abscess and define associated bone or disk infections, and it is particularly helpful in planning treatment.

MRI is the imaging modality of choice. Gadolinium-enhanced studies provide the highest known accuracy for this diagnosis by reducing the incidence of false-negative results. MRI has the additional benefit of providing detailed regional anatomy as well as investigating the presence of coexistent vertebral column infections. The abscess appears iso- or hypointense on T1-weighted images (Fig. 6, *center*). It is usually hyperintense on T2-weighted images. The addition of gadolinium tends to further intensify the signal (Fig. 6, *right*).

Epidural abscesses are most common in the thoracic spine, followed by the lumbar spine. Cervical lesions are uncommon, representing less than 18% of all cases. The epidural space is most generous in the lumbar spine, followed by the thoracic spine. There is little or no epidural fat in the cervical spine. Lesions are typically dorsal in the thoracic and lumbar spinal and are more commonly ventral in the cervical spine. When associated with intervertebral diskitis or osteomyelitis, abscesses tend to occur ventrally. They tend to span two to four vertebral levels but may extend along virtually the entire spinal canal. The microbiology of epidural abscesses parallels that of other spinal infections. Three fourths of infections are caused by gram-positive cocci, and > 50% are *S aureus.* The remaining organisms are predominantly gram negative, but some aerobes have been cultured. The spectrum of organisms reflects that associated with remote sites of infection, which have been documented as hematogenous sources of spread in at least one half of cases. The initial antibiotic treatment should be broad spectrum with drugs that readily penetrate the blood–brain barrier. The choice of drugs may be further refined once culture and sensitivity data are available.

The differential diagnosis is broad. Other vertebral column infections have similar initial presenting complaints. The physician must also consider intraspinal tumors, especially epidural metastases; spontaneous epidural hematomas; intraspinal vascular anomalies; disk herniations; subdural or intramedullary abscesses; acute transverse myelitis; and meningitis. The history, physical examination, imaging studies, and CSF analysis should rapidly limit the diagnostic possibilities.

Treatment of epidural abscess is a medical and surgical emergency. Because the prognosis is directly related to the speed of diagnosis and intervention, delay in treatment should be avoided at all costs. Once the location of the abscess is known, it should be surgically decompressed; institution of antibiotic treatment should not be delayed. Laminectomy usually provides effective decompression because most thoracic and lumbar abscesses are dorsal. Every attempt should be made to preserve the facet joints and capsules. If extensive decompression is required, a supplemental arthrodesis is advised, either acutely or delayed. Anterior epidural abscesses should be approached anteriorly, especially when they are associated with disk space infections or vertebral osteomyelitis. The procedure should include resection of all involved spinal column tissues. The nature of the compressive mass will range from purulent material to granulation tissue depending on the causative organism and duration of infection. Anterior vertebral column deficiencies should be reconstructed acutely with autogenous bone graft. Anterior spinal instrumentation is controversial and not routinely recommended. Resections of two or more vertebral bodies may necessitate supplemental posterior stabilization. Certain contraindications to surgical intervention have been proposed.

The prognosis for epidural abscesses is favorable provided the diagnosis is timely and intervention rapid. Poor prognostic factors include rapidly progressing paralysis and complete paralysis or neurologic deficits present for more than 36 hours. Other factors felt to prejudice the probability of recovery include diabetes, advanced age, immunosuppression (eg, AIDS), and possibly associated osteomyelitis. The probability of survival has changed dramatically during the antibiotic era. However, combined analysis of modern clinical series still suggests a mortality rate in excess of 12%.

Postoperative Infections of the Spine

All invasive diagnostic and therapeutic spinal procedures have an associated risk of infection (Fig. 7). The magnitude of risk varies with the type of procedure. Timely diagnosis and prompt intervention will minimize any comorbidity. The risk of infection varies in proportion to the magnitude of the operation performed. Lumbar laminotomy and diskectomy following the administration of prophylactic antibiotics carries an infection risk of 0.5% or less. The addition of a fusion without instrumentation increases the risk of infection to 2% or less. Instrumentation further increases the risk of spinal wound infection, but the reported incidences are highly variable. In the absence of certain predisposing risk factors, postoperative wound infections can be expected in 2% to 5% of complex instrumented spinal reconstructions.

Appropriate administration of prophylactic antibiotics significantly reduces the incidence of infection associated with spinal surgery. The literature for laminectomy/diskectomy suggests that the infection risk has been reduced from 1% to 2% to less than 0.5%. Similar reduction of risk has been documented for lumbar fusions. The role of prophylactic antibiotics in diagnostic procedures is unclear. For percutaneous biopsy procedures, administration of antibiotics may be unwise because an infection may be part of the differential diagnosis. However, consideration should be given to prophylactic antibiotics for diskography when adverse risk factors are present.

Factors known to increase the risk of postoperative infections are malnutrition, obesity, poorly controlled diabetes, immunosuppression, long-term steroid therapy, advanced age, remote synchronous infections, and prolonged preoperative hospitalization. If surgery is nonemergent, attempts should be made to modify these risk factors preoperatively. Additionally, the patient and family should be counseled in regard to their increased morbidity risk. For patients who have received local radiation preoperatively, especially within 6 weeks of surgery, the possibility of wound dehiscence and secondary infection should be discussed. Treatment of wound infections begins with prevention. Delicate tissue handling during surgery minimizes tissue necrosis. The presence of foreign material and necrotic tissue increases the risk of infection. Meticulous hemostasis and avoidance of hematoma formation further reduce the incidence of wound infection. More extensive procedures should involve routine irrigation and debridement of

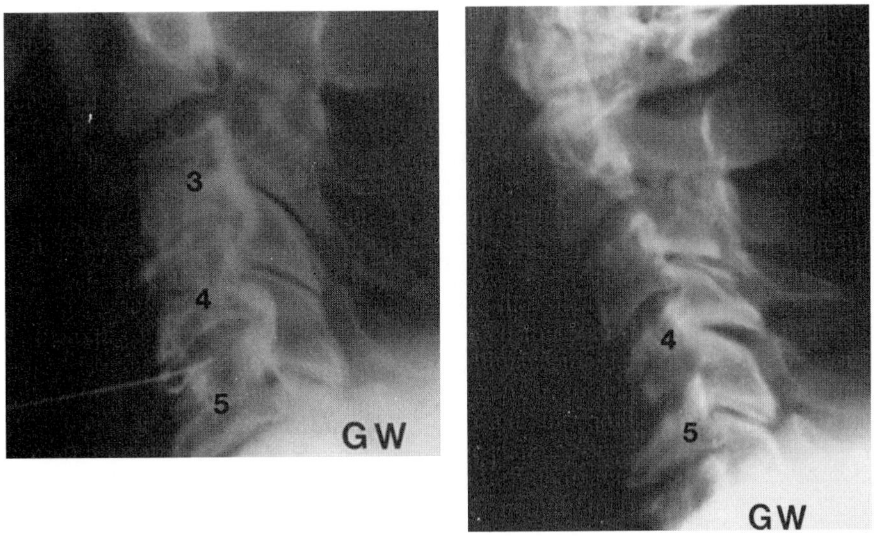

Fig. 7 Lateral diskogram image (**left**) obtained during evaluation of neck pain. The patient's pain worsened significantly following the procedure. A lateral film made 2 months later (**right**) shows evidence of cervical osteomyelitis at C4-C6. (Reproduced with permission from Heller JG: Infections of the cervical spine, in An HS, Simpson JM (eds): *Surgery of the Cervical Spine.* London, UK, Martin Dunitz, 1994, pp 335–356.)

devitalized tissues prior to closure. A high threshold of suspicion for infection should be maintained postoperatively.

Postoperative diskitis following laminotomy/diskectomy may be difficult to recognize. The diagnosis is often delayed. The patient's wound appears deceptively normal. The principal complaint is increasing back pain, often out of proportion to the physical findings and wound appearance. Patients are frequently distraught, and a propensity to consider their behavior hysterical has been noted. The physical examination usually reveals local tenderness and paraspinal spasm. Straight leg raise provokes back pain and, occasionally, leg pain. Significant neurologic deficit is an ominous finding suggestive of either an associated epidural abscess or massive recurrent disk herniation. Fever is relatively infrequent. Constitutional symptoms suggestive of infection are the exception for postoperative diskitis. Rarely, patients may be septic. Laboratory data are of limited help: the WBC count is frequently normal, and the ESR is universally elevated. Plain radiographs are of little help in the immediate postoperative period. Weeks later, the hallmarks of intervertebral disk space infection may evolve (Fig. 8). Radionuclide imaging is of some value, although the images are delayed, lack anatomic detail, and are nonspecific. MRI, the imaging modality of choice, has the added benefit of excluding some of the other more important considerations in the differential diagnosis. MRI characteristics are as described for primary intervertebral diskitis. The addition of gadolinium-enhanced studies is probably wise, given the small but finite possibility of false negative images in the presence of epidural abscesses.

The treatment of postoperative intervertebral diskitis must be individualized. Percutaneous biopsy may yield culture positive material. If not, surgical biopsy, culture, and debridement should be undertaken. In the absence of neurologic deficit, nonsurgical treatment may suffice. Medical management consists of bed rest, spinal immobilization, and appropriate antibiotic coverage for 2 weeks or more. Indications for surgical treatment include recurrent or progressive neurologic deficits, clinical sepsis, intractable pain, vertebral collapse or deformity with associated osteomyelitis, failed medical management, and the presence of an associated epidural abscess. Strong consideration should be given to surgical management for any infection in the cervical or thoracic spine.

Postoperative wound infections have been categorized as superficial or deep. Superficial infections are more easily found; deep wound infections are more deceptive. The wound frequently appears normal despite the patient's clinical course. Local pain is invariably the chief complaint. Deep wound infections tend to have more associated constitutional symptoms: the patients feel ill, complain of fever, chills, diaphoresis, and anorexia. There is a greater propensity for fever, leukocytosis, and greater elevations of the ESR than in intervertebral diskitis. Delay in diagnosis should be avoided. Clinical suspicion begets appropriate investigation, including surgical exploration of the wound.

Treatment of postoperative wound infections, superficial or deep, is surgical. The wound should be approached one layer at a time. Following submission of fluid and tissue samples for culture, each layer is thoroughly debrided and vigorously irrigated. All the devitalized tissue is removed. Bone graft material should be left in place unless it is dislodged by the irrigant, and spinal instrumentation should be left in place unless it is grossly loose. The wound is then closed in layers over closed suction drains. Inflow-

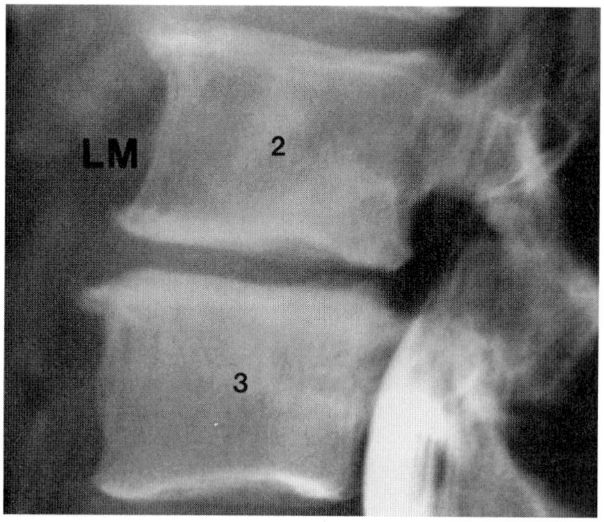

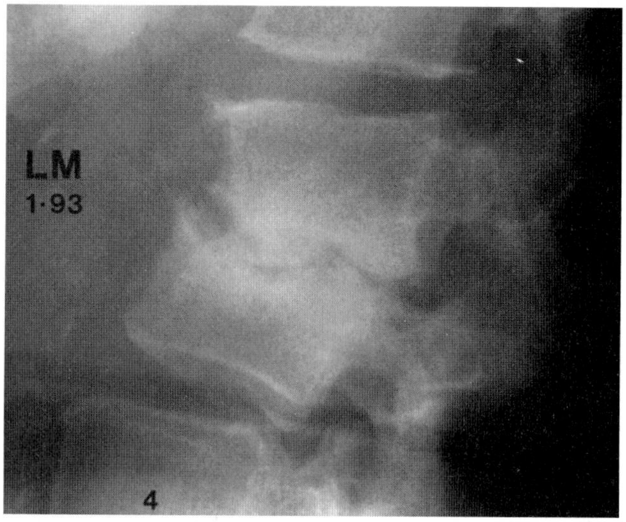

Fig. 8 Patient underwent L2–3 laminotomy and diskectomy for the large disk herniation demonstrated on the preoperative myelogram (**left**). Although symptoms were initially relieved, intense back pain recurred in the months following surgery. Follow-up radiograph (**right**) demonstrates findings consistent with an established postoperative intervertebral diskitis and associated osteomyelitis.

outflow catheters have also been used with some success, but carry a risk of superinfection. Rarely is it necessary to leave the wound open. In such cases, the patient's protein losses are massive, and nutritional support will be required. Consideration should be given to routine reexploration of deep wound infections 48 to 72 hours later to ensure that they have been rendered culture negative. This reexploration is particularly important if the patient remains febrile. Antibiotic coverage should be broad initially, then subsequently refined on the basis of culture and sensitivity data. The duration of treatment should be 2 weeks or more for a laminectomy patient. Wound infections in the presence of an attempted fusion should receive 4 to 6 weeks of intravenous antibiotic therapy. The ESR is a useful measure of response to treatment.

Complications associated with deep wound infections include progression to vertebral osteomyelitis, associated epidural abscesses, enhanced risk of pseudarthroses, chronic pain, and disability. Early and aggressive treatment helps reduce the co-morbidity risk.

Classic Bibliography

General References

An HS, Vaccaro AR, Dolinskas CA, et al: Differentiation between spinal tumors and infections with magnetic resonance imaging. *Spine* 1991;16(suppl 8):S334-S338.

Currier BL, Eismont FJ: Infections of the spine, in Rothman RH, Simeone FA (eds): *The Spine,* ed 3. Philadelphia, PA, WB Saunders, 1992, pp 1319–1380.

Heller JG: Infections of the cervical spine, in An HS, Simpson JM (eds): *Surgery of the Cervical Spine.* London, England, Martin Dunitz, 1994, pp 335–356.

Post MJ, Sze G, Quencer RM, et al: Gadolinium enhancing MR in spinal infection. *J Comput Assist Tomogr* 1990;14:721–729.

Van Lom KJ, Kellerhouse LE, Pathria MN, et al: Infection versus tumor in the spine: criteria for distinction with CT. *Radiology* 1988;166:851–855.

Vincent KA, Benson DR: Differential diagnosis and conservative treatment of infectious diseases, in Frymoyer JW (ed): *The Adult Spine: Principles and Practice.* New York, NY, Raven Press, 1991, vol 1, pp 763–786.

Vincent KA, Benson DR: Infectious diseases of the spine: Surgical treatment, in Frymoyer JW (ed): *The Adult Spine: Principles and Practice.* New York, NY, Raven Press, 1991, pp 787–810.

Whalen JL, Brown ML, McLeod R, et al: Limitations of Indium leukocyte imaging for the diagnosis of spine infections. *Spine* 1991;16:193–197.

Pyogenic Vertebral Osteomyelitis

Eismont FJ, Bohlman HH, Soni PL, et al: Pyogenic and fungal vertebral osteomyelitis with paralysis. *J Bone Joint Surg* 1983;65A:19–29.

Eismont FJ, Green BA, Brown MD, et al: Coexistent infection and tumor of the spine: A report of three cases. *J Bone Joint Surg* 1987;69A:452–458.

Emery SE, Chan DP, Woodward HR: Treatment of hematogenous pyogenic vertebral osteomyelitis with anterior debridement and primary bone grafting. *Spine* 1989;14:284–291.

Modic MT, Feiglin DH, Piraino DW, et al: Vertebral osteomyelitis: Assessment using MR. *Radiology* 1985;157:157–166.

Tuberculous Vertebral Osteomyelitis

Ho EKW, Leong JCY: Tuberculosis of the spine, in Weinstein SL (ed): *The Pediatric Spine: Principles and Practice.* New York, NY, Raven Press, 1994, vol 1, pp 837–850.

Hodgson AR, Skinsnes OK, Leong CY: The pathogenesis of Pott's paraplegia. *J Bone Joint Surg* 1967;49A:1147–1156.

Hsu LC, Cheng CL, Leong JC: Pott's paraplegia of late onset: The cause of compression and results after anterior decompression. *J Bone Joint Surg* 1988;70B:534–538.

Hsu LCS, Leong JC: Tuberculosis of the lower cervical spine (C2 to C7): A report on 40 cases. *J Bone Joint Surg* 1984;66B:1–5.

Smith AS, Weinstein MA, Mizushima A, et al: MR imaging characteristics of tuberculous spondylitis v. vertebral osteomyelitis. *Am J Roentgenol* 1989;153:399–405.

Childhood Diskitis/Osteomyelitis

Crawford AH, Kucharzyk DW, Ruda R, et al: Diskitis in children. *Clin Orthop* 1991;266:70–79.

Du Lac P, Panuel M, Devred P, et al: MRI of disk space infection in infants and children: Report of 12 cases. *Pediatr Radiol* 1990;20:175–178.

Hoffer FA, Strand RD, Gebhardt MC: Percutaneous biopsy of pyogenic infection of the spine in children. *J Pediatr Orthop* 1988;8:442–444.

Sartoris DJ, Moskowitz PS, Kaufman RA, et al: Childhood diskitis: Computed tomographic findings. *Radiology* 1983;149:701–707.

Schofferman L, Schofferman J, Zucherman J, et al: Occult infections causing persistent low-back pain. *Spine* 1989;14:417–419.

Szypryt EP, Hardy JG, Hinton CE, et al: A comparison between magnetic resonance imaging and scintigraphic bone imaging in the diagnosis of disk space infection in an animal model. *Spine* 1988;13:1042–1048.

Wenger DR, Bobechko WP, Gilday DL: The spectrum of intervertebral disk-space infection in children. *J Bone Joint Surg* 1978;60A:100–108.

Wenger DR, Davids JR, Ring D: Discitis and osteomyelitis, in Weinstein SL (ed): *The Pediatric Spine: Principles and Practice.* New York, NY, Raven Press, 1994, pp 813–836.

Epidural Abscesses

Angtuaco EJ, McConnell JR, Chadduck WM, et al: MR imaging of spinal epidural sepsis. *Am J Roentgenol* 1987;149:1249–1253.

Bertino RE, Porter BA, Stimac GK, et al: Imaging spinal osteomyelitis and epidural abscess with short TI inversion recovery (STIR). *Am J Neuroradiol* 1988;9:563–564.

Danner RL, Hartman BJ: Update of spinal epidural abscess: 35 cases and review of the literature. *Rev Infect Dis* 1987;9:265–274.

Postoperative Infections

Dempsey R, Rapp RP, Young B, et al: Prophylactic parenteral antibiotics in clean neurosurgical procedures: A review. *J Neurosurg* 1988;69:52–57.

Heller JG: Postoperative infections of the spine, in Rothman RH, Simeone FA (eds): *The Spine,* ed 3. Philadelphia, PA, WB Saunders, 1992, vol 2, pp 1817–1837.

Lee JT Jr, Ahrenholz DH, Nelson RD, et al: Mechanisms of the adjuvant effect of hemoglobin in experimental peritonitis: V. The significance of the coordinated iron component. *Surgery* 1979;86:41–48.

Petty W, Spanier S, Shuster JJ, et al: The influence of skeletal implants on incidence of infection. *JBone Joint Surg* 1985;67A:1236–1244.

Ritter MA: Surgical wound environment. *Clin Orthop* 1984;190:11–13.

55

Tumors of the Spine

Introduction

Differentiating neoplastic spine symptoms from those of the common and self-limited processes can be difficult. A carefully detailed initial history and physical examination will identify candidates appropriate for early screening studies. The natural history of acute self-limited disorders will eliminate the need for further investigation. Patients whose symptoms progress or fail to respond in an appropriate period of time warrant further evaluation. Delayed diagnoses are to be avoided; however, evaluation should be undertaken in a cost-effective manner.

Diagnosis

History and Physical Examination

During the initial history, certain clinical features should heighten the physician's suspicion of a tumor. The chief complaint, pain, occurs in 85% of patients with tumors, as with most other spinal conditions. However, tumor pain differs qualitatively from the pain of other spinal disorders. Tumor pain frequently occurs at night, often waking the patient. This pain tends to be progressive rather than self-limited. It is not clearly related to activity, nor is it predictably relieved by rest. A history of trauma is either absent or is trivial at best. Weakness is noted by 40% of patients with spinal tumors, but it can be difficult to distinguish true motor weakness from listlessness. Such subjective complaints are worth investigating. A detailed review of symptoms is essential. Unintentional weight loss, anorexia, or fatigue should be identified. Smokers should be questioned about frequency and type of cough, hemoptysis, or increasing dyspnea with exertion. Gastrointestinal malignancies are suggested by a change in the character, quality, or diameter of the stool; bleeding from the rectum; constipation; or incontinence. Genitourinary tumors should be suspected with changes in urinary patterns, such as frequency, hesitancy, incontinence, or hematuria. A change in appearance of the breast, the presence of masses or discharge, or a positive family history should be sought in women.

Suspicious historic features help focus the physical examination. During the examination, note any spinal deformities, evidence of cachexia, or changes in breast appearance. Paraspinal masses are rare. The examination should include the breasts, abdomen, and regional lymph nodes. Percussion over bony prominences of the spine may elicit focal pain. Detailed neurologic examination should be conducted of the extremities. Sensory, motor, or reflex changes, particularly pathologic reflexes, should be carefully documented. A rectal examination is performed to rule out rectal masses and prostate nodules, and to quantify rectal tone. The stool should be tested for occult blood.

Laboratory Studies

Screening laboratory studies, starting with a complete blood count with a differential, a platelet count, and a sedimentation rate, are a cost effective way to screen patients at risk for tumor. Serum chemistry profiles and a urinalysis should be considered. Prostate specific antigen levels should be checked in males if prostatic carcinoma is in the differential diagnosis. These studies, combined with the physical examination, chest radiograph, and a hemoccult test, will identify many primary tumors.

Radiology

If a spinal tumor is suspected, anteroposterior (AP) and lateral radiographs should be obtained to evaluate spinal alignment, bone integrity, and soft-tissue contours. Indirect evidence of mass lesions can be inferred from these studies. Destructive lesions of bone are not usually detectable until 30% to 50% of the vertebral bone mass has been destroyed. An initial clue in the AP radiograph is the "winking owl sign," which reflects a unilateral destruction of the pedicle. In the elderly, the physician often has to distinguish new from old compression fractures, as well as those due to osteopenia from more serious (tumors/infections) pathologic fractures. Whenever possible, old radiographs should be obtained for comparison. Preservation of the adjacent disk spaces can help exclude the possibility of vertebral osteomyelitis. However, plain radiographs have limited ability to distinguish early infections from fractures due to metabolic bone diseases or tumors. Finally, posteroanterior (PA) and lateral chest radiographs of patients with a history of cigarette smoking or increasing dyspnea can rule out a lung primary tumor or pulmonary metastases from a remote primary tumor.

Technetium bone scans, which demonstrate osteoblastic activity and provide a panoramic skeletal survey for areas of bone injury and repair, are an effective screening tool for spinal neoplasms. They can locate isolated occult lesions and disclose patterns of widespread metastatic disease. If there are multiple lesions, a bone scan can indicate the most convenient biopsy site. Two cautions are in order: (1) technetium bone scans cannot distinguish areas of destruction due to tumor from those due to infections or fractures, and (2) there is a high false negative rate in the

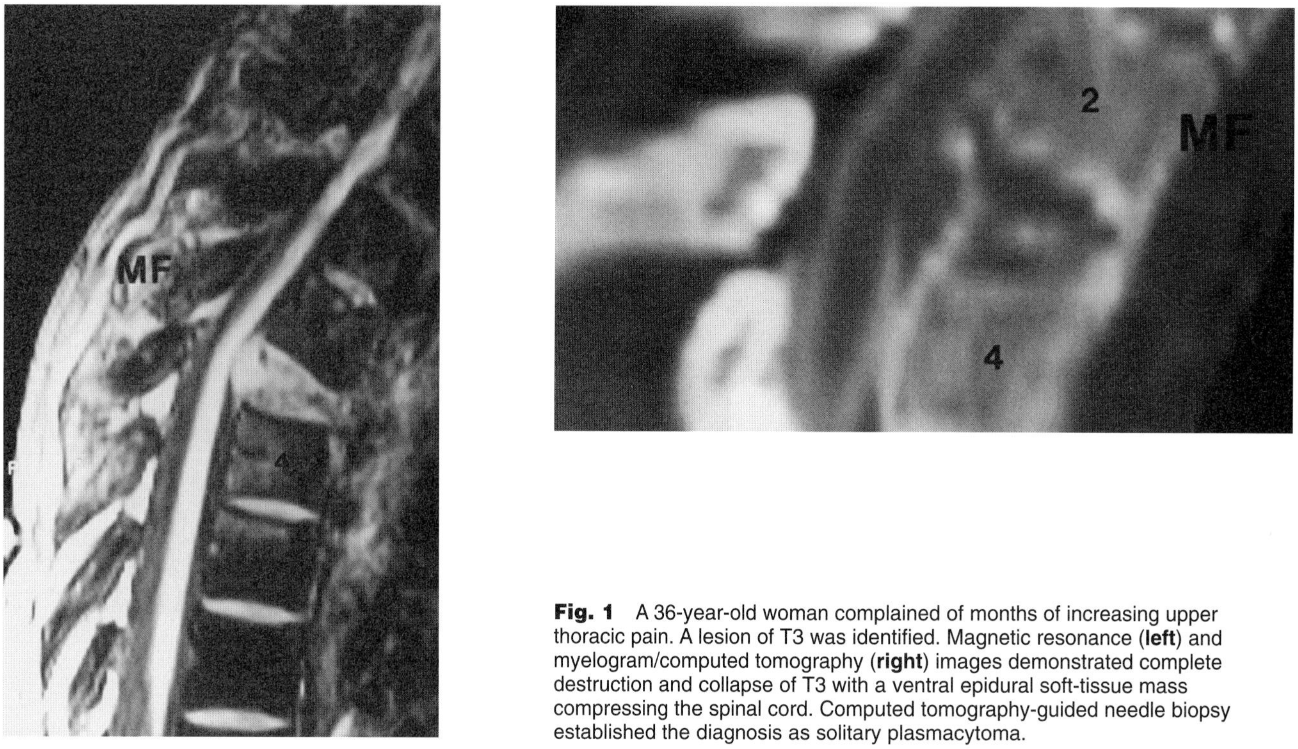

Fig. 1 A 36-year-old woman complained of months of increasing upper thoracic pain. A lesion of T3 was identified. Magnetic resonance (**left**) and myelogram/computed tomography (**right**) images demonstrated complete destruction and collapse of T3 with a ventral epidural soft-tissue mass compressing the spinal cord. Computed tomography-guided needle biopsy established the diagnosis as solitary plasmacytoma.

presence of multiple myeloma. Nonetheless, the bone scan in combination with screening laboratory studies and physical examination will identify approximately 95% of spinal tumors early in their course.

Known lesions merit further study. The primary imaging for anatomic definition of spinal tumors is magnetic resonance imaging (MRI). This noninvasive technology is capable of multiplanar imaging of not only the lesion itself but the regional anatomy (Fig. 1, *left*). MRI readily defines the relationship of the lesion to the spinal cord, meninges, and paravertebral tissues. It is the most sensitive tool for identifying marrow changes caused by primary or metastatic disease. Unfortunately, because of its sensitivity to marrow changes, MRI tends to overestimate vertebral destruction. Diffuse marrow replacement can occur in the absence of significant bone destruction. Unlike technetium bone scans, the MRI can differentiate most spinal infections from neoplasms. However, it is limited in distinguishing acute osteoporotic or traumatic fractures from neoplastic fractures. Either biopsy or follow-up MRI 6 to 8 weeks later may be appropriate in a given circumstance.

Spinal computed tomography (CT) scans with or without intrathecal contrast remain an important part of the evaluation and treatment of spinal neoplasia. Unlike plain radiographs, CT scans accurately localize and quantify vertebral destruction. Its unique ability to image bone detail makes CT of great importance in assessing the need for surgical care and in planning surgical intervention. CT scans without intrathecal contrast complement MRI when it is necessary to quantify the degree of bone destruction and plan surgical intervention. When MRI has not been obtained, CT with intrathecal contrast (Fig. 1, *right*) is a useful alternative. Imaging of neural structures and meninges is indirect but sufficient in most cases. Myelography also provides cerebrospinal fluid (CSF) for analysis. Samples should be sent for cytology, culture, and determination of glucose and protein levels.

Goals of Treatment

The first goal of the treating physician is to establish a definitive diagnosis. The physician must first determine whether the lesion is primary or metastatic in origin. Often this question is answered during the history, physical examination, and initial screening evaluation. However, if the primary tumor is still unknown, the metastatic workup should proceed. In addition to the laboratory studies ordered above, patients should be evaluated by CT scan with intravenous and oral contrast to include the chest, abdomen, and pelvis. Females should undergo mammography. If these studies do not detect the primary lesion, further investigations are neither cost-effective nor likely to locate the primary tumor site. At this point, the lesion should be biopsied. The most accessible site should be biopsied. However, for isolated spinal lesions, alternative sites are not available. CT guided biopsy is preferable in most circumstances. It is safe and effective for virtually all spinal levels. Incisional biopsies may be necessary for inaccessible lesions or if a percutaneous biopsy was nondiagnostic. Excisional biopsies may be performed occasionally if there is high probability of a benign lesion amenable to intralesional or marginal excision. A few cautions are in order with regard to biopsy. Specimens should be sent for both pathologic and microbiologic study, because the differential diagnosis frequently includes both neoplastic and infectious processes. Needles or incisions should be carefully placed, so the entire wound can be excised during definitive treatment of primary spinal malignacies. Meticulous hemostasis and tissue-handling techniques will minimize contiguous spread of tumor.

Once the diagnosis is established, the treating physician must initiate the appropriate therapy. Medical therapy may include chemotherapy, radiation therapy, or both, with or without the use of supplemental spinal orthoses. In certain circumstances, surgical treatment will be definitive. In other circumstances it is an adjunct to medical therapy. Indications for surgical treatment include: (1) lack of a definitive diagnosis, (2) failed medical therapy, (3) tumors known to be resistant to medical therapy, (4) the presence or threat of significant spinal instability, (5) progressive or significant neurologic deficits, and (6) intractable pain or disability. Quite often the goal of medical and surgical therapy is palliative. Surgery may be used to restore or preserve the structural integrity and stability of the spine, to minimize discomfort, and to maximize function for the patient's remaining life span.

Primary Lesions

Benign Tumors

Benign primary spinal tumors are less common than malignancies. However, there is a clear relationship between the age at onset and the likelihood of benignity. Spinal tumors in patients younger than 21 years of age are usually benign. Only one third of these tumors are malignant, while more than 80% of primary tumors of the spine are malignant in patients older than 21. Tumor location is equally important. Less than one third of lesions occurring in the posterior elements are malignant, while more than 75% of lesions arising in the vertebral body prove to be malignant.

Osteoid Osteoma Perhaps the most common benign primary bone tumor of the spine, osteoid osteoma has a peak incidence between the ages of 6 and 17 years. Osteoid osteomas represent 11% of all primary bone tumors, and 10% of osteoid osteomas occur in the spine. More than half of these lesions are in the lumbar spine. Osteoid osteoma is the most common cause of painful scoliosis in adolescence. The presenting complaint, relentless pain, is often dramatically relieved by aspirin, but failure to relieve the pain with aspirin does not exclude the diagnosis. Technetium bone scans are the most sensitive diagnostic test used to localize the tumor (Fig. 2, *left*). Plain radiographs can be difficult to interpret because of overlapping shadows next to the posterior elements. The diagnosis should be suspected in the presence of a focal area of osteosclerosis in the posterior elements. Thin sectioned CT scans will demonstrate the radiolucent nidus surrounded with dense sclerotic reactive bone margins (Fig. 2, *right*). Osteoid osteomas are generally self-limited and remit spontaneously within 3 to 4 years. If the pain can be managed with nonsteroidal anti-inflammatory drugs (NSAIDs), medical treatment may suffice. However, the pain frequently is intolerable. En bloc excision is curative with rapid relief of pain, and painful scoliosis caused by the lesion will correct spontaneously if surgical excision is performed within 15 months of onset. Excision beyond this time risks persistence of a structural curve.

Osteoblastoma These tumors are histologically similar to osteoid osteomas from which they are differentiated primarily by their size, history, and clinical course. Incidence of osteoblastoma peaks between the ages of 10 and 15 years. Osteoblastomas account for 1% of all primary bone tumors; 40% occur in the spine, most commonly the thoracic and lumbar spine. As with osteoid osteoma, the presenting complaint is pain, but the pain is not as reliably relieved with aspirin. Painful scoliosis occurs in up to two thirds of patients with spinal osteoblastoma. Myelopathy is uncommon, but radiculopathy is frequent. The lesions arise from the posterior elements as expansile destructive lesions with a thin shell of reactive bone. They often displace surrounding tissues, and extension into the vertebral body can be seen. Treatment consists of complete surgical excision; recurrence rates following excision approach 10%. Malignant transformation has been reported. Radiation therapy is not recommended.

Aneurysmal Bone Cysts Nearly 20% of aneurysmal bone cysts (ABCs) occur in the spine, usually between the ages of 10 and 20 years. Most spinal ABCs occur in the posterior elements; two thirds involve the cervical and thoracic spine (Fig. 3). As with osteoblastoma, they are destructive lesions with a thin shell of surrounding reactive bone. However, ABCs typically have a soap bubble appearance on radiographs. They are highly vascular, and surgical excision may involve significant intraoperative blood loss. Preoperative angiography and embolization may facilitate resection. Recurrences, common following incomplete excision, should be treated by re-excision. Radiation therapy is not recommended.

Giant Cell Tumors Giant cell tumors (GCTs) are relatively common in the appendicular skeleton, but rarely occur in the spine. Most common during the fourth or fifth decades of life, these lesions tend to affect the vertebral body. GCTs are destructive lesions with variable amounts of reactive bone at their margin; they have a benign, but locally aggressive behavior. As with other GCTs, successful treatment requires complete surgical excision. The

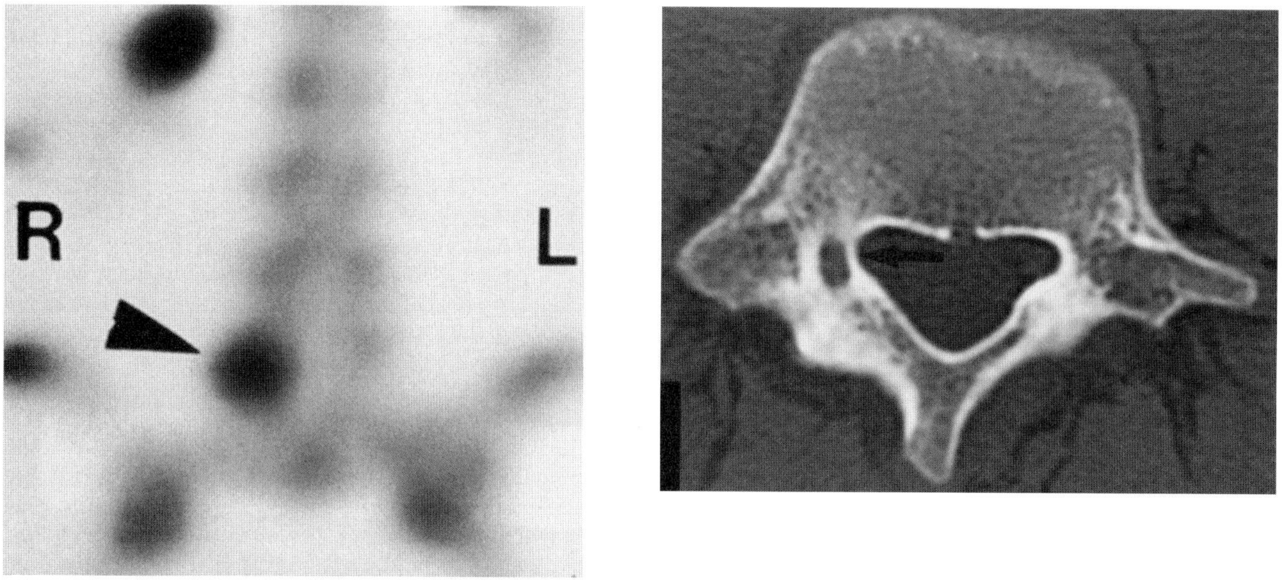

Fig. 2 A 16-year-old boy complained of spontaneous right sided low back pain and sciatica. Plain radiographs had been unremarkable. Bone scan revealed an isolated area of tracer activity in the right L5 pedicle (**left**), which appeared consistent with an osteoid osteoma on computed tomography scan (**right**). The diagnosis was confirmed following en bloc excision.

proximity of critical structures in the spine makes complete excision difficult. Recurrence is common and is best treated with re-resection. Tumors deemed unresectable or incompletely resectable may be treated with radiation therapy; however, there is a risk of sarcomatous degeneration. Theoretically, this risk is reduced if the total dose of radiation is less than 30 Gy, but patients receiving radiotherapy for GCTs should be followed sequentially for evidence of this complication.

Eosinophilic Granuloma Eosinophilic granuloma is part of a spectrum of disease entities known as histiocytoses that afflict the reticuloendothelial system. The clinical syndromes range from isolated lesions to multiple lesions seen in Hand-Schüller-Christian disease or the more fulminant Letterer-Siwe disease. The lesions are usually seen in children less than 10 years of age, and 10% to 15% of them occur in the spine and usually affect the vertebral body. Patients usually complain of pain, local muscle spasm, and, occasionally, neurologic deficit. The radiographic appearance is affected by the patient's age. In younger children, there is a tendency toward complete collapse of the vertebral body, a vertebra plana appearance. In older children, with more mature vertebrae, the destruction may be focal, tending towards angulation rather than complete collapse. The differential diagnosis includes osteomyelitis, leukemia, metastases, and Ewing's sarcoma. Biopsy confirms the diagnosis. Most neurologically intact children with isolated lesions may be treated with rest, bracing, and observation. Surgical treatment is rarely indicated.

Hemangioma Hemangiomas are common, usually incidental findings seen in up to 10% of normal people. MRI technology has revealed the widespread occurrence of small, asymptomatic hemangiomas. Larger ones are visible on plain radiographs as coarse vertical striations within the vertebral body. Axial CT scans show a characteristic coarse speckled trabecular pattern. Their signal characteristics on MRI are diagnostic. These well-defined, often lobular lesions occur within the vertebral bodies and are hyperintense on both T1 and T2 images. Intraosseous hemangiomas are rarely symptomatic. They may cause pathologic fractures and/or neurologic deficits.

Neurofibromas Spinal neurofibromas may be isolated or occur in association with neurofibromatosis. Two subtypes of neurofibromatosis have been recognized, each with autosomal dominant inheritance. The more typical syndrome, von Recklinghausen's disease, is distinguished by multiple neurofibromas in association with café-au-lait spots. In the second subtype, neurofibromas occur in association with acoustic neuromas. Patients with neurofibromatosis have an increased risk for meningiomas and astrocytomas. Spinal neurofibromas generally arise from the nerve root or nerve root sheath. In most cases, the tumor is both intradural and extradural. The extradural extension distinguishes them from meningiomas. Lesions that extend through the neural foramen give rise to the classic dumb-bell lesion (Fig. 4). Radiographic diagnostic clues include sharp angular scoliosis, rib thinning, or enlarged vertebral foramen. CT scans with intrathecal con-

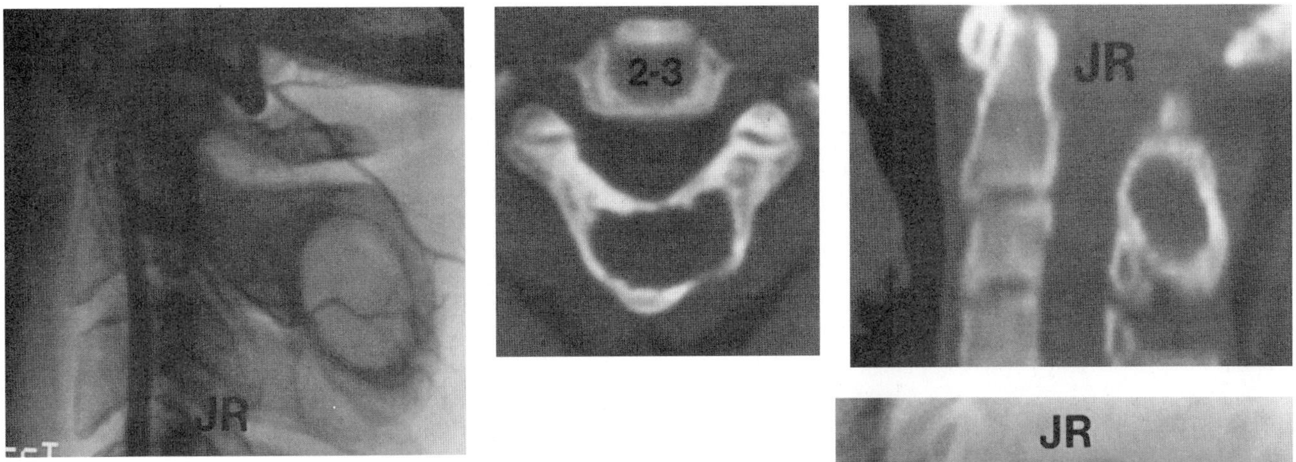

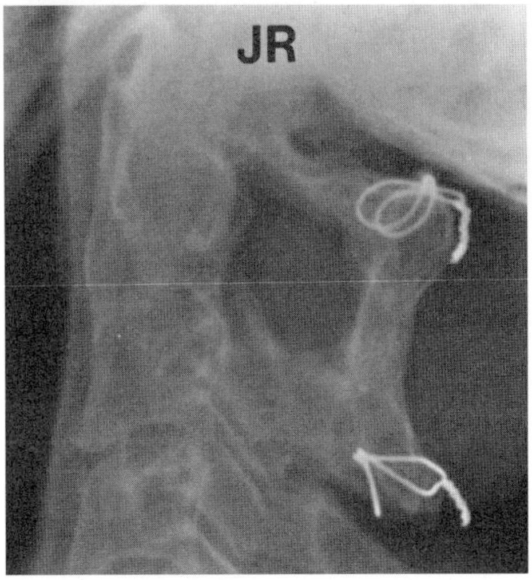

Fig. 3 Lateral cervical view obtained during a preoperative vertebral angiogram of a 45-year-old man with neck pain, which reveals an expansile mass arising from the posterior arch of C2 with a well-defined reactive osseous margin (**left**). Axial computed tomography and sagittal reformation (**center and right**) defined the mass, facilitating surgical planning. Radiograph 4 years following en bloc excision of an aneurysmal bone cyst and C1-C3 arthrodesis (**bottom**), without evidence of recurrence.

trast and/or MRI will characterize these lesions more fully before treatment. Malignant degeneration is possible in up to 20%. Symptomatic lesions should be excised, and those associated with noncritical nerve roots should be resected en bloc. Lesions involving a functionally significant nerve root require microdissection techniques to attempt dissection of the lesion from the nerve fascicles. When these lesions occur in association with scoliosis, they should be treated early because the curve tends to progress rapidly.

Malignant Tumors

Multiple Myeloma Multiple myeloma is the most common primary malignancy of bone (and of the spine), with an incidence of 2.5 per 100,000 people. The disease is clinically distinct from the solitary plasmacytoma. Multiple myeloma is a systemic process characterized by malignant plasma cells, which are responsible for local bone destruction and aberrant immunoglobulin production. Spinal lesions are common, given the preponderance of hematopoietic marrow within the axial skeleton. Elderly patients often present with pain and spontaneous vertebral fractures (Fig. 5). Early in the disease, radiographs may be normal. A lateral skull film may show multiple punched-out lesions. A skeletal survey is used to identify other lesions within the appendicular skeleton, pelvis, and so forth. Technetium bone scans have a high false negative rate in this disease because of the lack of local bone reaction to the lesions. Screening laboratory studies revealing concurrent anemia, thrombocytopenia, hyperproteinemia, and hypoalbuminemia suggest the diagnosis, which is confirmed by a serum protein electrophoresis and serum immunoglobulin electrophoresis.

Chemotherapy is used to treat the systemic disease. Spinal lesions should be imaged with CT scans to determine the amount of vertebral destruction. Symptomatic lesions with less than 50% vertebral body destruction may be treated with bracing and radiation therapy in addition to the chemotherapy. If pathologic fractures are present, particularly in the presence of a neurologic deficit, or if a vertebral lesion is determined to be at high risk for pathologic fracture, surgical intervention is warranted. Prior to fracture, posterior segmental instrumentation and fusion should be performed with supplemental radiation 6 to 8

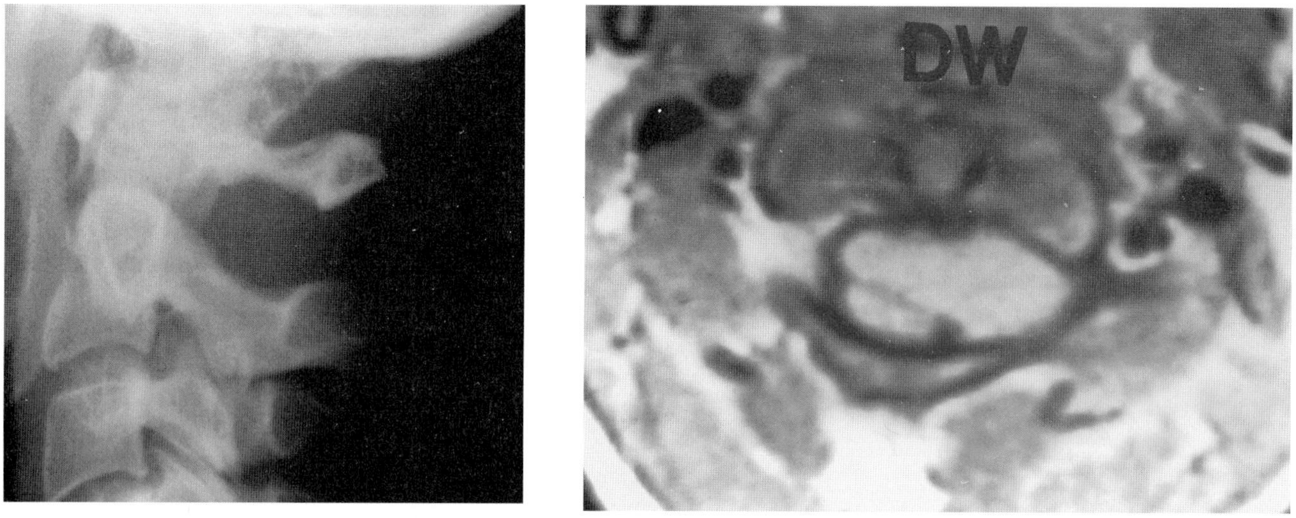

Fig. 4 Lateral cervical radiograph of a woman with neck pain and headaches. **Left,** the posterior C1–2 interlaminar gap appeared too wide. Magnetic resonance imaging (**right**) identified a high signal intensity mass anterior to and compressing the cord at this level. The classic "dumbbell shape" was consistent with a neurofibroma, which was confirmed at the time of excision.

weeks postoperatively. In the presence of fracture, kyphosis, or canal compromise, anterior procedures may be indicated. The prognosis for patients with multiple myeloma is guarded. Approximately 20% of patients achieve 5-year survival, and mean survival is only 28 months.

Solitary Plasmacytoma Solitary plasmacytomas are rare, making up 3% of all plasma cell tumors. Fifty percent of patients ultimately develop multiple myeloma. Patients are somewhat younger than those with multiple myeloma, but the peak incidence is still in middle age. Plasmacytomas are by definition isolated plasma cell lesions that affect the vertebral body. They must be considered in the differential diagnosis of isolated vertebral body lesions and/or pathologic fractures (Fig. 1). The diagnosis is established by biopsy. Because the tumors are exquisitely radiosensitive, they may be treated by bracing and radiotherapy in the absence of pathologic fracture or neurologic compromise. En bloc excision is indicated for patients with pathologic fractures, kyphosis, and/or spinal cord compression. Reconstruction, segmental instrumentation, and fusion should be performed, and adjunctive radiotherapy added 6 to 8 weeks postoperatively. The prognosis for solitary plasmacytomas is better than for multiple myeloma. It is also better for patients with spinal lesions than for those with lesions elsewhere in the skeletal system. Approximately 60% of patients survive 5 years, with a mean survival of 92 months. All patients should be followed with serum protein electrophoresis to observe for the evolution of multiple myeloma.

Osteosarcoma At least one third of spinal osteosarcomas are of a secondary variety, high-grade sarcomas that usually occur after radiation. Those arising in the setting of Paget disease usually present in the sixth decade of life; those following radiotherapy for other diseases tend to occur in the fourth or fifth decade. Patients with a history of radiation therapy near the spine, or with Paget disease, should be worked up aggressively when presenting with new complaints of back pain. As with the treatment of other sarcomas, successful outcome requires an aggressive approach. In general, a confirmatory biopsy should be performed by the team undertaking the resection. Biopsy technique and placement are critical. Preoperative adjuvant chemotherapy and radiation therapy are frequently recommended. Preoperative angiography, with embolization of the tumor, can reduce intraoperative blood loss. Although the goal is to achieve en bloc excision of the tumor, this is rarely possible in the spine. Recently reported techniques have suggested good results following excision of these high-grade malignancies. Postoperative chemotherapy and/or additional radiotherapy may be appropriate in certain circumstances. Pulmonary metastases should be resected, if possible, when they occur. Historically, the prognosis for patients with spinal osteosarcomas has been poor. Spinal lesions carry a worse prognosis than appendicular lesions because of the lack of a distinct anatomic compartment in the spine and because their proximity to vital structures limits reasonable margins of resection.

Chordoma These rare lesions usually occur in the fifth or sixth decade of life, but they can occur at any age. These malignant tumors arise from notochord remnants with a preponderance for the base of the skull, the sacrum, and the coccyx. Chordomas rarely involve the thoracic or lum-

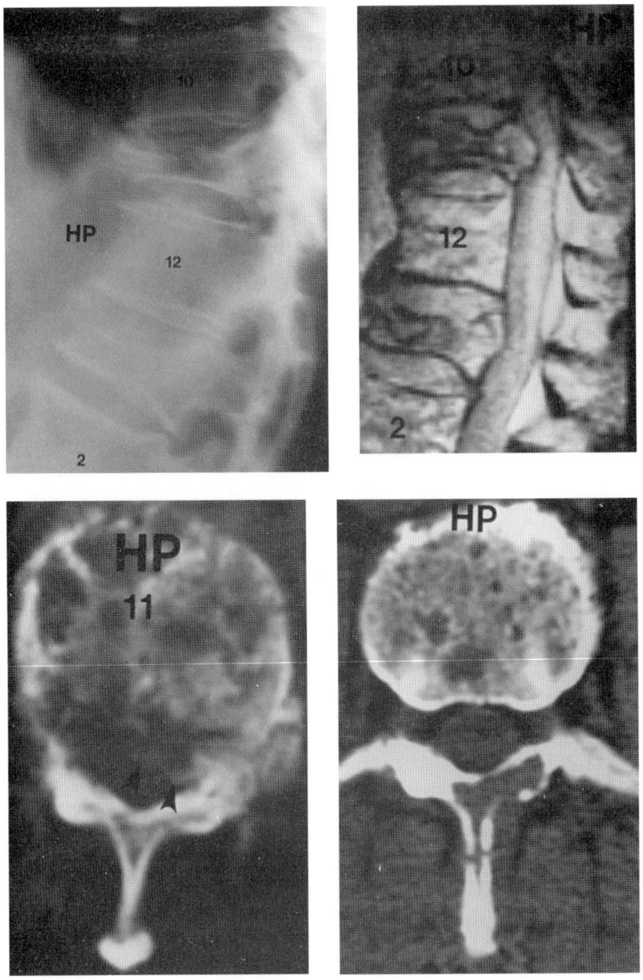

Fig. 5 An elderly man presented with acute progressive paraparesis following months of increasingly severe thoracolumbar pain. **Top left,** Lateral radiograph with pathologic burst fractures at T11 and L1. His admission laboratory studies were consistent with multiple myeloma. Magnetic resonance (**top right**) and myelogram/computed tomography (**bottom**) images demonstrated two noncontiguous areas of spinal cord compression. Note the multiple "punched out" lesions on the CT scans, even at intact levels (**bottom right**).

bar spine, are characterized by relentless local growth, and have some potential to metastasize. Patients typically present with complaints of pain and neurologic deficit, depending on the location of the lesion. Lesions in the sacrum or coccyx may lead to bowel or bladder problems from direct local compression or by neurogenic dysfunction from terminal cauda equina compression. Chordoma should be considered in the differential diagnosis of coccydynia. When performing a rectal exam for complaints in this area, the physician should take careful note to exclude any palpable masses posterior to the rectum arising from the sacrum or coccyx.

Successful treatment of chordomas requires wide local excision following appropriate preoperative staging. The diagnosis is confirmed by biopsy. The biopsy incision or needle tract should be excised with the specimen at the time of definitive resection. Continence can be preserved with sacral amputation if the S3 nerve roots are spared during resection. Unfortunately, chordomas are often diagnosed late and require more aggressive resection. Thoracic and lumbar lesions should also be treated with en bloc resection if possible. The prognosis for long-term survival depends directly on the surgical margins. Local recurrence is a poor prognostic sign.

Metastatic Lesions of the Spine Metastatic spinal tumors are important in the differential diagnosis of progressive spinal pain. Metastatic lesions of the spine are identified at autopsy in over 80% of patients who die of cancer. Clinically significant spinal metastases are far less common, although they are the most frequent type of clinically significant skeletal metastases. Tumors most likely to metastasize to the spine include lung, prostate, breast, renal, and gastrointestinal. Thyroid metastases are now unusual due to early diagnosis and successful treatment of primary thyroid carcinoma. In children, leukemia should be considered in the differential diagnosis of vertebral fractures because it is the most common childhood cancer and 10% to 15% of patients will develop a pathologic vertebral fracture. Evaluation of the patient suspected to have spinal metastases proceeds as described above. If the primary tumor is not discovered by the history, physical examination, screening laboratory studies, chest radiograph, and CT scan of the trunk, then biopsy is indicated. If the need for surgical intervention is clear, the biopsy may be done at the time of definitive intervention.

A treatment plan for spinal metastases must take many variables into account. Factors to be weighed include: (1) the patient's life expectancy and overall condition; (2) the primary tumor type; (3) the integrity of the spinal column; (4) the patient's neurologic status; (5) capabilities of the treating team of physicians; and (6) the wishes of the patient and his or her family. Harrington's classification of metastatic lesions is a useful framework for choosing among treatment options for a given tumor. Five general classes of tumors have been described (Fig. 6): class I, tumor is present without significant bony destruction or canal compromise; class II, bone destruction is present in less than half the vertebral body, without any evidence of fracture or instability, and with no compromise of the spinal canal or neurologic deficit; class III, spinal canal compromise due to epidural disease without significant bone involvement; class IV, pathologic fracture with or without spinal deformity, but without significant neurologic compromise; and class V, pathologic fracture with collapse, instability, and significant neurologic compromise due to either epidural tumor, retropulsed bony debris, and/or kyphosis.

In addition to classifying the lesions, the physician must consider the susceptibility of the primary tumor to chemo-

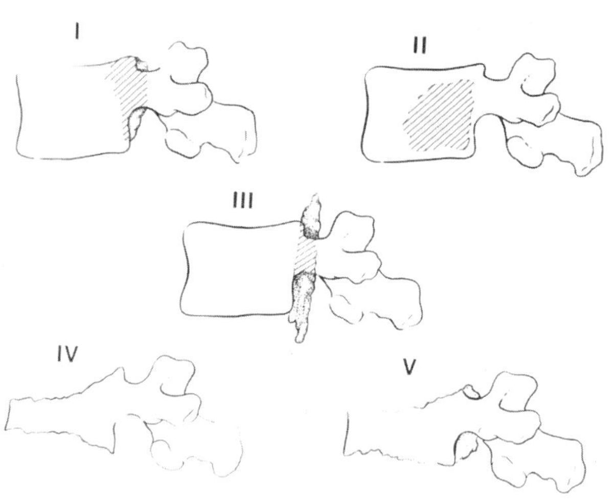

Fig. 6 Schematic drawing after Harrington's classification of spinal metastases.

therapy and radiation therapy. For tumor types refractory to radiation and chemotherapy, surgery is indicated for all but class I disease. For susceptible tumor types, medical management often suffices for classes I and II, and probably for class III. Surgical treatment of class III disease may be appropriate for certain patients, especially if rapid response to medical therapy is not evident. Surgery is essential in the management of classes IV and V disease, provided the patient's medical status and life expectancy do not preclude general anesthesia. In general, with life expectancy of greater than 3 months, surgical intervention should be considered to enhance quality of life and facilitate nursing care of the patient.

The goals of treatment for spinal metastases are: (1) to enhance quality of life through pain relief and maintenance of personal independence; (2) to restore or preserve neurologic function; (3) to maintain or restore spinal column integrity; and (4) to establish definitive diagnosis if not otherwise available. Because vertebral metastases often involve the vertebral body, surgical treatment is usually via anterior decompression and reconstruction (Fig. 7). For metastases that involve the posterior arch alone, posterior decompression and stabilization seems advisable (Fig. 8). For circumferential involvement of the vertebral segment, combined anterior and posterior surgery may be indicated. Additionally, corpectomies of two or more levels may necessitate supplemental posterior segmental instrumentation and fusion. The choice of reconstructive techniques depends on the patient's life expectancy. In general, patients anticipated to survive 2 or more years, as with breast carcinoma, prostate carcinoma, or multiple

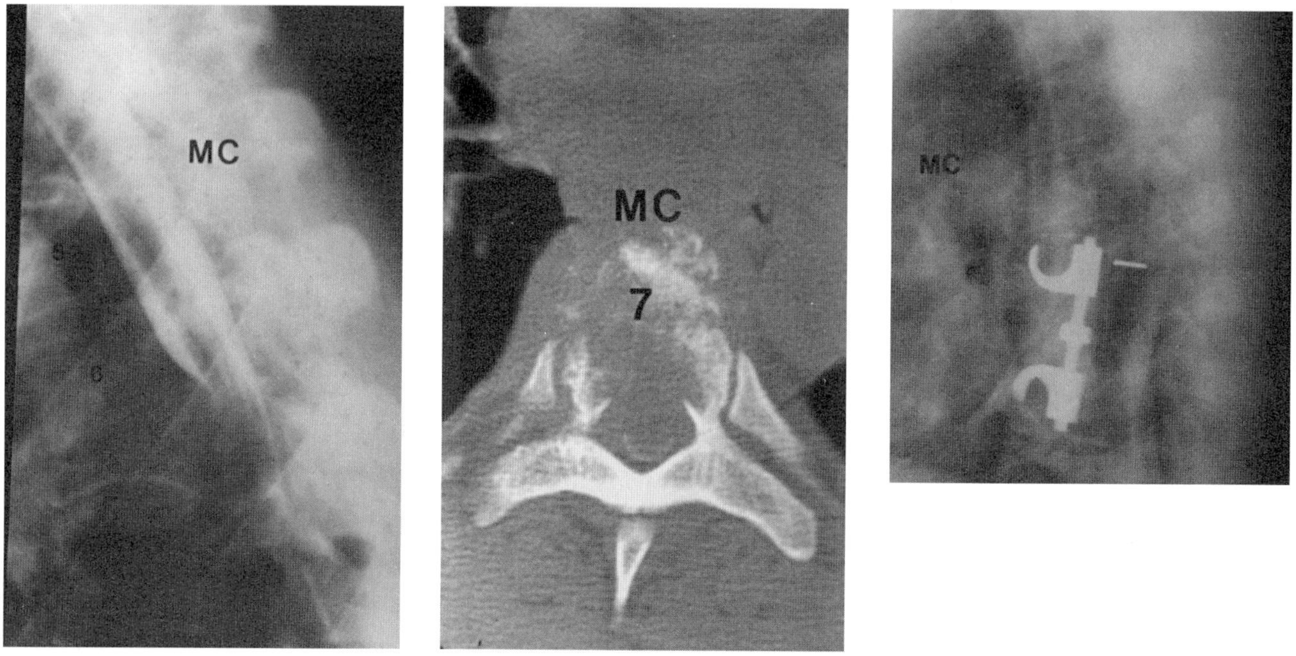

Fig. 7 A 29-year-old smoker presented with acute severe thoracic pain and leg weakness, as well as a lung mass on his chest radiograph. The lateral thoracic myelogram (**left**) illustrates a pathologic fracture with cord compression. The post-myelogram computed tomography (**center**) shows near complete osteolysis of T7 and associated ventral tumor mass with nearly complete myelographic block. This class V metastasis was treated with anterior corpectomy and reconstruction with Knodt rods and methylmethacrylate (**right**).

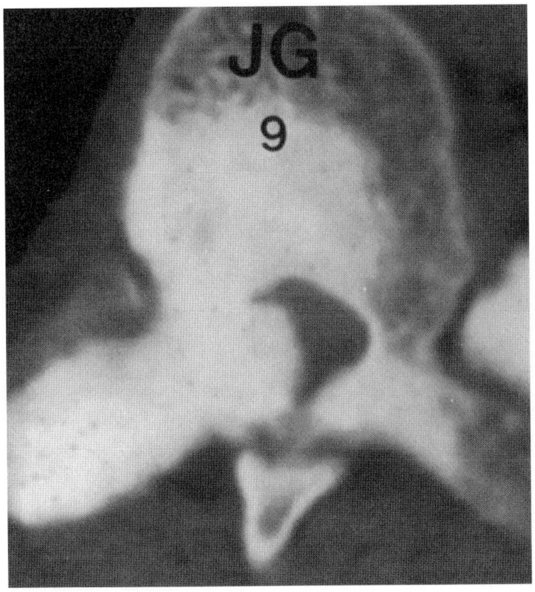

Fig. 8 This patient with metastatic carcinoid tumor developed symptomatic spinal cord compression from an osteoblastic metastasis in the T9 pedicle. Because the spinal cord compression is posterolateral, this lesion is best approached posteriorly.

myeloma, should be reconstructed with autogenous bone graft so that their reconstruction is durable. For patients with shorter life expectancies, vertebral column spacers, such as polymethylmethacrylate, provide adequate short-term spinal stability (Fig. 7).

The findings on a preoperative bone scan may significantly influence the choice of surgical technique. For patients with diffuse spinal involvement, the surgeon must choose between nonsurgical management and multi-level segmental stabilization. If surgical treatment is chosen, despite the fact that compression is generally anterior, posterior segmental instrumentation with supplemental posterolateral decompression is favored. The surgeon should also note any asymptomatic lesions disclosed on the preoperative diagnostic studies that may border the intended surgical segments. Such lesions may need to be included in the postoperative radiation field. If there is significant bone destruction at the border zones, the segments of stabilization should be extended beyond known lesions. Surgical treatment usually does not obviate the need for medical treatment. If the patient is to receive chemotherapy or hormonal therapy for the systemic disease, this should continue. Radiosensitive lesions should receive postoperative irradiation over the entire operative field; however, it should be delayed for at least 2 weeks to allow early wound healing. When bone graft is used in the reconstruction and arthrodesis is intended, radiation should be delayed for 6 to 8 weeks to permit the critical early phases of graft revascularization.

In counseling patients and their families regarding their options, the doctor must help them choose among the various approaches. It should be stressed that medical and surgical intervention for spinal metastases will not alter life expectancy. The primary purpose of care is enhanced quality of life, comfort, and independence. The risks associated with these procedures are noteworthy, particularly given the general state of a patient with metastatic disease. However, the enhancement to the quality of the patient's remaining months or years may be dramatic.

Annotated Bibliography

Emery SE, Brazinski MS, Koka A, et al: The biological and biomechanical effects of irradiation on anterior spinal bone grafts in a canine model. *J Bone Joint Surg* 1994;76A:540–548.

A canine model was used to compare the effects of the timing of adjunctive radiation therapy on anterior vertebral autograft strut healing and biomechanics. The results suggest that postoperative radiation be delayed so as not to impair graft strength and union rates.

Harrington KD: Metastatic tumors of the spine: Diagnosis and treatment. *J Am Acad Orthop Surg* 1993;1:76–86.

This is a thorough review of the evaluation and treatment of spinal metastases. The differential diagnosis, imaging, technologies, and treatment options are discussed. References are excellent.

Kneisl JS, Simon MA: Medical management compared with operative treatment for osteoid-osteoma. *J Bone Joint Surg* 1992;74A:179–185.

This is a retrospective comparison of 15 osteoid osteoma patients treated by surgical excision with nine patients managed with only long-term oral NSAIDs. The authors concluded that surgery is not always necessary in managing osteoid osteomas.

Rougraff BT, Kneisl JS, Simon MA: Skeletal metastases of unknown origin: A prospective study of a diagnostic strategy. *J Bone Joint Surg* 1993;75A:1276–1281.

The authors prospectively evaluate a diagnostic strategy for patients presenting with skeletal metastases of unknown origin.

Eighty-five percent of primary tumors were identified by the combination of history and physical examination; routine laboratory studies; chest radiographs; bone scans; and computed tomography of the chest, abdomen, and pelvis. Further medical workup was not cost-effective. Biopsy is recommended if the origin is still undisclosed.

Tomita K, Kawahara N, Baba H, et al: Total en bloc spondylectomy for solitary spinal metastases. *Int Orthop* 1994;18:291–298.

The authors describe a promising surgical technique that may yield improved cure rates for primary vertebral tumors.

Classic Bibliography

An HS, Vaccaro AR, Dolinskas CA, et al: Differentiation between spinal tumors and infections with magnetic resonance imaging. *Spine* 1991;16(suppl 8):S334-S338.

Azouz EM, Kozlowski K, Marton D, et al: Osteoid osteoma and osteoblastoma of the spine in children: Report of 22 cases with brief literature review. *Pediatr Radiol* 1986;16:25–31.

Bouchard JA, Koka A, Bensusan JS, et al: Effects of irradiation on posterior spinal fusions: A rabbit model. *Spine* 1994;19:1836–1841.

Dahlin DC: Giant-cell tumor of vertebrae above the sacrum: A review of 31 cases. *Cancer* 1977;39:1350–1356.

Delamarter RB, Sachs BL, Thompson GH, et al: Primary neoplasms of the thoracic and lumbar spine: An analysis of 29 consecutive cases. *Clin Orthop* 1990;256:87–100.

Healey JH, Ghelman B: Osteoid osteoma and osteoblastoma: Current concepts and recent advances. *Clin Orthop* 1986;204:76–85.

Huvos AG, Woodard HQ, Cahan WG, et al: Postradiation osteogenic sarcoma of bone and soft tissues: A clinicopathologic study of 66 patients. *Cancer* 1985;55: 1244–1255.

Kostuik JP, Weinstein JN: Differential diagnosis and surgical treatment of metastatic spine tumors, in Frymoyer JW, Ducker TB, Hadler NM, et al (eds): *The Adult Spine: Principles and Practice.* New York, NY, Raven Press, 1991, vol 1, pp 861–888.

Mankin HJ, Lange TA, Spanier SS: The hazards of biopsy in patients with malignant primary bone and soft-tissue tumors. *J Bone Joint Surg* 1982;64A:1121–1127.

McClain RF, Weinstein JN: Solitary plasmacytomas of the spine: A review of 84 cases. *J Spinal Disord* 1989;2: 69–74.

Rogalsky RJ, Black GB, Reed MH: Orthopaedic manifestations of leukemia in children. *J Bone Joint Surg* 1986;68A:494–501.

Shives TC, McLeod RA, Unni KK, et al: Chondrosarcoma of the spine. *J Bone Joint Surg* 1989; 71A:1158–1165.

Shives TC, Dahlin DC, Sim FH, et al: Osteosarcoma of the spine. *J Bone Joint Surg* 1989;68A:660–668.

Siegal T, Siegal T: Current considerations in the management of neoplastic spinal cord compression. *Spine* 1989;14:223–228.

Sim FH, Dahlin DC, Stauffer RN, et al: Primary bone tumors simulating lumbar disc syndrome. *Spine* 1977; 2:65–74.

Vergel De Dios AM, Bond JR, Shives TC, et al: Aneurysmal bone cyst: A clinicopathologic study of 238 cases. *Cancer* 1992;69:2921–2931.

Weinstein JN: Spine neoplasms, in Weinstein SL (ed): *The Pediatric Spine: Principles and Practice.* New York, NY, Raven Press, 1994, vol 1, pp 887–916.

Weinstein JN, McLain RF: Primary tumors of the spine. *Spine* 1987;12:843–851.

Weinstein JN: Differential diagnosis and surgical treatment of primary benign and malignant neoplasms, in Frymoyer JW, Ducker TB, Hazdler NM, et al (eds): *The Adult Spine: Principles and Practice.* New York, NY, Raven Press, 1991, vol 1, pp 829–860.

Weinstein JN, McLain RF: Tumors of the spine, in Rothman RH, Simeone FA (eds): *The Spine,* ed 3. Philadelphia, PA, WB Saunders, 1992, vol 2, pp 1279–1318.

56
Adult Rheumatoid Arthritis

Rheumatoid Arthritis

Rheumatoid arthritis (RA) in the adult spine primarily affects the cervical spine. The anatomic abnormalities of the cervical spine involved in RA are a consequence of synovitic destruction in joints, ligaments, and bone. The synovitis in articular cartilage causes direct destruction and extension of rheumatoid pannus into adjacent structures. Ligamentous laxity and rupture can result in instability. Bony osteoporosis, cyst formation, and erosion may result in destruction with loss of skeletal integrity. The subluxations that result from synovitic destruction depend on the specific cervical anatomy destroyed. Pain and neurologic abnormality result from spinal cord and nerve root compression and distortion. Vertebral artery involvement may occur in the presence of cervical subluxation. The activity of RA in the cervical spine appears to begin early in the disease process in a given patient and progresses in relationship to peripheral involvement. Eighty-three percent of patients with anterior atlantoaxial subluxation studied prospectively developed their subluxation within 2 years of disease onset. Cervical spine subluxation has been shown to correlate with damage to metacarpal, phalangeal, and carpal bones. The degree of cervical destruction strongly correlates with that of peripheral erosive disease. A history of corticosteroid therapy, seropositivity, the presence of rheumatoid subcutaneous nodules, and the presence of erosive and mutilating articular disease correlate with a progression of atlantoaxial subluxation. Male patients are more frequently affected by subluxations, although the prevalence of RA is clearly higher in females than in males, with a ratio of about 2.5:1.

Subluxations

Atlantoaxial subluxation (AAS) can be anterior, posterior, and/or lateral. Anterior AAS is the most common subluxation observed and has been found in 11% to 46% of cases studied at postmortem examination. Most anterior AAS seen in RA is greater than the 3.5-mm limit of normal flexion in adults. Overall, 43% to 86% of RA patients exhibit subluxations, and anterior AAS is present in 19% to 71% of patients surveyed radiologically. A study of RA patients undergoing total joint replacement revealed 61% had anterior AAS, but only 50% had any symptoms or signs. Anterior AAS may be reducible (Fig. 1), with the subluxation corrected in extension; unreducible, remaining fixed in position; or uncorrectable to within a normal degree of subluxation. Posterior AAS accounts for 6.7% of all AAS and usually is not associated with spinal cord compression. Myelopathy may be seen in association with posterior AAS as a result of a kyphotic configurational abnormality of the spinal cord, rather than direct compression. Lateral AAS is defined as 2 mm or more of subluxation of the lateral masses of the atlas on the axis. Rotational deformity often accompanies lateral AAS. Unreducible head tilt has been found in 10% of RA patients with lateral AAS. It is frequently combined with other deformities.

Atlantoaxial impaction (AAI) is also described as cranial settling, upward migration of the odontoid, pseudobasilar invagination, and/or vertical subluxation of the atlas. AAI has been found in 5% to 32% of RA patients and accounts for 22% of all upper cervical subluxations. AAI results from bone and cartilage loss in the occipitoatlanto and atlantoaxial joints.

The subaxial cervical spine is affected by rheumatoid involvement of the facets, interspinous ligaments, and intervertebral disks (spondylodiskitis). Pathophysiologic mechanisms leading to instability are synovitic destruction of the neurocentral joints in which erosion of adjacent disk and bone causes subluxation and facet RA and ligamentous laxity, which causes chronic diskovertebral injury and destructive changes. Spinal cord responses to subluxations are pachymeningitis, arachnoiditis, and medullary compression. Subaxial subluxations are most often found at the C2–C3 and C3–C4 segments, typically lack osteophyte formation, and often occur at multiple levels, causing a stepladder appearance of subluxations. Subaxial subluxations are found in 10% to 20% of patients. Subaxial disease having neurologic consequence includes subluxations below higher cervical fusions, anterior spondylodiskitis with

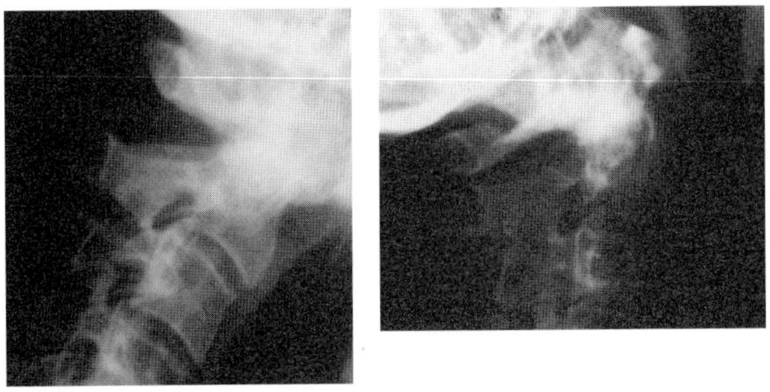

Fig. 1 A lateral radiograph in flexion (**left**) shows the forward subluxation of C1 on C2; in extension (**right**), it is reducible to within a normal degree of subluxation.

direct spinal cord compression, intracanal rheumatoid granulations, and a hyperlordotic subaxial spine.

Clinical Manifestations and Natural History

Cervical spine RA manifests by pain, neurologic disturbance, and death. Pain is typically in the neck and in particular at the craniocervical junction, where it is experienced as occipital headache. Neurologic symptoms can be multiple and may be obscure. Subjective symptoms of paresthesias in the hands, Lhermitte's sign, and symptoms of weakness or loss of endurance may occur. Objective weakness and upper motor neuron signs may be found in overt myelopathy. Vertebrobasilar insufficiency, especially in AAI, may cause loss of equilibrium, tinnitus, vertigo, dysphagia, visual disturbance, and diplopia. Physical examination of a debilitated RA patient may be confounded by peripheral rheumatoid disease causing weakness from articular involvement, tenosynovitis, tendon rupture, rheumatoid myopathy, and rheumatoid vasculitic peripheral neuropathy. A high index of suspicion for a symptomatic subluxation must be maintained.

Pain is a common finding in cervical RA, occurring in 40% to 88% of affected patients. Neurologic signs are noted in 7% to 34% of patients. In order to determine the likelihood of severe neurologic progression or death in an RA patient with cervical involvement, it is necessary to examine the natural history of the disease. This information is fundamental to the decision as to whether surgical intervention is necessary and will be effective. A 10% incidence of fatal medullary compression leading to sudden death has been reported. Survival is not influenced by subluxation in RA, but RA patients have a significantly shorter life expectancy than the general population. A series of RA patients studied over 5 years revealed a 17% mortality rate, 10% higher than the general population. Although AAS did not cause death in this series, subluxations did worsen in 80% of patients and new subluxations were noted in 27% of patients. The data gathered from clinical series lead to the conclusion that adult RA patients have a shortened life expectancy, which may be contributed to by subluxations, which may worsen, but the subluxations alone do not reliably lead to death.

Neurologic progression has been noted in 2% to 36% of patients with cervical spine subluxations. Once cervical myelopathy is established, mortality is a common outcome, if the myelopathy is untreated. RA patients with cervical myelopathy are at risk for a premature death, most commonly due to infection and comorbid conditions. Severe extra-articular manifestations and most especially interstitial lung disease constitute major factors of risk for an early postoperative death in RA patients undergoing cervical spine surgery.

Radiologic Imaging

Plain radiographs with flexion-extension views are necessary for initial assessment of involvement, localization of instabilities, and identification of cervical areas that require further study. A study of RA patients undergoing total joint replacement demonstrated that 61% had radiographic evidence of anterior AAS, but only 50% of these patients had any signs or symptoms of their cervical disease. On the basis of plain radiographs, risk factors identified that predisposed a patient to cord compression and neurologic compression are male gender, anterior AAS > 9 mm, and the presence of AAI. The presence of lateral AAS is a lesser factor. The atlantodental distance is measured from the base of the odontoid to the base of the anterior arch of the atlas and is abnormal in adults when it is > 3.5 mm.

The posterior atlantodental interval (if < 14 mm) has been shown to have a high sensitivity in predicting paralysis. AAI may be measured on plain radiographs in a variety of methods. McGregor's line measures the distance of the tip of the odontoid above a line drawn from the hard palate to the base of the occiput on a lateral view. The tip should not project more than 4.5 mm above this line. The most commonly used method, among many, is the Ranawat index, measured on a lateral radiograph where a line is connected between the midpoints of the anterior and posterior arches of the atlas. A point at the center of the pedicles of the axis is selected, and a line is drawn perpendicular from this point to the mid-atlas line. When this line is < 13 mm in height, AAI is present.

Computed tomography (CT) may provide valuable information as to the extent of erosions, spinal cord compression, and axial and sagittal relationships. Bone detail has been shown to be superior in conventional tomography compared to sagittally reformatted CT images. Sagittal imaging with either CT or contrast-enhanced lateral tomography can demonstrate configurational change in the spinal cord. The degree of medullary compression noted on CT scan correlates with the presence of upper

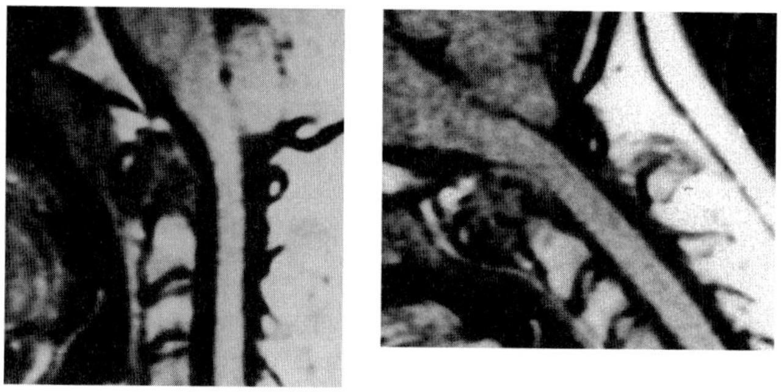

Fig. 2 A sagittal MRI in a patient with anterior atlantoaxial subluxation. In extension (**left**), the spinal cord does not undergo compression and sits behind the dens, which is involved with rheumatoid pannus. In flexion (**right**), the spinal cord abuts the pannus involved at the dens and drapes itself over it, causing compression.

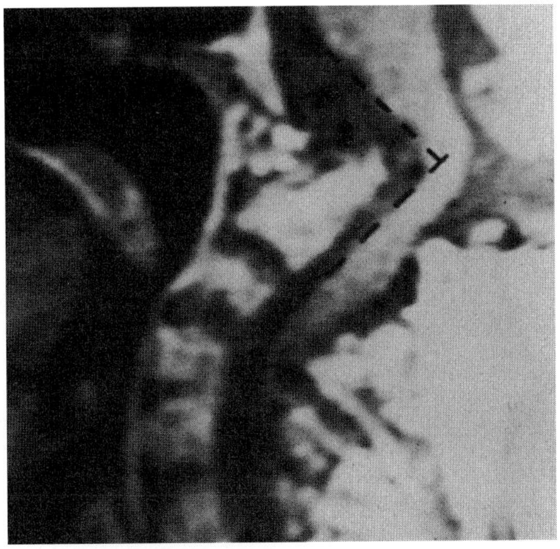

Fig. 3 A sagittal MRI with atlantoaxial impaction demonstrating a decreased cervicomedullary angle of less than 90°.

motor neuron signs. CT with intrathecal contrast increases the ability to demonstrate the role of pannus in cord compression.

Magnetic resonance imaging (MRI) permits further definition of pathologic anatomy in RA patients with involvement of the cervical spine. MRI has the advantage of requiring no contrast and may be reformatted in any plane. The craniomedullary junction and the entire length of the cervical spinal cord may be visualized. Erosion, pannus, and inflammation of soft tissues may be demonstrated. Flexion-extension MRI may display kinking of the spinal cord over the pannus behind the dens (Fig. 2). Distortion of the spinal cord correlates with signs of myelopathy. The cervicomedullary angle (Fig. 3) is normally 135° to 175°. When the angle is less than 135°, it is correlated with clinical evidence of myelopathy and provides another measurement for AAI as an underlying source of myelopathy.

Nonsurgical Management

Because cervical spine involvement in RA starts early in the course of a patient's disease and correlates with the extent and severity of the disease, early aggressive and continued medical management of a given patient's RA is of importance. Nonsurgical management is supportive. Cervical collars have been used commonly, but do not protect against subluxation or neurologic progression. Cervical collars may be used for emotional support, pain relief, warmth, and a feeling of stability. A study of rigid cervical collars showed that they limit anterior AAS but block spontaneous reduction of the anterior AAS in extension. Rigid orthoses are often not helpful, and may be poorly tolerated by RA patients with temporal mandibular joint involvement, dental problems, and/or skin sensitivity.

Surgical Management

The indications for surgical intervention in cervical spine RA are neurologic abnormality and severe pain. Because subluxations are highly prevalent, the mere existence of a subluxation does not constitute an absolute indication for surgery. The definition of impending neurologic deficit, ie, subluxations of a degree likely to result in paralysis, determined by radiologic studies, permits the selection of patients at risk for the onset of neurologic abnormality. Patients appear to have a better outcome if operated on before severe neurologic deficits develop.

A major problem confronting the orthopaedic surgeon initially is the patient who tends to be severely affected by RA with debilitation; deformity; poor skin; poorly healing wounds; osteopenic bone, making fixation of the spine difficult; bone graft that is mechanically inadequate to hold internal fixation, such as wires; high rates of nonunion in arthrodesis; and an increased susceptibility to infection. RA patients undergoing cervical spine surgery have difficulty with anesthesia in terms of upper airway obstruction and perioperative management. A 14% incidence of upper airway obstruction has been reported following standard intubation. Fiberoptically assisted intubation reduces the incidence to 1%.

Preoperative skeletal traction is necessary to reduce subluxation and improve myelopathic neurologic losses. Constant skeletal traction is recommended by most surgeons. Halo traction may be incorporated postoperatively into a halo vest if desired. A halo vest may present difficulties in a given patient because of debilitation, poor skin, and poor mobility. Preoperatively, a halo wheelchair is of benefit because it allows continuous traction while the patient is sitting or in bed. A halo wheelchair improves tolerance and comfort while avoiding the skin and infection problems of prolonged bed rest and the need for frames or special beds. Reduction of subluxations permits reversal of more recent onset myelopathy and a skeletal alignment that is surgically more approachable, and therefore, safer (Fig. 4).

Atlantoaxial arthrodeses are often performed using the Gallie-type or Brooks-type procedures. If alignment can be obtained and bone quality is adequate, posterior C_2 to C_1 facet screws and fusions are recommended by same. Occipitocervical fusions have undergone an evolution from original onlay techniques to wired bone graft, wires and methylmethacrylate cement, metal mesh wired in place with and without cement (Fig. 5), contoured metal loops wired in place, and, most recently, plates affixed with screws. Implants may provide immediate internal splinting and minimize the need for halo vests. The posterior foramen magnum and posterior arch of the atlas may be resected at the time of arthrodesis, if needed. Posterior

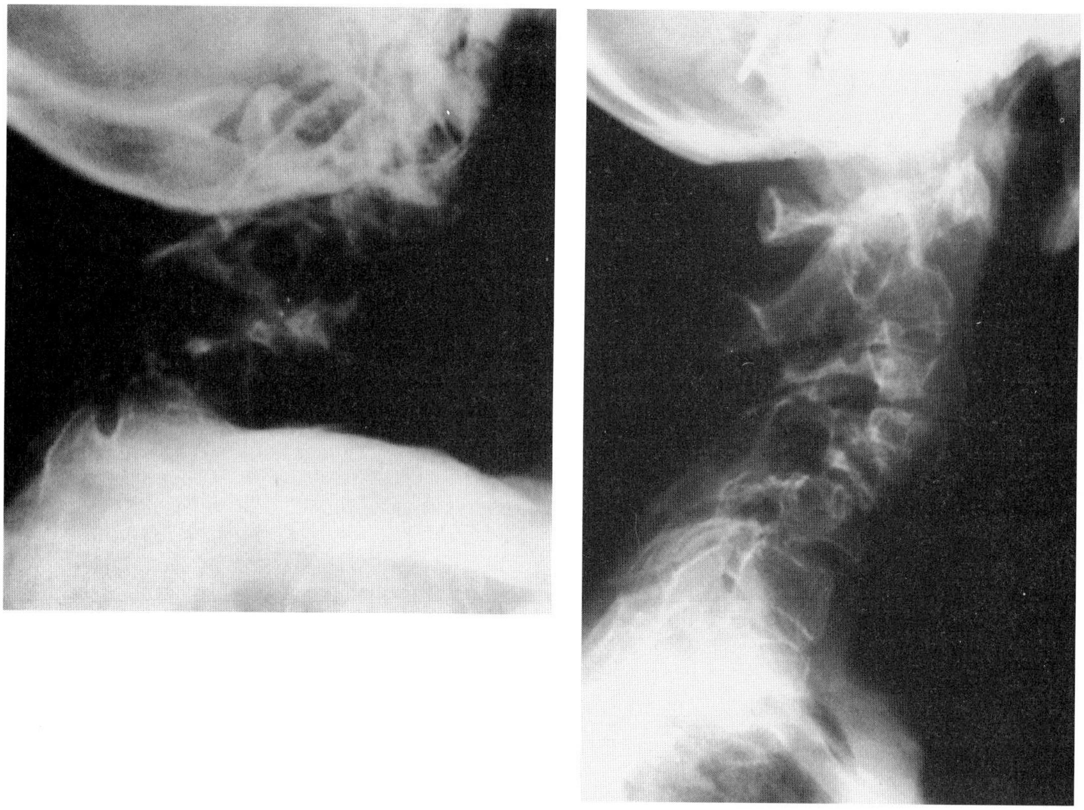

Fig. 4 A patient with severe subaxial subluxation (**left**) had marked deformity that corrected significantly after being placed in halo traction (**right**), demonstrating improvement in skeletal alignment.

arthrodesis at the craniocervical level has resulted in reported nonunion rates ranging from 0 to 50%. Postoperative mortality ranges from 0 to 33%, but recent reports indicate a less than 10% mortality. The reduction in perioperative mortality results from earlier intervention and improvements in anesthetic and perioperative management. Neurologic improvement has been noted in 42% to 100% of patients. Marked pain relief is generally anticipated.

Death at a time outside of the perioperative period is significant. It is not known whether surgery alters the long-term survival of RA, although it appears that survival in RA cervical myelopathy is improved by surgery. It has been reported the probability of survival following operation is 1 year in 74% and 5 years in 57% of patients. In this series, all patients with interstitial lung disease died within 28 months of surgery. In another study, of patients with severe neurologic involvement, 87% had an early death or failure; whereas, of those patients with less neurologic involvement, 80% had good results. Early diagnosis and intervention are important in avoiding worsening myelopathy. Decompression of the spinal cord has not been systematically studied, but if done, should be accompanied by arthrodesis.

Complications of cervical spine surgery of any type in RA patients include infection, wound dehiscence, nonunion, and late subaxial subluxation below a fused segment. All anatomically involved levels should be incorporated into the arthrodeses. Previously asymptomatic levels can develop subluxation below rigid segments, emphasizing the need for long-term follow-up.

Juvenile Rheumatoid Arthritis

Juvenile rheumatoid arthritis (JRA) is characterized by chronic synovial inflammation of unknown cause. The disease may develop at any age during childhood, with girls more often affected than boys. Ten percent of children with JRA have a systemic onset. Arthritis in five or more joints occurs in approximately 40% of children with JRA. Cervical spine involvement, most often at the C2–C3 apophyseal joints, is frequent in the polyarticular type of JRA found in 40% of children, but can be found in the systemic onset subtype found in 10% of JRA patients. Extensive fusion of the posterior articulations of the cervical spine may result in a loss of cervical lordosis and limitation of motion. Cervical myelopathy is not common; occa-

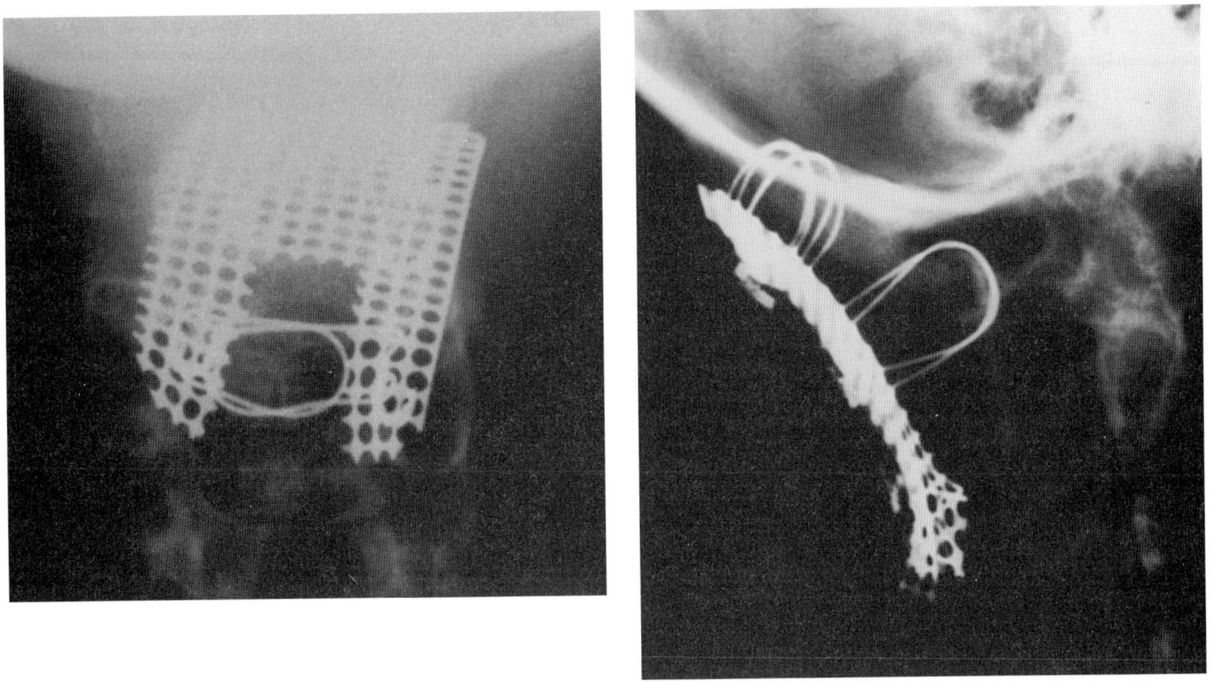

Fig. 5 An occiput to C2 arthrodesis utilizing metal mesh backing of bone graft seen on anteroposterior (**left**) and lateral (**right**) views. Bone from the occiput to C2 is located anterior to the metal mesh.

sionally atlantoaxial subluxation occurs, which may require arthrodesis.

Seronegative Spondyloarthropathies

Seronegative spondyloarthropathies are an interrelated group of multisystem inflammatory disorders. The structures affected are the spine, peripheral joints, periarticular structures, or all three, and are variably associated with extra-articular manifestations. The recognized entities include ankylosing spondylitis (AS), reactive arthritis, Reiter's syndrome, spondylitis and peripheral arthritis associated with psoriasis and inflammatory bowel disease, juvenile spondyloarthropathy, and undifferentiated spondyloarthropathies. AS is the most common type encountered involving spinal disorders.

AS is a chronic systemic inflammatory rheumatic disorder that primarily affects the axial skeleton, with sacroiliac joint involvement (sacroiliitis) as its hallmark. The most common and characteristic early complaint is chronic low back pain of insidious onset, usually beginning in late adolescence or early adulthood. Back stiffness, which is worse in the morning and is eased by mild physical activity or a hot shower, is the second most common early symptom. Stiffness and pain in the cervical spine and tenderness of the spinous processes occur in early stages of the disease in some patients, but generally tend to occur after some years. The entire spine becomes increasingly stiff after many years of disease progression, with continued flattening of the lumbar spine and gentle thoracic kyphosis. Involvement of the cervical spine results in progressive limitation of neck motion and a forward cervical stoop. Back pain and stiffness generally diminish over years with a persistence of some degree of inflammatory pain being usual. Spinal ankylosis develops at a variable rate and pattern. The disease may be confined to one part of the spine. Typical deformities tend to evolve after 10 years or more of disease. Functional impairment is more likely in those patients with hip involvement or a completely ankylosed cervical spine with kyphosis.

Cervical spine involvement may lead to marked impairment of neck motion in all directions. The atlantooccipital and atlantoaxial joints do not usually completely ankylose. Anterior atlantoaxial subluxation may occur through laxity of the transverse ligament. When it does, atlantoaxial arthrodesis is required. The ankylosed osteoporotic spine in AS is susceptible to fracture, even with minor trauma. The fracture is usually transverse and the cervical spine is the most common site, usually at C5–C6 or C6–C7. The fracture may not be easily apparent on plain radiographs and further imaging with bone scan and MRI may be helpful in its detection. A patient with AS who complains of a change in head position can be assumed to have a fracture. A complaint of neck or back pain, even without significant trauma, may be assumed to have an origin in an underlying fracture. The fracture may result in spondylodiskitis with diskovertebral destruction and pseudarthrosis. The reported incidence of spondylodiskitis in AS is 5% to 6%, and the most common level is T11 to L1. Spondylodiskitis may be asymptomatic in about one half of patients and have a benign clinical course. Some patients may require bed rest and localized immobilization in order to allow spontaneous bony ankylosis.

A patient with an AS cervical spine fracture with subluxation should have an attempt at reduction to his/her previous head position through halo traction and a trial of halo vest immobilization to allow arthrodesis. If union fails, surgical arthrodesis is indicated. Surgical arthrodesis of a thoracic or lumbar spondylodiskitis may be useful if a painful nonunion persists. AS deformity in the spine may be corrected through a cervical osteotomy for a chin-on-chest deformity and a lumbar wedge osteotomy for severe kyphosis.

Annotated Bibliography

Boden SD, Dodge LD, Bohlman HH, et al: Rheumatoid arthritis of the cervical spine: A long-term analysis with predictors of paralysis and recovery. *J Bone Joint Surg* 1993;75A:1282–1297.

A posterior atlantodental interval (PADI) of $\leq$ 14 mm is more sensitive than the anterior atlantodental interval in predicting the risk of paralysis. The role of pannus cannot be assessed in plain radiographs. Patients with a PADI of $<$ 10 mm preoperatively have a poor prognosis for motor recovery, while those with a PADI of $>$ 14 mm have a more likely recovery.

Clark CR, Goetz DD, Menezes AH: Arthrodesis of the cervical spine in rheumatoid arthritis. *J Bone Joint Surg* 1989;71A:381–392.

Forty-one patients with rheumatoid arthritis were treated with cervical arthrodesis. Atlantoaxial, occipitocervical, and subaxial arthrodeses were included. Eighty-eight percent had union, with nonunion isolated to C1–C2 arthrodeses. Sixty-six percent of patients improved and nearly all lost their preoperative pain. Impending neurologic deficit is a valid indication for early surgery.

Crockard HA, Calder I, Ransford AO: One-stage transoral decompression and posterior fixation in rheumatoid atlanto-axial subluxation. *J Bone Joint Surg* 1990;72B:682–685.

Sixty-eight rheumatoid arthritics with irreducible anterior craniocervical cord compression underwent a combined anterior transoral decompression combined with posterior occipitocervical fixation. Fiberoptic laryngoscopy was less hazardous than tracheostomy. A contoured wire loop was used for occipitocervical stabilization, and no bone graft was recommended.

Peppelman WC, Kraus DR, Donaldson WF III, et al: Cervical spine surgery in rheumatoid arthritis: Improvement of neurologic deficit after cervical spine fusion. *Spine* 1993;18:2375–2379.

Rheumatoid arthritis with cervical myelopathy improved by at least one Ranawat class in 95% of C1–C2 arthrodeses, 76% of occipitocervical arthrodeses, 94% of subaxial arthrodeses, and 71% of combined arthrodeses. Early surgery is encouraged. Immediate halo immobilization is recommended for all Ranawat III B patients.

Rana NA: Natural history of atlanto-axial subluxation in rheumatoid arthritis. *Spine* 1989;14:1054–1056.

Atlantoaxial subluxation in rheumatoid arthritis was followed in 41 patients for 10 years. Sixty-one percent remained unchanged radiographically, 27% progressed, and 12% demonstrated a decrease in subluxation. Twelve patients died, two with neurologic damage. Only three patients were surgically stabilized. Atlantoaxial subluxation is compatible with life, with only some patients requiring surgery.

Ranawat CS, O'Leary P, Pellicci P, et al: Cervical spine fusion in rheumatoid arthritis. *J Bone Joint Surg* 1979;61A:1003–1010.

In a study of 33 patients with atlantoaxial subluxation, superior migration of the odontoid and subaxial subluxation, the authors devised a classification of pain and neurologic involvement that has become a standard of assessment. A method of measuring superior migration on plain radiographs is presented.

Wattenmaker I, Concepcion M, Hibberd P, et al: Upper-airway obstruction and perioperative management of the airway in patients managed with posterior operations on the cervical spine for rheumatoid arthritis. *J Bone Joint Surg* 1994;76A:360–365.

A review of 128 posterior cervical operations for rheumatoid arthritis was done to examine perioperative complications related to the airway. Fourteen percent of patients intubated without fiberoptic assistance experienced upper airway obstruction after extubation versus 1% of those intubated fiberoptically.

Weissman BN, Aliabadi P, Weinfeld MS, et al: Prognostic features of atlantoaxial subluxation in rheumatoid arthritis patients. *Radiology* 1982;144:745–751.

An anterior atlantodental distance of 9 mm or more on plain radiographs placed rheumatoid arthritis patients at risk for neurologic compromise over a 5-year period of observation. Atlantoaxial impaction and being male are additional risk factors for paralysis.

Classic Bibliography

Bundschuh C, Modic MT, Kearney F, et al: Rheumatoid arthritis of the cervical spine: Surface-coil MR imaging. *Am J Roentgenol* 1988;151:181–187.

Conaty JP, Mongan ES: Cervical fusion in rheumatoid arthritis. *J Bone Joint Surg* 1981;63A:1218–1227.

Dvorak J, Grob D, Baumgartner H, et al: Functional evaluation of the spinal cord by magnetic resonance imaging in patients with rheumatoid arthritis and instability of upper cervical spine. *Spine* 1989;14: 1057–1064.

Lipson SJ: Cervical myelopathy and posterior atlanto-axial subluxation in patients with rheumatoid arthritis. *J Bone Joint Surg* 1985;67A:593–597.

Lipson SJ: Rheumatoid arthritis of the cervical spine. *Clin Orthop* 1984;182:143–149.

Lipson SJ: Rheumatoid arthritis in the cervical spine. *Clin Orthop* 1989;239:121–127.

Morizono Y, Sakou T, Kawaida H: Upper cervical involvement in rheumatoid arthritis. *Spine* 1987;12: 721–725.

Pellicci PM, Ranawat CS, Tsairis P, et al: A prospective study of the progression of rheumatoid arthritis of the cervical spine. *J Bone Joint Surg* 1981;63A:342–350.

Santavirta S, Slatis P, Kankaanpaa U, et al: Treatment of the cervical spine in rheumatoid arthritis. *J Bone Joint Surg* 1988;70A:658–667.

Zoma A, Sturrock RD, Fisher WD, et al: Surgical stabilisation of the rheumatoid cervical spine: A review of indications and results. *J Bone Joint Surg* 1987;69B:8–12.

Zygmunt S, Saveland H, Brattstrom H, et al: Reduction of rheumatoid periodontoid pannus following posterior occipito-cervical fusion visualised by magnetic resonance imaging. *Br J Neurosurg* 1988;2:315–320.

57

Spinal Instrumentation

Introduction

Spinal instrumentation was originally developed for the treatment of scoliosis. The instrumentation was devised as a temporary reduction system and an adjunct to spinal fusion. Shortly after introduction of the Harrington rod for scoliosis, its use was expanded to include spinal trauma. Since that time, the indications for spinal instrumentation have broadened, and it now serves as an adjunct to the treatment of not only scoliosis and spinal trauma, but also degenerative conditions, tumors, and salvage spine surgery. Overall, the advantages of spinal instrumentation are that it can (1) reduce spinal deformity and provide reduction of scoliosis, spondylolisthesis, and kyphosis; (2) provide stability to the spine to maintain reduction and to prevent increasing deformity during healing; and (3) increase the chances for successful fusion.

The general types of instrumentation used in the spine include screws only (used in compression as lag screws), wire only (used as a tension band), and combinations of rods and hooks, rods and wires, rods and screws, or plates and screws. Rod-screw and plate-screw combinations can be further subdivided into those that are constrained or nonconstrained; ie, having a rigid locking mechanism between plate and screw versus a toggling connection; and those that are constrained and flexible or rigid, ie, threaded or solid rods. Spinal instrumentation can also be divided into segmental (attaching to each vertebra in sequence) and nonsegmental (attaching only at the upper and lower ends of the instrumentation). Nonsegmental instrumentation, such as Harrington or Knodt rods, while still helpful in traumatic and some deformity disorders, has limited use in degenerative lumbar conditions.

Cervical Instrumentation

The use of bone screws alone in the cervical spine is primarily for the treatment of upper cervical spine instabilities. The posterior transarticular C1-C2 screw technique was developed by Magerl. It leads to a high degree of rigidity of the C1-C2 complex and, theoretically, augments atlantoaxial fusions. A halo orthosis usually is not necessary when C1-C2 screws are successfully placed. However, the C1-C2 transarticular screw technique is anatomically demanding and should be used only by surgeons with advanced training. Relative indications include those patients who have pseudarthrosis of previous C1-C2 posterior fusion, those patients with absent or fractured posterior elements at C1 or C2, and those patients in whom a halo should be avoided.

Anterior bone screws can be used in the axis for the treatment of type II odontoid fractures. This technique leads to a high rate of healing and to maintenance of reduction without using a halo device. Anterior fixation of the odontoid is indicated for displaced type II fractures, in patients for whom it is best not to use a halo vest, and in those patients in whom preservation of C1-C2 motion is important. This technique is anatomically demanding and requires thorough evaluation of the odontoid using computed tomography (CT) scanning and radiography to ensure adequate reduction and space for the placement of the screws. Current biomechanical and clinical data suggest that a single screw may be as effective as two screws.

Wiring of the posterior cervical spine is a time-honored technique for the maintenance of spinal reduction and the attainment of posterior fusion. Posterior Rogers wiring has stood the test of time and remains the standard for posterior fusions. Enhancements of this technique, such as the Bohlman triple wire and posterior cable techniques, have increased the rigidity of posterior wire fixation. However, posterior wire–bone graft fusion is primarily a tension-band technique and is not indicated when posterior elements are either fractured or absent, or when a high degree of torsional or sagittal instability exists. Posterior wiring techniques are less rigid than lateral mass plate fixation in torsion and extension, and external rigid orthotic support is recommended when posterior wiring techniques are used. Indications for posterior wiring include instability of the cervical spine, either acute or chronic, with intact posterior elements, as an adjunct to anterior bone grafting in cases of instability and/or burst fracture, and in posterior occipital–cervical or C1-C2 fusions.

Posterior rod and lamina/facet hook devices can be used in the cervical spine. These include posterior cervical clamps or pediatric hook-rod systems. A posterior clamp is indicated primarily for one-level cervical instabilities. The clamp systems have not been found to be as rigid as screw techniques in the upper cervical spine. In the mid-to-lower cervical spine, the clamps may encroach on the spinal canal and should be used cautiously in cases of spinal canal compromise. Posterior rod-hook devices are indicated primarily for cervical extension of scoliosis, tumor reconstruction, and upper thoracic trauma. Because these hooks are sublaminar and do encroach on the spinal canal, they must be used carefully in the cervical spine, particularly when any preexisting spinal canal compromise exists.

Anterior cervical plates have been used for decades to treat cervical trauma. Biomechanically, anterior plating provides equal rigidity to posterior wiring in torsion, lateral bending, and extension. In flexion with posterior instability, anterior plating may not be optimal. However, clinical studies have shown that anterior plating and bone grafting is effective in the treatment of burst fractures following corpectomy, cervical subluxations with disk herniations, and cervical tumors. Anterior cervical plate application may also prove useful as an adjunct to anterior fusion for repair of a pseudarthrosis or for multilevel fusions. The routine use of anterior cervical plating in one- or two-level anterior cervical diskectomy and fusion has not yet been shown to be advantageous over noninstrumented fusion. Current indications for anterior plating in trauma are cervical disk herniation associated with subluxation, extension-type tear-drop fractures, burst fractures, and as an adjunct to anterior-posterior fusion in severe rotational-type injuries. Applications in degenerative conditions include multilevel instability in rheumatoid arthritis, multilevel corpectomy, pseudarthrosis repair, and degenerative disk disease following cervical laminectomy. Anterior plating is also useful for reconstruction following resection of cervical vertebral body tumors.

Posterior cervical plates are fixed to bone by attachment to the lateral mass with bone screws.* When attaching to the upper cervical spine, a screw can be placed either transarticularly across C1-C2 or in the C2 pedicle. From C3 to C6 the lateral mass is used for fixation. At C7, either the lateral mass or the C7 pedicle can be used. Before surgery, the surgeon should examine each patient's anatomy on radiographs and CT scan to determine the correct site for placement of each screw. Caution should be exercised in the placement of lateral mass screws because of the anatomic proximity of the vertebral arteries, the spinal cord, and the cervical roots.

Indications for lateral mass plating in trauma include burst fractures that do not require corpectomy, cervical dislocation/subluxation with fractured posterior elements, and severe torsional deformities that require anterior and posterior fusion. Indications for posterior lateral mass plating in degenerative conditions include multilevel fusions following laminectomy, postlaminectomy instability, adjunct fixation following corrective osteotomy, and certain cases of occipital and upper cervical fusions in which a goal is to avoid the use of halo devices. Lateral mass plating can be extended up to the occiput in cases of severe occipital cervical instability. However, the occipital bone laterally can be thin. Cerebrospinal fluid leaks, venous sinus tears, and cerebellar injuries can occur with penetration of the occipital inner cortex.

Thoracolumbar Instrumentation/Posterior

Bone screws used posteriorly in the lumbar spine are primarily for the repair of spondylolytic defects (Buck technique), and as used with transfacet fixation (Magerl technique).* In most reported series of direct repair of spondylolytic defects, results are fair to good when narrow indications for repair are followed. Direct repair may be indicated for patients with no or minimal spondylolisthesis, persistent backache, and relief of back pain following lidocaine infiltration of the pars defect, when there is not an associated severely degenerated disk at the same level. Transfacet screws are used primarily for one- or two-level posterolateral lumbar fusions. These screws serve as an adjunct to fusion when rigid instrumentation and/or reduction are not required. Although several authors have reported high rates of fusion using translaminar facet screw techniques, others have shown this technique to be inferior to pedicle instrumentation.

Simple posterior wiring is rarely indicated in the thoracic or lumbar spine. Segmental posterior rod-wire fixation was introduced by Luque. The Luque instrumentation system represented the first segmental fixation system for use in the spine. Excellent reduction of scoliosis and correction of thoracic hypokyphosis are possible using the Luque system. However, wire passage carries some neurologic risk, which can be minimized by the use of cables rather than wires. Current indications for sublaminar wiring include neuromuscular scoliosis, scoliosis with thoracic lordosis, and idiopathic scoliosis. Contraindications include spinal canal stenosis and kyphosis. There are few indications at present for sublaminar wiring in the lumbar spine.

Posterior rod-hook devices for use in the thoracic and lumbar spine can be categorized as segmental and nonsegmental. Nonsegmental systems include the Harrington rod and the Knodt rod. The Harrington rod is rarely indicated for the treatment of lumbar scoliosis. Posterior distraction alone often leads to flat-back syndrome and failure to maintain lumbar lordosis. Harrington rods with rod sleeves may be useful in the treatment of burst fractures. This technique, which obtains three-point fixation (two hooks and intervening sleeve) has been shown to reduce the retropulsed fragment, and it provides rigidity across a burst fracture. Recommendations are to place the hooks 3 to 5 cm above and below sleeves that nestle over the injured segment. Simple rod-hook compression systems are indicated for flexion-distraction injuries such as a Chance fracture.

Segmental rod-hook devices were first described by Cotrel, with the introduction of the Cotrel-Dubousset (CD) system. By attaching multiple hooks along a rod, both segmental fixation and derotation of scoliotic deformities can be accomplished. Segmental hook systems allow attachment of both screws and hooks to a rod and are indicated primarily for the treatment of scoliosis and trauma. Sublaminar hooks attached to rods often function poorly in the lumbar spine because they do not allow the ability to gain sufficient lumbar lordosis, particularly over lower lumbar segments. In general, for lumbar scoliosis or trauma (particularly low lumbar), transpedicular fixation is preferred. Most authors recommend a dual rod construct, including at least two cross-links between rods, in the treatment of scoliosis. Occasionally, a single-rod, multiple-hook construct may be used.

There has been extensive basic science research on spinal instrumentation. Data from animal studies have shown that the use of posterior spinal fixation increases the chances of obtaining a successful posterior bony fusion. Additionally, when the rigidity of the fixation system is increased, the rigidity of the ensuing fusion mass also increases. With too great an increase in rigidity, however, device-related osteopenia may occur, ie, loss of bone in the underlying vertebral bodies. Whether this device-related osteoporosis is clinically significant is not known.

In vitro biomechanical testing has shown that spinal instrumentation increases the stiffness of spinal constructs. In general, spinal instrumentation systems can be divided into constrained and nonconstrained groups. A constrained system implies a rigid linkage between the longitudinal (plate or rod) and the spinal attachment (screw or hook) members. Nonconstrained systems are those that allow some toggling motion between the longitudinal member and the spine affixing member. Constrained systems have a higher construct stiffness than nonconstrained systems. The nonconstrained systems have a longer fatigue life and fail by loosening, rather than by instrumentation breakage.

Pedicle screw instrumentation was first used by Harrington and popularized by Roy-Camille. Pedicle screw fixation constructs have been shown to be more rigid than hook or wire systems. Using screws placed in the pedicle, the surgeon has the ability to reduce spondylolisthesis, neutralize a vertebral motion segment, correct lumbar scoliosis, and reduce the kyphotic deformity associated with fracture. In addition, the fusion rate for degenerative posterolateral fusions is higher when rigid transpedicular instrumentation is utilized. All of these advantages, however, must be balanced against a higher complication rate. Increased blood loss, operating time, and infection rate occur with spinal instrumentation compared to noninstrumental fusion. Pedicle screw fixation requires advanced training and a high degree of anatomic knowledge to reduce the incidence of complications, such as pedicle fracture, dural tear, nerve root injury, spinal cord injury, and vascular injuries. Current considerations for the use of transpedicular instrumentation include reduction of spondylolisthesis, fusion for degenerative spondylolisthesis, reduction of lumbar scoliosis, repair of posterolateral pseudarthrosis, three-level or greater lumbar fusion, mid to low lumbar burst fracture with instability, and posttumor resection reconstruction.

Anterior Thoracolumbar Instrumentation

Anterior vertebral body screws and rods have been useful for the correction of thoracolumbar scoliosis. Anterior vertebral body derotation and scoliosis correction, which was developed initially by Dwyer and modified by Hall and Zielke, can be performed by placing a rod on the convexity of a thoracolumbar curve and connecting it by screws and staples to each vertebral body. Compression and derotation can then be accomplished, reducing the deformity. This technique allows preservation of mid to low lumbar levels and correction of short thoracolumbar curves, and it avoids posterior hardware. Cable and threaded rod systems tend to have a higher breakage rate, whereas solid rod systems tend to have a higher profile off the vertebral body. In adult scoliosis, anterior instrumentation may be included in a circumferential (anterior and posterior) fusion.

Anterior or lateral thoracolumbar instrumentation is also useful in reconstruction after trauma or tumor surgery. Following corpectomy and strut grafting, anterior instrumentation can help provide reduction of kyphosis, stability, and graft compression. Modern, third generation anterior lateral devices have a low profile, provide the ability to distract or compress, and provide excellent stability. When used correctly, they lead to a high percentage of fusions and a low percentage of hardware failures. However, these systems require familiarity with anterior approaches and vertebral anatomy and should be used primarily by experienced spine surgeons. Current indications for short segment anterolateral instrumentation include reconstruction after burst fracture with neurologic compression, reconstruction of unstable burst fractures with loss of the weightbearing column, and reconstruction after vertebral body resection for tumor.

Biomechanical testing has shown that constrained anterior stabilizing devices can return spinal stiffness to that of the intact spine. Instrumentation one level above and below an unstable segment is equivalent in stiffness to posterior pedicle screw fixation two levels above and below. The decision regarding whether to instrument unstable burst fractures and, if so, whether to stabilize anteriorly or posteriorly is difficult. Relative indications for an anterior approach include neurologic deficit and severe vertebral comminution or displacement.*

*At the time of this writing, bone screws placed posteriorly into vertebral elements have not been cleared for general use in this specific manner by the Food and Drug Administration (FDA). These are Class III devices. This category includes screws placed transfacetally, within pedicles, or in articular, lateral masses. Some screws for use within the sacrum have been approved as Class II devices. Some companies have received Class II clearance for use of screws in lumbar pedicles specifically to supplement fusions in the treatment of grade III and IV spondylolisthesis with the proviso that these devices are removed after the arthrodesis has healed. Anterior vertebral body screws (cervical, thoracic, and lumbar) are Class II devices and can be used as labeled in vertebral bodies. Many of the posterior screw-based devices have been shown in laboratory and clinical testing to be useful and can be used in an off-label manner if the physician feels this is appropriate and important for the treatment of the patient. As with all surgeries, informed consent should explain the procedure and why a particular technique has been chosen, as well as its risks and benefits. The question of whether informed consent regarding pedicle screws must include a discussion of the device's FDA clearance status is currently being litigated in several jurisdictions.

Annotated Bibliography

Anderson PA, Henley MB, Grady MS, et al: Posterior cervical arthrodesis with AO reconstruction plates and bone graft. *Spine* 1991;16(suppl 3):S72–S79

The standard technique of application of lateral mass plates and screws is described. In 30 patients with cervical spine injuries, there were no neurologic or vascular complications, and all had solid fusion.

Kaneda K, Abumi K, Fujiya M: Burst fractures with neurologic deficits of the thoracolumbar-lumbar spine: Results of anterior decompression and stabilization with anterior instrumentation. *Spine* 1984;9:788–795.

This paper reviews the clinical results of the treatment of patients with burst fractures and neurologic deficit by anterior corpectomy, strut grafting, and anterior stabilization using the Kaneda device. A high percentage of successful fusions, a low percentage of hardware failure, and excellent neurologic recovery results are reported.

Kostuik JP: Anterior fixation for burst fractures of the thoracic and lumbar spine with or without neurological involvement. *Spine* 1988;13:286–293.

This paper reports a series of 80 cases of burst injuries of the thoracic and lumbar spine treated with anterior instrumentation. At follow-up there were two cases of nonunion and 11 cases with hardware failure, but no early or late vascular or neurologic complications. All incomplete paraplegics recovered at least one grade.

Lorenz M, Zindrick M, Schwaegler P, et al: A comparison of single-level fusions with and without hardware. *Spine* 1991;16(suppl 8):S455–S458.

A prospective study of 68 patients undergoing single-level posterolateral lumbar fusion was performed in which no instrumentation was compared to pedicle screw fixation. Pseudoarthroses were demonstrated in 59% of the noninstrumented group and 0% of the instrumented patients. Thirty-one percent of the noninstrumented patients returned to work compared to 72% of the instrumented patients. Significant improvement in results was associated with pedicle screw instrumentation.

McAfee PC, Farey ID, Sutterlin CE, et al: 1989 Volvo award in basic science: Device-related osteoporosis with spinal instrumentation. *Spine* 1989;14:919–926.

In an animal model of lumbar fusion, the authors noted that increasing the rigidity of the instrumentation system resulted in an increased fusion rate and increased stiffness of the resulting fusion with an associated device-related osteoporosis occurring in the underlying vertebral body.

Montesano PX, Juach EC, Anderson PA, et al: Biomechanics of cervical spine internal fixation. *Spine* 1991;16(suppl 3):S10–S16.

The authors describe the relative biomechanical benefits of screw fixation of the odontoid, C1-C2 arthrodesis, and anterior and posterior cervical plates.

Steffee AD, Brantigan JW: The variable screw placement spinal fixation system: Report of a prospective study of 250 patients enrolled in Food and Drug Administration clinical trials. *Spine* 1993;18:1160–1172.

Clinical success was obtained in 80% and fusion success in 92% of patients who had the underlying diagnosis of postsurgical failed back syndrome and had posterolateral fusion augmented with pedicle screw fixation. Clinical success was obtained in 86% and fusion success in 91% of patients with spondylolisthesis.

Sutterlin CE III, McAfee PC, Warden KE, et al: A biomechanical evaluation of cervical spinal stabilization methods in a bovine model: Static and cyclical loading. *Spine* 1988;13:795–802.

The authors of this biomechanics paper compare commonly used cervical spine implants. Improved rigidity is seen with the posterolateral mass screw construct. Anterior cervical plates performed well except in flexion.

Zdeblick TA: A prospective, randomized study of lumbar fusion: Preliminary results. *Spine* 1993;18:983–991.

In a prospective, randomized study of patients undergoing posterolateral fusion, significantly higher clinical success rates and fusion rates were obtained when rigid pedicle screw fixation was used compared to no fixation.

Classic Bibliography

An HS, Vaccaro A, Cotler JM, et al: Low lumbar burst fractures: Comparison among body cast, Harrington rod, Luque rod, and Steffee plate. *Spine* 1991;16(suppl 8): S440–S444.

Ani N, Keppler L, Biscup RS, et al: Reduction of high-grade slips (grades III–V) with VSP instrumentation: Report of a series of 41 cases. *Spine* 1991;16(suppl 6): S302–S310.

Esses SI, Sachs BL, Dreyzin V: Complications associated with the technique of pedicle screw fixation: A selected survey of ABS members. *Spine* 1993;18:2231–2239.

Panjabi MM: Biomechanical evaluation of spinal fixation devices: Part I. A conceptual framework. *Spine* 1988;13: 1129–1134.

Panjabi MM, Abumi K, Duranceau J, et al: Biomechanical evaluation of spinal fixation devices: Part

II. Stability provided by eight internal fixation devices. *Spine* 1988;13:1135–1140.

Roy-Camille R, Saillant G, Berteaux D, et al: Osteosynthesis of thoraco-lumbar spine fractures with metal plates screwed through the vertebral pedicles. *Reconstr Surg Trauma* 1976;15:2–16.

Tippets RH, Apfelbaum RI: Anterior cervical fusion with the Caspar instrumentation system. *Neurosurgery* 1988;22:1008–1013.

Truchly G, Thompson WA: Posterolateral fusion of the lumbosacral spine. *J Bone Joint Surg* 1962;44A:505–512.

Zdeblick TA, Shirado O, McAfee PC, et al: Anterior spinal fixation after lumbar corpectomy: A study in dogs. *J Bone Joint Surg* 1991;73A:527–534.

VI
Rehabilitation

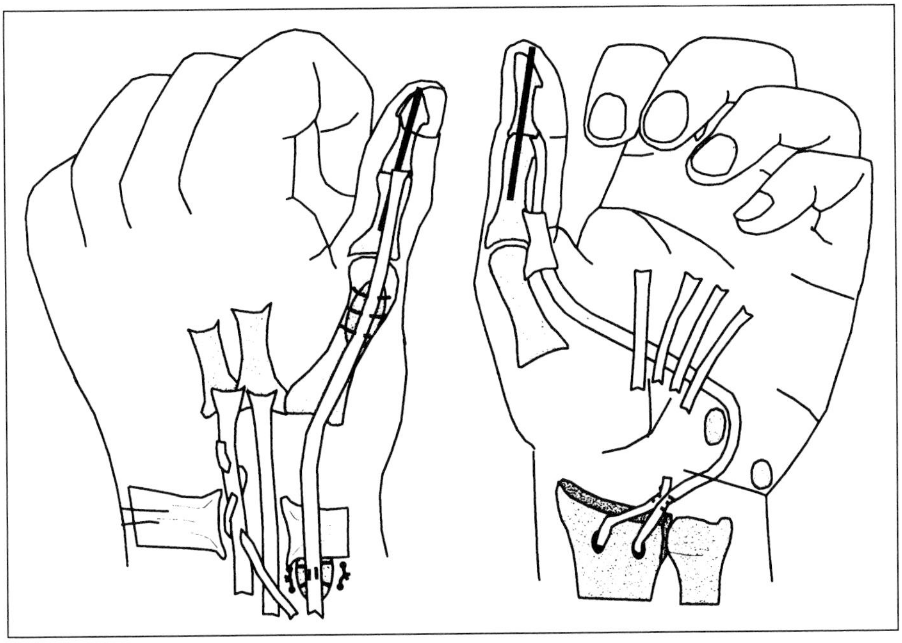

58

Spinal Cord Injuries and Miscellaneous Neurologic Diseases

Spinal Cord Injuries

The annual incidence of acute spinal cord injury in the United States is difficult to estimate accurately because it is not a reportable condition, but it is believed that this injury occurs at an annual incidence of about 30 per million population. The etiology of traumatic spinal cord injury has varied; however, a survey of spinal cord injury patients treated at regional trauma centers indicated that 85% were due to blunt trauma (motor vehicle accidents, falls) and 15% were due to penetrating injuries (gunshot wounds). The majority of spinal cord injuries occur in young males (79%, average age: 33.5 years). The incidence of polytrauma, including traumatic brain injury with associated spinal cord injury, is significant, and the overall mortality after acute spinal cord injury is about 17%.

The rehabilitation of patients with spinal cord injury should begin at the time of the initial injury. It is important to be able to document accurately the neurologic status of the patient, because changing neurologic examination is one indication for surgical intervention. The American Spinal Injury Association (ASIA) standards for neurologic and functional classification of spinal cord injury are most commonly used to document neurologic deficits in spinal cord injury. The efficacy of surgical decompression and stabilization to achieve neurologic recovery after a spinal cord injury is controversial. However, early surgical stabilization, once the patient is medically stable, does improve rehabilitation.

In cervical spinal cord injury patients, the autonomic nervous system is impaired and systemic hypotension may occur without hypovolemia. The systolic blood pressure should be maintained at at least 70 mm Hg to ensure adequate vascular supply to the spinal cord. The histologic and vascular changes that occur in the spinal cord following traumatic injury include a shift to anaerobic glycolysis with a resultant accumulation of lipid peroxides and free radicals at the site of injury and loss of vascular autoregulation. Systemic and local hypotension occur, mediated in part by endogenous endorphins. High-dose methylprednisolone (30 mg/kg given as a bolus, maintenance of 5.4 mg/kg/hour for 23 hours) given within 8 hours of injury has been shown to improve neurologic function (motor and sensory) at 6 weeks and 6 months postinjury, even in complete spinal cord injuries.

Patients with spinal cord injury, as well as patients with other acquired neurologic diseases, should have early stabilization of extremity fractures and careful repeat evaluation to rule out occult injuries not detected in the initial evaluation. In addition, patients with spinal cord injury are at significant risk for deep vein thrombosis, and appropriate prophylaxis is indicated. Patients with spinal cord injury require management of the neurogenic bladder as well as a bowel program. Pressure sores are a significant problem in both the acute period following the injury and in later rehabilitation. Skin capillary pressure averages 32 mm Hg, and the pressure over the ischial tuberosities with sitting can exceed 300 mm Hg. In addition to excessive pressure over bony prominences, shear also increases the risk of pressure sores in these patients. Smoking and poor nutrition (decreased serum albumin and decreased total lymphocyte count), heterotopic ossification, and psychosocial problems are also factors in the development of pressure sores. In the acute period following a spinal cord injury, pressure sore prevention requires bed positioning and frequent turning. In later rehabilitation, patient education and various devices, such as wheelchair cushions, are used to distribute pressure evenly for the prevention of pressure sores.

The prognosis for functional outcome after spinal cord injury depends on multiple variables including psychosocial status, concomitant injuries, and most importantly, the degree of residual motor function. The level of bony injury to the spinal column does not always correlate with the residual neurologic function. In consideration of tendon transfers in the upper extremity for tetraplegia, it is important to assess accurately the strength of muscles to be transferred and to assess carefully sensation of the hand. Two-point discrimination in the hand should be less than 10 mm to allow cutaneous sensibility (if two-point discrimination is greater than 10 mm, ocular sensibility is required). There have been several classifications of residual function of the upper extremity in tetraplegia, but the most commonly used is the Modified International Classification of the Hand in Tetraplegia, which has allowed determination of functional potential and comparison of outcome following tendon transfers. However, it is useful to discuss in general terms a neurologic level of injury with appropriate rehabilitation goals.

C1 to C4 Quadriplegia

Rehabilitation of patients with high-level quadriplegia requires extensive, sophisticated equipment. These patients often require ventilator support for respiration. High cervical quadriplegics are totally dependent for activities of daily living (ADL). Equipment that may be necessary includes an emergency call system, computer, speaker telephone, electric page turner, and an environmental control unit (ECU). These devices can be activated with breath control (sip and puff) or mouth stick. Implantable muscle stimulation for voluntary grasp (ie, neuroprosthetics) is available in a very few select centers for patients in this group.

C5 Quadriplegia

C5 quadriplegics have functional shoulder abduction and elbow flexion. These patients require assistance for ADL. Function may be enhanced by a balanced forearm orthosis attached to a wheelchair to position the arm for such activities as eating and typing. Tendon transfers used at this level of tetraplegia include a deltoid-to-triceps transfer. This provides elbow extension, thereby potentially allowing bed-to-wheelchair transfers. The most common tendon transfer for upper extremity tetraplegia is the Moberg key grip procedure (Fig. 1). The procedure requires a functional brachioradialis (difficult to access because of lack of independent function of the brachioradialis). The brachioradialis is transferred to the extensor carpi radialis brevis to provide wrist extension. The flexor pollicis longus (FPL) is then tenodesed to the volar radius and the interphalangeal joint of the thumb is fused. The metacarpophalangeal joint of the thumb is then stabilized by dorsal tenodesis of the extensor pollicis longus and extensor pollicis brevis to the first metacarpal. The patient can then perform a lateral key pinch by dorsiflexing the wrist, with the volar distal thumb pinching the lateral second ray by the tenodesed FPL. An alternative to the Moberg procedure for C5 quadriplegia to provide a lateral key pinch is a tenodesis orthosis. With tendon transfers or assistive devices, C5 quadriplegics should be able to feed themselves, perform oral hygiene, participate in table top activities, and assist in upper extremity dressing. Usually a powered wheelchair is necessary for locomotion. Transfers from bed to wheelchair are dependent.

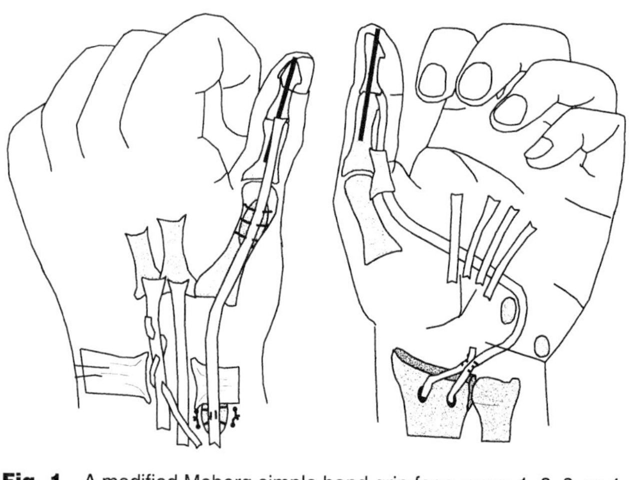

Fig. 1 A modified Moberg simple hand grip for a group 1, 2, 3, or 4 patient.

C6 Quadriplegia

The C6 quadriplegic has active wrist extension, which in some circumstances allows independent living. Similarly to the C5 quadriplegic, a deltoid to triceps transfer can be done in the C6 quadriplegic to achieve elbow extension. Hand function can be enhanced to achieve pinch strength, allowing such tasks as self-catheterization by wrist-driven flexor-hinged orthosis. If these patients have a pronator teres function or a demonstrable extensor carpi radialis longus (ECRL), hand function can be enhanced by transfers of the ECRL to the flexor digitorum profundus, the brachioradialis to the thumb flexor, and digital intrinsic tenodesis. The digital extensors are tenodesed to the dorsal radius. Potential independent ADL achievable in C6 quadriplegics include self-feeding, oral hygiene, upper extremity dressing, assistant or independent lower extremity dressing, and bladder/bowel programs with either orthoses or tendon transfers. Wheelchair locomotion is usually independent manually at this level of injury. Transfers are independent with a sliding board.

C7-8 Quadriplegia

C7 quadriplegics have functional triceps allowing elbow extension, which facilitates transfers. They also have finger extension and wrist flexion which enhance grip strength. In addition, C8 quadriplegics have flexor digitorum profundi function, thereby improving hand function. Tendon transfers useful at these levels of injury include surgical transfers to restore intrinsic function of the hand. Patients with C7-8 quadriplegia can be independent in most ADL.

Thoracic and Lumbar Paraplegia

Patients with thoracic and lumbar paraplegia have normal upper extremity function and should be independent in a wheelchair. At this level of spinal cord injury, the major functional gain is orthotic-assisted ambulation. Standard metal upright knee-ankle-foot orthoses (KAFO) or reciprocating gait orthoses (RGO-LSU orthoses) are used. In addition, functional electric stimulation for external stimulation of paralytic muscles has been used experimentally to facilitate ambulation. The feasibility of orthotic-assisted gait in paraplegics depends on the cardiopulmonary reserve of the patient, the presence of spasticity, the cost, and the availability of a support team to monitor care.

Pediatric Patients

Spinal cord injury in pediatric patients is relatively rare. In pediatric patients with immature bony spinal columns (below the age of 9 years), there is increased mobility of the cervical space because of ligamentous laxity, underdevelopment of neck and paraspinous muscles, incompletely ossified vertebral bodies, and high head-to-torso weight radio. Spinal cord injuries in this group tend to be high cervical injuries with a significant incidence of spinal cord injuries without radiologic abnormality (SCIWORA). The acute rehabilitation program for pediatric patients with spinal cord injury is generally comparable to adult spinal cord injury rehabilitation programs. The long-term outcome for neurologic recovery in pediatric patients with spinal cord injuries is much better than the potential recovery for adults.

Miscellaneous Neurologic Diseases

Post-Polio Syndrome

Post-polio syndrome is a recently recognized syndrome that occurs in patients who initially had acute anterior poliomyelitis 30 to 40 years ago. It has been estimated that there are about 1.63 million survivors of the polio epidemics of the 1950s and 1960s, and about one half of these patients will ultimately develop post-polio syndrome. Through epidemiologic studies, an attempt has been made to establish a profile of polio survivors likely to develop post-polio syndrome. Patients who had more severe cases of initial poliomyelitis as evidenced by longer hospitalization and more extensive neurologic deficits and those patients who were older at the onset of disease are more likely to develop post-polio syndrome.

Post-polio syndrome is varied in its clinical presentation, but commonly includes increased fatigability, joint pain, atrophy of muscles, respiratory insufficiency, dysphasia, and sleep apnea. One consistent symptom of post-polio syndrome is increasing muscle weakness, both in muscles already paretic from the initial polio episode and in muscles previously thought to be normal. There have been a number of theories concerning the etiology of post-polio syndrome, including activation of latent polio virus in the anterior horn cells, an immune process, progression of polio to a variant of amyotrophic lateral sclerosis, premature aging of overworked residual anterior horn cells, defective neuromuscular transmission, and even depression. Weakness of the muscle groups following the initial infection with the polio virus resulted from destruction of anterior horn cells. After the initial illness, some recovery of muscle strength was obtained by physiologic adaptation such as terminal axonal sprouting and reinnervation or myofibril hypertrophy. The most accepted theory of the etiology of post-polio syndrome is dysfunction of surviving motor neurons that causes a slow disintegration of terminals of individual nerve axons. This dysfunction may be caused by premature exhaustion or "aging" of the new sprouts that developed after the acute polio episode. In addition, there is energy inefficient muscle usage during polio paretic gait, with resultant muscle fiber damage from chronic overuse of weakened muscles.

The most important component of treatment of post-polio syndrome is recognition of the pathophysiology of the disease. Usually the treatment of musculoskeletal weakness is rehabilitation through strenuous exercise. In post-polio syndrome, vigorous exercise is likely detrimental to enhancing muscle strength. Nonfatiguing resistive exercises or modified aerobic training may enhance endurance and reduce fatigue in patients with post-polio syndrome, but should not be done to extreme. The mainstays of orthopaedic management of post-polio syndrome are modification of lifestyle to reduce the demands on symptomatic muscles and orthotic management.

Charcot-Marie-Tooth Disease

A syndrome of progressive symmetric distal muscular atrophy of the extremity was described independently by Charcot-Marie-Tooth in 1886. This syndrome is characterized by initial weakness in the peroneal muscles of the foot, followed by progressive weakness of the intrinsic muscles of the foot, dorsiflexors of the foot and toes, and finally, the ankle plantarflexors. Clinically, at the end of presentation of Charcot-Marie-Tooth disease, the foot has toe clawing, forefoot varus, cavus deformity, and equinus of the ankle. In addition, there is often associated weakness of the intrinsic muscles of the hand.

Treatment of Charcot-Marie-Tooth disease consists of initial orthotic management to support the foot in a plantigrade position. Because this disease is a sequela of weakness of muscles, the lightweight plastic ankle-foot orthosis (AFO) may more easily allow limb advancement than a heavier metal hinged AFO.

In the past, surgical management consisted of early triple arthrodesis, Achilles tendon lengthening, and plantar fasciotomy. Recently, soft-tissue procedures consisting of Achilles tendon lengthening, split anterior tibial tendon transfers, plantar fascial release, and claw toe procedures done early in the disease process may preclude a later need for arthrodesis. However, once a significant fixed deformity is present, more extensive procedures, including osteotomies, are needed.

Annotated Bibliography

Spinal Cord Injury

American Spinal Injury Association: *Standards for Neurological and Functional Classification of Spinal Cord Injury.* Chicago, IL, American Spinal Injury Association, 1992.

This is a description of the ASIA standards for the documentation of spinal cord injuries. The ASIA Motor Score uses standard manual muscle testing on a scale of zero to five. Assessment of sensory function requires testing of pin-prick discrimination and light touch for a designated key area in each of 28 dermatomes bilaterally. The neurologic level of injury refers to the most caudal segment of the spinal cord with normal sensory and motor function bilaterally.

Bracken MB, Shepard MJ, Collins WF, et al: A randomized, controlled trial of methylprednisolone or naloxone in the treatment of acute spinal-cord injury: Results of the Second National Acute Spinal Cord Injury Study. *N Engl J Med* 1990;322:1405–1411.

The Second National Acute Spinal Cord Injury Study (NASCIS II) showed the efficacy of high-dose methylprednisolone in improving neurological outcome.

Burney RE, Maio RF, Maynard F, et al: Incidence, characteristics, and outcome of spinal cord injury at trauma centers in North America. *Arch Surg* 1993; 128:596–599.

This reports an epidemiologic study of spinal cord injured patients treated at regional trauma centers.

Freehafer AA: Tendon transfers in patients with cervical spinal cord injury. *J Hand Surg* 1991;16A:804–809.

This is a retrospective review of 85 procedures on 32 patients with tetraplegia. There were 124 transfers in this group. All but three patients were improved (91%). None were made worse. The author's classification system is used.

Garfin SR, Shackford SR, Marshall LF, et al: Care of the multiply injured patient with cervical spine injury. *Clin Orthop* 1989;239:19–29.

This is a description of medical, radiologic, and surgical management of acute spinal cord injury.

Hamilton M, Myles S: Pediatric spinal injury. *J Neurosurg* 1992;77:700.

In this review of 174 pediatric patients with spine injuries, the incidence of spinal cord injury without radiologic abnormality was 42% in patients younger than 9 years of age and only 8% in patients between the ages of 14 and 17 years. Neurologic improvement occurred in 74% of patients with incomplete spinal cord injuries, and 59% of these patients had complete resolution of their neurologic deficits.

McDowell CL, Moberg EA, House JH: The Second International Conference on surgical rehabilitation of the upper limb in tetraplegia (quadriplegia). *J Hand Surg* 1986;11A:604–608.

This is a description of the Modified International Classification for Surgery of the Hand in Tetraplegia. This is a system that provides the functional potential of quadriplegics by classifying sensory function retained as well as residual motor function.

Mohammed KD, Rothwell AG, Sinclair SW, et al: Upper-limb surgery for tetraplegia. *J Bone Joint Surg* 1992;74B: 873–879.

This is a retrospective review of the results of surgical reconstruction in 97 consecutive limbs in 57 tetraplegics with an average follow-up of 37 months. A subjective good or excellent result was obtained in 70%. Revisions were necessary for 14 cases (14%). Complications were minor.

Murphy CP, Chuinard RG: Management of the upper extremity in traumatic tetraplegia. *Hand Clin* 1988;4: 201–209.

General tetraplegia care, sensory and motor evaluation, and a variety of classification systems are described and compared. Appropriate transfers for each classification group are briefly described.

Waters RL, Adkins R, Yakura J, et al: Prediction of ambulatory performance based on motor scores derived from standards of the American Spinal Injury Association. *Arch Phys Med Rehabil* 1994;75:756–760.

Strength, gait performance, and energy expenditure were measured in 36 spinal cord injured patients. Patients with lower extremity ASIA scores less than 20 were limited ambulators with slower average velocities at higher heart rates, greater energy expenditure, and greater peak axial load on assisted devices than patients with lower extremity ASIA scores greater than 30, who were community ambulators. The ASIA motor score correlated with walking ability in paraplegics.

Wuolle KS, Van Doren CL, Thrope GB, et al: Development of a quantitative hand grasp and release test for patients with tetraplegia using a hand neuroprosthesis. *J Hand Surg* 1994;19A:209–218.

The authors report an objective functional outcome study on the use of a neuroprosthesis for C5 and C6 quadriplegics. A neuroprosthesis electrically stimulates paralyzed hand and forearm muscles via percutaneous or implanted electrodes. The stimulation typically is controlled by movement of the contralateral part using electronics.

Post Polio Syndrome

Dalakas MC, Elder G, Hallett M, et al: A long-term follow-up study of patients with post-poliomyelitis neuromuscular symptoms. *N Engl J Med* 1986;314: 959–963.

Neuromuscular function in post-polio patients was assessed by muscle biopsy, electromyography, quantitative muscle strength testing, and serologic and virologic testing of cerebrospinal fluid.

Jubelt B, Drucker J: Post-polio syndrome: An update. *Semin Neurol* 1993;13:283–290.

The authors report an epidemiologic study of post-polio syndrome, including a profile of those patients at risk for developing the disorder.

Moore T, Lin R (eds): *Atlas of Orthotics.* St. Louis, MO, Mosby-Year Book, 1995.

This is a description of orthotic management in post-polio syndrome.

Perry J, Mulroy SJ, Renwick SE: The relationship of lower extremity strength and gait parameters in patients with post-polio syndrome. *Arch Phys Med Rehabil* 1993;74: 165–169.

This is an analysis of specific muscle group weakness and the effect on gait.

Classic Bibliography

Gould N: Surgery in advanced Charcot-Marie-Tooth Disease. *Foot Ankle* 1984;4:267–273.

Perry J, Barnes G, Bronley J: The Post-Polio Syndrome: An overuse phenomenon. *Clin Orthop* 1988;223:145–159.

Waring W, Karunas R: Acute spinal cord injury and the incidence of clinically occurring thromboembolic disease. *Paraplegia* 1991;29:8–16.

59
Stroke

The majority of stroke survivors have the potential for return to functional and useful lives. Approximately 2 million stroke patients reside in the United States. The average life expectancy for patients surviving the first months after a stroke is 6 years.

Neurologic Recovery of Motor and Sensory Function

Motor recovery following a stroke follows a fairly typical pattern. The size of the lesion and the amount of collateral circulation determine the amount of permanent damage. The majority of recovery occurs within 6 months of the stroke. Functional improvement may continue as a result of further sensorimotor reeducation.

The legs and arms are usually flaccid immediately after a stroke. This flaccidity is followed by a gradual increase in muscle tone. In the arm, the shoulder adductor and internal rotator muscles become tight. The elbow, wrist, and finger flexors also develop marked tone. In the leg, the hip adductors, knee extensors, and ankle plantarflexors develop spasticity. These changes are usually evident within 48 hours after the stroke.

Motor control is graded in the extremity using a clinical scale (Table 1). The extremity may be hypotonic or flaccid and without any volitional movement. A spastic extremity may be held rigidly without any volitional or reflexive movement. Patterned or synergistic motor control is defined as a mass flexion or extension response involving the entire extremity. A mass flexion pattern in the upper extremity consists of shoulder abduction, forearm pronation, and flexion of the elbow, wrist, and fingers. A mass extension pattern in the lower extremity consists of extension of the hip and knee with equinovarus of the foot and ankle. This mass patterned movement may be reflexive in response to a stimulus, but without volitional control. The mass movement can also be volitionally initiated by some patients. Selective motor control with pattern overlay is defined as the ability to move a single joint or digit with minimal movement in the adjacent joints when performing an activity slowly. Rapid movements or physiologic stress make the mass pattern more pronounced. Selective motor control is the ability to volitionally move a single joint or digit independently of the adjacent joints. Spasticity can mask underlying motor control.

Even when patterned movement can be initiated volitionally, it is a neurologically primitive form of motor control and of no functional use in the upper extremity. The hand requires some selective control for functional use.

Table 1. Clinical scale of motor control

Motor Control	Description
Flaccid	Hypotonic, no active motion
Rigid	Hypertonic, no active motion
Reflexive mass pattern (synergy)	Mass flexion or extension in response to stimulation
Volitional mass pattern	Patient-initiated mass flexion or extension movement
Selective with pattern overlay	Slow volitional movement of specific joints Physiologic stress results in mass action
Selective	Volitional control of individual joints

However, the lower extremity can more successfully use synergistic motions for functional activities, such as transfers or walking. The patient can be taught to use the flexion movement to advance the limb and the extension pattern to provide limb stability during stance.

The final processes in sensory perception occur in the cerebral cortex, where basic sensory information is integrated to complex sensory phenomena such as proprioception, spatial relationships, shape, sight, and texture. Patients with severe parietal dysfunction and sensory loss may lack sufficient perception of space and awareness of the involved segment of their body to ambulate. Patients with severe perceptual loss may lack balance to sit, stand, or walk.

Management of Spasticity

Lower Extremity

In order to walk, the hemiplegic patient requires the following: (1) adequate balance reactions, (2) volitional hip flexion to advance the limb, and (3) stability of the involved limb during the stance phase of gait. Good balance requires sufficient muscle control to respond quickly to perturbances and intact proprioception to be aware of the limb's position in space. A cane or hemiwalker can be used to improve balance. A leg can be made more stable by supporting weak muscles with a brace or by surgically correcting muscle imbalance.

Surgical procedures to correct limb deformities should be delayed for 6 months after a stroke to allow spontaneous neurologic recovery to occur. After this time, surgery can be performed to rebalance muscle forces and improve function of the spastic limb. In limbs without volitional movement, surgery is indicated to correct contractures caused by spasticity.

Hip Adduction Most hemiplegics have hip abductor and extensor weakness. A quad cane or hemiwalker is used to provide support. Limb scissoring due to overactive hip adductors is a common problem. Hip adductor release or anterior obturator neurectomy can be done to widen the base of support and improve standing balance. If there is scissoring of the legs while standing but no fixed contracture, transection of the anterior branch of the obturator nerve will correct the problem. If the adduction deformity has been present for a longer time and there is a fixed adduction contracture, then tenotomy of the hip adductor muscles is needed (Fig. 1).

Hip Flexion Hip flexor spasticity causes a crouched gait with compensatory knee flexion and lumbar hyperlordosis. The hip and knee flexion posture causes an increased demand on the hip and knee extensors during standing and walking; this demand is extremely energy consuming.

Release of the spastic iliopsoas muscle at the level of the lesser trochanter diminishes the deforming force. The iliopsoas muscle retains its surrounding capsular attachments and reattaches in a more proximal position. Therefore, the iliopsoas is weakened yet maintains the ability to advance the limb during gait.

Stiff Knee Gait Inadequate knee flexion due to inappropriate quadriceps activity in the terminal stance phase and early swing phase of gait may block knee flexion during swing. The patient must compensate by hiking the pelvis and circumducting the leg so that the foot clears the floor during swing. Electromyographic studies have shown that the abnormal activity in the different heads of the quadriceps is often restricted to the rectus femoris muscle. When this pattern of activity is seen, the rectus femoris can be transferred to the sartorius or gracilis. Following the transfer, the rectus femoris will provide active knee flexion at the time of hip flexion for limb advancement during swing.

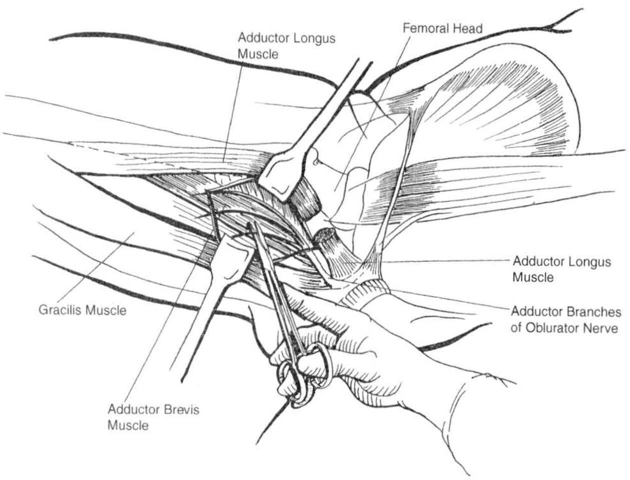

Fig. 1 Release of the adductor longus and neurectomy of the anterior branches of the obturator nerve to correct a hip adduction deformity. (Reproduced with permission from Keenan MAE, Kozin SH, Berlet A: *Manual of Orthopaedic Surgery for Spasticity.* New York, NY, Raven Press, 1993.)

Knee Flexion Excessive hamstring spasticity causes a dynamic knee flexion deformity. In the ambulatory patient, a flexed-knee position during stance increases the quadriceps requirement necessary to stabilize the knee in order to maintain an upright posture. This increase decreases the efficiency of gait and increases the energy consumption during ambulation. A KAFO (knee ankle foot orthosis) may be used temporarily as a training aid but is difficult for the stroke patient to don and wear for permanent use.

Surgical lengthening of the spastic hamstring muscles corrects the dynamic knee flexion deformity while preserving hamstring function. If the knee flexion deformity is greater than 45°, a complete release of the distal hamstring tendons should be done. This procedure eliminates the dynamic component of the flexion deformity. There is usually a residual joint contracture that is corrected by postoperative serial casting. Hamstring function at the knee is not a requirement for ambulation.

Equinovarus Foot A spastic varus deformity of the foot interferes with ambulation and renders brace wear difficult or impossible. This deformity is usually accompanied by an equinus deformity of the foot and toe flexion.

Gait analysis with dynamic, multichannel electromyography is useful to supplement the physical examination and to delineate the spastic muscle groups. The tibialis anterior muscle frequently demonstrates continuous electromyographic activity, which contributes to the forefoot varus. The posterior tibialis is usually inactive or minimally active in the adult stroke patient. When a spastic equinus deformity is present, the gastrocnemius and soleus exhibit premature and often prolonged activity in late swing. In addition, spasticity of the flexor hallucis longus, flexor digitorum longus, and the intrinsic toe flexors is frequently evident, causing toe curling and contributing to the ankle equinus.

Surgical correction of varus is indicated when varus is not corrected by an ankle-foot orthosis (AFO) or when the patient has the potential to walk without a brace following surgery. The anterior tibialis is the key muscle responsible for varus. The split anterior tibialis transfer (SPLATT) diverts the inverting deforming force of the anterior tibialis to a corrective force (Fig. 2). One half of the tendon is transferred laterally to the cuboid or peroneus brevis tendon. The anterior tibialis is secured sufficiently taut to hold the foot in a neutral plantigrade position. Surgical correction of equinus is indicated most commonly when the foot cannot be maintained in the neutral position with

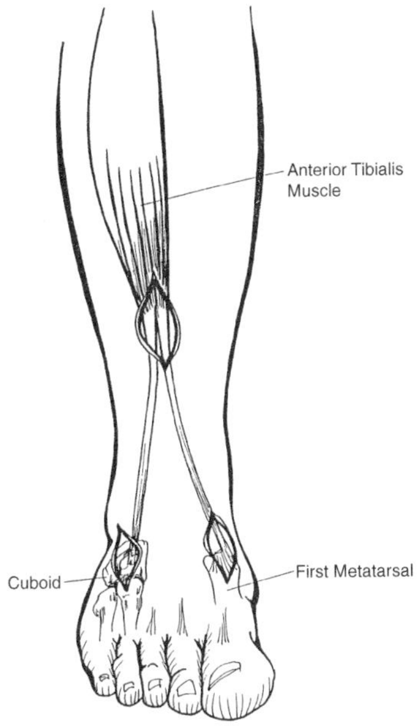

Fig. 2 The split anterior tibial tendon transfer (SPLATT) is used to correct a spastic varus deformity of the foot. (Reproduced with permission from Keenan MAE, Kozin SH, Berlet A: *Manual of Orthopaedic Surgery for Spasticity.* New York, NY, Raven Press, 1993.)

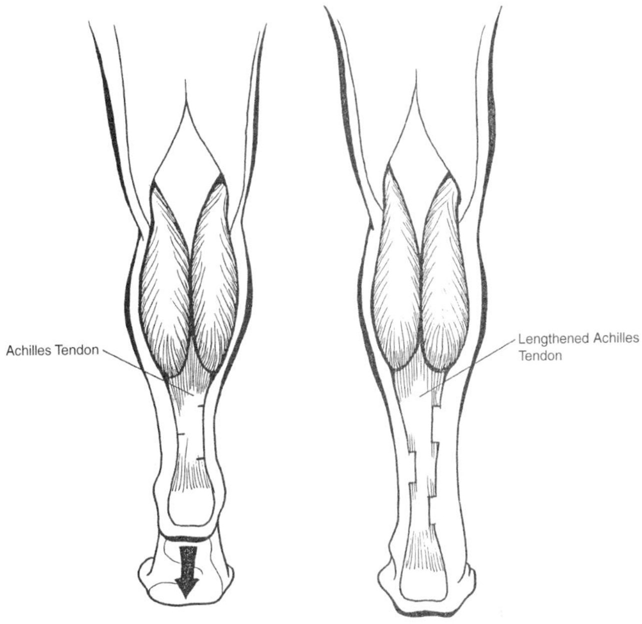

Fig. 3 Three percutaneous hemisections combined with a dorsiflexion force will lengthen the Achilles tendon. (Reproduced with permission from Keenan MAE, Kozin SH, Berlet A: *Manual of Orthopaedic Surgery for Spasticity.* New York, NY, Raven Press, 1993.)

the heel in firm contact with the sole of the shoe in a well-fitted, rigid AFO (ankle foot orthosis). An Achilles tendon lengthening (TAL) using the triple hemisection tenotomy technique is performed (Fig. 3). Both long and short flexors are responsible for excessive toe flexion. Treatment consists of dividing the long and short flexors via longitudinal incisions over the volar aspect of each toe or by releasing the flexor hallucis longus and flexor digitorum longus through the medial incision used to divide the anterior tibial tendon. Spastic muscles are weak muscles. In order to improve calf strength and improve the likelihood of the patient becoming ambulatory without an AFO, the flexor hallucis longus and flexor digitorum longus tendons can be transferred to the os calcis.

The patient is placed in a short leg walking cast or rigid cam walker brace to hold the foot in a neutral position postoperatively. Gait training can be started on the first postoperative day, allowing the patient to bear full weight on the foot. The cast is kept on the foot for 6 weeks and then the patient must use a rigid AFO for an additional 4 to 5 months.

Upper Extremity

The first objective in treating the spastic upper extremity following stroke is to prevent contracture. Severe deformities at the shoulder, elbow, and wrist are seen in the neglected or noncompliant stroke patient. Assistive equipment can be used to position the upper extremity, to aid in prevention of contractures, and to support the shoulder. Positioning extends spastic muscles but does not subject them to sudden postural changes that trigger the stretch reflex and aggravate spasticity. Brief periods should be scheduled when the upper extremity is not suspended to allow for range of motion therapy and hygiene.

An overhead suspension sling attached to the wheelchair is used for patients with adductor and internal rotator spasticity of the shoulder. An alternative is an arm trough attached to the wheelchair. It is usually not possible to maintain the wrist in neutral position with a wrist-hand orthosis (WHO) when wrist flexion spasticity is severe or if the wrist is flaccid.

Shoulder Subluxation In an arm with flaccid paralysis from a stroke, the shoulder will often develop a painful inferior subluxation. This subluxation is usually self-limiting but occasionally, the shoulder will chronically be subluxated, causing pain. The shoulder can be surgically reduced using the tendon of the long head of the biceps. The biceps tendon is detached distally from the muscle, leaving the proximal origin intact at the superior rim of the glenoid. The tendon is passed through a tunnel developed in the humeral head just posterior to the biceps tendon groove and woven back on itself to created a suspensory ligament. An alternative surgical procedure for a painful inferiorly subluxated shoulder in the stroke patient is a glenohumeral fusion.

Shoulder Contracture An adduction and internal rotation contracture of the shoulder may cause hygiene problems in the axilla and result in difficulty in dressing and positioning. Commonly, this contracture is painful. Shoulder adduction and internal rotation is caused by spasticity and myostatic contracture of the pectoralis major, subscapularis, latissimus dorsi, and teres major muscles. In a nonfunctional extremity, surgical release of all four muscles is usually necessary to resolve the deformity (Fig. 4). In a functional extremity, only those muscles most involved, usually the pectoralis major and the subscapularis muscles, are released. The joint capsule is not released as this could result in anterior instability.

Elbow Flexion Selected control of elbow flexion and extension is frequently impaired in the stroke patient. This impairment limits the patient's ability to perform activities of daily living, even when good hand control is present. Dynamic electromyographic analysis of stroke patients shows that the brachioradialis has severe spasticity, the biceps has moderate spasticity, and the brachialis has only mild spasticity. The triceps generally has normal activity. Surgical release of the severely spastic brachioradialis muscle combined with lengthening of the less spastic biceps and brachialis muscles will improve elbow motion and hand placement. In a contracted, nonfunctional arm, the biceps tendon and brachioradialis muscle are released completely. The brachialis is lengthened or released as needed. The joint capsule is not released. Any residual flexion contracture can be treated by serial casting or physical therapy.

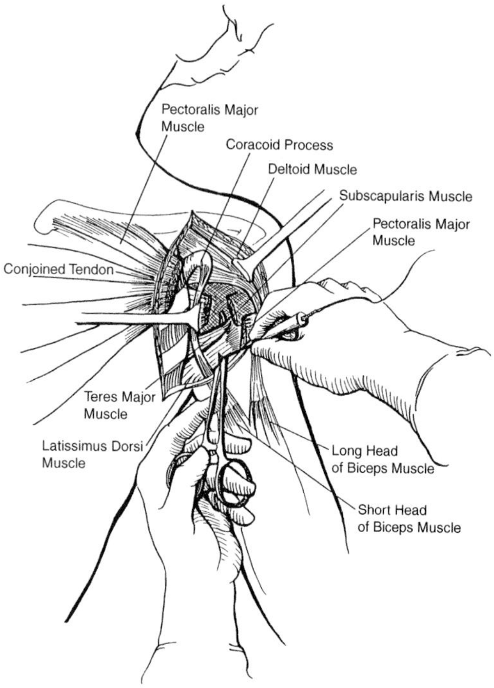

Fig. 4 Release of the adductor and internal rotator muscles of the shoulder to correct a contracture. (Reproduced with permission from Keenan MAE, Kozin SH, Berlet A: *Manual of Orthopaedic Surgery for Spasticity.* New York, NY, Raven Press, 1993.)

Wrist And Finger Flexion Flexor spasticity results in no extension or limited extension of the fingers. The patient is unable to open the hand and release objects. A wrist flexion deformity is often seen as well. Lengthening of the spastic flexor muscles decreases their overreactive stretch response and rebalances the forces between the flexor and extensor muscle groups. This procedure results in improved hand opening while maintaining a functional grasp.

Clenched Fist Contracture A spastic clenched fist deformity in a nonfunctional hand causes palmar skin breakdown and hygiene problems. Recurrent infections of the fingernail beds are common. Adequate flexor tendon lengthening to correct the clenched hand deformity cannot be attained by fractional lengthening without causing discontinuity at the musculotendinous junction. Transection of the flexor tendons is not recommended because any remaining extensor muscle tone may result in an unopposed hyperextension deformity of the wrist and digits. A superficialis-to-profundus (STP) tendon transfer provides sufficient flexor tendon lengthening with preservation of a passive tether to prevent a hyperextension deformity.

Intrinsic spasticity and contracture are masked by the presence of extrinsic flexor spasticity or contracture. To prevent an intrinsic plus deformity, a neurectomy of the motor branches of the ulnar nerve in Guyon's canal is routinely done in conjunction with the STP transfer. If there is an intrinsic contracture, the intrinsic tendons are released at the metacarpophalangeal joints.

Severe wrist flexion deformities usually accompany a clenched fist deformity. Median nerve compression results. The wrist flexor tendons are transected and a carpal tunnel release is done at the time of the STP. A wrist arthrodesis may be done to prevent a wrist flexion deformity and eliminate the need for a splint.

Thumb-In-Palm Spasticity of the thumb musculature causes the thumb to assume a position of flexion and adduction within the palm. This deformity interferes with function because the ability to grasp and oppose is severely limited. In addition, skin maceration and breakdown occurs as proper hygiene is prevented.

Generally, all of the thenar muscles are spastic or contracted and a proximal myotomy is required to reposition the thumb and decrease the underlying tone in order to improve pinch function. Distal releases are to be avoided because these often result in a hyperextension deformity of the metacarpophalangeal joint of the thumb.

Annotated Bibliography

Keenan M, Perry J, Jordan C: Factors affecting balance and ambulation following stroke. *Clin Orthop* 1984;182: 165–172.

Ninety consecutive patients evaluated for ambulation potential following a stroke were evaluated for the variables most important to achieve ambulation. Intact truncal balance reaction was the most important variable to predict ambulation potential. Lower extremity weakness, spasticity, or imbalance can be compensated for by orthotics or surgery.

Waters R, Frazier J, Garland D, et al: Electromyographic gait analysis before and after operative treatment for hemiplegic equinus and equinovarus deformity. *J Bone Joint Surg* 1982;64A:284–292.

Dynamic gait analysis was done on 27 hemiplegic patients before and after a surgical procedure to correct the abnormal gait. Abnormal patterns of muscle activity (out of phase contractions) were found in the gastrocnemius, soleus, posterior tibial, anterior tibial, flexor hallucis longus, flexor digitorum longus, and peroneus brevis muscles. Surgeries to treat equinovarus deformities of the foot in acquired neurologic spasticity (split anterior tibial tendon transfer, Achilles tendon lengthening) achieve their effect by weakening muscles, by lengthening tendons, or by changing the direction of action of the muscle. The muscles maintained their abnormal phasic activity following surgical intervention.

Classic Bibliography

Botte MJ, Waters RL, Keenan MA, et al: Approaches to senior care: 2. Orthopaedic management of the stroke patient: Part I. Pathophysiology, limb deformity, and patient evaluation. *Orthop Rev* 1988;17:637–647.

Botte MJ, Waters RL, Keenan MA, et al: Approaches to senior care: 3. Orthopaedic management of the stroke patient: Part II. Treating deformities of the upper and lower extremities. *Orthop Rev* 1988;17:891–910.

Botte MJ, Keenan MA, Jordan C: Stroke, in Nickel VL, Botte MJ (eds): *Orthopaedic Rehabilitation.* New York, NY, Churchill Livingstone, 1992, pp 337–360.

Garraway WM, Whisnant JP, Drury I: The changing pattern of survival following stroke. *Stroke* 1983;14: 699–703.

Keenan MA, Ure K, Smith CW, et al: Hamstring release for knee flexion contracture in spastic adults. *Clin Orthop* 1988;236:221–226.

Keenan MAE, Waters RL: Surgical treatment of the upper extremity after stroke or brain injury, in Chapman MW, Madison M (eds): *Operative Orthopaedics,* ed 2. Philadelphia, PA, JB Lippincott, 1993, vol 2, pp 1529–1544.

Keenan MAE, Waters RL: Surgical treatment of the lower extremity after stroke, in Chapman MW, Madison M (eds): *Operative Orthopaedics,* ed 2. Philaelphia, PA, JB Lippincott, 1993, vol 4, pp 3449–3465.

Keenan MAE, Kozin SH, Berlet AC (eds): *Manual of Orthopaedic Surgery for Spasticity.* New York, NY, Raven Press, 1993.

Ough JL, Garland DE, Jordan C, et al: Treatment of spastic joint contractures in mentally disabled adults. *Orthop Clin North Am* 1982;12:143–151.

60

Traumatic Brain Injury

Adult

More than two million significant traumatic brain injuries occur in the United States each year, with approximately one-half million of those affected requiring hospitalization. About 70,000 patients with acute traumatic brain injuries die from the initial injury, and about 150,000 are left with substantial neurologic deficits. Several modalities, including the initial Glasgow coma scale (GCS), the computed tomography findings, and the duration of coma have been used to predict the eventual neurologic outcome. Although no modality is absolutely accurate in predicting neurologic outcome following traumatic brain injury, the initial GCS value correlates with eventual outcome. Patients with GCS values of 13 to 15 have a 99% chance of good neurologic recovery, whereas patients with a GCS value of less than 9 have only a 35% chance of good recovery. Patients with traumatic brain injury and musculoskeletal injury should be treated orthopaedically with the expectation that neurologic recovery will occur.

In patients with traumatic brain injury and fractures, optimal care usually requires surgical stabilization. These patients may be comatose, agitated, or spastic. Closed treatment of fractures is therefore difficult. With proper anesthetic monitoring of patients with traumatic brain injury, especially intracranial pressure, surgical stabilization of extremity fractures can be done safely. However, patients with traumatic brain injury can have medical problems, such as neurogenic pulmonary edema or electrolyte imbalance, which will affect surgical intervention for fractures. In addition, about 10% of patients with traumatic brain injury have a coagulopathy, initiated by release of thromboplastin from damaged brain tissue. Fractures in these patients heal with abundant callus when compared to fractures in patients without brain injury. An in vivo study of cultured osteoblasts in serum of patients with traumatic brain injury showed an osteogenic factor to be present.

Patients with traumatic brain injury may have significant problems with spasticity. Untreated spasticity in these patients can result in contracture of limbs in a nonfunctional position in a relatively short period of time. Even a 15° plantar contracture of the foot can result in a cascade of pathologic gait abnormalities, with increased weight-bearing over the metatarsal heads, compensatory knee recurvatum, forward trunk lean, and increased tone in the paravertebral muscles. The prevention of contractures requires the use of orthoses or inhibitory casts with the limb in a position of function. Phenol injections into the motor branches of peripheral nerves can be used to temporarily decrease spasticity with no sensory loss until either neurologic recovery occurs or definitive surgical treatment can be undertaken.

Clinically significant periarticular neurogenic heterotopic ossification occurs in 10% to 20% of patients with traumatic brain injury. Concomitant trauma to a joint results in a higher incidence of heterotopic ossification. There also is an increased incidence of heterotopic ossification following internal fixation of acetabular fractures in these patients.

The treatment of heterotopic ossification in patients with traumatic brain injury consists of prophylaxis, manipulation, and surgical resection. Various modalities of prophylaxis that have been used to prevent heterotopic ossification in these patients include diphosphonates, nonsteroidal anti-inflammatory drugs (particularly indomethacin), and radiation. Joint manipulation, once heterotopic ossification has formed, has variable success. Surgical resection of periarticular heterotopic ossification in ankylosed joints will result in satisfactory functional outcome, provided the procedure is done at least 18 months after the traumatic brain injury, the heterotopic ossification is radiographically mature, the patient is at a relatively high cognitive status, and the patient has some selective motor control of the involved extremity.

Pediatric

Traumatic brain injury is a common occurrence in the pediatric population and is the most frequent cause of traumatic death and disability in this age group in the United States. The acute rehabilitation of pediatric patients with head injuries is similar to that of adult patients. Long-bone fractures frequently require surgical stabilization, because the usual closed treatment of pediatric fractures becomes difficult in the presence of impaired cognition and spasticity. The long-term rehabilitation of pediatric patients with head injuries requires a multidisciplinary approach. Surgical procedures for residual spasticity should be delayed until at least 1 year following the head injury. Common surgical procedures for residual spasticity or contractures in pediatric head injured patients include thumb-web space release, flexor digitorum sublimis release, wrist flexor release, shoulder adductor releases, hip adductor tenotomy or obturator neurectomy, psoas tenotomy, hamstring lengthening, Achilles tendon lengthening, and toe flexor release.

The potential for neurologic recovery is much better in pediatric patients with traumatic brain injury than in adults with traumatic brain injury. In a series of pediatric patients with major traumatic brain injuries treated at John Hopkins, 29% were normal at final follow-up (both cognitively and physically) and 53% were able to return to school with mild behavior or cognitive problems. Improvement in speech and cognitive function can occur over several years in the pediatric population with head injuries.

Annotated Bibliography

Bidner SM, Rubins IM, Desjardins JV, et al: Evidence for a humoral mechanism for enhanced osteogenesis after head injury. *J Bone Joint Surg* 1990;72A:1144–1149.

This study demonstrated that the serum of patients who have a head injury has growth factor activity increased for cells of the osteoblast phenotype, suggesting a humeral mechanism for the enhanced osteogenesis that occurs with traumatic brain injury.

Garland DE: A clinical perspective on common forms of acquired heterotopic ossification. *Clin Orthop* 1991;263: 13–29.

This review article describes the etiology, diagnosis, location, and treatment of heterotopic ossification in patients with traumatic brain injury.

Gennarelli TA: Mechanisms of brain injury. *J Emerg Med* 1993;11(suppl 1):5–11.

This is a study of the epidemiology of traumatic brain injury as well as the physiologic changes that occur as a result of a head injury.

Malisano LP, Stevens D, Hunter GA: The management of long bone fractures in the head-injured polytrauma patient. *J Orthop Trauma* 1994;8:1–5.

In this retrospective study of 108 patients with traumatic brain injury and concomitant extremity fractures, 88 of the 108 patients were treated surgically for their fracture, and fracture outcome was satisfactory with no systemic complications from anesthesia.

Moore TJ: Functional outcome following surgical excision of heterotopic ossification in patients with traumatic brain injury. *J Orthop Trauma* 1993;7:11–14.

The author reports a retrospective study of heterotopic ossification resection of 20 ankylosed joints in patients with traumatic brain injury. Satisfactory functional results were obtained if the surgery was 18 months after the traumatic brain injury, the heterotopic ossification was radiographically mature, the patient was at a high cognitive status, and the patient had some selective control of the involved extremity.

Moore TJ, Anderson RB: The use of open phenol blocks to the motor branches of the tibial nerve in adult acquired spasticity. *Foot Ankle* 1991;11:219–221.

The authors report a retrospective study of the indications and results of open injections of phenol into the motor branches of the tibial nerve in 19 patients with traumatic brain injuries. The indication for injection of phenol into the motor branches of the tibial nerve is lower extremity spasticity with the foot in significant equinovarus that is refractory to conventional treatment (splints, physical therapy). The phenol injection into the motor branches of the tibial nerve spares normal sensation and decreases spasticity, thereby preventing contracture. The effect lasts for about 14 weeks, thereby allowing potential neurologic recovery without permanent sequelae to the tibial nerve.

Perkins R, Skirving AP: Callus formation and the rate of healing of femoral fractures in patients with head injuries. *J Bone Joint Surg* 1987;69B:521–524.

This study is a retrospective review of 22 patients with traumatic brain injury and concomitant femur fractures matched with 22 patients without head injury but with a similar femur fracture (matched by Winquist classification).The patients with traumatic brain injury had a significant radiographic increase in callus formation.

Perry J: Contractures: A historical perspective. *Clin Orthop* 1987;219:8–14.

This review article describes the historic treatment of spasticity and the biomechanical alterations of normal gait by lower extremity contractures.

Teasdale G, Jennett B: Assessment of coma and impaired consciousness: A practical scale. *Lancet* 1974;2:81–84.

This article provides the initial description of the Glasgow coma scale (GCS), in which three aspects of neurologic status (motor responsiveness, verbal performance, and eye opening) are used to assess the severity of traumatic brain injury.

Webb LX, Bosse MJ, Mayo KA, et al: Results in patients with craniocerebral trauma and an operatively managed acetabular fracture. *J Orthop Trauma* 1990;4:376–382.

This multicenter study demonstrates the increased incidence of heterotopic ossification in patients with traumatic brain injury and concomitant acetabular fracture that requires surgical reconstruction.

61

Amputations and Prosthetics

Amputation of all or part of a limb is performed for trauma, peripheral vascular disease, tumor, infection, or congenital anomaly. Amputation is often a reasonable alternative to limb salvage. Because of the psychologic implications of amputation and the alteration of body self-image, a multidisciplinary team approach should be taken to return patients to their maximum levels of independent function. An appropriately done amputation should be considered the first step in the rehabilitation of the patient, rather than a concluding event in failure.

Metabolic Cost of Amputation

The metabolic cost of walking, which is inversely proportional to the length of the residual limb and the number of joints preserved, is increased with proximal level amputations. With more proximal amputation, patients have decreased self-selected and maximum walking speeds, with a corresponding increase in oxygen consumption. This metabolic cost of walking becomes so great that the geriatric transfemoral amputee with peripheral vascular disease has almost no energy reserve, using virtually maximum energy expenditure during normal walking.

Load Transfer (Weightbearing)

The soft-tissue envelope acts as an interface between the bone of the residual limb and the prosthetic socket. Ideally, it should be composed of a mobile, nonadherent muscle mass, and full-thickness skin that will tolerate the direct pressures and shearing forces associated with residual limb pistoning within the prosthetic socket. It is rare for the prosthetic socket to achieve a perfect intimate fit. A nonadherent soft-tissue envelope will allow some degree of mobility, or pistoning, of the bone within the soft-tissue envelope, thus negating the shear forces on adherent skin that produce tissue breakdown and ulceration.

Weightbearing is accomplished by either direct or indirect load transfer. Direct load transfer, ie, end weightbearing, is accomplished with knee disarticulation (through-knee amputation) or ankle disarticulation (through-ankle, Syme's amputation). When the amputation is performed through a long bone, ie, transfemoral or transtibial, the terminal residual limb must be unloaded and the load transferred indirectly over the entire residual limb surface area by the total contact method. This requires an intimate prosthetic socket fit combined with 7° to 10° of flexion of the tibia below, or adduction of the femur above the knee joint.

Amputation Wound Healing

Oxygenated blood is a prerequisite for all wound healing. Amputation wounds generally heal by collateral flow, so arteriography is rarely a useful preoperative test to predict wound healing. The ultrasound Doppler, which measures arterial systolic pressures, has historically been used as the determinant of vascular inflow to the ischemic limb. The area of the Doppler waveform measures blood flow at the level being tested in the limb. The ischemic index is the ratio of the Doppler pressure at the level being tested to the brachial systolic pressure. The most commonly measured value is the ischemic index recorded at the ankle level, the ankle-brachial index (ABI). An absolute Doppler pressure of 70 mm Hg, or an ischemic index of 0.45, has been accepted as the minimum measure of inflow to support wound healing. These values are falsely elevated, and nonpredictive in at least 15% of patients with peripheral vascular disease, because of the noncompressibility and limited compliance of the calcified peripheral arteries, especially in diabetics.

Transcutaneous oximetry, or measurement of the transcutaneous partial pressure of oxygen ($TcPO_2$) at the level of potential amputation is presently the "gold standard" measurement of vascular inflow. It actually records the capacity of the vascular system to deliver oxygen to the level of proposed surgery. Values of 20 to 30 mm Hg are correlated with acceptable wound healing rates, without the false positive values seen in noncompliant peripheral vascular diseased vessels as determined by Doppler pressures.

Amputation wound healing is not solely dependent on vascular inflow. Patients with malnutrition or immune deficiency have a high rate of wound failure or infection. Patients with serum albumin below 3.5 g/dl are malnourished, and those with total (absolute) lymphocyte counts below 1,500 are immunodeficient. If possible, surgery in these patients should be delayed until these values can be improved by nutritional supplement or hyperalimentation (usually oral) to support wound healing. When infection or gangrene dictates urgent surgery, drainage of infection or open amputation at the most distal viable level, followed by open wound care, can be carried out until wound healing potential can be optimized.

Pediatric Considerations

Pediatric amputations are typically the result of congenital limb deficiencies, trauma, or tumors. The traditional method of describing congenital amputations is based on the premise that the limb, or limb segment, was lost before birth, as opposed to the concept of failure of formation. The present system is based on the original work of a 1991 Conference of the International Society for Prosthetics and Orthotics (ISPO) Deficiencies are either longitudinal or transverse, with the potential for intercalary deficits. Preaxial refers to the radial or tibial side, and postaxial to the ulnar or fibular side.

Amputation is rarely indicated in the case of a congenital upper limb deficiency, because even rudimentary appendages can be functionally useful. In the lower limb, amputation of an unstable segment may allow direct load transfer and enhanced prosthetic walking. In the growing child, disarticulations should be performed whenever possible to maintain maximal residual limb length and prevent terminal bony overgrowth. Terminal bony overgrowth occurs most commonly in the humerus, fibula, tibia, and femur, in that order, and occurs most commonly in diaphyseal amputations. Numerous surgical procedures have been described to resolve this problem, but the best method is surgical revision of the residual limb with adequate resection of bone or autogenous osteochondral stump capping.

Considerations in Trauma

The absolute indication for amputation in trauma remains an ischemic limb with nonreconstructable vascular injury. Recent studies in severe open tibia fractures (Gustillo-Anderson grades IIIB and IIIC) reveal that limb salvage is often associated with a higher rate of morbidity from sepsis, poor end functional results, and decreased potential to return to work. Early amputation in the appropriate trauma patient may prevent emotional, marital, financial, and addictive disorders.

Guidelines for immediate or early amputation of mangled limbs differ between upper and lower limbs. When a salvaged upper limb remains sensate and maintains some prehension, it will function better than a prosthesis. Sensation is not as crucial in the lower limb, where current prostheses can effectively protect insensate limbs. The salvaged lower extremity with an insensate plantar weightbearing surface is unlikely to provide a long-term durable limb for stable walking and is likely to be a source of recurrent sepsis. The grading scales for evaluating mangled extremities are not absolute predictors for amputation, but act as a reasonable guideline for determining whether salvage is appropriate.

Considerations in Peripheral Vascular Disease

In order for patients to learn to walk with a prosthesis and care for their residual limb and prosthesis, they must possess certain cognitive capacities: (1) memory, (2) attention, (3) concentration, and (4) organization. Patients with cognitive deficits or psychiatric disease have a low likelihood of becoming successful prosthetic users.

About half of lower extremity amputees are diabetic, with inherent immune deficiency and malnourishment. If these patients have peripheral vascular disease of sufficient magnitude to require amputation, vascular disease is probably present in their coronary and cerebral vasculature. Appropriate consultation with physical therapists, social workers, and psychologists is valuable to maximize rehabilitation potential. Medical consultation should evaluate cardiopulmonary reserve. The vascular surgeon should determine if vascular reconstruction is feasible or appropriate.

The biologic amputation level is the most distal functional amputation level with a high probability of supporting wound healing. This level is determined according to whether the patient has adequate viable local tissue to construct a residual limb capable of supporting weightbearing, adequate vascular inflow. In addition, serum albumin and total lymphocyte count, indicating nutritional status, should be compatible with wound healing. Amputation level is selected by combining the biologic amputation level with the rehabilitation potential to determine the amputation level that maximizes ultimate functional outcome.

Musculoskeletal Tumors

Recent advances in perioperative chemotherapy and allograft or prosthetic reconstruction have made limb salvage a viable option in extremity tumors. The primary goal in musculoskeletal oncology surgery is to provide adequate surgical margins for patient survival. If adequate margins can be achieved with limb salvage and residual muscle and nerves are compatible with function, the decision can be made to attempt limb salvage. When limb salvage is compared to amputation, significant controversy exists in the literature regarding energy expenditure to ambulate and quality of life measures. Expected functional outcome should include the psychosocial and body image values associated with limb salvage and amputation. These concerns should be balanced with the apparent improved task performance and decreased worry of late mechanical injury associated with amputation and prosthetic limb fitting.

Gas Gangrene

There are three types of common gas-forming extremity infections. With clostridial myonecrosis, patients are acutely critically ill with sepsis, pain, and disorientation. They have a typical brownish discharge from their wounds and have crepitus of the soft tissues when examined. Treatment requires open amputation above the level of infection. Adjunctive treatment is with penicillin and hyperbaric oxygen therapy.

Streptococcal myonecrosis is actually a tissue-plane infection. Development is slower, and patients are not quite as septic as patients with clostridial myonecrosis. Treatment requires excision of the involved compartments, combined with open wound management and penicillin.

Anaerobic gas-forming infections caused by gram negative bacilli are common in diabetics. Frequently, infections in diabetics are polymicrobial, and treatment consists of open drainage and parenteral antibiotics. If systemic sepsis is present, an open amputation may be necessary.

Technical Considerations

Handling of the soft tissues is critical to wound healing and ultimate functional outcome in amputation surgery. The skin often is fragile due to impaired circulation or recent trauma. Flaps should be full thickness, avoiding unnecessary dissection between the skin, subcutaneous, fascial, and muscle planes. Periosteum should not be stripped proximal to the level of the bone transection to prevent regenerative bony overgrowth. Wounds should never be closed under tension. In children, excision of 0.5 cm of the distal periosteum may limit bony overgrowth. All bone edges should be rounded and smooth.

Muscles should be secured at their normal resting length to either bone, ie, myodesis, or to periosteum, fascia, or antagonist muscle fascia, ie, myoplasty. Stable residual limb muscle mass can improve function by preventing atrophy, by providing counterbalance to antagonist muscle forces, and by establishing a stable soft-tissue envelope over the end of the bone for prosthetic fitting.

All transected nerves form neuromas. To prevent these neuromas from being painful, the nerve should be gently retracted distally and transected as far proximally as possible with a fresh scalpel blade. The nerve should not be crushed with a clamp prior to transection, because this crush injury may predispose to postoperative phantom or residual limb pain that mimics reflex sympathetic dystrophy. Ligation, crushing, cauterization, capping, perineural closures, and end-loop anastomoses have not been shown to be more effective in preventing painful neuromas than gentle traction and proximal transection and allowing the nerve to retract deep within the muscle mass. Occasionally, ligature or careful cauterization of a perineural vessel from a large peripheral nerve is necessary to achieve hemostasis in traumatic or tumor amputations.

Split-thickness skin grafts are discouraged in amputation surgery except in the presence of a mobile resilient muscle mass when skin grafting is essential to preserve a more distal amputation level. If grafted skin provides insufficient durability, reconstructive procedures, such as free tissue transfer or tissue expansion, can be done at a later date following maturation of the residual limb.

Postoperative Care

Residual limb care in the early postoperative period can enhance or detract from functional outcome in amputation surgery. Specific wound care is related to the circumstances of the surgery. Traumatic amputations are simply grade IIIC open fractures and should be managed accordingly with open-wound treatment. Skin traction is no longer recommended because it applies a stress to already compromised tissues. Skin contracture is not a problem because the retained soft tissues can be returned to their functional resting lengths at the time of early delayed wound closure.

When foot or ankle amputations are performed for diabetic foot infection or gangrene, surgery should be staged, with primary open amputation or incision and drainage procedures, followed by definitive amputation surgery after the surrounding soft-tissue infection, ie, cellulitis, is resolved. A safe method of decreasing retained debris or bacterial inoculation at the amputation site is the use of closed wound irrigation by means of a percutaneous small bore catheter combined with loose wound closure, allowing drainage through the wound. At 1 to 3 days following surgery, the catheter can be removed and a short leg cast applied.

The use of rigid postoperative plaster dressings in transtibial or knee disarticulation amputations controls swelling, decreases postoperative pain, and protects the limb from trauma. Early postoperative prosthetic limb fitting is initiated between 5 and 21 days following surgery. Immediate postoperative prosthetic fitting (IPOP) should be reserved for patients with very stable, secure residual limbs, usually young traumatic amputees. Because weightbearing is not an issue in the upper limb amputee, very early prosthetic fitting can be accomplished without the same concerns for wound trauma, and early prosthetic fitting in upper extremity amputations enhances long-term prosthetic usage.

Complications

Pain

Phantom limb sensation, the feeling that all or part of an amputated limb is present, occurs in virtually all adults following an amputation. It usually diminishes with time. Phantom pain is a burning, painful sensation in the distribution of the amputated part. It is present in less than 10% of adults with acquired amputations. Noninvasive treatments, such as increased prosthetic limb use, physical therapy modalities, intermittent compression, and transcutaneous electrical nerve stimulation, often will decrease symptoms.

A more common cause of residual limb pain is a condition that is similar to reflex sympathetic dystrophy. In this condition, the pain is within the residual limb. The pain is described as burning, tearing, throbbing, or piercing. These patients frequently underwent amputation following a crush injury and, therefore, have symptoms much like those of a major causalgia. The personality traits of these patients often mirror those of the reflex sympathetic dystrophy population.

Localized residual limb pain is often related to an incompetent soft-tissue envelope, prominent underlying bony projection, or scarred deep structures. An etiology of pain not directly related to the amputation should be considered. Ischemia of the residual limb is an occasional etiology of pain in the patient with peripheral vascular disease. Nerve entrapment, disk herniation, proximal arthritis, or visceral etiologies occasionally cause pain in the residual limb.

Edema

Postoperative residual limb edema is common following amputation. It is uncomfortable for the patient, and it may impede wound healing by increasing tissue and venous pressures. Rigid dressings help reduce this problem. If soft dressings are used, they should be combined with compression stump wrapping. Compression stump wrappings, if too tight proximally, can produce bulbous distal swelling and a residual limb that is difficult to encase within a prosthetic socket. Compression wraps in transfemoral residual limbs fall off if not suspended about the waist.

Late residual limb swelling can be produced by proximal constriction of the prosthetic socket, thus causing congestion in the stump. In its most severe form, verrucous hyperplasia develops in transtibial amputations when distal total contact is not achieved. This condition is characterized by a wart-like overgrowth of skin combined with darkened pigmentation, fissuring, and a serous discharge, which often becomes secondarily infected. The cellulitis is treated with broad spectrum antibiotics and avoidance of socket wear. The prosthetic socket needs to be altered on an ongoing basis to provide total contact, until a volume stable residual limb with a healthy soft-tissue envelope is achieved.

Joint Contractures

Joint contractures usually occur between amputation surgery and prosthetic fitting. They are best avoided by early prosthetic fitting and weightbearing, combined with an aggressive physical therapy program. Hip flexion contractures in transfemoral amputation can be produced at the time of surgery by performing myodesis or myoplasty with the retained muscles tensioned with the hip in a flexed position.

Preoperative, static joint contractures need to be corrected at the time of surgery, because they rarely can be corrected postoperatively. The transfemoral amputee should be encouraged to lie prone after surgery to prevent hip flexion contracture. The transtibial amputee should not sit for long periods with the residual tibia unsupported in a flexed knee position.

Wound Failure

Wound failure following amputation is not uncommon, especially in diabetic and ischemic limbs. Open wound care can be used for small wounds. Even larger wounds can be managed with total contact plaster or plastic sockets and continued weightbearing, as long as the bone is not exposed. When localized wound failure is larger, or the bone is exposed, or the soft-tissue envelope is tight (as long as the vascular inflow remains adequate), the residual limb can be revised by shortening the bone, resection of a wedge of soft tissue, and nontensioned wound closure.

Dermatologic Problems

Many skin problems can be prevented by good hygiene, which includes keeping both the residual limb and socket clean, dry, and free of any residual soap. Epidermoid cysts can occur at the socket brim. They are best managed by modification of the socket to relieve localized pressure. Contact dermatitis can be confused with infection. It is often caused by retained detergents or soaps. Treatment involves good hygiene practices and topical steroid creams. Folliculitis or acneform hidradenitis is common. Meticulous hygiene, sweat-absorbing stump socks made from natural fibers, and occasional courses of oral tetracycline therapy can usually control this problem.

Amputation Levels and Prosthetic Principles

Upper Limb

The shoulder provides the center of the radius of the functional sphere of the upper limb. The elbow acts as the caliper to position the hand at a workable distance from that center to perform tasks. People normally perform multiple joint segment tasks simultaneously. Upper limb prostheses perform these same tasks sequentially; thus, limb length and joint salvage are directly correlated with functional outcome. Motion at the retained joints is essential to maximize that function. Residual limb length is valuable for both prosthetic socket suspension and providing the lever arm necessary to drive the prosthesis through space.

Limb salvage is more critical in the upper limb than the lower limb, because sensation is critical to upper extremity function. An insensate prosthesis provides less function than a partially sensate, partially functional salvaged limb. This fact is in contradistinction to the retained lower limb in which function is not as dependent on sensation.

When upper limb amputation is necessary, prosthetic fitting should be initiated as soon as possible, even before the wound is healed. Outcomes of prosthetic limb usage vary from 70% to 85% when prosthetic fitting is initiated within 30 days of amputation, as opposed to less than 50% when prosthetic fitting occurs late.

Myoelectric prostheses are promising, but are slow to perform tasks. Increased speed and power requires increased weight for the motor and battery pack. These prostheses appear to be most successful in the midlength transradial amputee, in whom only the terminal device needs to be controlled.

Hand Amputation Surgical reconstruction to obtain prehension can be accomplished with pollicization, ray transposition, central ray resection, or toe-to-hand transfer. Functional static partial hand prostheses can provide a stable post for opposition from remaining digits or the palm. Cosmetic partial hand prostheses may be psychologically beneficial because they retain body image.

Wrist Disarticulation Wrist disarticulation has two advantages over transradial amputation: (1) preservation of more forearm rotation due to preservation of the distal radioulnar joint, and (2) improved prosthetic suspension due to the flare of the distal radius. However, wrist disarticulation provides challenges to the prosthetist that may outweigh its benefits. Cosmetically, the prosthetic limb will be longer than the contralateral remaining limb, and, if myoelectric componentry is used, the motor and battery cannot be hidden within the prosthetic shank.

Transradial Amputation High levels of function can be obtained at this level of amputation (Fig. 1). Forearm rotation and strength are directly related to the length of the residual limb, with the optimum length being at the junction of the middle and distal thirds of the forearm. At this level, the soft-tissue envelope can be constructed with adequate muscle myoplasty or myodesis, and the components of a myoelectric prosthesis can be hidden within the prosthetic shank. Because function at this level is accomplished prosthetically only by opening and closing the terminal device, elbow joint function is essential. When the residual forearm is so short as to preclude an adequate lever arm for driving the prosthesis through space, supracondylar suspension (the Munster socket) and step-up hinges can be used to augment function.

Krukenberg's Amputation This kineplastic operation transforms the transradial residual limb into radial and ulnar pincers capable of strong prehension and excellent manipulative ability due to the retention of sensation. Due to psychologic considerations, it is generally restricted to blind bilateral amputees who cannot use visual cues to operate their prostheses (Fig. 2).

Elbow Disarticulation/Transhumeral Amputation Functionally, both levels require two acts to develop prehension, making these amputations significantly less functional and making the prosthesis heavier than the prosthesis for amputation at the transradial level. The length and shape of elbow disarticulation provides improved suspension and lever arm capacity compared to the transhumeral amputation. The drawback is cosmetic, because the elbow will be too far distal and the forearm shank too short for the limbs to be of equal length. Prosthetically, the best function with the least weight at the lowest cost is provided by hybrid prosthetic systems combining myoelectric, traditional body-powered, and body-driven switch componentry for elbow disarticulation or transhumeral amputation.

Patients with a complete unreconstructable brachial plexus injury can achieve function by amputation of the insensate dead-weight arm, leaving a sensate residual limb which can be fitted with a prosthesis. If no voluntary shoulder motion remains, shoulder fusion allows scapulothoracic motion to drive the prosthesis.

Shoulder Disarticulation/Forequarter Amputation These levels of amputation provide minimal function, because the patient must sequentially control two joints and a terminal device. Limited function can be achieved with a manual universal shoulder joint positioned by the opposite hand, combined with a lightweight hybrid prosthetic components.

Lower Limb

Two major recent advances in lower limb prosthetics are socket design and fabrication, and dynamic-response feet. New plastics allow sockets to be lighter and more flexible,

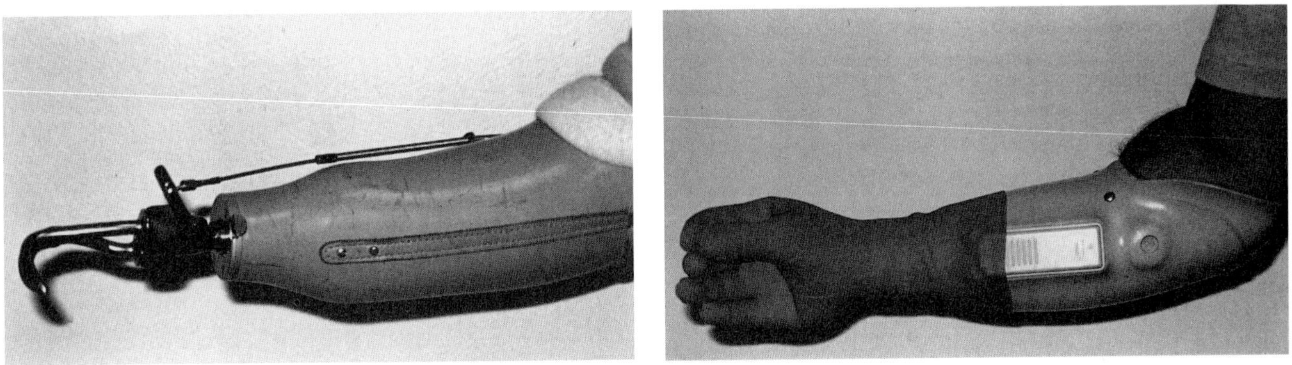

Fig. 1 **Left,** Standard, below-elbow shoulder-powered conventional prosthesis. The terminal device is a canted finger voluntary opening split hook. Closure occurs passively through rubber bands. A friction wrist allows passive pronation and supination placement with the other hand. **Right,** Below-elbow myoelectric prosthesis with the standard glove. Suspension is by suction fit. The removable battery is visible just at the edge of the glove.

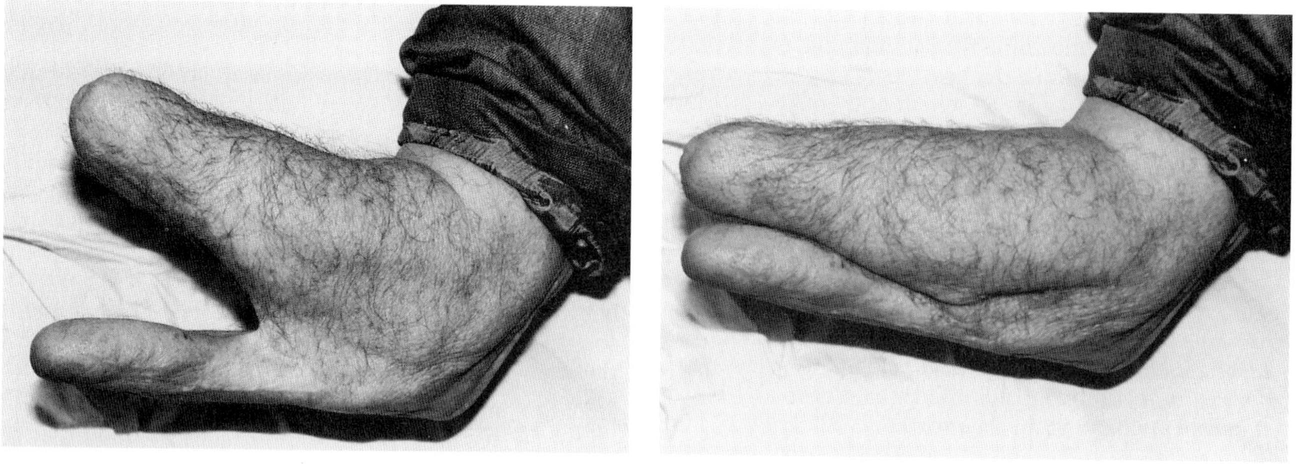

Fig. 2 The Krukenberg procedure. In a medium-length to long below-elbow amputation, the radius and ulna can be separated to produce a strong, sensate pincer grip without the need for a prosthesis.

and therefore, more comfortable. Computer-assisted design and fabrication allow more efficient fabrication with the newer materials. The standard quadrilateral prosthetic socket for transfemoral amputees is gradually being replaced by the newer ischial containment socket designs, which more efficiently transfer load by total contact. Silicone sleeves, used primarily in transtibial levels, improve comfort and suspension. Dynamic response feet now provide spring and push-off to the amputee's gait, probably lessening the energy demands for walking or running.

Toes The great toe, primarily, and the lesser toes act as stabilizers during stance phase. Ischemic patients generally ambulate with an apropulsive gait pattern, so they suffer little disability from toe amputation. Traumatic amputees will lose some late stance-phase stability with toe amputation. When amputation of the great toe is necessary, an attempt should be made to salvage the proximal aspect of the proximal phalanx with the insertion of the flexor hallucis brevis in order to maintain some stabilizing function. Isolated second toe amputation should be amputated just distal to the proximal phalanx metaphyseal flare to act as a buttress that prevents late hallux valgus.

Ray Resection Single outer (first or fifth) ray resection functions well in standard shoes. Resection of more than one ray leaves a narrow forefoot that is difficult to fit in shoes. Central ray resections are complicated by prolonged wound healing, and rarely outperform midfoot amputation.

Midfoot Amputation There is little functional difference between transmetatarsal and tarsal-metatarsal (Lisfranc) amputation. The long plantar flap used in these amputations acts as a myocutaneous flap and is preferred to fish-mouth dorsal-plantar flaps. Transmetatarsal amputation should be performed in the distal shaft to retain lever arm length, or through the proximal metaphyses to prevent late plantar pressure ulcers under the residual bone ends. A percutaneous Achilles tendon lengthening should be performed with the Lisfranc amputation to balance the foot to prevent the late development of equinus or equinovarus. Late dynamic varus occurring during stance phase of gait can be corrected with lateral transfer of the tibialis anterior tendon. Midfoot amputees rarely require the stability of high-topped shoes, generally being sufficiently stable with standard tie shoes.

Hindfoot Amputation Whereas some authors have reported reasonable functional outcomes with hindfoot amputation, ie, Chopart's or Boyd's, especially in children, the functional outcome is generally poor at these levels. Most patients with hindfoot amputation retain an inadequate lever arm, and are prone to develop significant equinus. In addition, they lack push-off at terminal stance.

Ankle Disarticulation (Through-Ankle, Syme's) This is a durable amputation level that allows direct load transfer and is rarely complicated by late residual limb ulcers or tissue breakdown in young traumatic amputees. It provides a stable gait pattern that rarely requires postoperative gait training. Previously, it had been suggested that a Syme's amputation be done in two stages. However, recent data suggest that it can be performed in one stage, even in ischemic limbs with insensate heel pads. The malleoli and metaphyseal flares should be removed from the tibia and fibula, but the remaining tibial articular surface should be retained to provide a resilient residual limb. The heel pad should be secured to the tibia via drill holes, either anteriorly or posteriorly.

Transtibial (Below-Knee) The long posterior myocutaneous flap is preferred to sagittal flaps in transtibial amputation. Optimal bone length is 12 to 15 cm below the knee joint, or longer if adequate gastrocnemius or soleus can be used to construct a functional soft-tissue envelope comprising a mobile muscle mass and full-thickness skin. Posterior muscle should be secured to the beveled anterior tibia by myoplasty or myodesis. Rigid dressings should be used during the early postoperative period, and weightbearing should be initiated between 5 and 21 days following surgery if the residual limb is capable of transferring load. Young active transtibial amputees have the greatest benefit from the new technology, including flexible sockets, silicone liner suction, suspension, and dynamic response feet.

Knee Disarticulation (Through-Knee) Knee disarticulation is performed using sagittal skin flaps and covering the end of the femur with gastrocnemius to act as a soft-tissue envelope end pad. This level is generally performed in the nonambulator who can support wound healing at the transtibial, or distal level. This level is muscle-balanced, and it provides an excellent weightbearing platform and lever arm for transfer. When performed in a potential walker, it provides a direct load transfer residual limb that can take advantage of the intrinsically stable polycentric four-bar linkage prosthetic knee joint.

Transfemoral (Above-Knee) This level provides significant problems in energy cost for walking. Transfemoral amputees who have peripheral vascular disease are unlikely to be prosthetic ambulators. Salvaging the limb at the knee disarticulation, or transtibial level is essential to allow potential prosthetic ambulation in geriatric, dysvascular amputees. The optimal transfemoral bone length is 12 cm above the knee joint to accommodate the prosthetic knee. Adductor myodesis maintains normal femoral adduction during stance phase, allowing optimum prosthetic function.

Ischial containment sockets improve comfort and suspension, but waist belts of various types are frequently necessary. Although suction suspension remains the primary mode of suspension, silicone liners, much like those used in transtibial amputation, may be used.

Hip Disarticulation Few hip disarticulation amputees will become functional walkers due to the high energy cost of prosthetic ambulation. Posttrauma or tumor patients will occasionally use a prosthesis for limited activity. These patients sit in their prostheses and must use their torsos to achieve momentum to throw the limb forward and advance the limb.

Pediatric Prosthetics

Prosthetic fitting for growing children is challenging because frequent adjustments are needed. Prosthetic fitting should be initiated to closely coincide with normal skill development. In the upper limb, this development begins at the time of sitting balance, usually 4 to 6 months of age. Initially, a passive rubberized terminal device with blunt rounded edges is used. Active cable control and a voluntary opening terminal device are added when the child exhibits initiative in placing objects in the terminal device, usually in the second or third year of life. Myoelectric prostheses are not usually prescribed until the child has mastered body-powered componentry.

In the lower limb, prosthetic fitting usually coincides with crawling and pulling to stand at 8 to 12 months of age. Knee control at the transfemoral level cannot be expected until the child demonstrates proficiency in walking with a locked knee. Children will have unusual gait patterns, and formal gait training should be delayed until age 5 to 6 years.

Annotated Bibliography

Harris IE, Leff AR, Gitelis S, et al: Function after amputation, arthrodesis, or arthroplasty for tumors about the knee. *J Bone Joint Surg* 1990;72A:1477–1485.

The authors report an objective study measuring the function of 22 patients who underwent amputation (seven), arthrodesis (nine), and arthroplasty (six) for malignant tumors about the knee. Patients were evaluated with 0_2 consumption studies, psychologic effects, and overall satisfaction. There was little difference in the psychologic and physical function in the three groups of patients.

Pinzur M: New concepts in lower limb amputation and prosthetic management, in Greene WB (ed): *Instructional Course Lectures XXXIX.* Park Ridge, IL, American Academy of Orthopaedic Surgeons, 1990, pp 361–366.

This is an overview of preoperative evaluation of ischemic limbs, and of surgical and prosthetic management of different levels of lower-extremity amputations.

Silcox DH III, Rooks MD, Vogel RR, et al: Myoelectric prostheses: A long-term follow-up and a study of the use of alternate prostheses. *J Bone Joint Surg* 1993;75A: 1781–1789.

This is a detailed evaluation of long-term prosthetic usage in 46 patients with myoelectric prostheses, 40 of whom also have conventional prostheses. Follow-up averaged 5 years. Fifty percent of patients rejected the myolectric prosthesis; 32% rejected the conventional prosthesis. Factors associated with the rejection of the myolectric prosthesis were occupations requiring heavy lifting (more than 10 pounds) or occupations requiring repetitive manual labor.

Waters RL, Perry J, Antonelli D, et al: Energy cost of walking of amputees: The influence of level of amputation. *J Bone Joint Surg* 1976;58A:42–46.

Seventy amputees with transfemoral amputations, transtibial amputations, and Symes amputations were compared to 40 nonamputees in regards to gait velocity and metabolic cost of amputation. The oxygen uptake per meter walked determines the energy cost of amputation, and hence the efficiency of prosthetic ambulation correlates with the level of amputation: the more distal the amputation, the more energy efficient the gait.

Classic Bibliography

Bernd L, Blasius K, Lukoschek M, et al: The autologous stump plasty: Treatment for bony overgrowth in juvenile amputees. *J Bone Joint Surg* 1991;73B:203–206.

Bowker JH, Michael JW (eds): *Atlas of Limb Prosthetics: Surgical, Prosthetic, and Rehabilitation Principles,* ed 2. St. Louis, MO, Mosby Year-Book, 1992.

Day HJB: The ISO/ISPO classification of congenital limb deficiency, in Bowker JH, Michael JW, (eds): *Atlas of Limb Prosthetics: Surgical, Prosthetic, and Rehabilitation Principles,* ed 2. St. Louis, MO, Mosby Year-Book, 1992, pp 743–748.

DeHaven KE, Evarts CM: The continuing problem of gas gangrene: A review and report of illustrative cases. *J Trauma* 1971;11:983–991.

Gottschalk FA, Kourosh S, Stills M, et al: Does socket configuration influence the position of the femur in above-knee amputation? *J Prosthet Orthot* 1989;2:94–102.

Kay HW (ed): *The Proposed International Terminology for the Classification of Congenital Limb Deficiencies: The Recommendations of a Working Group of the International Society for Prosthetics and Orthotics.* London, England, W Heinemann, 1975.

Lagaard SW, McElfresh EC, Premer RF: Gangrene of the upper extremity in diabetic patients. *J Bone Joint Surg* 1989;71A:257–264.

Light TR: Kinesiology of the upper limb, in Bunch WH (ed): *Atlas of Orthotics,* ed 2. St. Louis, MO, CV Mosby, 1985, pp 126–138.

Pinzur MS: Knee disarticulation: Surgical procedures, in Bowker JH, Michael JW, (eds): *Atlas of Limb Prosthetics: Surgical, Prosthetic, and Rehabilitation Principles,* ed 2. St. Louis, MO, Mosby Year-Book, 1992, pp 479–486.

Pinzur MS, Gold J, Schwartz D, et al: Energy demands for walking in dysvascular amputees as related to the level of amputation. *Orthopedics* 1992;15:1033–1037.

Pinzur MS, Sage R, Stuck R, et al: Transcutaneous oxygen as a predictor of wound healing in amputations of the foot and ankle. *Foot Ankle* 1992;13:271–272.

Wagner FW Jr: A classification and treatment program for diabetic, neuropathic, and dysvascular foot problems, in Cooper RR (ed): *Instructional Course Lectures XXVIII.* St. Louis, MO, CV Mosby, 1979, pp 143–165.

Wyss CR, Harrington RM, Burgess EM, et al: Transcutaneous oxygen tension as a predictor of success after an amputation. *J Bone Joint Surg* 1988;70A:203–207.

Index